Handbook of Antioxidants

OXIDATIVE STRESS AND DISEASE

Series Editors

LESTER PACKER, PH.D.
ENRIQUE CADENAS, M.D., PH.D.
University of Southern California School of Pharmacy
Los Angeles, California

1. Oxidative Stress in Cancer, AIDS, and Neurodegenerative Diseases, *edited by Luc Montagnier, René Olivier, and Catherine Pasquier*
2. Understanding the Process of Aging: The Roles of Mitochondria, Free Radicals, and Antioxidants, *edited by Enrique Cadenas and Lester Packer*
3. Redox Regulation of Cell Signaling and Its Clinical Application, *edited by Lester Packer and Junji Yodoi*
4. Antioxidants in Diabetes Management, *edited by Lester Packer, Peter Rösen, Hans J. Tritschler, George L. King, and Angelo Azzi*
5. Free Radicals in Brain Pathophysiology, *edited by Giuseppe Poli, Enrique Cadenas, and Lester Packer*
6. Nutraceuticals in Health and Disease Prevention, *edited by Klaus Krämer, Peter-Paul Hoppe, and Lester Packer*
7. Environmental Stressors in Health and Disease, *edited by Jürgen Fuchs and Lester Packer*
8. Handbook of Antioxidants: Second Edition, Revised and Expanded, *edited by Enrique Cadenas and Lester Packer*

Related Volumes

Vitamin E in Health and Disease: Biochemistry and Clinical Applications, *edited by Lester Packer and Jürgen Fuchs*

Vitamin A in Health and Disease, *edited by Rune Blomhoff*

Free Radicals and Oxidation Phenomena in Biological Systems, *edited by Marcel Roberfroid and Pedro Buc Calderon*

Biothiols in Health and Disease, *edited by Lester Packer and Enrique Cadenas*

Handbook of Antioxidants, *edited by Enrique Cadenas and Lester Packer*

Handbook of Synthetic Antioxidants, *edited by Lester Packer and Enrique Cadenas*

Vitamin C in Health and Disease, *edited by Lester Packer and Jürgen Fuchs*

Lipoic Acid in Health and Disease, *edited by Jürgen Fuchs, Lester Packer, and Guido Zimmer*

Flavonoids in Health and Disease, *edited by Catherine Rice-Evans and Lester Packer*

Additional Volumes in Preparation

Handbook of Antioxidants

Second Edition
Revised and Expanded

edited by

Enrique Cadenas
Lester Packer

University of Southern California School of Pharmacy
Los Angeles, California

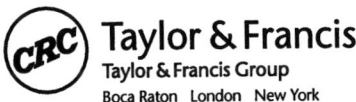
Taylor & Francis Group
Boca Raton   London   New York

A CRC title, part of the Taylor & Francis imprint, a member of the Taylor & Francis Group, the academic division of T&F Informa plc.

ISBN: 0-8247-0547-5

This book is printed on acid-free paper.

Headquarters
Marcel Dekker
270 Madison Avenue, New York, NY 10016
tel: 212-696-9000; fax: 212-685-4540

World Wide Web
http://www.dekker.com

The publisher offers discounts on this book when ordered in bulk quantities. For more information, write to Special Sales/Professional Marketing at the headquarters address above.

Copyright © 2002 by Marcel Dekker   All Rights Reserved.

Neither this book nor any part may be reproduced or transmitted in any form or by any means, electronic or mechanical, including photocopying, microfilming, and recording, or by any information storage and retrieval system, without permission in writing from the publisher.

Current printing (last digit):
10 9 8 7 6 5 4 3 2

PRINTED IN THE UNITED STATES OF AMERICA

Series Introduction

Oxygen is a dangerous friend. Overwhelming evidence indicates that oxidative stress can lead to cell and tissue injury. However, the same free radicals that are generated during oxidative stress are produced during normal metabolism and thus are involved in both human health and disease.

> Free radicals are molecules with an odd number of electrons. The odd, or unpaired, electron is highly reactive as it seeks to pair with another free electron.
>
> Free radicals are generated during oxidative metabolism and energy production in the body.
>
> Free radicals are involved in:
>
> Enzyme-catalyzed reactions
>
> Electron transport in mitochondria
>
> Signal transduction and gene expression
>
> Activation of nuclear transcription factors
>
> Oxidative damage to molecules, cells, and tissues
>
> Antimicrobial action of neutrophils and macrophages
>
> Aging and disease

Normal metabolism is dependent on oxygen, a free radical. Through evolution, oxygen was chosen as the terminal electron acceptor for respiration. The two unpaired electrons of oxygen spin in the same direction; thus, oxygen is a biradical, but not a very dangerous free radical. Other oxygen-derived free radical species, such as superoxide or hydroxyl radicals, formed during metabolism or by ionizing radiation are stronger oxidants and are therefore more dangerous.

In addition to research on the biological effects of these reactive oxygen species, research on reactive nitrogen species has been gathering momentum. NO, or nitrogen monoxide (nitric oxide), is a free radical generated by NO synthase (NOS). This enzyme modulates physiological responses such as vasodilation or signaling in the brain. However, during inflammation, synthesis of NOS (iNOS) is induced. This iNOS can result in the overproduction of NO, causing damage. More worrisome, however, is the fact that excess NO can react with superoxide to produce the very toxic product peroxynitrite. Oxidation of lipids, proteins, and DNA can result, thereby increasing the likelihood of tissue injury.

Both reactive oxygen and nitrogen species are involved in normal cell regulation, in which oxidants and redox status are important in signal transduction. Oxidative stress is increasingly seen as a major upstream component in the signaling cascade involved in inflammatory responses, stimulating adhesion molecule and chemoattractant production. Hydrogen peroxide, which breaks down to produce hydroxyl radicals, can also activate NF-κB, a transcription factor involved in stimulating inflammatory responses. Excess production of these reactive species is toxic, exerting cytostatic effects, causing membrane damage, and activating pathways of cell death (apoptosis and/or necrosis).

Virtually all diseases thus far examined involve free radicals. In most cases, free radicals are secondary to the disease process, but in some instances free radicals are causal. Thus, there is a delicate balance between oxidants and antioxidants in health and disease. Their proper balance is essential for ensuring healthy aging.

The term oxidative stress indicates that the antioxidant status of cells and tissues is altered by exposure to oxidants. The redox status is thus dependent on the degree to which a cell's components are in the oxidized state. In general, the reducing environment inside cells helps to prevent oxidative damage. In this reducing environment, disulfide bonds (S—S) do not spontaneously form because sulfhydryl groups kept in the reduced state (SH) prevent protein misfolding or aggregation. This reducing environment is maintained by oxidative metabolism and by the action of antioxidant enzymes and substances, such as glutathione, thioredoxin, vitamins E and C, and enzymes such as superoxide dismutase (SOD), catalase, and the selenium-dependent glutathione and thioredoxin hydroperoxidases, which serve to remove reactive oxygen species.

Changes in the redox status and depletion of antioxidants occur during oxidative stress. The thiol redox status is a useful index of oxidative stress mainly because metabolism and NADPH-dependent enzymes maintain cell glutathione (GSH) almost completely in its reduced state. Oxidized glutathione (glutathione disulfide, GSSG) accumulates under conditions of oxidant exposure, and this changes the ratio of oxidized to reduced glutathione; an increased ratio indicates oxidative stress. Many tissues contain large amounts of glutathione, 2–4 mM in erythrocytes or neural tissues and up to 8 mM in hepatic tissues. Reactive oxygen and nitrogen species can directly react with glutathione to lower the levels of this substance, the cell's primary preventative antioxidant.

Current hypotheses favor the idea that lowering oxidative stress can have a clinical benefit. Free radicals can be overproduced or the natural antioxidant system defenses weakened, first resulting in oxidative stress, and then leading to oxidative injury and disease. Examples of this process include heart disease and cancer. Oxidation of human low-density lipoproteins is considered the first step in the progression and eventual development of atherosclerosis, leading to cardiovascular disease. Oxidative DNA damage initiates carcinogenesis.

Compelling support for the involvement of free radicals in disease development comes from epidemiological studies showing that an enhanced antioxidant status is associated with reduced risk of several diseases. Vitamin E and prevention of cardiovascular disease is a notable example. Elevated antioxidant status is also associated with decreased incidence of cataracts and cancer, and some recent reports have suggested an inverse correlation between antioxidant status and occurrence of rheumatoid arthritis and diabetes mellitus. Indeed, the number of indications in which antioxidants may be useful in the prevention and/or the treatment of disease is increasing.

Oxidative stress, rather than being the primary cause of disease, is more often a secondary complication in many disorders. Oxidative stress diseases include inflammatory bowel diseases, retinal ischemia, cardiovascular disease and restenosis, AIDS, ARDS, and neurodegenerative diseases such as stroke, Parkinson's disease, and Alzheimer's disease. Such indications may

Series Introduction

prove amenable to antioxidant treatment because there is a clear involvement of oxidative injury in these disorders.

In this new series of books, the importance of oxidative stress in diseases associated with organ systems of the body will be highlighted by exploring the scientific evidence and the medical applications of this knowledge. The series will also highlight the major natural antioxidant enzymes and antioxidant substances such as vitamins E, A, and C, flavonoids, polyphenols, carotenoids, lipoic acid, and other nutrients present in food and beverages.

Oxidative stress is an underlying factor in health and disease. More and more evidence indicates that a proper balance between oxidants and antioxidants is involved in maintaining health and longevity and that altering this balance in favor of oxidants may result in pathological responses causing functional disorders and disease. This series is intended for researchers in the basic biomedical sciences and clinicians. The potential for healthy aging and disease prevention necessitates gaining further knowledge about how oxidants and antioxidants affect biological systems.

Rapid progress in the application of antioxidant substances and other micronutrients warranted a revision and update of *Handbook of Antioxidants*, highlighting new fundamental studies on food-derived antioxidants and biomarkers, vitamins E and C, coenzyme Q, carotenoids, flavonoids and other polyphenols, antioxidants in beverages and herbal products, the thiol antioxidants glutathione and lipoic acid, melatonin, selenium, and nitric oxide. *Handbook of Antioxidants: Second Edition, Revised and Expanded*, is an authoritative volume regarding the chemical, biological, and clinical aspects of antioxidant molecules. The individual chapters provide an in-depth account of the current knowledge of vitamins or other naturally occurring antioxidant compounds and discuss critically the new aspects of antioxidant therapy. We are delighted to have been involved with this project and are grateful to the authors in this volume for their outstanding contributions.

Lester Packer
Enrique Cadenas

Preface

The *Handbook of Antioxidants: Second Edition, Revised and Expanded*, is an authoritative treatise on the chemical, biological, and clinical aspects of antioxidant molecules. Each chapter provides an in-depth account of the current knowledge of vitamins or other naturally occurring antioxidant compounds and discusses critically the new aspects of antioxidant therapy.

About 100 million Americans are now using food supplements that have antioxidant activity, and there is an urgent need for providing the scientific community and the general public with the most current information available.

The biochemistry of reactive oxygen species is an important field with vast implications. Whereas oxygen is an essential component for living organisms, the generation of reactive oxygen species seems to be commonplace in aerobically metabolizing cells. Cells convene substantial resources to protect themselves against the potentially damaging effects of reactive species. The first line of defense against these free radicals is composed by enzymes, such as superoxide dismutase, glutathione peroxidase, and catalase, and several vitamins and micronutrients, which actively quench these free radical species or are required as cofactors for antioxidant enzymes. The cellular antioxidant status and its role in fighting progression of certain disease processes associated with oxidative stress have gained potential therapeutic significance in view of the beneficial effects of free-radical-scavenging drugs or antioxidants. Likewise, epidemiological studies emphasize the relevance of antioxidant vitamins and nutrients in health issues and/or prevention of chronic and degenerative diseases of aging.

Rapid progress in the application of antioxidant substances and other micronutrients warranted a revision of *Handbook of Antioxidants*. This updated edition highlights new fundamental studies on food-derived antioxidants and biomarkers, vitamins E and C, coenzyme Q, carotenoids, flavonoids and other polyphenols, antioxidants in beverages and herbal products, the thiol antioxidants glutathione and lipoic acid, and melatonin, selenium, and nitric oxide.

We are delighted to have been involved with this project and thank the contributors to this volume for their outstanding efforts.

Enrique Cadenas
Lester Packer

Contents

Series Introduction (Lester Packer and Enrique Cadenas)	*iii*
Preface	*vii*
Contributors	*xiii*

I. General Topics

1. Food-Derived Antioxidants: How to Evaluate Their Importance in Food and In Vivo — *Barry Halliwell* — 1

2. Measurement of Total Antioxidant Capacity in Nutritional and Clinical Studies — *Guohua Cao and Ronald L. Prior* — 47

3. Quantification of Isoprostanes as Indicators of Oxidant Stress In Vivo — *Jason D. Morrow, William E. Zackert, Daniel S. Van der Ende, Erin E. Reich, Erin S. Terry, Brian Cox, Stephanie C. Sanchez, Thomas J. Montine, and L. Jackson Roberts* — 57

II. Vitamin E

4. Efficacy of Vitamin E in Human Health and Disease — *Sharon V. Landvik, Anthony T. Diplock, and Lester Packer* — 75

5. Vitamin E Bioavailability, Biokinetics, and Metabolism — *Maret G. Traber* — 99

6. Biological Activity of Tocotrienols — *Stefan U. Weber and Gerald Rimbach* — 109

III. Vitamin C

7. Vitamin C: From Molecular Actions to Optimum Intake 117
   Sebastian J. Padayatty, Rushad Daruwala, Yaohui Wang, Peter K. Eck,
   Jian Song, Woo S. Koh, and Mark Levine

8. Vitamin C and Cardiovascular Diseases 147
   Anitra C. Carr and Balz Frei

9. Epidemiological and Clinical Aspects of Ascorbate and Cancer 167
   James E. Enstrom

IV. Carotenoids

10. Carotenoids: Linking Chemistry, Absorption, and Metabolism to Potential
    Roles in Human Health and Disease 189
    Denise M. Deming, Thomas W.-M. Boileau, Kasey H. Heintz,
    Christine A. Atkinson, and John W. Erdman, Jr.

11. Antioxidant Effects of Carotenoids: Implication in Photoprotection in Humans 223
    Wilhelm Stahl and Helmut Sies

12. Oxidative Breakdown of Carotenoids and Biological Effects of
    Their Metabolites 235
    Werner G. Siems, Olaf Sommerburg, and Frederik J. G. M. van Kuijk

13. Carotenoids in the Nutrition of Infants 251
    Olaf Sommerburg, Werner G. Siems, Kristina Meissner, and
    Michael Leichsenring

14. Human Studies on Bioavailability and Serum Response of Carotenoids 265
    Elizabeth J. Johnson

V. Polyphenols and Flavonoids

15. Caffeic Acid and Related Antioxidant Compounds: Biochemical and
    Cellular Effects 279
    João Laranjinha

16. Polyphenols and Flavonoids Protect LDL Against Atherogenic Modifications 303
    Bianca Fuhrman and Michael Aviram

Contents

17. Phytoestrogen Content in Foods and Their Role in Cancer ... 337
    Anna H. Wu and Malcolm C. Pike

18. Peroxynitrite Scavenging by Mitochondrial Reductants and Plant Polyphenols ... 351
    Alberto Boveris, Silvia Alvarez, Silvia Lores Arnaiz, and Laura B. Valdez

VI. Antioxidants in Beverages and Herbal Products

19. Antioxidant and Other Properties of Green and Black Tea ... 371
    Philip J. Rijken, Douglas A. Balentine, C. A. J. van Mierlo,
    I. Paetau-Robinson, F. van de Put, Paul T. Quinlan, Ute M. Weisgerber,
    and Sheila A. Wiseman

20. The Phenolic Wine Antioxidants ... 401
    Andrew L. Waterhouse

21. French Maritime Pine Bark: Pycnogenol ... 417
    Gerald Rimbach, Fabio Virgili, and Lester Packer

22. Spices as Potent Antioxidants with Therapeutic Potential ... 437
    Bharat B. Aggarwal, Nihal Ahmad, and Hasan Mukhtar

VII. Lipoic Acid and Glutathione

23. Lipoic Acid: Cellular Metabolism, Antioxidant Activity, and
    Clinical Relevance ... 473
    Oren Tirosh, Sashwati Roy, and Lester Packer

24. Cellular Effects of Lipoic Acid and Its Role in Aging ... 489
    Régis Moreau, Wei-Jian Zhang, and Tory M. Hagen

25. Vascular Complications in Diabetes: Mechanisms and the Influence
    of Antioxidants ... 511
    Peter Rösen, Hans-Jürgen Tritschler, and Lester Packer

26. Therapeutic Effects of Lipoic Acid on Hyperglycemia and
    Insulin Resistance ... 535
    Erik J. Henriksen

27. Bioavailability of Glutathione ... 549
    Dean P. Jones

VIII. Melatonin

28. Antioxidant Capacity of Melatonin — 565
    Russel J. Reiter, Dun-xian Tan, Lucien C. Manchester, and Juan R. Calvo

29. Radical and Reactive Intermediate-Scavenging Properties of Melatonin in Pure Chemical Systems — 615
    Maria A. Livrea, Luisa Tesoriere, Dun-xian Tan, and Russel J. Reiter

IX. Selenium

30. Selenium: An Antioxidant? — 633
    Regina Brigelius-Flohé, Matilde Maiorino, Fulvio Ursini, and Leopold Flohé

31. Selenium Status and Prevention of Chronic Diseases — 665
    Paul Knekt

X. Nitric Oxide

32. Antioxidant Properties of Nitric Oxide — 689
    Homero Rubbo and Rafael Radi

Index — 707

Contributors

Bharat B. Aggarwal, Ph.D. Professor of Medicine and Chief, Cytokine Research Section, Department of Bioimmunotherapy, The University of Texas M.D. Anderson Cancer Center, Houston, Texas

Nihal Ahmad, Ph.D. Assistant Professor, Department of Dermatology, Case Western Reserve University, Cleveland, Ohio

Silvia Alvarez, Ph.D. Laboratory of Free Radical Biology, School of Pharmacy and Biochemistry, University of Buenos Aires, Buenos Aires, Argentina

Silvia Lores Arnaiz, Ph.D. Laboratory of Free Radical Biology, School of Pharmacy and Biochemistry, University of Buenos Aires, Buenos Aires, Argentina

Christine A. Atkinson Division of Nutritional Sciences, University of Illinois, Urbana, Illinois

Michael Aviram, D.Sc. Head, Lipid Research Laboratory, Rambam Medical Center, Haifa, Israel

Douglas A. Balentine, Ph.D. Department of Tea Research, Lipton, Englewood Cliffs, New Jersey

Thomas W.-M. Boileau, Ph.D. Division of Nutritional Sciences, University of Illinois, Urbana, Illinois

Alberto Boveris, Ph.D. Laboratory of Free Radical Biology, School of Pharmacy and Biochemistry, University of Buenos Aires, Buenos Aires, Argentina

Regina Brigelius-Flohé, Ph.D. Professor and Head, Department of Vitamins and Atherosclerosis, German Institute of Human Nutrition, Potsdam–Rehbrücke, Germany

Juan R. Calvo, M.D., Ph.D. Professor, Department of Medical Biochemistry and Molecular Biology, University of Seville School of Medicine, Seville, Spain

Guohua Cao, M.D., Ph.D. Assistant Professor, Jean Mayer USDA Human Nutrition Research Center on Aging at Tufts University, Boston, Massachusetts

Anitra C. Carr, Ph.D. Assistant Professor (Senior Research), Linus Pauling Institute, Oregon State University, Corvallis, Oregon

Brian Cox Departments of Medicine and Pharmacology, Vanderbilt University School of Medicine, Nashville, Tennessee

Rushad Daruwala, Ph.D. Molecular and Clinical Nutrition Section, National Institute of Diabetes and Digestive and Kidney Diseases, National Institutes of Health, Bethesda, Maryland

Denise M. Deming Division of Nutritional Sciences, University of Illinois, Urbana, Illinois

Anthony T. Diplock United Medical and Dental Schools, University of London, and Guy's Hospital, London, England

Peter K. Eck, Ph.D. Molecular and Clinical Nutrition Section, National Institute of Diabetes and Digestive and Kidney Diseases, National Institutes of Health, Bethesda, Maryland

James E. Enstrom, Ph.D., M.P.H. Research Professor, School of Public Health, University of California, Los Angeles, California

John W. Erdman, Jr., Ph.D. Division of Food Science and Human Nutrition, University of Illinois, Urbana, Illinois

Leopold Flohé, M.D. Professor and Head, Department of Biochemistry, Technical University of Braunschweig, Braunschweig, Germany

Balz Frei, Ph.D. Professor and Director, Linus Pauling Institute, Oregon State University, Corvallis, Oregon

Bianca Fuhrman, D.Sc. Lipid Research Laboratory, Rambam Medical Center, Haifa, Israel

Tory M. Hagen, Ph.D. Assistant Professor of Biochemistry and Biophysics, Linus Pauling Institute, Oregon State University, Corvallis, Oregon

Barry Halliwell, D.Sc. Professor, Department of Biochemistry, National University of Singapore, Singapore

Kasey H. Heintz Division of Nutritional Sciences, University of Illinois, Urbana, Illinois

Erik J. Henriksen, Ph.D. Department of Physiology, University of Arizona College of Medicine, Tucson, Arizona

Elizabeth J. Johnson, Ph.D. Assistant Professor, Jean Mayer USDA Human Nutrition Research Center on Aging at Tufts University, Boston, Massachusetts

Contributors

Dean P. Jones, Ph.D. Professor, Department of Biochemistry, Emory University, Atlanta, Georgia

Paul Knekt, Ph.D. Department of Health and Disability, National Public Health Institute, Helsinki, Finland

Woo S. Koh, Ph.D. Molecular and Clinical Nutrition Section, National Institute of Diabetes and Digestive and Kidney Diseases, National Institutes of Health, Bethesda, Maryland

Sharon V. Landvik Vitamin E Research and Information Service, Edina, Minnesota

João Laranjinha, Ph.D. Assistant Professor, Laboratory of Biochemistry, Faculty of Pharmacy and Center for Neurosciences, University of Coimbra, Coimbra, Portugal

Michael Leichsenring, M.D., Ph.D. University Children's Hospital, Ulm, Germany

Mark Levine, M.D. Molecular and Clinical Nutrition Section, National Institute of Diabetes and Digestive and Kidney Diseases, National Institutes of Health, Bethesda, Maryland

Maria A. Livrea, Ph.D. Professor of Biochemistry, Department of Pharmaceutical, Toxicological, and Biological Chemistry, University of Palermo, Palermo, Italy

Matilde Maiorino Department of Biological Chemistry, University of Padua, Padua, Italy

Lucien C. Manchester, Ph.D. Professor, Department of Biological Science, St. Mary's University, San Antonio, Texas

Kristina Meissner, M.D. University Children's Hospital, Würzburg, Germany

Thomas J. Montine Departments of Medicine and Pharmacology, Vanderbilt University School of Medicine, Nashville, Tennessee

Régis Moreau, Ph.D. Linus Pauling Institute, Oregon State University, Corvallis, Oregon

Jason D. Morrow, M.D. F. Tremaine Billings Professor of Medicine, Department of Medicine, Vanderbilt University School of Medicine, Nashville, Tennessee

Hasan Mukhtar, Ph.D. Professor and Director of Research, Department of Dermatology, Case Western Reserve University, Cleveland, Ohio

Lester Packer, Ph.D. Department of Molecular Pharmacology and Toxicology, University of Southern California School of Pharmacy, Los Angeles, California

Sebastian J. Padayatty, F.F.A.R.C.S., M.R.C.P., Ph.D. National Institute of Diabetes and Digestive and Kidney Diseases, National Institutes of Health, Bethesda, Maryland

I. Paetau-Robinson Lipton, Englewood Cliffs, New Jersey

Malcolm C. Pike, Ph.D.   Professor, Department of Preventive Medicine, University of Southern California, Los Angeles, California

Ronald L. Prior, Ph.D.   Research Chemist, Arkansas Children's Nutrition Center, USDA-ARS, Little Rock, Arkansas

Paul T. Quinlan, B.Sc., Ph.D.   Unilever Health Institute, Unilever Research, Vlaardingen, The Netherlands

Rafael Radi, M.D., Ph.D.   Professor, Department of Biochemistry, School of Medicine, Universidad de la República, Montevideo, Uruguay

Erin E. Reich   Department of Pharmacology, Vanderbilt University School of Medicine, Nashville, Tennessee

Russel J. Reiter, Ph.D.   Professor, Department of Cellular and Structural Biology, The University of Texas Health Science Center, San Antonio, Texas

Philip J. Rijken, Ph.D.   Unilever Health Institute, Unilever Research, Vlaardingen, The Netherlands

Gerald Rimbach   Department of Molecular and Cell Biology, University of California, Berkeley, California

L. Jackson Roberts, M.D.   Professor, Departments of Pharmacology and Medicine, Vanderbilt University School of Medicine, Nashville, Tennessee

Peter Rösen, Ph.D.   Professor, Department of Clinical Biochemistry, Diabetes Research Institute, Düsseldorf, Germany

Sashwati Roy   Department of Molecular and Cell Biology, University of California, Berkeley, California

Homero Rubbo, Ph.D.   Department of Biochemistry, School of Medicine, Universidad de la República, Montevideo, Uruguay

Stephanie C. Sanchez   Department of Clinical Pharmacology, Vanderbilt University School of Medicine, Nashville, Tennessee

Werner G. Siems, M.D., Ph.D.   Herzog-Julius Hospital, Bad Harzburg, Germany

Helmut Sies, M.D.   Head, Institut für Physiologische Chemie I, Heinrich-Heine-Universität, Düsseldorf, Germany

Olaf Sommerburg, M.D.   Department of Pediatrics, University Children's Hospital, Ulm, Germany

Jian Song, M.D., Ph.D.   Molecular and Clinical Nutrition Section, National Institutes of Diabetes and Digestive and Kidney Diseases, National Institutes of Health, Bethesda, Maryland

Contributors

Wilhelm Stahl, Ph.D. Institut für Physiologische Chemie I, Heinrich-Heine-Universität, Düsseldorf, Germany

Dun-xian Tan, M.D. Department of Cellular and Structural Biology, The University of Texas Health Science Center, San Antonio, Texas

Erin S. Terry Department of Pharmacology, Vanderbilt University School of Medicine, Nashville, Tennessee

Luisa Tesoriere, M.D. Dipartimento di Scienze Farmacologiche, University of Palermo, Palermo, Italy

Oren Tirosh Department of Molecular and Cell Biology, University of California, Berkeley, California

Maret G. Traber, Ph.D. Associate Professor, Linus Pauling Institute, Oregon State University, Corvallis, Oregon, and University of California, Davis, School of Medicine, Sacramento, California

Hans-Jürgen Tritschler, Ph.D. Asta Medica AG, Frankfurt Am Main, Germany

Fulvio Ursini Department of Biological Chemistry, University of Padua, Padua, Italy

Laura B. Valdez, Ph.D. Laboratory of Free Radical Biology, School of Pharmacy and Biochemistry, University of Buenos Aires, Buenos Aires, Argentina

F. van de Put, Ph.D. Unilever Health Institute, Unilever Research, Vlaardingen, The Netherlands

Daniel S. Van der Ende Departments of Medicine and Pharmacology, Vanderbilt University School of Medicine, Nashville, Tennessee

Frederik J. G. M. van Kuijk Department of Ophthalmology and Visual Sciences, University of Texas Medical Branch, Galveston, Texas

C. A. J. van Mierlo, M.Sc. Unilever Health Institute, Unilever Research, Vlaardingen, The Netherlands

Fabio Virgili Department of Molecular and Cell Biology, University of California, Berkeley, California

Yaohui Wang, M.D. Molecular and Clinical Nutrition Section, National Institute of Diabetes and Digestive and Kidney Diseases, National Institutes of Health, Bethesda, Maryland

Andrew L. Waterhouse, Ph.D. Department of Viticulture and Enology, University of California, Davis, California

Stefan U. Weber Department of Molecular and Cell Biology, University of California, Berkeley, California

Ute M. Weisgerber, Ph.D.   Unilever Health Institute, Unilever Research, Vlaardingen, The Netherlands

Sheila A. Wiseman, Ph.D.   Unilever Health Institute, Unilever Research, Vlaardingen, The Netherlands

Anna H. Wu, Ph.D.   Professor, Department of Preventive Medicine, University of Southern California, Los Angeles, California

William E. Zackert   Department of Clinical Pharmacology, Vanderbilt University School of Medicine, Nashville, Tennessee

Wei-Jian Zhang, Ph.D., M.D.   Research Associate, Linus Pauling Institute, Oregon State University, Corvallis, Oregon

# 1
Food-Derived Antioxidants: How to Evaluate Their Importance in Food and In Vivo

Barry Halliwell
National University of Singapore, Singapore

I. INTRODUCTION

Antioxidants in food are of interest for at least four reasons. First, endogenous or added antioxidants may protect components of the food itself against oxidative damage. For example, spices rich in antioxidants have been used for centuries to delay oxidative deterioration of foods (especially lipid peroxidation and consequent development of off-flavors and rancidity) during storage or cooking. Indeed, dietary supplementation of livestock with vitamin E can improve the keeping properties of their meat (1). The use of synthetic food antioxidant additives such as butylated hydroxytoluene (BHT), butylated hydroxyanisole (BHA), and propyl gallate is under increasing regulatory scrutiny (2), and so attention is turning to the possibility that "natural" antioxidants may replace them for at least some food applications. Examples include antioxidants from rosemary (3,4), hydroxytyrosol, a phenolic antioxidant from olives (5,6), the tocopherols, tocotrienols, and flavonoids. Most antioxidants in dietary plants are phenols, which act as chain-breaking antioxidants because their $-OH$ group scavenges reactive radicals such as peroxyl radicals ($RO_2^\bullet$)

$$-OH + RO_2^\bullet \rightarrow R-O^\bullet + ROOH$$

The resulting phenoxyl radical ($R-O^\bullet$) tends to be poorly reactive because of electron delocalization into the aromatic ring, so that the reactive $RO_2^\bullet$ radical is replaced by one of limited reactivity. Phenols sometimes have additional mechanisms of antioxidant action, e.g., by chelating transition metal ions (7).

Second, dietary antioxidants may be absorbed into the human body and might exert beneficial effects. This has been established most clearly for α-tocopherol and vitamin C. Specific uptake mechanisms for L-ascorbate exist in the human gastrointestinal tract. Absorption of all tocopherols in the diet occurs, but the liver selectively secretes α-tocopherol into the plasma (8). Evidence for the absorption of other plant phenolics is growing (9). For example, quercetin and catechins can be absorbed to some extent in humans; they and their metabolites can reach plasma concentrations in the range of 0.1–1 μM (9–14). Such concentrations can, in vitro, delay the process of lipid peroxidation in liposomes, microsomes, and low-density lipoproteins (LDLs).

Third, food-derived antioxidants could exert beneficial effects, without being absorbed, in the gastrointestinal tract itself (15). For example, saliva is rich in nitrite (16), as are many foods (e.g., preserved meats and kimchi) (17,18). Nitrite is frequently used in meat preservation, because NO_2^-/oxides of nitrogen have powerful antibacterial actions (18,19). Nitric oxide can also prevent rancidity, as it can inhibit lipid peroxidation by at least two mechanisms. It can scavenge reactive peroxyl radicals that propagate the chain reaction (20)

$$RO_2^{\cdot} + NO^{\cdot} \rightarrow ROONO$$

Lipid peroxidation in meat can be promoted by release of iron ions and by heme compounds, such as myoglobin, and $NO^{\cdot}$ antagonizes these actions (21–23). By contrast to these beneficial actions, ingested nitrite reacts with gastric acid to produce nitrous acid (HNO_2), which decomposes to oxides of nitrogen, such as N_2O_3. This can lead to nitrosation of amines, nitration of aromatic compounds, and deamination of DNA bases, especially guanine (15). Several phenolic compounds found in plants are powerful inhibitors of HNO_2-dependent tyrosine nitration and DNA base deamination in vitro, inhibiting much more effectively than does ascorbate (24). Hence, phenols in fruits, vegetables, wines, tea, and other beverages could conceivably exert a gastroprotective effect in situations of excess production of reactive nitrogen species (a term defined in Table 1). Perhaps this is one reason why green tea might protect against cancer: some of its constituents may remove potentially DNA-damaging reactive nitrogen species in the stomach. This assumes that any products (e.g., nitrated or oxidized phenols) resulting from the interactions of phenols with reactive species (25) are not themselves toxic.

To consider the other end of the gastrointestinal tract, unabsorbed dietary phenolics will end up in the colon. It is perhaps fortunate that the human colon is hypoxic, as feces incubated under aerobic conditions generate oxygen radicals at a high rate by reactions involving iron ions (26), which are poorly absorbed in the small intestine and thus usually found in the colonic contents of subjects on iron-replete diets. The ability of unabsorbed dietary phenolics to pass into the colon, where they may chelate iron ions and scavenge any "reactive species" (see Table 1) that are formed may thus be beneficial when transient rises in intracolonic oxygen tension occur and allow production of such species. Several flavonoids can inhibit cyclooxygenase and lipoxygenase enzymes, which may be important in the development of colon cancer (27,28).

Fourth, there is considerable interest in plant extracts for therapeutic use (e.g., as anti-inflammatory, anti-ischemic, and antithrombotic agents). An extract of the ornamental tree *Ginkgo biloba* has been used in herbal medicine for thousands of years: the extract has antioxidant properties in vitro, apparently largely from the flavonoids present, which include rutin, kaempferol, quercetin, and myricetin (29). Traditional Japanese Kampo medicines are extracts of multiple herbs and contain a complex mixture of phenols and other compounds, including glycyrrhizin from roots of the licorice plant, *Glycyrrhiza glabra* (30,31). Extracts of propolis, a resinous substance collected by bees, have often been used in herbal medicine, and contain many phenolic compounds (32). Pycnogenol, an extract of pine bark, shows several antioxidant effects in vitro (33).

Not all the biological effects of plant phenols need be related to antioxidant activity: estrogen antagonism, antiangiogenic effects, promotion of apoptosis, inhibition of cytochromes P450, protein kinases and telomerase, and up-regulation of the expression of genes encoding enzymes that detoxify xenobiotics are additional mechanisms of action. These effects will not be explored further here.

Table 1 The "Reactive Species"

Radicals	Nonradicals
Reactive oxygen species (ROS)	
Superoxide, $O_2^{\cdot-}$ [a]	Hydrogen peroxide, H_2O_2 [a]
Hydroxyl, $OH^{\cdot}$ [a]	Hypobromous acid, HOBr
Hydroperoxyl, $HO_2^{\cdot}$ [a]	Ozone O_3
Lipid peroxyl, $LO_2^{\cdot}$ [a]	Singlet oxygen $(O_2{}^1\Delta g)$ [a]
Lipid alkoxyl, $LO^{\cdot}$ [a]	Lipid peroxides, LOOH [a]
	Maillard reaction products [a]
Reactive chlorine species (RCS)	
Atomic chlorine, $Cl^{\cdot}$	Hypochlorous acid, HOCl [a]
	Nitryl (nitronium) chloride NO_2Cl [b]
	Chloramines
Reactive nitrogen species (RNS)	
Nitric oxide, $NO^{\cdot}$ [a]	Nitrous acid, HNO_2 [a]
Nitrogen dioxide, $NO_2^{\cdot}$ [a]	Nitrosyl cation, NO^+
	Nitroxyl anion, NO^-
	Dinitrogen tetroxide, N_2O_4
	Dinitrogen trioxide, N_2O_3
	Peroxynitrite, $ONOO^-$
	Peroxynitrous acid, ONOOH
	Nitronium (nitryl) cation, NO_2^+
	Alkyl peroxynitrites, ROONO
	Nitryl (nitronium) chloride, NO_2Cl [b]

Reactive oxygen species (ROS) is a collective term that includes both oxygen radicals and certain nonradicals that are oxidizing agents or are easily converted into radicals (HOCl, O_3, $ONOO^-$, $^1O_2$, H_2O_2). RNS is also a collective term including nitric oxide and nitrogen dioxide radicals, as well as such nonradicals as HNO_2 and N_2O_4. $ONOO^-$ is often included in both categories. *Reactive* is not always an appropriate term: H_2O_2, $NO^{\cdot}$, and $O_2^{\cdot-}$ react quickly with only a few molecules, whereas $OH^{\cdot}$ reacts quickly with almost everything. $RO_2^{\cdot}$, $RO^{\cdot}$, HOCl, $NO_2^{\cdot}$, $ONOO^-$, and O_3 have intermediate reactivities.
HOBr could also be considered a "reactive bromine species."
[a] Reactive species particularly relevant to foods.
[b] NO_2Cl is a chlorinating and nitrating species produced by reaction of HOCl with NO_2.

II. HOW TO DEFINE AN ANTIOXIDANT

The major interest of antioxidants to the food industry is in the prevention of off-flavors, rancidity, and similar phenomena (34). These undesirable characteristics are related to lipid peroxidation, either nonenzymic peroxidation or peroxidation initiated by the action of lipoxygenase enzymes in the plant (35). Hence, food scientists often equate antioxidants with "inhibitors of lipid peroxidation and consequent food deterioration." By contrast, in the human gastrointestinal tract as well as within the body tissues, oxidative damage to proteins and DNA is just as important as damage to lipids, if not more so (36). Indeed, oxidative DNA damage may be a major risk factor for the development of cancer, so that dietary antioxidants able to decrease such damage in vivo would be expected to have an anticancer effect (36). Hence, a broader definition (36) of an *antioxidant* is *any substance that, when present at low concentrations compared with those of an oxidizable substrate, significantly delays or prevents oxidation of that substrate.* The term *oxidizable substrate* encompasses almost everything (except H_2O) found in foods and in living tissues and includes proteins, lipids, carbohydrates, and DNA.

The foregoing definition does not include all possibilities for mechanisms of antioxidant action, but it does have the virtue of emphasizing the importance of the target chosen for study and the source of reactive species employed when characterizing an antioxidant. The "rank order" or "relative importance" of antioxidants is not an absolute: it depends on which reactive species are being generated, in which environment, and what target of damage is examined. For example, if human blood plasma is tested for its ability to inhibit iron ion-dependent lipid peroxidation, transferrin and ceruloplasmin are the most important protective agents (37). If plasma is exposed to the toxic free radical gas nitrogen dioxide, uric acid is the most important protective antioxidant (38), whereas urate plays little protective role against damage by hypochlorous acid (HOCl) in plasma (39). Similarly, if the source of reactive species is kept the same, but a different *target* of oxidative damage is measured, the results can be different. For example, when human blood plasma is exposed to gas-phase cigarette smoke in vitro, lipid peroxidation occurs and ascorbate inhibits this process (40). By contrast, ascorbic acid has no effect on formation of plasma protein carbonyls, an index of oxidative protein damage, caused by cigarette smoke (41). In a recent in vivo study, consumption of blackcurrant and apple juice by human volunteers appeared to decrease lipid peroxidation, but to *increase* oxidative protein damage (42).

Hence, it is possible for an antioxidant to protect in one biological or food system, but to fail to protect (or even sometimes to promote damage) in others. For example, antioxidant inhibitors of lipid peroxidation may not protect other molecular targets (such as DNA and protein) against oxidative damage, and may sometimes aggravate such damage (43). This may not matter a great deal in foods, because damage to DNA and proteins, unless extensive, will (unlike lipid peroxidation) not normally alter the taste or texture of food or affect nutritional quality. However, essential amino acids, such as tryptophan and methionine, are destroyed by certain reactive species (44), and oxidative damage to sulfur-containing amino acids can sometimes create off-flavors (45). By contrast to foods, oxidative DNA and protein damage are of the greatest importance in the cells of the human gastrointestinal tract and within the body. Oxidative DNA damage is a risk factor for cancer development, and protein damage by reactive species is involved in cancer, cardiovascular, and neurodegenerative diseases (36,44,46,47).

Hundreds of compounds have been suggested to act as antioxidants. Proposed antioxidants range from carotenoids and metallothioneins, to histidine-containing dipeptides (carnosine, homocarnosine, anserine), mucus, phytic acid, taurine, bilirubin, estrogens, creatinine, lipoic acid, polyamines, melatonin, quercetin, carnosol, thymol, carnosic acid, hydroxytyrosol, gallic acid derivatives, tannins, catechins, rutin, morin, ellagic acid, eugenol, and rosemarinic acids. These individual compounds, as well as complex plant extracts such as *G. biloba*, pycnogenol, and Kampo medicines have antioxidant activity in vitro. But how should such "antioxidant activity" be quantitated for comparative purposes (e.g., for "standardization" of herbal medicine preparations)? Could compounds that are excellent antioxidants in vitro work as such in vivo? If absorbed into the body, will they be safe? Could they cause damage in the gastrointestinal tract, or will they protect it? Characterizing antioxidants only on the basis of ability to inhibit lipid peroxidation is inadequate. For example, the established carcinogen diethylstilbestrol is a powerful inhibitor of lipid peroxidation in vitro (48), while being a DNA-damaging agent in vivo (49). Butylated hydroxytoluene is a powerful inhibitor of lipid peroxidation,

FOOD-DERIVED ANTIOXIDANTS

yet large doses of it can induce oxidative DNA damage and cancer development in the rat forestomach (2,50).

III. ANTIOXIDANT CHARACTERIZATION IN VITRO

A compound might exert antioxidant actions in vivo or in food by inhibiting generation of reactive species, or by directly scavenging them. An additional mechanism by which an antioxidant might act in vivo is by raising the levels of endogenous antioxidant defenses (e.g., by up-regulating expression of the genes encoding SOD, catalase, or glutathione peroxidase). Section IV will be devoted to a consideration of how to evaluate antioxidant action in vivo. The aim of the present section is to outline simple experiments that are able to assess direct antioxidant ability in vitro and to test for possible pro-oxidant effects on different molecular targets. This "screening" approach can be used to rule out direct antioxidant activity in vivo: a compound that is a poor antioxidant in vitro is unlikely to be any better as a direct antioxidant in vivo. Screening can also alert one to the possibility of damaging effects.

During in vitro testing, it is essential to examine the action of a putative antioxidant over a concentration range that is relevant. For example, if compound X is present in vivo at concentrations less than 1 μM, its ability to inhibit lipid peroxidation in vitro only at concentrations greater than 10 μM is irrelevant unless there is good reason to suspect that X concentrates at a particular site in vivo. One must also bear in mind that, if a compound acts as a scavenger of free radicals, an "antioxidant" may itself give rise to damaging radical species, because reaction of a free radical with a nonradical always generates a new free radical (radicals beget radicals). It is also important to use relevant reactive oxygen, nitrogen, or chlorine species and sources generating such species (see Table 1); the choice will depend on whether effects in vivo (including the gastrointestinal tract) or effects in foods are being considered.

A. Assays of "Total Antioxidant Activity"

Several attempts have been made to assess the "total antioxidant activity" (TAA) of plant extracts, foods, or body fluids, rather than go to the trouble of specifically identifying each antioxidant present. The first assay of this type to become popular was the total (peroxyl) radical-trapping antioxidant parameter (TRAP) assay (51). The system under study is incubated with the azo compound azobis(2-amidinopropane) hydrochloride (AAPH), which decomposes to form carbon-centered radicals that then react with oxygen to generate peroxyl radicals ($RO_2^{\cdot}$)

$$AAPH \rightarrow N_2 + 2R^{\cdot}$$
$$2R^{\cdot} + 2O_2 \rightarrow 2RO_2^{\cdot}$$

Peroxyl radicals are scavenged by antioxidants in the system under test: only when these antioxidants have been depleted will the $RO_2^{\cdot}$ radicals attack lipids (lipids in the system under test, or lipids added to it) to cause peroxidation. By measuring the lag period before onset of peroxidation (e.g., assayed by O_2 uptake) and calibrating the assay with a known antioxidant (usually the water-soluble vitamin E analogue, Trolox C), a value for TRAP can be obtained as the number of micromoles of peroxyl radicals trapped per liter of body fluid or food extract. Trolox can trap two $RO_2^{\cdot}$ per molecule. It is essential to ensure that O_2 uptake does not cause substantial O_2 depletion during the TRAP assay because the carbon-centered radicals ($R^{\cdot}$) generated from AAPH can themselves react with certain antioxidants (52).

Several variations on the TRAP assay exist. One is to use alternative peroxyl radical generators (e.g., the lipid-soluble compound AMVN). Another is to use different detection methods, such as luminol-enhanced chemiluminescence or bleaching of crocetin. Similar assays have been developed using different sources of free radicals and different types of detector molecule: they include ORAC, FRAP (53), and the ABTS assay (54). The ABTS assay has proved especially suitable for application to beverages and food extracts (54–56). The compound ABTS (2,2-azinobis [3-ethyl-benzothiazoline-6-sulfonate]) is chemically oxidized (54) to a stable, colored free radical cation, ABTS$^{\cdot+}$. Scavenging of this radical is easily followed by loss of its characteristic absorbance. For example, Table 2 shows an application of the ABTS assay to compare the "total antioxidant" content of various seasonings. Other stable radicals, employed for antioxidant characterization include 1,1-diphenyl-2-picrylhydrazyl (DPPH) (57) and galvinoxyl. For example, Shi and Niki (58) examined the antioxidant activity of *G. biloba* extracts by measuring their ability to quench the galvinoxyl radical and concluded that 1 g of the extract used contained 6.62×10^{19} "active hydrogens," each able to quench a single galvinoxyl radical.

Total antioxidant activity assays are useful in obtaining a global picture of relative antioxidant activities in different body fluids, foods, and drinks, and how they change (e.g., in disease or after food processing or storage). They may also help detect synergistic interactions of antioxidants. For example, not all the TAA of human plasma is accounted for by known antioxidants: it is not known whether the "unidentified" part is due to synergistic antioxidant interactions or to antioxidant molecules that have not yet been identified (59). Nevertheless, the results of TAA assays should be interpreted in the light of the chemistry of the assay and can sometimes be misleading. Urate is a major contributor to the TAA of human plasma in most assays (60); rises in plasma urate levels could obscure depletions of ascorbate and other

Table 2 Trolox Equivalent Antioxidant Capacities (TEAC) of Seasonings Used in Asian Cooking

Seasoning	TEAC (mM) (mean ± SD, $n = 3$)
Dark soy sauce (Tiger brand)	147.33 ± 9.45
Dark soy sauce (Tai Hua brand)	127.33 ± 4.93
Dark soy sauce (Woh Hup brand)	47.1 ± 1.93
HP sauce	9.80 ± 0.53
Tomato sauce	3.23 ± 0.06
Kung Bo sauce	9.17 ± 0.91
Black vinegar	10.37 ± 1.00
Chinese cooking wine	6.17 ± 0.35
Chinese rice wine	0.36 ± 0.13
Chili sauce	11.10 ± 1.51
Sweet dark soy sauce (Zara)	28.73 ± 2.54
Sweet soy sauce	35.43 ± 1.60
Oyster sauce	5.58 ± 2.75
Plum sauce	3.53 ± 1.27
Hoisin sauce	13.60 ± 2.16
Sweet flour sauce	10.40 ± 0.53
Soba sauce	9.27 ± 0.64
Sesame oil	3.27 ± 1.08

Note the high antioxidant ability of dark soy sauces.
Source: Ref. 56.

antioxidants in certain diseases if only TAA is examined. Preservatives added to foods and beverages can also contribute to TRAP [e.g., sulfites added to white wines (56) and ascorbate to fruit juices].

B. Scavenging of Reactive Nitrogen Species

Several reactive nitrogen species are relevant to the food matrix, to the gastrointestinal tract, and to the rest of the human body. Nitrogen is present in foods as nitrates, amines, nitrites, peptides, proteins, and amino acids, and its metabolites in vivo include nitric oxide, higher oxides of nitrogen, and peroxynitrite (61,62). Indeed, generation of HNO_2 and oxides of nitrogen in the stomach by reaction of salivary (and dietary) NO_2^- with gastric acid may be an important antibacterial mechanism (16). However, excess intragastric production of reactive nitrogen species (e.g., as a result of *Helicobacter pylori* infection, chronic inflammation, or excessive consumption of NO_2^--rich foods), may enhance the risk of gastric cancer by mechanisms involving formation of *N*-nitroso compounds and possibly also deamination of DNA (15,24,62–65). Similarly, excess production of reactive nitrogen species may be a risk factor for cancer development in hepatitis and other chronic inflammatory processes (62,66).

Although nitric oxide ($NO^{\cdot}$) is a free radical, it is probably insufficiently reactive to attack DNA directly. By contrast, dinitrogen trioxide (N_2O_3), nitrous acid (HNO_2), and peroxynitrite ($ONOO^-$) can lead to deamination and nitration of DNA (62). Living organisms, therefore, have evolved enzymes that can remove deamination products of cytosine (uracil), adenine (hypoxanthine), and guanine (xanthine) from DNA to decrease the risk of mutagenicity (67–69). Estimates of total daily endogenous production of oxides of nitrogen in the healthy human body are about 1 mmol/day, based on steady-state levels of plasma NO_3^- and NO_2^- in subjects placed on diets free of these substances (70).

1. Nitrous Acid

It follows from the foregoing that agents able to interfere with nitrosation, nitration, and deamination reactions may be important in gastroprotection, and possibly also in helping to protect food constituents against damage by any oxides of nitrogen generated in the food matrix (15). For example, studies in vitro show that catechins and several other phenolic compounds can inhibit the nitration of tyrosine and the deamination of DNA bases induced by addition of HNO_2 (24) (although possible biological effects of any nitrated or oxidized phenols generated during such reactions must be considered). γ-Tocopherol has been reported to react with various reactive nitrogen species, including peroxynitrite and $NO_2^{\cdot}$, faster than does α-tocopherol (71,72). Although the significance of such reactions in the human body is uncertain (73), γ-tocopherol may help protect against deleterious effects of oxides of nitrogen in plants (74).

Methodology that enables the "screening" of compounds for the ability to prevent deamination and nitration in vitro has been recently reviewed (75). In essence, it involves examining effects on 3-nitrotyrosine formation from tyrosine, or formation of xanthine and hypoxanthine (deamination products of guanine and adenine, respectively) from DNA, after exposure to HNO_2. All these products can be measured by high-performance liquid chromatography (HPLC) or by gas chromatography–mass spectrometry (GC–MS) (75).

2. Peroxynitrite

Peroxynitrite is a cytotoxic species that can be generated in several ways, most usually by the rapid addition of superoxide and nitric oxide radicals (61).

$$O_2^{\cdot -} + NO^{\cdot} \rightarrow ONOO^-$$

Peroxynitrite anion ($ONOO^-$) is stable at highly alkaline pH, but undergoes reaction with CO_2, protonation, isomerization, and decomposition at physiological pH to give noxious products that deplete antioxidants and oxidize and nitrate lipids, proteins, and DNA (61,76–79). These noxious products may include $NO_2^·$, NO_2^+, and $OH^·$ (76–82). The detailed mechanisms by which $ONOO^-$ and species derived from it cause modification of biomolecules are still controversial and incompletely understood, but there is little doubt about the ability of $ONOO^-$ to be cytotoxic at physiological pH (61,79). Indeed, formation of $ONOO^-$ has been suggested to contribute to tissue injury in a wide range of human diseases, usually on the basis of detection of 3-nitrotyrosine in the injured tissues (79,80,82). Nitrotyrosine is generated when $ONOO^-$ is added to tyrosine itself or to proteins containing tyrosine residues, and the rate of nitration can be increased if transition metal ions or certain metalloproteins [e.g., copper, zinc-superoxide dismutase (Cu,Zn-SOD)] are present (61,81). Detection of 3-nitrotyrosine is most often achieved by antibody immunostaining of tissues, but HPLC- and GC–MS-based techniques have also been described (80). However, caution must be used in interpreting nitration of tyrosine as definitive evidence for $ONOO^-$ formation, because other tyrosine-nitrating reactions can occur (79,80,82). Nevertheless, the substantial evidence that the cytotoxic actions of $ONOO^-$ (or species derived from it) contribute to the damage that can be caused by overproduction of $NO^·$ in vivo has led to considerable interest in the development of agents that can scavenge $ONOO^-$, or toxic species derived from $ONOO^-$.

Need for Different Types of Assay. The chemistry of $ONOO^-$ is complex; addition of $ONOO^-$ to biological material leads to oxidation of different biomolecules by different mechanisms (76–81). Use of a single assay method can thus give misleading results about the efficacy of scavengers. Hence, I recommend use of at least two different in vitro assays as a preliminary "screen" of putative $ONOO^-$ "scavengers."

Ability to Protect Against $ONOO^-$-Dependent Tyrosine Nitration. This assay is chosen because nitration of tyrosine occurs in vivo. Peroxynitrite is added to tyrosine in vitro, and the formation of 3-nitrotyrosine is measured by HPLC. Good scavengers of $ONOO^-$ (or of the tyrosine-nitrating species derived from $ONOO^-$) will inhibit the production of 3-nitrotyrosine. Powerful inhibitors of $ONOO^-$-dependent tyrosine nitration present in plants include ergothionine (83), ascorbate (84), and phenolic compounds, including flavonoids (85–87). A major fate of $ONOO^-$ in vivo is reaction with CO_2/HCO_3^-, which alters its nitrating ability and reactivity with antioxidants (88,89). Hence, assays of $ONOO^-$ scavengers intended for in vivo use should include HCO_3^- in the assay system (90).

Ability to Affect $ONOO^-$-Dependent Inactivation of α_1-Antiprotease. This protein target has been selected because damage to α_1-antiprotease occurs at sites of chronic inflammation, and the generation of $ONOO^-$ may be involved. Inactivation of α_1-antiprotease by $ONOO^-$ appears to occur by oxidation of methionine residues (91). α_1-Antiprotease is the major plasma inhibitor of serine proteases, such as elastase, in humans. It is assayed by its ability to inhibit elastase, the activity of which, in turn, is determined by the ability of elastase to hydrolyze the synthetic substrate N-succinyl(ala)$_3$-p-nitroanilide (92). One advantage of this assay is that α_1-antiprotease is susceptible to inactivation by a wide range of free radicals. Peroxynitrite reacts with several biomolecules to generate free radicals that can inactivate α_1-antiprotease. Hence, this protein is a useful "screen" for formation of such secondary radicals from putative "peroxynitrite scavengers." One example is the detection of cytotoxic products formed by the interaction of $ONOO^-$ with sulfite (SO_3^{2-}), an agent added to many foodstuffs as a preservative (93). Several other "detector molecules" for $ONOO^-$ are available for use in screening putative scavengers (94).

C. Scavenging of Reactive Oxygen Species

1. Superoxide Radical ($O_2^{\cdot-}$) and Hydrogen Peroxide (H_2O_2)

Superoxide radical is produced in vivo, and the superoxide dismutase enzymes are an important protective antioxidant defense (36,95). Superoxide may also be produced by autoxidation (or metal-catalyzed oxidation) of several food constituents, including flavonoids, fragrant components of soy sauce, sulfite, hydroxyhydroquinone and other phenolics in coffee, and food additives, such as the colorant carminic acid (96–99). Photochemical generation of $O_2^{\cdot-}$ can occur in light-exposed foods (see Sec. III.F). Superoxide generated both in vivo and in foods can undergo several reactions, including dismutation to give H_2O_2.

$$O_2^{\cdot-} + O_2^{\cdot-} + 2H^+ \to H_2O_2 + O_2$$

Dismutation occurs spontaneously at a rate that decreases with a rise in pH, but the rate can be accelerated enormously by addition of superoxide dismutase (SOD) enzymes, which are present in essentially all body tissues (95) and in most uncooked foods (100).

Other sources of H_2O_2 in vivo include such enzymes as glycollate oxidase and monoamine oxidases (36). Hydrogen peroxide is generated in many foods and beverages, including black tea, green tea, and coffee. Instant coffee is especially effective in producing H_2O_2, often generating concentrations in the hundreds of micromolar range (99,101). This H_2O_2 appears to arise by oxidation of some of the phenols present (99,101). Hydrogen peroxide has been used in the food industry as a sterilizing agent (e.g., for poultry carcasses) (102) and it has been detected in human urine, often in substantial quantities (103).

Fortunately, neither $O_2^{\cdot-}$ nor H_2O_2 is very reactive. H_2O_2 can cross membranes readily, which $O_2^{\cdot-}$ is unable to do; the charged natured of $O_2^{\cdot-}$ renders it membrane-impermeable unless there is a transmembrane channel through which it can move, such as the anion channel in erythrocytes (104). Only a few compounds, other than specific enzymes such as SOD and catalase, are able to react with $O_2^{\cdot-}$ and H_2O_2 at rapid rates (one exception is the very fast reaction of $O_2^{\cdot-}$ with $NO^{\cdot}$ to give $ONOO^-$). For example, many thiols have been claimed to react with H_2O_2 and with $O_2^{\cdot-}$, but the rate constants for these reactions are low (105–107). However, H_2O_2 can form highly reactive hydroxyl radicals ($OH^{\cdot}$) in the presence of transition metal ions (108), such as iron.

$$Fe^{2+} + H_2O_2 \to \text{intermediate species} \to OH^{\cdot} + OH^- + Fe^{3+}$$

Superoxide reacts with several enzymes that possess iron–sulfur clusters at their active sites, including mammalian aconitase, and such reactions can lead to transition metal ion release, which could conceivably facilitate hydroxyl radical formation (109). Superoxide can also release some iron from ferritin (110). As well as promoting Fenton chemistry by iron release, superoxide can reduce Fe(III) to Fe^{2+} to accelerate Fenton chemistry by regenerating Fe^{2+}.

$$Fe^{3+} + O_2^{\cdot-} \rightleftharpoons Fe^{2+} + O_2$$

Ascorbate in foods can have a similar pro-oxidant effect (111).

Assessment of Superoxide Scavenging. Superoxide can be produced by exposure of water to ionizing radiation, and the technique of pulse radiolysis allows examination of the absorbance spectrum of any products formed when $O_2^{\cdot-}$ reacts with a putative antioxidant (112). However, pulse radiolysis is unsuitable for measuring most reactions of $O_2^{\cdot-}$ in aqueous solution, because the reaction rates are usually lower than the overall rate of nonenzymic dismutation of $O_2^{\cdot-}$ (105). This limits measurements of rate constants to those of 10^5 M^{-1} s^{-1} or greater. Unfortunately, the rate constants for the reaction of $O_2^{\cdot-}$ with most biological molecules, exceptions being ascorbate (113), NO·, and SOD, are less than this. Stopped-flow methods can be used to study these slower reactions. However, provided that suitable control experiments are done, good approximations to rate constants may be achieved using simple test tube systems (114). For example, a mixture of hypoxanthine (or xanthine) and xanthine oxidase at pH 7.4 generates $O_2^{·-}$ that reacts with cytochrome c and nitroblue tetrazolium (NBT) with defined rate constants, namely 2.6×10^5 and 6×10^4 M^{-1} s^{-1}, respectively (105). Any added antioxidant that reacts with $O_2^{·-}$ will decrease the rates of cytochrome c or NBT reduction, and analysis of the inhibition produced allows calculation of an approximate rate constant for reaction of X with $O_2^{·-}$ (114). This approach has been widely used to establish rate constants for the reactions of $O_2^{·-}$ with various molecules. However, some controls are essential.

1. It must be checked that the putative $O_2^{·-}$ scavenger does not inhibit $O_2^{·-}$ generation (e.g., by inhibiting xanthine oxidase). Several plant phenolics have been reported to inhibit this enzyme (115). This possibility is often examined by measuring uric acid formation as the rise in absorbance at 290 nm. However, many compounds absorb strongly at 290 nm, making spectrophotometric assessment of xanthine oxidase activity inaccurate. HPLC analysis of uric acid production, or measurement of O_2 uptake in an O_2 electrode, are alternative assays of xanthine oxidase that are not subject to his artifact.

2. It must be checked that the substance does not itself reduce cytochrome c or NBT, or react with $O_2^{·-}$ to initiate an autoxidation reaction that leads to further $O_2^{·-}$ generation. Direct reduction is a particular problem with cytochrome c (e.g., it is easily reduced by ascorbic acid and thiols).

Assessment of Hydrogen Peroxide Formation and Scavenging. H_2O_2 is easily and sensitively measured by using peroxidase-based assay systems. One popular system uses horseradish peroxidase, and follows the oxidation of scopoletin by H_2O_2 to form a nonfluorescent product (116). Other peroxidase substrates can also be used (e.g., oxdiation of guaiacol gives a brown chromogen, and oxidation of 4-aminoantipyrine has been used to measure low levels of H_2O_2 in noodles, fish paste, dried fish, and herring roe) (117). Thus, if a putative peroxide scavenger is incubated with H_2O_2 and the reaction mixture sampled for analysis of H_2O_2 at various times by addition of an aliquot to peroxidase and peroxidase substrate, the rate of loss of H_2O_2 can be measured to allow calculation of rate constants for reaction of the scavenger with H_2O_2. An essential control is to check that the scavenger being tested is not itself oxidizable by peroxidase; if it is, it might compete with the peroxidase substrate and cause an artifactual inhibition. For example, ascorbic acid and flavonoids can be oxidized by horseradish peroxidase, and in the presence of H_2O_2 they have the potential to interfere with peroxidase-based assay systems. Superoxide radical can react with peroxidase to convert it to the less active compound III, thus potentially compromising measurement of H_2O_2 in systems generating $O_2^{·-}$. This can be avoided by adding SOD to the assay mixture (118).

If the compound or extract under test does interfere with peroxidase-based systems, other assays for H_2O_2 can be used. Thus, H_2O_2 can be estimated by simple titration with acidified potassium permanganate ($KMnO_4$) or by measuring the O_2 release (1 mol of O_2 per 2 mol of H_2O_2) when a sample of the reaction mixture is injected into an O_2 electrode containing buffer and a large amount of catalase. Varma (119) has described a sensitive radiochemical assay for H_2O_2, based on its ability to decarboxylate ^{14}C-labeled 2-oxoglutarate to $^{14}CO_2$ (measured by scintillation counting). Another method that can easily measure H_2O_2 (although with a lower degree of sensitivity) is the ferrous-oxidation xylenol orange (FOX) assay. Peroxides oxidize Fe^{2+} to Fe^{3+}, which forms a colored complex with the dye xylenol orange (120).

This method has been used to measure rates of H_2O_2 generation in beverages (101), but a control with added catalase is needed to show that the oxidizing species is H_2O_2 (which will be degraded by catalase, thus abolishing color development). The FOX assay can also measure lipid peroxides (120).

2. Hydroxyl Radical

Much of the damage that can be done by $O_2^{\cdot-}$ and H_2O_2 in vivo is thought to be due to their conversion into more reactive species (108), probably the most important of which is hydroxyl radical, $OH^{\cdot}$.

Formation of $OH^{\cdot}$ in vivo and in foods can be achieved by at least four different mechanisms. One requires traces of transition metal ions, of which iron and copper seem likely to be the most important in vivo (see Sec. III.C.1). Iron and copper ions become available to catalyze such reactions when human tissues are damaged (36,108,121,122). Iron and copper ions can also be liberated during processing and cooking of foods, especially of meats (18,21,123–125). Vitamin C in foods can reduce transition metal ions, facilitating $OH^{\cdot}$ generation.

$$Fe^{3+} + ascorbate \rightarrow ascorbate\ radical + Fe^{2+}$$

$$Cu^{2+} + ascorbate \rightarrow ascorbate\ radical + Cu^{+}$$

A second mechanism is exposure to ionizing radiation, which causes $OH^{\cdot}$ formation by homolysis of water (126).

$$H_2O_2 \xrightarrow{energy} \underset{\substack{\text{hydrogen} \\ \text{radical} \\ \text{(atom)}}}{H^{\cdot}} + \underset{\substack{\text{hydroxyl} \\ \text{radical}}}{OH^{\cdot}}$$

This mechanism is particularly relevant to food irradiation. If water is present in the food (as it usually is), $OH^{\cdot}$ can be generated, leading to formation of secondary free radicals—which are often stable enough to be detected by electron spin resonance (ESR) in bone and cuticle—as well as oxidative damage to DNA, lipids, and proteins (127–129). Indeed, $OH^{\cdot}$-dependent formation of such products as thymine glycol from DNA and *ortho*-tyrosine from phenylalanine residues in proteins has been measured as "biomarkers" of $OH^{\cdot}$ generation in irradiated foods (129). Stadler et al. (130) used the formation of 8-oxocaffeine from caffeine as a means of monitoring hydroxyl radical formation in coffee and other foods.

A third source of some $OH^{\cdot}$ is the decomposition of $ONOO^{-}$ (as described in Sec. III.B.2), although only small amounts of $OH^{\cdot}$ appear to be formed. Finally, reaction of hypochlorous acid (HOCl) with $O_2^{\cdot-}$ can make some $OH^{\cdot}$ (131).

$$HOCl + O_2^{\cdot-} \rightarrow OH^{\cdot} + O_2 + Cl^{-}$$

Reactions of Hydroxyl Radical. The hydroxyl radical is highly reactive: it can react with essentially all molecules found in foods or in vivo, with rate constants of 10^9–10^{10} M^{-1} s^{-1} (132). Thus, almost everything in food or in vivo is potentially an $OH^{\cdot}$ scavenger: no specific molecule has evolved for this role in living organisms. Hence, suggestions that diet-derived or synthetic antioxidants can scavenge $OH^{\cdot}$ within the human body are unlikely. Their rate constants for reaction with $OH^{\cdot}$ in vitro may be high, but the molar concentrations of these substances achieved in vivo are usually far less than that of endogenous molecules that are also capable of rapid reaction with $OH^{\cdot}$. For example, blood plasma albumin [concentration $\sim$ 0.5 mM) is an excellent $OH^{\cdot}$ scavenger (rate constant $> 10^{10}$ M^{-1} s^{-1}) (133). Glucose is not quite as good an $OH^{\cdot}$ scavenger (rate constant about 10^9 M^{-1} s^{-1}) (132), but it is present at relatively high concentrations (4–10 mM) in plasma. Nevertheless, the very high concentrations of sugars present in certain foods could represent a powerful potential for scavenging OH·.

Antioxidants Affecting Hydroxyl Radical Formation. Agents that inhibit damage caused by OH· in vivo are more likely to act by scavenging or blocking formation of the precursors of OH· ($O_2^{·-}$, H_2O_2, HOCl, $ONOO^-$) or by binding the transition metal ions needed for OH· formation from H_2O_2. Metal ion chelation can inhibit OH· generation by two general mechanisms. First, binding of the ion to the chelator may so alter the redox potential or accessibility of the ion that it cannot participate in OH· formation from H_2O_2. This occurs for iron ions bound to the iron-binding proteins, transferrin and lactoferrin, for example (134). Second, the binding of a transition metal ion to an "antioxidant" may not prevent redox reactions, but the OH· formed can be directed onto the antioxidant, so protecting an external target (108,135,136). For example, when copper ions bind to albumin, Fenton-type reactions can still occur at the binding sites, and the albumin is damaged by OH· (136). However, albumin is a much less important target of damage than are plasma lipoproteins and the membranes of blood cells and vascular endothelial cells. Thus, the binding of copper ions to albumin may represent a protective mechanism, because the damaged albumin can be replaced quickly (137). Histidine-containing dipeptides such as carnosine, which are found in many mammalian tissues and in foods of animal origin, might also act as antioxidants by metal ion chelation (138). Citrate is frequently added to foods: one of its advantages is that it can chelate iron ions in forms that are poorly reactive (139)—although not completely unreactive (140)—in catalyzing free radical damage.

Assessment of Hydroxyl Radical Scavenging. The definitive technique for measuring the rate constant for reaction of a substance with OH·, and for studying the products of that reaction, is pulse radiolysis (112,132). If pulse radiolysis facilities are not available, approximate rate constants can often be obtained using several simpler assays. In the author's laboratory, the "deoxyribose method" is often used (141). Hydroxyl radicals are generated by a mixture of ascorbic acid, H_2O_2, and Fe(III)–EDTA

$$Fe(III)\text{–}EDTA + ascorbate \rightarrow Fe^{2+}\text{–}EDTA + ascorbate\ radical$$
$$Fe^{2+}\text{–}EDTA + H_2O_2 \rightarrow Fe(III)\text{–}EDTA + OH· + OH^-$$

Those OH· radicals that are not scavenged by other components of the reaction mixture (e.g., the EDTA) attack the sugar deoxyribose. They degrade it into a series of fragments, some of which react on heating with thiobarbituric acid (TBA) at low pH to give a chromogen, which is an adduct of TBA with malondialdehyde. If a scavenger (X) of OH· is added to the reaction mixture, it will compete with deoxyribose for the OH· radicals and inhibit deoxyribose degradation. Competition plots allow the rate constant for the reaction of X with OH· to be calculated, assuming that deoxyribose reacts with OH· with a rate constant of 3.1×10^9 M^{-1} s^{-1} (141). Essential controls include checking that X does not interfere with the production of OH·, for example, by reacting rapidly with H_2O_2, or by chelating iron (the latter is unlikely as iron is already chelated to EDTA). One must also check that attack of OH· on X does not produce a chromogen (by carrying out a control in which deoxyribose is omitted from the reaction mixture), or that X does not interfere with measurement of products (it should not inhibit if it is added to the reaction mixture at the end of the incubation with the TBA and acid).

Ferric–EDTA is frequently used to fortify foods with iron (142). This represents a potential source of oxidative damage if H_2O_2 is generated in the food. However, although EDTA usually accelerates iron-dependent OH· generation from H_2O_2, an excess of EDTA inhibits iron-dependent lipid peroxidation under most reaction conditions (143).

The deoxyribose method can also be used to examine the ability of a putative antioxidant to chelate Fe^{3+} iron ions, by replacing the EDTA normally used in the assay by $FeCl_3$. When unchelated iron ions are added to the reaction mixture, some of them bind to deoxyribose. The bound iron ions still participate in a Fenton reaction, but any OH˙ radicals formed attack deoxyribose and are not released into free solution. Hydroxyl radical scavengers, at moderate concentrations, do not inhibit this deoxyribose degradation because they cannot compete with the deoxyribose for this "site-specific" OH˙ generation by iron ions (139). Better inhibitors are compounds that chelate iron ions strongly enough to withdraw them from the deoxyribose, provided that the resulting chelates are poorly redox-active, or redox-inactive, or that the chelator efficiently absorbs any OH˙ generated by reacting with it in a "site-specific" manner (135).

Detection of Hydroxyl Radicals. The most specific technique for detecting any free radical is *electron spin resonance* (ESR; sometimes called *electron paramagnetic resonance*; EPR), simply because this method detects the presence of unpaired electrons. A radical can be identified from its ESR spectrum by examining the g value, hyperfine structure, and line shape. The sensitivity of ESR is sufficient to detect radicals derived from such antioxidants as ascorbate and vitamin E in biological tissues, body fluids, foods, and beverages. For example, ESR has been used to detect long-lived radicals formed in bone or cuticle of irradiated foods (127) and for quality control of milk powder (144). However, ESR is insufficiently sensitive to directly detect highly reactive radicals such as OH˙, RO_2˙, or alkoxyl (RO˙) radicals. For example, OH˙ formed within food or in vivo reacts at once with adjacent molecules (i.e., its steady-state concentration is effectively zero). *Spin-trapping* is usually employed to detect OH˙ and other reactive radicals, such as peroxyl (RO_2˙). The radical is allowed to react with a trap to produce a long-lived radical. Reaction of nitroso (R–NO) compounds with radicals often produces *nitroxide* radicals that have a long lifetime

$$R-N=O \ + \ R'˙ \ \longrightarrow \ \underset{\underset{R'}{|}}{\overset{\overset{R}{|}}{N}}-O˙$$

| R symbolizes | reactive | nitroxide radical |
| 'rest of molecule' | radical | (fairly stable) |

Nitrone traps also produce nitroxide radicals

$$\underset{+}{\overset{H \ \ O^-}{\underset{|\ \ \ |}{R-C=N-R'}}} \ + \ R'''˙ \ \rightarrow \ \overset{H \ \ O˙}{\underset{\underset{R''}{|}}{\underset{|\ \ \ |}{R-C-N-R'}}}$$

The chemistry of spin-trapping is well-described in the literature and need not be reiterated here, but one problem is worth comment. The nitroxide radical adducts of several spin traps, including the frequently used 5,5-dimethylpyrroline-*N*-oxide (DMPO), can be reduced by several reducing agents present in food and in vivo, to give "ESR-silent" species (i.e., species that no longer give an ESR signal). This can be misinterpreted as scavenging of the radical that initially reacted with the DMPO. Ascorbate is especially effective at reducing DMPO spin adducts.

Another useful method to detect OH˙ employs aromatic compounds (145). Both decarboxylation and hydroxylation reactions of aromatic compounds have been used to detect OH˙. For example, decarboxylation of benzoic acid (which is added to many foods as a preservative), labeled with ^{14}C in the carboxyl group, has been used to measure generation of OH· in biochemical systems (146). The assay is sensitive, as small amounts of $^{14}CO_2$ can be trapped in alkaline solutions and measured by scintillation counting. An alternative approach is to use benzoic acid labeled with ^{13}C in the carboxyl group and measure production of $^{13}CO_2$ with a mass spectrometer (146). However, decarboxylation is often only a minor reaction pathway when OH· reacts with aromatic compounds (i.e., only a small fraction of the OH· is measured). Also, RO_2· radicals can decarboxylate benzoate (146). Hence, aromatic hydroxylation products are usually measured, often by HPLC with electrochemical or diode array detection (145). Suitable aromatic "detectors" include salicylate; attack of OH· upon salicylate (2-hydroxybenzoate) produces two dihydroxylated products (2,3- and 2,5-dihydroxybenzoates), together with a small amount of the decarboxylation product catechol. Attack of OH· on phenylalanine produces three dihydroxylated products: 2-hydroxyphenylalanine (*o*-tyrosine), 3-hydroxyphenylalanine (*m*-tyrosine), and 4-hydroxyphenylalanine (*p*-tyrosine). Both the D- and L-isomers of phenylalanine react with OH· (145). Formation of *ortho*-tyrosine from phenylalanine residues in food proteins has been used as a detection method for irradiated food (129). Table 3 summarizes several other methods that are available to detect OH·.

3. Peroxyl Radicals

Formation of peroxyl radicals (RO_2·) is the major chain-propagating step in lipid peroxidation, but RO_2· can also be formed in nonlipid systems, such as proteins (44). Decomposition of both lipid and protein peroxides on heating or by addition of transition metal ions can generate peroxyl and alkoxyl (RO·) radicals.

Reaction of OH·, RO_2·, or transition metal ions with thiols in foods (e.g., cysteine; GSH) or in vivo can produce thiyl radicals (RS·), which can then combine with oxygen to give reactive oxysulfur radicals, such as RSO· and RSO_2· (thiyl peroxyl): the chemistry of these reactions is complex (126,147,148). An illustration of their potential importance in vivo is that oxysulfur radicals resulting from attack of OH· on the drug penicillamine appear to be capable of inactivating α_1-antiprotease (149). Peroxynitrite can oxidize several thiol compounds into free radicals (150). Oxidative damage to sulfur-containing compounds in foods can sometimes lead to generation of abnormal smells and flavors (151,152).

One antioxidant property of nitric oxide in vivo and in foods may be its ability to react quickly with RO_2· radicals,

$$RO_2· + NO· \rightarrow ROONO$$

so preventing them from causing damage (20). The rate constant for this reaction is $> 10^9$ M^{-1} s^{-1} (153). However, the biological and toxicological significance of any nitrated or nitrosylated lipids so produced remains to be established.

Peroxyl Radical Scavenging. Scavengers able to remove peroxyl radicals might be effective in the aqueous phase (e.g., dealing with radicals from DNA, thiols, and proteins). For example, reduced glutathione (GSH) reacts rapidly (rate constants about 10^7 to 10^8 M^{-1} s^{-1}) with radicals resulting from attack of OH· on DNA (126,154), although if thiols donate hydrogen, then RS· radicals will be formed. Ascorbate is also a good scavenger of RO_2· in the aqueous phase (51,155). Peroxyl radical scavengers could also operate in hydrophobic (e.g., food lipid, membrane, lipoprotein interior) phases and act as chain-breaking inhibitors of lipid peroxidation. Such hydrophobic peroxyl radical scavengers will slow or stop lipid peroxidation, provided they are able to react more quickly with lipid peroxyl radicals than these radicals react with fatty acid residues.

Table 3 Some Methods for Detection of Hydroxyl Radicals

Method	Principle of method	Comments
Conversion of methional ($CH_3SCH_2CH_2CHO$) and related compounds (methionine, or 2-keto-4-methylthiobutanoic acid, $CH_3SCH_2CH_2COCOOH$) into ethylene gas ($H_2C=CH_2$)	Measurement of ethylene by GC.	Not specific for $OH^\bullet$; these compounds are oxidized by $RO_2^\bullet$, decomposing $ONOO^-$ and some peroxidase enzymes; confirmatory evidence for role of $OH^\bullet$ required.
Coumarin fluorescence	Coumarin-3-carboxylic acid (CCA) is hydroxylated at position 7 to a fluorescent product.	CCA has been covalently linked to various biomolecules and fluorescence changes used to measure $OH^\bullet$ generation in their vicinity (Int J Rad Biol 1993; 63:445). For example, $OH^\bullet$ generation by copper ions bound to DNA could not be decreased by adding DMSO, methanol, or ethanol, but could be by histidine (which chelates copper). This is typical of a "site-specific" reaction (Free Radic Biol Med 1995; 18:669).
Conversion of caffeine to 8-oxocaffeine	Caffeine is hydroxylated at position 8; product analyzed by HPLC with electrochemical detection.	Formation of 8-oxocaffeine from endogenous caffeine has been used to measure free radical generation during roasting and brewing of coffee (J Agric Food Chem 1995; 43:1332).

(*continued*)

Table 3 (*Continued*)

Method	Principle of method	Comments
Dimethylsulfoxide (DMSO) method	OH· radicals react with DMSO, generating, among other products, methane gas, measured by gas chromatography (Biochemistry 1981; 20:6006) or formaldehyde, measured colorimetrically $$(CH_3)_2SO + OH· \rightarrow CH_3SO_2H + ·CH_3$$ $$·CH_3 + O_2 \rightarrow CH_3OO·$$ $$2CH_3OO· \rightarrow HCHO + CH_3OH + O_2$$ $$·CH_3 + R-H \rightarrow CH_4 + R·$$	Babbs et al. (Free Radic Biol Med 1989; 6:493) have suggested that oxidation of DMSO to CH_3SO_2H, methanesulfinic acid (measured colorimetrically or by HPLC) is a means of detecting OH· in vivo (also see Anal Biochem 1993; 269:273). Another approach is to trap the CH_3· radicals (Anal Chem 1997; 69:4295).
Benzoate fluorescence	Reaction of benzoic acid with OH· gives 3- and 4-hydroxybenzoates, which are fluorescent at 407 nm when excited at 305 nm.	Sensitive method (Biochem J 1987; 243:709); confirmatory evidence for role of OH· required. Benzene-1,4-dicarboxylic acid (terephthalic acid) is reported to give a product with superior fluorescence properties (Free Radic Res 1999; 31:429).
Spin trapping/HPLC	A combination of the principles of spin trapping and aromatic hydroxylation; HPLC is used to separate radical adducts of a spin trap, such as DMPO.	Electrochemical detection can allow high sensitivity (e.g., Anal Biochem 1991; 196:111).

Where AOH is the antioxidant the reaction can be written as

$$RO_2^{\cdot} + AOH \rightarrow RO_2H + AO^{\cdot}$$

The fate of the AO$^{\cdot}$ radical must be considered: does it react with another radical (e.g., by addition)

$$RO_2^{\cdot} + AO^{\cdot} \rightarrow ROOOA$$

does it dimerize

$$AO^{\cdot} + AO^{\cdot} \rightarrow AOOA$$

or does it react with another molecule, for example, the "recycling" of α-tocopherol (α-TOH)-derived radicals by ascorbate?

$$\alpha TOH + RO_2^{\cdot} \rightarrow \alpha TO^{\cdot} + RO_2H$$

$$\alpha TO^{\cdot} + \text{ascorbate} \rightarrow \alpha TOH + \text{ascorbate}^{\cdot}$$

Semidehydroascorbate (ascorbate$^{\cdot}$) radicals can disproportionate to regenerate some ascorbate:

$$2 \text{ ascorbate}^{\cdot} \rightarrow \text{ascorbate} + \text{semidehydroascorbate}$$

In vivo, several enzyme systems that convert ascorbate radicals back to ascorbate have been described (36), but these are not relevant to the food matrix, so that the ascorbate present is often slowly lost, especially if O_2 and transition metal ions are present. Iron, and especially copper, ions promote rapid loss of ascorbate. Oxidizing ascorbate can modify proteins by taking part in Maillard-type reactions (156). Hence, ascorbate can have a paradoxical effect in foods: it can both inhibit and promote browning reactions (157).

Assessment of Peroxyl Radical Scavenging Peroxyl radicals can easily be generated by allowing O_2 to add to carbon-centered radicals

$$\geqslant C^{\cdot} + O_2 \rightarrow \geqslant C\text{--}OO^{\cdot}$$

and their reaction with scavengers examined by following absorbance changes or by ESR (158,159). Another method of examining reactions of antioxidants with peroxyl radicals is related to the TRAP assay (see Sec. III.A). Peroxyl radicals are generated at a controlled rate by the thermal decomposition of a water-soluble "azo initiator," such as AAPH. This yields carbon-centered radicals, which react quickly with O_2 to give peroxyl radicals. These are allowed to react with a target, such as a lipid (causing lipid peroxidation). Thus by analyzing the effect of an antioxidant on the rate of peroxidation, a relative rate for its reaction with peroxyl radicals can be measured (51,160). Radicals derived from AAPH also inactivate the enzyme lysozyme, which provides a different (protein) target for studies of protection by antioxidants (161). The carbon-centered radicals produced by AAPH decomposition can do direct damage (e.g., to DNA) (162) and can react with antioxidants (52). Thus, it must be ensured that reaction mixtures contain enough O_2 to convert these carbon radicals completely into peroxyl radicals.

Another approach to assessment of peroxyl radical scavenging has been to use a model lipid-soluble radical, *trichloromethylperoxyl* (TMP) (163,164), which can be formed by exposing a mixture of carbon tetrachloride (CCl_4), propan-2-ol, and buffer to ionizing radiation, so producing hydrated electrons (e^-_{aq}) and $OH^\cdot$.

$$e^-_{aq} + CCl_4 \to {}^\cdot CCl_3 + Cl^-$$

$$OH^\cdot + CH_3CHOHCH_3 \to H_2O + CH_3{}^\cdot COHCH_3$$

$$CH_3{}^\cdot COHCH_3 + CCl_4 \to CH_3COCH_3 + {}^\cdot CCl_3 + H^+ + Cl^-$$

$$^\cdot CCl_3 + O_2 \to \underset{\text{trichloromethylperoxyl}}{CCl_3O_2{}^\cdot}$$

Rate constants for reactions of several antioxidants with $CCl_3O_2{}^\cdot$ have been published (158,164,165). However, $CCl_3O_2{}^\cdot$ is more reactive than nonhalogenated peroxyl radicals (164), and so the results should be taken as only approximations of relative reactivity with the peroxyl radicals that are generated during lipid peroxidation in vivo or in foods.

4. Pro-Oxidant Effects of Chain-Breaking Antioxidants

Many lipid-soluble chain-breaking antioxidants can exert pro-oxidant properties (i.e., they appear to stimulate oxidative damage to the target molecule being used) in certain assay systems in vitro. Often this occurs because they are capable of reducing Fe(III) or Cu^{2+} ions, to Fe^{2+} or Cu^+. This property has been demonstrated for propyl gallate, Trolox C, and for several plant phenolics, including flavonoids and α-tocopherol (166–170). When α-tocopherol reduces metal ions, the tocopheroxyl radical is generated, for example,

$$\alpha TOH + Cu^{2+} \to \alpha TO^\cdot + Cu^+ + H^+$$

This radical is capable of abstracting H atoms from polyunsaturated fatty acids, although it does so at a rate that is an order of magnitude slower than the rate for $H^\cdot$ abstraction by peroxyl radicals (74,171). Hence, if peroxyl radicals are present in a lipid system, any α-tocopherol present will scavenge them and would normally decrease the rate of lipid peroxidation. However, if copper (and possibly iron) ions are added to unperoxidized lipids containing α-tocopherol, $\alpha TO^\cdot$ can be produced and act as a weak initiator of peroxidation (169,172). The pro-oxidant properties of α-tocopherol probably occur rarely (if ever) in vivo because this radical is quickly reduced by such agents as ubiquinol and ascorbate (173). They could occur in certain food matrices, if reducing agents able to convert $\alpha TO^\cdot$ back to α-tocopherol were absent (174).

5. Action of Antioxidants on Lipoxygenase

Damage to plant tissues (e.g., during food processing) often leads to the activation of lipoxygenase enzymes, which catalyze the O_2-dependent stereospecific peroxidation of fatty acids. The resulting hydroperoxides can be cleaved to aldehydes and other products, both nonenzymically in the presence of transition metal ions and by the action of specific "cleavage enzymes" within plants (175,176). The control of lipoxygenase activity is essential in the food industry, both in the processing of plant material and in the preservation of fish, which are rich in lipoxygenase (177–179). Several antioxidants can inhibit lipoxygenases from both plants and animals (27,180). For example, 12-lipoxygenase from fish gills is inhibited by micromolar levels of fisetin and quercetin (179). Lipoxygenases can be assayed by the rate of O_2 uptake in the presence of their fatty acid substrates (179) or by the rate of formation of end-products (27). There is increasing evidence that lipoxygenase enzymes are involved in atherosclerosis, so it is possible that their inhibition could delay this process (180,181).

6. Direct Studies of the Effects of Antioxidants on Lipid Peroxidation

Several factors in addition to efficiency in peroxyl radical scavenging influence the ability of antioxidants to inhibit peroxidation in "real" lipids (membranes, lipoproteins, food lipids). Examples include partition coefficients (which govern the distribution of the antioxidant between the aqueous and lipid phases), and the ability to interact with any transition metal ions present. Thus, a direct test of antioxidant ability toward the lipid substrate of interest is often more informative than tests of the ability of an antioxidant to scavenge $RO_2\cdot$ radicals in isolation. Lipid substrates that can be used include emulsions of, or liposomes made from, fatty acids or fatty acid esters. Oils and melted fats, ground meat, or other food homogenates can also be used. Biological systems can include erythrocytes, isolated lipoproteins (most often low-density lipoproteins [LDL] or high-density lipoproteins [HDL]); tissue homogenates, and mitochondrial, nuclear, or microsomal fractions made from such homogenates.

Tens of thousands of measurements of lipid peroxidation are performed each year in laboratories throughout the world, but several points must be considered in interpreting them. In most assays the lipid systems are maintained under ambient pO_2, although some putative antioxidants (e.g., β-carotene) appear more effective at the lower O_2 concentrations that often exist in vivo (182). For example, the kinetics of Cu^{2+}-dependent LDL oxidation are different when assayed under physiological O_2 levels rather than under ambient air (183). During peroxidation assays, variable results could arise if rapid peroxidation depleted the O_2 content of reaction mixtures. A second factor to be considered is the content of endogenous antioxidants in the lipid substrate and their interaction with added antioxidants. For example, ascorbate usually stimulates iron ion-dependent peroxidation of phospholipid liposomes (143), but it can inhibit peroxidation of LDL, in part by recycling tocopheryl radicals back to α-tocopherol (183). The dithiol antioxidant dihydrolipoic acid does not inhibit iron ion-dependent peroxidation in liposomes (184), but can do so in microsomes, again probably by recycling tocopheryl radicals (185). This is an important concept in the food industry: can added antioxidants help to preserve food levels of vitamin E, which is essential in the human diet, by "recycling" it as it becomes oxidized?

7. Assays of Lipid Peroxidation

Lipid peroxidation is a complex process and occurs in multiple stages. Hence, many techniques are available for measuring the rate of peroxidation of membranes, food lipids, lipoproteins, or fatty acids. Each technique measures something different, and no one method by itself can be said to be the gold standard for measurement of lipid peroxidation. Table 4 summarizes various methods, together with my comments on some of the more widely used tests.

Loss of Substrates. Lipid peroxidation causes loss of unsaturated fatty acid side chains, so a simple way (in principle) of measuring the extent of peroxidation is to examine the loss of fatty acids. The system under study must be disrupted (e.g., lipids extracted from foods, cells, or lipoproteins) and the lipids hydrolyzed to release the fatty acids, which are then usually converted into volatile products (e.g., by formation of methyl esters) and analyzed by gas chromatography. Care must be taken to avoid further peroxidation during the hydrolysis and extraction procedures (e.g., by adding antioxidants and carrying out the procedures under nitrogen). Additional information can be gained by separating the different classes of lipids before hydrolysis to release the fatty acids.

The other substrate for peroxidation is oxygen. Hence, measurement of the rate of O_2 uptake is another overall index of peroxidation.

Table 4 Some of the Methods Used to Detect and Measure Lipid Peroxidation in Biological Material and Food Systems

Method	What is measured	Remarks
A. Loss of substrates		
Analysis of fatty acids by gas chromatography or HPLC	Loss of unsaturated fatty acids.	Useful for assessing lipid peroxidation stimulated by different pro-oxidants that give different product distributions.
Oxygen electrode	Uptake of O_2 by carbon-centered radicals and during peroxide-decomposition reactions.	Dissolved O_2 concentration is measured; useful when spectrophotometric interference occurs or toxic chemicals interfere with enzymic technique. Not very sensitive. Sometimes used in studies of food lipid peroxidation.
B. Peroxide assays: simple total peroxide measurements		
Iodine liberation	Lipid peroxides	One of the oldest methods, widely used in the food industry; lipid peroxides oxidize I^- to I_2. $$ROOH + 2I^- + 2H^+ \rightarrow I_2 + ROH + H_2O$$ In the presence of excess I^- the tri-iodide ion (I_3^-) can be measured at 358 nm. Useful for bulk lipids. H_2O_2 and protein peroxides also oxidize I_2. Method can be applied to extracts of biological samples if other oxidizing agents are absent. Levels of peroxides in human blood plasma reported to be 2.1–4.6 μM (Anal Biochem 1989; 176:360).
FOX (ferrous oxidation xylenol orange) assay	Absorbance change	Simple, easy to use, works well in vitro (e.g., for LDL peroxidation). Oxidation of Fe^{2+} to $Fe(III)$ is detected by xylenol orange (ΔA at 560 nm). 3–4 μM "lipid peroxide" is measured in normal human plasma. Sensitivity low μM

		range (Anal Biochem 1994; 220:403). Also detects H_2O_2 and probably protein peroxides. Addition of triphenylphosphine reduces lipid peroxide to allow measurement of H_2O_2. Has been used to measure peroxides in cooking oils and H_2O_2 in beverages (see text).
Glutathione peroxidase (GPX)	Fatty acid peroxides (GPX does not act on peroxidized fatty acids within membrane or LDL lipids)	GPX reacts with H_2O_2 and organic peroxides, oxidizing GSH to GSSG. Addition of glutathione reductase and NADPH to reduce GSSG back to GSH results in stoichiometric consumption of NADPH. Alternatively, GSSG can be determined directly (e.g., by HPLC; Chem Res Toxicol 1989; 2:295; Anal Biochem 1990; 186:108). Cannot measure peroxides within membranes unless phospholipases are first used. Phospholipid hydroperoxide GP could be employed for this. Peroxide levels in human blood plasma quoted as approx. 1 μM (Chem Res Toxicol 1989; 2:295).
Cyclooxygenase (COX)	Lipid peroxides (rate of COX-1 oxidation of arachidonic acid stimulated by traces of lipid hydroperoxides)	Stimulation of COX-1 activity (usually assayed as O_2 uptake) can measure trace amounts of peroxide in biological fluids (Anal Biochem 1985; 192; 1991; 193:55). Assay relates the presence of peroxides to their potential biological actions (i.e., stimulation of eicosanoid synthesis). Human blood plasma levels measured are ~0.5 μM. The assay cannot be used to identify individual peroxides and value for "total peroxide" will depend to some extent on what species are present (different peroxides stimulate COX to different extents).

(continued)

Table 4 (*Continued*)

Method	What is measured	Remarks
C. Peroxide assays: separation of products		
Heme degradation of peroxides (after HPLC separation)	Lipid peroxides (HPLC allows separation of phospholipid, cholesterol ester peroxides, etc.)	Heme and heme proteins decompose lipid peroxides to form products that react with isoluminol to produce light. For example, microperoxidase, a heme-peptide produced by proteolytic degradation of cytochrome *c* is often used. HPLC method measures ~40 nM levels of peroxides in human plasma (e.g., Anal Biochem 1988; 175:120. Methods Enzymol 1994; 233, 319, and 324). Electrochemical or redox-dye detections of peroxide have also been described (e.g., Free Radic Biol Med 1996; 20:365). The identity of peroxides after HPLC separation must be confirmed; diode array detection which records the absorbance spectrum of each peak, is a good validation method. Another method of detecting peroxides after HPLC is to react them with derivatives of diphenylphosphine, oxidized to fluorescent phosphine oxides (Anal Chim Acta 1995; 307:97).
GC–mass spectrometry	Lipid peroxides (also aldehydes, isoprostanes, cholesterol/cholesterol ester peroxides)	Peroxides are extracted, usually reduced (e.g., by borohydride) to alcohols, separated by GC, and identified by mass spectrometry. Several methodological variations exist (e.g., Methods Enzymol 1994; 233:332; Anal Biochem 1991; 198:104). Controls are needed to show that the alcohols were not present in the system *before* reduction (e.g., alcohols generated by the action of glutathione peroxidase on peroxides).

D. Miscellaneous methods
   Spin trapping — Intermediate radicals — Spin traps (e.g., PBN, POBN, DMPO) intercept radicals intermediate to the chain reaction. They have been used in whole animals to detect carbon radicals as well as RO$^{\cdot}$ and RO$_2^{\cdot}$ radicals. They are also important in mechanistic studies. (Proc Natl Acad Sci USA 1981; 78:7346; J Biol Chem 1992; 267:5743).

   Light emission — Excited carbonyls, singlet oxygen, many other light-emitting systems — Complex chemistry, but fairly simple to carry out.

   Diene conjugation — See text

E. Measurement of end products
   TBA test — TBA-reactive material (TBARS) — See text
   GC, HPLC, or antibody techniques — Cytotoxic aldehydes — Hydroxynonenal frequently measured by immunostaining or chemical techniques (186).
   Hydrocarbon gases — Pentane and ethane — See text. Potentially a noninvasive measure of peroxidation in vivo. Results using mammals have been variable; some authors have found that the technique works well, but others have abandoned it. Many GC columns do not separate pentane from isoprene. Ethane can result from free radical attack on certain amino acids (Biochem Pharmacol 1990; 39:1347).
   F$_2$-isoprostanes (and related products from other fatty acids). — Fatty acid peroxides (GC/negative ion chemical ionization mass spectrometry) — Peroxidation of PUFAs produces a complex mixture of isoprostranes. Found at low levels (both free and esterified to lipids) in human and animal tissues and body fluids (e.g., ~30–40 pg/mL in fresh human plasma, ~2 ng/mg creatinine in human urine).

Measurement of Peroxides. Several methods exist for measurement of lipid peroxides: they can be classified into those that measure "total peroxides" (e.g., iodine liberation, methylene blue test, the FOX assay, cyclooxygenase, glutathione peroxidase) and those that separate different types of peroxide (see Table 4). The amount of peroxide present at a given time during lipid peroxidation depends on both the rate of initiation of peroxidation and on how quickly peroxides break down. Lipid peroxides are fairly stable at room temperature, but break down quickly on heating to give a complex mixture of aldehydes and other products (186,187). However, the presence of transition metal ions, especially iron or copper ions, promotes peroxide breakdown even at room temperature. Both lipid peroxides and aldehydes can be absorbed, to some extent, through the gastrointestinal tract, and so their presence in food is an area of concern (187–190), although intestinal glutathione peroxidase and glutathione S-transferase enzymes appear to detoxify most of them (189). Excessive peroxidation usually confers rancidity and other off-flavor on foods, making them unlikely to be eaten. Nevertheless, the peroxidation of lipoproteins, such as LDL, in vitro in the presence of copper ions requires low levels of "seeding peroxides," and these peroxides could conceivably originate from the diet (191).

Diene Conjugation. The oxidation of polyunsaturated fatty acids (PUFAs) is accompanied by the formation of conjugated diene structures that absorb UV light in the wavelength range 230–235 nm. Measurement of this UV absorbance is a useful index of the early stages of peroxidation in studies with pure lipids and isolated lipoproteins (190). Diene conjugation measurements can rarely be carried out directly on foods, animal tissues, or body fluids, because many other substances present absorb strongly in the UV. Extraction of lipids into organic solvents (e.g., chloroform:methanol mixtures) before analysis is a common approach to this problem.

Nevertheless, it is dangerous to assume that diene-conjugated material equates with lipid peroxidation. Separation of the UV-absorbing "diene conjugate" material from human body fluids revealed that most or all of it consists of a non–oxygen-containing isomer of linoleic acid, octadeca-9(*cis*),11(*trans*)-dienoic acid. This and similar UV-absorbing products are found in several foods (red meat, meat products, butter, lard, cream, ice-cream, cheese, milk, and yogurt) and can also be produced by bacterial metabolism (192,193). Thus, the diene conjugated material detected in human tissues and body fluids may be absorbed from food or produced by the metabolism of bacteria, such as those present in the gut, lung, and cervical mucus. It follows that application of diene conjugation assays to foods, animal tissues, or body fluids, is a questionable index of lipid peroxidation. Nevertheless, diene conjugation methods are still useful for isolated lipid or lipoprotein fractions, such as LDL. HPLC can be used to separate octadeca-9,11-dienoic acid from what appear to be "real" conjugated diene products of lipid peroxidation (194).

Ethane and Pentane Measurement. The measurement of these hydrocarbon gases is based on their formation as a product of the decomposition of peroxides produced by nonenzymic (195,196) or by lipoxygenase-catalyzed (197) lipid peroxidation. Ethane is derived from (n-3) PUFAs and pentane from (n-6) PUFAs. The latter PUFAs predominate in the human body, suggesting that pentane would be produced in greater amounts if all PUFAs peroxidize equally. Both gases are easily measured by gas chromatography. For hydrocarbon exhalation studies in whole animals, breath is passed through an adsorbent at low temperature to concentrate the hydrocarbons, which are then desorbed and assayed (195). One potential problem is that hydrocarbons are minor end products of peroxidation, and their formation depends on the decomposition of peroxides by heating, peroxide cleavage enzymes, or the presence of transition metal ions. In both nonenzymic and lipoxygenase-dependent peroxidation, the amount of pentane produced is affected by the O_2 concentration (196,197). Pentane production has been used to examine the deterioration of foods on storage (e.g., raw chicken) (198,199).

Some problems have arisen in attempting to use hydrocarbon gas exhalation as an index of "whole-body" lipid peroxidation in humans and other animals. Pentane is metabolized in the liver, by some cytochromes P450. This can introduce artifacts (e.g., drugs or toxins that affect liver metabolism might decrease pentane metabolism by liver P450, thereby increasing pentane excretion). This might be mistakenly thought to be elevating the rate of lipid peroxidation in vivo. Another problem is that many GC columns fail to separate pentane from isoprene (2-methyl-1,3-butadiene), a hydrocarbon present in large amounts in human breath that is apparently a side product of cholesterol biosynthesis (195). Thus, several reported "breath pentane" levels are artifactually high, and some reports suggest that healthy humans exhale little, if any, pentane (200). Perhaps, therefore, ethane should receive more attention as a biomarker of in vivo lipid peroxidation (195,201).

Care must be taken in human and other animal experiments to control for hydrocarbon production from the bacteria always present (e.g., on the skin and in the gut). The atmosphere in large cities is contaminated with hydrocarbons from combustion processes (e.g., in motor vehicles and environmental tobacco smoke). Hydrocarbons probably partition into body fat stores and must first be flushed out by breathing hydrocarbon-free air before reliable measurements can be made (201).

The Thiobarbituric Acid Test. The thiobarbituric acid (TBA) test is one of the oldest and most frequently used tests for measuring the peroxidation of fatty acids, membranes, and foods (198,202). Its advantage is its simplicity: the material under test is simply heated with TBA at low pH, and the formation of a pink color is measured at (or close to) 532 nm or by fluorescence at 553 nm. Unfortunately, the simplicity of performing the TBA test belies its chemical complexity.

Small amounts of "free" malondialdehyde (MDA; sometimes called malonaldehyde) are formed during the peroxidation of many lipid-containing systems, especially microsomes, and react with TBA to generate an MDA–$(TBA)_2$ adduct, the pink chromogen (186). However, the amount of free MDA produced in most peroxidizing lipid systems is too low to account for more than a small part of the color in the TBA test. Indeed, most of the MDA that reacts in the TBA test is created during the assay by decomposition of lipid peroxides during heating at low pH (203). Peroxide decomposition generates $RO_2{}^{\cdot}$ radicals that can oxidize more lipid (i.e., the TBA test amplifies peroxidation and subsequent MDA formation). Peroxide breakdown during the assay is accelerated by the presence of iron salts in the sample or in the reagents used in the TBA test, and chelation of such iron salts decreases the detected TBA reactivity (204). This can lead to artifacts in studies of the action of metal-chelating agents on lipid peroxidation: they will also affect color development in the TBA test itself. Attempts to overcome this problem have included addition of excess iron with the TBA reagents or, alternatively, the addition of chain-breaking antioxidants (usually butylated hydroxytoluene; BHT) to suppress peroxidation during the test itself. Thus the TBA-reactivity (or TBA reactive material; TBARS) content measured in a sample will differ according to the assay conditions used (203,204). Another problem is that several compounds other than MDA give products that absorb at, or close to, 532 nm on heating with TBA. These include sucrose, bile pigments, and some amino acids (203). One approach to avoid this has been to separate the $(TBA)_2$–MDA adduct from other chromogens, usually by HPLC; multiple HPLC methods applicable to foods and biological material have been described (205,206). Gas chromatographic analysis of MDA and other aldehydes is also possible (207,208). However, authentic MDA can arise from products other than lipids, including sorbic acid (a preservative added to many foods) (209). Application of the TBA assay to human body fluids will also measure MDA produced enzymically during eicosanoid synthesis (210).

Despite these problems, TBA tests (preferably linked to HPLC to remove interfering chromogens) are useful "screening" methods for examining large numbers of biological or food samples for lipid peroxidation. However, it is difficult to use them to *compare* levels of peroxidation between tissues or foods with a different fatty acid composition, for not all fatty acids generate MDA on oxidation. MDA largely arises from peroxidation of polyunsaturated fatty acids with more than two double bonds, especially linolenic, arachidonic, and docosahexenoic acids. Basal levels of MDA in human plasma were reported as 25–38 nM using a GC–MS method (208), and the HPLC-based method of Chirico et al. (206) gives values of 100 nM or less in plasma from healthy subjects.

Isoprostanes. Animal tissues and body fluids (including urine) contain low levels of F_2-isoprostanes, and their metabolites. F_2-isoprostanes are prostaglandin isomers that are specific end products of the peroxidation of phospholipids containing arachidonic acid. Isoprostanes in plasma are largely esterified to phospholipids, rather than being "free," and sensitive GC–MS assays to measure them have been described (211,212). Isoprostane levels in vivo are increased under conditions of oxidative stress (e.g., in plasma and urine of cigarette smokers, in breath from asthma patients, in diabetic patients, in lung lining fluid of rats exposed to elevated O_2, in plasma of iron-overloaded rats, and in animals treated with CCl_4) (211–213). Other PUFAs (including eicosapentaenoic and docosahexenoic acids) give rise to different families of isoprostane-like compounds on peroxidation (214–216). Measurement of different families of isoprostanes might be an approach to assessing the relative rates of peroxidation of different PUFAs in vivo and in food material. For example, it is well known that increasing the number of double bonds in a PUFA increases its propensity to oxidize in vitro (36), but it is unclear if this is true in vivo. Isoprostanes may also form in foods, but dietary intake seems to contribute little to plasma levels in humans (217). Families of E_2 and D_2 isoprostanes, as well as "isothromboxanes" and "isoleukotrienes," have also been described (211,212).

Conclusion. There is no "best method" to measure lipid peroxidation, either in foods or in biological material. Each assay measures something different. For example, diene conjugation can give information about the early stages of peroxidation (e.g., in LDL), as does direct measurement of lipid peroxides. In the absence of metal ions, enzymic cleavage systems, or high temperatures to decompose lipid peroxides there will be limited formation of decomposition products such as hydrocarbon gases or carbonyl compounds; lack of observation of these, therefore, does not mean the absence of peroxidation. Whereas most scientists studying peroxidation in isolated lipid systems add an excess (50–200 μM) of iron salt or iron chelates, the availability of metal ions to decompose lipid peroxides in the human body is very limited (36). It is probably also limited in most foods, although iron availability can be increased by its release during cooking or grinding and when food is fortified with iron salts or iron chelates. The most specific assays of peroxidation (unfortunately also the most difficult to do) involve HPLC, GC–MS, or antibody-based determinations of such individual products as specific aldehydes (MDA and others), isoprostanes, or peroxides. One issue that needs resolution is the disagreement over "basal" levels of peroxides (e.g., in human blood plasma) using different assays that all allegedly measure them (see Table 4).

Whatever method is chosen, one should think clearly *what* is being measured and *how* it relates to the overall lipid peroxidation process. Whenever possible, two or more different assay methods should be used, especially when antioxidants are being characterized. One should be alert for interference with the assay, especially with diene conjugation and the TBA test. For example, much of the apparent antioxidant effect of carnosine and anserine in inhibiting lipid peroxidation in vitro is due to their ability to interfere with the TBA test (218).

D. Effects of Antioxidants on Phagocytes

On activation, neutrophils, macrophages, eosinophils, and monocytes produce $O_2^{\cdot-}$ and H_2O_2. Most, if not all, of the H_2O_2 arises by dismutation of $O_2^{\cdot-}$, the first product of oxygen reduction by the NADPH oxidase enzyme complex (219). Rodent phagocytes readily produce $NO^{\cdot}$; human phagocytes can also do so under certain circumstances (220,221). If $O_2^{\cdot-}$ and $NO^{\cdot}$ are coproduced, $ONOO^-$ may form.

If phagocyte-derived $O_2^{\cdot-}$, H_2O_2, and reactive nitrogen species are involved in producing damage to tissues, antioxidant protection could be achieved not only by scavenging these species, but also by agents that block their formation by the phagocyte. For example, it has been suggested that several anti-inflammatory drugs interfere with phagocyte function. However, few of these claims meet the criteria that the drug at the concentrations achieved in vivo during therapy must inhibit a respiratory burst that is triggered by using physiologically relevant stimuli, such as opsonized bacteria. Artifacts can also arise when assessing effects of agents on phagocyte production of reactive oxygen species, especially using assays based on cytochrome c or nitroblue tetrazolium reduction for $O_2^{\cdot-}$, or peroxidase-based assays for H_2O_2. For example, some thiols have been claimed to decrease phagocyte production of ROS, but thiols readily reduce cytochrome c and can interfere with peroxidase-based measurement of H_2O_2 (see Sec. III.C.1).

1. Hypochlorous Acid

Activated neutrophils contain and secrete the enzyme myeloperoxidase, which uses H_2O_2 to oxidize chloride ions into the powerful oxidizing and chlorinating agent hypochlorous acid (HOCl) (222). Myeloperoxidase in the presence of H_2O_2 is capable of oxidizing many other substrates (including guaiacol, nitrite ions, and the amino acid tyrosine) (223), that is, it has "nonspecific" peroxidase activity. Human eosinophils contain a similar enzyme that utilizes bromide (Br^-) ions as a substrate and produces HOBr (224). The hypohalous acids are part of the mechanism by which neutrophils and eosinophils attack microorganisms, and HOCl produced outside the phagocyte may also contribute to tissue damage at sites of inflammation. For example, HOCl oxidizes an essential methionine residue in α_1-antiprotease, and inactivates it (222). Hypochlorous acid is widely used in bleaches (as the sodium salt, NaOCl) and can be generated during irradiation of materials containing chloride ions (225).

Assays for Scavengers of Hypochlorous Acid. Compounds that decrease tissue damage caused by HOCl could act by scavenging HOCl or by inhibiting HOCl production by myeloperoxidase (MPO). Myeloperoxidase can be assayed in several ways, including "standard" peroxidase activity assays (e.g., its ability to oxidize guaiacol to a brown chromogen in the presence of H_2O_2) (226). Myeloperoxidase can also be assayed by measuring HOCl production (e.g., by allowing HOCl to react with monochlorodimedon to produce an absorbance change) (227). When testing for MPO inhibitors, the former type of assay may be less prone to artifact, because an HOCl scavenger could also inhibit by competing with monochlorodimedon for the HOCl generated by the enzyme. If a compound appears to inhibit myeloperoxidase, it should be checked whether the compound is an inhibitor or is simply a competing substrate for the enzyme.

Scavenging of HOCl can be examined directly; HOCl can be made by acidifying commercial sodium hypochlorite (Na^+OCl^-) to pH 6.2 and using its molar absorption coefficient at

235 nm to calculate the concentration (228). Thus, the ability of a putative antioxidant to protect a target against attack by HOCl can be examined. Targets that have been used include thiols (229) and α_1-antiprotease (230). A good scavenger of HOCl should protect α_1-antiprotease against inactivation when HOCl is added. If a substance fails to protect α_1-antiprotease, it may be that its reaction with HOCl is too slow or is nonexistent. However, it is also possible that the substance reacts with HOCl to form a "long-lived" oxidant that is also capable of inactivating α_1-antiprotease (231). For example, taurine reacts with HOCl to give chloramines that can inactivate α_1-antiprotease (231). Both HOCl and chloramines are particularly reactive with thiol compounds and with methionine (222,230,232), but chloramines are generally less reactive with biomolecules than is HOCl.

Several papers have examined the ability of drugs to scavenge HOCl (229,230,232). Many therapeutic agents are capable of reacting with HOCl in vivo, but few are present in vivo at the concentrations that would enable them to protect important biological targets from attack by the highly reactive HOCl. Even if antioxidants could scavenge HOCl in vivo, the possibility of forming toxic oxidation or chlorination products must be considered (233). Myeloperoxidase can also oxidize some drugs directly to toxic products (233). The plant product 4-hydroxy-3-methoxyacetophenone (apocynin) inhibits neutrophil $O_2^{\cdot -}$ release in vitro, apparently because it is oxidized by myeloperoxidase to a product damaging to the phagocytes (234).

E. Heme Proteins as Pro-Oxidants

Mixtures of H_2O_2 or organic peroxides with many heme proteins, including cytochrome c, hemoglobin, and myoglobin, oxidize many bimolecules, including lipids (235–238). Reactions of heme proteins with peroxides generate amino acid radicals on the protein, and higher oxidation states of the iron in the heme ring (236–239). Amino acid radicals and heme ferryl species can both participate in the oxidation of substrates. Once lipid peroxidation has begun, heme proteins can further facilitate peroxidation by promoting degradation of lipid peroxides into peroxyl and alkoxyl radicals. Oxidative damage involving reactions of heme proteins with peroxides has been suggested to contribute to ischemia–reperfusion injury, atherosclerosis, crush injury, and chronic inflammation (238,239). Analogous damage can also occur in meat products (18,21). Indeed, crush injury to human tissues has some similarities in this context to the disruption of muscle tissue that occurs during meat processing.

The ability of a substance to react with activated heme proteins can be examined spectrophotometrically by looking for loss of the ferryl myoglobin (or hemoglobin) spectrum as the compound reduces it from Fe(IV) to the ferrous or ferric state (240). A good "quencher" of ferryl species and protein radicals, such as ascorbate, will inhibit heme protein-dependent peroxidation of fatty acids or membrane lipids (235,240). Hydroxamate antioxidants acting in this way have been described (241).

Exposure of heme proteins to a large molar excess of peroxides causes release from the protein of both heme and of "free" iron ions resulting from heme breakdown (242–244). Some antioxidants, such as ascorbic acid, prevent this process (240).

F. Singlet Oxygen

Oxygen has two singlet states, but the $^1\Delta g$ state is probably the most important in biological and food systems. Singlet O_2 $^1\Delta g$ has no unpaired electrons and, therefore, is not a free radical, but it is a powerful oxidizing agent, able to rapidly oxidize many molecules (including PUFAs) that are unreactive with ground-state O_2 (245).

Singlet oxygen can be produced in the laboratory, in vivo, and in foods by photosensitization reactions (45,245,246). A photosensitizing agent absorbs light, enters a higher electronic excitation state, and transfers energy onto "ground-state" O_2 to generate singlet O_2. For example, sunlight can damage milk by photosensitization reactions involving the riboflavin present (246). Many plants, including celery and St. John's wort, contain photosensitizers (247,248). Singlet O_2 is formed when ozone reacts with several biomolecules, including thiols and proteins (249) and during lipid peroxidation, where it seems to arise largely by the self-reaction of peroxyl radicals (250).

Singlet O_2 can be generated in the laboratory by photosensitization reactions employing such molecules as methylene blue and rose bengal (245). In assessing $^1O_2$ quenching or scavenging by putative antioxidants using photochemical systems, it is important to ensure that any damage caused to a target molecule is due to singlet O_2 and is not caused by direct interaction with the excited state of the sensitizer, or by reactions involving other ROS (such as $O_2^{\cdot -}$ and $OH^{\cdot}$), that are often generated in illuminated pigment-containing systems. A technique has been described in which singlet O_2 is generated by an immobilized sensitizer and allowed to diffuse a short distance to react with the target molecule (251); it has been used to study the mutagenicity of singlet O_2 (252). Singlet O_2 can also be generated by the thermal decomposition of endoperoxides, such as 3,3'-(1,4-naphthylidene) dipropanoate, and such sources have been used to examine the reactions of singlet O_2 with human plasma (253).

Singlet O_2 can be identified by several mechanisms (245). As it returns to the ground state, singlet O_2 emits light in two ways: a weak monomol emission at 1270 nm and a dimol emission resulting from collision of two $^1O_2$ molecules, which produces light at 630 and 701 nm. The 1270 nm (infrared) emission has been much used to study $^1O_2$ chemistry, but special detectors are needed. The dimol emission wavelengths are prone to interference by other light-emitting reactions. The mere observation of "light emission" from a living organism or chemical reaction does not implicate $^1O_2$ generation, unless the characteristic emission spectrum can be demonstrated. Many free radical reactions produce light, including Fenton reactions and reactions of certain heme proteins with H_2O_2. Another approach to implicating singlet O_2 is the use of deuterium oxide. The lifetime of singlet O_2 is longer in D_2O than in H_2O by a factor of 10–15 (245). Thus, if a reaction in aqueous solution is dependent on singlet O_2, carrying it out in D_2O instead of H_2O should potentiate the effect.

IV. WHAT DO WE LEARN FROM IN VITRO ANTIOXIDANT CHARACTERIZATION?

The battery of tests outlined in the foregoing enables us to examine *the possibility* that a given compound could act as an antioxidant in one or more ways in vivo or in the food matrix. The tests may show that a direct antioxidant action is unlikely (e.g., because the compound is simply too inefficient as an antioxidant). Alternatively, they could show that an antioxidant action is *feasible*, in that the compound shows protective action in vitro at concentrations within the range present in foods or in vivo. Nevertheless, even an excellent in vitro antioxidant will not necessarily work in vivo (e.g., it may not be absorbed, not reach the correct site of action, or be rapidly metabolized to inactive products). In addition, some compounds may exert indirect antioxidant actions (e.g., by up-regulating the levels of endogenous antioxidant defenses such as SOD or glutathione peroxidase). How then can the effectiveness of antioxidants be evaluated in vivo?

The methodology available for detecting oxidative damage has improved rapidly in recent years, especially for damage to lipids and DNA (36,254). Particularly encouraging is the establishment of "quality-control circles" to compare methodology among laboratories (255–257).
Where do we stand currently?

A. DNA

Oxidative damage to DNA occurs in vivo, in that low levels of DNA base oxidation products such as 8-hydroxyguanine have been detected in DNA isolated from all human cells and tissues yet examined (257). The chemical pattern of damage to the purine and pyrimidine bases in isolated cellular DNA resembles the pattern produced by OH$\cdot$ attack, suggesting that OH$\cdot$ formation occurs within the cell nucleus in vivo, even in healthy subjects (36). It is widely believed that oxidative DNA damage is an important factor in the age-related development of the common cancers, so that agents able to decrease its levels should hinder cancer development.

There are two types of measurement of oxidative DNA damage. *Steady-state damage* is measured when DNA is isolated from human cells and tissues and analyzed for base damage products: it reflects the balance between damage and DNA repair. Hence, a rise in steady-state oxidative DNA damage could be due to increased damage or to decreased repair. Another approach attempts to assess total ongoing oxidative DNA damage in vivo, usually by estimating the rate of repair of DNA that has been damaged by reactive species. This is most often done by measurement of urinary excretion of DNA base oxidation products, especially 8-hydroxy-2'-deoxyguanosine (8OHdG) (257–260). Recent articles have examined all these methods in detail (254–259). Their application to nutritional studies has provided some unexpected results. For example, the "classic" antioxidants vitamin C, β-carotene, and vitamin E may make little, if any, contribution to the ability of diets rich in fruits and vegetables to decrease either oxidative DNA damage in vivo or cancer incidence (15,254,260–263). This is especially true for β-carotene: no convincing evidence exists that β-carotene can significantly decrease oxidative DNA damage in vivo, perhaps consistent with its lack of protective effect against cancer as revealed in intervention trials (260,264). Administering ascorbic acid supplements to well-nourished humans does not appear to decrease total oxidative DNA damage, and may transiently increase it (261,264,265). By contrast, low intakes of vitamin C seem associated with increased oxidative DNA damage (265–267). Therefore, there may be an optimal intake of ascorbate, perhaps in the range of 50–200 mg/day (267).

B. Lipids: Lipid Peroxidation

Lipid peroxidation is important in vivo for several reasons, in particular because it contributes to the development of atherosclerosis (181,190) and probably of diabetes (268). Hence, a common test of the effectiveness of antioxidants is to measure their effects on the "peroxidizability" of LDL isolated from blood plasma after administration of the antioxidant to human subjects. For example, Esterbauer et al. (269) showed that supplementation of humans with vitamin E increased the length of the "lag period" before onset of peroxidation when LDL subsequently isolated from their plasma, was incubated with copper ions in vitro. For example, supplementation with 1200 International Units (IU) of α-tocopherol daily increased the lag period by about 75%. By contrast, administering green or black tea to humans was reported to have no effect on the resistance of LDL to subsequent oxidation in vitro, even though some of the tea phenolics were absorbed (270,271). Several studies (272) have reported that consumption of red wine by volunteers decreases the peroxidizability of their LDL, although some data are conflicting (273).

One factor that must be considered is that lipoproteins are usually isolated by a lengthy centrifugation procedure, and phenolic compounds soluble even to a limited extent in water could leach out during isolation (i.e., they could interact with lipoproteins in vivo, but appear to have no effect in vitro). Another factor to be considered is the exact experimental conditions used to study LDL peroxidation in vitro; usually this is done by adding copper ions, but other biologically relevant mechanisms of LDL peroxidation (e.g., lipoxygenase, heme protein addition, HOCl, $ONOO^-$) could give different results when examining the effect of antioxidants (274). For example, there is evidence that lipoxygenases contribute to LDL peroxidation in vivo, and this enzyme can be inhibited by several plant phenolics (see Sec. III.C.5).

Lipid peroxidation is also important because its end products (particularly cytotoxic aldehydes, such as malondialdehyde and 4-hydroxynonenal) can cause damage to proteins and to DNA (186,275,276). Adducts of these aldehydes with DNA and with proteins have been detected in vivo (186,275–277) (e.g., a deoxyguanosine–MDA adduct has been identified in human and rat urine; 278).

1. Measuring Lipid Peroxidation In Vivo

Several assays for measurement of lipid peroxides in plasma have been described, but they give different values (see Table 4). Simple "total peroxide" assays give values in the micromolar range, but HPLC-based methods give lower values, usually less than 100 nM. Do the latter assays cause peroxide loss, or are the simpler assays less specific? Are there peroxides in plasma that do not arise from lipids that could be detected in simple colorimetric assays? All these questions need resolution.

Animal body fluids also contain F_2-isoprostanes, largely esterified to phospholipids (see under Sec. III.C.7). Isoprostane levels appear to be a balance between generation and metabolism–excretion (i.e., plasma isoprostane levels represent the "steady state" of a dynamic equilibrium) (279). Because isoprostanes are measured by chemically rigorous techniques, appear to arise largely or entirely from lipid peroxidation, and appear not to be confounded by dietary lipid oxidation products, the view is growing that they are the best currently available biomarker of lipid peroxidation in vivo, especially as their levels are elevated in situations of oxidative stress, and can be lowered by supplementation with antioxidants, such as vitamin E (211–213).

2. Measuring "Total" Lipid Peroxidation In Vivo

The levels of lipid peroxidation products in cells, tissues, and body fluids represent a steady-state balance between their rates of formation and metabolism, excretion, or decomposition. Can some measure of "total" peroxidation (i.e., the input side of the balance equation) be obtained?

One approach to this question has been to measure hydrocarbon gases (ethane or pentane) in exhaled air (see under Sec. III.C.7). Another has been to assess urinary excretion of MDA and its metabolites (280,281), but unfortunately this assay can be confounded by diet: much of the MDA and MDA metabolites in urine appear to arise from lipid peroxides or aldehydes in ingested food (282,283). Hence, urinary MDA or TBARS is not a suitable assay to assess whole-body lipid peroxidation in response to changes in dietary composition, although it could be used to look at effects of antioxidant supplementation of persons on a "fixed" diet (281). Another problem in applying the TBA test (rather than specific measurements of MDA) to urine is that much urinary TBARS is not lipid-derived or arises from aldehydes other than MDA (284,285). Some or all of the MDA–guanine adduct detected in urine (278) could conceivably also arise from diet.

Isoprostanes and their metabolites can be measured in urine (211–213,279,283,286,287), and this may prove to be a valuable assay of whole-body lipid peroxidation.

C. Proteins: Damage by Reactive Species

Oxidative damage to proteins may be important in vivo both in its own right (affecting the function of receptors, enzymes, antibodies, cell-signaling mechanisms and transport proteins) (44), and perhaps, generating new antigens that provoke immune responses (288), and because protein damage can lead to secondary damage to other biomolecules (e.g., by inactivation of DNA repair enzymes). Measuring oxidative protein damage is intrinsically difficult, because 20 different amino acid residues in proteins can be attacked by reactive species, generating a vast range of end-products (44).

Attack of reactive species on proteins can often generate amino acid radicals, which react with O_2 to give peroxyl radicals, that can abstract hydrogen to give protein peroxides, which in turn, may decompose in complex ways, facilitated by heat (e.g., in cooking) or transition metal ions (44). Assays of human tissues and body fluids by simple "peroxide determinations" (see Table 4) could conceivably measure protein peroxides, as well as lipid peroxides.

Because there are so many end-products of damage to proteins by reactive species, it is unlikely that any one of them is a generally applicable biomarker for oxidative protein damage. Products for which assays exist include methionine sulfoxide, dihydroxyphenylalanine (DOPA, produced by tyrosine hydroxylation), 2-amino-adipic semialdehyde, γ-glutamyl semialdehyde, valine hydroxides (produced by reduction of valine hydroperoxides), tryptophan hydroxylation and ring-opening products, 2-oxohistidine, dityrosine, *ortho*- and *meta*-tyrosines, 3-nitrotyrosine, and 3-chlorotyrosine (44,82,289–295). 3-Chlorotyrosine is a minor end product of attack of reactive chlorine species on tyrosine residues in proteins (294,296). Attack of reactive nitrogen species on tyrosine residues can generate both nitrotyrosine and bityrosine (79,223,296,297).

In principle, the levels of one (or preferably of several) of these products in proteins could be used to assess the steady-state level of oxidative protein damage in vivo (i.e., the balance between rates of damage and rates of repair, or of hydrolytic removal of damaged proteins). The products most exploited to date have been 3-nitrotyrosine, methionine sulfoxide, the hydroxylated phenylalanines, and bityrosine. For example, levels of *ortho*-tyrosine and dityrosine in human lens proteins have been reported in relation to age (291). Dityrosine has been measured in human atherosclerotic lesions (297). The measurement of 3-nitrotyrosine in tissues and body fluids is subject to some artifacts, which have been discussed in recent reviews and so need not be repeated here (79,80). A GC–MS-based method that avoids these artifacts has been described (298).

1. Carbonyl Assay

The carbonyl assay has been used as a "general" assay of oxidative protein damage to assess steady-state levels of protein damage in foods, tissues, and body fluids. It is based on the ability of several reactive species to attack amino acid residues in proteins (particularly histidine, arginine, lysine, and proline) to produce carbonyl functions that can be measured after reaction with 2,4-dinitrophenylhydrazine (299,300). The carbonyl assay has become widely used, and many laboratories have developed individual protocols for it (301), which may account for the widely variable results in the literature about levels of protein carbonyls in animal tissues. By contrast, most groups seem to obtain broadly comparable values for protein carbonyls in human plasma, of about 0.4–1.0 nmol/mg protein, so that plasma protein carbonyls might be a useful "general" marker of oxidative protein damage. However, Davies and Dean (44) have suggested that carbonyl levels are an overestimate of steady-state levels of oxidative protein damage.

More research is needed to identify the molecular nature of the carbonyls (i.e., which amino acid residues have been damaged and on which proteins). HPLC, ELISA, and Western-blotting assays have been developed in an attempt to identify oxidatively damaged proteins in cells, tissues, and body fluids (300,302–305). Carbonyls need not always arise by oxidation of amino acid residues. Thus, binding of certain aldehydes (including HNE and MDA) to proteins can generate "carbonyls" (41,186). Glycation of proteins can also generate carbonyls (306), which precludes the application of the carbonyl assay to cooked foods, where Maillard browning has occurred.

2. *Measuring the Rate of Total Protein Damage In Vivo*

Several modified amino acids or their metabolites can be detected in urine, including bityrosine, a lysine–MDA adduct (307), and 4-hydroxy-3-nitrophenylacetic acid, a metabolite of 3-nitrotyrosine (63). Much more research is required in this area, and the possible confounding effects of oxidized proteins or amino acids in the diet (e.g., in cooked or irradiated foods) must be investigated.

V. CONCLUSION

In this review, I have discussed in some detail the techniques needed for in vitro evaluation of antioxidants, and the even more difficult task of proving that good antioxidants in vitro can act as such in vivo. Given the increasing interest in the role of antioxidants in food preservation, nutraceuticals, herbal medicines, and health maintenance (9,308–310), the methodologies described are likely to be increasingly used in the future. More attention should be given to their further development and validation, with the eventual aim of setting up internationally agreed quality-controlled procedures.

REFERENCES

1. Liu Q, Lanari MC, Schaefer DM. A review of dietary vitamin E supplementation for improvement of beef quality. J Anim Sci 1995; 73:3131–3140.
2. Life Sciences Research Office. Evaluation of evidence for the carcinogenicity of butylated hydroxyanisole (BHA). Bethesda, MD: FASEB, 1994.
3. Geoffroy M, Lambelet P, Richert P. Radical intermediates and antioxidants: an ESR study of radicals formed on carnosic acid in the presence of oxidized lipids. Free Radic Res 1994; 21:247–258.
4. Cuppett SL, Hall CA III. Antioxidant activity of the labiatae. Adv Food Nutr Res 1998; 42:245–271.
5. Salami M, Galli C, De Angelis L, Visioli F. Formation of F_2-isoprostanes in oxidized low density lipoprotein: inhibitory effect of hydroxytyrosol. Pharmacol Res 1995; 31:275–279.
6. Deiana M, Aruoma OI, de Lourdes M, Bianchi P, Spencer JPE, Kaur H, Halliwell B, Aeschbach R, Banni S, Dessi MA, Corongiu FP. Inhibition of peroxynitrite dependent DNA base modification and tyrosine nitration by the extra virgin olive oil-derived antioxidant hydroxytyrosol. Free Radic Biol Med 1999; 26:762–769.
7. Halliwell B. Antioxidant activity and other biological effects of flavonoids. In: Rice-Evans C, ed. Wake up to Flavonoids. London: Royal Society of Medicine, 2000:13–23.
8. Traber MG. Regulation of human plasma vitamin E. Adv Pharmacol 1997; 38:49-63.
9. Rice–Evans C, ed. Wake up to Flavonoids. London: Royal Society of Medicine, 2000.
10. Hollman PC, Tijburg LB. Bioavailability of flavonoids from tea. Crit Rev Food Sci Nutr 1997; 37:719–738.

11. de Vries JH, Hollman PC, Meyboom S, Buysman MN, Zock PL, van Staveren WA, Katan MB. Plasma concentrations and urinary excretion of the antioxidant flavonols quercetin and kaempferol as biomarkers for dietary intake. Am J Clin Nutr 1998; 68:60–65.
12. Manach C, Morand C, Crespy V, Demigne C, Texier O, Regerat F, Remesy C. Quercetin is recovered in human plasma as conjugated derivatives that retain antioxidant properties. FEBS Lett 1998; 426:331–336.
13. Paganga G, Rice–Evans C. The identification of flavonoids as glycosides in human plasma. FEBS Lett 1997; 401:78–82.
14. Donovan JL, Bell JR, Kasim–Karakas S, et al. Catechin is present as metabolites in human plasma after consumption of red wine. J Nutr 1999; 129:1662–1668.
15. Halliwell B, Zhao K, Whiteman M. The gastrointestinal tract: a major site of antioxidant action? Free Rad Res 2000; 33:819–830.
16. McKnight GM, Smith LM, Drummond RS, Duncan CW, Golden M, Benjamin N. Chemical synthesis of nitric oxide in the stomach from dietary nitrate in humans. Gut 1997; 40:211–214.
17. Cheigh HS, Park KY. Biochemical, microbiological and nutritional aspects of kimchi. Crit Rev Food Sci Nutr 1994; 34:175–189.
18. Igene JO, King JA, Pearson AM, Gray JI. Influence of heme pigments, nitrates and non-heme iron on development of warmed-over flavor (WOF) in cooked meat. J Agric Food Chem 1979; 27:832–842.
19. Cammack R, Ioannou CL, Cui XY, Torres Martinez C, Maraj SR, Hughes MN. Nitrite and nitrosyl compounds in food preservation. Biochim Biophys Acta 1999; 1411:475–488.
20. Rubbo H, Parthasarathy S, Barnes S, Kirk M, Kalyanaraman B, Freeman BA. Nitric oxide inhibition of lipoxygenase-dependent liposome and LDL oxidation: termination of radical chain propagation reactions and formation of nitrogen-containing oxidized lipid derivatives. Arch Biochem Biophys 1995; 324:15–25.
21. Kanner J, Shegalovich I, Harel S, Hazan B. Muscle lipid peroxidation dependent on oxygen and free metal ions. J Agric Food Chem 1988; 36:409–417.
22. Gorbunov NV, Osipov AN, Day BW, Zayas–Rivera B, Kagan VE, Elsayed NM. Reduction of ferrylmyoglobin and ferrylhemoglobin by nitric oxide: a protective mechanism against ferryl hemoprotein-induced oxidations. Biochemistry 1995; 34:6689–6699.
23. Kanner J, Harel S, Granit R. Nitric oxide as an antioxidant. Arch Biochem Biophys 1991; 289:130–136.
24. Oldreive C, Zhao K, Paganga G, Halliwell B, Rice–Evans C. Inhibition of nitrous acid-dependent tyrosine nitration and DNA base deamination by flavonoids and other phenolic compounds. Chem Res Toxicol 1998; 11:1574–1579.
25. Pannala AS, Razaq R, Halliwell B, Singh S, Rice–Evans CA. Inhibition of peroxynitrite dependent tyrosine nitration by hydroxycinnamates: nitration or electron donation? Free Radic Biol Med 1998; 24:594–606.
26. Babbs CF. Free radicals and etiology of colon cancer. Free Radic Biol Med 1990; 8:191–200.
27. Laughton MJ, Evans PJ, Moroney MA, Hoult JR, Halliwell B. Inhibition of mammalian 5-lipoxygenase and cyclo-oxygenase by flavonoids and phenolic dietary additives. Relationship to antioxidant activity and to iron ion-reducing ability. Biochem Pharmacol 1991; 42:1673–1681.
28. Ikawa H, Kamitani H, Calvo BF, Foley JF, Eling TE. Expression of 15-lipoxygenase-1 in human colorectal cancer. Cancer Res 1999; 59:360–366.
29. Droy–Lefaix MT, Packer L. Antioxidant properties of *Ginkgo biloba* extract: EGb 761. In: Packer L, Hiramatsu M, Yoshikawa T, eds. Antioxidant Food Supplements in Human Health. San Diego: Academic Press, 1999; 343–357.
30. Ondrias K, Stasko A, Gergel D, Hromadova M, Benes L. Formation of stable free radicals from kampo medicines TJ-9, TJ-15, TJ-23, TJ-96, TJ-114 and their antioxidant effect on low-density lipoproteins. Free Radic Res Commun 1992; 16:227–237.
31. Vaya J, Belinky PA, Aviram M. Antioxidant constituents from licorice roots: isolation, structure elucidation and antioxidative capacity towards LDL oxidation. Free Radic Biol Med 1997; 23:302–313.
32. Burdock GA. Review of the biological properties and toxicity of bee propolis. Food Chem Toxicol 1998; 36:347–363.
33. Drehsen G. From ancient pine bark uses to pycnogenol. In: Packer L, Hiramatsu M, Yoshikawa T, eds. Antioxidant Food Supplements in Human Health. San Diego: Academic Press, 1999:311–322.

34. Löliger J. The use of antioxidants in foods. In: Aruoma OI, Halliwell B, eds. Free Radicals and Food Additives. London: Taylor & Francis, 1991:121–150.
35. Halliwell B. Food-derived antioxidants. Evaluating their importance in food and in vivo. Food Sci Agric Chem 1999; 1:67–109.
36. Halliwell B, Gutteridge JMC. Free Radicals in Biology and Medicine. 3rd ed. Oxford: Oxford University Press, 1999.
37. Gutteridge JMC, Quinlan GJ. Antioxidant protection against organic oxygen radicals by normal human plasma: the important primary role for iron-binding and iron-oxidising proteins. Biochim Biophys Acta 1992; 1159:248–254.
38. Halliwell B, Hu ML, Louie S, Duvall TR, Tarkington BR, Motchnik P, Cross CE. Interaction of nitrogen dioxide with human plasma. Antioxidant depletion and oxidative damage. FEBS Lett 1992; 313:62–66.
39. Hu ML, Louie S, Cross CE, Motchnik P, Halliwell B. Antioxidant protection against hypochlorous acid in human plasma. J Lab Clin Med 1992; 121:257–262.
40. Frei B, Forte TM, Ames BN, Cross CE. Gas phase oxidants of cigarette smoke induce lipid peroxidation and changes in lipoprotein properties in human blood plasma. Biochem J 1991; 247:133–138.
41. Reznick AZ, Cross CE, Hu M, Suzuki YJ, Khwaja S, Safadi A, Motchnik PA, Packer L, Halliwell B. Modification of plasma proteins by cigarette smoke as measured by protein carbonyls. Biochem J 1992; 286:607–611.
42. Young JF, Nielsen SE, Haraldsdottir J, et al. Effect of fruit juice on urinary quercetin excretion and biomarkers of antioxidative status. Am J Clin Nutr 1999; 69:87–94.
43. Halliwell B. Antioxidants: the basics—what they are and how to evaluate them. Adv Pharmacol 1996; 38:3–20.
44. Davies MJ, Dean RT. Radical-Mediated Protein Oxidation. From Chemistry to Medicine. Oxford: Oxford University Press, 1997.
45. Korycka–Dahl M, Richardson T. Initiation of oxidative changes in foods. J Dairy Sci 1980; 63:1181–1198.
46. Hazen SL, Heinecke JW. 3-Chlorotyrosine, a specific marker of myeloperoxidase-catalyzed oxidation, is markedly elevated in LDL isolated from human atherosclerotic intima. J Clin Invest 1997; 99:2075–2081.
47. Feig DI, Loeb LA. Mechanisms of mutation by oxidative DNA damage: reduced fidelity of mammalian DNA polymerase β. Biochemistry 1993; 32:4466–4473.
48. Wiseman H, Halliwell B. Carcinogenic antioxidants: diethylstilboestrol, hexoestrol and 17α-ethynyl-oestradiol. FEBS Lett. 1993; 322:159–163.
49. Roy D, Liehr JG. Elevated 8-hydroxydeoxyguanosine levels in DNA of diethylstilboestrol-treated Syrian hamsters: covalent DNA damage by free radicals generated by redox cycling of diethylstilboestrol. Cancer Res 1991; 51:3882–3885.
50. Schildermann PAEL, ten Vaarwerk FJ, Lutgerink JT, Van der Wurff A, ten Hoor F, Kleinjans JCS. Induction of oxidative DNA damage and early lesions in rat gastro-intestinal epithelium in relation to prostaglandin H synthase-mediated metabolism of butylated hydroxyanisole. Food Chem Toxicol 1995; 33:99–109.
51. Wayner DDM, Burton GW, Ingold KU. The antioxidant efficiency of vitamin C is concentration-dependent. Biochim Biophys Acta 1986; 884:119–123.
52. Soriani M, Pietraforte D, Minetti M. Antioxidant potential of anaerobic human plasma: role of serum albumin and thiols as scavengers of carbon radicals. Arch Biochem Biophys 1994; 312:180–188.
53. Benzie IFF, Strain J. The ferric reducing ability of plasma (FRAP) as a measure of "antioxidant power": the FRAP assay. Anal Biochem 1996; 239:70–76.
54. Re R, Pellegrini N, Proteggente A, Pannala A, Yang M, Rice–Evans C. Antioxidant activity applying an improved ABTS radical cation decolorization assay. Free Radic Biol Med 1999; 26:1231–1237.
55. Paganga G, Miller N, Rice–Evans CA. The polyphenolic content of fruits and vegetables. What does a serving constitute? Free Radic Res 1999; 30:153–162.
56. Long LH, Kwee DCT, Halliwell B. The antioxidant activities of seasonings used in Asian cooking. Powerful antioxidant activity of dark soy sauce revealed using the ABTS assay. Free Radic Res 2000; 32:181–186.

57. Ratty AK, Sunamoto J, Das NP. Interaction of flavonoids with 1,1-diphenyl-2-picrylhydrazyl free radical, liposomal membranes and soybean lipoxygenase-1. Biochem Pharmacol 1988; 37:989–995.
58. Shi H, Niki E. Stoichiometric and kinetic studies on *Ginkgo biloba* extract and related antioxidants. Lipids 1998; 33:365–370.
59. Aejmelaeus R, Ketela TM, Pirttila T, Hervonen A, Alho H. Unidentified antioxidant defences of human plasma in immobilized patients: a possible relation to basic metabolic rate. Free Radic Res 1997; 26:335–341.
60. Rice–Evans C. Measurement of total antioxidant activity as a marker of antioxidant status in vivo: procedures and limitations. Free Radic Res 2000; 33:S59–S66.
61. Beckman JS, Chen J, Ischiropoulos H, Crow JP. Oxidative chemistry of peroxynitrite. Methods Enzymol 1994; 233:229–240.
62. Felley–Bosco E. Role of nitric oxide in genotoxicity: implication for carcinogenesis. Cancer Metastasis Rev 1998; 17:25–37.
63. Ohshima H, Friesen M, Brouet I, Bartsch H. Nitro-tyrosine as a new marker for endogenous nitrosation and nitration of proteins. Food Chem Toxicol 1990; 28:647–652.
64. Shephard SE, Schlatter C, Lutz WK. Assessment of the risk of formation of carcinogenic *N*-nitroso compounds from dietary precursors in the stomach. Food Chem Toxicol 1987; 25:91–108.
65. Ohshima H, Bartsch H. Quantitative assessment of endogenous nitration in humans by measuring excretion of *N*-nitrosoproline in the urine. Cancer Res 1981; 41:3658–3662.
66. Ohshima H, Bartsch H. Chronic infections and inflammatory processes as cancer risk factors: possible role of nitric oxide in carcinogenesis. Mutat Res 1994; 305:253–264.
67. Savva R, McAuley–Hecht K, Brown T, Pearl L. The structural basis of specific base-excision repair by uracil–DNA glycosylase. Nature 1995; 373:487–493.
68. Wilson DM III, Thompson LH. Life without DNA repair. Proc Natl Acad Sci USA 1997; 94:12754–12757.
69. Demple B, Harrison L. Repair of oxidative damage to DNA: enzymology and biology. Annu Rev Biochem 1994; 63:915–948.
70. Wennmalm A, Benthin G, Jungersten L, Edlund A, Petersson AS. Nitric oxide formation in man as reflected by plasma levels of nitrate, with special focus on kinetics, confounding factors and response to immunological challenge. In: Moncada S, Feelish M, Busse R, Higgs EA, eds. The Biology of Nitric Oxide. Vol. 4. Portland Press, UK, 1994:474–476.
71. Wolf G. gamma-Tocopherol: an efficient protector of lipids against nitric oxide-initiated peroxidative damage. Nutr Rev 1997; 55:376–378.
72. Christen S, Woodall AA, Shigenaga MK, Southwell–Keely PT, Duncan MW, Ames BN. gamma-Tocopherol traps mutagenic electrophiles such as NO(X) and complements alpha-tocopherol: physiological implications. Proc Natl Acad Sci USA 1997; 94:3217–3222.
73. Goss SP, Hogg N, Kalyanaraman B. The effect of α-tocopherol on the nitration of α-tocopherol by peroxynitrite. Arch Biochem Biophys 1999; 363:333–340.
74. Kamal–Eldin A, Appelqvist LA. The chemistry and antioxidant properties of tocopherols and tocotrienols. Lipids 1996; 31:671–701.
75. Zhao K, Whiteman M, Spencer JPE, Halliwell B. DNA damage by nitrite and peroxynitrite: protection by dietary phenols. Methods Enzymol 2001 (in press).
76. Lymar SV, Hurst JK. Carbon dioxide: physiological catalyst for peroxynitrite-mediated cellular damage or cellular protectant? Chem Res Toxicol 1996; 9:845–850.
77. Merenyi G, Lind J. Free radical formation in the peroxynitrous acid (ONOOH)/peroxynitrite ($ONOO^-$) system. Chem Res Toxicol 1998; 11:243–246.
78. Kaur H, Whiteman M, Halliwell B. Peroxynitrite-dependent aromatic hydroxylation and nitration of salicylate and phenylalanine. Is hydroxyl radical involved? Free Radic Res 1997; 26:71–82.
79. Van der Vliet A, Eiserich JP, Shigenaga MK, Cross CE. Reactive nitrogen species and tyrosine nitration in the respiratory tract. Am J Respir Crit Care Med 1999; 159:1–9.
80. Halliwell B, Zhao K, Whiteman M. Nitric oxide and peroxynitrite. The ugly, the uglier and the not so good. Free Radic Res 1999; 31:651–669.
81. Ischiropoulos H, Zhu L, Chen J, Tsai M, Martin JC, Smith CD, Beckman JS. Peroxynitrite-mediated tyrosine nitration catalyzed by superoxide dismutase. Arch Biochem Biophys 1992; 298:431–437.
82. Halliwell B. What nitrates tyrosine? Is nitrotyrosine specific as a biomarker of peroxynitrite formation in vivo? FEBS Lett 1997; 411:157–160.

83. Aruoma OI, Whiteman M, England TG, Halliwell B. Antioxidant action of ergothioneine: assessment of its ability to scavenge peroxynitrite. Biochem Biophys Res Commun 1997; 231:389–391.
84. Whiteman M, Halliwell B. Protection against peroxynitrite-dependent tyrosine nitration and α_1-antiproteinase inactivation by ascorbic acid. A comparison with other biological antioxidants. Free Radic Res 1996; 25:275–283.
85. Pannala AS, Rice–Evans CA, Halliwell B, Singh S. Inhibition of peroxynitrite-mediated tyrosine nitration by catechin polyphenols. Biochem Biophys Res Commun 1997; 232:164–168.
86. Kato Y, Ogino Y, Aoki T, Uchida K, Kawakishi S, Osawa T. Phenolic antioxidants prevent peroxynitrite-derived collagen modification in vitro. J Agric Food Chem 1997; 45:3004–3009.
87. Haenen GR, Paquay JB, Korthouwer RE, Bast A. Peroxynitrite scavenging by flavonoids. Biochem Biophys Res Commun 1997; 236:591–593.
88. Radi R, Denicola A, Freeman BA. Peroxynitrite reactions with carbon dioxide–bicarbonate. Methods Enzymol 1999; 301:353–367.
89. Gow A, Duran D, Thom SR, Ischiropoulos H. CO_2 enhancement of peroxynitrite-mediated protein tyrosine nitration. Arch Biochem Biophys 1996; 333:42–48.
90. Ketsawatsakul U, Whiteman M, Halliwell B. A reevaluation of the peroxynitrite scavenging activity of some dietary phenolics. Biochem Biophys Res Commun 2000; 279:692–699.
91. Moreno JJ, Pryor WA. Inactivation of alpha 1-proteinase inhibitor by peroxynitrite. Chem Res Toxicol 1992; 5:425–431.
92. Halliwell B, Whiteman M. Assessment of peroxynitrite scavengers in vitro. Methods Enzymol 1999; 301:333-342.
93. Reist M, Marshall KA, Jenner P, Halliwell B. Toxic effects of sulphite in combination with peroxynitrite on neuronal cells. J Neurochem 1998; 71:2431–2438.
94. Kooy NW, Royal JA, Ischiropoulos H. Oxidation of $2',7'$-dichlorofluorescin by peroxynitrite. Free Radic Res 1997; 27:245–254.
95. Fridovich I. Superoxide dismutases. An adaptation to a paramagnetic gas. J Biol Chem 1989; 264:7761–7764.
96. Hiramoto K, Sekiguchi K, Ayuka K, Aso-o R, Moriya N, Kato T, Kikugawa K. DNA breaking activity and mutagenicity of soy sauce: characterization of the active components and identification of 4-hydroxy-5-methyl-3(2H)-furanone. Mutat Res 1996; 359:119–132.
97. McCord JM, Fridovich I. The utility of SOD in studying free radical reactions. I Radicals generated by the interaction of sulfite, dimethyl sulfoxide and oxygen. J Biol Chem 1969; 244:6056–6063.
98. Gutteridge JMC, Quinlan GJ. Carminic acid-promoted oxygen radical damage to lipid and carbohydrate. Food Addit Contam 1986; 3:289–293.
99. Hiramoto K, Li X, Makimoto M, Kato T, Kikugawa K. Identification of hydroxyhydroquinone in coffee as a generator of reactive oxygen species that break DNA single strands. Mutat Res 1998; 419:43–51.
100. Donnelly JK, Robinson DS. Superoxide dismutase. In: Robinson DS, Eskin NAM, eds. Oxidative Enzymes in Foods. London: Elsevier, 1991:49–91.
101. Long LH, Lan ANB, Hsuan TTY, Halliwell B. Generation of H_2O_2 by "antioxidant" beverages and the effect of milk addition. Is cocoa the best beverage? Free Radic Res 1999; 31:67–71.
102. Mulder RW, van der Hulst MC, Bolder NM. *Salmonella* decontamination of broiler carcasses with lactic acid, L-cysteine and H_2O_2. Poultry Sci 1987; 66:1555-1557.
103. Long LH, Evans PJ, Halliwell B. Hydrogen peroxide in human urine: implications for antioxidant defense and redox regulation. Biochem Biophys Res Commun 1999; 262:605–609.
104. Lynch RE, Fridovich I. Permeation of the erythrocyte stroma by superoxide radicals. J Biol Chem 1978; 253:4697–4699.
105. Bielski BHJ. Reactivity of HO_2/O_2^- radicals in aqueous solution. J Phys Chem Ref Data 1985; 14:1041–1100.
106. Aruoma OI, Akanmu D, Cecchini R, Halliwell B. Evaluation of the ability of the angiotensin-converting enzyme inhibitor captopril to scavenge reactive oxygen species. Chem Biol Interact 1991; 77:303–314.
107. Winterbourn CC, Metodiewa C. Reactivity of biologically important thiol compounds with superoxide and H_2O_2. Free Radic Biol Med 1999; 27:322–328.
108. Halliwell B, Gutteridge JMC. Role of free radicals and catalytic metal ions in human disease: an overview. Methods Enzymol 1990; 186:1–85.

109. Liochev S. The role of iron–sulfur clusters in in vivo hydroxyl radical production. Free Radic Res 1996; 25:369–384.
110. Bolann BJ, Ulvik RJ. On the limited ability of superoxide to release iron from ferritin. Eur J Biochem 1990; 193:899–904.
111. Ahn DU, Kim SM. Effect of superoxide and superoxide-generating systems on the prooxidant effect of iron in oil emulsion and raw turkey homogenates. Poultry Sci 1998; 77:1428–1435.
112. Butler J, Hoey BM, Lea JS. The measurement of radicals by pulse radiolysis. In: Rice–Evans C, Halliwell B, eds. Free Radicals, Methodology and Concepts. London: Richelieu Press, 1988:457–479.
113. Som S, Raha C, Chatterjee IB. Ascorbic acid: a scavenger of superoxide radical. Acta Vitam Enzymol 1983; 5:243–250.
114. Halliwell B. Use of desferrioxamine as a probe for iron-dependent formation of hydroxyl radicals. Evidence for a direct reaction between desferal and the superoxide radical. Biochem Pharmacol 1985; 34:229–233.
115. Hayashi T, Sawa K, Kawasaki M, Arisawa M, Shimazu M, Morita N. Inhibition of cow's milk xanthine oxidase by flavonoids. J Natl Prod 1988; 51:345–348.
116. Corbett JT. The scopoletin assay for hydrogen peroxide. A review and a better method. J Biochem Biophys Methods 1989; 18:297–308.
117. Ito Y, Tonogai Y, Suzuki H, Ogawa S, Yokoyama T, Hashizume T, Santo H, Tanaka KI, Nishigaki K, Iwaida M. Improved 4-aminoantipyrine colorimetry for detection of residual H_2O_2 in noodles, fish paste, dried fish, and herring roe. J Assoc Offic Anal Chem 1981; 64:1448–1452.
118. Kettle AJ, Carr AC, Winterbourn CC. Assays using horseradish peroxidase and phenolic substrates require superoxide dismutase for accurate determination of hydrogen peroxide production by neutrophils. Free Radic Biol Med 1994; 17:161–164.
119. Varma SD. Radio-isotopic determination of subnanomolar amounts of peroxide. Free Radic Res Commun 1989; 5:359–368.
120. Nourooz-Zadeh J, Tajaddini-Sarmadi J, Wolff SP. Measurement of plasma hydroperoxide concentrations by the ferrous-oxidation xylenol orange (FOX) assay in conjunction with triphenylphosphine. Anal Biochem 1994; 220:403–409.
121. Berenshtein E, Mayer B, Goldberg C, Kitrossky N, Chevion M. Patterns of mobilization of copper and iron following myocardial ischemia: possible predictive criteria for tissue injury. J Mol Cell Cardiol 1997; 29:3025–3034.
122. Evans PJ, Smith C, Mitchinson MC, Halliwell B. Metal ion release from mechanically-disrupted arterial wall. Implications for the development of atherosclerosis. Free Radic Res 1995; 23:465–469.
123. Ramanathan L, Das NP. Effect of natural copper chelating compounds on the pro-oxidant activity of ascorbic acid in steam-cooked ground fish. Int J Food Sci Technol 1993; 28:279–288.
124. Kimura M, Itokawa Y. Cooking losses of minerals in foods and its nutritional significance. J Nutr Sci Vitaminol 1990; 36(suppl 1):S25–S32.
125. Miller DK, Smith VL, Kanner J, Miller DD, Lawless HT. Lipid oxidation and warmed-over aroma in cooked ground pork from swine fed increasing levels of iron. J Food Sci 1994; 59:751–756.
126. von Sonntag C. The Chemical Basis of Radiation Biology. London: Taylor & Francis, 1987.
127. Dodd NJ. Free radicals and food irradiation. Biochem Soc Symp 1995; 61:247–258.
128. Grootveld M, Jain R. Recent advances in the development of a diagnostic test for irradiated foodstuffs. Free Radic Res Commun 1989; 6:271–292.
129. Karam LR, Bertgold DS, Simic MG. Biomarkers of OH radical damage in vivo. Free Radic Res Commun 1991; 12:11–16.
130. Stadler TH, Turesky RJ, Welti DM, Fay LB. Oxidation of caffeine and related methylxanthines in ascorbate and polyphenol-driven Fenton-type oxidations. Free Radic Res 1996; 24:225–230.
131. Candeias LP, Patel KB, Stratford MRL, Wardman P. Free hydroxyl radicals are formed on reaction between the neutrophil-derived species superoxide anion and hypochlorous acid. FEBS Lett 1993; 333; 151–153.
132. Anbar M, Neta P. A compilation of specific bi-molecular rate constants for the reactions of hydrated electrons, hydrogen atoms and hydroxyl radicals with inorganic and organic compounds in aqueous solution. Int J Appl Radiat Isot 1965; 18:495–523.
133. Smith CA, Halliwell B, Aruoma OI. Protection by albumin against pro-oxidant actions of phenolic dietary components. Food Chem Toxicol 1992; 30:483–489.

134. Aruoma OI, Halliwell B. Superoxide-dependent and ascorbate-dependent formation of hydroxyl radicals from hydrogen peroxide in the presence of iron. Are lactoferrin and transferrin promoters of hydroxyl radical generation? Biochem J 1987; 241:273–278.
135. Gutteridge JMC, Nagy I, Maidt L, Floyd RA. ADP-iron as a Fenton reactant: radical reactions detected by spin trapping, hydrogen abstraction and aromatic hydroxylation. Arch Biochem Biophys 1990; 277:422–428.
136. Marx G, Chevion M. Site-specific modification of albumin by free radicals. Reaction with copper(II) and ascorbate. Biochem J 1986; 236:397–400.
137. Halliwell B. Albumin—an important extracellular antioxidant? Biochem Pharmacol 1988; 37:569–571.
138. Kohn R, Yamamoto Y, Cundy KC, Ames BN. Antioxidant activity of carnosine, homocarnosine and anserine present in muscle and brain. Proc Natl Acad Sci USA 1988; 85:3175–3179.
139. Aruoma OI, Halliwell B. The iron-binding and hydroxyl radical scavenging actions of anti-inflammatory drugs. Xenobiotica 1988; 18:459–470.
140. Gutteridge JMC. Superoxide-dependent formation of hydroxyl radicals from ferric-complexes and H_2O_2: an evaluation of fourteen iron chelators. Free Radic Res Commun 1990; 9:119–125.
141. Halliwell B, Gutteridge JMC, Aruoma OI. The deoxyribose method: a simple "test tube" assay for determination of rate constants for reactions of hydroxyl radicals. Anal Biochem 1987; 165:215–219.
142. Martinez–Torres C, Romano EL, Renzi M, Layrisse M. Fe(III)–EDTA complex as iron fortification. Further studies. Am J Clin Nutr 1979; 32:809–816.
143. Gutteridge JMC, Richmond R, Halliwell B. Inhibition of iron-catalysed formation of hydroxyl radicals from superoxide and of lipid peroxidation by desferrioxamine. Biochem J 1979; 184:469–472.
144. Stapelfeldt H, Nielsen BR, Skibsted LH. Towards use of ESR in quality control of milk powder. Milchwissenschaft 1997; 52:682–685.
145. Kaur H, Halliwell B. Detection of hydroxyl radicals by aromatic hydroxylation. Methods Enzymol 1994; 233:67–82.
146. Lamrini R, Lacan P, Francina A, Guilluy R, Desage M, Michon J, Becchi M, Brazier JL. Oxidative decarboxylation of benzoic acid by peroxyl radicals. Free Radic Biol Med 1998; 24:280–289.
147. Asmus KD. Sulfur-centered free radicals. In: Slater TF, ed. Radio-Protectors and Anticarcinogens. London: Academic Press, 1987:24–42.
148. Wardman P, von Sonntag C. Kinetic factors that control the fate of thiyl radicals in cells. Methods Enzymol 1995; 251:31–45.
149. Aruoma OI, Halliwell B, Butler J, Hoey BM. Apparent inactivation of α_1-antiproteinase by sulphur-containing radicals derived from penicillamine. Biochem Pharmacol 1989; 38:4353–4357.
150. Karoui H, Hogg N, Frejaville C, Tordo P, Kalyanaraman B. Characterization of sulfur-centered radical intermediates formed during the oxidation of thiols and sulfite by peroxynitrite—an ESR study. J Biol Chem 1996; 271:6000–6009.
151. Aylward F, Coleman G, Haisman DR. Catty odours in food: the reaction between mesityl oxide and sulphur compounds in foodstuffs. Chem Ind 1967; 37:1563–1564.
152. Christensen KR, Reineccius GA. Gas chromatographic analysis of volatile sulfur compounds from heated milk. J Dairy Sci 1992; 75:2098-2104.
153. Padmaja S, Huie RE. The reaction of nitric oxide with organic peroxyl radicals. Biochem Biophys Res Commun 1993; 195:539–544.
154. Fahey RC. Protection of DNA by thiols. Pharmacol Ther 1988; 39:101–108.
155. Irwin JA, Ostdal H, Davies MJ. Myoglobin-induced oxidative damage: evidence for radical transfer from oxidized myoglobin to other proteins and antioxidants. Arch Biochem Biophys 1999; 362:94–104.
156. Miyata T, Inagi R, Asahi K, Yamada Y, Horie K, Sakai H, Uchida K, Kurokawa K. Generation of protein carbonyls by glycoxidation and lipoxidation reactions with autoxidation products of ascorbic acid and polyunsaturated fatty acids. FEBS Lett 1998; 437:24–28.
157. Davies CG, Wedzicha BL. Kinetics of the inhibition of ascorbic acid browning by sulphite. Food Addit Contam 1992; 9:471–477.
158. Willson RL. Organic peroxy free radicals as ultimate agents in oxygen toxicity. In: Sies H, ed. Oxidative Stress. London: Academic Press, 1985:41–72.

159. Greenley TL, Davies MJ. Detection of radicals produced by reaction of hydroperoxides with rat liver microsomal fractions. Biochim Biophys Acta 1992; 1116:192–203.
160. Darley-Usmar VM, Hershey A, Garland LG. A method for the comparative assessment of antioxidants as peroxyl radical scavengers. Biochem Pharmacol 1989; 38:1465–1469.
161. Lissi EA, Clavero N. Inactivation of lysozyme by alkylperoxyl radicals. Free Radic Res Commun 1990; 10:177–184.
162. Hiramoto K, Johkoh H, Sako K, Kikugawa K. DNA breaking activity of the carbon-centered radical generated from 2,2′-azobis(2-aminidopropane) hydrochloride (AAPH). Free Radic Res Commun 1993; 19:323–332.
163. Alfassi ZB, Huie RE, Neta P. Rate constants for reaction of perhaloalkyl peroxyl radicals with alkanes. J Phys Chem 1993; 97:6835–6838.
164. Lal M, Schoneich C, Monigh J, Asmus KD. Rate constants for the reactions of halogenated organic radicals. Int J Rad Biol 1988; 54:773–785.
165. Aruoma OI, Spencer JP, Butler J, Halliwell B. Reaction of plant-derived and synthetic antioxidants with trichloromethylperoxyl radicals. Free Radic Res 1995; 22:187–190.
166. Gutteridge JMC, Xaio-Chang F. Enhancement of bleomycin–iron free radical damage to DNA by antioxidants and their inhibition of lipid peroxidation. FEBS Lett 1981; 123:71–74.
167. Laughton MJ, Halliwell B, Evans PJ, Hoult JRS. Antioxidant and pro-oxidant actions of the plant phenolics quercetin, gossypol and myricetin. Biochem Pharmacol 1989; 38:2859–2865.
168. Aruoma OI, Evans PJ, Kaur H, Sutcliffe L, Halliwell B. An evaluation of the antioxidant and potential pro-oxidant properties of food additives and of Trolox C, vitamin E, and probucol. Free Radic Res Commun 1990; 10:143–157.
169. Maiorino M, Zamburtini A, Roveri A, Ursini F. Pro-oxidant role of vitamin E in copper induced lipid peroxidation. FEBS Lett 1993; 330:174–176.
170. Yamamoto K, Niki E. Interaction of α-tocopherol with iron: antioxidant and pro-oxidant effects of α-tocopherol in the oxidation of lipids in aqueous dispersions in the presence of iron. Biochim Biophys Acta 1998; 958:19–23.
171. Mukai K, Morimoto H, Okauchi Y, Nagaoka S. Kinetic study of reactions between tocopheroxyl radicals and fatty acids. Lipids 1993; 28:753–756.
172. Neuzil J, Thomas SR, Stocker R. Requirement for promotion or inhibition by α-tocopherol of radical-induced initiation of plasma lipoprotein lipid peroxidation. Free Radic Biol Med 1997; 22:57–71.
173. Thomas SR, Neuzil J, Mohr D, Stocker R. Co-oxidants make α-tocopherol an efficient antioxidant for LDL. Am J Clin Nutr 1995; 62(suppl 6):1357S–1364S.
174. Cillard J, Cillard P. Prooxidant effect of α-tocopherol on essential fatty acids in aqueous media. Ann Nutr Alim 19; 34:579–591.
175. Galliard T. Lipolytic and lipoxygenase enzymes in plants and their action in wounded tissue. In: Kahl G, ed. Biochemistry of Wounded Plant Tissues. Berlin: Walter de Gruyter, 1978.
176. Hatanaka A. The biogeneration of green odour by green leaves. Phytochemistry 1993; 34:1201–1205.
177. Ramanathan L, Das NP. Studies on the control of lipid oxidation in ground fish by some polyphenolic natural products. J Agric Food Chem 1992; 40:17–21.
178. Ramanathan L, Das NP. Natural products inhibit oxidative rancidity in salted cooked ground fish. J Food Sci 1993; 58:318–320.
179. Hsieh RJ, German JB, Kinsella JE. Relative inhibitory potencies of flavonoids on 12-lipoxygenase of fish gill. Lipids 1988; 23:322–326.
180. Devaraj S, Jialal I. alpha-Tocopherol decreases interleukin-1 beta release from activated human monocytes by inhibition of 5-lipoxygenase. Arterioscler Thromb Vasc Biol 1999; 19:1125–1133.
181. Cornicelli JA, Trivedi BK. 15-Lipoxygenase and its inhibition: a novel therapeutic target for vascular disease. Curr Pharm Design 1999; 5:11–20.
182. Burton GW, Ingold KU. β-Carotene, an unusual type of lipid antioxidant. Science 1984; 224:569–573.
183. Hatta A, Frei B. Oxidative modification and antioxidant protection of human LDL at high and low oxygen partial pressures. J Lipid Res 1995; 36:2383–2393.
184. Scott BC, Aruoma OI, Evans PJ, O'Neill C, van der Vliet A, Cross CE, Tritschler H, Halliwell B. Lipoic and dihydrolipoic acids as antioxidants. A critical evaluation. Free Radic Res 1994; 20:119–133.

185. Scholich H, Murphy ME, Sies H. Antioxidant activity of dihydrolipoate against microsomal lipid peroxidation and its dependence on α-tocopherol. Biochim Biophys Acta 1989; 1001:256–261.
186. Esterbauer H, Schaur RG, Zollner H. Chemistry and biochemistry of 4-hydroxynonenal, malonaldehyde and related aldehydes. Free Radic Biol Med 1991; 11:81–128.
187. Haywood RM, Claxson AW, Hawkes GE, Richardson DP, Naughton DP. Detection of aldehydes and their conjugated hydroperoxy diene precursors in thermally-stressed culinary oils and fats: investigations using high resolution proton NMR spectroscopy. Free Radic Res 1995; 22:441–482.
188. Grootveld M, Atherton MD, Sheerin AN, Hawkes J, Blake DR, Richens TE, Silwood CJ, Lynch E, Claxson AW. In vivo absorption, metabolism, and urinary excretion of α,β-unsaturated aldehydes in experimental animals. J Clin Invest 1998; 101:1210–1218.
189. Aw TY. Determinants of intestinal detoxication of lipid hydroperoxides. Free Radic Res 1998; 28:637–646.
190. Esterbauer H, Gebicki J, Puhl H, Jurgens G. The role of lipid peroxidation and antioxidants in oxidative modification of LDL. Free Radic Biol Med 1992; 13:341–390.
191. Darley–Usmar V, Halliwell B. Blood radicals. Reactive nitrogen species, reactive oxygen species, transition metal ions and the vascular system. Pharm Rev 1996; 13:649–662.
192. Britton M, Fory C, Wickens D, Yudkin J. Diet as a source of phospholipid esterified 9,11-octadecadienoic acid. Clin Sci 1992; 83:97–101.
193. Chin SF, Storkson JM, Liu W, Albright KJ, Pariza MW. Conjugated linoleic acid (9,11- and 10,12-octadecadienoic acid) is produced in conventional but not germ-free rats fed linoleic acid. J Nutr 1994; 124:694–701.
194. Banni S, Contini MS, Angioni E, Deiana M, Dessi MA, Melis MP, Carta G, Corongiu FP. A novel approach to study linoleic acid autoxidation: importance of simultaneous detection of the substrate and its derivative oxidation products. Free Radic Res 1996; 25:43–53.
195. Kneepkens CMF. Assessment of oxidative stress and antioxidant status in humans: the hydrocarbon breath test. In: Aruoma OI, ed. Antioxidant Methodology. Indianapolis: AOCS, 1997:23.
196. Reiter R, Burk RF. Effect of oxygen tension on the generation of alkanes and MDA by peroxidizing rat liver microsomes. Biochem Pharmacol 1987; 36:925–929.
197. Sanders JH, Pattee HE, Singleton JA. Aerobic pentane production by soybean lipoxygenase enzymes. Lipids 1975; 10:568–570.
198. Zallen EM, Hitchcock MJ, Goertz GE. Chilled food systems. Effects of chilled holding on quality of beef loaves. J Am Diet Assoc 1975; 67:552–557.
199. Eilamo M, Kinnunen A, Latva–Kala K, Ahvenainen R. Effects of packaging and storage conditions on volatile compounds in gas-packed poultry meat. Food Addit Contam 1988; 15:217–228.
200. Mendis S, Sobotka PA, Euler DE. Expired hydrocarbons in patients with acute myocardial infarction. Free Radic Res 1995; 23:117–122.
201. Knutson MD, Lim AK, Viteri FE. A practical and reliable method for measuring ethane and pentane in expired air from humans. Free Radic Biol Med 1999; 27:560–571.
202. Wills ED. Lipid peroxide formation of microsomes. The role of non-haem iron. Biochem J 1969; 113:325-332.
203. Gutteridge JMC. Aspects to consider when detecting and measuring lipid peroxidation. Free Radic Res Commun 1986; 1:173–184.
204. Gutteridge JMC, Quinlan GJ. MDA formation from lipid peroxides in the TBA test: the role of lipid radicals, iron salts, and metal chelators. J Appl Biochem 1983; 5:293–299.
205. Bird RP, Hung SS, Hadley M, Draper HH. Determination of malonaldehyde in biological materials by HPLC. Anal Biochem 1983; 128:240–244.
206. Chirico S, Smith C, Marchant C, Mitchinson MJ, Halliwell B. Lipid peroxidation in hyperlipidaemic patients. A study of plasma using an HPLC-based thiobarbituric acid test. Free Radic Res Commun 1993; 19:51–57.
207. Miyake T, Shibamoto T. Simultaneous determination of acrolein, malonaldehyde and 4-hydroxy-2-nonenal produced from lipids oxidized with Fenton's reagent. Food Chem Toxicol 1996; 34:1009–1011.
208. Yeo HC, Helbock HJ, Chyu DW, Ames BN. Assay of MDA in biological fluids by gas chromatography–mass spectrometry. Anal Biochem 1994; 220:391–396.
209. Lau OW, Luk SF, Lam RK. Spectrophotometric method for the determination of sorbic acid in various food samples with iron (III) and 2-thiobarbituric acid as reagents. Analyst 1989; 114:217–219.

210. Shimizu T, Kondo K, Hayaishi O. Role of prostaglandin endoperoxides in the serum thiobarbituric acid reaction. Arch Biochem Biophys 1981; 206:271–276.
211. Roberts LJ II, Morrow JD. The generation and actions of isoprostanes. Biochim Biophys Acta 1997; 1345:121–135.
212. Lawson JA, Rokach J, FitzGerald GA. Isoprostanes: formation, analysis and use as indices of lipid peroxidation in vivo. J Biol Chem 1999; 275:24441–24444.
213. Halliwell B. Lipid peroxidation, antioxidants and cardiovascular disease: how should we move forwards? Cardiovasc Res 2000; 47:410–418.
214. Roberts JL II, Montine TJ, Markesbery WR, Tappert AR, Hardy P, Chemtob S, Dettbarn WD, Morrow JD. Formation of isoprostane-like compounds (neuroprostanes) in vivo from docosahexaenoic acid. J Biol Chem 1998; 273:13605–13612.
215. Nourooz–Zadeh J, Halliwell B, Änggård EE. Evidence for the formation of F_3-isoprostanes during peroxidation of eicosapentaenoic acid. Biochem Biophys Res Commun 1997; 236:467–472.
216. Nourooz–Zadeh J, Liu EHC, Änggård EE, Halliwell B. F_4-isoprostanes: a novel class of prostanoids formed during peroxidation of docosahexaenoic acid. Biochem Biophys Res Commun 1998; 242:338–344.
217. Gopaul NK, Halliwell B, Änggård EE. Measurement of plasma F_2-isoprostanes as an index of lipid peroxidation does not appear to be confounded by diet. Free Radic Res 2000; 33:115–127.
218. Aruoma OI, Laughton MJ, Halliwell B. Carnosine, homocarnosine and anserine. Could they act as antioxidants in vivo? Biochem J 1989; 264:863–869.
219. Curnutte JT, Babior BM. Chronic granulomatous disease. Adv Hum Genet 1987; 6:229–297.
220. Wheeler MA, Smith SD, Garcia–Cardena G, Nathan CF, Weiss RM, Sessa WC. Bacterial infection induces nitric oxide synthase in human neutrophils. J Clin Invest 1997; 99:110–116.
221. Evans TJ, Buttery LD, Carpenter A, Springall DR, Polak JM, Cohen J. Cytokine-treated human neutrophils contain iNOS that produces nitration of ingested bacteria. Proc Natl Acad Sci USA 1996; 93:9553–9558.
222. Weiss SJ. Tissue destruction by neutrophils. N Engl J Med 1989; 320:365–376.
223. Van der Vliet A, Eiserich JP, Halliwell B, Cross CE. Formation of reactive nitrogen species during peroxidase-catalysed oxidation of nitrite. J Biol Chem 1997; 272:7617–7625.
224. Mayeno AN, Curran AJ, Roberts RL, Foote CS. Eosinophils preferentially use bromide to generate halogenating agents. J Biol Chem 1989; 264:5660–5668.
225. Czapski G, Goldstein S, Andorn N, Aronovitch J. Radiation-induced generation of chlorine derivatives in N_2O-saturated phosphate buffered saline: toxic effects on *Escherichia coli* cells. Free Radic Biol Med 1992; 12:353–364.
226. Iwamoto H, Kobayashi T, Hasegawa E, Morita Y. Reactions of human myeloperoxidase with hydrogen peroxide and its true catalase activity. J Biochem (Tokyo) 1987; 101:1407–1412.
227. Kettle AJ, Winterbourn CC. The mechanism of myeloperoxidase-dependent chlorination of monochlorodimedon. Biochim Biophys Acta 1988; 957:185–191.
228. Green TR, Fellman JH, Eicher AL. Myeloperoxidase oxidation of sulfur-centered and benzoic acid hydroxyl radical scavengers. FEBS Lett 1985; 192:33–36.
229. Ching TL, de Jong J, Bast A. A method for screening HOCl scavengers by inhibition of the oxidation of 5-thio-2-nitrobenzoic acid: application to anti-asthmatic drugs. Anal Biochem 1994; 218:377–381.
230. Wasil M, Halliwell B, Moorhouse CP, Hutchison DCS, Baum H. Biologically-significant scavenging of the myeloperoxidase-derived oxidant hypochlorous acid by some anti-inflammatory drugs. Biochem Pharmacol 1987; 36:3847–3850.
231. Weiss SJ, Lampert MB, Test ST. Long-lived oxidants generated by human neutrophils: characterization and bioactivity. Science 1983; 222:625–628.
232. Cuperus RA, Muijsers AO, Wever R. Anti-arthritic drugs containing thiol groups scavenge hypochlorite and inhibit its formation by myeloperoxidase from human leukocytes. Arthritis Rheum 1985; 28:1228–1233.
233. Uetrecht JP. Idiosyncratic drug reactions: possible role of reactive metabolites generated by leukocytes. Pharmacol Rev 1983; 6:265–273.
234. Hart BAT, Simons JM, Knaan–Shanzer S, Bakker NPM, Labadie RP. Antiarthritic activity of the newly developed neutrophil oxidative burst antagonist apocynin. Free Radic Biol Med 1990; 9:127–131.

235. Evans PJ, Akanmu D, Halliwell B. Promotion of oxidative damage to arachidonic acid and α_1-antiproteinase by anti-inflammatory drugs in the presence of the haem proteins myoglobin and cytochrome c. Biochem Pharmacol 1994; 48:2173–2179.
236. Kelman DJ, De Gray JA, Mason RP. Reaction of myoglobin with hydrogen peroxide forms a peroxyl radical which oxidizes substrates. J Biol Chem 1994; 269:7458–7463.
237. Rao SI, Wilks A, Hamberg M, Ortiz de Montellano P. The lipoxygenase activity of myoglobin: oxidation of linoleic acid by the ferryl oxygen rather than protein radical. J Biol Chem 1994; 269:7210–7216.
238. Galaris D, Cadenas E, Hochstein P. Glutathione-dependent reduction of peroxides during ferryl and met-myoglobin interconversion: a potential protective mechanism in muscle. Free Radic Biol Med 1989; 6:473–478.
239. Paganga G, Rice–Evans C, Rule R, Leake D. The interaction between ruptured erythrocytes and low-density lipoproteins. FEBS Lett 1992; 303:154–158.
240. Rice–Evans C, Okunade G, Khan R. The suppression of iron release from activated myoglobin by physiological electron donors and by desferrioxamine. Free Radic Res Commun 1989; 7:45–54.
241. Cooper CE, Green ES, Rice–Evans CA, Davies MJ, Wrigglesworth CM. A hydrogen-donating monohydroxamate scavenges ferryl myoglobin radicals. Free Radic Res 1994; 20:219–227.
242. Gutteridge JMC. Iron promoters of the Fenton reaction and lipid peroxidation can be released from haemoglobin by peroxides. FEBS Lett 1986; 201:291–295.
243. Harel S, Salan MA, Kanner J. Iron release from metmyoglobin, methaemoglobin and cytochrome c by a system generating hydrogen peroxide. Free Radic Res Commun 1988; 5:11–19.
244. Prasad MR, Engelman RM, Jones RM, Das DK. Effect of oxyradicals on oxymyoglobin. Deoxygenation, haem removal and iron release. Biochem J 1989; 263:731–736.
245. Foote CS, Clennan EL. Properties and reactions of singlet O_2. In: Foote CS et al., eds. Active Oxygen in Chemistry. London: Blackie, 1995:105.
246. Aurand LW, Singleton JA, Noble BW. Photoxidation reactions in milk. J Dairy Sci 1966; 49:138–143.
247. Ljunggren B. Severe phototoxic burn following celery ingestion. Arch Dermatol 1990; 126:1334–1336.
248. Ebermann R, Alth G, Kreitner M, Kubin A. Natural products derived from plants as potential drugs for the photodynamic destruction of tumor cells. J Photochem Photobiol B 1996; 36:95–97.
249. Kanofsky JR, Sima PD. Singlet-oxygen generation at gas-liquid interfaces: a significant artefact in the measurement of singlet oxygen yields from ozone–biomolecule reactions. Photochem Photobiol 1993; 58:335–340.
250. Wefers H. Singlet oxygen in biological systems. Bioelectrochem Bioenerg 1987; 18:91–104.
251. Midden WR, Wang SY. Singlet oxygen generation for solution kinetics: clean and simple. J Am Chem Soc 1983; 105:4129–4135.
252. Dahl TA, Midden WR, Hartman PE. Pure exogenous singlet oxygen: nonmutagenicity in bacteria. Mut Res 1988; 201:127–136.
253. Wagner JR, Motchnik PA, Stocker R, Sies H, Ames BN. The oxidation of blood plasma and LDL components by chemically generated singlet O_2. J Biol Chem 1993; 268:18502–18506.
254. Halliwell B. Establishing the significance and optimal intake of dietary antioxidants: the biomarker concept. Nutr Rev 1999; 57:104–113.
255. Lunec J. ESCODD: European Standards Committee on oxidative DNA damage. Free Radic Res 1998; 29:601–608.
256. ESCODD. Comparison of different methods of measuring 8-oxoguanine as a marker of oxidative DNA damage. Free Radic Res 2000; 32:333–341.
257. Special issue. DNA damage. Measurement and mechanism. Free Radic Res 1988; 29:461–624.
258. Bogdanov MB, Beal MF, McCabe DR, Griffin RM, Matson WR. A carbon column-based LC-electrochemical approach to routine 80HdG measurements in urine and other biologic matrices: a one year evaluation of methods. Free Radic Biol Med 1999; 27:647–666.
259. Ravanat JL, Guicherd P, Tuce Z, Cadet J. Simultaneous determination of five oxidative DNA lesions in human urine. Chem Res Toxicol 1999; 12:802–808.
260. Von Poppel G, Poulsen H, Loft S, Verhagen H. No influence of beta carotene on oxidative DNA damage in male smokers. J Natl Cancer Inst 1995; 87:310–311.
261. Podmore ID, Griffiths HR, Herbert KE, Mistry N, Mistry P, Lunec J. Vitamin C exhibits pro-oxidant properties. Nature 1998; 392:559.

262. Priemé H, Loft S, Nyysssonen K, Salonen JT, Poulsen HE. No effect of supplementation with vitamin E, ascorbic acid or coenzyme Q10 on oxidative DNA damage estimated by 8-oxo-7,8-dihydro-2′-deoxyguanosine excretion in smokers. Am J Clin Nutr 1997; 65:503–507.
263. Cadenas S, Barja G, Poulsen HE, Loft S. Oxidative DNA damage estimated by oxo^{8}dG in the liver of guinea-pigs supplemented with graded dietary doses of ascorbic acid and α-tocopherol. Carcinogenesis 1997; 18:2373–2377.
264. Beatty ER, England TG, Geissler CA, Aruoma, OI, Halliwell B. Effect of antioxidant vitamin supplementation on markers of DNA damage and plasma antioxidants. Proc Nutr Soc 1999; 58:44A (abstract).
265. Rehman A, Collis CS, Yang M, Kelly M, Diplock AT, Halliwell B, Rice–Evans C. The effects of iron and vitamin C co-supplementation on oxidative damage to DNA in healthy volunteers. Biochem Biophys Res Commun 1998; 246:293–298.
266. Halliwell B. Vitamin C: poison, prophylactic or panacea? Trends Biochem Sci 1999; 24:255-259.
267. Fraga CG, Motchnik PA, Shigenaga MK, Helbock HJ, Jacob RA, Ames BN. Ascorbic acid protects against endogenous oxidative DNA damage in human sperm. Proc Natl Acad Sci USA 1991; 88:11003–11006.
268. Oranje WA, Wolffenbuttel BHR. Lipid peroxidation and atherosclerosis in type II diabetes. J Lab Clin Med 1999; 134:19–32.
269. Esterbauer H, Puhl H, Dieber–Rotheneder M, Waeg G, Rabl H. Effect of antioxidants on oxidative modification of LDL. Ann Med 1991; 23:573–581.
270. Van Het Hof KH, de Boers HS, Wiseman SA, Lien N, Westrate JA, Tijburg LB. Consumption of green or black tea does not increase resistance of LDL to oxidation in humans. Am J Clin Nutr 1997; 66:1125–1132.
271. Cherubini A, Beal MF, Frei B. Black tea increases the resistance of human plasma to lipid peroxidation in vitro, but not ex vivo. Free Radic Biol Med 1999; 27:381–387.
272. Aviram M. Review of human studies on oxidative damage and antioxidant protection related to cardiovascular diseases. Free Rad Res 2000; 33:S85–S97.
273. de Rijke YB, Demacher PN, Assen NA, Sloots LM, Katan MB, Stalenhof AF. Red wine consumption does not affect oxidizability of LDL in volunteers. Am J Clin Nutr 1996; 63:329–334.
274. Rice–Evans C, Leake D, Bruckdorfer KR, Diplock AT. Practical approaches to LDL oxidation: whys, wherefores and pitfalls. Free Radic Res 1996; 25:285–311.
275. Bartsch H, Nair J, Velic I. Etheno-DNA base adducts as tools in human cancer aetiology and chemoprevention. Eur J Cancer Prevent 1997; 6:529–534.
276. Chaudhary AK, Nokubo M, Reddy GR, et al. Detection of endogenous malondialdehyde–deoxyguanosine adducts in human liver. Science 1994; 265:1580–1582.
277. Vaca CE, Fang JL, Mutanen M, Valsta L. ^{32}P-postlabelling determination of DNA adducts of malonaldehyde in humans: total white blood cells and breast tissue. Carcinogenesis 1995; 16:1847–1851.
278. Agarwal S, Wee JJ, Hadley M, Draper HH. Identification of a deoxyguanosine-malondialdehyde adduct in rat and human urine. Lipids 1994; 29:429–432.
279. Basu S. Metabolism of 8-iso-prostaglandin $F_{2\alpha}$. FEBS Lett 1998; 428:32–36.
280. McGirr LG, Hadley M, Draper HH. Identification of N^α-acetyl-ε-(2-propenal) lysine as a urinary metabolite of malondialdehyde. J Biol Chem 1985; 260:15427–15431.
281. Dhanakoti SN, Draper HH. Response of urinary malondialdehyde to factors that stimulate lipid peroxidation in vivo. Lipids 1987; 22:643–646.
282. Brown ED, Morris VC, Rhode DG, et al. Urinary excretion of malondialdehyde in subjects fed meat cooked at high or low temperatures. Lipids 1995; 30:1053–1056.
283. Richelle M, Turini ME, Guidoux R, Tavazzi I, Metairon S, Fay LB. Urinary isoprostane excretion is not confounded by the lipid content of the diet. FEBS Lett 1999; 459:259–262.
284. Gutteridge JMC, Tickner TR. The thiobarbituric acid-reactivity of bile pigments. Biochem Med 1978; 19:127–132.
285. Kosugi H, Kojima T, Kikugawa K. Characteristics of the thiobarbituric acid reactivity of human urine as possible consequence of lipid peroxidation. Lipids 1993; 28:337–343.
286. Wang Z, Ciabattoni G, Creminon C, et al. Immunological characterization of urinary 8-epi-prostaglandin $F_2\alpha$ excretion in man. J Pharmacol Exp Ther 1995; 275:94–100.
287. Holt S, Reeder B, Wilson M, Harvey S, Morrow JD, Roberts LJ II, Moore K. Increased lipid peroxidation in patients with rhabdomyolysis. Lancet 1999; 353:1241.

288. Halliwell B. Biochemical mechanisms accounting for the toxic action of oxygen on living organisms: the key role of superoxide dismutase. Cell Biol Int Rep 1978; 2:113–128.
289. Daneshvar B, Frandsen H, Autrup H, Dragsted LO. γ-Glutamyl semialdehyde and 2-amino-adipic semialdehyde: biomarkers of oxidative damage to protein. Biomarkers 1997; 2:117–123.
290. Uchida K, Kawakishi S. 2-Oxo-histidine as a novel biological marker for oxidatively modified proteins. FEBS Lett 1993; 332:208–210.
291. Wells–Knecht MC, Huggins TG, Dyer DG, et al. Oxidized amino acids in lens proteins with age. Measurement of o-tyrosine and dityrosine in the aging human lens. J Biol Chem 1993; 268:12348–12352.
292. Giulivi C, Davies KJA. Dityrosine and tyrosine oxidation products are endogenous markers for the selective proteolysis of oxidatively modified red blood cell hemoglobin by (the 19S) proteasome. J Biol Chem 1993; 268:8752–8759.
293. Khan J, Brennand DM, Bradley N, Gao B, Bruckdorfer R, Jacobs M, Brennand DM. 3-Nitrotyrosine in the proteins of human plasma determined by an ELISA method. Biochem J 1998; 330:795–801.
294. Kettle AJ. Neutrophils convert tyrosyl residues in albumin to chlorotyrosine. FEBS Lett 1996; 379:103–106.
295. Levine RL, Berlett BS, Moskovitz J, Mosoni L. Methionine residues may protect proteins from critical oxidative damage. Mech Age Dev 1999; 107:323–332.
296. Eiserich JP, Cross CE, Jones DA, Halliwell B, van der Vliet A. Formation of nitrating and chlorinating species by reaction of nitrite with hypochlorous acid. A novel mechanism for nitric oxide-mediated protein modification. J Biol Chem 1996; 271:19199–19208.
297. Leeuwenburgh C, Rassmussen JE, Hsu FF, Muller DM, Pennathur S, Heinecke JW. Mass spectrometric quantitation of markers for protein oxidation by tyrosyl radical, copper, and hydroxyl radical in LDL isolated from human atherosclerotic plaques. J Biol Chem 1997; 272:3520–3526.
298. Frost M, Halliwell B, Moore K. Analysis of free and protein-bound nitrotyrosine in human plasma by a GC–MS method that avoids artifactual nitration. Biochem J 2000; 345:453–458.
299. Amici A, Levine RL, Tsai L, Stadtman ER. Conversion of amino acid residues in proteins and amino acid homopolymers to carbonyl derivatives by metal-catalyzed oxidation reactions. J Biol Chem 1989; 264:3341–3346.
300. Levine RL, Garland D, Oliver CN, Amici A, Climent I, Lenz AG, Ahn BW, Shaltiel S, Stadtman ER. Determination of carbonyl content in oxidatively modified protein. Methods Enzymol 1990; 186:464–487.
301. Evans P, Lyras L, Halliwell B. Measurement of protein carbonyls in human brain tissue. Methods Enzymol 1999; 300:145–156.
302. Shacter E, Williams JA, Lim M, Levine RL. Differential susceptibility of plasma proteins to oxidative modification: examination by Western blot immunoassay. Free Radic Biol Med 1994; 17:429–437.
303. Yan LJ, Orr WC, Sohal RS. Identification of oxidized proteins based on SDS gel electrophoresis, immunochemical detection, isoelectric focusing and microsequencing. Anal Biochem 1998; 263:67–71.
304. Keller J, Halmes NC, Hinson JA, Pumford NR. Immuno-chemical detection of oxidized proteins. Chem Res Toxicol 1993; 6:430–433.
305. Winterbourn CC, Buss IH. Protein carbonyl measurement by enzyme-linked immunosorbent assay. Methods Enzymol 1999; 300:106–111.
306. Liggins J, Furth AJ. Role of protein-bound carbonyl groups in the formation of advanced glycation end-products. Biochim Biophys Acta 1997; 1361:123–130.
307. Mahmoodi H, Hadley M, Chang YX, Draper HH. Increased formation and degradation of malondialdehyde-modified proteins under conditions of peroxidative stress. Lipids 1995; 30:963–966.
308. Anton R. Flavonoids and traditional medicine. In: Cody V, Middleton E, Harborne JB, Bertez A, eds. Plant Flavonoids in Biology and Medicine: Biochemical, Cellular and Medicinal Properties. New York: Alan R Liss, 1988:423–438.
309. Ho CT, Osawa T, Huang M-T, Rosen RT, eds. Food Phytochemicals for Cancer Prevention II, Teas, Spices and Herbs. ACS Symposium Series 547. Washington, DC: American Chemical Society, 1994.
310. Huang MT, Osawa T, Ho CT, Rosen RT, eds. Food Phytochemicals for Cancer Prevention I, Fruits and Vegetables. ACS Symposium Series 546. Washington, DC: American Chemical Society, 1994.

2
Measurement of Total Antioxidant Capacity in Nutritional and Clinical Studies

Guohua Cao

Jean Mayer USDA Human Nutrition Research Center on Aging at Tufts University, Boston, Massachusetts

Ronald L. Prior

Arkansas Children's Nutrition Center, USDA-ARS, Little Rock, Arkansas

I. INTRODUCTION

There has been intense interest recently among the public and the media in the possibility that increased intake of dietary antioxidants may protect against chronic diseases, which include cancers, cardiovascular, and cerebrovascular diseases. Antioxidants are substances that, when present at low concentrations, compared with those of an oxidizable substrate, significantly prevent or delay a pro-oxidant–initiated oxidation of the substrate (1). A pro-oxidant is a toxic substance that can cause oxidative damage to lipids, proteins, and nucleic acids, resulting in various pathological events or diseases. Examples of pro-oxidants include reactive oxygen and nitrogen species (ROS and RNS), which are products of normal aerobic metabolic processes. ROS include superoxide ($O_2^{-\cdot}$), hydroxyl ($OH^{\cdot}$), and peroxyl ($ROO^{\cdot}$) radicals, and hydrogen peroxide (H_2O_2). RNS include nitric oxide ($NO^{\cdot}$) and nitrogen dioxide ($NO_2^{\cdot}$). There is a considerable body of biological evidence that ROS and RNS can be damaging to cells and, thereby, they might contribute to cellular dysfunction and diseases. The existence and development of cells in an oxygen-containing environment would not be possible without the presence of a complicated antioxidant defense system that includes enzymatic and nonenzymatic components.

The nonenzymatic antioxidants, most of which have low molecular weights and are able to directly and efficiently quench ROS and RNS, constitute an important aspect of the body's antioxidant system. The interaction among these antioxidants and the difficulty in measuring

---

Mention of a trade name, proprietary product, or specific equipment does not constitute a guarantee by the U. S. Department of Agriculture and does not imply its approval to the exclusion of other products that may be suitable.

all of them individually prompted the development of assays for measuring total antioxidant capacity. The measurement of total antioxidant capacity from all these nonenzymatic antioxidants is necessary and important in evaluating in vivo antioxidant status in many clinical and nutritional studies. The aim of this chapter is to help readers in understanding, selecting, and performing total antioxidant capacity measurement in these studies.

II. OVERVIEW OF TOTAL ANTIOXIDANT CAPACITY ASSAY METHODOLOGY

All the methods developed for measuring total antioxidant capacity of a biological sample involve oxidants or oxidizing agents that accept electrons from reductants, which are often treated as the antioxidants being measured. On the basis of the oxidants used, these methods can be divided into two groups: one using oxidants that are not necessarily pro-oxidant, and the other using oxidants that are pro-oxidants.

A. Methods Using Oxidants That Are Not Necessarily Pro-Oxidants

The methods that use oxidants that are not necessarily pro-oxidants include the ferric reducing–antioxidant power (FRAP) assay (2,3), the Trolox equivalent antioxidant capacity (TEAC) assay (4–7), and a cyclic voltammetry procedure (8). The FRAP assay was originally defined as ferric-reducing ability of plasma (2). It depends on the reduction of a ferric tripyridyltriazine (Fe^{3+}-TPTZ) complex to the ferrous tripyridyltriazine (Fe^{2+}–TPTZ) by a reductant at low pH. Fe^{2+}–TPTZ has an intensive blue color and can be monitored at 593 nm. What this method really measures is the ability of a compound or compounds to reduce Fe^{3+} (the oxidant in the assay system) to produce Fe^{2+}.

The TEAC assay is based on the inhibition by reductants of the absorbance of the radical cation of 2,2′-azinobis(3-ethylbenzothiazoline 6-sulfonate) (ABTS), which has a characteristic long-wavelength absorption spectrum showing maxima at 660, 734, and 820 nm. The ABTS radical cation in the original version (4,5) is formed by the interaction of ABTS with the ferrylmyoglobin radical species, generated by the activation of metmyoglobin with H_2O_2. This original TEAC assay measures the ability of a compound in reducing the ABTS radical, although the compound under analysis can also reduce ferrylmyoglobin radicals. The modified or improved TEAC assay uses ABTS radicals preformed by oxidation of ABTS with potassium persulfate (6) or 2,2′-azobis(2-amidinopropane) dihydrochloride (AAPH) (7).

The cyclic voltammetry procedure uses three electrodes: the working electrode (e.g., glassy carbon), the reference electrode (Ag–AgCl), and the auxiliary electrode (platinum wire). The potential is applied to the working electrode at a constant rate (100 mV/s). During operation of the cyclic voltammetry, a potential current curve is recorded (cyclic voltammogram). The reducing power of a sample is composed of two parameters: the peak potential [$E_{p(a)}$] and the anodic current (AC). The $E_{p(a)}$ is measured at the half increase of the current at each anodic wave (AW) and is referred as $E_{1/2}$. The $E_{1/2}$ correlates with the type of reductant: the lower the $E_{1/2}$, the higher the ability of the tested compounds to donate electrons to the working electrode. The AC is measured from the y axis of each AW and correlates with the overall concentration of the reductants.

"Reducing capacity or power" is probably a better term than "antioxidant capacity or power" for describing the results obtained by using the FRAP, TEAC, or cyclic voltammetry procedures. As we discussed in the foregoing, antioxidants are substances that can efficiently

MEASUREMENT OF TOTAL ANTIOXIDANT CAPACITY

reduce pro-oxidants (i.e., oxidants of pathological importance), with the formed products having no or low toxicity. However, the oxidants used in the FRAP (Fe^{3+}) do not directly cause oxidative damage to lipids, proteins, or nucleic acids. On the contrary, the Fe^{2+} produced from Fe^{3+} is a well-known "pro-oxidant"; it can react with H_2O_2 to produce $OH^{\cdot}$, the most harmful free radical found in vivo. There is no evidence that the oxidant (ABTS radical) used in the TEAC assay has any pathological importance. It is unlikely that ABTS radical, which is not found in the body, causes oxidative damage to lipids, protein, or nucleic acids because it is stable for at least 2 days when stored in the dark at room temperature (6). The oxidant or electron acceptor used in the cyclic voltammetry procedure is glass carbon electrode, which is obviously of no pathological importance. Additionally, neither the FRAP assay nor the cyclic voltammetry procedure using glass carbon electrode measures GSH and other −SH−containing compounds, an important group of antioxidants in the body.

B. Methods Using Oxidants That Are Pro-Oxidants

Most total antioxidant capacity assays using pro-oxidants also use an oxidizable substrate. The pro-oxidants induce oxidative damage (to the substrate), which is inhibited in the presence of antioxidants. This inhibition is measured and related to antioxidant capacity of the antioxidants. The measured antioxidant capacity may have physiological importance, because the pro-oxidants used in these systems are pathologically important. The total radical-trapping parameter (TRAP) assay was one of the earliest methods for measuring total antioxidant capacity of plasma or serum. The TRAP assay uses peroxyl radicals generated from AAPH and peroxidizable materials contained or added in plasma or other biological fluids (9,10). After adding AAPH to the plasma, the oxidation of the oxidizable materials is monitored by measuring the oxygen consumed during the reaction. During an induction period, this oxidation is inhibited by the antioxidants in the plasma. The length of the induction period (lag phase) is compared with that of an internal standard, Trolox (6-hydroxyl-2,5,7,8-tetramethylchroman-2-carboxylic acid), and then quantitatively related to the antioxidant capacity of the plasma. The major problem with the original TRAP assay lies in the oxygen electrode endpoint; an oxygen electrode will not maintain its stability over the period of time required (5). Other total antioxidant capacity assays that also use peroxyl radicals include the chemiluminescence-based TRAP assay) (11), the dichlorofluorescein-diacetate (DCFH-DA)-based TRAP assay (12), the total oxyradical scavenging capacity (TOSC) assay (13), the crocin-based assays (14,15), and the phycoerythrin (PE)-based assays (16–18). The chemiluminescence-based TRAP assay uses luminol as an oxidizable substrate; the oxidized luminol (luminol radicals) emits the light that can be detected by a luminometer. The DCFH-DA-based TRAP assay uses DCFH-DA as an oxidizable substrate. The oxidation of DCFH-DA by peroxyl radicals produces dichlorofluorescein, which can be monitored either fluorometrically or spectrophotometrically. The TOSC assay uses α-keto-γ-methiolbutyric acid (KMBA) as an oxidizable substrate. The oxidation of KMBA produces ethylene, which is monitored by gas chromatography. The crocin-based assays use crocin as an oxidizable substrate. The oxidation of crocin can be monitored by measuring its absorbance at 443 nm. The traditional and modified TRAP assays (9–12) all require the determination of a lag phase for quantification, which is usually not an easy job. The TOSC assay integrates the area from the curve defining the sample or control reaction for result quantification, although the system is an "open" system in terms of area integration (the production of ethylene should increase continuously after the consumption of antioxidants) (13). The crocin-based procedures use either competition kinetics (14) or inhibition percentage (15) for quantifying antioxidant capacity.

The PE-based assays include the Glazer's method (16), the "TRAP" assay reported by Ghiselli et al. (17), and the ORAC assay (18–20). PE is a mixture of fluorescent proteins. Glazer's method represents the first antioxidant capacity assay that uses the natural protein as an oxidizable substrate. The "TRAP" assay reported by Ghiselli et al. is basically a duplicate of that part of Glazer's method that uses peroxyl radicals. Glazer et al. used either AAPH or Cu^{2+}-ascorbate to produce the pro-oxidants and a lag phase for quantitation. However, the kinetics of PE fluorescence quenching are not linear in the presence of peroxyl or hydroxyl radicals, which makes the lag phase determination difficult, particularly when a plasma or serum sample is analyzed. The ORAC assay is based on the work of Glazer et al. It is, to date, the only method that takes free radical action to completion and uses an area-under-curve (AUC) technique for quantitation, and thus combines both inhibition percentage and the length of inhibition time of the free radical action by antioxidants into a single quantity. The ORAC assay has been used by different laboratories and has provided significant information on the antioxidant capacity of various biological samples from pure compounds to complex matrices (1).

III. APPLICATION OF TOTAL ANTIOXIDANT CAPACITY ASSAYS IN NUTRITIONAL AND CLINICAL STUDIES

All the foregoing methods may be used to assess the total antioxidant capacity, although what is actually measured by some of them is total capacity of a sample in reducing a specific oxidant, which is not necessarily a pro-oxidant. Such a total reducing capacity of a sample may reflect its ability in reducing pro-oxidants or reactive species. For example, we observed a significant, but weak, correlation between serum FRAP and serum ORAC in one clinical study (21). However, in this chapter we will focus on the ORAC assay, which we have been using for several years (18–20). Other methods are described in detail in the cited references.

A. Sample Preparation

The samples used for ORAC analysis in nutritional and clinical studies include plasma, serum, urine, and other biological fluids, as well as fruits, vegetables, oils, and various dietary supplements. Possible correlations found between dietary intake of total antioxidants and in vivo antioxidant status, oxidative stress, diseases, or disease risks will provide strong evidence to support antioxidant-related hypotheses. The ORAC assay, but not other assays, has been widely used for the determination of total antioxidant capacity in fruits, vegetables, and dietary supplements (22–28).

Blood plasma is prepared by using heparin, which has no effect on the ORAC assay. Blood plasma or serum needs to be diluted 100- to 200-fold with 75 mM phosphate buffer (pH 7.0) before it is used in the ORAC assay. To measure the ORAC in the nonprotein fraction of plasma or serum, dilute serum with 0.5-M perchloric acid (PCA) (1:1, v/v) or acetone (1:4, v/v), centrifuge at 4°C for 10 min, and recover the supernatant for the ORAC assay after suitable dilution with the buffer. Plasma, serum, or PCA-treated plasma or serum can be stored at −80°C for at least 6 months. Other biological fluids, including urine, can be used in the ORAC assay either directly after suitable dilution or after removing their protein components.

The edible portion of a fresh fruit or vegetable is weighed and then homogenized by adding deionized water (e.g., 1:2 w/v). A dried fruit, vegetable, or dietary supplement is soaked in deionized water (e.g., 1:9 w/v) for a certain period, depending on the sample analyzed, and then

MEASUREMENT OF TOTAL ANTIOXIDANT CAPACITY

homogenized. The homogenate is then centrifuged and the supernatant (water-soluble fraction) is recovered. The pulp is washed with deionized water, and the recovered supernatant is pooled with the supernatant obtained from the first centrifugation step. The pooled supernatant is measured for its volume and used directly for the ORAC assay after suitable dilution with phosphate buffer. The pulp is then further extracted by using pure acetone (1:4 w/v) with shaking at room temperature for 30 min. The acetone extract is recovered after centrifugation and used for the ORAC assay after suitable dilution with phosphate buffer. The ORAC activity is calculated by adding the activity from the water-soluble fraction and the activity from the acetone-extracted fraction. Fruits and vegetables can also be extracted by using a mixture of acetone, water, and acetic acid (70:29.5:0.5, v/v/v) without separating the water-soluble fraction from the acetone-extracted fraction. Acetonitrile, containing 4% acetic acid, was also used by us to extract antioxidants from fresh blueberries (27). However, water needs to be added when dried fruits or vegetables are extracted by using this acetonitrile procedure. Wine and fruit or vegetable juices can be used in the ORAC assay directly after suitable dilution, if there are no obvious precipitates; otherwise, these samples need to be centrifuged before use.

Oils can also be analyzed for their total antioxidant capacities by the ORAC assay. An oil sample needs to be diluted with acetone (e.g., 1:9, v/v) first and then with the phosphate buffer for the ORAC analysis. No antioxidant activity was detected in common corn oils. However, some specific oils, such as corn fiber oil and some fruit seed oils have strong antioxidant activities. There is much less interference from colored extracts or compounds with fluorescence measurement used in the ORAC assay compared with an absorbance measurement used in other total antioxidant capacity assays. It will be difficult, if not impossible, for those other assays to analyze oil samples. This is an important factor to consider, particularly when oils, fruits, vegetables, and natural product supplements are analyzed for their antioxidant capacities.

B. Automated Procedure on Cobas Fara II

A Cobas Fara II centrifugal analyzer (Roche Diagnostic System, Inc., Branchburg, NJ) is used for the automated procedure. The Cobas Fara II is programmed to maintain a temperature of 37°C and a two-reagent system (Reaction Mode 3, P-I-SRI-A) is used. This reaction mode pipettes and transfers sample (20 μL), phosphate buffer (5 μL), and the main reagent (PE) (365 μL, 3.73 mg/L, prepared with the phosphate buffer) in parallel (P) into the primary reagent wells of their respective cuvette rotor positions, spins, mixes, and incubates (I) for the programmed time of 1 min, and records the initial fluorescence (F_0) (E_x 540 nm; E_m 565 nm). When the rotor stops spinning, a start reagent (SRI) consisting of 5 μL of AAPH (320 mM, prepared with the phosphate buffer) plus 5 μL of the phosphate buffer is pipetted into the appropriate start reagent wells in the cuvette rotor. Between transfers, sample and reagent transfer pipettes are washed with buffer to eliminate sample cross-contamination. When the analyzer starts spinning, it causes mixing of sample–PE with AAPH and the reaction starts. Fluorescence readings are then taken again every 2 min (F_2, F_4, F_6, $\cdots$) for up to 70 min. If the fluorescence of the last reading does not decline to less than 5% of the first reading, the dilution of the sample analyzed is adjusted accordingly and the sample is reanalyzed. The reaction direction is selected as a "decrease" and the conversion factor is set to "1." To determine the maximum voltage for the photomultiplier tube (PM adjust), AAPH is omitted, replaced with buffer, and the analyzer is run for 10 min using the ORAC assay program. The PM adjustment procedure should be performed when different PE or the same PE with different lot number is used. The phosphate buffer is used as a blank and Trolox (20 μM) is used as a standard, which is added in a manner similar to the samples to give a final concentration of 1 μM. The final results (ORAC value) are expressed using Trolox equivalents.

$$\text{ORAC value } (\mu M) = 20k(S_{\text{Sample}} - S_{\text{Blank}})/(S_{\text{Trolox}} - S_{\text{blank}}) \quad (1)$$

Where k = sample dilution factor, and S = the area under the fluorescence decay curve of the sample, Trolox, or blank, which are calculated as follows:

$$S = (0.5 + f_2/f_0 + f_4/f_0 + f_6/f_0 + \cdots + f_{68}/f_0 + f_{70}/f_0) \times 2 \quad (2)$$

Where f_0 = initial fluorescence at 0 min and f_i = fluorescence measurement at time i.

Use of multiple concentrations of Trolox to obtain a standard curve reduces the intra- and intersystem variables, but also reduces the number of samples that can be handled by the machine. Samples and standards are always analyzed in duplicate using a "forward-then-reverse" ordering to correct for the signal "drift" that correlated with the position of each sample in the Cobas Fara II cuvettes. Data generated from the Cobas Fara II are sent electronically through the RS-232 serial interface to a PC computer system running Crosstalk (Digital Communications Associates, Alpharetta, GA) or other similar communication software. The data are then analyzed using Microsoft Excel (Microsoft Corporation, Roselle, IL 60172) to apply Eq. (2) to the area under the fluorescence decay curve (AUC) and Eq. (1) to the final ORAC value.

C. Manual Procedure

For a manual procedure, the following reagents are used: the phosphate buffer, 1750 μL; PE (68 mg/L), 100 μL; AAPH (160 mM), 50 μL; and sample, 100 μL. The assay is carried out at 37°C in fluorimeter cuvettes. A blank and a standard are assayed during each run. For the blank, 100 μL of buffer instead of sample is used. For the standard, 100 μL of 20 μM Trolox solution instead of sample is used. The reaction is started by the addition of AAPH. Once AAPH is added, the cuvette is vortexed briefly and the fluorescence is measured immediately (E_m 565 nm, E_x 540 nm) using a fluorescence spectrophotometer (e.g., Perkin-Elmer LS-5). The fluorescence is recorded every 5 min until the fluorescence of the last reading has declined to less than 5% of the first reading. One blank, one standard, and a maximum of eight samples can be analyzed at the same time, when a cuvette rack is used. The cuvette rack should be kept at 37°C in a waterbath. For calculation of the results, Eq. (2) is modified as follows:

$$S = (0.5 + f_5/f_0 + f_{10}/f_0 + f_{15}/f_0 + \cdots + f_{65}/f_0 + f_{70}/f_0) \times 5 \quad (3)$$

Where f_0 = initial fluorescence at 0 min and f_i = fluorescence measurement at time i.

D. Using H_2O_2–Cu^{2+} as Pro-oxidants in the ORAC Assay

The automated and manual ORAC procedures using H_2O_2–Cu^{2+} as pro-oxidants are similar to those using AAPH. For the automated procedure, the Cobas pipettes and transfers 20 μL of sample, 5 μL of phosphate buffer, and 360 μL of main reagent (PE, 3.78 mg/L) into the main reagent wells, and 10 μL of the H_2O_2–Cu^{2+} mixture and 5 μL of buffer into the start reagent wells. H_2O_2 (24%) and cupric sulfate (0.72 mM) are mixed (1:1, v/v) before loading into the Cobas reagent rack. For the manual procedure, the following reagents and volumes are used: phosphate buffer, 1750 μL; PE (68 mg/L), 100 μL; H_2O_2–Cu^{2+} mixture, 50 μL; and sample, 100 μL. The reaction is started by the addition of 50 μL of H_2O_2–Cu^{2+} mixture.

The fluorescence intensity and the sensitivity to peroxyl radical damage can be different even for the same PE with different lot numbers. The ORAC assay procedures described earlier are based on using B- or R-PE that loses more than 90% of its fluorescence within 30 min in the presence of 4-mM AAPH. When PE is relatively resistant to peroxyl radical damage, the concentration of AAPH and Trolox standard can be increased accordingly in the ORAC assay.

E. ORAC Measured in Plasma or Serum: Effects of PCA or Acetone Treatment

Treating plasma or serum with PCA or acetone removes proteins. The PCA treatment of a plasma or serum sample before storage at $-80°C$ also preserves ascorbate. Contribution of albumin, uric acid, α-tocopherol, ascorbic acid, bilirubin, and other antioxidants to total ORAC measured in serum without any treatments was 27.8, 7.1, 0.8, 1.3, 0.3, and 62.7%, respectively. These contributions to total ORAC measured in serum treated with PCA were 0, 39.2, 0, 7.2, 1.3, and 52.3%, respectively. The contributions to ORAC measured in serum treated with acetone were 0, 45.4, 6.1, 10.5, 1.9, and 36.1, respectively. It is recommended that both untreated and PCA (or acetone)-treated plasma or serum be analyzed for the total antioxidant capacity (21).

IV. FACTORS TO BE CONSIDERED IN TOTAL ANTIOXIDANT CAPACITY ASSESSMENT

A. Diets

Diet has significant effects on the total antioxidant capacity measured in plasma, serum, and urine, even when the diet does not contain antioxidants. We found in healthy elderly women, who resided in a metabolic research unit, that serum total antioxidant capacity, measured as ORAC and FRAP increased significantly following the consumption of lunch and dinner meals. These meals were designed to contain as minimal amounts of antioxidant components as possible. Serum ORAC and FRAP did not increase until after the consumption of the dinner when lunch was not provided. Among the individual antioxidants examined, serum uric acid was the only one that showed a significant postprandial increase, which was also parallel with the postprandial response in serum total antioxidant capacity (Cao G, Prior RL, unpublished data). The results indicate the importance of controlling the diets in nutritional and clinical studies.

B. Physical Activity

Physical activity can also affect the total antioxidant capacity measurement. In young subjects, a graded aerobic exercise to exhaustion significantly increased serum ORAC (Cao G, et al., unpublished data). Aerobic exercise increases oxygen consumption, which is directly related to ROS production. The increased serum antioxidant capacity after aerobic exercise can be viewed as an adaptive response in the antioxidant defense system.

C. Diseases and Genetics

Kidney dysfunction increases the uric acid concentration and thus total antioxidant capacity in plasma or serum (29). The plasma or serum total antioxidant capacity may be altered in many other diseases, but has not been fully investigated. Serum total antioxidant capacity in healthy humans is tightly regulated. Fasting plasma ORAC varies markedly between subjects but is stable for the same subject over several months (30).

V. INTERPRETATION OF PLASMA OR SERUM TOTAL ANTIOXIDANT CAPACITY

The interpretation of the changes in plasma or serum antioxidant capacity depends not only on the method used in detecting these changes but also on the conditions under which the plasma or serum antioxidant capacity is determined, because the determined antioxidant capacity reflects outcomes in a dynamic system. The increase in total antioxidant capacity in plasma or serum after consumption of antioxidants should indicate an absorption of the antioxidants and an improved in vivo antioxidant defense status (30,31). An increased plasma or serum antioxidant capacity could also be an adaptation to an increased oxidative stress at an early stage. In addition, an increased antioxidant capacity in plasma or serum may not necessarily be a desirable condition, as we mentioned earlier in the patients with chronic renal failure (29). An increased serum antioxidant capacity observed in rats exposed to hyperoxia is simply a result of an increase in capillary permeability that causes the redistribution of antioxidants between tissues (32).

Similarly, a decrease in plasma or serum antioxidant capacity is not necessarily an undesirable condition when the production of reactive species decreases (e.g., when rats are food-restricted) (33). Because of these complications, a single measurement of total antioxidant capacity in plasma or serum is not going to be sufficient, but a "battery" of measurements, which should include measurements of oxidative damage, will be necessary to adequately assess oxidative stress in vivo.

REFERENCES

1. Prior RL, Cao G. In vivo total antioxidant capacity: comparison of different analytical methods. Free Radic Biol Med 1999; (in press).
2. Benzie IFF, Strain JJ. The ferric reducing ability of plasma (FRAP) as a measure of "antioxidant power": the FRAP assay. Anal Biochem 1996; 239:70–76.
3. Benzie IFF, Strain JJ. Ferric reducing/antioxidant power assay: direct measure of total antioxidant activity of biological fluids and modified version for simultaneous measurement of total antioxidant power and ascorbic acid concentration. Methods Enzymol 1999; 299:15–27.
4. Miller NJ, Rice–Evans C, Davies MJ, Gopinathan V, Milnen A. A novel method for measuring antioxidant capacity and its application to monitoring the antioxidant status in premature neonates. Clin Sci 1993; 84:407–412.
5. Rice–Evans C, Miller NJ. Total antioxidant status in plasma and body fluids. Methods Enzymol 1994; 234:279–293.
6. Re R, Pellegrini N, Proteggente A, Pannala A, Yang M, Rice–Evans C. Antioxidant activity applying an improved ABTS radical cation decolorization assay. Free Radic Biol Med 1999; 26:1231–1237.
7. Van den Berg R, Haenen GRMM, Van den Berg H, Bast A. Application of an improved Trolox equivalent antioxidant capacity (TEAC) assay for evaluation of antioxidant capacity measurements of mixtures. Food Chem 1999; 66:511–517.
8. Kohen R, Beit–Yannai E, Berry EM, Tirosh O. Overall low molecular weight and antioxidant activity of biological fluids and tissues by cyclic voltammetry. Methods Enzymol 1999; 300:285–296.
9. Wayner DDM, Burton GW, Ingold KU, Locke S. Quantitative measurement of the total, peroxyl radical-trapping antioxidant capacity of human blood plasma by controlled peroxidation. FEBS Lett 1985; 187:33–37.
10. Wayner DDM, Burton GW, Ingold KU. The antioxidant efficiency of vitamin C is concentration-dependent. Biochim Biophys Acta 1986; 884:119–123.
11. Alho H, Leinonen J. Total antioxidant activity measured by chemiluminescence methods. Methods Enzymol 1999; 299:3–14.
12. Valkonen M, Kuusi T. Spectrophotometric assay for total peroxyl radical-trapping antioxidant potential in human serum. J Lipid Res 1997; 38:823–833.

13. Winston GW, Regoli F, Dugas AJ Jr, Fong JH, Blanchard KA. A rapid gas chromatographic assay for determining oxyradical scavenging capacity of antioxidants and biological fluids. Free Radic Biol Med 1998; 24:480–493.
14. Tubaro F, Ghiselli A, Papuzzi P, Maiorino M, Ursini F. Analysis of plasma antioxidant capacity by competition kinetics. Free Radic Biol Med 1998; 24:1228–1234.
15. Lussignoli S, Fraccaroli M, Andrioli G, Brocco G, Bellavite P. A microplate-based colorimetric assay of the total peroxyl radical trapping capability of human plasma. Anal Biochem 1999; 269:38–44.
16. Glazer AN. Phycoerythrin fluorescence-based assay for reactive oxygen species. Methods Enzymol 1990; 186:161–168.
17. Ghiselli A, Serafini M, Maiani G, Assini E, Ferro–Luzzi A. A fluorescence-based method for measuring total plasma antioxidant capability. Free Radic Biol Med 1994; 18:29–36.
18. Cao G, Alessio HM, Cutler RG. Oxygen-radical absorbance capacity assay for antioxidants. Free Radic Biol Med 1993; 14:303–311.
19. Cao G, Verdon CP, Wu AHB, Wang H, Prior RL. Automated oxygen radical absorbance capacity assay using the COBAS FARA II. Clin Chem 1995; 41:1738–1744.
20. Cao G, Prior RL. The measurement of oxygen radical absorbance capacity in biological samples. Methods Enzymol 1999; 299:50–62.
21. Cao G, Prior RL. Comparison of different analytical methods for assessing total antioxidant capacity of human serum. Clin Chem 1998; 44:1309–1315.
22. Cao G, Sofic E, Prior RL. Antioxidant capacity of tea and common vegetables. J Agric Food Chem 1996; 44:3426–3431.
23. Wang H, Cao G, Prior RL. Total antioxidant capacity of fruits. J Agric Food Chem 1996; 44:701–705.
24. Prior RL, Cao G. Antioxidant capacity and polyphenolic components of teas: implications for altering in vivo antioxidant status. Proc Soc Exp Biol Med 1999; 220:255–261.
25. Lin YL, Juan IM, Chen YL, Liang YC, Lin JK. Composition of polyphenols in fresh tea leaves and associations of their oxygen–radical-absorbing capacity with antiproliferative actions in fibroblast cells. J Agric Food Chem 1996; 44:1387–1394.
26. Sharma HM, Hanna AN, Kauffman EM, Newman HAI. Effect of herbal mixture student rasayana on lipoxygenase activity and lipid peroxidation. Free Radic Biol Med 1995; 18:687–697.
27. Prior GL, Cao G, Martin A, Sofic E, McEwen J, O'Brien C, Lischner N, Ehlenfeldt M, Kalt W, Krewer G, Mainland CM. Antioxidant capacity as influenced by total phenolic and anthocyanin content, maturity, and variety of *Vaccinium* species. J Agric Food Chem 1998; 46:2686–2693.
28. Prior RL, Cao G. Variability in dietary antioxidant related natural product supplements: the need for methods of standardization. J Am Nutraceut Assoc 1999; 2:36–46.
29. Jackson P, Loughrey CM, Lightbody JH, McNamee PT, Young IS. Effect of hemodialysis on total antioxidant capacity and serum antioxidants in patients with chronic renal failure. Clin Chem 1995; 41:1135–1138.
30. Cao G, Booth SL, Sadowski JA, Prior RL. Increases in human plasma antioxidant capacity following consumption of controlled diets high in fruits and vegetables. Am J Clin Nutr 1998; 68:1081–1087.
31. Cao G, Russell RM, Lischner N, Prior RL. Serum antioxidant capacity is increased by consumption of strawberries, spinach, red wine or vitamin C in elderly women. J Nutr 1998; 128:2383–2390.
32. Cao G, Shukitt–Hale B, Bickford PC, Joseph JA, McEwen J, Prior RL. Hyperoxia-induced changes in antioxidant capacity and the effect of dietary antioxidants. J Appl Physiol 1999; 86:1817–1822.
33. Cao G, Prior RL, Cutler RG, Yu BP. Effect of dietary restriction on serum antioxidant capacity in rats. Arch Gerontol Geriatr 1997; 25:245–253.

3

Quantification of Isoprostanes as Indicators of Oxidant Stress In Vivo

Jason D. Morrow, William E. Zackert, Daniel S. Van der Ende, Erin E. Reich, Erin S. Terry, Brian Cox, Stephanie C. Sanchez, Thomas J. Montine, and L. Jackson Roberts

Vanderbilt University School of Medicine, Nashville, Tennessee

I. INTRODUCTION

Free radicals derived from molecular oxygen have been implicated in a variety of human diseases, ranging from atherosclerosis, to cancer, to neurodegenerative disorders (1–4). It is postulated that the pathophysiological sequelae of oxidant stress result partly from damage to tissue biomolecules. Understanding the role that oxidant stress plays in human disease has been hampered, however, by the lack of reliable methods to assess oxidant injury (5). The development of accurate methods for measuring oxidative stress in humans is essential to establish a means for quantifying the role of free radical injury in disease processes.

A well-recognized result of oxidant injury is peroxidation of lipids. Nearly a decade ago, we reported that a series of prostaglandin (PG)-like compounds are produced by the free radical-catalyzed peroxidation of arachidonic acid, independently of the cyclooxygenase enzyme, which had previously been considered obligatory for endogenous prostanoid synthesis (6). Since then, we and others have accumulated a large body of evidence indicating that quantification of these unique products of lipid peroxidation, now termed isoprostanes (IsoPs), provides a reliable marker of oxidant injury both in vitro and in vivo (7–9). Furthermore, several of these compounds possess potent biological activity and thus may be mediators of oxidant injury (7–9). It is the purpose herein to summarize selected aspects of our knowledge about the IsoPs. This chapter will (1) highlight mechanisms involved in IsoP formation, (2) summarize methods of analyzing IsoPs, (3) examine the usefulness of quantifying IsoPs in selected animal models of oxidant stress, and (4) explore their use as markers of oxidant injury in association with human disease.

II. HISTORICAL PERSPECTIVES

In the 1960s and 1970s, it was shown that PG-like compounds can be formed by the autoxidation of purified polyunsaturated fatty acids (10–13). Seminal and elegant studies performed by Pryor, Porter, and others led to a proposed mechanism by which these compounds were generated by bicycloendoperoxide intermediates (11). However, this work was never carried beyond in vitro studies. Moreover, it was not determined whether PG-like compounds could be formed in biological fluids containing unsaturated fatty acids.

In the 1980s, we showed that PGD_2 derived from cyclooxygenase is primarily metabolized in vivo in humans to form $9\alpha,11\beta\text{-}PGF_2$ by the enzyme 11-ketoreductase (14). In aqueous solutions, however, PGD_2 is an unstable compound that undergoes isomerization of the lower side chain, and these isomers can be likewise reduced by 11-ketoreductase to yield isomers of $9\alpha,11\beta\text{-}PGF_2$ (15). In studies undertaken to further characterize these compounds utilizing a gas chromatographic–mass spectrometric (GC–MS) assay, we found that when plasma samples from normal volunteers that were processed and analyzed immediately, a series of peaks were detected possessing characteristics of F-ring PGs (Fig. 1). Interestingly, however, when plasma samples that had been stored at $-20°C$ for several months were reanalyzed, identical chromatographic peaks were detected, but levels of putative PGF_2-like compounds were up

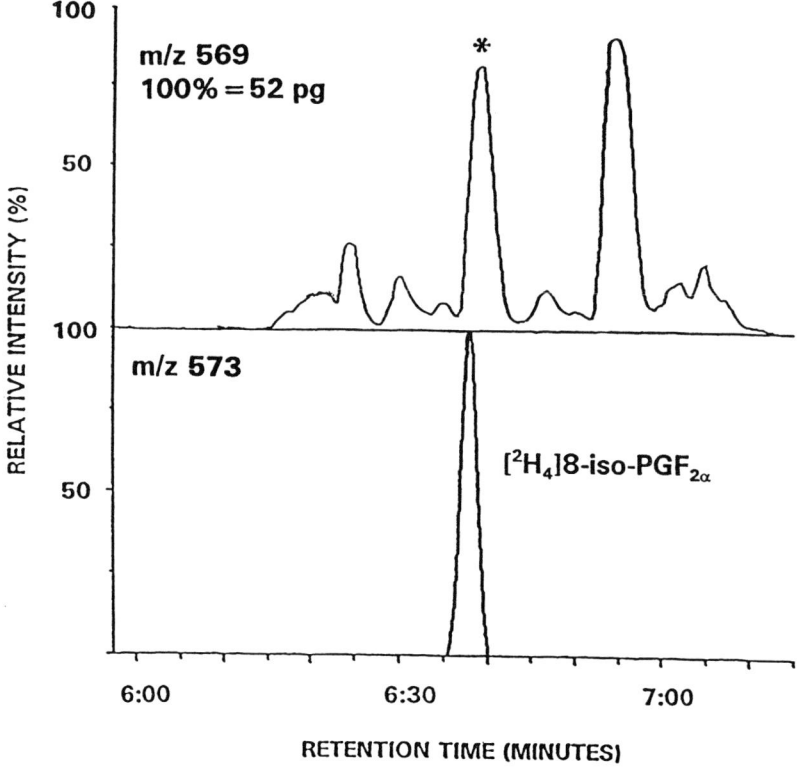

Figure 1 Analysis of F_2-IsoPs in a plasma sample from a normal human volunteer: The m/z 569 ion current chromatogram represents endogenous F_2-IsoPs. The m/z 573 chromatogram represents the $[^2H_4]8\text{-iso-}PGF_{2\alpha}$ internal standard. The peak represented by the star (*) is the one routinely quantified for F_2-IsoPs. The concentration of F_2-IsoPs in this plasma sample was 47 pg/mL.

to 100-fold higher (6). Subsequent experiments led to the finding that these PGF_2-like compounds were generated in both freshly processed and stored plasma, not by a cyclooxygenase derived mechanism, but nonenzymatically by autoxidation of plasma arachidonic acid (6,16). Because these compounds contain F-type prostane rings, they are referred to as F_2-isoprostanes (F_2-IsoPs).

III. MECHANISM OF FORMATION OF THE ISOPROSTANES

A mechanism to explain the formation of the F_2-IsoPs is outlined in Figure 2 and is based on that proposed by Pryor for the generation of bicycloendoperoxide intermediates resulting from the peroxidation of other polyunsaturated fatty acids (11). Precursor arachidonic acid at the top of the figure initially undergoes abstraction of an allylic hydrogen atom to yield an arachidonyl carbon-centered radical. Subsequently, there is insertion of oxygen to yield peroxyl radicals. Depending on the site of hydrogen abstraction and oxygen insertion, four different peroxyl radical isomers are formed. Endocyclization of the radicals occurs, followed by the addition of another molecule of oxygen to yield four bicycloendoperoxide (PGG_2-like) regioisomers. These intermediates are then reduced to F_2-IsoPs. Each of the four regioisomers can theoretically comprise eight racemic diastereomers. Thus, a total of 64 different compounds can be generated by this process, although as discussed later, the formation of some is favored over others. Regioisomers are denoted as either 5-, 12-, 8-, or 15-series compounds, depending on the carbon atom to which the side-chain hydroxyl is attached (17). In support of the proposed mechanism of formation, we have obtained direct evidence both in vitro and in vivo utilizing various mass spectrometric methods that each of the four classes of regioisomers are formed (18). An alternative pathway for isoprostane formation has been proposed by FitzGerald and colleagues involving a dioxetane–endoperoxide mechanism that would lead to the formation of the same regioisomers as the endoperoxide pathway (9). The extent to which this latter mechanism is responsible for formation of IsoPs in vivo is unknown.

In addition to IsoPs containing F-type prostane rings, IsoP bicycloendoperoxide intermediates can also undergo rearrangement to D_2 or E_2-IsoPs containing ring structures analogous to PGD_2 and PGE_2, and to thromboxane-like compounds termed isothromboxanes. A further discussion of these compounds is outside the scope of this chapter and the reader is referred to the references cited for further information (19,20).

Two structural aspects of the F_2-IsoPs should be noted in comparison with cyclooxygenase-derived PGs. Because F-ring compounds derive from the reduction of endoperoxide intermediates, the hydroxyls on the prostane ring must be oriented *cis*, although they can be α,α or β,β (6,13). In addition, unlike cyclooxygenase-derived PGs, nonenzymatic generation of the IsoPs favors compounds in which the side chains are predominantly oriented *cis* in relation to the prostane ring.

IV. FORMATION OF ISOPROSTANES IN VIVO

We initially discovered IsoPs as products of the oxidation of plasma arachidonic acid that had been stored at $-20°C$ (6). Because these compounds are readily formed in vitro, we sought to determine whether they might also be generated in vivo. Several observations suggested that this would be true. First, we were able to detect measurable quantities of F_2-IsoPs in fresh human plasma from normal volunteers analyzed immediately at levels of 35 ± 6 pg/mL ($n = 12$) (16,21). However, as large quantities of IsoPs can be generated ex vivo, we were concerned whether these amounts represented true endogenous levels or whether they were formed ex vivo

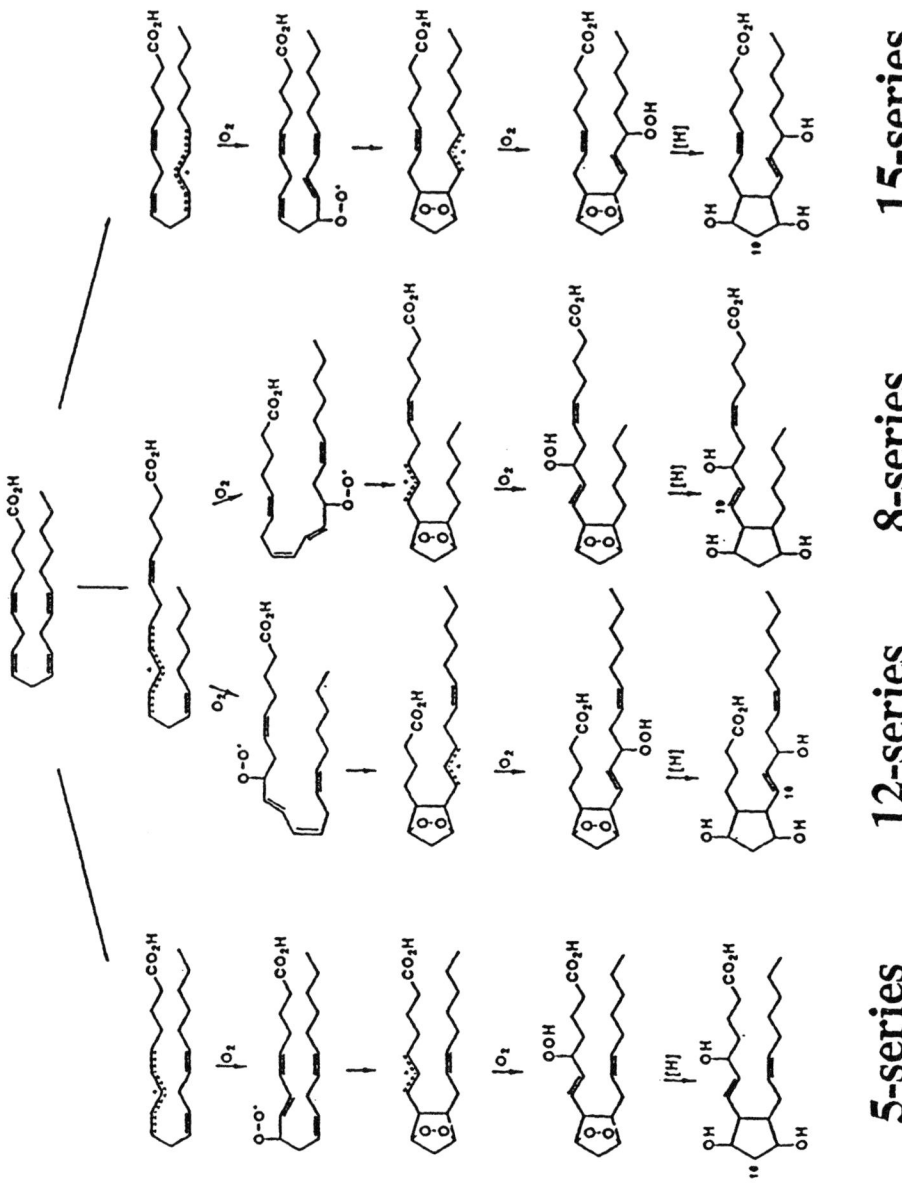

Figure 2 Mechanism of formation of the F_2-IsoPs: This pathway leads to the formation of four regioisomers. For simplicity, stereochemical orientation is not indicated. Each regioisomer theoretically comprises a mixture of eight racemic diastereomers. (From Ref. 6.)

by autoxidation of plasma lipids. This latter possibility seemed unlikely for several reasons. First, plasma contains significant quantities of antioxidants, and it has been reported that lipid peroxidation is inhibited until endogenous ascorbate is nearly entirely consumed (22,23). Second, drawing blood into syringes containing the antioxidant butylated hydroxytoluene (BHT) or the reducing agent triphenylphosphine, failed to reduce levels (16,24). Third, levels of F_2-IsoPs in urine from normal human volunteers were high (1.6 ± 0.6 ng/mg creatinine) (24). Urine contains only minute amounts of arachidonate and thus it was unlikely that such substantial levels of these compounds would be generated ex vivo. Further support for this was the finding that urinary IsoP levels did not increase when urine was incubated at 37°C for up to 5 days (16,24). Definitive evidence that IsoPs are formed in vivo was demonstrated by showing that levels of compounds detected in the plasma of rats treated with either CCl_4 or the herbicide diquat to induce an oxidant injury were increased up to 200 times the levels measured in untreated rats (16,25).

A second aspect related to the formation of isoprostanes is that they are formed in situ esterified to phospholipids in vivo. Only trivial amounts of arachidonic acid are present in the unesterified state and the vast majority is esterified to phospholipids (26). Thus, we examined whether F_2-IsoPs are initially formed esterified to phospholipids and are subsequently released in the free form by phospholipases. This was important because it counters the accepted dogma that prostanoids do not exist esterified in phospholipids. Thus, to determine this, we examined the time course for appearance of increases in levels of F_2-IsoPs esterified in liver phospholipids and free in the circulation following administration of CCl_4 to rats to induce an oxidant injury (25). Levels of esterified IsoPs increased rapidly, reaching half maximum concentrations in the liver within 15 min, whereas the appearance of increases in the circulation was delayed significantly up to several hours (25). Direct evidence for the formation of F_2-IsoPs esterified to phospholipids was obtained when a lipid extract of liver tissue from rats treated with CCl_4 was subjected to high-performance liquid chromatographic (HPLC) purification using a straight phase system that separates phosphatidylcholine from less polar lipids (26). Fractions collected were then subjected to chemical hydrolysis and analyzed for free F_2-IsoPs to detect those that contained esterified F_2-IsoPs; Fractions containing presumed esterified F_2-IsoPs eluted in a region that was more polar than unoxidized phosphatidylcholine (26). Analysis of these fractions by fast atom bombardment MS definitely identified phosphatidylcholine species with palmitate or stearate esterified at the sn-1 position and an F_2-IsoP at the sn-2 position. More detailed analyses of phospholipid-containing F_2-IsoPs have since been carried out utilizing collision-induced dissociation tandem MS (27).

After the administration of CCl_4 to rats, increased concentrations of F_2-IsoPs esterified in liver tissue can be detected, followed by increased levels in the circulation (25). This suggests that free compounds derive, at least in part, from the hydrolysis of IsoPs from phospholipids in vivo. It is reasonable to assume that the hydrolysis is catalyzed by phospholipases. In vitro, bee (Apis mellifera) venom phospholipase A_2 efficiently hydrolyzes IsoPs from lipids (26), although the phospholipase(s) responsible for the hydrolysis of IsoPs in vivo remains to be firmly established.

After determining that IsoPs are initially formed by peroxidation of arachidonic acid esterified to tissue lipids, we have analyzed a variety of normal rodent tissues for levels of esterified F_2-IsoPs, including liver, testes, heart, brain, skeletal muscle, kidney, and lung, and found detectable levels in all of these tissues (Table 1). Analysis of human tissues has been limited to gastric biopsies and arteries, where levels of F_2-IsoPs in the nanogram per gram tissue are present (Table 2). In addition, F_2-IsoPs are detectable in human cerebrospinal fluid at picogram per milliliter concentrations and are significantly increased in patients with Alzheimer's disease,

Table 1 Basal Levels of F_2-Isoprostanes in Body Fluids or Tissues from Various Animal Species

Body fluid or tissue	Animal species	Level (mean ± 1 s.d.)
Plasma (free)	Rat	22 ± pg/mL
Plasma (esterified)	Rat	168 ± 41 pg/mL
Urine	Rat	2.6 ± 1.4 ng/mg creatinine
Bile	Rat	0.77 ± 0.36 ng/kg min^{-1}
Liver tissue	Rat	6.1 ± 0.7 ng/g
Kidney	Rat	1.2 ± 0.4 ng/g
Lung	Rat	0.7 ± 0.2 ng/g
Skeletal muscle	Rat	0.5 ± 0.2 ng/g
Heart	Rat	2.5 ± 0.5 ng/g
Brain	Rat	1.0 ± 0.1 ng/g
Brain	Mouse (3 months old)	1.0 ± 0.2 ng/g
Brain	Mouse (12 months old)	1.7 ± 0.2 ng/g
Testes	Mouse	0.9 ± 0.1 ng/g
Thymus	Mouse	3.7 ± 0.4 ng/g

Source: Refs. 25, 46, 80, and unpublished data.

a chronic neurodegenerative disorder associated with increased oxidant stress in the central nervous system (28). Interestingly, increases in cerebrospinal fluid IsoPs correlate with increases in cortical atrophy and decreases in brain weight, two sensitive indices of Alzheimer's disease severity. These findings, taken together, are consistent with the fact that detectable levels of unesterified F_2-IsoPs are present in all normal biological fluids from both animals and humans that have been tested to date.

V. RELEVANCE OF THE DISCOVERY OF ISOPROSTANES

A. Analytical Ramifications

The discovery of IsoPs is important for several reasons. First, that they can be generated in biological fluids in vitro has potentially important analytical ramifications for the analysis of

Table 2 Basal Levels of F_2-Isoprostanes in Various Body Fluids and Tissues from Normal Humans

Body fluid or tissue	Level (mean ± 1 s.d.)
Plasma (free)	35 ± 6 pg/mL
Plasma (esterified)	119 ± 22 pg/mL
Urine	1.6 ± 0.6 ng/mg creatinine
Cerebrospinal fluid	23 ± 1.0 pg/mL
Lateral ventricular fluid	46 ± 4 pg/mL
Gastric biopsy	4.3 ± 1.4 ng/g
Human umbilical vein	1.4 ± 0.7 ng/g

Source: Refs. 16, 21, 24, 28, 64, 78, and unpublished data.

prostanoids (6). This applies to both physical and immunological methods of analysis. Precautions, such as storage of fluids at $-70°C$ or addition of antioxidants to extraction solutions, must be taken to avoid generation of IsoPs in lipid-containing biological fluids before analysis (24,29). F_2-IsoPs have chromatographic properties on TLC, HPLC, and GC similar to those of $PGF_{2\alpha}$, and thus can confound an interpretation of whether a PGF_2 compound measured by physical methods (e.g., GC–MS) is enzymatically or nonenzymatically generated (6). Furthermore, antibodies used in immunoassays for cyclooxygenase-derived PGF_2 compounds can cross-react with F_2-IsoPs. For example, an antibody obtained commercially (Amersham Life Science) to the PGD_2 metabolite, $9\alpha,11\beta$-PGF_2, exhibits significant cross-reactivity with the complex mixture of F_2-IsoPs, even though the prostane ring hydroxyls in F_2-IsoPs are predominantly oriented in a *cis* configuration (6).

B. The Isoprostanes as an Index of Endogenous Lipid Peroxidation

A second important aspect of the discovery of IsoPs relates to the use of measurement of IsoPs as an index of lipid peroxidation or oxidant stress in vivo. One of the greatest needs in the field of free radical research is the availability of a reliable noninvasive method to assess oxidative stress status in vivo in humans. This is because most techniques available to assess oxidant stress in vivo have suffered from a lack of specificity or sensitivity, or are unreliable (5). However, evidence has been obtained that indicates measurement of IsoPs in urine or plasma provides a reliable noninvasive approach to assess lipid peroxidation in vivo and, thus, a major advance in our ability to assess oxidative stress status in humans. Furthermore, the sensitivity of the mass spectrometric method of analysis appears sufficient to quantify levels of F_2-IsoPs in small biopsies of human tissue, which should permit an assessment of oxidant injury in key tissues of interest.

The ability to quantify F_2-IsoPs, therefore, will potentially permit exploration of the role of free radicals in the pathophysiology of a wide range of human diseases. It also provides a valuable tool to define the clinical pharmacology of antioxidant agents. There are trials either planned or underway examining the effect of antioxidants, such as vitamin C or vitamin E, to prevent or ameliorate some of the pathology of diseases in which free radicals have been implicated. However, such studies are hampered by insufficient information on what doses and combinations of antioxidants are maximally effective. Measurement of IsoPs should provide a valuable approach to define the clinical pharmacology of antioxidants. We have previously shown that the formation of F_2-IsoPs increases significantly in animals deficient in vitamin E or selenium (16,30). In addition, administration of antioxidants inhibits the formation of IsoPs in animal models of oxidant injury (31). More recently, we have found that the administration of a combination of antioxidants at high doses (4 g/day of vitamin C, 3200 IU/day of vitamin E, and 300 mg/day of β-carotene) to normal volunteers for a period of 2 weeks inhibited the formation of F_2-IsoPs esterified to plasma lipids by a mean 37% (32). In addition, we assessed the effect of administration of 200 mg of d-α-tocopherol alone, 500 mg of vitamin C alone, and the two agents in combination, in a cohort of 100 men enrolled in the "Antioxidant Supplementation in Atherosclerosis Prevention" trial (32). After 1 year of treatment, plasma concentrations of F_2-IsoPs were measured to determine the effect of treatment regimens on endogenous lipid peroxidation. Vitamin E administration significantly reduced plasma concentrations of F_2-IsoPs by 20–30% ($p = 0.003$). Vitamin C supplementation alone had no effect. In addition, in the group of men administered both agents, levels of F_2-IsoPs were not suppressed further with the addition of vitamin C to vitamin E and, in fact, vitamin C appeared to diminish the IsoP decrease observed with vitamin E alone. The reasons for this latter observation are unclear. Nonetheless, these data suggest that measurement of IsoPs can be used to quantitatively define the effects of antioxidants to inhibit free radical processes in vivo in humans.

Levels of IsoPs in normal human plasma and urine exceed levels of cyclooxygenase-derived PGs and thromboxane by at least an order of magnitude, suggesting that the formation of IsoPs is a major pathway of arachidonic acid disposition (16). Additionally, it is important to consider the relevance of the finding that levels of F_2-IsoPs are sufficient to be detected in every normal biological fluid and tissue that has been assayed. Previously, using other methods to assess lipid peroxidation, there had been little definitive evidence indicating lipid peroxidation occurs in vivo except under abnormal circumstances of marked oxidative stress. However, the finding of detectable levels of F_2-IsoPs in all normal animal and human biological fluids and esterified in normal animal tissues indicates that there is ongoing lipid peroxidation that is incompletely suppressed by antioxidant defenses, even in normal individuals. This finding may lend support to the hypothesis that the normal-aging process is due to enhanced oxidant damage of important biological molecules over time (4). It has been reported that there is a trend for the formation of F_2-IsoPs to increase with age in humans (33), although a more recent study refutes this (34).

VI. METHOD OF ANALYSIS OF THE ISOPROSTANES

The method that we have used for measurement of F_2-IsoPs is a GC–negative-ion chemical ionization MS assay (16,24,29). It is highly sensitive with a lower limit of detection in the low picogram range. Moreover, it is highly accurate (precision = ±6%; accuracy = 96%). Previously we have used either $[^2H_7]9\alpha,11\beta$-PGF_2 synthesized in our laboratory or commercially available $[^2H_4]PGF_{2\alpha}$ as an internal standard, but recently $[^2H_4]$8-iso-$PGF_{2\alpha}$ (15-F_{2t}-IsoP), one of the more abundant F_2-IsoPs produced in vivo (35), has become available commercially. Measurement of esterified levels of F_2-IsoPs in tissues is accompanied by measurement of free compounds following alkaline hydrolysis of a lipid extract of tissue (29). IsoPs are analyzed following conversion to pentafluorobenzyl ester trimethylsilylether derivatives. For quantification purposes, we quantify the starred (*) peak shown in the m/z 569 chromatogram in Figure 1. We have previously shown that one IsoP, 8-iso-$PGF_{2\alpha}$, (15-F_{2t}-IsoP) constitutes a significant proportion of the F_2-IsoPs represented by this chromatographic peak (35). The reader is referred the cited reference for a further detailed discussion of methods to measure the F_2-IsoPs (29).

Other investigators, including FitzGerald and colleagues, have developed similar GC–MS methods for the analysis of IsoPs (9,36). In addition, it is likely that sensitive electrospray ionization MS approaches will become available in the future for the analysis of IsoPs (9). The potential attractiveness of this latter approach may be that compound derivatization will be rendered unnecessary.

Although highly accurate, the mass spectrometric method of assay is labor-intensive, and the technology is not widely available. However, both commercial enterprises and academic investigators have developed immunoassays for specific F_2-IsoPs (37), which should expand research in this area. Currently, at least three immunoassay kits are commercially available. One potential drawback of these immunoassay methods, however, is that they appear to require significant sample processing (such as Sep-Pak purification) before sample analysis for accurate quantification of IsoPs. Furthermore, there is limited information on direct quantitative comparisons of these immunoassays with mass spectrometry.

VII. QUANTIFICATION OF ISOPROSTANES AS AN INDEX OF OXIDANT STRESS

A. In Vitro Studies

Several studies have been carried out involving the quantification of F_2-IsoPs in in vitro systems of lipid peroxidation, and F_2-IsoP formation has been compared with other markers of lipid peroxidation. This work has demonstrated the usefulness of measuring these compounds as a reliable index of lipid peroxidation in vitro and has provided a scientific basis to explore their role as markers of oxidant stress in vivo. Some of these in vitro studies are briefly summarized in the following.

The formation of F_2-IsoP has been compared with malondialdehyde (MDA) in Fe/ADP/ascorbate-induced peroxidation of rat liver microsomes (38). MDA is one of the most commonly used measures of lipid peroxidation and was quantified in these studies by measuring thiobarbituric acid-reacting substances. Both F_2-IsoP and MDA formation increased in parallel in a time-dependent manner and correlated with the loss of arachidonic acid and with increasing oxygen concentrations up to 21%. Although the formation of F_2-IsoP correlated with other measures of lipid peroxidation in this in vitro model, as discussed below, measurement of F_2-IsoPs is superior to measurements of MDA as an index of lipid peroxidation in vivo.

We and others have carried out studies examining the formation of F_2-IsoP in low-density lipoproteins (LDL) exposed to various oxidizing conditions in vitro. Much of the interest in examining this stems from the hypothesis that oxidization of LDL in vivo converts it to an atherogenic form that is taken up by macrophages in the vessel wall. Subsequent activation of these cells may play an important role in the development and progression of atherosclerotic lesions in humans (39). Thus, we have performed studies examining the formation of F_2-IsoP in LDL that is oxidized to determine whether measurement of F_2-IsoP esterified to lipoproteins may provide an approach to assess lipoprotein oxidation in vivo (22). These studies are also of interest because one F_2-IsoP, 15-F_{2t}-IsoP (8-iso-$PGF_{2\alpha}$) is a vasoconstrictor and induces mitogenesis in vascular smooth-muscle cells (16); these effects may be of relevance to the pathophysiology associated with atherosclerosis. In these studies, either plasma lipids or purified LDL from humans was peroxidized with Cu^{2+} or the water-soluble oxidizing agent 2,2-azobis(2-amidinopropane) (AAPH) (22). The formation of F_2-IsoPs was compared with other markers of lipid peroxidation, including formation of cholesterol ester hydroperoxides, phospholipid hydroperoxides, loss of antioxidants, and changes in the electrophoretic mobility of LDL. In plasma oxidized with AAPH, increases in the formation of F_2-IsoP paralleled increases in lipid hydroperoxide formation and occurred only after depletion of the antioxidants ascorbate and ubiquinol-10. In purified LDL that was oxidized, formation of F_2-IsoP again correlated with increases in lipid hydroperoxides and increases in the electrophoretic mobility of LDL. Additionally, increased F_2-IsoP formation occurred only after depletion of the antioxidants α-tocopherol and ubiquinol-10. Similar findings have been reported by Gopual and colleagues (40) when LDL is oxidized in the presence of endothelial cells or Cu^{2+}. FitzGerald and colleagues (41) have reported large increases in F_2-IsoPs in LDL oxidized in vitro in the presence of macrophages stimulated with zymosan. This enhanced formation of IsoPs may be due to activation of superoxide production.

There has been significant interest in the role that the macrophage 15-lipoxygenase enzyme might play in the oxidation of lipoproteins in the vascular wall and the relation to atherosclerosis (42). In support of a role for this enzyme in the oxidation of LDL in vivo, 15-F_{2t}-IsoP formation in LDL incubated with stimulated macrophages, isolated from mice genetically engineered with a targeted disruption of the 15-lipoxygenase gene, was significantly less than when LDL was incubated with macrophages isolated from control animals (43).

There has also been interest in the potential role of the oxidant peroxynitrite in LDL oxidation. Peroxynitrite is the coupling product of nitric oxide and superoxide. We examined the formation of F_2-IsoPs in LDL exposed to peroxynitrite and found that peroxynitrite catalyzed the formation of F_2-IsoPs in a concentration-dependent fashion that correlated with increases in the electrophoretic mobility of LDL (44).

Taken together, these studies suggest that quantification of F_2-IsoP esterified to lipoproteins may provide a useful approach to assessing oxidation of LDL in vivo.

B. F_2-Isoprostane Quantification in Animal Models of Oxidant Stress

Evidence that measurement of IsoPs provides a valuable approach to assess oxidative stress status in vivo emerged from early studies that we carried out related to the discovery of these compounds (16,25). Importantly, we have detected measurable levels of IsoPs in virtually every animal and human biological fluid and tissue that has been analyzed. This allows the definition of a normal range, and even small increases in IsoP formation can be accurately quantified (7). Furthermore, overproduction of IsoPs has been well documented to occur in settings of oxidant injury. Initial work in vivo with the IsoPs employed two models of liver injury in rats in which lipid peroxidation had been implicated as an important factor: (1) administration of CCl_4 to normal rats and (2) administration of diquat to selenium (Se)-deficient rats.

1. CCl_4-Induced Lipid Peroxidation

Administration of hepatotoxic doses of CCl_4 to rats caused hepatic lipid-esterified IsoPs to increase 200-fold within 1 h, with a subsequent decline over 24 h (25,45). Plasma-free and lipid-esterified IsoP concentrations increased after liver levels and peaked at 4–8 h after CCl_4 administration (25). Elevated IsoP levels were also documented in the bile (46). Increased formation of F_2-IsoPs is proportional to the CCl_4 dose administered (45). Moreover, animals administered agents such as isoniazid or phenobarbital, which induce hepatic cytochrome P-450 enzymes and increase CCl_4 metabolism, have IsoP levels higher than animals administered only CCl_4 (25). In addition, depletion of endogenous glutathione stores markedly increases F_2-IsoP levels after the administration of CCl_4 (25). On the other hand, circulating and tissue levels of F_2-IsoP can be decreased compared with those of animals administered CCl_4 alone by pretreatment of rats with the antioxidant lazaroid U-78517 or cytochrome P-450 inhibitors such as 4-methylpyrazole or proadifenhydrochloride (SK&F-525-A) (25,31).

Studies carried out with CCl_4 to induce oxidant injury in the rat have also illustrated that quantification of F_2-IsoP provides a much more sensitive and accurate method to assess lipid peroxidation in vivo compared with other markers. As an example, following administration of CCl_4 to rats, levels of F_2-IsoPs esterified to lipids increased more than 80-fold, whereas levels of MDA in the liver increased only 2.7-fold (38). In another study, measurement F_2-IsoP afforded a more sensitive indicator of CCl_4-induced lipid peroxidation compared with measurement of lipid hydroperoxides by mass spectrometry (31).

2. Diquat-Induced Hepatic and Renal Toxicity

Diquat is a dipyridyl herbicide that undergoes redox cycling in vivo generating large amounts of the superoxide anion. This compound causes hepatic and renal injury in rats, an effect that is markedly augmented in animals deficient in Se, a trace element that is required for the enzymatic activities of glutathione peroxidase and other antioxidant proteins (47). Previous studies have suggested that lipid peroxidation might be involved in the tissue damage associated with this agent. To study whether F_2-IsoPs were generated in increased amounts in association with diquat administration to Se-deficient animals, levels of F_2-IsoPs were quantified in plasma and tissues from Se-deficient rats following diquat administration. Se-deficient rats administered diquat showed 10- to 200-fold increases in plasma F_2-IsoPs, and the sources of the IsoPs were determined to be primarily the kidney and liver (45). Additional studies have also shown that GSH depletion increases IsoP levels significantly after the administration of diquat to rats (48).

3. Nutritional Antioxidant Deficiency

We have carried out numerous studies examining the role of the antioxidant micronutrients vitamin E and Se in IsoP formation. Rats raised on a diet deficient in both Se and vitamin E from weaning begin to lose weight and can die of massive hepatic necrosis (49). In vitro studies demonstrating that vitamin E blocks propagation of lipid peroxidation, suggested that uncontrolled lipid peroxidation might be responsible for the liver injury seen in vitamin E–Se-deficient animals, although clearcut data supporting this hypothesis were scant (50). In an effort to examine the role of oxidant injury in combined vitamin E–Se deficiency, we quantified F_2-IsoP in plasma and tissues of deficient rats without any exogenous oxidant stress.

Interestingly, plasma F_2-IsoPs in rats raised on a doubly deficient diet were sixfold higher than in rats raised on a control diet (30). In addition, there were significant increases in phospholipid esterified F_2-IsoP levels in the tissues of deficient animals, including the liver, lung, kidney, heart, and skeletal muscle. These data support the contention that lipid peroxidation is increased in animals deficient in both vitamin E and selenium (45).

In additional studies, we have also found markedly increased baseline levels of isoprostanes both in plasma and tissues of animals deficient in vitamin E alone (30). On the other hand, animals deficient in Se alone do not have significantly increased F_2-IsoP levels in tissues or plasma when compared with Se-replete animals unless they are exposed to an oxidant stress (30).

4. F_2-Isoprostane Levels in Other Animal Models of Oxidant Injury

A role for free radicals and lipid peroxidation in alcoholic liver damage has been controversial for many years. Previously, Nanji and colleagues reported increased plasma and lipid isoprostanes in rats fed ethanol continuously (51). In a separate study, cimetidine given to rats to inhibit ethanol metabolism prevented the increase in F_2-IsoP formation and also prevented ethanol-induced liver injury (52).

In rats rendered Cu-deficient by reduction of dietary Cu, Cu/Zn superoxide dismutase (SOD) activity is markedly reduced. In these animals, we found significantly increased levels of F_2-IsoPs esterified in plasma lipoproteins (mean 2.5-fold increased) compared with normal control animals (53). In addition, there was a strong correlation between increased IsoP levels and vascular dysfunction. These data suggest a role for superoxide and its coupling product formed with nitric oxide, peroxynitrite, in lipoprotein oxidation and vascular function in vivo. More recently, we have also found a marked decrease in urinary F_2-IsoP levels in rats with a targeted deletion of the gene encoding inducible nitric oxide synthase (JD Morrow, unpublished data).

Organophosphate poisoning is associated with muscle endplate necrosis, and increased levels of IsoPs esterified to muscle tissue have been demonstrated in animals poisoned with organophosphates (54). Administration of a lazaroid antioxidant suppressed both levels of IsoPs and protected against organophosphate-induced muscle necrosis, suggesting that free radicals are involved in the pathological changes that occur in the muscle in association with organophosphate poisoning.

Increased formation of IsoPs has also been demonstrated in settings of ischemia–reperfusion injury to both the liver and kidney (55). Dietary iron overload is associated with increased levels of F_2-IsoPs esterified to lipids in the livers of rats (56). The anesthetic halothane can induce liver injury, especially under hypoxic conditions, which is thought to involve the production of free radicals by the reductive metabolism of halothane (57). We have demonstrated that in rats given halothane, even under normoxic conditions, increased levels of F_2-IsoPs are present esterified to hepatic lipids, indicative of free radical-induced peroxidation of hepatic lipids (58).

C. Quantification of F_2-Isoprostanes to Assess the Role of Oxidant Injury in Human Diseases

From the foregoing examples, measurement of IsoPs appears to be a reliable index of lipid peroxidation in vivo and thus potentially provides us with a tool to assess the role of free radicals in the pathophysiology of human disease. We and others have carried out numerous studies examining the role of oxidant stress in human diseases. Elevations in IsoPs in human body fluids and tissues are present in several disorders, including the hepatorenal renal syndrome (59), scleroderma (60), Alzheimer's disease (28), rhabdomyolysis (61), and various pulmonary disorders (9,62). Recently, FitzGerald and colleagues reported that humans with alcoholic hepatitis have excessive IsoP formation in vivo (63). On the other hand, IsoPs are not increased in neurodegenerative disorders, such as amyotrophic lateral sclerosis or unstable coronary syndromes (64,65). Additionally, dietary fat intake, at least in the short-term, does not appear to influence IsoP formation (16,66). The reader is referred to the cited references for further discussions of IsoP formation in these situations.

As noted, over the past decade, there has been considerable interest in the role that oxidation of LDL plays in the development and progression of atherosclerosis in humans (39). We and others have previously reported that oxidation of LDL in vitro results in the formation of significant increases in IsoP formation (23,41). It has been reported that ApoE-deficient mice, which develop atherosclerosis, levels of IsoPs in plasma and atherosclerotic vascular tissue are increased compared with control mice and can be suppressed with vitamin E (67). These data suggest that IsoPs may be a useful marker of atherosclerotic risk in humans. Recently, we and others have sought to determine whether this is so. The following studies outline research that has been carried out examining the formation of IsoPs in humans with various risk factors for atherosclerosis and provide an example of how measurement of IsoPs has provided insight into the association of oxidant stress and IsoP formation with human disease.

1. Isoprostane Formation in Long-Term Smokers

A link between cigarette smoking and risk of cardiovascular disease is well established (68). However, the underlying mechanism(s) for this effect is not fully understood. The gaseous phase of cigarette smoke contains several oxidants, and exposure of LDL to the gaseous phase of cigarette smoke in vitro induces oxidation of the LDL lipids (69). Thus, we explored the hypothesis that smoking induces an oxidative stress, and we specifically determined whether lipoproteins in individuals who smoke contain higher levels of F_2-IsoPs, indicative of a greater degree of oxidative modification. Ten individuals who smoked heavily (more than 30 cigarettes per day) and ten age- and sex-matched nonsmoking normal volunteers were studied (70). Plasma concentrations of free and esterified F_2-IsoPs were significantly elevated in the smokers compared with the nonsmokers ($p = 0.02$ and $p = 0.03$, respectively). Confirmation that these differences in levels of F_2-IsoPs between smokers and nonsmokers were due to cigarette smoking was obtained by measuring levels of F_2-IsoPs following 2 weeks of abstinence from smoking in eight of the ten smokers who successfully abstained. In all subjects, levels of F_2-IsoPs both free in the circulation and esterified to plasma lipoproteins were significantly lower following 2 weeks of abstinence from smoking ($p = 0.03$ and $p = 0.02$, respectively). The occurrence of enhanced formation of IsoPs in smokers has also been subsequently confirmed in studies by FitzGerald and others (71). Collectively, these findings suggest strongly that smoking causes an oxidative stress, and the observation that smokers have elevated levels of F_2-IsoPs esterified in plasma lipids also supports the hypothesis that the link between smoking and risk of cardiovascular disease may be attributed to enhanced oxidation of LDL.

2. Isoprostanes in Patients with Polygenic Hypercholesterolemia

Patients with hypercholesterolemia have an increased risk for the development of atherosclerosis. Thus, it was of interest to determine whether levels of F_2-IsoPs are increased in patients with hypercholesterolemia.

Levels of F_2-IsoPs esterified in plasma lipids were determined in seven patients with polygenic hypercholesterolemia (32). Levels in patients with hypercholesterolemia were significantly increased a mean of 3.4-fold (range 1.7–7.5-fold) above levels measured in normal controls ($p < 0.001$). Interestingly, in these patients, there was no correlation between levels of F_2-IsoPs and serum cholesterol, triglycerides, or LDL–cholesterol. In addition, plasma arachidonic acid content was measured in three of these patients and six normal controls. Again, no correlation between IsoP and arachidonate levels was found. Thus, these data suggest that the finding of high levels of F_2-IsoPs in patients with hypercholesterolemia is not due simply to the presence of more lipid (i.e., arachidonic acid substrate). Rather, it is suggested that hypercholesterolemia is associated with enhanced oxidative stress. The underlying basis for this observation, however, remains unclear. Interestingly, a recent report also found that the urinary excretion of F_2-IsoPs was increased in patients with type II hypercholesterolemia by a mean of 2.5-fold, which was suppressed by approximately 60% with vitamin E treatment (600 mg/day) (72). A third study has also documented increases in F_2-IsoP formation in diabetics (73). In this latter report, however, increases in IsoP levels correlated with increased LDL cholesterol levels.

3. Isoprostanes in Patients with Diabetes

Patients with diabetes have an increased incidence of atherosclerotic vascular disease. Interestingly, the formation of F_2-IsoPs is induced in vascular smooth muscle cells in vitro by elevated glucose concentrations (74). Thus, we explored whether there was evidence for enhanced oxidative stress in vivo in patients with diabetes (75). In this study, levels of F_2-IsoPs esterified in plasma lipids were quantified in 61 patients who underwent coronary angiography. There were 15 patients with diabetes in this group. The extent of coronary atherosclerosis in the diabetic patients was similar to that in the 46 nondiabetic individuals. Plasma esterified levels of F_2-IsoPs measured in the diabetic patients (33.4 ± 4.8 pg/mL, mean $\pm$ SEM) were significantly increased compared with levels measured in the nondiabetic patients (22.2 ± 1.9 pg/mL) ($p < 0.02$). Similar findings have also been reported by Gopaul et al. in which they found a mean 3.3-fold increase in free F_2-IsoP concentrations in plasma of diabetic patients, compared with nondiabetic healthy control subjects (76). In addition, it has been reported that urinary IsoP levels in diabetics are suppressed by vitamin E and by control of hyperglycemia (9).

4. Correlation Between Plasma Concentrations of Homocysteine and Isoprostanes

High plasma levels of homocysteine are an independent risk factor for cardiovascular disease (77). The mechanism by which hyperhomocysteinemia induces atherosclerosis is not fully understood, but promotion of LDL oxidation has been suggested. The relation between total plasma concentrations of homocysteine and F_2-IsoPs in 100 Finnish male participants in the "Antioxidant Supplementation in Atherosclerosis Prevention" study was recently explored (32). The mean plasma total homocysteine and F_2-IsoP concentrations were 11.1 μmol/L and 29.6 ng/L, respectively. The simple correlation coefficient for association between plasma concentrations of homocysteine and F_2-IsoPs was 0.40 ($p < 0.0001$). Plasma concentrations of F_2-IsoPs increased linearly across quintiles of homocysteine levels. The finding of a positive correlation between plasma concentrations of F_2-IsoPs and homocysteine supports the suggestion that the mechanism underlying the link between high homocysteine levels and risk for cardiovascular disease may be attributed to enhanced lipid peroxidation.

5. Isoprostanes in Human Atherosclerotic Plaques

In accordance with the LDL oxidation hypothesis of atherosclerosis, levels of F_2-IsoPs should be higher in atherosclerotic plaques than in normal vascular tissue. To address this issue, levels of F_2-IsoPs were measured in fresh advanced atherosclerotic plaque tissue removed during arterial thrombarterectomy ($n = 10$) and compared with levels measured in normal human umbilical veins removed from the placenta immediately after delivery ($n = 10$) (78). Levels of F_2-IsoPs esterified in vascular tissue normalized to both wet weight and dry weight were significantly higher in atherosclerotic plaques compared with normal vascular tissue. A better measure of the actual extent of oxidation, however, would be obtained by normalizing the data to the amount of arachidonic acid present in the tissue because it is the substrate for IsoP formation. When the data was normalized to arachidonic acid content, the F_2-IsoP/arachidonic acid ratio was about fourfold higher than the ratio in normal vascular tissue ($p = 0.009$). This finding indicates that unsaturated fatty acids in atherosclerotic plaques are more extensively oxidized than lipids in normal vascular tissue. These observations are also in accord with data from FitzGerald and colleagues, who have shown increased amounts of F_2-IsoPs in human atherosclerotic lesions including the localization of F_2-IsoPs in atherosclerotic plaque tissue to foam cells and vascular smooth-muscle cells (79).

VIII. SUMMARY

The quantification of IsoPs appears to be an important advance in our ability to explore the role of oxidative stress in human physiology and pathophysiology. Increases in IsoP formation can be documented in many situations associated with enhanced oxidant stress both in vitro and in vivo. These include several human disorders, including atherosclerosis which is the most common cause of mortality in the Western world. Thus, studies delineating the role of oxidant injury in the pathophysiology of atherosclerosis may have important implications for the treatment of this disorder and other diseases associated with oxidant injury.

Currently, the IsoPs are most accurately quantified by mass spectrometric approaches. Despite the usefulness of these methods, mass spectrometry is unavailable to a large number of investigators. The development of immunoassay methods, if proved reliable, will one hopes allow a larger group of researchers to utilize IsoPs to assess oxidant stress.

In summary, considerable information has been obtained on the usefulness of quantifying IsoPs as an accurate index of oxidant injury since the initial report of their discovery. With continued research in this area, we believe that much new information will emerge that will open up additional important new areas for future investigation.

ACKNOWLEDGMENTS

Supported by NIH grants DK 48831, GM42056, GM15431, CA77839, Dk26657, and CA68485. JDM is the recipient of a Burroughs Wellcome Fund Clinical Scientist Award in Translational Research.

REFERENCES

1. Halliwell B, Gutteridge JMC. Role of free radicals and catalytic metal ions in human disease. Methods Enzymol 1990; 186:1–85.
2. Southorn PA, Powis G. Free radicals in medicine. II. Involvement in human disease. Mayo Clin Proc 1988; 63:390–408.
3. Ames BN. Dietary carcinogens and anticarcinogens. Science 1983; 221:1256–1264.
4. Harman D. The aging process. Proc Natl Acad Sci USA 1981; 78:7124–7128.
5. Halliwell B, Grootveld M. The measurement of free radical reactions. FEBS Lett 1987; 213:9–14.
6. Morrow JD, Harris TM, Roberts LJ. Noncyclooxygenase oxidative formation of a series of novel prostaglandins: analytical ramifications for the measurement of eicosanoids. Anal Biochem 1990; 184:1–10.
7. Morrow JD, Roberts LJ. The isoprostanes: unique bioactive products of lipid peroxidation. Prog Lipid Res 1997; 36:1–21.
8. Morrow JD, Chen Y, Brame CJ, Yang J, Sanchez SC, Xu J, Zackert WE, Awad JA, Roberts LJ. The isoprostanes: unique prostaglandin-like products of free radical-initiated lipid peroxidation. Drug Metab Rev 1999; 31:117–139.
9. Lawson JA, Rokach J, Fitzgerald GA. Isoprostanes: formation, analysis and use as indices of lipid peroxidation in vivo. J Biol Chem 1999; 274:24441–24444.
10. Nugteren DH, Vonkeman H, Van Dorp DA. Non-enzymic conversion of all cis-8,11,14-eicosatrienoic acid into prostaglandin E_1. Recl Trav Chim Pays-Bas 1967; 86:1237–1245.
11. Pryor WA, Stanley JP, Blair E. Autoxidation of polyunsaturated fatty acids: II. A suggested mechanism for the formation of TBA-reactive materials from prostaglandin-like endoperoxides. Lipids 1975; 30:370–379.
12. Porter NA, Funk MO. Peroxy radical cyclization as a model for prostaglandin biosynthesis. J Org Chem 1975; 40:3614–3915.
13. O'Connor DE, Mihelich ED, Coleman MC. Stereochemical course of the autoxidative cyclization of lipid hydroperoxides to prostaglandin-like bicycloendoperoxides. J Am Chem Soc 1984; 106:3577–3584.
14. Liston TE, Roberts LJ. Metabolic fate of radiolabeled prostaglandin D_2 in a normal human male volunteer. J Biol Chem 1985; 260:13172–13180.
15. Wendelborn DF, Seibert K, Roberts LJ. Isomeric prostaglandin F_2 compounds arising from prostaglandin D_2: a family of icosanoids produced in vivo in humans. Proc Natl Acad Sci USA 1988; 85:304–308.
16. Morrow JD, Hill KE, Burk RF, Nammour TM, Badr KF, Roberts LJ. A series of prostaglandin F_2-like compounds are produced in vivo in humans by a non-cyclooxygenase, free radical catalyzed mechanism. Proc Natl Acad Sci USA 1990; 87:9383–9387.
17. Taber DF, Morrow JD, Roberts LJ. A nomenclature system for the isoprostanes. Prostaglandins 1997; 53:63–67.
18. Waugh RJ, Morrow JD, Roberts LJ, Murphy RC. Identification and relative quantitation of F_2-isoprostane regioisomers formed in vivo in the rat. Free Radic Biol Med 1997; 23:943–954.
19. Morrow JD, Minton TA, Mukundan CR, Campbell MD, Zackert WE, Daniel VC, Badr KF, Blair IA, Roberts LJ. Free radical-induced generation of isoprostanes in vivo: evidence for the formation of D-ring and E-ring isoprostanes. J Biol Chem 1994; 269:4317–4326.
20. Morrow JD, Awad JA, Wu A, Zackert WE, Daniel VC, Roberts LJ. Nonenzymatic free radical-catalyzed generation of thromboxane-like compound (isothromboxanes) in vivo. J Biol Chem 1996; 271:23185–23190.
21. Morrow JD, Frei B, Longmire AW, Gaziano M, Lynch SM, Shyr Y, Strauss WE, Oates JA, Roberts LJ. Increase in circulating products of lipid peroxidation (F_2-isoprostanes) in smokers. N Engl J Med 1995; 332:1198–1203.

22. Lynch SM, Morrow JD, Roberts LJ, Frei B. Formation of non-cyclooxygenase-derived prostanoids (F_2-isoprostanes) in plasma and low density lipoprotein exposed to oxidative stress in vitro. J Clin Invest 1994; 93:998–1004.
23. Frei B, Stocker R, Ames BN. Antioxidant defenses and lipid peroxidation in human blood plasma. Proc Natl Acad Sci USA 1988; 85:9478–9752.
24. Morrow JD, Roberts LJ. Mass spectrometry of prostanoids: F_2-isoprostanes produced by non-cyclooxygenase free radical-catalyzed mechanism. Methods Enzymol 1994; 233:163–174.
25. Morrow JD, Awad JA, Kato T, Takahashi K, Badr KF, Roberts LJ, Burk RF. Formation of novel non-cyclooxygenase-derived prostanoids (F_2-isoprostanes) in carbon tetrachloride hepatotoxicity. J Clin Invest 1992; 90:2502–2507.
26. Morrow JD, Awad JA, Boss HJ, Blair IA, Roberts LJ. Noncyclooxygenase-derived prostanoids (F_2-isoprostanes) are formed in situ on phospholipids. Proc Natl Acad Sci USA 1992; 89:10721–10725.
27. Kayganich–Harrison KA, Rose DM, Murphy RC, Morrow JD, Roberts LJ. Collision-induced dissociation of F_2-isoprostane-containing phospholipids. J Lipid Res 1993; 34:1229–1235.
28. Montine TJ, Markesbery WR, Morrow JD, Roberts LJ. Cerebrospinal fluid F_2-isoprostane levels are increased in Alzheimer's disease. Ann Neurol 1998; 44:410–413.
29. Morrow JD, Roberts LJ. Mass spectrometric quantification of F_2-isoprostanes in biological fluids and tissues as measure of oxidant stress. Methods Enzymol 1999; 300:3–12.
30. Awad JA, Morrow JD, Hill KE, Roberts LJ, Burk RF. Detection and localization of lipid peroxidation in selenium- and vitamin E-deficient rats using F_2-isoprostanes. J Nutr 1994; 12:810–816.
31. Matthews WR, McKenna R, Guido DM, Petry TW, Jolly RA, Morrow JD, Roberts LJ. Formation of lipid peroxidation products (isoprostanes) in an animal model of oxidant injury. Proceeding, 41st ASMS Conference on Mass Spectrometry and Allied Topics. 1993:865a.
32. Roberts LJ, Morrow JD. Isoprostanes as markers of lipid peroxidation in atherosclerosis. In: Serhan CN, Ward PA, eds. Molecular and Cellular Basis of Inflammation. Totowa, NJ: Humana Press, 1999:141–163.
33. Pratico D, Reilly M, Lawson J, Delanty N, Fitzgerald GA. Formation of 8-iso-prostaglandin $F_{2\alpha}$ by human platelets. Agents Actions 1995; 45(suppl):27–31.
34. Feillet–Coudray C, Tourtauchaux R, Niculescu M, Rock E, Tauveron I, Alexandre–Gouabau M, Rayssiguier Y, Jalenques I, Mazur A. Plasma levels of 8-epiPGF2α, an in vivo marker of oxidative stress, are not affected by aging or Alzheimer's disease. Free Radic Biol Med 1999; 27:463–469.
35. Morrow JD, Minton TA, Badr KF, Roberts LJ. Evidence that the F_2-isoprostane, 8-epi-$PGF_{2\alpha}$, is formed in vivo. Biochim Biophys Acta 1994; 1210:244–248.
36. Mori TA, Croft KD, Puddey IB, Beilin LJ. An improved method for the measurement of urinary and plasma F_2-isoprostanes using gas chromatography–mass spectrometry. Anal Biochem 1999; 268:117–125.
37. Wang Z, Ciabattoni G, Creminon C, Lawson J, Fitzgerald GA, Patrono C, Maclouf J. Urinary characterization of 8-epi-PGF_2alpha excretion in man. J Pharm Exp Ther 1995; 275:94–100.
38. Longmire AW, Swift LL, Roberts LJ, Awad JA, Burk RF, Morrow JD. Effect of oxygen tension on the generation of F_2-isoprostanes and malondialdehyde in peroxidizing rat liver microsomes. Biochem Pharm 1994; 47:1173–1177.
39. Steinberg D, Parthasarathy S, Carew TE, Khoo JC, Witztum JL. Beyond cholesterol: modifications of low density lipoprotein that increase its atherogenicity. N Engl J Med 1989; 86:915–924.
40. Gopaul NK, Nourooz–Zadeh J, Malle AI, Anggard EE. Formation of F_2-isoprostanes during aortic endothelial cell-mediated oxidation of low density lipoprotein. FEBS Lett 1994; 348:297–300.
41. Pratico D, Smyth EM, Violi F, FitzGerald GA. Generation of 8-epi-prostaglandin $F_{2\alpha}$ by human monocytes: discriminate production by reactive oxygen species and prostaglandin endoperoxide synthase-2. J Biol Chem 1996; 271:8919–8924.
42. Parthasarathy S, Wieland E, Steinberg E. A role for endothelial cell lipoxygenase in the oxidative modification of low density lipoprotein. Proc Natl Acad Sci USA 1989; 86:1046–1050.
43. Sun D, Funk CD. Disruption of 12/15-lipoxygenase expression in peritoneal macrophages: enhanced utilization of the 5-lipoxygenase pathway and diminished oxidation of low density lipoprotein. J Biol Chem 1996; 271:24055–24062.
44. Moore KP, Darley-Usmar V, Morrow JD, Roberts LJ. Formation of F_2-isoprostanes during oxidation of human low-density lipoprotein and plasma by peroxynitrite. Circ Res 1995; 77:335–341.
45. Awad JA, Roberts LJ, Burk RF, Morrow JD. Isoprostanes—prostaglandin-like compounds formed in vivo independently of cyclooxygenase. Gastroenterol Clin North Am 1996; 25:409–427.

46. Awad JA, Morrow JD. Excretion of F_2-isoprostanes in bile: a novel index of hepatic lipid peroxidation. Hepatology 1995; 22:962–968.
47. Burk RF, Lawrence RA, Lane JM. Liver necrosis and lipid peroxidation in the rat as a result of paraquat and diquat administration: effect of selenium deficiency. J Clin Invest 1980; 65:1024–1031.
48. Awad JA, Burk RF, Roberts LJ. Effect of selenium deficiency and glutathione-modulating agents on diquat toxicity and lipid peroxidation in rats. J Pharmacol Exp Ther 1994; 270:858-864.
49. Schwarz K. Studies on vitamin E deficiency in rodents. Vitam Horm 1962; 20:463–488.
50. Tappel AL. Vitamin E and free radical peroxidation of lipids. Ann NY Acad Sci 1972; 203:12–28.
51. Nanji AA, Kwaja S, Tahan SR, Sadrzadeh SRM. Plasma levels of a novel noncyclooxygenase-derived prostanoid (8-isoprostane) correlate with severity of liver injury in experimental alcohol liver disease. J Pharmacol Exp Ther 1994; 269:1280–1285.
52. Nanji AA, Zhao S, Khwaja S, Sadrzadeh SRM. Cimetidine prevents alcoholic hepatic injury in the intragastric feeding rat model. J Pharmacol Exp Ther 1994; 269:827–832.
53. Lynch SM, Frei B, Morrow JD, Roberts LJ, Xu A, Jackson T, Reyna R, Klevay LM, Vita JA, Keaney JF. Vascular superoxide dismutase deficiency impairs endothelial vasodilator function through direct inactivation of nitric oxide and increased lipid peroxidation. Arterioscler Thromb Vasc Biol 1997; 17:2975–2981.
54. Yang ZP, Morrow JD, Wu A, Roberts LJ, Dettbarn WD. Diisopropylphosphorofluoridate-induced muscle hyperactivity associated with enhanced lipid peroxidation in vivo. Biochem Pharmacol 1996; 52:357–361.
55. Mathews WR, Guido DM, Fisher MA, Jaeschke H. Lipid peroxidation as a molecular mechanism of liver injury during reperfusion after ischemia. Free Radic Biol Med 1994; 16:763–770.
56. Dabbagh AJ, Mannion T, Lynch SM, Frei B. The effect of iron overload on rat plasma and liver oxidant status in vivo. Biochem J 1994; 300:799–803.
57. Gourlay GK, Adams JF, Cousins MJ, Hall P. Genetic differences in reductive metabolism and hepatotoxicity of halothane in three rat strains. Anesthesiology 1981; 55:96–103.
58. Awad JA, Horn JL, Roberts J, Franks JJ. Demonstration of halothane-induced hepatic lipid peroxidation in rats by quantification of F_2-isoprostanes. Anesthesiology 1996; 84:910–916.
59. Morrow JD, Moore KP, Awad JA, Ravenscraft MD, Marini G, Badr KF, Williams R, Roberts LJ. Marked overproduction of non-cyclooxygenase derived prostanoids (F_2-isoprostanes) in the hepatorenal syndrome. J Lipid Mediat 1993; 6:417–420.
60. Stein CM, Tanner SB, Awad JA, Roberts LJ, Morrow JD. Evidence of free radical-mediated injury (isoprostane overproduction) in scleroderma. Arthritis Rheum 1996; 39:1146–1150.
61. Holt S, Reeder B, Wilson M, Harvey S, Morrow JD, Roberts LJ, Moore K. Increased lipid peroxidation in patients with rhabdomyolysis. Lancet 1999; 353:1241.
62. Collins CE, Quaggiotto P, Wood L, O'Loughlin EV, Henry RL, Garg ML. Elevated plasma levels of F_2 alpha isoprostane in cystic fibrosis. Lipids 1999; 34:551–556.
63. Meagher EA, Barry OP, Burke A, Lucey MR, Lawson JA, Rokach J, FitzGerald GA. Alcohol-induced generation of lipid peroxidation products in humans. J Clin Invest 1999; 104:805–813.
64. Montine TJ, Beal MF, Robertson D, Cudkowicz ME, Biaggioni I, O'Donnell H, Zackert WE, Roberts LJ, Morrow JD. Cerebrospinal fluid F_2-isoprostane levels are elevated in Huntington's disease. Neurology 1999; 52:1104–1105.
65. Vita JA, Keaney JF, Raby KE, Morrow JD, Freedman JE, Lynch S, Koulouris SN, Hankin BR, Frei B. Low plasma ascorbic acid independently predicts the presence of an unstable coronary syndrome. J Am Coll Cardiol 1998; 31:980–986.
66. Richelle M, Turini ME, Guidox R, Tavazzi I, Metairon S, Fay LB. Urinary isoprostane excretion is not confounded by the lipid content of the diet. FEBS Lett 1999; 459:259–262.
67. Pratico D, Tangirala RK, Rader DJ, Rokach J, FitzGerald GA. Vitamin E suppresses isoprostane generation in vivo and reduces atherosclerosis in ApoE-deficient mice. Nat Med 1998; 4:1189–1192.
68. Kannel WB. Update on the role of cigarette smoking in coronary artery disease. Am Heart J 1981; 101:319–328.
69. Frei B, Forte TM, Ames BN, Cross CE. Gas phase oxidant of cigarette smoke induce lipid peroxidation and changes in lipoprotein properties in human blood plasma: protective effects of ascorbic acid. Biochem J 1991; 277:133–138.
70. Reilly M, Delanty N, Lawson JA, FitzGerald GA. Modulation of oxidant stress in vivo in chronic cigarette smokers. Circulation 1996; 94:19–25.

71. Obwegeser R, Oguogho A, Ulm M, Berghammer P, Sinzinger H. Maternal cigarette smoking increases F_2-isoprostanes and reduces prostacyclin and nitric oxide in umbilical vessels. Prostaglandins Other Lipid Mediat 1999; 57:269–279.
72. Davi G, Alessandrini P, Mezzetti A, Minotti G, Bucciarelli T, Costantini F, Cipollone F, Bon GB, Ciabattoni G, Patrono C. In vivo formation of 8-epi-prostaglandin $F_{2\alpha}$ is increased in hypercholesterolemia. Atheroscler Thromb Vasc Biol 1997; 117:3230–3235.
73. Reilly M, Pratico D, Delanty N, DiMinno G, Tremoli E, Rader D, Kapoor S, Rokach J, Lawson JA, FitzGerald GA. Increased formation of distinct F_2-isoprostanes in hypercholesterolemia. Circulation 1998; 98:2822–2828.
74. Natarajan R, Lanting L, Gonzales N, Nadler J. Formation of F_2-isoprostanes in vascular smooth muscle by elevated glucose and growth factors. Am J Physiol 1996; 271:J159–H165.
75. Koulouris S, Frei B, Morrow JD, Keaney JF, Vita JA. Increased oxidative stress in patients with diabetes mellitus. Circulation 1995; 92(suppl 1):I-102.
76. Gopaul NK, Anggard EE, Mallet AI, Beteridge DJ, Wolff SP, Nourooz–Zadey J. Plasma 8-epi-$PGF_{2\alpha}$ is elevated in individuals with non-insulin dependent diabetes mellitus. FEBS Lett 1995; 368:225–229.
77. Boushey CJ, Beresford SA, Omenn GS, Motulsky AG. A quantitative assessment of plasma homocysteine as a risk factor for vascular disease: probable benefits of increasing folic acid intakes. JAMA 1995; 274:1049–1057.
78. Gniwotta C, Morrow JD, Roberts LJ, Kuhn H. Prostaglandin F_2-like compounds (F_2-isoprostanes) are present in increased amounts in human atherosclerotic lesions. Arterioscler Thromb Vasc Biol 1997; 17:3236–3241.
79. Pratico D, Iuliano L, Mauriello A, Spagnoli L, Lawson JA, Rokach J, Maclouf J, Violi F, FitzGerald GA. Localization of distinct F-isoprostanes in human atherosclerotic lesions. J Clin Invest 1997; 100:2028–2034.
80. Barlow C, Dennery PA, Shigenega MK, Smith MA, Morrow JD, Roberts LJ, Wynshaw–Boris A, Levine RL. Loss of ataxia-telangiectasia gene product causes oxidative damage in target organs. Proc Natl Acad Sci USA 1999; 96:9915–9919.

4
Efficacy of Vitamin E in Human Health and Disease

Sharon V. Landvik
Vitamin E Research and Information Service, Edina, Minnesota

Anthony T. Diplock
United Medical and Dental Schools, University of London, and Guy's Hospital, London, England

Lester Packer
University of Southern California School of Pharmacy, Los Angeles, California

I. INTRODUCTION

Since the discovery of vitamin E in 1922 by Evans and Bishop, its role in human health has been extensively investigated. Vitamin E refers to a group of eight naturally occurring compounds—α-, β-, γ-, δ-tocopherols and tocotrienols. α-Tocopherol, especially the naturally occurring d-α-tocopherol, has the highest biological activity (1,2).

Vitamin E is the major chain-breaking antioxidant in body tissues, and it is considered the first line of defense against lipid peroxidation, protecting cell membranes at an early stage of free radical attack (3,4). Unchecked by an antioxidant, highly unstable free radicals attack cell constituents, particularly those containing polyunsaturated fatty acids, and can damage both the structure and function of cell membranes. Nucleic acids and electron-dense regions of proteins also come under attack (5,6). There is evidence to implicate free radicals in development of degenerative diseases and conditions (7,8). This chapter discusses vitamin E functions, requirements, and clinical deficiency states, and current research findings on the protective role of vitamin E in preventing or minimizing free radical damage associated with cancer, cardiovascular disease, premature aging, cataracts, air pollution, and strenuous exercise.

II. FUNCTIONS

Vitamin E is nature's most effective lipid-soluble antioxidant, protecting unsaturated fatty acids in cell membranes that are important for membrane function and structure (4,6,9). Increased vitamin E intake may enhance the immune response. Vitamin E regulates platelet aggregation by inhibiting prostaglandin (thromboxane) production. It also has a role in the regulation of protein kinase C (PKC) activation, mitochondrial function, nucleic acid and protein metabolism, and hormonal production. Vitamin E protects vitamin A from destruction in the body and spares selenium (10,11).

III. CLINICAL DEFICIENCY STATES

Clinical vitamin E deficiency states have been observed in individuals with a chronic malabsorption syndrome, premature infants, and patients receiving total parenteral nutrition (3). Conditions interfering with normal digestion, absorption, or transport of dietary fat have been associated with low serum vitamin E concentrations (12). In patients with malabsorption syndromes, such as celiac disease, biliary atresia, and cystic fibrosis, serum vitamin E concentrations can be less than 20% of normal. Serum vitamin E levels are often too low to measure in patients with abetalipoproteinemia. Hemolysis and a shortened life span of red blood cells have been reported at vitamin E plasma concentrations below 0.5 mg/dL (11).

Severe and chronic vitamin E deficiency in patient with fat malabsorption can lead to a progressive neurological syndrome, indicating the importance of vitamin E in optimal development and maintenance of the function and integrity of the nervous system and skeletal muscle (13). Characteristics of the neurological syndrome include progressive neuropathy with absent or altered reflexes, limb weakness, ataxia, and sensory loss in the legs and arms. Improvement of neurological function has been documented with appropriate vitamin E therapy; progressive neurological damage may be prevented in children with prolonged cholestatic disease by early initiation of vitamin E therapy (14,15).

Low birth weight premature infants are vulnerable to vitamin E deficiency owing to inadequate body stores, impaired absorption, and reduced transport capacity in the blood because of low levels of low-density lipoproteins (LDL) at birth (16). Plasma vitamin E levels are also frequently low in patients on a total parenteral nutrition regime. Parenteral lipid emulsions contain primarily γ- and δ-tocopherol homologues, which are much less biologically active forms than α-tocopherol. Plasma vitamin E levels cannot be maintained with high intakes of γ- and δ-isomers; thus α-tocopherol supplementation is required for patients receiving total parenteral nutrition (17,18).

IV. REQUIREMENTS

Depending on dietary and lifestyle habits or tissue composition from previous intake patterns, vitamin E requirements of normal adults may vary at least fivefold. Even greater variability in vitamin E requirements has been demonstrated in animals with a high polyunsaturated fatty acid intake (3) (Table 1). Serum or plasma vitamin E concentrations are usually considered to be the most convenient and useful measurement of vitamin E status. It is generally accepted that individuals with plasma vitamin E levels of less than 0.5 mg/dL are vitamin E-deficient (11). Daily dietary vitamin E intakes of 10–30 mg in healthy adults will maintain serum vitamin E concentrations in the normal range (11). In a study of well-nourished adults, mean plasma vitamin E concentrations were 1.06 mg/dL at baseline and doubled to 2.03 mg/dL after daily supplementation with 800 IU vitamin E for 8 weeks (19).

Determination of vitamin E requirements must consider whether requirements should reflect vitamin E intakes that are adequate to prevent deficiency symptoms and allow normal physiological function, or the higher intakes necessary to prevent oxidative damage (3,20).

Table 1 Relation of Vitamin E Requirement with Calculated Relative Susceptibility of Muscle Tissue Lipid to Peroxidation in Rats Fed Diets of Varying Fatty Acid Composition

Number of double bonds	Relative oxidative rate	Vitamin E requirement[a]
1	0.025	0.3
2	1	2
3	2	3
4	4	4
5	6	5
6	8	6

[a]Proportional to number of double bonds in muscle lipids, except for monounsaturated fatty acids.

A study of healthy adults showed that daily supplementation of 1000 IU vitamin E for 10 days significantly decreased breath pentane excretion. Based on these results, it may be inferred that there are undesirably high levels of lipid peroxidation in the body, which can be reduced by vitamin E supplementation (21). These results may be significant in light of research evidence showing involvement of free radical damage in normal body processes and certain diseases and the role of vitamin E in controlling or preventing lipid peroxidation (4,21).

V. CANCER

Cancer is believed to be the result of external factors combined with a hereditary disposition to cancer. Most human cancers are considered to be environmentally induced, based on lifestyle patterns, including diet. Free radicals frequently have a role in the process of cancer initiation and promotion. From cell culture and animal studies, it appears that vitamin E and other antioxidants may alter cancer incidence and growth through their action as anticarcinogens, quenching free radicals or reacting with their products, although this is a considerable oversimplification. Although studies do not provide conclusive documentation and a significant effect of vitamin E is not seen in all experimental models, the majority of studies show a protective effect of vitamin E relative to cancer risk in some sites (22–34).

Although controlled human studies on the antioxidants and cancer are limited, most available epidemiological evidence suggests that vitamin E and other antioxidants decrease the incidence of certain cancers (Table 2). However, because the range of dietary vitamin E intake within a population may be quite narrow, a protective effect of vitamin E may not be fully demonstrated in all epidemiological studies evaluating serum vitamin E levels and cancer risk (35).

An inverse correlation between serum antioxidant levels and subsequent cancer risk was demonstrated in several epidemiological studies in Finland (35–38). In a mortality follow-up study in Switzerland, low blood levels of β-carotene, vitamin C, and vitamin E were associated with increased risk for certain types of cancer (39). In additional follow-up of the same study, low plasma vitamin E levels were associated with significantly increased risk for prostate cancer mortality in smokers after exclusion of mortality during the first 2 years of follow-up (40). Low plasma concentrations of vitamin C and E were associated with an increased risk for lung cancer (41).

Table 2 Human Epidemiological Studies of Vitamin E and Other Antioxidants and Subsequent Cancer Risk

Cancer site	Country	Number of subjects with cancer	Findings	Ref.
All sites	Finland	453 males	0.7 adjusted relative risk of cancer in two highest quintiles of blood vitamin E levels	35
All sites	Finland	51	11.4-fold adjusted relative risk of fatal cancer with low blood vitamin E and selenium levels	36
Upper gastrointestinal tract	Finland	150	Relative cancer risk of 2.2 in the three lowest quintiles of serum vitamin E and 3.3 in the lowest quintile of serum selenium	37
Colorectal			No inverse association between serum vitamin E and selenium levels and colorectal cancer risk	
Reproductive organs	Finland	313 females	1.5-fold higher cancer risk with serum vitamin E levels in the lowest quintile, tenfold higher selenium and vitamin E levels	38
Stomach	Switzerland	129 males	Blood levels of β-carotene, vitamin C, and vitamin E were lower in cancer cases than in controls	39
Colon			Vitamin E blood levels were lower in cancer cases compared with controls	
All sites	Switzerland	290 males	Low blood vitamin E levels associated with increased risk for prostate cancer mortality in smokers; no association between plasma α- and β-carotene levels and prostate cancer mortality	40
			Low vitamin C and vitamin E plasma levels associated with increased lung cancer risk	41
All sites	United States	111	No relation between blood antioxidant levels and subsequent cancer risk	42
Lung	United States	284 males	3.4-fold relative risk of lung cancer with serum β-carotene levels in the lowest quintile	43
Bladder, gastrointestinal tract			No association between serum vitamin A or E levels and cancer risk	
Nine primary sites	United States	436	Serum β-carotene and vitamin E had a protective association with lung cancer	44

Site	Country	N	Findings	Ref
All sites	England	271 males	Serum vitamin E levels were significantly lower in subjects diagnosed with cancer within 1 year after blood collection, but not in other cancer subjects	45
Breast	England	39 females	Five times greater cancer risk for women with vitamin E blood levels in the lowest fifth than in the highest fifth	46
All sites	India	101	Plasma levels of vitamins A, C, and E and β-carotene were significantly lower in cancer patients than in the controls	47
Lung	United States	99	2.5 times higher cancer risk with serum vitamin E levels in the lowest quintile than in the highest quintile	48
Lung	United States	59	Serum vitamin E and carotenoid levels were significantly lower in cancer patients than in controls	49
Lung	Japan	37	Mean blood vitamin E and selenium levels were significantly lower in cancer patients than in controls	50
Lung	Finland	117 males	Adjusted risk of cancer in nonsmokers in the lowest tertile of intake compared with the highest tertile was 2.5 for carotenoids and 3.1 for vitamins C and E	51
Lung	United Kingdom	171	Serum β-carotene, vitamin A, and vitamin E levels were lower in cancer patients than in controls	52
Lung	United States	328	Inverse correlation between upper lobe location of cancer and intake of vitamin E and yellow–orange vegetables	53
Lung	Uruguay	541	Cancer risk was 57% lower in the highest quintile of total carotenoid intake and 50% lower in the highest quintile of vitamin E intake	54
Lung	United States	413 nonsmokers	β-Carotene intake was associated with a significant reduction in cancer risk; vitamin E supplementation was also protective against cancer	55
Cervix	United States	10 females	Blood β-carotene and vitamin E levels were significantly lower in cancer cases than in controls	56
Cervix	United States	189 females	High vitamin C and vitamin E intake were associated with a significantly reduced risk of cancer	57
Cervix	United States	27 females	Plasma carotenoid and α-tocophenol levels lower in cancer cases	58
Ovaries	United States	35 females	No association between serum carotenoid and vitamin E levels and cancer risk	59

(continued)

Table 2 (*Continued*)

Cancer site	Country	Number of subjects with cancer	Findings	Ref.
Breast	United States	105 females	Inverse association between serum lycopene levels, but not other antioxidants and cancer risk	60
Breast	Italy	2569 females	Inverse association between dietary β-carotene and vitamin E intake and cancer risk	61
Breast	United States	297 females	Cancer risk in highest quartile of intake was 45% lower for vitamin E and β-carotene, and 53% lower for lutein and zeaxanthin	62
Mouth and pharynx	United States	190	Lower cancer risk was associated with increased intake of fiber, carotene, and vitamins C and E in males and of vitamin C and fiber in women	63
Mouth and pharynx	United States	1103	Use of vitamin E supplements was associated with a significantly reduced risk of cancer	64
Oral cavity	India	24	Plasma vitamin C and vitamin E levels lower in cancer cases	65
Oral cavity, pharynx, larynx	The Netherlands	86	Serum levels of vitamins A and E lower in patients with a second primary tumor	66
Upper gastrointestinal tract	United States	59 females	Lower cancer risk associated with higher intake of carotene and vitamins C and E	67
Stomach	Italy	1016	Fivefold difference in cancer risk between high vitamins C and E intake and low protein and nitrite intake and low vitamins C and E intake and high protein and nitrite intake	68
Colon	United States	212	68% lower relative risk of cancer for subjects in the highest quintile of total vitamin E intake compared with the lowest quintile	69
Stomach	Korea	59	Serum levels of vitamin C, vitamin E, and β-carotene lower in cancer cases	70
Thyroid	Italy	399	Cancer risk was 33% lower for vitamin E and 42% lower for β-carotene in the highest quartile of intakes compared with the lowest quartile	71
Leukemia, lymphoma	India	NA	Serum vitamin E levels lower in cancer cases	72
Prostate	Uruguay	175 males	60, 40, and 50% lower cancer risk with high intakes of vitamin C, vitamin E, and fruits and vegetables, respectively	73

In a follow-up of a blood pressure risk study in United States, it was concluded that there was no association between blood antioxidant concentrations and subsequent cancer risk, although blood vitamin E levels were somewhat lower in subjects who later developed cancer, but the vitamin E levels seemed to relate to blood cholesterol levels (42).

In a study of men of Japanese ancestry in Hawaii, there was a significant association between serum β-carotene concentrations and subsequent lung cancer risk, but not between serum vitamin A or vitamin E concentrations and subsequent risk of lung, bladder, or gastrointestinal cancers (43). Serum β-carotene and vitamin E levels showed a protective association with lung cancer in another study in The United States (44). In the two studies in England, men who had a diagnosis of cancer within 1 year after blood collection had significantly lower mean serum vitamin E levels than controls, and women with low plasma vitamin E concentrations had a significantly increased risk of breast cancer (45,46). In a case–control study in India of patients with cancer at various sites, plasma levels of vitamin A and E and β-carotene were significantly lower in the cancer patients (47).

Blood vitamin E levels were significantly lower in subjects who subsequently developed lung cancer than in controls in a study in the United States (48). Results of another U. S. study showed that newly diagnosed lung cancer patients had significantly lower average serum levels of vitamin E and carotenoids than controls (49). Mean blood vitamin E and selenium concentrations were also significantly lower in a group of patients in Japan with lung cancer than in controls (50). Using dietary intake data based on dietary history interviews in a study in Finland, the age-adjusted relative risk of lung cancer in the lowest tertile of intake compared with the highest tertile was 2.5 for carotenoids and 3.1 for vitamin C and vitamin E (51). In a case–control study in United Kingdom, serum β-carotene, vitamin A, and vitamin E levels were lower in lung cancer patients than in controls (52).

A U. S. study that examined the association between diet and tumor location in patients with lung cancer showed a strong inverse correlation between upper lobe location of cancer and intake of vitamin E and yellow–orange vegetables (53). Results of a study in Uruguay showed a 57 and 50% decrease in lung cancer risk with intakes in the highest quartile versus the lowest quartile for total carotenoids and vitamin E, respectively (54). In a study of nonsmokers in the United States, dietary β-carotene intake was associated with a significant reduction in lung cancer risk, and use of vitamin E supplements was also protective against lung cancer (55).

There was a significant reduction in average plasma vitamin E and β-carotene levels in women with cervical dysplasia or cancer compared with controls in a U.S. study (56). In a study of the relation of diet to risk of invasive cervical cancer, a high dietary intake of vitamins C and E was associated with a significantly lower risk of cervical cancer. Use of vitamin A and vitamin E supplements was associated with a slight decrease in cervical cancer risk (57). Plasma levels of carotenoids and α-tocopherol, but not γ-tocopherol, were lower in patients with cervical cancer than in patients with cervical precancer or noncancerous diseases in a U. S. study (58). Serum carotenoid and vitamin E levels were not associated with cancer risk in a U. S. study of patients with ovarian cancer (59).

In another U. S. study, serum lycopene levels were inversely associated with breast cancer risk. There was no evidence for a protective effect for vitamin E, α- and β-carotene, vitamin A, or selenium (60). However, there was a significant inverse association between dietary vitamin E and β-carotene intake and breast cancer risk in a study in Italy (61). A U. S. study of premenopausal women demonstrated a 45% lower breast cancer risk for women in the highest quartile of vitamin E intake compared with those in the lowest quartile. Breast cancer risk was 33% lower for α-carotene, 54% lower for β-carotene and 53% lower for lutein plus zeaxanthin in the highest quartile of intake compared with the lowest quartile (62).

A multicenter study evaluated the association between diet and incidence of oral and pharyngeal cancer among African Americans. A lower risk of oral and pharyngeal cancer was associated with an increased intake of fiber, carotene, and vitamins C and E in men and of vitamin C and fiber in women (63). In another study in the United States, individuals who took vitamin E supplements had a significantly reduced risk of oral and pharyngeal cancer (64). Plasma vitamin C and vitamin E concentrations were significantly lower in patients with oral cancer than in controls in a study in India (65). Serum levels of vitamins A and E were significantly lower in patients with a second primary tumor than in patients with a single head and neck cancer in a study in The Netherlands. Serum β-carotene levels were depressed in both groups of patients (66). High dietary intakes of carotene and vitamins C and E were related to decreased risk of both oral/pharyngeal/esophageal and stomach cancer in a U. S. study of postmenopausal women. A higher vitamin A intake was associated with a lower risk of stomach cancer only (67).

In a study in Italy, the risk of gastric cancer increased with increasing intake of nitrites and protein and decreased in proportion to increased intake of vitamin C and E, β-carotene, and vegetable fat (68). In a U. S. study, the relative risk was largely associated with the use of supplemental vitamin E (69). Serum levels of vitamin C, vitamin E, and β-carotene were significantly lower in patients with stomach cancer than in controls in a Korean study (70).

In a study that investigated the relation between micronutrient intake and thyroid cancer in Italy, the risk of cancer was 33% lower for vitamin E and 42% lower for β-carotene in the highest quartile of intakes compared with the lowest quartile (71). Serum vitamin E concentrations were significantly lower in leukemia and lymphoma patients than in controls in a study in India (72). In a case–control study in Uruguay, prostate cancer risk was decreased 60, 40, and 50% with high intakes of vitamin C, vitamin E, and fruits and vegetables, respectively (73).

From results of animal and human studies, it was concluded by the authors that vitamin E and other antioxidants merit continued active research evaluation utilizing epidemiological studies and randomized placebo-controlled clinical trials to evaluate the role of antioxidant supplements in cancer prevention (74). A limited number of intervention trials have evaluated the role of vitamin E and other antioxidants in cancer prevention, with mixed results. In a nutrition intervention trial of 29,584 adults from Linxian, China, cancer mortality was 13% lower, and the mortality rate from stomach and esophageal cancers combined was 10% lower in the group supplemented with β-carotene, vitamin E, and selenium for 5 years (75). A clinical trial in the United States of 864 patients who had had a colorectal adenoma removed before entering the study did not demonstrate a benefit of vitamins C and E or β-carotene in decreasing the incidence of new colorectal adenomas over 4 years (76).

In a primary prevention trial of 29,133 male smokers, aged 50–69 years, in Finland (ATBC study), there was no reduction in lung cancer incidence among men supplemented with 50 mg of synthetic vitamin E per day for 5–8 years compared with those who were not. Lung cancer incidence was 18% higher in the group supplemented with 20 mg synthetic β-carotene per day (77). This effect may be associated with heavier cigarette smoking and higher intake of alcohol (78). In contrast, prostate cancer incidence was 32% lower and prostate cancer mortality was decreased by 41% among vitamin E-supplemented men. Among β-carotene supplemental subjects, prostate cancer incidence was 23% higher and mortality owing to prostate cancer was 15% higher (79). There was a 19% decrease in lung cancer incidence in the highest versus the lowest quartile of baseline serum vitamin E levels in the ATBC study population (80).

In a study that evaluated the effects of antioxidant supplementation (800 IU vitamin E, 30 mg β-carotene, and 1000 mg vitamin C per day for 9 months) in 79 patients with oral leukoplakia (precancerous lesions of the oral cavity), 90% of subjects who decreased their use of tobacco or alcohol showed clinical improvement. Approximately 50% of the patients who did not change their use of tobacco or alcohol also showed clinical improvement of lesions (81). In a multicenter trial of the efficacy of vitamin E supplements (800 IU/day for 24 weeks) in patients with oral leukoplakia, 20 of the 43 patients had clinical responses (disappearance or significant decrease in size of lesions) and 9 had histological responses (improvement in the degree of dysplasia) (82).

VI. CARDIOVASCULAR DISEASE

It is well established that cholesterol deposited in arteries originates primarily from LDLs and that elevated LDL levels are associated with an increased risk for atherosclerosis. One of the earliest stages in development of atherosclerosis is accumulation in the arteries of foam cells, which are macrophages that have taken up oxidized LDL. These foam cells are filled with liquid droplets of cholesterol and are a key component of the fatty streak lesion (83). LDL is an important target of free radicals, and oxidation of LDL is believed to be an important event in development of atherosclerosis (84). Results of cell and animal research support the hypothesis that oxidative modification of LDL results in an enhanced uptake by macrophages, leading to conversion of macrophages into foam cells, and that antioxidants may protect against LDL oxidation (85–87).

In isolated cell studies in which high amounts of vitamin E were added to the culture medium, cell-mediated oxidation of LDL was largely prevented over 24 h. Supplementation of plasma with increasing vitamin E concentrations before isolation of LDL resulted in a proportional increase in the duration of the lag phase during which there was no detectable oxidative modification of LDL (83,88). In a study of the oxidation of LDL separated from plasma of healthy subjects, the results demonstrated that vitamins E and C act synergistically as antioxidants to suppress LDL oxidation (84).

In studies of healthy, nonsmoking subjects supplemented with vitamin E, there was a significant increase in resistance of LDL isolated from plasma to induced oxidation (89–92). Resistance of LDL to oxidation also increased significantly in a group of smokers supplemented with vitamin E (93).

Research in animals has also investigated possible protective effects of vitamin E on the development and progression of atherosclerosis. In studies of specific types of hens and rabbits that are susceptible to development of atherosclerosis, early aortic lesion development was significantly inhibited by vitamin E supplementation (94–97). Prevention and regression of induced atherosclerosis by vitamin E were studied in male monkeys on an atherosclerosis-promoting diet. Stenosis progressed more rapidly and to a greater extent in unsupplemented monkeys compared with vitamin E-treated monkeys. Stenosis in the group of animals with established atherosclerosis significantly decreased from 33 to 8% after 8 months of vitamin E therapy. According to the researchers, their results show that vitamin E may be effective in both prevention and treatment of atherosclerosis (98). Extensive additional research is required to establish the clinical relevance of the experimental data. The relation between plasma antioxidant levels and incidence of coronary heart disease has been investigated in a number of recent studies in adult populations. In the WJO/MONICA study, comparison was made of plasma antioxidant concentrations of middle-aged men (40–59 years of age) from different European populations. There was a high inverse correlation between age-specific mortality from ischemic heart disease and lipid-standardized plasma vitamin E levels (99). In contrast, there was no consistent association between serum selenium, vitamin A, or vitamin E levels and risk of death from coronary heart disease in prospective epidemiological studies in Finland and The Netherlands (100,101). However, it was noted that the data from the two studies in Finland and The Netherlands must be considered with reservation owing to methodological problems, including lack of standardization for cholesterol and triglycerides (102). The relative risk of heart disease was 32% lower for men and 65% lower for women in the highest tertile of vitamin E intake compared with the lowest tertile in a study in Finland (103).

In a U. S. study that evaluated the association between serum antioxidant levels and risk of myocardial infarction, a protective association with serum vitamin E levels was suggested only among individuals with high serum cholesterol concentrations (104). In a study in Poland, plasma vitamin E levels were significantly lower in patients with stable and unstable angina compared with healthy controls, whereas vitamin E levels in red blood cells were significantly lower only in patients with unstable angina (105). In a population case–control study in the United Kingdom, there was a significant inverse association between plasma vitamin E concentrations and angina risk. According to the researchers, the results suggest that some populations with a high coronary heart disease incidence may benefit from a diet rich in antioxidants, particularly vitamin E (106).

Serum and LDL vitamin E levels were significantly lower in patients with coronary artery disease than in controls in a study in Sweden (107). In a U. S. study of postmenopausal women with no evidence of coronary heart disease, the relative risk of death from coronary heart disease was 58% lower in the two highest quartile of dietary vitamin E intake than in the lowest quartile (108). In a group of subjects 67–105 years of age in the United States, use of vitamin E supplements decreased the risk of coronary heart disease mortality by 47% (109). Vitamin E supplementation was associated with a decreased incidence of ischemic heart disease in a study of men in Canada (110). In middle-aged men with previous coronary bypass graft surgery who were placed on a cholesterol-lowering diet and randomized to receive colestipol–niacin or placebo, those who took at least 100 IU vitamin E per day from supplements showed significantly less coronary artery disease progression for all lesions and for mild to moderate lesions than men who took less than 100 IU vitamin E per day (111).

In the Harvard-based study of 39,910 male health professionals in the United States, a 36% lower relative risk of coronary heart disease was demonstrated in men who consumed more than 60 IU vitamin E per day compared with men consuming less than 7.5 IU daily. Men who took at least 100 IU vitamin E per day for at least 2 years had a 37% lower relative risk of coronary heart disease than men who did not take vitamin E supplements (112).

In the Harvard-based 8-year study of 87,245 healthy nurses in the United States, women in the top fifth of vitamin E intake had a 34% lower relative risk of major coronary disease than women in the lowest fifth, after adjustment for age and smoking. The relative risk of coronary heart disease (CHD) was 48% lower in women taking vitamin E supplements of more than 100 mg/day for at least 2 years. No protective effect was seen in women whose only source of vitamin E was dietary intake. The researchers in both of the Harvard-based studies noted that these data and other evidence suggest that vitamin E supplements may reduce risk of heart disease (113).

In the ATBC study of male smokers in Finland, there was little difference in total incidence or mortality from CHD between the vitamin E-supplemented subjects (56 vs. 67 cases), and rates of hemorrhagic stroke were slightly increased compared with the placebo group (66 vs. 44 cases). However, implications of this study are limited because a criterion for entry into the study was that the study population had smoked at least 20 cigarettes daily for 36 years before the study was begun. (Smoking is an extremely strong risk factor for CHD, stroke, and many cancers.) The dose of vitamin E was lower than that observed to be protective in prospective studies, and the length of follow-up was relatively short (5–8 years). The baseline plasma levels of vitamin E among the participants in the study were also quite high, which suggests that any benefit derived from vitamin E may have been achieved during the development of the disease (77). Mortality from cerebrovascular disease was 10% lower among subjects supplemented with vitamin E, β-carotene, and selenium in the intervention trial in Linxian, China of 29,584 adults (75). A clinical trial in Italy of 11,324 patients who had survived a recent myocardial infarction evaluated the effects of daily supplementation of 1 g of n-3 polyunsaturated fatty acids (fish oil), 300 IU synthetic vitamin E, fish oil and vitamin E, or no supplementation on morbidity and mortality over 3 1/2 years. Treatment with fish oil, but not vitamin E, significantly decreased the risk of reaching the primary combined endpoint of death, nonfatal myocardial infarction, and stroke during the study period. The effect of the combined treatment of fish oil and vitamin E was similar to the effect for fish oil alone. However, a subgroup analysis of cardiovascular deaths showed a decreased risk for individual components (ranging from a 20% lower risk for all cardiovascular deaths to a 35% lower risk of sudden death) in the vitamin E-supplemented group that was similar to the effects of fish oil supplements (114). The Cambridge Heart Antioxidant Study (CHAOS) evaluated the effect of supplementation with natural source vitamin E (400 or 800 IU/day) or placebo on the risk of myocardial infarction in 2002 patients with angiographic evidence of atherosclerosis. The risk of nonfatal myocardial infarction was reduced by 77% in the vitamin E-supplemented group (115).

Increasing research evidence that chronic diseases, such as atherosclerosis, are more easily prevented than cured has led to particular interest in defining the antiatherosclerotic effect of vitamin E and other antioxidants (116). Results of recent research suggest that vitamin E and other antioxidants may be expected to be important factors or even preventers of coronary heart disease (102). The specific protective role of the antioxidants against which subjects with low plasma antioxidant levels are supplemented with vitamin E and other antioxidants is documented (102,106).

VII. AGING

Approximately 40% of the factors influencing life expectancy can be controlled, suggesting not only that length of life can be extended, but also that quality of life, particularly in the later years, can be enhanced through better health. One area of aging research implicates free radical-mediated cell damage in development of the pathological changes associated with aging (116). It has been suggested that free-radical generation associated with aging may be a contributory factor in the depressed immune response documented in aged rodents and that improved antioxidant status may have an immunostimulatory effect (117).

In a study that evaluated the effect of vitamin E supplementation (800 mg/day for 30 days) or placebo on cell-mediated immune response in 32 healthy adults 60 years of age or older, there was a significant improvement in delayed-type hypersensitivity skin test response in the vitamin E-supplemented group. Vitamin E supplementation also resulted in enhanced response of isolated lymphocytes to concanavalin A. Immune response was enhanced in most, but not all, of the vitamin E-supplemented subjects (118).

Effects on immune response of daily vitamin and trace element supplementation (vitamins A, C, D, and E, B vitamins, β-carotene, folate, iron, zinc, copper, selenium, iodine, calcium, and magnesium), or placebo, were investigated in a group of 96 healthy elderly individuals. There was a significant improvement in several immune-response parameters in the supplemented group. Infection-related illness was significantly less frequent in the supplemented group than in the group on placebo. It was concluded that supplementation with modest physiological doses of micronutrients improves immune response and the incidence of infection in the elderly (119).

A study of 30 elderly patients who had been hospitalized for over 3 months assessed cell-mediated immune function before and following daily antioxidant supplementation (8000 IU vitamin A, 100 mg vitamin C, and 50 mg vitamin E) or placebo for 28 days. There was an improvement in cell-mediated immune function in the antioxidant-supplemented group, but immune function was unchanged in the group receiving placebo. As noted by the researchers, the results suggest that supplementation with slightly higher than RDA levels of the antioxidant vitamins can improve cell-mediated immunity. Additional research is required to determine whether these benefits continue with long-term supplementation and are associated with decreased morbidity in long-stay patients (120).

A study of 30 older women in Spain assessed the effect of antioxidants (1000 mg vitamin C and 200 mg vitamin E per day for 16 weeks) on immune function. Antioxidant supplementation resulted in a significant improvement in parameters of immune function and a significant decrease in lipid peroxide levels in healthy older women and also in older women with coronary heart disease or major depression disorders (121). Vitamin E supplements (200 or 800 mg/day for 235 days) improved certain clinical relevant indexes of cell-mediated immunity in a study of 88 healthy elderly subjects in the United States. The researchers noted that because age-associated decline in immune response is associated with increased incidence of morbidity and mortality, recommendations to increase vitamin E intake should be considered for the elderly (122).

The effects of antioxidants on free radical levels were evaluated in a study in Poland of 100 subjects 60–100 years of age. Average blood malondialdehyde (MDA) levels (which may give an index of lipid peroxidation) decreased 26% in subjects receiving 200 IU vitamin E, 13% in the group supplemented with 400 mg vitamin C, and 25% for combined administration of vitamins E and C (123).

In a study in Finland, concentrations of serum thiobarbituric acid (TBA) reactants (which may also give an index of lipid peroxidation) were initially higher in a group of elderly nursing home patients, but declined to concentrations found in younger controls after supplementation with vitamins E, C, and B6, selenium, β-carotene, and zinc for 3 months. A slight improvement in several psychological tests was observed in the antioxidant-supplemented subjects (124). In another study of nursing home patients in Finland, there was a marked improvement in general condition after 2 months in the vitamin E- and selenium-supplemented subjects, which continued throughout the 1-year study (125).

As research continues on the protective role of the antioxidants in the aging process, study results suggest that free radicals have a significant influence on aging, that free radical-mediated damage can be controlled with adequate antioxidant defenses, and that optimal antioxidant intake can lead to a longer, healthier life.

VIII. CATARACTS

Age is considered a major risk factor in cataract development. It is unclear whether cataract development is the result of cumulative insults of a lifetime or whether decreased resistance or repair capacity of the lens—or the aging process itself—increases susceptibility to cataract formation (126–128). The lens of the eye is very susceptible to light-induced lipid peroxidation, and oxidation is believed to be an early and significant event in development of the majority of cases of senile cataract (126,129).

Results of animal research have shown that vitamin E can arrest and reverse cataract development to some extent, suggesting that lipid peroxidation is involved in the process. In isolated animal lenses and in a number of animal models, vitamin E delayed or minimized cataract development induced by experimental oxidative stress (Table 3; 130–139). Recent epidemiological research has also suggested an association between risk of cataract and antioxidant status.

In a comparison of self-reported vitamin supplementation by 175 subjects with cataracts and 175 individually matched cataract-free subject, significantly more supplementary vitamins C and E were taken by the cataract-free group than the group with cataracts. In the group who took only vitamin E supplements, cataract risk was 56% lower than in the group who did not take vitamin E. There was a 70% decrease in cataract risk in subjects using vitamin C supplements alone compared with subjects who did not take vitamin C (129).

Results of a study of the correlation between antioxidant status and senile cataract in 112 subjects 40–70 years of age suggest that high plasma levels of at least two of the three antioxidant vitamins (vitamins E and C and carotenoids) were associated with a significantly reduced risk of cataract development, compared with low plasma levels of at least one of these vitamins. The odds ratio for senile cataract (controlled for age, race, sex, and diabetes) was 0.2 for subjects with a high serum antioxidant status. The researchers noted that the study results

Table 3 Effects of Vitamin E on Induced Cataract Development

Study	Results	Ref.
Isolated rat lenses exposed to glucose	Vitamin E protected lenses from extensive swelling and degenerative changes	130
Irradiated isolated rat lenses	Vitamin E reduced the degree and extent of cataract development	131
Isolated rat lenses exposed to heat	Vitamin E prevented cataract development	132
Isolated rat lenses exposed to galactose	Vitamin E partially prevented degeneration typical of mature cataracts	133
Streptozocin-induced diabetic rats	Vitamin E-supplemented animals had only slight lens changes compared with extensive cataractous degeneration in unsupplemented rats	134
Isolated rat lenses exposed to corticosteroids	Vitamin E decreased the incidence of cataract development	135
Rats fed 50% galactose diet	Vitamin E supplementation had no significant effect on cataract incidence, but there appeared to be less lens damage	133
Rats fed 30% galactose diet	Vitamin E supplementation reduced rate of cataract formation and delayed appearance of various cataract stages	136
Cataract-prone mice	Vitamin E-supplemented animals had substantially lower incidence of lens opacities	137
Oxidant-treated rabbits	Vitamin E supplementation arrested cataract progression in 50% of animals	138
Rats exposed to single brief doses of neutron or gamma irradiation	Vitamin E pretreatment decreased cataractogenic damage to lenses induced by irradiation	139

appear to support the hypothesis that the lens antioxidant defense may be a factor in cataract development (140).

In a case–control study in Finland that evaluated the association between serum levels of vitamin E, β-carotene, and selenium and subsequent risk of senile cataract over a 15-year period, low serum vitamin E and β-carotene levels predicted an increased risk of senile cataract. The odds ratio for cataract risk was 2.6 for patients with serum vitamin E and β-carotene levels in the lowest third (141). In another study in Finland of 410 male subjects, aged 44–63 years at baseline, there was an inverse association between plasma vitamin E levels and progression of cortical lens opacities. Plasma vitamin E concentrations in the lowest quartile were associated with a 3.7-fold increased risk of progression of early cortical lens opacities compared with the highest quartile (142). Results of the longitudinal study of cataract in the United States, which included 764 participants, showed that the risk of nuclear opacification was decreased by 57% in subjects who regularly used vitamin E supplements (143). In the Beaver Dam Eye Study in the United States, the relation between serum vitamin E and carotenoid levels and cataract incidence was evaluated in 252 subjects 50–86 years of age. Subjects with serum vitamin E levels in the highest tertile had a 60% decrease in cataract risk. Although serum carotenoid levels were not significantly inversely related to cataract risk, there were marginal inverse correlations between serum cryptoxanthin and lutein levels and cataract risk in individuals 65 years of age and older (144). Although most research evidence suggests a beneficial effect of vitamin E and other antioxidants against cataract development, controlled clinical trials are recommended to more precisely define the protective role of antioxidants in prevention of cataracts.

IX. AIR POLLUTION

Ozone and nitrogen dioxide are present in very high concentrations in polluted environments and can initiate free radical reactions that lead to lung damage. Cigarette smoke contains numerous substances known to be oxidants or free radicals; smoking also initiates a significant increase in lung inflammatory cells (potent producers of free radicals) (145). A protective role for vitamin E against the damaging effects of smoke and smog has been demonstrated in a number of studies in animals (146–149).

Studies in humans have also shown protective effects of vitamin E against pollution damage. In a study of the effects of daily vitamin E supplementation (600 mg) on red blood cell susceptibility to ozone-related free radical damage in 12 adults, vitamin E significantly protected red blood cells at the highest levels of hydrogen peroxide-induced stress, but not at lower levels (150). In other studies of Los Angeles residents exposed to photochemical smog, vitamin E supplementation was not protective against biological responses to short-term exposure to ozone. However, the researchers noted that their results do not rule out the possibility that vitamin E supplementation may have a protective effect on human lung tissue, where free radical levels may be higher than in the blood (151,152).

Because smokers inhale high levels of free radicals in the gaseous and tar phases of tobacco use, an increased antioxidant intake may be beneficial (153). A study of young adult smokers demonstrated that the lower respiratory tract fluid of smokers was deficient in vitamin E compared with nonsmokers. Vitamin E supplementation (2400 IU/day for 3 weeks) resulted in increased vitamin E concentrations in lower than baseline levels of nonsmokers, providing clear evidence that vitamin E utilization may be increased in lung cells of smokers. As noted by the researchers, vitamin E may be an important antioxidant in the lung's defense against free radical damage by cigarette smoke (145).

In another study, red blood cells of smokers showed increased peroxidation when incubated with hydrogen peroxide compared with nonsmokers. This effect was inhibited in smokers supplemented with vitamin E (1000 IU/day for 2 weeks). Levels of free radical products in plasma were much higher in unsupplemented smokers than in vitamin E-supplemented smokers or nonsmokers. According to the researchers, their results suggest that smoking leads to changes in antioxidant status (153).

Initial breath pentane output, which may provide an index of lipid peroxidation in vivo, was significantly higher in a group of smokers than in healthy nonsmokers, although plasma vitamin E concentrations were similar in both groups. When smokers were supplemented with 800 mg vitamin E per day for 2 weeks, breath pentane excretion decreased significantly, but remained significantly higher than in nonsmokers. It was concluded that a normal plasma vitamin E concentration does not prevent the increased peroxidation observed in smokers but that vitamin E supplementation will significantly reduce lipid peroxidation and that the recommended daily allowance for vitamin E may be insufficient for individuals exposed to cigarette smoke (154). Until the causative agents of air pollution are completely eliminated, it is likely that vitamin E can help protect the lungs from damage and disease.

X. STRENUOUS EXERCISE

There is increased uptake and utilization of oxygen during exercise, and two- to threefold higher free radical levels are observed in muscle and liver of exercise-exhausted animals (155). During exhaustive exercise, muscle damage occurs even in highly trained athletes. In a study of marathon runners, men had significantly greater skeletal muscle damage (estimated by analysis of serum concentrations of the intramuscular enzyme creatine kinase) than women after a 42-km race, with or without correction for body surface area. Although creatine kinase release from skeletal muscle results from muscle cell injury, it is yet to be determined if it is related to reversible or irreversible damage (156). As exercise is associated with free radical-mediated tissue damage, there should be a greater demand for antioxidants during exercise. Results of animal studies suggest an increased vitamin E requirement during endurance training (157,158).

In a study of male college students, exhaustive exercise led to a significant rise in serum lipid peroxide levels immediately following exercise. Leakage of enzymes from tissues to the blood increased significantly with exercise and was considered to be indicative of exercise-induced, free radical-mediated tissue damage. When the students were supplemented with vitamin E (300 mg/day for 4 weeks), serum MDA levels significantly decreased immediately after exhaustive exercise and the increase in serum enzyme activities was lower. It was concluded by the investigators that lipid peroxidation associated with strenuous exercise can be inhibited by vitamin E supplementation (159).

Another study of young, healthy males investigated the effects of antioxidant supplementation (vitamin C, vitamin E, and β-carotene) on breath pentane output and serum MDA levels before and after exercise (treadmill running). Antioxidant supplementation resulted in significantly lower resting and postexercise concentrations of expired pentane and serum MDA, but did not prevent the exercise-induced rise in indices of lipid peroxidation (160).

Another study evaluated the modulating effects of daily antioxidant supplementation (100 mg vitamin E and 500 mg vitamin C for 15 weeks) or placebo on the short-term effects of ozone in 38 Dutch cyclists. Relatively low ozone concentrations were associated with a decrease in two lung function parameters (FEUI and FUC) after cycling. Ozone had a significant effect on these parameters of lung function during exercise in the placebo group, but not in the antioxidant-supplemented group (161).

In a study of male volunteers in two age groups (22–29 and 55–74 years), subjects were randomized to receive 800 IU vitamin E per day for 48 days or placebo before eccentric exercise (running downhill on an inclined treadmill). All vitamin E-supplemented subjects excreted fewer urinary TBA adducts after an intense bout of eccentric exercise than subjects who received placebo at 12 days postexercise. Muscle lipid-conjugated dienes tended to increase after exercise in the young group of subjects taking placebo, but the vitamin E-supplemented group showed no change in this index of lipid peroxidation. The researchers noted that study results are consistent with the concept that vitamin E provides protection against exercise-induced oxidative injury (162).

In two studies evaluating the effects of vitamin E on performance of trained swimmers, swimming speed did not differ significantly between vitamin E-supplemented swimmers and those receiving placebo (163,164). Effects of vitamin E on physical performance and tissue damage were also evaluated in a group of mountain climbers. In unsupplemented mountain climbers, prolonged exposure to physical exertion at high altitudes while climbing resulted in significantly increased breath pentane output and decreased physical performance, as demonstrated by a significant decrease in anaerobic threshold. In contrast, vitamin E supplementation (400 IU/day) prevented the increase in breath pentane exhalation and the decrease in anaerobic threshold. The researchers concluded that vitamin E has a beneficial effect on cell protection and physical performance, at least at high altitude (165).

As research continues on the protective role of vitamin E in exercise, study results have shown an increased requirement for vitamin E to prevent lipid peroxidation associated with strenuous exercise.

XI. SUMMARY

Increasing evidence implicates free radical-mediated cell damage in the development of various degenerative diseases and conditions. Susceptibility of the body to free radical stress and peroxidative damage is related to the balance between the free radical load and the adequacy of antioxidant defenses. Levels of antioxidants shown to be protective against free radical damage are substantially higher than intakes readily obtainable from normal diets. As studies continue on the beneficial effects of vitamin E and other antioxidants in counteracting peroxidative damage in the body, increased intakes of vitamin E and other antioxidant nutrients can provide protection from the increasingly high free radical loads deriving from environmental sources and associated with current lifestyle habits.

REFERENCES

1. Bjorneboe A, Bjorneboe GE, Drevon CA. Absorption, transport and distribution of vitamin E. J Nutr 1990; 120:233–242.
2. Brigelius–Flohe R, Traber MG. Vitamin E: function and metabolism. FASEB J 1999; 13:1145–1155.
3. Horwitt MK. Interpretations of requirements for thiamin, riboflavin, niacin–tryptophan, and vitamin E plus comments on balance studies and vitamin B-6. Am J Clin Nutr 1986; 44:973–985.
4. Van Gossum A, Shariff R, Lemoyne M, Kurian R, Jeejeebhoy K. Increased lipid peroxidation after lipid infusion as measured by breath pentane output. Am J Clin Nutr 1988; 48:1394–1399.
5. Fritsma GA. Vitamin E and autoxidation. Am J Med Technol 1983; 49:453–456.
6. Maxwell SR. Prospects for the use of antioxidant therapies. Drugs 1995; 49:345–361.
7. Cross CE, Halliwell B, Borish ET, Pryor WA, Ames BN, Saul RL, McCord JM, Harman D. Oxygen radicals and human disease [clinical conference]. Ann Intern Med 1987; 107:526–545.

8. Aruoma OI. Nutrition and health aspects of free radicals and antioxidants [published erratum appears in Food Chem Toxicol 1994 Dec; 32:1185]. Food Chem Toxicol 1994; 32:671–683.
9. Inhibition of free radical chain oxidation by alpha-tocopherol and other plasma antioxidants. Nutr Rev 1988; 46:206–207.
10. Watson RR, Leonard TK. Selenium and vitamins A, E, and C: nutrients with cancer prevention properties. J Am Diet Assoc 1986; 86:505–510.
11. Machlin LJ. Vitamin E. In: Handbook of Vitamins. 2nd ed. New York: Marcel Dekker, 1991:99–144.
12. Carpenter D. Vitamin E deficiency. Semin Neurol 1985; 5:238–247.
13. Sokol RJ. Vitamin E deficiency and neurologic disease. Annu Rev Nutr 1988; 8:351–373.
14. Satya–Murti S, Howard L, Krohel G, Wolf B. The spectrum of neurologic disorder from vitamin E deficiency. Neurology 1986; 36:917–921.
15. Vitamin E deficiency and neurologic dysfunction. Nutr Rev 1986; 44:268–269.
16. Lloyd JK. The importance of vitamin E in human nutrition. Acta Pediatr Scand 1990; 79:6–11.
17. Vandewoude MG, Vandewoude MF, De Leeuw IH. Vitamin E status in patients on parenteral nutrition receiving Intralipid. JPEN J Parenter Enteral Nutr 1986; 10:303–305.
18. Kelly FJ, Sutton GL. Plasma and red blood cell vitamin E status of patients on total parenteral nutrition. JPEN J Parenter Enteral Nutr 1989; 13:510–515.
19. Willett WC, Stampfer MJ, Underwood BA, Taylor JO, Hennekens CH. Vitamins A, E, and carotene: effects of supplementation on their plasma levels. Am J Clin Nutr 1983; 38:559–566.
20. Jacobson HN. Dietary standards and future developments. Free Radic Biol Med 1987; 3:209–213.
21. Lemoyne M, Van Gossum A, Kurian R, Ostro M, Axler J, Jeejeebhoy KN. Breath pentane analysis as an index of lipid peroxidation: a functional test of vitamin E status. Am J Clin Nutr 1987; 46:267–272.
22. Borek C, Ong A, Mason H, Donahue L, Biaglow JE. Selenium and vitamin E inhibit radiogenic and chemically induced transformation in vitro via different mechanisms. Proc Natl Acad Sci USA 1986; 83:1490–1494.
23. Prasad KN, Edwards–Prasad J. Effect of tocopherol (vitamin E) acid succinate on morphological alterations and growth inhibition in melanoma cells in culture. Cancer Res 1982; 42:550–555.
24. Horvath PM, Ip C. Synergistic effect of vitamin E and selenium in the chemoprevention of mammary carcinogenesis in rats. Cancer Res 1983; 43:5335–5341.
25. Cook MG, McNamara P. Effect of dietary vitamin E on dimethylhydrazine-induced colonic tumors in mice. Cancer Res 1980; 40:1329–1331.
26. Toth B, Patil K. Enhancing effect of vitamin E on murine intestinal tumorigenesis by 1,2-dimethylhydrazine dihydrochloride. J Natl Cancer Inst 1983; 70:1107–1111.
27. Odeleye OE, Eskelson CD, Mufti SI, Watson RR. Vitamin E inhibition of lipid peroxidation and ethanol-mediated promotion of esophageal tumorigenesis. Nutr Cancer 1992; 17:223–234.
28. Odukoya O, Hawach F, Shklar G. Retardation of experimental oral cancer by topical vitamin E. Nutr Cancer 1984; 6:98–104.
29. Trickler D, Shklar G. Prevention by vitamin E of experimental oral carcinogenesis. J Natl Cancer Inst 1987; 78:165–169.
30. Shklar G, Schwartz J. Tumor necrosis factor in experimental cancer regression with alphatocopherol, beta-carotene, canthaxanthin and algae extract. Eur J Cancer Clin Oncol 1988; 24:839–850.
31. Shklar G, Schwartz J, Trickler D, Reid S. Regression of experimental cancer by oral administration of combined alpha-tocopherol and beta-carotene. Nutr Cancer 1989; 12:321–325.
32. Shklar G, Schwartz J, Trickler D, Reid S. Regression of experimental cancer by oral administration of combined alpha-tocopherol and beta-carotene. Nutr Cancer 1989; 12:321–325.
33. Perchellet JP, Abney NL, Thomas RM, Guislain YL, Perchellet EM. Effects of combined treatments with selenium, glutathione, and vitamin E on glutathione peroxidase activity, ornithine decarboxylase induction, and complete and multistage carcinogenesis in mouse skin. Cancer Res 1987; 47:477–485.
34. Shklar G, Schwartz JL, Trickler DP, Reid S. Prevention of experimental cancer and immunostimulation by vitamin E (immunosurveillance). J Oral Pathol Med 1990; 19:60–64.
35. Knekt P, Aromaa A, Maatela J, Aaran RK, Nikkari T, Hakama M, Hakulinen T, Peto R, Saxen E, Teppo L. Serum vitamin E and risk of cancer among Finnish men during a 10-year follow-up. Am J Epidemiol 1988; 127:28–41.

36. Salonen JT, Salonen R, Lappetelainen R, Maenpaa PH, Alfthan G, Puska P. Risk of cancer in relation to serum concentrations of selenium and vitamins A and E: matched case–control analysis of prospective data. Br Med J (Clin Res Ed) 1985; 290:417–420.
37. Knekt P, Aromaa A, Maatela J, Alfthan G, Aaran RK, Teppo L, Hakama M. Serum vitamin E, serum selenium and the risk of gastrointestinal cancer. Int J Cancer 1988; 42:846–850.
38. Knekt P. Serum vitamin E level and risk of female cancers. Int J Epidemiol 1988; 17:281–286.
39. Stahelin HB, Rosel F, Buess E, Brubacher G. Cancer, vitamins, and plasma lipids: prospective Basel study. J Natl Cancer Inst 1984; 73:1463–1468.
40. Eichholzer M, Stahelin HB, Ludin E, Bernasconi F. Smoking, plasma vitamins C, E, retinol, and carotene, and fatal prostate cancer: seventeen-year follow-up of the prospective Basel study. Prostate 1999; 38:189–198.
41. Eichholzer M, Stahelin HB, Gey KF, Ludin E, Bernasconi F. Prediction of male cancer mortality by plasma levels of interacting vitamins: 17-year follow-up of the prospective Basel study. Int J Cancer 1996; 66:145–150.
42. Willett WC, Polk BF, Underwood BA, Stampfer MJ, Pressel S, Rosner B, Taylor JO, Schneider K, Hames CG. Relation of serum vitamins A and E and carotenoids to the risk of cancer. N Engl J Med 1984; 310:430–434.
43. Nomura AM, Stemmermann GN, Heilbrun LK, Salkeld RM, Vuilleumier JP. Serum vitamin levels and the risk of cancer of specific sites in men of Japanese ancestry in Hawaii. Cancer Res 1985; 45:2369–2372.
44. Comstock GW, Helzlsouer KJ, Bush TL. Prediagnostic serum levels of carotenoids and vitamin E as related to subsequent cancer in Washington County, Maryland. Am J Clin Nutr 1991; 53:260S–264S.
45. Wald NJ, Thompson SG, Densem JW, Boreham J, Bailey A. Serum vitamin E and subsequent risk of cancer. Br J Cancer 1987; 56:69–72.
46. Wald NJ, Boreham J, Hayward JL, Bulbrook RD. Plasma retinol, beta-carotene and vitamin E levels in relation to the future risk of breast cancer. Br J Cancer 1984; 49:321–324.
47. Singh RB, Niaz MA, Rastogi V, Beegom R, Singh NK. Diet, antioxidants and risk of cancer: a case–control study. J Nutr Environ Med (Abingdon) 1997; 7:267–274.
48. Menkes MS, Comstock GW, Vuilleumier JP, Helsing KJ, Rider AA, Brookmeyer R. Serum beta-carotene, vitamins A and E, selenium, and the risk of lung cancer. N Engl J Med 1986; 315:1250–1254.
49. LeGardeur BY, Lopez A, Johnson WD. A case–control study of serum vitamins A, E, and C in lung cancer patients. Nutr Cancer 1990; 14:133–140.
50. Miyamoto H, Araya Y, Ito M, Isobe H, Dosaka H, Shimizu T, Kishi F, Yamamoto I, Honma H, Kawakami Y. Serum selenium and vitamin E concentrations in families of lung cancer patients. Cancer 1987; 60:1159–1162.
51. Knekt P, Jarvinen R, Seppanen R, Rissanen A, Aromaa A, Heinonen OP, Albanes D, Heinonen M, Pukkala E, Teppo L. Dietary antioxidants and the risk of lung cancer [see comments]. Am J Epidemiol 1991; 134:471–479.
52. Harris RW, Key TJ, Silcocks PB, Bull D, Wald NJ. A case–control study of dietary carotene in men with lung cancer and in men with other epithelial cancers. Nutr Cancer 1991; 15:63–68.
53. Lee BW, Wain JC, Kelsey KT, Wiencke JK, Christian DC. Association between diet and lung cancer location. Am J Respir Crit Care Med 1998; 158:1197–1203.
54. Stefani ED, Boffetta P, Deneo-Pellegrini H, Mendilaharsu M, Carzoglio JC, Ronco A, Olivera L. Dietary antioxidants and lung cancer risk: a case–control study in Uruguay. Nutr Cancer 1999; 34:100–110.
55. Mayne ST, Janerich DT, Greenwald P, Chorost S, Tucci C, Zaman MB, Melamed MR, Kiely M, McKneally MF. Dietary beta carotene and lung cancer risk in U. S. nonsmokers. J Natl Cancer Inst 1994; 86:33–38.
56. Palan PR, Mikhail MS, Basu J, Romney L. Plasma levels of antioxidant beta-carotene and alpha-tocopherol in uterine cervix dysplasias and cancer. Nutr Cancer 1991; 15:13–20.
57. Verreault R, Chu J, Mandelson M, Shy K. A case–control study of diet and invasive cervical cancer. Int J Cancer 1989; 43:1050–1054.
58. Peng YM, Peng YS, Childers JM, Hatch KD, Roe DJ, Lin Y, Lin P. Concentrations of carotenoids, tocopherols, and retinol in paired plasma and cervical tissue of patients with cervical cancer, precancer, and noncancerous diseases. Cancer Epidemiol Biomarkers Prev 1998; 7:347–350.

59. Helzlsouer KJ, Alberg AJ, Norkus PE, Morris JS, Hoffman SC, Comstock GW. Prospective study of serum micronutrients and ovarian cancer [see comments]. J Natl Cancer Inst 1996; 88:32–37.
60. Dorgan JF, Sowell A, Swanson CA, Potischman N, Miller R, Schussler N, Stephenson HE Jr. Relationships of serum carotenoids, retinol, alpha-tocopherol, and selenium with breast cancer risk: results from a prospective study in Columbia, Missouri (United States). Cancer Causes Control 1998; 9:89–97.
61. Negri E, La Vecchia C, Franceschi S, Levi F, Parazzini F. Intake of selected micronutrients and the risk of endometrial carcinoma. Cancer 1996; 77:917–923.
62. Freudenheim JL, Marshall JR, Vena JE, Laughlin R, Brasure JR, Swanson MK, Nemoto T, Graham S. Premenopausal breast cancer risk and intake of vegetables, fruits, and related nutrients. J Natl Cancer Inst 1996; 88:340–348.
63. Gridley G, McLaughlin JK, Block G, Blot WJ, Winn DM, Greenberg RS, Schoenberg JB, Preston-Martin S, Austin DF, Fraumeni JF Jr. Diet and oral and pharyngeal cancer among blacks. Nutr Cancer 1990; 14:219–225.
64. Gridley G, McLaughlin JK, Block G, Blot WJ, Gluch M, Fraumeni JF Jr. Vitamin supplement use and reduced risk of oral and pharyngeal cancer. Am J Epidemiol 1992; 135:1083–1092.
65. Manoharan S, Nagini S. Lipid peroxidation and antioxidant status in oral cancer patients. Med Sci Res 1994; 22:291–292.
66. de Vries N, Snow GB. Relationships of vitamins A and E and beta-carotene serum levels to head and neck cancer patients with and without second primary tumors. Eur Arch Otorhinolaryngol 1990; 247:368–370.
67. Zheng W, Sellers TA, Doyle TJ, Kushi LH, Potter JD, Folsom AR. Retinol, antioxidant vitamins, and cancers of the upper digestive tract in a prospective cohort study of postmenopausal women. Am J Epidemiol 1995; 142:955–960.
68. Buiatti E, Palli D, Decarli A, et al. A case–control study of gastric cancer and diet in Italy: II. Association with nutrients. Int J Cancer 1990; 45:896–901.
69. Bostick RM, Potter JD, McKenzie DR, Sellers TA, Kushi LH, Steinmetz KA, Folsom AR. Reduced risk of colon cancer with high intake of vitamin E: the Iowa Women's Health Study. Cancer Res 1993; 53:4230–4237.
70. Choi MA, Kim BS, Yu R. Serum antioxidative vitamin levels and lipid peroxidation in gastric carcinoma patients. Cancer Lett 1999; 136:89–93.
71. D'Avanzo B, Ron E, La Vecchia C, Francaschi S, Negri E, Zleglar R. Selected micronutrient intake and thyroid carcinoma risk. Cancer 1997; 79:2186–2192.
72. Dasgupta J, Sanyal U, Das S. Vitamin E—its status and role in leukemia and lymphoma. Neoplasma 1993; 40:235–240.
73. Deneo–Pellegrini H, De Stefani E, Ronco A, Mendilaharsu M. Foods, nutrients and prostate cancer: a case–control study in Uruguay. Br J Cancer 1999; 80:591–597.
74. Hennekens CH, Stampfer MJ, Willett W. Micronutrients and cancer chemoprevention. Cancer Detect Prev 1984; 7:147–158.
75. Blot WJ, Li JY, Taylor PR, et al. Nutrition intervention trials in Linxian, China: supplementation with specific vitamin/mineral combinations, cancer incidence, and disease-specific mortality in the general population [see comments]. J Natl Cancer Inst 1993; 85:1483–1492.
76. Greenberg ER, Baron JA, Tosteson TD, et al. A clinical trial of antioxidant vitamins to prevent colorectal adenoma. Polyp Prevention Study Group [see comments]. N Engl J Med 1994; 331:141–147.
77. The effect of vitamin E and beta carotene on the incidence of lung cancer and other cancers in male smokers. The alpha-Tocopherol, beta-Carotene Cancer Prevention Study Group [see comments]. N Engl J Med 1994; 330:1029–1035.
78. Albanes D, Heinonen OP, Taylor PR, et al. alpha-Tocopherol and beta-carotene supplements and lung cancer incidence in the alpha-Tocopherol, beta-Carotene Cancer Prevention Study: effects of base-line characteristics and study compliance [see comments]. J Natl Cancer Inst 1996; 88:1560–1570.
79. Heinonen OP, Albanes D, Virtamo J, et al. Prostate cancer and supplementation with alpha-tocopherol and beta-carotene: incidence and mortality in a controlled trial [see comments]. J Natl Cancer Inst 1998; 90:440–446.
80. Woodson K, Tangrea JA, Barrett MJ, Virtamo J, Taylor PR, Albanes D. Serum alpha-tocopherol and subsequent risk of lung cancer among male smokers. J Natl Cancer Inst 1999; 91:1738–1743.

81. Kaugars GE, Silverman S Jr, Lovas JG, Brandt RB, Riley WT, Dao Q, Singh VN, Gallo J. A clinical trial of antioxidant supplements in the treatment of oral leukoplakia. Oral Surg Oral Med Oral Pathol 1994; 78:462–468.
82. Benner SE, Winn RJ, Lippman SM, Poland J, Hansen KS, Luna MA, Hong WK. Regression of oral leukoplakia with alpha-tocopherol: a community clinical oncology program chemoprevention study. J Natl Cancer Inst 1993; 85:44–47.
83. Esterbauer H, Dieber-Rotheneder M, Waeg G, Striegl G, Jurgens G. Biochemical, structural, and functional properties of oxidized low-density lipoprotein. Chem Res Toxicol 1990; 3:77–92.
84. Sato K, Niki E, Shimasaki H. Free radical-mediated chain oxidation of low density lipoprotein and its synergistic inhibition by vitamin E and vitamin C. Arch Biochem Biophys 1990; 279:402–405.
85. Esterbauer H, Jurgens G, Quehenberger O, Koller E. Autoxidation of human low density lipoprotein: loss of polyunsaturated fatty acids and vitamin E and generation of aldehydes. J Lipid Res 1987; 28:495–509.
86. Esterbauer H, Rotheneder M, Striegl G, Waeg G, Ashy A, Sattler W, Jurgens G. Vitamin E and other lipophilic antioxidants protect LDL against oxidation. Fat Sci Technol 1989; 91:316–324.
87. Steinberg D, Parthasarathy S, Carew TE, Khoo JC, Witzum JL. Beyond cholesterol-modifications of low-density lipoprotein that increase to its atherogenicity. N Engl J Med 1989; 320:915–924.
88. Jessup W, Rankin SM, De Whalley CV, Hoult JR, Scott J, Leake DS. alpha-Tocopherol consumption during low-density-lipoprotein oxidation. Biochem J 1990; 265:399–405.
89. Abbey M, Nestel PJ, Baghurst PA. Antioxidant vitamins and low-density-lipoprotein oxidation. Am J Clin Nutr 1993; 58:525–532.
90. Rifici VA, Khachadurian AK. Dietary supplementation with vitamins C and E inhibits in vitro oxidation of lipoproteins. J Am Coll Nutr 1993; 12:631–637.
91. Jialal I, Grundy SM. Effect of combined supplementation with alpha-tocopherol, ascorbate, and beta carotene on low-density lipoprotein oxidation [see comments]. Circulation 1993; 88:2780–2786.
92. Reaven PD, Khouw A, Beltz WF, Parthasarathy S, Witztum JL. Effect of dietary antioxidant combinations in humans. Protection of LDL by vitamin E but not by beta-carotene. Arterioscler Thromb 1993; 13:590–600.
93. Princen HM, van Poppel G, Vogelezang C, Buytenhek R, Kok FJ. Supplementation with vitamin E but not beta-carotene in vivo protects low density lipoprotein from lipid peroxidation in vitro. Effect of cigarette smoking. Arterioscler Thromb 1992; 12:554–562.
94. Smith TL, Kummerow FA. Effect of dietary vitamin E on plasma lipids and atherogenesis in restricted ovulator chickens. Atherosclerosis 1989; 75:105–109.
95. Wojcicki J, Rozewicka L, Barcew-Wisniewska B, Samochowiec L, Juzwiak S, Kadlubowska D, Tustanowski S, Juzyszyn Z. Effect of selenium and vitamin E on the development of experimental atherosclerosis in rabbits. Atherosclerosis 1991; 87:9–16.
96. Williams RJ, Motteram JM, Sharp CH, Gallagher PJ. Dietary vitamin E and the attenuation of early lesion development in modified Watanabe rabbits. Atherosclerosis 1992; 94:153–159.
97. Willingham AK, Nolanos C, Bohannan E, Canedella RJ. The effects of high levels of vitamin E on the progression of atherosclerosis in the Watanabe heritable hyperlipidemic rabbit. J Nutr Biochem 1993; 4:651–654.
98. Verlangieri AJ, Bush MJ. Effects of *d*-alpha-tocopherol supplementation on experimentally induced primate atherosclerosis. J Am Coll Nutr 1992; 11:131–138.
99. Gey KF, Puska P. Plasma vitamins E and A inversely correlated to mortality from ischemic heart disease in cross-cultural epidemiology. Ann NY Acad Sci 1989; 570:268–282.
100. Salonen JT, Salonen R, Penttila I, Herranen J, Jauhiainen M, Kantola M, Lappetelainen R, Maenpaa PH, Alfthan G, Puska P. Serum fatty acids, apolipoproteins, selenium and vitamin antioxidants and the risk of death from coronary artery disease. Am J Cardiol 1985; 56:226–231.
101. Kok FJ, de Bruijn AM, Vermeeren R, Hofman A, van Laar A, de Bruin M, Hermus RJ, Valkenburg HA. Serum selenium, vitamin antioxidants, and cardiovascular mortality: a 9-year follow-up study in The Netherlands. Am J Clin Nutr 1987; 45:462–468.
102. Gey KF, Puska P, Jordan P, Moser UK. Inverse correlation between plasma vitamin E and mortality from ischemic heart disease in cross-cultural epidemiology. Am J Clin Nutr 1991; 53:326S–334S.
103. Knekt P, Reunanen A, Jarvinen R, Seppanen R, Heliovaara M, Aromaa A. Antioxidant vitamin intake and coronary mortality in a longitudinal population study. Am J Epidemiol 1994; 139:1180–1189.

104. Street DA, Comstock GW, Salkeld RM, Schuep W, Klag MJ. Serum antioxidants and myocardial infarction. Are low levels of carotenoids and alpha-tocopherol risk factors for myocardial infarction? Circulation 1994; 90:1154–1161.
105. Sklodowska M, Wasowicz W, Gromadzinska J, Miroslaw W, Strzelcyk M, Malczyk J, Goch JH. Selenium and vitamin E concentrations in plasma and erythrocytes of angina pectoris patients. Trace Elem Med 1991; 8:113–117.
106. Riemersma RA, Wood DA, MacIntyre CC, Elton RA, Gey KF, Oliver MF. Risk of angina pectoris and plasma concentrations of vitamins A, C, and E and carotene [see comments]. Lancet 1991; 337:1–5.
107. Regnstrom J, Nilsson J, Moldeus P, Strom K, Bavenholm P, Tornvall P, Hamsten A. Inverse relation between the concentration of low-density-lipoprotein vitamin E and severity of coronary artery disease. Am J Clin Nutr 1996; 63:377–385.
108. Kushi LH, Folsom AR, Prineas RJ, Mink PJ, Wu Y, Bostick RM. Dietary antioxidant vitamins and death from coronary heart disease in postmenopausal women [see comments]. N Engl J Med 1996; 334:1156–1162.
109. Losonczy KG, Harris TB, Havlik RJ. Vitamin E and vitamin C supplement use and risk of all-cause and coronary heart disease mortality in older persons: the Established Populations for Epidemiologic Studies of the Elderly. Am J Clin Nutr 1996; 64:190–196.
110. Meyer F, Bairati I, Dagenais GR. Lower ischemic heart disease incidence and mortality among vitamin supplement users. Can J Cardiol 1996; 12:930–934.
111. Hodis HN, Mack WJ, La Bree L, Cashin–Hemphill L, Sevanian A, Johnson R, Azen SP. Serial coronary angiographic evidence that antioxidant vitamin intake reduces progression of coronary artery atherosclerosis. JAMA 1995; 273:1849–1854.
112. Rimm EB, Stampfer MJ, Ascherio A, Giovannucci E, Colditz GA, Willett WC. Vitamin E consumption and the risk of coronary heart disease in men [see comments]. N Engl J Med 1993; 328:1450–1456.
113. Stampfer MJ, Hennekens CH, Manson JE, Colditz GA, Rosner B, Willett WC. Vitamin E consumption and the risk of coronary disease in women [see comments]. N Engl J Med 1993; 328:1444–1449.
114. Dietary supplementation with n-3 polyunsaturated fatty acids and vitamin E after myocardial infarction: results of the GISSI-Prevenzione trial. Gruppo Italiano per lo Studio della Sopravvivenza nell'Infarto miocardico [see comments]. Lancet 1999; 354:447–455.
115. Stephens NG, Parsons A, Schofield PM, Kelly F, Cheeseman K, Mitchinson MJ. Randomised controlled trial of vitamin E in patients with coronary disease: Cambridge Heart Antioxidant Study (CHAOS) [see comments]. Lancet 1996; 347:781–786.
116. Harman D. Free radical theory of aging: the free radical diseases. Age 1984; 7:111–131.
117. Meydani SN, Meydani M, Barklund PM, Liu S, Miller RA, Cannon JG, Rocklin R, Blumberg JB. Effect of vitamin E supplementation on immune responsiveness of the aged. Ann NY Acad Sci 1989; 570:283–290.
118. Meydani SN, Barklund MP, Liu S, Meydani M, Miller RA, Cannon JG, Morrow FD, Rocklin R, Blumberg JB. Vitamin E supplementation enhances cell-mediated immunity in healthy elderly subjects [see comments]. Am J Clin Nutr 1990; 52:557–563.
119. Chandra RK. Effect of vitamin and trace-element supplementation on immune responses and infection in elderly subjects [see comments]. Lancet 1992; 340:1124–1127.
120. Penn ND, Purkins L, Kelleher J, Heatley RV, Mascie-Taylor BH, Belfield PW. The effect of dietary supplementation with vitamins A, C and E on cell-mediated immune function in elderly long-stay patients: a randomized controlled trial. Age Ageing 1991; 20:169–174.
121. de la Fuente M, Ferrandez MD, Burgos MS, Soler A, Prieto A, Miquel J. Immune function in aged women is improved by ingestion of vitamins C and E. Can J Physiol Pharmacol 1998; 76:373–380.
122. Meydani SN, Meydani M, Blumberg JB, Leka LS, Siber G, Loszewski R, Thompson C, Pedrosa MC, Diamond RD, Stollar BD. Vitamin E supplementation and in vivo immune response in healthy elderly subjects. A randomized controlled trial [see comments]. JAMA 1997; 277:1380–1386.
123. Wartanowicz M, Panczenko–Kresowska B, Ziemlanski S, Kowalska M, Okolska G. The effect of alpha-tocopherol and ascorbic acid on the serum lipid peroxide level in elderly people. Ann Nutr Metab 1984; 28:186–191.

124. Tolonen M, Sarna S, Halme M, Tuominen SE, Westermarck T, Nordberg UR, Keinonen M, Schrijver J. Anti-oxidant supplementation decreases TBA reactants in serum of elderly. Biol Trace Elem Res 1988; 17:221–228.
125. Tolonen M, Halme M, Sarna S. Vitamin E and selenium supplementation in geriatric patients. Biol Trace Elem Res 1985; 7:161–168.
126. Bunce GE, Hess JL. Cataract—what is the role of nutrition in lens health? Nutr Today 1988; 23:6–12.
127. Taylor A. Associations between nutrition and cataract. Nutr Rev 1989; 47:225–234.
128. Gerster H. Antioxidant vitamins in cataract prevention. Z Ernahrungsswiss 1989; 28:56–75.
129. Robertson JM, Donner AP, Trevithick JR. Vitamin E intake and risk of cataracts in humans. Ann NY Acad Sci 1989; 570:372–382.
130. Trevithick JR, Creighton MO, Ross WM, Stewart–DeHaan PJ, Sanwal M. Modelling cortical cataractogenesis: 2. In vitro effects on the lens of agents preventing glucose- and sorbitol-induced cataracts. Can J Ophthalmol 1981; 16:32–38.
131. Ross WM, Creighton MO, Inch WR, Trevithick JR. Radiation cataract formation diminished by vitamin E in rat lenses in vitro. Exp Eye Res 1983; 36:645–653.
132. Stewart–DeHaan PJ, Creighton MO, Sanwal M, Ross WM, Trevithick JR. Effects of vitamin E on cortical cataractogenesis induced by elevated temperature in intact rat lenses in medium 199. Exp Eye Res 1981; 32:51–60.
133. Creighton MO, Ross WM, Stewart–DeHaan PJ, Sanwal M, Trevithick JR. Modelling cortical cataractogenesis VII: Effects of vitamin E treatment on galactose-induced cataracts. Exp Eye Res 1985; 40:213–222.
134. Ross WM, Creighton MO, Stewart–DeHaan PJ, Sanwal M, Hirst M, Trevithick JR. Modelling cortical cataractogenesis: 3. In vivo effects of vitamin E on cataractogenesis in diabetic rats. Can J Ophthalmol 1982; 17:61–66.
135. Creighton MO, Sanwal M, Stewart–DeHaan PJ, Trevithick JR. Modelling cortical cataractogenesis. V. Steroid cataracts induced by solumedrol partially prevented by vitamin E in vitro. Exp Eye Res 1983; 37:65–76.
136. Gupta PP, Pandey DJ, Sharma AL, Srivastava RK, Mishra SS. Prevention of experimental cataract by alpha-tocopherol. Indian J Exp Biol 1984; 22:620–622.
137. Varma SD, Chand D, Sharma YR, Kuck JF Jr, Richards RD. Oxidative stress on lens and cataract formation: role of light and oxygen. Curr Eye Res 1984; 3:35–57.
138. Bhuyan KC, Bhuyan DK, Podos SM. The role of vitamin E in therapy of cataract in animals. Ann NY Acad Sci 1982; 393:169–171.
139. Ross WM, Creighton MO, Trevithick JR. Radiation cataractogenesis induced by neutron or gamma irradiation in the rat lens is reduced by vitamin E. Scan Microsc 1990; 4:641–650.
140. Jacques PF, Chylack LT Jr, McGandy RB, Hartz SC. Antioxidant status in persons with and without senile cataract. Arch Ophthalmol 1988; 106:337–340.
141. Knekt P, Heliovaara M, Rissanen A, Aromaa A, Aaran RK. Serum antioxidant vitamins and risk of cataract. Br Med J 1994; 305:1392–1394.
142. Rouhiainen P, Rouhiainen H, Salonen JT. Association between low plasma vitamin E concentration and progression of early cortical lens opacities. Am J Epidemiol 1996; 144:496–500.
143. Leske MC, Chylack LT Jr, He Q, Wu SY, Schoenfeld E, Friend J, Wolfe J. Risk factors for nuclear opalescence in a longitudinal study. LSC Group. Longitudinal Study of Cataract. Am J Epidemiol 1998; 147:36–41.
144. Lyle BJ, Mares–Perlman JA, Klein BE, Klein R, Palta M, Bowen PE, Greger JL. Serum carotenoids and tocopherols and incidence of age-related nuclear cataract. Am J Clin Nutr 1999; 69:272–277.
145. Pacht ER, Kaseki H, Mohammed JR, Cornwell DG, Davis WB. Deficiency of vitamin E in the alveolar fluid of cigarette smokers. Influence on alveolar macrophage cytotoxicity. J Clin Invest 1986; 77:789–796.
146. Sevanian A, Hacke AD, Elsayed N. Influence of vitamin E and nitrogen dioxide on lipid peroxidation in rat lung and liver microsomes. Lipids 1982; 17:269–277.
147. Chow CK, Plopper CG, Dungworth DL. Influence of dietary vitamin E on the lungs of ozone-exposed rats: a correlated biochemical and histological study. Environ Res 1979; 20:309–317.
148. Chow CK, Chen LH, Thacker RR, Griffith RB. Dietary vitamin E and pulmonary biochemical responses of rats to cigarette smoking. Environ Res 1984; 34:8–17.

149. Elsayed NM, Kass R, Mustafa MG, Hacker AD, Ospital JJ, Chow CK, Cross CE. Effect of dietary vitamin E level on the biochemical response of rat lung to ozone inhalation. Drug Nutr Interact 1988; 5:373–386.
150. Calabrese EJ, Victor J, Stoddard MA. Influence of dietary vitamin E on susceptibility to ozone exposure. Bull Environ Contam Toxicol 1985; 34:417–422.
151. Posin CI, Clark KW, Jones MP, Buckley RD, Hackney JD. Human biochemical response to ozone and vitamin E. J Toxicol Environ Health 1979; 5:1049–1058.
152. Hackney JD, Linn WS, Buckley RD, Jones MP, Wightman LH, Karuza SK, Blessey RL, Hislop HJ. Vitamin E supplementation and respiratory effects of ozone in humans. J Toxicol Environ Health 1981; 7:383–390.
153. Duthie GG, Arthur JR, James WPT, Vint HM. Antioxidant status of smokers and nonsmokers—effects of vitamin E supplementation. Ann NY Acad Sci 1989; 570:435–438.
154. Hoshino E, Shariff R, Van Gossum A, Allard JP, Pichard C, Kurian R, Jeejeebhoy KN. Vitamin E suppresses increased lipid peroxidation in cigarette smokers. J Parenter Enteral Nutr 1990; 14:300–305.
155. Davies KJ, Quintanilha AT, Brooks GA, Packer L. Free radicals and tissue damage produced by exercise. Biochem Biophys Res Commun 1982; 107:1198–1205.
156. Apple FS, Rhodes M. Enzymatic estimation of skeletal muscle damage by analysis of changes in serum creatine kinase. J Appl Physiol 1988; 65:2598–2600.
157. Packer L. Vitamin E, physical exercise and tissue damage in animals. Med Biol 1984; 62:105–109.
158. Kumar CT, Reddy VK, Prasad M, Thyagaraju K, Reddanna P. Dietary supplementation of vitamin E protects heart tissue from exercise-induced oxidant stress. Mol Cell Biochem 1992; 111:109–115.
159. Sumida S, Tanaka K, Kitao H, Nakadomo F. Exercise-induced lipid peroxidation and leakage of enzymes before and after vitamin E supplementation. Int J Biochem 1989; 21:835–838.
160. Kanter MM, Nolte LA, Holloszy JO. Effects of an antioxidant vitamin mixture on lipid peroxidation at rest and postexercise. J Appl Physiol 1993; 74:965–969.
161. Grievink L, Zijlsra AG, Ke X, Brunekreef B. Double-blind intervention trial on modulation of ozone effects on pulmonary function by antioxidant supplements. Am J Epidemiol 1999; 149:306–314.
162. Meydani M, Evans WJ, Handelman G, Biddle L, Fielding RA, Meydani SN, Burrill J, Fiatarone MA, Blumberg JB, Cannon JG. Protective effect of vitamin E on exercise-induced oxidative damage in young and older adults. Am J Physiol 1993; 264:R992–R998.
163. Sharman IM, Down MG, Norgan NG. The effects of vitamin E on physiological function and athletic performance of trained swimmers. J Sports Med Phys Fitness 1976; 16:215–225.
164. Lawrence JD, Bower RC, Riehl WP, Smith JL. Effects of alpha-tocopherol acetate on the swimming endurance of trained swimmers. Am J Clin Nutr 1975; 28:205–208.
165. Simon–Schnass I, Pabst H. Influence of vitamin E on physical performance. Int J Vitam Nutr Res 1988; 58:49–54.

5
Vitamin E Bioavailability, Biokinetics, and Metabolism

Maret G. Traber
*Oregon State University, Corvallis, Oregon, and
University of California, Davis, School of Medicine, Sacramento, California*

I. INTRODUCTION

Vitamin E bioavailability, biokinetics, and metabolism are dependent on intestinal absorption, plasma lipoprotein transport, and hepatic metabolism of unoxidized vitamin E (1). Studies using stable isotopes of vitamin E, genetic analysis of vitamin E-deficient subjects, and techniques of biochemistry and molecular biology have been instrumental in providing a basis for assessing vitamin E status in humans.

The definition of vitamin E is critical to understanding these concepts. Vitamin E includes a family of tocopherols and tocotrienols that have chain-breaking antioxidant activity. The tocopherols and the tocotrienols include α-, β-, γ-, and δ-, which differ in the number of methyl groups on the chromanol ring. Tocopherols have a phytyl tail, whereas tocotrienols have an unsaturated tail. Importantly, α-tocopherol is the only form of vitamin E that reverses deficiency symptoms in humans. Synthetic α-tocopherol (*all rac*) is not identical with the naturally occurring form. The naturally occurring form, *RRR*-α-tocopherol, represents only one of the eight stereoisomers present in *all rac-α*-tocopherol (*RRR*-, *RRS*-, *RSR*-, *RSS*-, *SRR*-, *SSR*-, *SRS*-, and *SSS*-). The 2S-stereoisomers disappear from the plasma faster (2); therefore, when *RRR* and *all rac-α*-tocopheryl acetates are administered in equal amounts, plasma and tissue ratios of natural to synthetic α-tocopherol equal 2 (3). Thus, *RRR*-α-tocopherol is twice as effective as *all-rac-α*-tocopherol in achieving elevations of plasma α-tocopherol (2–7). The following discussion will highlight the factors involved in this preference for *RRR*-α-tocopherol.

II. FACTORS THAT INFLUENCE BIOAVAILABILITY

A. Intestinal Absorption

1. Vitamin E Absorption Requires Bile and Pancreatic Secretions

Vitamin E absorption is dependent on processes necessary for fat digestion. Bile acids aid in the formation of mixed micelles and are essential for vitamin E absorption (8,9). Pancreatic lipases and esterases are required for triglyceride hydrolysis and cleavage of tocopheryl esters (10), a common form of vitamin E in dietary supplements. Generally, these esterases are quite effective; the apparent absorption of deuterated *RRR*-α-tocopherol was similar whether administered as α-tocopherol, α-tocopheryl acetate, or α-tocopheryl succinate (11). In the absence of biliary secretions or pancreatic secretions, vitamin E absorption and secretion into the lymphatic system is poor. In the absence of both, only negligible amounts of vitamin E are absorbed (8,9,12,13). Thus, vitamin E deficiency occurs as a result of malabsorption in patients with biliary obstruction, cholestatic liver disease, pancreatitis, or cystic fibrosis (14).

Interference in vitamin E absorption by inhibitors of cholesterol or triglyceride absorption has been reported. Plant sterol-containing margarines decrease cholesterol absorption and simultaneously interfere with vitamin E absorption (15). Similarly, in humans consuming 20–40 g/day of sucrose polyester, a fat-replacer that inhibits cholesterol absorption, plasma α-tocopherol concentrations decreased. Orlistat, an inhibitor of pancreatic lipases, also inhibited the increase in plasma α-tocopherol by 60% following a 400-IU dose of vitamin E. These data suggest that orlistat inhibits hydrolysis of α-tocopheryl acetate, and thus it impairs vitamin E absorption. However, the limitation in fat absorption by orlistat may also impair free tocopherol absorption because plasma α-tocopherol levels of subjects consuming normal diets decrease (16). Therefore, consumers of these products should take vitamin E supplements with meals at times when these fat-absorption inhibitors are not consumed.

2. Vitamin E Absorption Requires Chylomicron Synthesis and Secretion

The movement of vitamin E through the absorptive cells remains poorly understood; no intestinal tocopherol transfer proteins have been described. In the intestinal mucosa, chylomicrons containing dietary fat and fat-soluble vitamins, carotenoids, and other fat-soluble dietary components are synthesized and secreted into the lymph (17). Even in healthy individuals, the efficiency of vitamin E absorption estimated using radioactively labeled α-tocopherol is low (about 15–45%) (18).

Often it is assumed that differences in plasma concentrations of various forms of vitamin E result from differences in the degree of intestinal absorption; but, this is not true. In studies using deuterated tocopherols, discrimination between forms of vitamin E does not occur during their absorption (19,20). Various forms of vitamin E, such as α- and γ-tocopherols (21,22), or *RRR*- and *SRR*-α-tocopherols (19,20), showed similar apparent efficiencies of intestinal absorption and secretion in chylomicrons. Thus, in humans it is likely that all dietary forms of vitamin E are equally well absorbed and secreted into chylomicrons, despite the subsequent low plasma concentrations of the non–2R-α-tocopherol forms (23).

3. Vitamin E Absorption Relative to Dose Size

Plasma α-tocopherol levels in normal subjects can be raised only about two- to fourfold—regardless of the duration, size (>100 mg), or frequency of vitamin E supplementation (24–28). Although this limitation could result from a limitation in vitamin E absorption, as has been found in rats (29), more recent studies in humans using deuterated (d_3) vitamin E suggest that fractional vitamin E absorption in humans is not limited. Traber et al. (30) found a linear increase in plasma d$_3$-*RRR*-α-tocopherol areas under the curve (AUCs) in response to increasing doses from 15 to 150 mg d$_3$-*RRR*-α-tocopheryl acetate, whereas total plasma α-tocopherol was unchanged. Although the absorptive rate was not estimated, a linear increase in chylomicron d$_3$-*RRR*-α-tocopherol area under the curve (AUC) was also observed. These data suggest that vitamin E incorporation into chylomicrons and its subsequent secretion into plasma does not decrease with increasing dose size up to 150 mg.

B. Plasma Transport

1. Distribution of Vitamin E to Tissues During Lipolysis

During chylomicron catabolism in the circulation, some of the newly absorbed vitamin E is transferred to circulating lipoproteins and some remains with the chylomicron remnants. During lipolysis, vitamin E is also transferred to high-density lipoproteins (HDL), which can distribute it to all of the circulating lipoproteins, a process that appears to be catalyzed by the phospholipid transfer protein (PLTP) (31). Importantly, PLTP can also transfer α-tocopherol from HDL to the endothelial lining of capillary walls (32). This may be an important mechanism for maintenance of vascular wall antioxidant defenses.

2. Preferential Secretion of α-Tocopherol from the Liver

With chylomicron remnant uptake by the liver, a variety of vitamin E forms are delivered to the liver. However, only one form of vitamin E, *RRR*-α-tocopherol, is preferentially secreted by the liver (19,33,34), and it is likely that the other 2*R*-forms behave similarly (35). Thus, the liver, not the intestine, discriminates between tocopherols. The α-tocopherol transfer protein (α-TTP) is a likely candidate for this function. But, unlike other fat-soluble vitamins, which are secreted from the liver bound to a transport protein, α-tocopherol is not bound to α-TTP, but rather is transported in circulating lipoproteins.

The American diet contains large amounts of γ-tocopherol owing to the high consumption of soy bean and corn oils. Despite the high dietary γ-tocopherol intake, plasma α-tocopherol in nonvitamin E-supplemented subjects is about tenfold higher than γ-tocopherol, demonstrating the preference of the sorting mechanism for α-tocopherol. Moreover, plasma γ-tocopherol decreases when α-tocopherol supplements are consumed (36,37).

C. Hepatic α-Tocopherol Transfer Protein

α-TTP (30.5 kDa) has been purified and characterized from rat liver (38,39) and from human liver cytosol (40), and its cDNA sequence has been reported (41). It is present in hepatocytes (39) and in brain, in or near Purkinje cells (42,43).

Purified α-TTP transfers α-tocopherol between liposomes and microsomes (38). Hosomi et al. (16) studied in detail the structural characteristics of vitamin E analogues required for α-TTP recognition. Ligand specificity was assessed by evaluating the competition of nonlabeled vitamin E analogues and α-[^{3}H]tocopherol for transfer from liposomes to crude rat liver mitochondria in vitro. Relative affinities were *RRR*-α-tocopherol, 100%; β-tocopherol, 38%; γ-tocopherol, 9%; δ-tocopherol, 2%; α-tocopherol acetate, 2%; α-tocopherol quinone, 2%; *SRR*-α-tocopherol, 11%; α-tocotrienol, 12%; and Trolox, 9%. Traber and Arai (44) suggested that three structural features containing α-TTP recognition could be concluded from these data: (1) The three methyl groups on the chromanol ring are needed, but the methyl group at position 5 is especially critical based on the differences between β- and γ-tocopherols; (2) the hydroxyl group on the chromanol ring is essential; and (3) the phytyl chain structure and its orientation is important, but a tocopherol analogue without a side chain still possesses 10%

α-TTP affinity. Thus, γ-tocopherol, *SRR*-α-tocopherol, α-tocotrienol, and Trolox have roughly 10% the activity of *RRR*-α-tocopherol, thereby explaining why these forms of vitamin E are at low concentrations in the plasma, despite generous intakes.

III. VITAMIN E BIOKINETICS

A model of plasma vitamin E biokinetics has been developed using data from studies with deuterium-labeled stereoisomers of α-tocopherol (*RRR*- and *SRR*-) (45). *SRR*-α-Tocopherol was used to model nonspecific transport, whereas *RRR*- was used to model α-TTP-mediated α-tocopherol transport. It was assumed that intestinal absorption and chylomicron secretion of the two deuterated tocopherols (*RRR*- and *SRR*-α-tocopherols) were similar and that the initial inputs into the plasma occur simultaneously for the two labels. In three patients with a defect in the α-TTP gene, the fractional plasma disappearance rates of deuterium-labeled *RRR*- and *SRR*-α-tocopherols were rapid and similar (1.4 ± 0.6 and 1.3 ± 0.3 pools per day, respectively). However, in control subjects the fractional disappearance rate of deuterium-labeled *RRR*-α-tocopherol (0.4 ± 0.1 pools per day) was significantly ($p < 0.01$) slower than for *SRR*- (1.2 ± 0.6). The differences (0.8 ± 0.6 pools per day) between the *RRR*- and *SRR*-α-tocopherol rates in controls estimate the rate that *RRR*-α-tocopherol was resecreted by the liver into the plasma. Because *RRR*-α-tocopherol is returned to the plasma from the liver, its apparent turnover is slow. This recirculation of *RRR*-α-tocopherol results in the daily replacement of nearly all of the plasma *RRR*-α-tocopherol.

Consistent with the "slow" disappearance of *RRR*-α-tocopherol from the plasma, its apparent half-life in normal subjects was approximately 48 h (45), in contrast with *SRR*-α-tocopherol half-life of approximately 13 h (45) and γ-tocopherol half-life of approximately 15 h (46).

IV. DISTRIBUTION TO TISSUES

Vitamin E is transported in plasma lipoproteins, and the mechanisms of lipoprotein metabolism determine the delivery of vitamin E to tissues. Tissues likely acquire vitamin E by lipoprotein lipase-mediated lipoprotein catabolism and transfer from lipoproteins to tissues and between lipoproteins and by LDL receptor-mediated LDL uptake.

A. Vitamin E Delivery to Tissues

Peripheral tissues can acquire dietary vitamin E during chylomicron catabolism and can acquire α-tocopherol following its preferential secretion by the liver and uptake by nascent very low-density lipoproteins (VLDL). Vitamin E delivery from both chylomicrons and VLDL are mediated by lipoprotein lipase (47). This mechanism may be particularly important for tissues that express lipoprotein lipase, such as adipose tissue, muscle, and brain (47). Indeed, Sattler et al. (48) demonstrated in mice that overexpression of lipoprotein lipase in muscle resulted in increased muscle vitamin E content. Vitamin E can also exchange between the lipoproteins during lipolysis, as discussed in the foregoing.

One other important mechanism for the delivery of tocopherols to tissues is by the LDL receptor. By using fibroblasts with and without LDL receptor activity, Traber and Kayden (49) demonstrated that LDL containing vitamin E is taken up more effectively by fibroblasts with functional than by those with nonfunctional LDL receptor activity. Cohn et al. (50) demonstrated that in vivo both LDL receptor-dependent and nondependent pathways are important for tissue uptake of tocopherols.

B. Tissue Vitamin E

Deuterated α-tocopherol has been used to assess the kinetics and distribution of α-tocopherol into various tissue both in rats and in guinea pigs (51,52). From these studies, it is apparent that a group of tissues are in rapid equilibrium with the plasma α-tocopherol pool. Tissues, such as erythrocytes, liver, and spleen, quickly replace "old" with "new" α-tocopherol (53). Other tissues, such as heart, muscle, and spinal cord, have slower α-tocopherol turnover times. By far the tissue with the slowest α-tocopherol turnover times appears to be the brain. In general, the vitamin E content of the nervous system is spared during vitamin E depletion (54–56). Recent data suggest that this may be due to the function of the α-TTP (42,43).

Limited studies of human tissue α-tocopherol uptake have been carried out. Burton et al. (57) gave equimolar amounts of *RRR*-α- and *all rac*-α-tocopherol acetates labeled with deuterium (d_3 and d_6, respectively) to test the hypothesis that the uptake of vitamin E by tissues is dependent on the amounts and forms of vitamin E present in plasma. In two terminally ill subjects who took the deuterated tocopherols, the 30-mg dose yielded 6% deuterated form both in plasma and tissues, whereas the 300-mg dose yielded a 60% deuterated form; thus, a tenfold increase in dose resulted in a tenfold increase in fractional labeling. Importantly, the 300-mg dose doubled plasma and tissue α-tocopherol concentrations (Fig. 1).

V. METABOLISM

A. Chroman Ring Oxidation

α-Tocopherol quinone is the result of a two-electron oxidation of α-tocopherol. It arises from the reaction of α-tocopherol with a peroxyl radical, forming the tocopheroxyl radical and its subsequent oxidation (58). Two tocopheryl radicals can also react together forming a dimer, a stable end-product. Reduction of α-tocopherol quinone to α-tocopherol hydroquinone by NAD(P)H-dependent microsomal and mitochondrial enzymes has also been described (59). Urinary metabolites (Simon metabolites) with an opened chroman ring and a shortened tail (e.g., α-tocopheronic acid and its lactone) (60,61). In general, oxidation products are in low abundance in vivo, suggesting that reduction of the tocopheryl radical by other antioxidants is a predominant reaction (62).

B. Unoxidized Metabolites

2,5,7,8-Tetramethyl-2(2′-carboxyethyl)-6-hydroxychroman (α-CEHC) is an unoxidized metabolite of α-tocopherol. α-CEHC has an intact chroman structure and a shortened side chain (63,64). γ-CEHC is the corresponding γ-tocopherol metabolite, detected as a natriuretic factor, named LLU-α, for Loma Linda University metabolite-α, (65). Despite the higher α-/γ-tocopherol ratio in human plasma, urinary γ-CEHC excretion is higher than that of α-CEHC (7,66). It has been suggested that most of the absorbed γ-tocopherol is converted to γ-CEHC (67). δ-CEHC has also been described; it was detected in the urine of rats given tritium-labeled δ-tocopherol intravenously (68).

In the liver, it likely that α-tocopherol is salvaged by α-TTP and secreted into plasma, whereas the other forms are metabolized. This hypothesis is supported by the observation that synthetic *all rac*-α-tocopherol is more readily converted to α-CEHC than is natural *RRR*-α-tocopherol (7). It seems likely that these metabolites are synthesized in the liver, transported in the plasma, and secreted in the urine. Stahl et al. (69) reported that plasma concentrations of α-CEHC in subjects were $0.007 \pm 0.003 \mu M$ and of γ-CEHC were $0.066 \pm 0.15 \mu M$, whereas plasma α-tocopherol concentrations were $43.3 \pm 17.3 \mu M$, and γ-tocopherol $2.6 \pm 1.3 \mu M$.

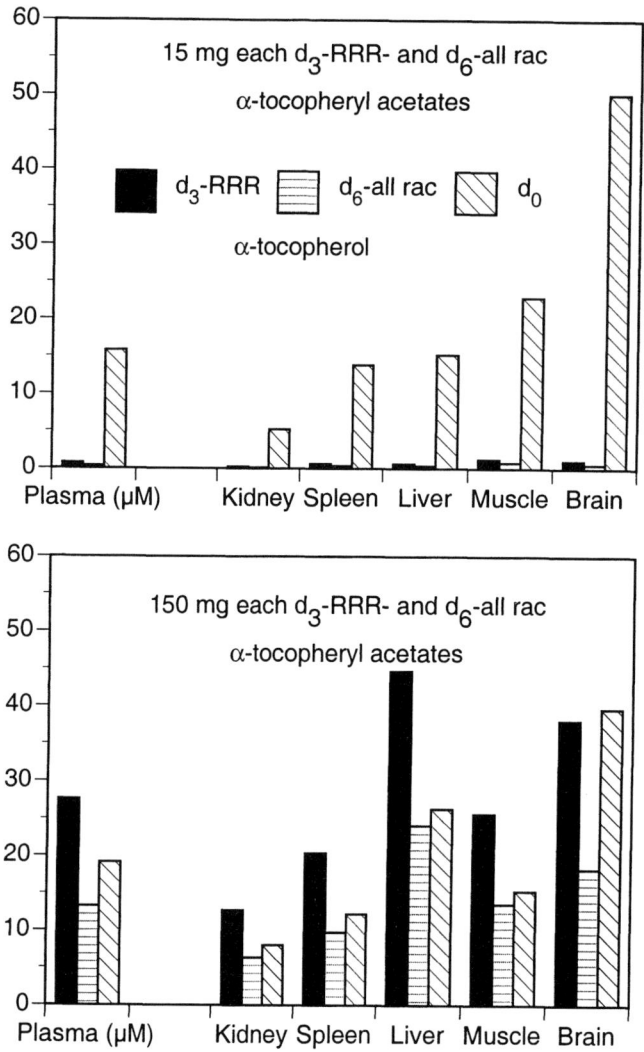

Figure 1 To obtain a variety of tissues following long-term consumption of deuterated α-tocopheryl acetates, two terminally ill subjects were enlisted to consume deuterated vitamin E (3). At death an autopsy was performed to obtain various tissues. One subject took 30 mg (15 mg d_3-*RRR*- and 15 mg d_6-*all-rac*-α-tocopheryl acetates) for 361 days; the other subject (A6690) took 300 mg (150 mg d_3-*RRR*- and 150 mg d_6-*all-rac*-α-tocopheryl acetates) for 615 days. Deuterated and unlabeled α-tocopherol concentrations in selected tissues (nmol/mg) and in plasma (μM) are shown.

VI. CONCLUSIONS

Vitamin E bioavailability, biokinetics, and metabolism have been discussed with an emphasis on α-tocopherol because α-tocopherol appears to be the form of vitamin E that is required by humans. α-TTP controls plasma α-tocopherol concentrations, and the plasma lipoproteins, in turn, deliver α-tocopherol to tissues. Increases in human plasma α-tocopherol result in increased tissue α-tocopherol. The preference for α-tocopherol, in contrast with other forms of vitamin E, is for some as yet unknown specific molecular function.

REFERENCES

1. Traber MG. Vitamin E. In Shils ME, Olson JA, Shike M, Ross AC, eds. Modern Nutrition in Health and Disease. Baltimore: Williams & Wilkins, 1999:347–362.
2. Kiyose C, Muramatsu R, Kameyama Y, Ueda T, Igarashi O. Biodiscrimination of alpha-tocopherol stereoisomers in humans after oral administration. Am J Clin Nutr 1997; 65:785–789.
3. Burton GW, Traber MG, Acuff RV, Walters DN, Kayden H, Hughes L, Ingold K. Human plasma and tissue α-tocopherol concentrations in response to supplementation with deuterated natural and synthetic vitamin E. Am J Clin Nutr 1998; 67:669–684.
4. Traber MG, Rader D, Acuff R, Brewer HB, Kayden HJ. Discrimination between *RRR*- and *all rac*-α-tocopherols labeled with deuterium by patients with abetalipoproteinemia. Atherosclerosis 1994; 108:27–37.
5. Acuff RV, Thedford SS, Hidiroglou NN, Papas AM, Odom TAJ. Relative bioavailability of *RRR*- and *all-rac*-alpha-tocopheryl acetate in humans: studies using deuterated compounds. Am J Clin Nutr 1994; 60:397–402.
6. Acuff RV, Dunworth RG, Webb LW, Lane JR. Transport of deuterium-labeled tocopherols during pregnancy. Am J Clin Nutr 1998; 67:459–464.
7. Traber MG, Elsner A, Brigelius–Flohe R. Synthetic as compared with natural vitamin E is preferentially excreted as α-CEHC in human urine; studies using deuterated α-tocopherol acetates. FEBS Lett 1998; 437:145–148.
8. Gallo–Torres H. Obligatory role of bile for the intestinal absorption of vitamin E. Lipids 1970; 5:379–384.
9. Sokol RJ, Heubi JE, Iannaccone S, Bove KE, Harris RE, Balistreri WF. The mechanism causing vitamin E deficiency during chronic childhood cholestasis. Gastroenterology 1983; 85:1172–1182.
10. Nakamura T, Aoyama Y, Fujita T, Katsui G. Studies on tocopherol derivatives: V. Intestinal absorption of several d,1-3,4-3H2-alpha-tocopheryl esters in the rat. Lipids 1975; 10:627–633.
11. Cheesemen KH, Holley AE, Kelly FJ, Wasil M, Hughes L, Burton G. Biokinetics in humans of *RRR*-α-tocopherol: the free phenol, acetate ester, and succinate ester forms of vitamin E. Free Radic Biol Med 1995; 19:591–598.
12. Harries JT, Muller DPR. Absorption of different doses of fat soluble and water miscible preparations of vitamin E in children with cystic fibrosis. Arch Dis Child 1971; 46:341–344.
13. Sokol RJ, Reardon MC, Accurso FJ, Stall C, Narkewicz M, Abman SH, Hammond KB. Fat-soluble-vitamin status during the first year of life in infants with cystic fibrosis identified by screening of newborns. Am J Clin Nutr 1989; 50:1064–1071.
14. Sokol RJ. Vitamin E deficiency and neurological disorders. In: Packer L, Fuchs J, eds. Vitamin E in Health and Disease. New York: Marcel Dekker, 1993:815–849.
15. Gylling H, Puska P, Vartiainen E, Miettinen TA. Retinol, vitamin D, carotenes and alpha-tocopherol in serum of a moderately hypercholesterolemic population consuming sitostanol ester margarine. Atherosclerosis 1999; 145:279–285.
16. Tonstad S, Pometta D, Erkelens DW et al. The effect of the gastrointestinal lipase inhibitor, orlistat, on serum lipids and lipoproteins in patients with primary hyperlipidaemia. Eur J Clin Pharmacol 1994; 46:405–410.
17. Cohn JS, McNamara JR, Cohn SD, Ordovas JM, Schaefer EJ. Plasma apolipoprotein changes in the triglyceride-rich lipoprotein fraction of human subjects fed a fat-rich meal. J Lipid Res 1988; 29:925–936.
18. Blomstrand R, Forsgren L. Labelled tocopherols in man. Int J Vitam Nutr Res 1968; 38:328–344.
19. Traber MG, Brown GW, Ingold KU, Kayden HJ. *RRR*- and *SRR*-α-tocopherols are secreted without discrimination in human chylomicrons, but *RRR*-α-tocopherol is preferentially secreted in very low density lipoproteins. J Lipid Res 1990; 31:675–685.
20. Traber MG, Burton GW, Hughes L, Ingold KU, Hidaka H, Malloy M, Kane J, Hyams J, Kayden HJ. Discrimination between forms of vitamin E by humans with and without genetic abnormalities of lipoprotein metabolism. J Lipid Res 1992; 33:1171–1182.

21. Traber MG, Kayden HJ. Preferential incorporation of α-tocopherol vs γ-tocopherol in human lipoproteins. Am J Clin Nutr 1989; 49:517–526.
22. Meydani M, Cohn JS, Macauley JB, McNamara JR, Blumberg JB, Schaefer EJ. Postprandial changes in the plasma concentration of α- and γ-tocopherol in human subjects fed a fat-rich meal supplemented with fat-soluble vitamins. J Nutr 1989; 119:1252–1258.
23. O'Byrne D, Traber MG, Packer L, Grundy S, Jialal I. Supplementation with alpha-tocotrienyl acetate enhances LDL oxidative resistance without lowering serum cholesterol in hypercholesterolemic humans. FASEB J 1999; 13:A536.
24. Dimitrov NV, Meyer C, Gilliland D, Ruppenthal M, Chenoweth W, Malone W. Plasma tocopherol concentrations in response to supplemental vitamin E. Am J Clin Nutr 1991; 53:723–729.
25. Reaven PD, Witztum JL. Comparison of supplementation of *RRR*-α-tocopherol and racemic α-tocopherol in humans. Effects on lipid levels and lipoprotein susceptibility to oxidation. Arterioscler Thromb 1993; 13:601–608.
26. Princen HMG, van Poppel G, Vogelezang C, Buytenhek R, Kok FJ. Supplementation with vitamin E but not β-carotene in vivo protects low density lipoprotein from lipid peroxidation in vitro. Effect of cigarette smoking. Arterioscler Thromb 1992; 12:554–562.
27. Princen HMG, van Duyvenvoorde W, Buytenhek R, van der Laarse A, van Poppel G, Leuven JAG, van Hinsbergh VWM. Supplementation with low doses of vitamin E protects LDL from lipid peroxidation in men and women. Arterioscler Thromb Vasc Biol 1995; 15:325–333.
28. Jialal I, Fuller CJ, Huet BA. The effect of α-tocopherol supplementation on LDL oxidation. A dose–response study. Arterioscler Thromb Vasc Biol 1995; 15:190–198.
29. Traber MG, Kayden HJ, Green JB, Green MH. Absorption of water miscible forms of vitamin E in a patient with cholestasis and in rats. Am J Clin Nutr 1986; 44:914–923.
30. Traber MG, Rader D, Acuff R, Ramakrishnan R, Brewer HB, Kayden HJ. Vitamin E dose response studies in humans using deuterated *RRR*-α-tocopherol. Am J Clin Nutr 1998; 68:847–853.
31. Kostner GM, Oettl K, Jauhiainen M, Ehnholm C, Esterbauer H, Dieplinger H. Human plasma phospholipid transfer protein accelerates exchange/transfer of alpha-tocopherol between lipoproteins and cells. Biochem J 1995; 305:659–667.
32. Desrumaux C, Deckert V, Athias A, Masson D, Lizard G, Palleau V, Gambert P, Lagrost L. Plasma phospholipid transfer protein prevents vascular endothelium dysfunction by delivering alpha-tocopherol to endothelial cells. FASEB J 1999; 13:883–892.
33. Traber MG, Sokol RJ, Burton GW, Ingold KU, Papas AM, Huffaker JE, Kayden HJ. Impaired ability of patients with familial isolated vitamin E deficiency to incorporate α-tocopherol into lipoproteins secreted by the liver. J Clin Invest 1990; 85:397–407.
34. Traber MG, Sokol RJ, Kohlschütter A, Yokota T, Muller DPR, Dufour R, Kayden HJ. Impaired discrimination between stereoisomers of α-tocopherol in patients with familial isolated vitamin E deficiency. J Lipid Res 1993; 34:201–210.
35. Ingold KU, Burton GW, Foster DO, Hughes L. Is methyl-branching in alpha-tocopherol's "tail" important for its in vivo activity? Rat curative myopathy bioassay measurements of the vitamin E activity of three 2*RS-n*-alkyl-2,5,7,8-tetramethyl-6-hydroxychromans. Free Radic Biol Med 1990; 9:205–210.
36. Handelman GJ, Machlin LJ, Fitch K, Weiter JJ, Dratz EA. Oral α-tocopherol supplements decrease plasma γ-tocopherol levels in humans. J Nutr 1985; 115:807–813.
37. Baker H, Handelman GJ, Short S, Machlin LJ, Bhagavan HN, Dratz EA, Frank O. Comparison of plasma α- and γ-tocopherol levels following chronic oral administration of either *all-rac*-α-tocopherol acetate or *RRR*-α-tocopheryl acetate in normal adult male subjects. Am J Clin Nutr 1986; 43:382–387.
38. Sato Y, Hagiwara K, Arai H, Inoue K. Purification and characterization of the α-tocopherol transfer protein from rat liver. FEBS Lett 1991; 288:41–45.
39. Yoshida H, Yusin M, Ren I, Kuhlenkamp J, Hirano T, Stolz A, Kaplowitz N. Identification, purification and immunochemical characterization of a tocopherol-binding protein in rat liver cytosol. J Lipid Res 1992; 33:343–350.
40. Kuhlenkamp J, Ronk M, Yusin M, Stolz A, Kaplowitz N. Identification and purification of a human liver cytosolic tocopherol binding protein. Protein Exp Purif 1993; 4:382–389.
41. Arita M, Sato Y, Miyata A, Tanabe T, Takahashi E, Kayden H, Arai H, Inoue K. Human alpha-tocopherol transfer protein: cDNA cloning, expression and chromosomal localization. Biochem J 1995; 306:437–443.

42. Hosomi A, Goto K, Kondo H, Iwatsubo T, Yokota T, Ogawa M, Arita M, Aoki J, Arai H, Inoue K. Localization of alpha-tocopherol transfer protein in rat brain. Neurosci Lett 1998; 256:159–162.
43. Copp RP, Wisniewski T, Hentati F, Larnaout A, Ben Hamida M, Kayden HJ. Localization of alpha-tocopherol transfer protein in the brains of patients with ataxia with vitamin E deficiency and other oxidative stress related neurodegenerative disorders. Brain Res 1999; 822:80–87.
44. Traber MG, Arai H. Molecular mechanisms of vitamin E transport. Annu Rev Nutr 1999; 19:343–355.
45. Traber MG, Ramakrishnan R, Kayden HJ. Human plasma vitamin E kinetics demonstrate rapid recycling of plasma *RRR*-α-tocopherol. Proc Natl Acad Sci USA 1994; 91:10005–10008.
46. Acuff RV, Webb LW, Brooks LJ, Papas AM, Lane JR. Pharmacokinetics of *RRR*-gamma-tocopherol in humans after a single dose administration of deuterium-labeled gamma-tocopherol in humans. FASEB J 1997; 11:A449.
47. Traber MG, Olivecrona T, Kayden HJ. Bovine milk lipoprotein lipase transfers tocopherol to human fibroblasts during triglyceride hydrolysis in vitro. J Clin Invest 1985; 75:1729–1734.
48. Sattler W, Levak–Frank S, Radner H, Kostner G, Zechner R. Muscle-specific overexpression of lipoprotein lipase in transgenic mice results in increased alpha-tocopherol levels in skeletal muscle. Biochem J 1996; 318:15–19.
49. Traber MG, Kayden HJ. Vitamin E is delivered to cells via the high affinity receptor for low density lipoprotein. Am J Clin Nutr 1984; 40:747–751.
50. Cohn W, Goss–Sampson M, Grun H. Plasma clearance and net uptake of alpha-tocopherol and low-density lipoprotein by tissues in WHHL and control rabbits. Biochem J 1992; 287:247–254.
51. Ingold KU, Burton GW, Foster DO, Hughes L, Lindsay DA, Webb A. Biokinetics of and discrimination between dietary *RRR*- and *SRR*-α-tocopherols in the male rat. Lipids 1987; 22:163–172.
52. Burton GW, Wronska U, Stone L, Foster DO, Ingold KU. Biokinetics of dietary *RRR*-α-tocopherol in the male guinea pig at three dietary levels of vitamin C and two levels of vitamin E. Evidence that vitamin C does not "spare" vitamin E in vivo. Lipids 1990; 25:199–210.
53. Burton GW, Traber MG. Vitamin E: antioxidant activity, biokinetics and bioavailability. Annu Rev Nutr 1990; 10:357–382.
54. Bourre J, Clement M. Kinetics of rat peripheral nerve, forebrain and cerebellum α-tocopherol depletion: comparison with different organs. J Nutr 1991; 121:1204–1207.
55. Vatassery GT. alpha-Tocopherol levels in various regions of the central nervous systems of the rat and guinea pig. Lipids 1978; 13:828–831.
56. Meydani M, Macauley JB, Blumberg JB. Influence of dietary vitamin E, selenium and age on regional distribution of α-tocopherol in the rat brain. Lipids 1986; 21:786–791
57. Burton GW, Traber MG, Acuff RV, Walters DN, Kayden H, Hughes L, Ingold KU. Human plasma and tissue alpha-tocopherol concentrations in response to supplementation with deuterated natural and synthetic vitamin E. Am J Clin Nutr 1998; 67:669–684.
58. Liebler DC. The role of metabolism in the antioxidant function of vitamin E. Crit Rev Toxicol 1993; 23:147–169.
59. Hayashi T, Kanetoshi A, Nakamura M, Tamura M, Shirahama H. Reduction of alpha-tocopherolquinone to alpha-tocopherolhydroquinone in rat hepatocytes. Biochem Pharmacol 1992; 44:489–493.
60. Simon EJ, Gross CS, Milhorat AT. The metabolism of vitamin E. I. The absorption and excretion of d-α-tocopheryl-5-methyl-C14-succinate. J Biol Chem 1956; 221:797–805.
61. Simon EJ, Eisengart A, Sundheim L, Milhorat AT. The metabolism of vitamin E. II. Purification and characterization of urinary metabolites of α-tocopherol. J Biol Chem 1956; 221:807–817.
62. Packer L. Vitamin E is nature's master antioxidant. Sci Am Sci Med 1994; 1:54–63.
63. Schultz M, Leist M, Petrzika M, Gassmann B, Brigelius–Flohe R. Novel urinary metabolite of alpha-tocopherol, 2,5,7,8-tetramethyl-2(2′-carboxyethyl)-6-hydroxychroman, as an indicator of an adequate vitamin E supply? Am J Clin Nutr 1995; 62(suppl):1527S–1534S.
64. Schultz M, Leist M, Elsner A, Brigelius–Flohé R. α-Carboxyethyl-6-hydroxychroman as an urinary metabolite of vitamin E. Methods Enzymol 1997; 282:297–310.
65. Wechter WJ, Kantoci D, Murray EDJ, D'Amico DC, Jung ME, Wang W-H. A new endogenous natriuretic factor: LLU-alpha. Proc Natl Acad Sci USA 1996; 93:6002–6007.
66. Lodge JK, Traber MG, Elsner A, Brigelius–Flohé R. A rapid method for the extraction and determination of vitamin E metabolites in human urine. J Lipid Res 2000; 41:148–154.

67. Swanson JE, Ben R, Burton GW, Parker RS. Urinary excretion of 2,7,8-trimethyl-2-(β-carboxyethyl)-6-hydroxychroman (γ-CEHC) represents a major pathway of elimination of γ-tocopherol in humans. FASEB J 1998; 12:A658.
68. Chiku S, Hamamura K, Nakamura T. Novel urinary metabolite of δ-tocopherol in rats. J Lipid Res 1984; 25:40–48.
69. Stahl W, Graf P, Brigelius–Flohe R, Wechter W, Sies H. Quantification of the alpha- and gamma-tocopherol metabolites 2,5,7,8-tetramethyl-2-(2′-carboxyethyl)-6-hydroxychroman and 2,7,8-trimethyl-2-(2′-carboxyethyl)-6-hydroxychroman in human serum. Anal Biochem 1999; 275:254–259.

6
Biological Activity of Tocotrienols

Stefan U. Weber and Gerald Rimbach
University of California, Berkeley, California

I. INTRODUCTION

Vitamin E was discovered by Evans in 1936 at the University of California at Berkeley (1), after Evans and Bishop had already described vitamin E deficiency in 1922 (2). Vitamin E was characterized as α-tocopherol (3). In the following years, other isoforms were isolated and characterized (4). Apart from other tocopherols, which are discussed in detail in Chapter 5, four tocotrienols were also discovered. When these forms of vitamin E were compared with α-tocopherol for their biopotency in a rat assay, which is based on the prevention of fetal resorption, none of them reached the biopotency of α-tocopherol. While d-α-tocotrienol still achieves 50% of the efficacy of *RRR*-α-tocopherol, which corresponds to 0.75 IU/mg (as compared with 1.49 IU/mg for *RRR*-α-tocopherol), the activity of d-β-tocotrienol is only 5% (0.08 IU/mg). The activities of γ- and δ-tocotrienol in the rat assay are unknown (5). This low biological activity of tocotrienols after oral supplementation has limited their practical use, although their antioxidant properties may be superior to tocopherols in certain applications.

The following will introduce the chemistry of tocotrienols, their redox properties, explain their metabolism and tissue distribution and will discuss different biological activities of tocotrienols as compared with tocopherols.

II. VITAMIN E ISOFORMS AND THEIR NATURAL SOURCES

The tocotrienols differ from the corresponding tocopherols only in their tail. Whereas tocopherols have a phytyl side chain attached to their chromanol nucleus, the tail of tocotrienols is unsaturated and forms an isoprenoid chain (Fig. 1) (6). This leaves the lipophilic tail shorter and more rigid, which may partly account for the functional differences between tocopherols and tocotrienols, as explained later in the chapter. The different isoforms of tocotrienols differ in their substituents on the chromanol nucleus. The α-form contains three methyl groups, the β- and γ- have two, and the δ-form only one (see Fig. 1) (7).

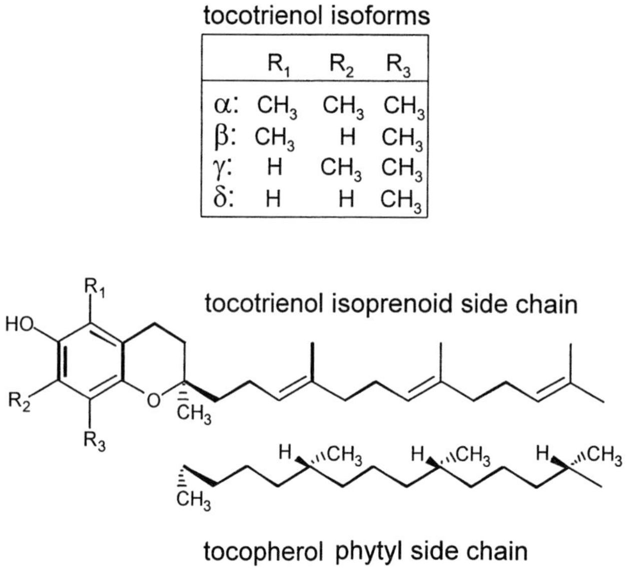
tocotrienol isoforms
R1 R2 R3
α: CH3 CH3 CH3
β: CH3 H CH3
γ: H CH3 CH3
δ: H H CH3
tocotrienol isoprenoid side chain
HO
R1
R2
R3
O
CH3
H CH3
tocopherol phytyl side chain

Figure 1 Chemical structures of tocotrienols: Isoforms differ in the methylation pattern on the chromanol nucleus.

Lipid-rich plant products are the main natural sources of vitamin E. Tocotrienols are found in high concentrations in palm oil and rice bran. Other natural sources include coconut oil, cocoa butter, soybean, barley, and wheat germ (Table 1). Moreover, tocotrienols have also been detected in meat and eggs. Sunflower, peanut, walnut, sesame, and olive oil, however contain only tocopherols (8,9).

III. ANTIOXIDANT ACTIVITY OF TOCOTRIENOLS

Vitamin E isoforms are potent antioxidants. The vitamin E molecule is incorporated into cellular lipid membranes, where it effectively inhibits the peroxidation chain of lipids. It scavenges the chain-propagation peroxyl radical (10). When comparing the effectiveness of different vitamin E homologues at least two factors need to be taken into account: the substituents on the chromanol nucleus and the properties of the side chain. In homogeneous solutions the reaction rate constant depends mainly on the number of methyl groups on the nucleus (11). In

Table 1 Vitamin E Content of Oils per 100 g Product

	Tocotrienols				Tocopherol	
Natural oil	α (mg)	β (mg)	γ (mg)	δ (mg)	α (mg)	Refs.
Palm	14.6	3.2	29.7	8.0	15.0	Ong/Sheppard
Rice bran	23.6	n.a.	34.9	—	32.4	Ong
Wheat germ	2.6	18.1	n.a.	n.a.	133.0	Sheppard
Coconut	0.5	0.1	—	—	0.5	Ong/Sheppard
Soy bean	0.2	0.1	0	0	7.5	Sheppard
Olive	0	0	0	0	11.9	Sheppard

membranes, the mobility of the molecule becomes important, which depends on the structure of the hydrophobic side chain.

Although no difference in radical-scavenging activity between α-tocopherol and α-tocotrienol was found in hexane, the activity of α-tocotrienol to scavenge peroxyl radicals is 1.5-fold higher in liposomes, when compared with α-tocopherol (12). In rat liver microsomes, the efficacy of α-tocotrienol to protect against Fe(II)+NADPH-induced lipid peroxidation was 40-fold higher than that of α-tocopherol. α-Tocotrienol also was 4.5 times more effective in the protection of cytochrome P450 against oxidative damage (12).

Several underlying reasons have been suggested to explain the raised efficacy of α-tocotrienol versus α-tocopherol, with the focus on the differences in tail structure. The chromanoxyl radical of α-tocotrienol is recycled faster than the corresponding α-tocopheroxyl radical. Nuclear magnetic resonance (NMR) studies have indicated, that α-tocotrienol is located closer to the membrane surface, which may facilitate recycling. Furthermore, α-tocotrienol had a stronger disordering effect on membranes than α-tocopherol, and was distributed more uniformly within the membrane. These properties likely enhance the interaction of chromanols with lipid radicals (13). In summary, there is substantial evidence that tocotrienols may be more efficient radicals scavengers in biomembranes than corresponding tocopherols.

IV. ABSORPTION AND DISTRIBUTION IN TISSUES

Although the efficacy of tocotrienols in membranes may be higher than that of tocopherols, uptake and distribution of tocotrienols after oral ingestion is less when compared with α-tocopherol. In hamsters fed with a mixture of vitamin E isoforms containing tocotrienols, α-tocopherol, was absorbed preferentially. However, tocotrienols could still be detected in the postprandial plasma of humans (14). Tocotrienols were found in all classes of lipoproteins (15). The liver contains a transfer protein that preferentially enriches very low-density lipoproteins (VLDL) with α-tocopherol (16,17). Therefore, α-tocopherol is secreted by the liver in a preferential manner, resulting in a decreased distribution of other vitamin E isoforms (18). For a more in-depth analysis of vitamin E transport please refer to Chapter 5.

The presence of a transfer protein that preferentially selects α-tocopherol may explain why all other forms of vitamin E have a lower biological activity in the gestation–resorption assay as compared with α-tocopherol. Even though tocotrienols have a higher radical-scavenging activity than tocopherols, they are less bioavailable after oral ingestion. It can be hypothesized, that tocotrienols are more effective antioxidants than tocopherols, if similar tissue levels are achieved. There is some evidence supporting this hypothesis. When supplementation was carried out such that comparable tissue concentrations of α-tocopherol and α-tocotrienol were reached in rats, the tocotrienol-supplemented heart tissues was more resistant to lipid peroxidation in vitro than the tocopherol-supplemented counterparts (11).

Interestingly, the distribution of vitamin E isoforms varies from tissue to tissue. In mouse skin, up to 15% of total vitamin E was composed of tocotrienols, whereas brain contained almost exclusively α-tocopherol (14,19). In the hamster also, tocotrienols were detected in all tissues except the brain. These results indicate that tissues may possess the ability to regulate the vitamin E homologue composition individually. Again, the α-TTP may play a major role. The message of the transfer protein was also found in the brain (20).

V. INHIBITION OF CHOLESTEROL SYNTHESIS

Vitamin E is attributed to a protective effect in cardiovascular diseases. In this scenario tocotrienols may exert protective effects exceeding those of tocopherols. In pigs with inherited hyperlipidemia, dietary tocotrienols from a tocotrienol-rich fraction (TRF) of palm oil reduced the concentrations of plasma cholesterol, apolipoprotein B, thromboxane B_2, and platelet factor 4, indicating a protective effect on endothelium and platelet aggregation (21). In a study carried out in rats fed with an atherogenic diet, both γ-tocotrienol and α-tocopherol lowered plasma lipid concentrations (22). In human studies conflicting results were obtained. TRF supplementation reduced cholesterol in an 8-week pilot study (23). In a 4-week trial these results were confirmed, and a carryover effect after the end of supplementation was reported (24). Interestingly, dietary α-tocopherol attenuated the cholesterol lowering effect of γ-tocotrienol in humans and chickens (24). In HepG2 cells γ-tocotrienol had a multifold enhanced hypercholesterolemic effect as compared with α-tocopherol (25). Although these studies had encouraging results, other studies reported conflicting effects. Even though antioxidant effects could be observed after tocotrienol supplementation of patients with hyperlipidemia and carotid stenosis, the cholesterol levels remained unchanged (26). Moreover, a recent double-blind placebo-controlled trial with 20 subjects found no effect of a vitamin E concentrate rich in tocotrienols (140 mg/day for 6 weeks) on serum lipids, lipoproteins, or platelet function in men with mildly elevated serum lipid concentrations (27).

Some of the conflicting results may be due to differing plasma levels of tocotrienols. The mechanism of lowering serum cholesterol is probably the regulation of cholesterol biosynthesis. An inhibitor of cholesterol synthesis was isolated from barley, which could be identified as α-tocotrienol (28). In HepG2 cells, 10 μM γ-tocotrienol increased the degradation of 3-hydroxy-3-methylglutaryl–coenzyme A reductase (HMG–CoA reductase), a key enzyme of the mevalonate pathway. Thus, γ-tocotrienol is believed to inhibit cholesterol synthesis by a posttranscriptional inhibition of HMG–CoA reductase (29). These in vitro studies suggest that tocotrienols are effective at 10 μM levels, which may not have been reached in all of the foregoing summarized human trials. In fact, the α-tocotrienol levels in the 1999 study reached only 0.17 μM after 6 weeks (27).

VI. INHIBITION OF LDL OXIDATION

The oxidation of LDL has been implicated in atherogenesis as a crucial step (30). Tocotrienols have been tested for their ability to protect against LDL oxidation. The ability of different vitamin E isoforms to spare vitamin C in ultraviolet (UV)-radiated solutions containing isolated LDL has been tested; vitamin C was spared more by α-tocotrienol then by α-tocopherol (31). Another study showed that α-tocotrienol inhibited LDL peroxidation as efficiently as α-tocopherol and more efficiently than γ-tocopherol or α-tocotrienol (15). Although several trials have shown protective effects of α-tocopherol against the progression of cardiovascular diseases, similar studies for tocotrienols are missing. The efficacy of tocotrienols may be restricted by their limited bioavailability.

VII. ANTICARCINOGENIC PROPERTIES

Tocotrienols belong to a phytochemical class of mixed and pure isoprenoids. These compounds share a common precursor, mevalonic acid (32). Tocotrienols are mixed isoprenoids, meaning that only a part, the lipophilic chain, is derived through the isoprenoid pathway. Isoprenoids exhibit anticarcinogenic properties. When different vitamin E isoforms were analyzed, it could be demonstrated that γ-tocotrienol and δ-tocotrienol inhibited tumor promotion in Raji cells most effectively (33). Tocotrienols from TRF inhibited the proliferation of human breast cancer cell lines (34,35). The inhibition was independent of the estrogen receptor status of the cell lines (36). Isoprenoids, among them tocotrienols, also suppressed the growth of murine B16 melanomas in vitro and in vivo (37). Recently, two groups have reported, that isoprenoids, including tocotrienols, induce cell cycle arrest in the G_1 phase and apoptosis in human and murine tumor cells (38,39). Because these effects can be observed with different isoprenoids, which are not antioxidants, it is likely that the anticancerigenic effects of tocotrienols are not necessarily related to their antioxidant properties.

VIII. NEUROPROTECTION

Glutamate is one of the main neurotransmitters in the central nervous system. Elevated levels of glutamate have been associated with a range of neurological disorders, including epilepsy, cerebral ischemia, Huntington's disease, and Parkinson's disease. In these disorders glutamate receptor-mediated cytotoxicity is believed to be one of the central mechanisms. Glutamate induces oxidative stress in C6 glial cells, and its toxicity can be mitigated by thiol antioxidants (40).

Recently, vitamin E isoforms were tested in a model of neuronal cell death, in which HT4 neuronal cells were challenged with glutamate (41). In this model tocotrienols inhibited the glutamate-induced cell death at much lower concentrations than tocopherols, indicating that this activity may not be related to antioxidant action. In fact, tocotrienols effectively inhibited the activation of pp60 c-src kinase, a kinase believed to be involved in glutamate-induced cell death.

Indications that vitamin E action may not necessarily be related to their antioxidant function have also been found earlier in other models, in which α-tocopherol, but not β-tocopherol, effectively inhibited protein kinase C (42). Recently, a new α-tocopherol-binding protein has been discovered, which may play an important role in mediation of the nonantioxidant actions of vitamin E (43).

IX. SKIN PROTECTION AGAINST OXIDANTS

Vitamin E isoforms are found in all layers of the skin and are an essential part of the antioxidant defense systems against environmental stressors. Surprisingly, murine skin contains relatively high levels of tocotrienols, compared with other organs (19). No tocotrienol was found in murine brain, as opposed to 5.4 nmol/mg tissue of α-tocopherol. In murine skin, however, 0.24 $\pm$ 0.2 nmol/mg tissue of α-tocotrienol and 0.76 $\pm$ 0.71 nmol/mg tissue of γ-tocotrienol were detected, whereas the α-tocopherol content remained the same as in brain tissue. Expressed as a percentage of total vitamin E, the α-tocotrienol content amounted to 3.4% and the γ-tocotrienol content to 10.4% (α-tocopherol, 85%). It is not clear why tocotrienols were preferentially distributed in the skin as opposed to other tissues.

When applied topically tocotrienols penetrate into the skin as readily as tocopherols. A tocotrienol-rich fraction of palm oil was used to explore the protective potential of vitamin E mixed against UV radiation and topical O_3. After UV exposure more vitamin E remained in the supplemented areas than in the vehicle-only–treated areas (44). The same was observed after O_3 exposure (45). Moreover, after O_3 exposure, lipid peroxidation, measured as malondialdehyde, was attenuated in the vitamin E-treated regions. These results point toward potential benefits of tocotrienols in models of environmental stress, even though further investigations are needed to characterize the protective effects in more detail.

X. CONCLUSIONS AND FUTURE DIRECTIONS

Tocotrienols make up a considerable portion of total vitamin E in many food sources. In vitro they exhibit enhanced antioxidant properties compared with tocopherols. Also, they exhibit cholesterol lowering, anticarcinogenic and neuroprotective properties, which may not be related to their antioxidant function. After oral ingestion, however, they are not recognized by their α-tocopherol transfer protein and thus have only a short half-life, which accounts for their low bioavailability. A more promising approach to utilize tocotrienols may be the topical application onto the skin. In this scenario, uptake and distribution within the skin does not depend on transfer proteins, thereby allowing active concentrations to be reached in the skin after topical exposure. The potential of tocotrienols in topical protection of the skin deserves further investigation.

ACKNOWLEDGMENT

The authors thank Celine Marquez for help with editing the manuscript.

REFERENCES

1. Evans HM, Emerson OH. The isolation from wheat germ oil of an alcohol, alpha-tocopherol, having the properties of vitamin E. J Biol Chem 1936; 113:319–332.
2. Evans HM, Bishop KS. On the existence of a hitherto unrecognized dietary factor essential for reproduction. Science 1922; 56:650–651.
3. Fernholz E. On the constitution of alpha-tocopherol. J Am Chem Soc 1938; 60:700–705.
4. Emerson OH, Emerson GA, Mohammed A, Evans HM. The chemistry of vitamin E: tocopherols from various soures. J Biol Chem 1937; 122:99–107.
5. Traber MG, Serbinova EA, Packer L. Biological activities of tocotrienols and tocopherols. In: Packer L, Hiramatsu M, Yoshikawa T, eds. Antioxidant Food Supplements in Human Health. New York: Academic Press, 1999:55–71.
6. Azzi A, Stocker A. Vitamin E: non-antioxidant roles. Prog Lipid Res 2000; 39:231–255.
7. Brigelius–Flohe R, Traber MG. Vitamin E: function and metabolism. FASEB J 1999; 13:1145–1155.
8. Sheppard AJ, Pennington JAT, Weihrauch JL. Analysis and distribution of vitamin E in vegetable oils and foods. In: Packer L, Fuchs J, eds. Vitamin E in Health and Disease. New York: Marcel Dekker, 1993.
9. Ong ASH. Natural sources of tocotrienols. In: Packer L, Fuchs J, eds. Vitamin E in Health and Disease. New York: Marcel Dekker, 1993:3–8.
10. Burton GW, Ingold KU. Autioxidation of biological molecules. I. The antioxidant activity of vitamin E and related chain-breaking phenolic antioxidants in vitro. J Am Chem Soc 1981; 103:6472–6477.
11. Serbinova EA, Packer L. Antioxidant properties of alpha-tocopherol and alpha-tocotrienol. Methods Enzymol 1994; 234:354–366.
12. Serbinova E, Kagan V, Han D, Packer L. Free radical recycling and intramembrane mobility in the antioxidant properties of alpha-tocopherol and alpha-tocotrienol. Free Radic Biol Med 1991; 10:263–275.
13. Suzuki YJ, Tsuchiya M, Wassall SR, Choo YM, Govil G, Kagan VE, Packer L. Structural and dynamic membrane properties of alpha-tocopherol and alpha-tocotrienol: implication to the molecular mechanism of their antioxidant potency. Biochemistry 1993; 32:10692–10699.
14. Hayes KC, Pronczuk A, Liang JS. Differences in the plasma transport and tissue concentrations of tocopherols and tocotrienols: observations in humans and hamsters. Proc Soc Exp Biol Med 1993; 202:353–359.
15. Suarna C, Hood RL, Dean RT, Stocker R. Comparative antioxidant activity of tocotrienols and other natural lipid-soluble antioxidants in a homogeneous system, and in rat and human lipoproteins. Biochim Biophys Acta 1993; 1166:163–170.

16. Ouahchi K, Arita M, Kayden H, Hentati F, Ben Hamida M, Sokol R, Arai H, Inoue K, Mandel JL, Koenig M. Ataxia with isolated vitamin E deficiency is caused by mutations in the alpha-tocopherol transfer protein. Nat Genet 1995; 9:141–145.
17. Arita M, Sato Y, Miyata A, Tanabe T, Takahashi E, Kayden HJ, Arai H, Inoue K. Human alpha-tocopherol transfer protein: cDNA cloning, expression and chromosomal localization. Biochem J 1995; 306:437–443.
18. Traber MG, Ramakrishnan R, Kayden HJ. Human plasma vitamin E kinetics demonstrate rapid recycling of plasma *RRR*-alpha-tocopherol. Proc Natl Acad Sci USA 1994; 91:10005–10008.
19. Podda M, Weber C, Traber MG, Packer L. Simultaneous determination of tissue tocopherols, tocotrienols, ubiquinols, and ubiquinones. J Lipid Res 1996; 37:893–901.
20. Hosomi A, Goto K, Kondo H, Iwatsubo T, Yokota T, Ogawa M, Arita M, Aoki J, Arai H, Inoue K. Localization of alpha-tocopherol transfer protein in rat brain. Neurosci Lett 1998; 256:159–162.
21. Qureshi AA, Qureshi N, Hasler–Rapacz JO, et al. Dietary tocotrienols reduce concentrations of plasma cholesterol, apolipoprotein B, thromboxane B_2, and platelet factor 4 in pigs with inherited hyperlipidemias. Am J Clin Nutr 1991; 53:1042S–1046S.
22. Watkins T, Lenz P, Gapor A, Struck M, Tomeo A, Bierenbaum M. gamma-Tocotrienol as a hypocholesterolemic and antioxidant agent in rats fed atherogenic diets. Lipids 1993; 28:1113–1118.
23. Qureshi AA, Qureshi N, Wright JJ, et al. Lowering of serum cholesterol in hypercholesterolemic humans by tocotrienols (palmvitee). Am J Clin Nutr 1991; 53:1021S–1026S.
24. Qureshi AA, Bradlow BA, Brace L, Manganello J, Peterson DM, Pearce BC, Wright JJ, Gapor A, Elson CE. Response of hypercholesterolemic subjects to administration of tocotrienols. Lipids 1995; 30:1171–1177.
25. Pearce BC, Parker RA, Deason ME, Qureshi AA, Wright JJ. Hypocholesterolemic activity of synthetic and natural tocotrienols. J Med Chem 1992; 35:3595–3606.
26. Tomeo AC, Geller M, Watkins TR, Gapor A, Bierenbaum ML. Antioxidant effects of tocotrienols in patients with hyperlipidemia and carotid stenosis. Lipids 1995; 30; 1179–1183.
27. Mensink RP, van Houwelingen AC, Kromhout D, Hornstra G. A vitamin E concentrate rich in tocotrienols had no effect on serum lipids, lipoproteins, or platelet function in men with mildly elevated serum lipid concentrations. Am J Clin Nutr 1999; 69:213–219.
28. Qureshi AA, Burger WC, Peterson DM, Elson CE. The structure of an inhibitor of cholesterol biosynthesis isolated from barley. J Biol Chem 1986; 261:10544–10550.
29. Parker RA, Pearce BC, Clark RW, Gordon DA, Wright JJ. Tocotrienols regulate cholesterol production in mammalian cells by post-transcriptional suppression of 3-hydroxy-3-methylglutaryl-coenzyme A reductase. J Biol Chem 1993; 268:11230–11238.
30. Steinberg D. Low density lipoprotein oxidation and its pathobiological significant. J Biol Chem 1997; 272:20963–20966.
31. Kagan VE, Serbinova EA, Forte T, Scita G, Packer L. Recycling of vitamin E in human low density lipoproteins. J Lipid Res 1992; 33:385–397.
32. Bach TJ. Some new aspects of isoprenoid biosynthesis in plants—a review. Lipids 1995; 30:191–202.
33. Goh SH, Hew NF, Norhanom AW, Yadav M. Inhibition of tumour promotion by various palm-oil tocotrienols. Int J Cancer 1994; 57:529–531.
34. Nesaretnam K, Guthrie N, Chambers AF, Carroll KK. Effect of tocotrienols on the growth of a human breast cancer cell line in culture. Lipids 1995; 30:1139–1143.
35. Guthrie N, Gapor A, Chambers AF, Carroll KK. Inhibition of proliferation of estrogen receptor-negative MDA-MB-435 and -positive MCF-7 human breast cancer cells by palm oil tocotrienols and tamoxifen, alone and in combination. J Nutr 1997; 127:544S–548S.
36. Nesaretnam K, Stephen R, Dils R, Darbre P. Tocotrienols inhibit the growth of human breast cancer cells irrespective of estrogen receptor status. Lipids 1998; 33:461–469.
37. He L, Mo H, Hadisusilo S, Qureshi AA, Elson CE. Isoprenoids suppress the growth of murine B16 melanomas in vitro and in vivo. J Nutr 1997; 127:668–674.
38. Yu W, Simmons–Menchaca M, Gapor A, Sanders BG, Kline K. Induction of apoptosis in human breast cancer cells by tocopherols and tocotrienols. Nutr Cancer 1999; 33:26–32.
39. Theriault A, Chao JT, Wang Q, Gapor A, Adeli K. Tocotrienol: a review of its therapeutic potential. Clin Biochem 1999; 32:309–319.
40. Han D, Sen CK, Roy S, Kobayashi MS, Tritscheler HJ, Packer L. Protection against glutamate-induced cytotoxicity in C6 glial cells by thiol antioxidants. Am J Physiol 1997; 273:R1771–1778.

41. Sen CK, Khanna S, Roy S, Packer L. Molecular basis of vitamin E action. Tocotrienol potently inhibits glutamate-induced pp60(c-Src) kinase activation and death of HT4 neuronal cells. J Biol Chem 2000; 275:13049–13055.
42. Tasinato A, Boscoboinik D, Bartoli GM, Maroni P, Azzi A. d-alpha-Tocopherol inhibition of vascular smooth muscle cell proliferation occurs at physiological concentrations, correlates with protein kinase C inhibition, and is independent of its antioxidant properties. Proc Natl Acad Sci USA 1995; 92:12190–12194.
43. Zimmer S, Stocker A, Sarbolouki MN, Spycher SE, Sassoon J, Azzi A. A novel human tocopherol-associated protein: cloning, in-vitro expression and characterization. J Biol Chem 2000;
44. Weber C, Podda M, Rallis M, Thiele JJ, Traber MG, Packer L. Efficacy of topically applied tocopherols and tocotrienols in protection of murine skin from oxidative damage induced by UV-irradiation. Free Radic Biol Med 1997; 22:761-769.
45. Thiele JJ, Traber MG, Podda M, Tsang K, Cross CE, Packer L. Ozone depletes tocopherols and tocotrienols topically applied to murine skin. FEBS Lett 1997; 401:167–170.

7
Vitamin C: From Molecular Actions to Optimum Intake

Sebastian J. Padayatty, Rushad Daruwala, Yaohui Wang, Peter K. Eck, Jian Song, Woo S. Koh, and Mark Levine
National Institute of Diabetes and Digestive and Kidney Diseases, National Institutes of Health, Bethesda, Maryland

I. DEFICIENCY OF VITAMIN C

A. Introduction

Vitamin C (ascorbic acid, ascorbate) is a water-soluble vitamin found widely in plants. Deficiency results in scurvy, a disease with an insidious onset, but fatal results. Vitamin C deficiency is now uncommon, although this was not always true. Scurvy was widespread until recent times, especially in northern latitudes whenever fruits and vegetables were scarce, and was endemic in many parts of Europe. More dramatic was its widespread occurrence whenever small or large bodies of men depended on stored rations, whether during military campaigns or ocean voyages. Large-scale fatalities from scurvy were often the limiting factor in these expeditions. It was so common during sea voyages that scurvy came to be regarded as the dread of sailors. After many false leads, it became clear that consumption of fruits and vegetables could prevent and cure this disease. However, preventive measures were only fitfully adopted by the merchant ships and navies. The widespread provision of antiscorbutic food, particularly citrus fruits, eventually eradicated this disease among sailors. Even so, scurvy was widespread among troops as recently as World War I. In fact, this was the impetus responsible for the studies that led to the identification of the antiscorbutic principle.

B. Scurvy and the Discovery of Ascorbic Acid

The earliest recorded descriptions of scurvy are probably bleeding from the gums and skin, described in Egyptian hieroglyphs circa 3000 BC. Hippocrates described the disease in 500 BC (1). Military campaigns from the Crusades to the Napoleonic wars, the American Civil War, and even World War I, were stymied by widespread and often fatal scurvy among troops. The explorer Robert Scott and his companions suffered from scurvy on the way back from the

South Pole and probably perished from it. Most sea voyages until recent times fell victim to it, despite early experience showing that it could be prevented by simple measures. For example, in 1600, 105 out of a total crew of 424 on the ships of the East India Company died of scurvy on the way to the Cape of Good Hope. However, none aboard the commander's ship died. He carried with him bottled lime juice and gave three teaspoons of it to any sailor with signs of scurvy.

Convincing evidence that fresh fruits and vegetables could prevent scurvy was gradually accepted after James Lind published his *Treatise on Scurvy*, in 1753 (2). Even then, scurvy was thought to be caused by many factors, including cold climate, dampness, lack of fresh air, foggy weather, and other unhealthy climatic or living conditions, in addition to the lack of fruits and vegetables. In the late 18th century, the Royal Navy made it mandatory to issue 1 oz. of lemon juice daily to every sailor after 2 weeks at sea, but this was enforced only in 1804. The term limey (for a British sailor) comes from the obligatory provision of lemon (after lime) juice to all sailors of the Royal Navy. Sailors in the merchant navies continued to suffer from scurvy for years later. Following the outbreak of scurvy during World War I, it was shown that germinating, but not dry, cereals and legumes were effective against scurvy in monkeys and guinea pigs. In 1928, Albert Szent-Gyorgyi isolated a six-carbon reducing substance from ox adrenals (3), oranges, and cabbages. In 1932, he (4) and C. C. King (5) showed this substance to be the antiscorbutic principle. Albert Szent-Gyorgyi named it ascorbic acid and was awarded the Nobel Prize in 1937.

C. Symptoms and Signs of Scurvy

Although vitamin C is concentrated in many tissues, these tissue stores are easily depleted. Lind reported the onset of the disease in sailors after 1 1/2 month at sea (2). The early symptoms are weakness, fatigue, listlessness, and lassitude. These were noted by Lind and confirmed others (6,7). Physical signs follow: these include perifollicular hyperkeratosis; erythema and purpura; bleeding into the skin, subcutaneous tissues, muscles, and joints; breakdown of wounds; swollen and friable gums; fever; and confusion. Untreated, scurvy is fatal. Although this disease is now rare, subclinical vitamin C deficiency may be common (8), especially because the first symptoms of deficiency are unremarkable and nonspecific. The more serious manifestations of scurvy, although rarely seen in clinical practice, serve to remind us to focus research on areas where vitamin C may have important roles.

The only proved function of vitamin C is the prevention of scurvy. Evidence suggests vitamin C may have many other functions in the body, albeit at concentrations higher than that required to prevent scurvy. However, whether vitamin C confers clear health benefits other than to prevent scurvy remains contentious. New data describing vitamin C absorption, bioavailability, dose–concentration relation, urinary excretion, cellular transport, tissue accumulation, and recycling throw light on the possible roles of this vitamin in human physiology and pathology.

II. PROPERTIES AND FUNCTIONS OF VITAMIN C

A. Ascorbic Acid as a Vitamin

Vitamin C (ascorbic acid, ascorbate) is a six-carbon lactone. Most animals synthesize it from glucose in the liver (mammals) or kidneys (birds and reptiles). Several species of animals, scattered throughout the evolutionary tree, are unable to synthesize vitamin C. These include human and nonhuman primates, guinea pigs, Indian fruit bats, bulbuls, and some fish. Primates (9) and guinea pigs (10) lack the terminal enzyme in the biosynthetic pathway, gulonolactone

VITAMIN C: NEW INSIGHTS

oxidase. In the human, the gene encoding this enzyme has extensive mutations, so that there is no protein product (11). For humans, the inability to synthesize ascorbic acid makes this otherwise ubiquitous chemical a vitamin. Other animals unable to synthesize vitamin C usually obtain sufficient amounts from their largely plant diet but, similar to humans, will rapidly develop scurvy when fed on processed diets in captivity (12). Vitamin C is synthesized by plants from several precursors and is abundant in leaves and, in particular, the chloroplast (13). It may play a role in photosynthesis, stress resistance, and plant growth and development (14).

B. Ascorbate Is an Electron Donor in Chemical Reactions

Ascorbate is an electron donor, and this property accounts for its known and postulated functions. As an antioxidant or reducing agent, it sequentially donates two electrons from the C2–C3 double bond, forming the intermediate free radical semidehydroascorbic acid (ascorbate free radical) (Fig. 1). The ascorbate free radical is unstable (10^{-5} s), but is relatively unreactive with other compounds to form potentially harmful free radicals, and can be reversibly reduced to ascorbate (15). These properties make ascorbate an ideal electron donor. Semidehydroascorbic acid, being unstable, undergoes further oxidation to form the more stable product, dehydroascorbic acid (DHA), which can exist in more than one structural form (see

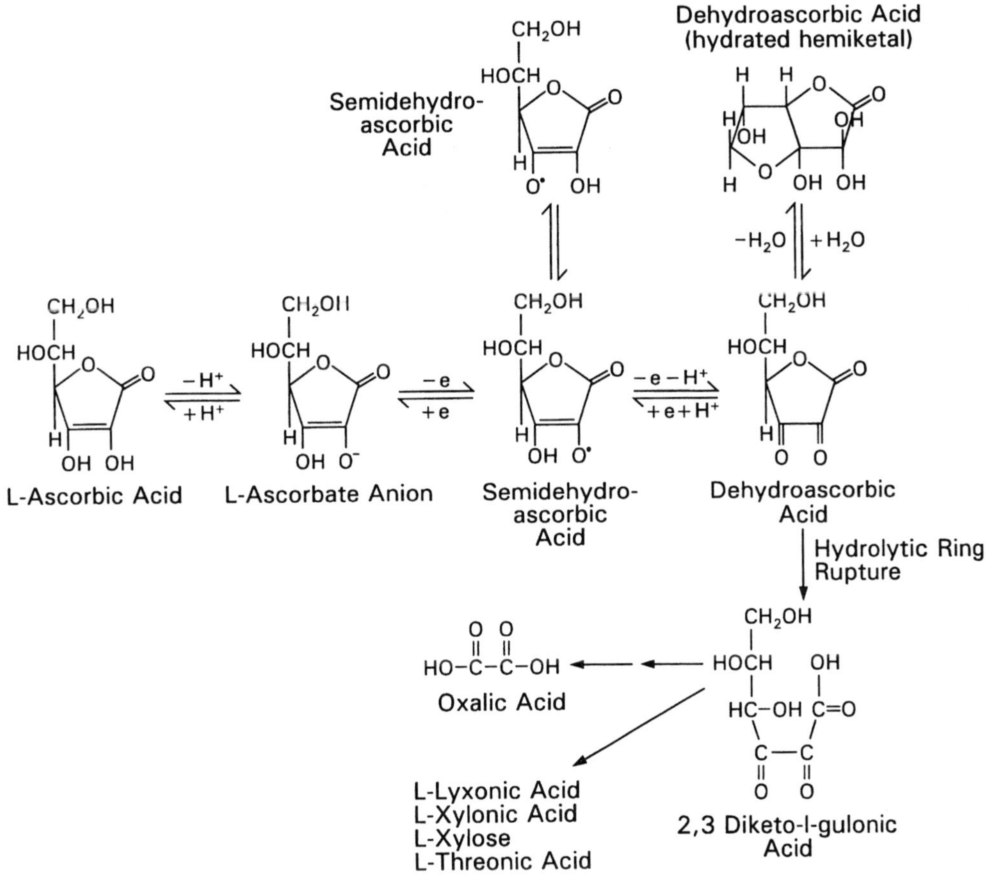

Figure 1 Ascorbic acid metabolism. (From Ref. 136.)

Fig. 1), but only a few minutes at physiological pH. DHA can be reduced back to ascorbate by glutathione, with formation of glutathione disulfide (16,17) or by enzymatic reduction mediated by at least three distinct proteins. If not reduced, DHA undergoes ring rupture and is irreversibly hydrolyzed to 2,3-diketogulonic acid. Diketogulonic acid is metabolized to xylose, xylonate, lyxonate, and oxalate, the last being a clinically significant end product of ascorbate metabolism. Although carbons from ascorbate contribute to expired carbon dioxide in some animals, this probably does not occur in humans (18,19). Molecular oxygen, with or without trace metals (iron, copper), superoxide, hydroxyl radical, and hypochlorous acid, all can oxidize ascorbic acid to DHA in biological systems.

C. Ascorbate Is a Cofactor for Enzymes

Ascorbate serves as a cofactor for eight different enzymes in mammals, and an additional three in yeast (Table 1) (20,21). It is assumed that scurvy is a result of impairment of these enzyme actions. Thus, the many signs related to wound dehiscence and friable gums may reflect impaired collagen synthesis. However, there is no experimental evidence that directly link the signs and symptoms of scurvy with specific enzyme actions.

D. Nonenzymatic Functions of Vitamin C

Vitamin C may have nonenzymatic functions, owing to its redox potential and free radical intermediate, and may be an electron donor in many intracellular and extracellular reactions (see Table 1). Intracellularly, vitamin C might act as an antioxidant to regulate gene expression, regulate mRNA translation, or prevent oxidant damage to intracellular proteins (37,38). Extracellular vitamin C might also be protective against oxidants and oxidant-mediated damage.

Many studies have described that vitamin C prevents low-density lipoprotein (LDL) oxidation in vitro (41,42). Although high LDL is a risk factor for atherosclerosis, it is atherogenic only when oxidized. It is possible that antioxidants inhibit LDL oxidation. In vitro, vitamin C inhibits metal-catalyzed LDL oxidation, possibly by quenching aqueous free radicals. Ascorbic acid protects LDL from oxidation at concentrations above 50 μM/L (43,44). Another potential protective mechanism is indirect, as vitamin C can regenerate oxidized α-tocopherol (vitamin E) in LDL. Whether vitamin C has these effects in vivo is unknown. Although cells in vessel walls may be affected by vitamin C in vivo, its action may be independent of its effect on metal-catalyzed LDL oxidation in vitro. This is because the high metal concentrations and the relatively long times needed to induce oxidation in vitro are unlikely to occur in the intact organism, especially as the relevant cations (iron, copper) in vivo are tightly bound to proteins. Furthermore, the oxidant itself may not be present at sufficient concentrations for these reactions to occur clinically. Additional effects of extracellular vitamin C in atherosclerosis could be due to its effects on adhesion of monocytes to endothelium or aggregation of platelets and leukocytes (45). Vitamin C may quench oxidants that leak from activated neutrophils or macrophages (46) that, in turn, may damage supporting tissues, such as collagen or surrounding fibroblasts (47). Although laboratory data show a protective role for vitamin C in atherosclerotic heart disease, epidemiological data are inconsistent (48–50).

Vitamin C may be the primary antioxidant in plasma for quenching aqueous peroxyl radicals and lipid peroxidation products (39). It is preferentially oxidized before other antioxidants in plasma, including uric acid, tocopherols, and bilirubin. However, all the foregoing studies on the antioxidant actions of vitamin C were conducted in vitro. These oxidation–reduction reactions may not specifically require vitamin C in vivo. Thus, it is unknown whether such effects demonstrated in vitro are relevant in vivo. Because ascorbic acid can donate electrons to

Table 1 Known and Postulated Functions of Vitamin C[a]

	Cofactor for enzymes		
	Enzymes	Function of enzyme	Ref.
Known roles	*Mammalian*		
	Prolyl 4-hydroxylase	Collagen hydroxylation	22–24
	Prolyl 3-hydroxylase		
	Lysyl hydroxylase		
	Trimethyllysine hydroxylase	Carnitine biosynthesis	25,26
	γ-Butyrobetaine hydroxylase		
	Dopamine β-monooxygenase	Norepinephrine biosynthesis	27,28
	Peptidyl-glycine α-amidating monooxygenase	Amidation of peptide hormones	29,30
	4-Hydroxyphenylpyruvate dioxygenase	Tyrosine metabolism	21,31
	Fungi		
	Deoxyuridine 1′-hydroxylase	Reutilization pathways for pyrimidines or the deoxyribose moiety of deoxynucleosides	32,33
	Thymine 7-hydroxylase		
	Pyridine deoxyribonucleoside 2′ hydroxylase		
	Reducing agent		
	Small intestine	Promote iron absorption	34,35
Postulated roles	*Antioxidant*		
	Cells	Regulate gene expression and mRNA translation, prevent oxidant damage to intracellular proteins	36–38
	Plasma	Quench aqueous peroxyl radicals and lipid peroxidation products	39
	Stomach	Prevent formation of N-nitroso compounds	40

[a] Its function as a cofactor for eight different enzymes in mammals and a further three in yeast are fairly well characterized. The postulated functions are all nonenzymatic and are based on the fact that vitamin C is a reducing agent. Postulated functions have been demonstrated in vitro; their relevance in vivo is unclear. Supporting data from animal or human experiments are sparse.

form semidehydroascorbic acid without the formation of reactive and harmful intermediaries, it remains the most potent water-soluble antioxidant in the body. Its physiological role in the intact organism relative to oxidation reactions is as yet uncertain.

Vitamin C can quench reactive oxygen metabolites in the stomach or duodenum, and prevent the formation of N-nitroso compounds that are mutagenic. In normal subjects, the concentration of vitamin C in gastric juice is three times higher than that of plasma (51). These properties make it an attractive candidate for the prevention of gastric cancer (52). However, gastric juice vitamin C concentrations are normal in patients at risk for familial gastric cancer (53). Ascorbic acid content is low in the gastric juice of patients with atrophic gastritis and *Helicobacter pylori* infection, a condition associated with gastric cancer. Eradication of the bacteria increases gastric ascorbic acid secretion (54). Whether this suggested antioxidant action has any significance in vivo is unclear. Formation of nitrosamines in the gastrointestinal tract can be reduced by foods high in ascorbic acid. This effect may be due to ascorbic acid as well as other chemicals in food. Whether this has any clinical benefit is unknown (40). Although high vitamin C dietary intake correlates with reduced gastric cancer risk (55), it is not certain what confers protection: vitamin C itself or other components of foods, particularly fruits and vegetables, that also happen to contain vitamin C. At doses of 20–60 mg, vitamin C promotes iron absorption in the small intestine (34,35). Absorption of soluble nonorganic iron is increased by vitamin C, which might keep iron in a reduced form. Amounts necessary for enhancing iron absorption are found in foods that are good sources of the vitamin. Although the effects of supplemental vitamin C on increased iron absorption have been shown in many (56,57), but not all studies (58,59), its effect on raising hemoglobin concentration is modest at best (57,60), particularly when studied under real-life conditions (61). Many of the studies on the effects of vitamin C on iron absorption and improvement in hematological parameters were conducted over short periods on small numbers of patients. Clinical trials, however, cannot detect significant changes in hematocrit or hemoglobin concentrations unless they are long-term studies with sufficient statistical power.

III. PHYSIOLOGY OF VITAMIN C

A. Tissue Distribution of Vitamin C

Ascorbic acid is widely distributed in the human and animals and is concentrated in many organs. The highest concentrations are found in adrenal and pituitary glands at 30–400 mg/100 g of tissue. Liver, spleen, pancreas, kidney, brain, and lens contain 10–50 mg/100 g (62). Assuming that 1 g of tissue is approximately equal to 1 mL, and since the molecular weight of ascorbic acid is 176, it is evident that many organs contain ascorbic acid in millimolar concentrations. By virtue of its mass, liver is the largest store of vitamin C. The choroid plexus actively secretes ascorbate into the cerebrospinal fluid, from where it is taken up and concentrated by many parts of the brain (63). Animal studies in the guinea pig (64) and other animals (62) show that tissue concentrations are related to intake, so that higher intake results in a higher tissue concentration. These studies were done before accurate ascorbic acid assays were available. Because it is labile, rapid loss can occur in isolated organs if samples are not processed rapidly. Therefore, the tissue concentrations of vitamin C reported in the literature may be inaccurate. Nevertheless, these studies indicate the wide range in ascorbic acid tissue concentration and its selective uptake by specific organs (65–67). The reason that many of these tissues concentrate vitamin C is unknown; it is also concentrated by white blood cells. These have been studied extensively owing to their easy availability and a possible link between vitamin C and infection. Neutrophils, lymphocytes, and monocytes have 1.3–4 mM internal concentrations of ascorbic acid (20- to 30-fold higher than plasma) (19). Mechanisms of ascorbic acid transport, described in the following section, were characterized based in part on studies of neutrophils (68).

B. Transport and Accumulation of Vitamin C

1. Vitamin C Recycling in Neutrophils

Neutrophils transport ascorbic acid from plasma and the extracellular milieu, probably utilizing the vitamin C transporter hSVCT2. When neutrophils are activated, superoxide and other oxidants are formed. Some oxidants diffuse out of the cell, and oxidize ascorbate to DHA. DHA enters neutrophils by glucose transporters, presumably the facilitative glucose transporters

GLUT1 and GLUT3. Once inside neutrophils, DHA is immediately reduced to ascorbic acid by the glutathione-dependent protein glutaredoxin (Fig. 2). Glutathione is oxidized by glutaredoxin to glutathione disulfide, and glutathione is regenerated by reducing equivalents from NADPH by the pentose shunt. Oxidation of extracellular ascorbate and its reduction intracellularly back to ascorbate is termed ascorbate recycling. It is likely that ascorbate recycling protects the neutrophil and surrounding tissues from oxidative damage by oxidants generated during

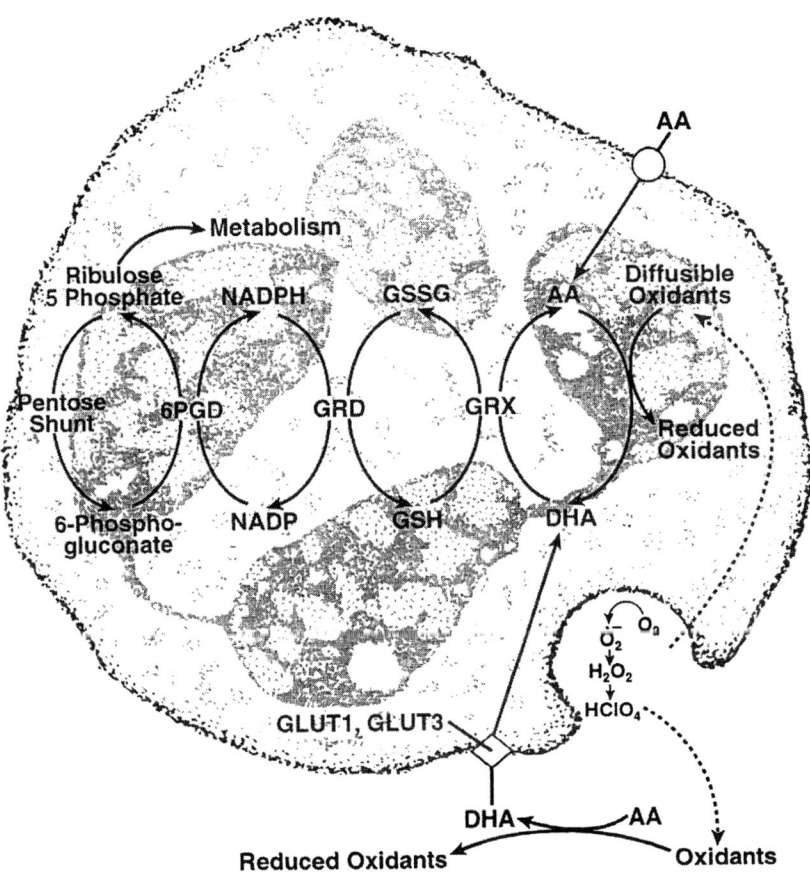

Figure 2 A model of dehydroascorbic acid and ascorbate transport and recycling in human neutrophils: Ascorbate and dehydroascorbic acid are transported differently (46,69,70,74,76,137). The ascorbate transporter (open circle), probably SVCT2, transports ascorbate and probably maintains millimolar concentrations of ascorbate inside neutrophils (46,76,98). With activation, neutrophils secrete reactive oxygen species that oxidize extracellular ascorbate to dehydroascorbic acid. Dehydroascorbic acid is rapidly transported by glucose transporter isoforms GLUT1 and GLUT3 (open diamond). Intracellular dehydroascorbic acid is immediately reduced to ascorbate. In neutrophils, glutaredoxin is responsible for most intracellular reduction (138). As a result of dehydroascorbic acid transport and reduction, as much as tenfold higher ascorbate internal concentrations are achieved compared with activity of the ascorbate transporter alone. The proposed mechanism of reduction could require glutathione, NADPH, and the enzymes shown (138). Abbrev: AA, ascorbate; DHA, dehydroascorbic acid; GRX, glutaredoxin; GSH, reduced glutathione; GSSG, oxidized glutathione; 6-PGD, 6-phosphogluconate dehydrogenase; GRD, glutathione reductase. (From Ref. 16.)

neutrophil activation and phagocytosis. Extracellular oxidants are quenched by ascorbic acid, which might protect surrounding tissue from oxidative damage from oxidants generated by neutrophil activation, and as a consequence, DHA is formed. DHA is then transported and reduced within the neutrophil, so that additional ascorbate is available to quench intracellular oxidants generated by neutrophil activation.

For neutrophils, the most potent activators of ascorbate recycling are bacteria (Fig. 3). Ascorbate recycling is induced by gram-positive and gram-negative bacteria as well as *Candida albicans* (68). However, bacteria lack mechanisms for ascorbate and DHA uptake, do not recycle ascorbate, and cannot use these mechanisms for oxidant protection. Thus, ascorbate recycling is a protective mechanism that is specific for the host, in this case humans, and is not utilized by pathogens, meaning bacteria and *Candida*.

It was predicted that ascorbate recycling would not occur in patients whose neutrophils do not make oxidants, as in chronic granulomatous disease (Fig. 4). Neutrophils from these patients have defective superoxide generation. Because superoxide generation is necessary for generating reactive oxidant, it was predicted and found that neutrophils from these patients cannot recycle ascorbate. This specifically is because, in the absence of oxidants, extracellular

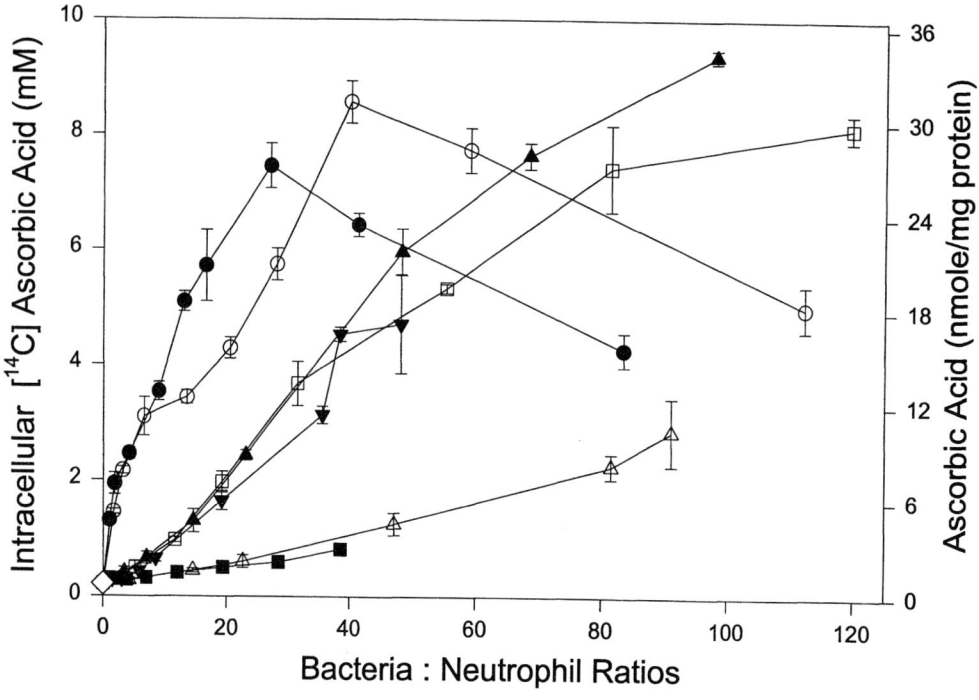

Figure 3 Induction of ascorbate recycling by different microorganisms (68): Neutrophils were incubated with 100 μM of ascorbate for 45 min with the indicated microorganism: neutrophils (effector/target) ratios for the following microorganisms: *Escherichia coli* CP9 (○) or CP922 (●); *Enterococcus faecalis* (■); *Moraxella catarrhalis* (□); *Klebsiella oxytoca* (▲); *Acinetobacter baumannii* (△); and *Candida albicans* (▲). Neutrophils incubated with ascorbate and no microorganisms are indicated by (◇) at the lower left hand corner of the figure. Intracellular ascorbate was measured by scintillation spectrometry and is shown as millimoles (mM) (left axis) and nanomoles (nmol per milligram of protein (right axis). (From Ref. 68.)

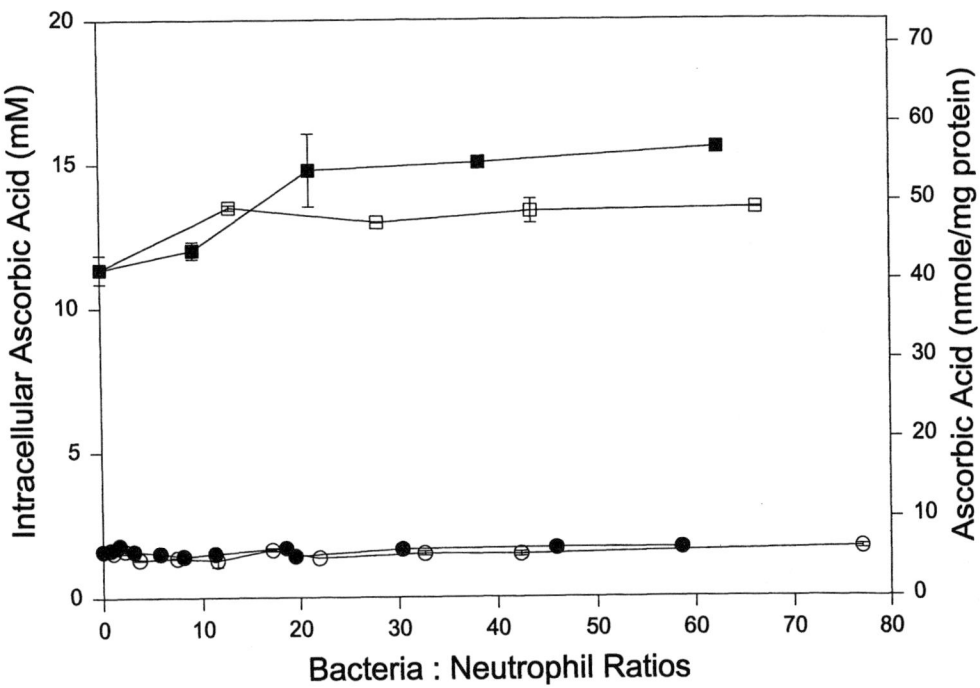

Figure 4 Ascorbate recycling in chronic granulomatous disease neutrophils: Chronic granulomatous disease neutrophils were incubated with 100 μM ascorbate (● and ○) for 45 min or 300 μM dehydroascorbic acid (□ and ■) for 5 min, and the indicated target/effector ratios for *E. coli* CP9 (● and ■) or *E. coli* CP922 (○ and □) were determined. Intracellular ascorbate was measured by HPLC and is shown as mM/mg (left axis) and nmol/mg protein (right axis). (From Ref. 68.)

ascorbic acid is not oxidized to DHA, which, therefore, is not available for transport by glucose transporters into neutrophils. When DHA is provided to neutrophils from patients with chronic granulomatous disease, DHA transport and reduction occurs efficiently.

2. *Vitamin C Transporters*

Two sodium-dependent vitamin C transporters, SVCT1 and SVCT2, have been identified (69,70). Properties of each transporter were measured using the *Xenopus laevis* oocyte expression system (Fig. 5). Both carrier proteins couple the transport of 2 Na$^+$:1 ascorbate. Kinetic analyses indicate that SVCT1 is a low-affinity (K_M 237 μM), high-velocity (V_{max} 15.8 pmol/min per oocyte) transporter (69). SVCT2 has a tenfold higher affinity for ascorbate (K_M 23 μM), but exhibits a lower rate of uptake (V_{max} 0.2 pmol/min per five oocytes). Northern blot analyses show that SVCT1 is primarily localized to the epithelium of the small intestine and kidney, consistent with a role in intestinal absorption and renal reabsorption of ascorbate. Other organs known to accumulate ascorbic acid, such as liver, ovary, and prostate, also have high levels of SVCT1. SVCT2 has a more general distribution, with mRNA found in most tissues, including the brain, retina, placenta, spleen, small intestine, and gonads (71,70). Neither of these transporters transport DHA (69). The gene for human (h)SVCT1 has been mapped (71) to chromosome 5q23 (72) and that of hSVCT2 to chromosome 20p12.3 (72).

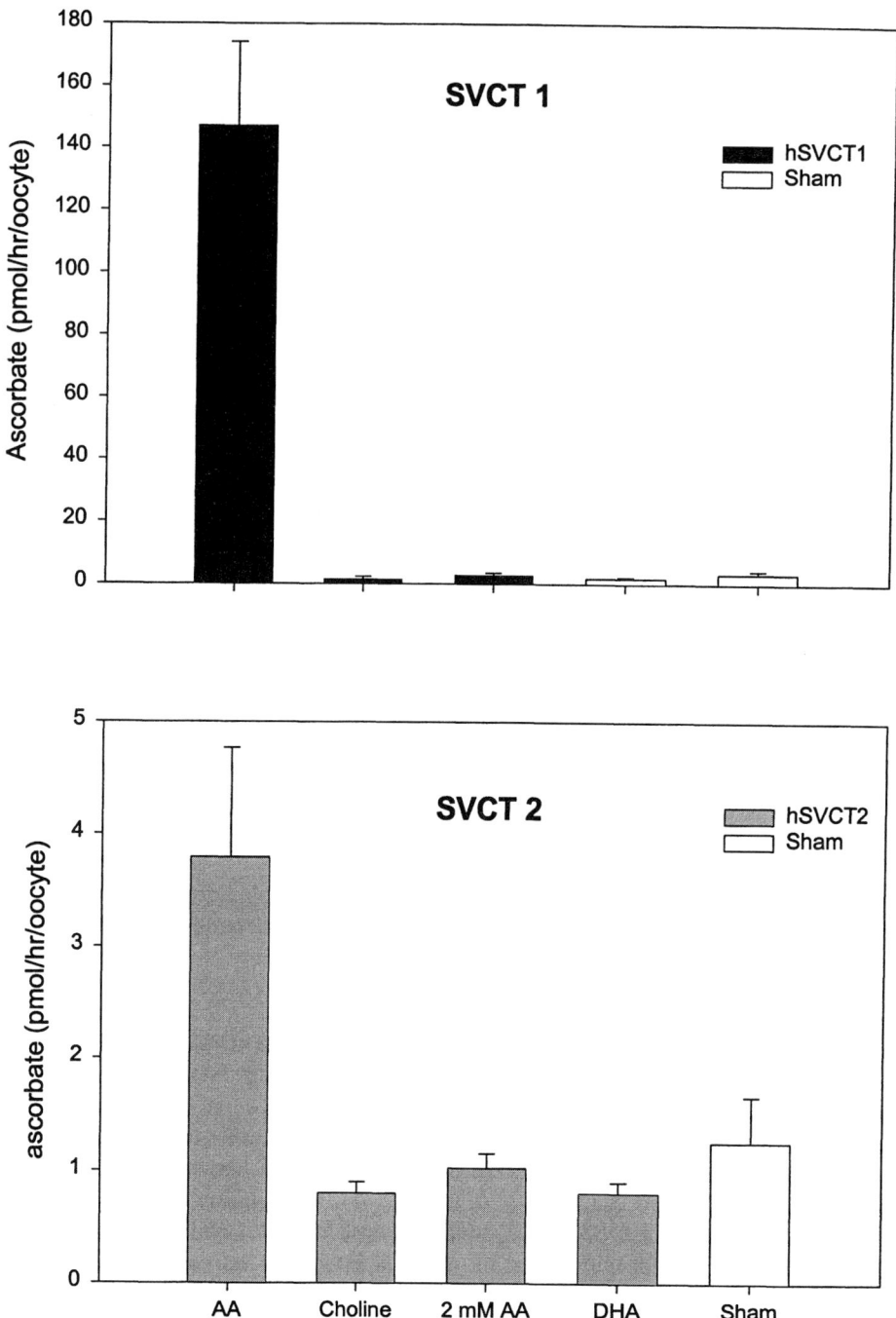

Figure 5 Functional expression of hSVCT1 and hSVCT2 in *Xenopus* oocytes: Oocytes were incubated in buffer containing 100 μM [^{14}C]ascorbate (AA), 500 μM dehydroascorbic acid (DHA), 2 mM unlabeled AA, choline, and [^{14}C]ascorbate. Sham oocytes were injected with sterile water. (From Ref. 69.)

3. DHA Transporters

Tissues transport DHA 10- to 20-fold faster than ascorbate. DHA is transported by facilitative glucose transporters GLUT1 and GLUT3 (73–75). GLUT1 and 3 transport DHA with an affinity similar to that for glucose (Fig. 6) (74). GLUT2, GLUT5, and SGLT1 do not transport DHA, and no glucose transporters transport ascorbic acid. DHA transport is inhibited by glucose and glucose analogues (74,76). Based on the interaction of DHA with some glucose transporters, it is possible that diabetes adversely affects ascorbate recycling in neutrophils. Other substances, such as endotoxin (77) and transforming growth factor beta (TGF-β) (78), also may have effects on DHA transport, but these remain uncertain.

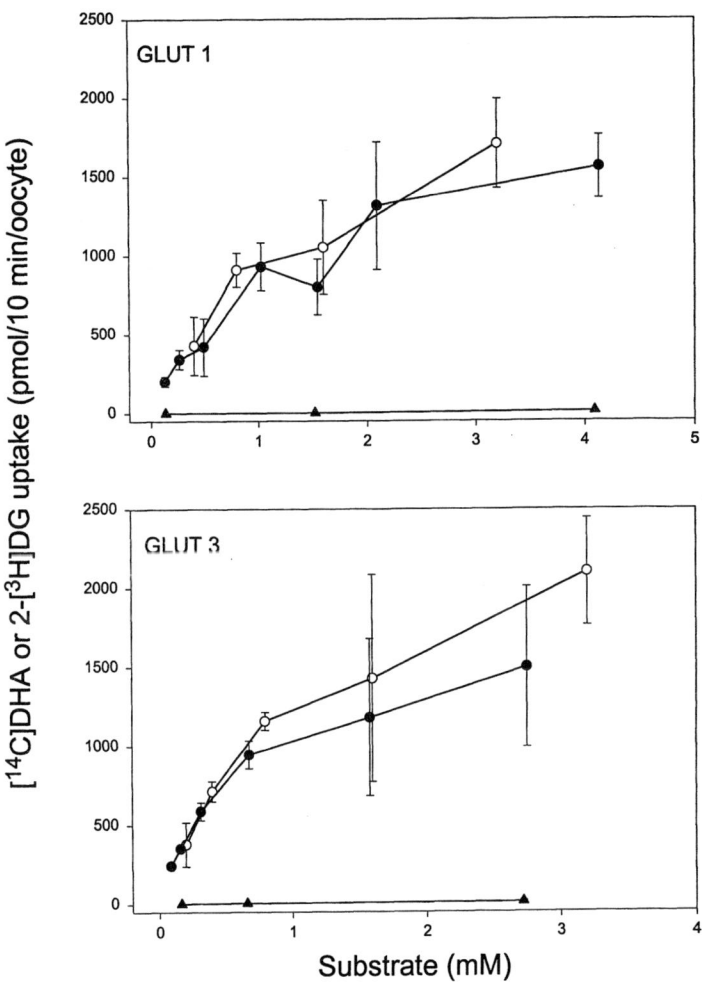

Figure 6 DHA transport by glucose transporter isoforms GLUT1 and GLUT3: *Xenopus* oocytes expressing individual glucose transporter isoforms GLUT1 and GLU3 were tested for [^{14}C]DHA transport activity. Oocytes were incubated with the concentrations shown of [^{14}C]DHA (●) or 2-[^{3}H]deoxyglucose (○), depending on the transport protein being tested, and the internalized radioactivity in individual oocytes was quantified. [^{14}C]DHA (▲) transport into sham water-injected oocytes is also shown. (From Ref. 74.)

4. *Studies of Vitamin C and DHA Transporters Using* Xenopus laevus *Oocytes*

The individual transporters that transport ascorbic acid and DHA can be studied singly or in combination using oocytes of the tropical frog *X. laevis*. mRNA for the appropriate transporter is microinjected into the surgically isolated oocyte, and the oocyte incubated in culture medium for 2–4 days. The transport proteins are translated from the injected mRNA, synthesized, and translocated to the oocyte membrane, where they are functionally active. When these oocytes are incubated with the appropriate substance, it is transported and concentrated in the oocyte, analogous to events in the human cell. These studies have demonstrated the specificity and the dynamics of each of the transporters for ascorbic acid and DHA and greatly increased our understanding of vitamin C transport (69,73,74).

5. *Ascorbate Recycling as a General Mechanism for Ascorbate Accumulation*

The contribution of ascorbate recycling to ascorbate accumulation in many tissues is unknown. DHA is not present in plasma of healthy persons, although it is uncertain whether DHA is found in plasma of ill patients. It is possible that DHA forms locally in the extracellular milieu, and that it is transported by glucose transporters and reduced internally to ascorbate. Ascorbic acid oxidizes to DHA outside of oxidant-generating cells, such as neutrophils. It is unknown whether low rates of ascorbic acid oxidation to DHA occur in the extracellular milieu of other tissues, and also whether such DHA contributes substantially to ascorbate accumulation in these tissues. It is possible for ascorbate recycling to occur, to some degree, in many tissues because most tissues contain GLUT1, GLUT3, or GLUT4, and glutaredoxin is also widely distributed. Because DHA formation is essential for recycling to occur, and because it is unknown if and how much DHA formation occurs locally, the contribution of ascorbate recycling to ascorbate accumulation remains to be determined.

Others have postulated that DHA transport is responsible for most of the ascorbate accumulated, especially in the brain and in tumors (79,80). Just as for ascorbate recycling, the mechanism of its accumulation depends on which substrates are available as well as which transporters are present. It is unrealistic to infuse completely unphysiological amounts of DHA into animals and then conclude that DHA transport is the major mechanism of ascorbate accumulation (80).

C. Biochemical Function in Relation to Concentration

Many experiments have shown varying biochemical roles of vitamin C, such as its role as cofactors for enzymes involved in collagen, carnitine, catecholamine, or peptide hormone synthesis, and perhaps in neutrophil function. However, we still do not know whether these functions are related to particular plasma or tissue concentrations of vitamin C. It is possible that many of these functions take place at maximal rates in vivo at low concentrations of vitamin C, perhaps as low as those resulting from doses of vitamin C that are just adequate to prevent scurvy. For example, catecholamine synthesis can occur efficiently as ascorbic acid is regenerated in chromaffin granules, where it is a cosubstrate for norepinephrine synthesis. The kinetics of this regenerating mechanism are such that reduction rates achieve V_{max} in situ (81). However, many other significant findings hint at a higher optimum plasma concentrations for vitamin C. For example, the V_{max} of vitamin C transporter hSVCT2 is 70 μM. LDL oxidation in vitro is inhibited by ascorbic acid at 40–50 μM. As described in detail later, plasma vitamin C concentrations in humans are tightly controlled at approximately 70 μM, and circulating white blood cells also saturate at this concentration. That physiological mechanisms involving vitamin C function optimally at 50–70 μM plasma concentrations may indirectly indicate some benefit to the organism if this plasma concentration is sustained.

D. Steady-State Plasma Concentration in Relation to Dose

To study the physiology, absorption, bioavailability, and the renal threshold of vitamin C, it is necessary to attain and maintain steady-state plasma concentrations of this vitamin. In the absence of a steady-state level, that is if plasma concentrations are decreasing or increasing, reliable measurements of dose–concentration relations and other dose- or concentration-related physiological functions cannot be made.

1. Vitamin C Assay and Sample Processing

For these experiments to be successfully carried out, the first prerequisite is a reliable method to measure ascorbic acid. It is now possible to measure it with a high degree of accuracy and precision using high-performance liquid chromatography (HPLC) with coulometric electrochemical detection (82,83). Optimal sample collection and handling are equally important, as ascorbate is labile and easily oxidized. Blood samples have to be carefully drawn to avoid hemolysis as ascorbate is oxidized in the presence of hemoglobin. In whole blood ascorbic acid is stable for 24–48 h if the sample is immediately placed on ice and then refrigerated, as long as no hemolysis occurs. Once the sample is centrifuged to remove red cells, white cells, and platelets, processing must not be interrupted. The sample is deproteinized, the precipitated protein removed by centrifugation, and the supernatant frozen at $-80°C$. The sample should be thawed immediately before assay. Under such careful conditions, the assay will reliably reflect plasma concentration. In healthy persons, all of the vitamin is present in the plasma in the form of ascorbic acid, and there is no detectable DHA in the circulation (84). There is still no direct assay for DHA. DHA is measured indirectly after reduction to ascorbic acid. Minute amounts of DHA, if present in the plasma, cannot be measured accurately by this method, as DHA will be masked by the much larger quantities of ascorbic acid present. Ascorbic acid is found in the plasma in a free form—it is not bound to plasma protein (84).

E. Vitamin C Intake Versus Plasma Concentration: Results of Dietary Surveys

When plasma ascorbic acid concentrations are correlated with estimated daily vitamin C intake derived from the number of fruit or vegetable servings per week, no relation is seen between the two (unpublished data). This is probably because of the inaccuracy of dietary surveys (85) and the inability of subjects to recall exactly what they ate and how much in the preceding days. Factors other than recall may also play a role—the type of fruits and vegetables eaten will have different amounts of vitamin C, the method of preparation may entail varying loss of vitamin C, and bioavailability might differ depending on the exact mix of diet consumed. The best way to eliminate these variables and study vitamin C dose–concentration relations is with precisely controlled intakes of known amounts of vitamin C.

F. Depletion–Repletion Studies

Depletion–repletion studies of vitamin C have been carried out for half a century. The early studies by the Royal Air Force (U. K.) showed that the dose of vitamin C necessary to prevent scurvy is probably less than 10 mg. The studies also concluded that body stores of vitamin C were sufficient to prevent scurvy for several months. Flaws of these studies are that dietary intake and vitamin C content were based on recall, without quantitation. A study conducted on prisoners (U. S.), in which four male prisoners were fed a vitamin C-free diet through a nasogastric tube, supported the finding that physical signs (what a physician finds on examination) of scurvy could be prevented by 10 mg of vitamin C daily (7,86). These findings were confirmed in a further five prisoners (87,88) and, for many years, formed the basis of the U. S. Recommended Dietary Allowance (RDA). The prisoner studies, however, indicated that body stores of vitamin C were much less than previously believed, and could prevent scurvy for less than 6 weeks. The prisoner studies unfortunately also suffer from defects (89). Vitamin C assays were unreliable and imprecise, the number of subjects were few and, in the prisoners study, the diet was deficient in not one, but many nutrients. Data collection was incomplete, as some of the prisoners escaped during the study. Other depletion studies carried out in outpatient settings demonstrated the ease with which plasma concentrations of ascorbic acid fell (90–97), consistent with Lind's observations more than 200 years ago.

The 1996 National Institutes of Health (NIH) study is the only one that determined steady-state concentration as a function of dose and used many different doses (19). This study used a repletion–depletion design with seven healthy men who were admitted to the NIH Clinical Center for an average period of 145 days (range 116–180) (Fig. 7). The subjects consumed

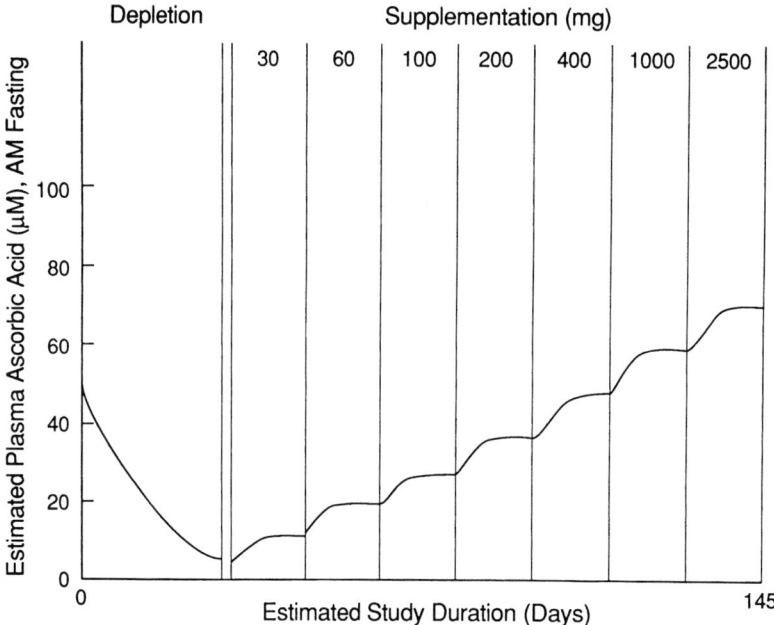

Figure 7 A schematic diagram of the 1996 NIH inpatient depletion–repletion study of seven healthy men. Note that the figure is not drawn to scale. The results of the study are presented in Table 2. To reduce inpatient time in the depletion phase, subjects were placed on a 60-mg vitamin C diet as outpatients for 3 weeks before admission. This led to a fall in plasma ascorbic acid concentration from 67 ± 17.6 μM (mean $\pm$ SD) at the time of prerecruitment screening to 23.0 ± 6.9 μM at the time of admission. After admission to the NIH Clinical Center, subjects were started on an inpatient vitamin C-free diet, containing < 5 mg/day of vitamin C. Blood samples were drawn fasting, in the morning, for vitamin C measurements daily, or several times per week. On this inpatient depletion diet, plasma vitamin C concentration fell to 6.9 ± 2 μM/L, at a rate of 1.3 ± 0.5 μM/L per day (100). Repletion, or supplementation, was started at this stage, with an initial dose of 30 mg daily in two divided doses until a steady-state concentration was reached. Bioavailability studies were carried out, and blood and white cell samples collected for vitamin C measurements. Subjects were given vitamin C in the following doses, and steady-state levels were attained at each dose: 30, 60, 100, 200, 400, 1000, and 2500 mg. The subjects were studied for a mean period of 145 days (range 116–180). (From Ref. 19.)

a diet containing less than 5 mg vitamin C daily, but with all other nutrients in adequate amounts. Blood samples were drawn fasting, in the morning, for vitamin C measurements daily or several times per week. When plasma levels of vitamin C fell to between 5 and 10 μM, the depletion phase was terminated. At this level, all subjects exhibited lassitude, but no signs of scurvy. It has to borne in mind that fatigue also was described by Lind in his treatise on scurvy in 1753 as the early symptom of impending scurvy. In the repletion or supplementation phase, subjects were commenced on graduated increases in vitamin C intake until they reached steady-state for each dose. The starting dose was 15 mg twice daily. On this dose (30 mg/day), most subjects reached steady-state levels in approximately 1 month. The steady-state level was defined as at least five consecutive measurements in which vitamin C concentrations of plasma samples obtained over at least 7 days had a SD of 10% or less: 85% of steady-state calculations were based on six or more plasma samples (per patient). An example of steady-state level for a single subject at the 60-mg dose is shown in Figure 8. At the steady-state level, bioavailability studies were performed, as will be described later. Blood samples were obtained for vitamin C measurements and isolation of neutrophils, and other white blood cells were obtained by apheresis (98,99). Subjects were then given the next higher dose of vitamin C (60 mg/day) until a new steady-state level was reached. Again, bioavailability studies were carried out, and blood and white cell samples collected for vitamin C measurements. In this fashion, patients were sampled for daily vitamin C doses of 30, 60, 100, 200, 400, 1000, and 2500 mg. Vitamin C was administered in fasted state, as pure vitamin C in water with pH adjusted to 6.5.

After the initiation of a vitamin C-free diet, plasma vitamin C concentrations fell to 6.9 ± 2 μM/L, at a rate of 1.3 ± 0.5 μM/L per day (100). Mean plasma steady-state concentrations attained at each of the vitamin C doses is given in Table 2. Different subjects required differing periods of time to deplete and to reach steady-state at each dose (Fig. 9). The underlying reasons for this interindividual variability are unknown. When the mean plasma steady-state concentrations for all subjects are plotted against dose, a sigmoidal dose–concentration curve results (Fig. 10). At the 30-mg dose, there is very little increase in plasma vitamin C concen-

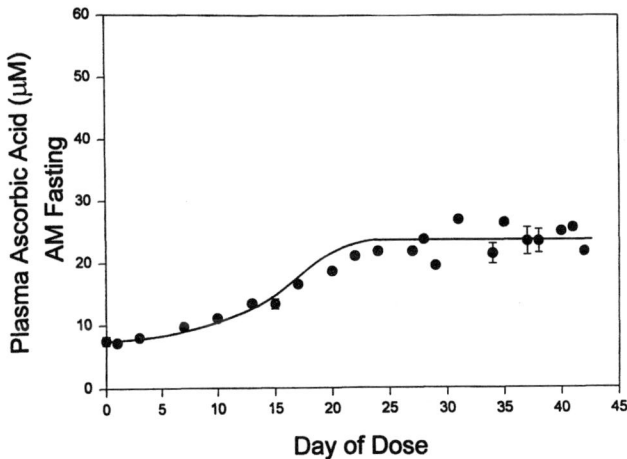

Figure 8 Steady-state fasting plasma ascorbic acid concentrations for a single subject at the 60-mg dose. Steady-state concentration was defined as five consecutive measurements in which vitamin C concentrations of plasma samples obtained over at least 7 days had a SD of 10% or less. (From Ref. 19.)

Table 2 Steady-State Plasma Concentration[a] of Vitamin C in an Inpatient Repletion–Depletion Study

Steady-state plasma concentration of vitamin C	
Oral dose (mg)	Plasma concentration (μM) mean (SD)
0 (depletion nadir)	7.6 (1.6)
30	8.7 (1.7)
60	24.8 (14.1)
100	56 (4.5)
200	65.8 (7.3)
400	70 (6.9)
1000	76.9 (5.3)
2500	85 (5.4)

[a] Seven healthy men consumed a diet containing < 5 mg vitamin C daily. Subjects were given vitamin C as daily oral doses of 30, 60, 100, 200, 400, 1000, and 2500 mg until a steady-state level was attained for each dose. Steady-state concentration was defined as at least five consecutive plasma measurements obtained over at least 7 days, with a SD of 10% or less. Samples were obtained in the morning in the fasted state.
Source: Ref. 19.

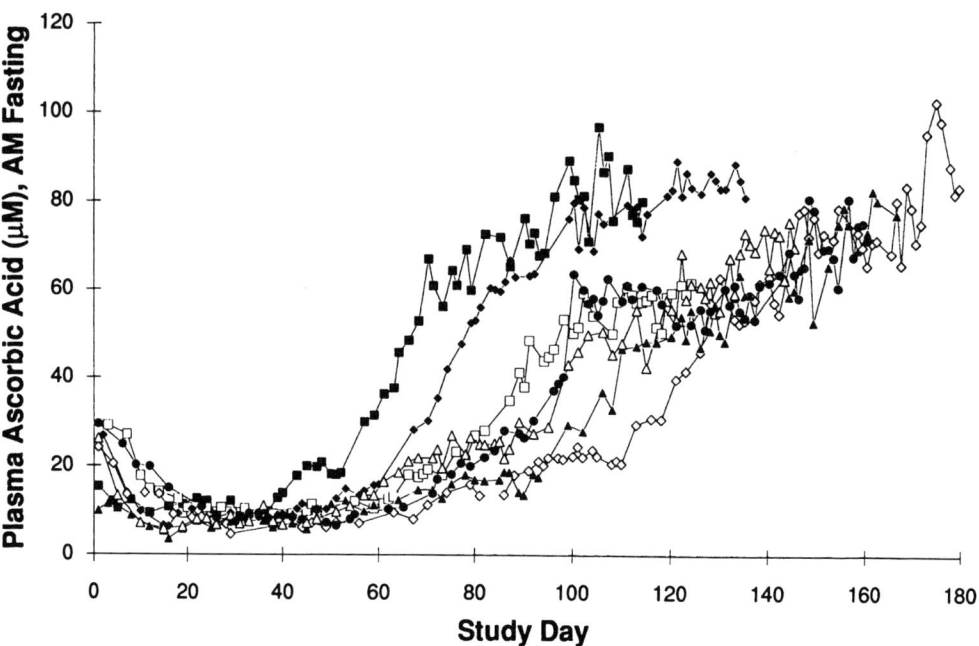

Figure 9 The relation between oral doses of vitamin C, inpatient time, and the fasting plasma ascorbic acid concentrations for each of the seven healthy men in the NIH inpatient depletion–repletion study. Different subjects required differing periods of time to deplete and to reach a steady-state level at each dose. (From Ref. 19.)

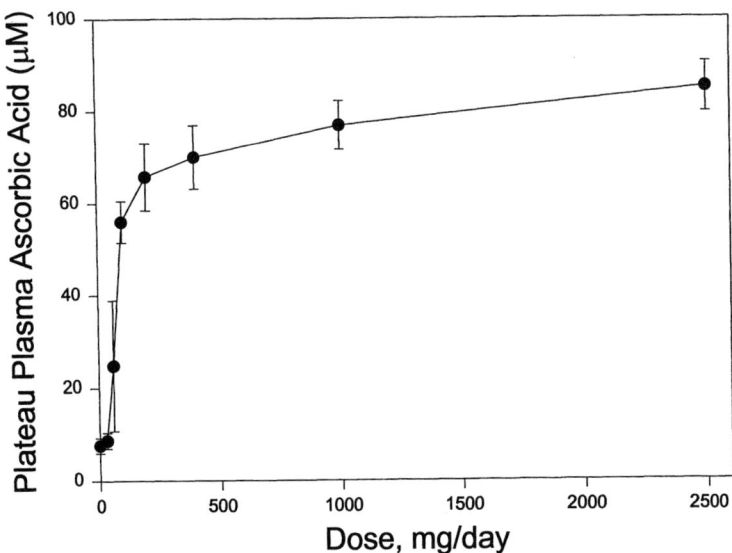

Figure 10 The relation between oral doses of vitamin C and the mean fasting steady-state plasma ascorbic acid concentration in seven healthy men from the NIH inpatient depletion–repletion study. The daily doses of vitamin C were 30, 60, 100, 200, 400, 1000, and 2500 mg. At the 30-mg dose, there is very little increase in plasma vitamin C concentration. Between 30 and 100 mg, there is a large increase, with the mean vitamin C concentration increasing from 8.7 to 56 μM. Further increase in oral intake results in relatively smaller increases in plasma concentration, so that a daily intake of 2500 mg produces only 85 μM. The dose–concentration curve is sigmoidal, with its steep portion between 30 and 100 mg of vitamin C daily. (From Ref. 19.)

tration. Between 30 and 100 mg, there is a large increase, with mean vitamin C concentrations increasing from 8.7 to 56 μM. Further increase in oral intake results in relatively smaller increases in plasma concentrations, so that a daily intake of 2500 mg produces only 85 μM. This steep portion of the sigmoid curve thus lies between 30 and 100 mg of vitamin C daily. As a consequence, small changes in intake in this range will result in large changes in plasma concentrations (19). This is of great public health importance, as well as in the study of vitamin C physiology, because accurate control over intake is necessary for meaningful experiments.

The foregoing data show that plasma is saturated at 1000 mg/day, a dose at which the plasma concentration was approximately 80 μM. Intracellular vitamin C concentrations in circulating blood cells (neutrophils, monocytes, and lymphocytes) also exhibit steep dose–concentration curves, but these cell saturate before plasma (Fig. 11). This is because they actively transport and concentrate vitamin C from the plasma, and the V_{max}s for these transporters are 60–70 μM.

1. Diet Used for Depletion–Repletion Studies

Previous studies used narrow vitamin C dose ranges or designs in which dietary intake of vitamin C could not be strictly controlled. As is apparent from the NIH study, the vitamin C dose–concentration relation is sigmoidal, so that small changes in oral intake produce a large change in plasma concentrations at low doses. Therefore, a consistently rigorous diet is essential to obtain meaningful data (85). In the NIH study, volunteers were admitted as inpatients for 4–6 months to ensure strict dietary control (19). A new diet was designed ensuring vitamin

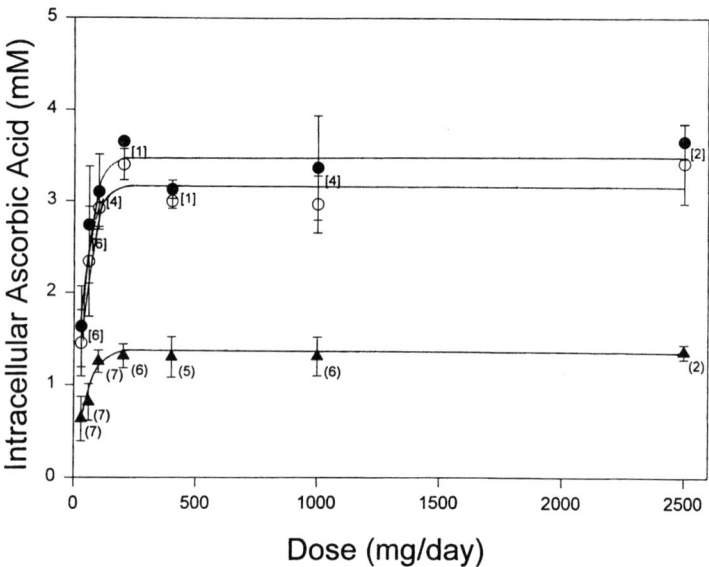

Figure 11 Intracellular ascorbic acid concentrations (mM) in circulating immune cells as a function of dose (mg/day) in seven healthy men in the NIH depletion–repletion study: Neutrophils (▲), monocytes (○), and lymphocytes (●) were isolated when the subjects were at steady state for each dose. Numbers in parenthesis ( ) at each dose indicate the number of volunteers from whom neutrophils were obtained; numbers in brackets [ ] at each dose indicate the number of volunteers from whom lymphocytes and monocytes were obtained. (From Ref. 19.)

C intake of less than 5 mg/day, but at the same time providing a varied fare (100). Patients could choose their diet from a computerized menu consisting of vitamin C-free foods. When the selected food contained vitamin C, it was weighed to ensure that daily intake of vitamin C was kept at less than 5 mg. All food consumed was weighed so that accurate daily amount of intake for each patient was known for vitamin C, calories, carbohydrates, fat, protein, and 18 vital nutrients. Nutrients that might possibly have been deficient were supplemented by daily vitamin and mineral tablets. The daily intake of vitamin C for all subjects from this vitamin C-deficient depletion diet was 3.87 ± 0.64 (mean $\pm$ SD) mg over the entire study period.

G. Bioavailability of Oral Vitamin C

The amount of vitamin C that has to be taken orally for optimum physiological function partly depends on its bioavailability. Oral consumption does not equate with availability to the tissues. A substance can be altered or destroyed in the gastrointestinal tract, be bound or otherwise made unabsorbable, destroyed by intestinal mucosal cells or by first-pass metabolism in the liver, or simply pass out of the gut unabsorbed. Previous studies of vitamin C bioavailability have compared oral absorption with urine excretion, and studied relative bioavailability by comparing vitamin C in food with that in supplements, but these studies were not performed at steady-state concentrations (97,101–104).

True bioavailability studies are more demanding and have to be done at a steady-state level for that dose. At steady-state, plasma and tissues are in equilibrium relative to the vitamin C dose. This avoids selective uptake of the vitamin by the liver or other tissues, producing misleadingly low plasma levels. Vitamin C is administered orally and plasma concentrations measured at frequent intervals. The same dose is administered intravenously at a different time (usually the next day). Again plasma concentrations are measured. Except for substances that are modified to their active form by first-pass hepatic metabolism, intravenous administration ensures complete bioavailability, as all the administered substance reaches the peripheral circulation. The areas under the curve (AUC) for oral administration (AUC_{po}) and for intravenous administration (AUC_{iv}) are calculated (Fig. 12). True bioavailability is given by the AUC_{po}/AUC_{iv} ratio. These calculations showed that bioavailability for oral vitamin C is approximately 100% for 200 mg, 73% for 500 mg, and 49% for 1250 mg (Fig. 13) (19).

Although these bioavailability data appear convincing, they suffer from some uncertainties. This is because bioavailability using the AUC calculations is accurate only if the test substance has a constant volume of distribution and a constant rate of clearance. As described earlier, vitamin C is distributed differently between plasma and blood cells. Many other compartments into which vitamin C is distributed, such as other tissues, cerebrospinal fluid, and so on, will have yet other distributions. Neither is excretion linear, as renal excretion starts only above the renal threshold, which occurs at a plasma concentration of approximately 60 μM. These objections are particularly relevant for doses less than 200 mg, and at these doses the AUC method cannot be used to calculate bioavailability. A mathematical model was developed to account for the nonlinearity in clearance and volume of distribution (105). By using this model, bioavailability was calculated to be 80% for 100 mg and 46% for 1250 mg. Values for bioavailability using these methods are shown in Table 3.

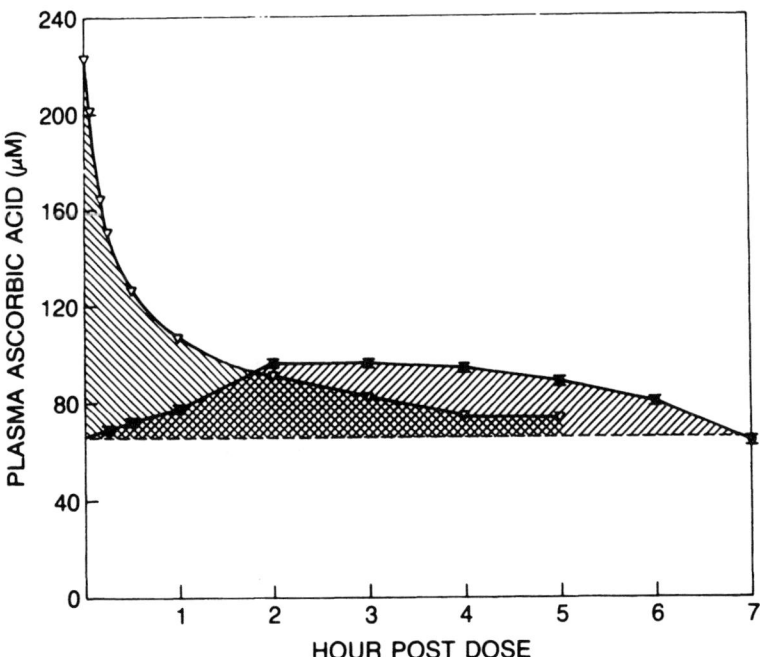

Figure 12 Schematic diagram of the method used to determine bioavailability of ascorbic acid: Bioavailability is determined by calculating the ratio of the areas under the curves (AUCs) of plasma concentrations, following oral (▲) or intravenous (▽) administration of the same dose of vitamin C on successive days. AUC is calculated by the linear trapezoidal method. The study is carried out at steady-state concentrations for that dose.

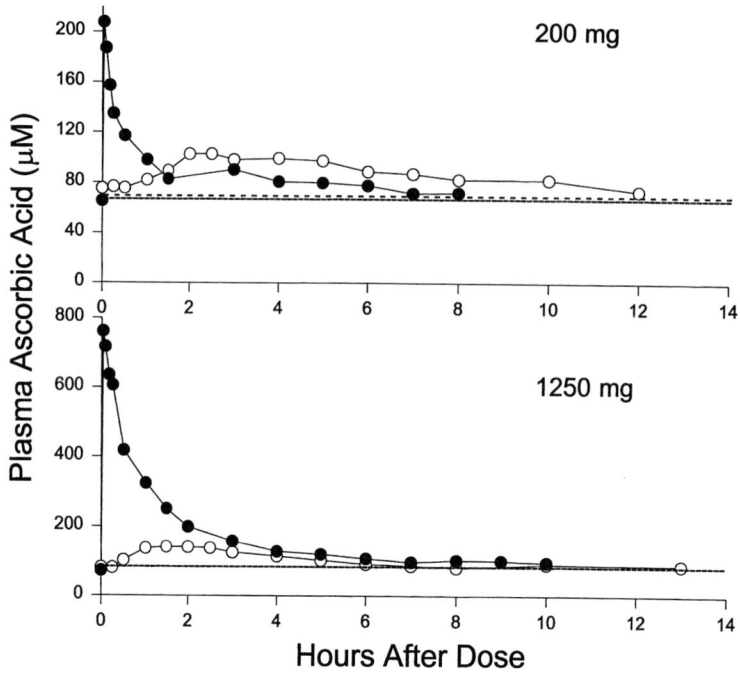

Figure 13 Ascorbic acid bioavailability in plasma: The upper figure displays bioavailability in a single subject for a 200-mg dose. The lower figure displays bioavailability for a single subject at the 1250-mg dose. For each dose ascorbic acid was administered at 0 time (8 AM) orally (○). The resulting plasma concentrations are shown for the times indicated. Baseline is indicated by a dashed line with large spaces (----). After 24 h, the same dose was given intravenously and samples were taken for the time indicated (●). Baseline is indicated by a dashed line with small spaces (----). For oral doses, samples taken before 0 time and between 13 and 24 h are not shown for clarity. AUCs were calculated using the linear trapezoidal method. Bioavailability was the ratio of the area of the oral dose (AUC$_{po}$) divided by the area of the intravenous dose (AUC$_{iv}$). AUC after the curve returned to baseline was assumed to equal zero. (From Ref. 19.)

These values were based on vitamin C administered as an aqueous solution on an empty stomach (fasted state). As the bioavailability for vitamin C is close to 100% when given in a chemically pure form, any alteration in bioavailability can mean only a decrease in bioavailability. It is not known what the bioavailability of vitamin C is when it is present in food or when administered as a supplement with food. Bioavailability may be substantially less than in its pure form as some food material might contain sequestered vitamin C, making it unavailable for absorption. Alternatively, other components of food, such as glucose (106) or flavonoids (107), might theoretically interfere with its absorption. Knowledge of bioavailability of vitamin C from food is critical to formulating recommendations for optimum dietary intake (108,109). Such information is currently unavailable.

H. Urinary Excretion of Vitamin C

As in bioavailability studies, accurate studies of urinary excretion can be done only at a steady state for that dose. The studies that previously demonstrated saturable tubular resorptive mechanisms were not done at steady-state levels. The prisoner's study stated that urinary

Table 3 Bioavailability of Vitamin C in 7 Healthy Men at Steady State

	Bioavailability of ascorbic acid[a]	
	Method using area under curve	Method using multicompartment mathematical model
Dose (mg)	Mean % (SD)	Median (%)
15	—	89
30	—	87.3
50	—	58
100	—	80
200	112 (25)	72
500	73 (27)	63
1250	49 (25)	46

[a]Subjects were given vitamin C as daily doses of 30, 60, 100, 200, 400, 1000, and 2500 mg until a steady-state level was attained for each dose. Bioavailability for 15 mg was determined at the nadir (that is at the end of depletion, but before starting repletion with vitamin C). Note that for some doses, the amount of vitamin C used for determining bioavailability was slightly different from the dose used to attain steady-state. Thus, when steady-state concentration was obtained for the 60-mg–daily dose, bioavailability for 50 mg was determined. Bioavailability using area under curves could not be determined when vitamin C did not have a constant volume of distribution or a constant rate of clearance. This is accounted for in the multicompartment mathematical model used to determine bioavailability.
Source: Refs. 19, 105.

excretion at oral doses occurred above 60 mg, but no data are available. Other studies have used a narrow-dose range or failed to use controlled vitamin C doses before measuring vitamin C excretion (110–114). Some of these studies also suffered from imprecise assays.

Studies of renal excretion carried out at steady-state levels for different doses of vitamin C show that no vitamin C appears in the urine until the oral dose is 100 mg, corresponding to a plasma concentration of approximately 60 μM. At higher doses, vitamin C appears in the urine in increasing amounts (Fig. 14). However, bioavailability falls with increasing oral doses, so that smaller and smaller amounts of vitamin C is absorbed. For example, when 1250 mg of vitamin C is given orally, less than half of it is absorbed, and this amount (approximately 600 mg) is excreted in the urine (see Fig. 14). If vitamin C is administered intravenously, renal excretion can be studied without the confounding effects of bioavailability. After intravenous administration, virtually all of the administered dose is excreted at 500 and 1250 mg (see Fig. 14B) (19). Vitamin C is not protein bound. It is, therefore, presumably filtered at the glomerulus and reabsorbed in the renal tubules. Reabsorption probably occur in a concentration-dependent manner, so that once the transport mechanism is saturated, vitamin C will be excreted in the urine. Whether additional mechanisms, such as active secretion, exist for the excretion of vitamin C is unknown. Vitamin C excretion may be similar to that of glucose, which appears in the urine when the ability of the kidney to reabsorb it is overwhelmed. In patients with renal failure, supplemental ascorbic acid can accumulate in the body, and large doses may produce hyperoxalemia (115–120), but there may not be a good correlation between the

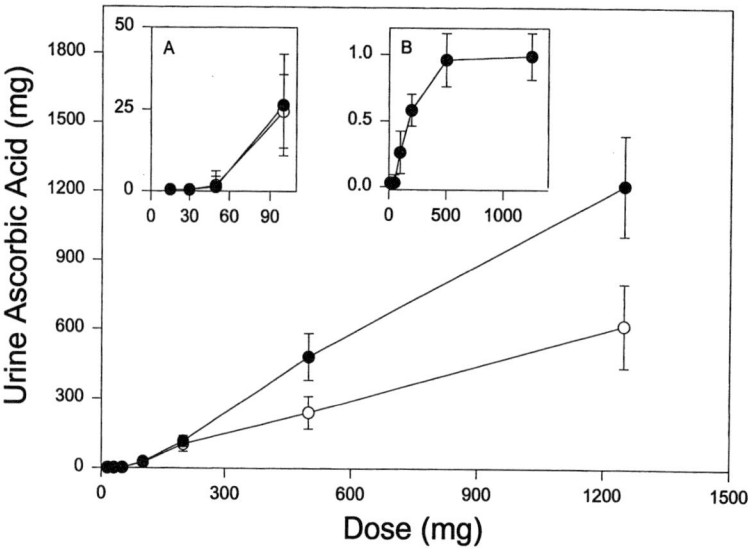

Figure 14 Ascorbic acid excretion as a function of single vitamin C doses: Ascorbic acid excretion in urine was determined after administration of single doses of vitamin C given either orally (○) or intravenously (●). Urine was collected during determination of ascorbic acid bioavailability for each dose. The collection time for oral sampling was 24 h, and the collection time for intravenous sampling was 9–10 h, the intervals required to be certain plasma ascorbate returned to baseline. (Inset A) Ascorbic acid excretion for 15–100 mg single oral (○) or intravenous (●) doses of vitamin C. x Axis indicates vitamin C dose and y axis indicates ascorbic acid excretion in the urine (mg). (Inset B) Fractional excretion (the fraction of the dose excreted) of ascorbic acid: Urine samples were collected after intravenous administration of single doses of vitamin C for bioavailability sampling. The minimum amount of ascorbate excreted was ≤ 0.4 mg. Fractional excretion was not determined for any dose of vitamin C administered orally, because of decreasing bioavailability at doses > 200 mg. x Axis indicates vitamin C dose and y axis indicates fractional excretion, defined as ascorbate excreted in urine (mg) divided by the dose administered intravenously. (From Ref. 19.)

plasma concentrations of ascorbate and oxalate (120). More commonly, patients with chronic renal failure lose ascorbic acid during dialysis. Its concentrations can fall by nearly half during a single dialysis session (120–124), so that these patients have chronically low plasma vitamin C concentrations (125,126) unless intake is adequate (127).

I. Food Sources of Vitamin C

Vitamin C is widely distributed in plant foods.

> *Fruits* containing large amounts of vitamin C include strawberries, papaya, oranges, kiwi, cantaloupe, grapefruit, mango, and honeydews.
>
> *Vegetables* rich in vitamin C are broccoli, brussel sprouts, red or green pepper, tomato, cabbage, potato, sweet potato, cauliflower, snow peas, and kale.
>
> *Fruit juices* such as orange juice, tomato juice, grapefruit juice, and fortified juices are also rich sources of vitamin C.

Five servings of a variety of fruits and vegetables per day will provide 210–280 mg of vitamin C, but consumption restricted to a narrow selection of fruits and vegetables may not provide the same amount of the vitamin (128). Vitamin C content varies to some extent depending on the season. Vitamin C may also be lost during food transportation and storage, or during cooking.

J. Vitamin C Intake in the United States

Several dietary surveys have examined vitamin C consumption in the U. S. population. The National Health and Nutrition Examination Survey (NHANHS) 3 study found that the median intake of vitamin C for males 20 years old or more, is 84 mg and for females 20 years old or more, it is 73 mg. Approximately 30% of adults consume less than 2.5 servings of fruits and vegetables per day. The estimated vitamin C intake is lower among many population subgroups including children (129,130). In one study of 9- and 10-year-old girls, approximately one-fourth had vitamin C ingestion less than the RDA of 45 mg for their age (131). Results of a survey of Latino children were that fewer than 15% ingested the recommended intake of fruits and vegetables (132). Data from the earlier nutritional survey NHANES 2 have been examined extensively. The analyses indicated that 20–30% of U. S. adults ingested less than 60 mg daily of vitamin C (129,130,133).

K. Recommended Dietary Allowance for Vitamin C

Recently U.S. RDAs for vitamin C were increased from 60 mg/day to 75 mg/day for women and 90 mg/day for men (134). These recommendations are based on the recent findings concerning the vitamin C intake necessary to saturate neutrophils. As a result of recent research into the varied actions of vitamin C, a wealth of biochemical, molecular, epidemiological, and clinical data have become available. From these data, the following criteria can serve as sound foundation for recommendations on optimum vitamin C intake.

- Dietary availability
- Steady-state concentrations in plasma in relation to dose
- Steady-state concentrations in tissue in relation to dose
- Bioavailability
- Urine excretion
- Adverse effects
- Biochemical and molecular function in relation to vitamin concentration
- Beneficial effects in relation to dose; direct effects and epidemiological observations
- Prevention of deficiency

When these criteria are applied to the Food and Nutrition Board's classification guidelines, the Dietary Reference Intakes, the Recommended Dietary Allowance has been proposed by us to be 100–120 mg daily (135). It is necessary to note that this value depends on the data selected for the new dietary reference intake classification, the Estimated Average Requirement. Adequate Intake, another new dietary reference intake classification, is used when data are considered insufficient for a recommended dietary allowance. Adequate Intake for vitamin C was estimated to be 200 mg daily, to be obtained from five servings of fruits and vegetables. The last new classification, Tolerable Upper Intake, is proposed to be less than 1 g of vitamin C daily (135). Physicians can tell patients now that five servings of fruits and vegetables provide sufficient vitamin C intake for healthy persons and are beneficial in preventing cancer, and that 1 g or more of vitamin C might have adverse consequences in some persons.

REFERENCES

1. Clemenston CAB. Classical scurvy: a historical review. In: Vitamin C. Vol. 1. Boca Raton, FL: CRC Press, 1989.
2. Lind J. The true causes of the disease, from observations made upon it, both at sea and land. In: Stewart CP, Guthrie D, eds. Lind's Treatise on Scurvy. Bicentenary Volume. Edinburgh: Edinburgh University Press, 1953:69–112.
3. Szent–Gyorgyi A. Observations on the function of peroxidase systems and chemistry of the adrenal cortex: description of a new carbohydrate derivative. Bioichem J 1928; 22:1387.
4. Svirbely JL, Szent–Gyorgyi A. The chemical nature of vitamin C. Biochem J 1932; 26:865–870.
5. King CG, Waugh WA. The chemical nature of vitamin C. Science 1932; 75:357.
6. Lind J. The diagnostics, or signs. In: Stewart CP, Guthrie D, eds. Lind's Treatise on Scurvy. Bicentenary Volume. Edinburgh: Edinburgh University Press, 1953:113–132.
7. Hodges RE, Baker EM, Hood J, Sauberlich HE, March SC. Experimental scurvy in man. Am J Clin Nutr 1969; 22:535–548.
8. Johnston CS, Thompson LL. Vitamin C status of an outpatient population. J Am Coll Nutr 1998; 17:366–370.
9. Ohta Y, Nishikimi M. Random nucleotide substitutions in primate nonfunctional gene for L-gulono-gamma-lactone oxidase, the missing enzyme in L-ascorbic acid biosynthesis. Biochim Biophys Acta 1999; 1472:408–411.
10. Nishikimi M, Kawai T, Yagi K. Guinea pigs possess a highly mutated gene for L-gulono-gamma-lactone oxidase, the key enzyme for L-ascorbic acid biosynthesis missing in this species. J Biol Chem 1992; 267:21967–21972.
11. Nishikimi M, Fukuyama R, Minoshima S, Shimizu N, Yagi K. Cloning and chromosomal mapping of the human nonfunctional gene for L-gulono-gamma-lactone oxidase, the enzyme for L-ascorbic acid biosynthesis missing in man. J Biol Chem 1994; 269:13685–13688.
12. Ratterree MS, Didier PJ, Blanchard JL, Clarke MR, Schaeffer D. Vitamin C deficiency in captive nonhuman primates fed commercial primate diet. Lab Anim Sci 1990; 40:165–168.
13. Wheeler GL, Jones MA, Smirnoff N. The biosynthetic pathway of vitamin C in higher plants. Nature 1998; 393:365–369.
14. Smirnoff N. Ascorbic acid: metabolism and functions of a multi-faceted molecule. Curr Opin Plant Biol 2000; 3:229–235.
15. Buettner GR, Moseley PL. EPR spin trapping of free radicals produced by bleomycin and ascorbate. Free Radic Res Commun 1993; 19:S89–S93.
16. Rumsey SC, Levine M. Absorption, transport, and disposition of ascorbic acid in humans. Nutr Biochem 1998; 9:116–130.
17. Winkler BS, Orselli SM, Rex TS. The redox couple between glutathione and ascorbic acid: a chemical and physiological perspective. Free Radic Biol Med 1994; 17:333–349.
18. Baker EM, Halver JE, Johnsen DO, Joyce BE, Knight MK, Tolbert BM. Metabolism of ascorbic acid and ascorbic-2-sulfate in man and the subhuman primate. Ann NY Acad Sci 1975; 258:72–80.
19. Levine M, Conry–Cantilena C, Wang Y, Welch RW, Washko PW, Dhariwal KR, Park JB, Lazarev A, Graumlich JF, King J, Cantilena LR. Vitamin C pharmacokinetics in healthy volunteers: evidence for a recommended dietary allowance. Proc Natl Acad Sci USA 1996; 93:3704–3709.
20. Levine M. New concepts in the biology and biochemistry of ascorbic acid. N Engl J Med 1986; 314:892–902.
21. Englard S, Seifter S. The biochemical functions of ascorbic acid. Annu Rev Nutr 1986; 6:365–406.
22. Prockop DJ, Kivirikko KI. Collagens: molecular biology, diseases, and potentials for therapy. Annu Rev Biochem 1995; 64:403–434.
23. Kivirikko KI, Myllyla R. Post-translational processing of procollagens. Ann NY Acad Sci 1985; 460:187–201.
24. Peterkofsky B. Ascorbate requirement for hydroxylation and secretion of procollagen: relationship to inhibition of collagen synthesis in scurvy. Am J Clin Nutr 1991; 54:1135S–1140S.
25. Rebouche CJ. Ascorbic acid and carnitine biosynthesis. Am J Clin Nutr 1991; 54:1147S–1152S.
26. Dunn WA, Rettura G, Seifter E, Englard S. Carnitine biosynthesis from gamma-butyrobetaine and from exogenous protein-bound 6-N-trimethyl-L-lysine by the perfused guinea pig liver. Effect of ascorbate deficiency on the in situ activity of gamma-butyrobetaine hydroxylase. J Biol Chem 1984; 259:10764–10770.

27. Levine M, Dhariwal KR, Washko PW, Butler JD, Welch RW, Wang YH, Bergsten P. Ascorbic acid and in situ kinetics: a new approach to vitamin requirements. Am J Clin Nutr 1991; 54:1157S–1162S.
28. Kaufman S. Dopamine-beta-hydroxylase. J Psychiatr Res 1974; 11:303–316.
29. Eipper BA, Milgram SL, Husten EJ, Yun HY, Mains RE. Peptidylglycine alpha-amidating monooxygenase: a multifunctional protein with catalytic, processing, and routing domains. Protein Sci 1993; 2:489–497.
30. Eipper BA, Stoffers DA, Mains RE. The biosynthesis of neuropeptides: peptide alpha-amidation. Annu Rev Neurosci 1992; 15:57–85.
31. Lindblad B, Lindstedt G, Lindstedt S. The mechanism of enzymic formation of homogenisate from p-hydroxyphenylpyruvate. J Am Chem Soc 1970; 92:7446–7449.
32. Wondrack LM, Hsu CA, Abbott MT. Thymine 7-hydroxylase and pyrimidine deoxyribonucleoside $2'$-hydroxylase activities in *Rhodotorula glutinis*. J Biol Chem 1978; 253:6511–6515.
33. Stubbe J. Identification of two alpha-ketoglutarate-dependent dioxygenases in extracts of *Rhodotorula glutinis* catalyzing deoxyuridine hydroxylation. J Biol Chem 1985; 260:9972–9975.
34. Hallberg L, Brune M, Rossander-Hulthen L. Is there a physiological role of vitamin C in iron absorption? Ann NY Acad Sci 1987; 498:324–332.
35. Hallberg L. Wheat fiber, phytates and iron absorption. Scand J Gastroenterol Suppl 1987; 129:73–79.
36. Hitomi K, Tsukagoshi N. Role of ascorbic acid in modulation of gene expression. Subcell Biochem 1996; 25:41–56.
37. Toth I, Roger JT, McPhee JA, Elliott SM, Abramson SL, Bridges KR. Ascorbic acid enhances iron-induced ferritin translation in human leukemia and hepatoma cells. J Biol Chem 1995; 270:2846–2852.
38. Stadtman ER, Berlett BS. Reactive oxygen-mediated protein oxidation in aging and disease. Chem Res Toxicol 1997; 10:485–494.
39. Frei B, Stocker R, England L, Ames BN. Ascorbate: the most effective antioxidant in human blood plasma. Adv Exp Med Biol 1990; 264:155–163.
40. Helser MA, Hotchkiss JH, Roe DA. Influence of fruit and vegetable juices on the endogenous formation of N-nitrosoproline and N-nitrosothiazolidine-4-carboxylic acid in humans on controlled diets. Carcinogenesis 1992; 13:2277–2280.
41. Gokce N, Frei B. Basic research in antioxidant inhibition of steps in atherogenesis. J Cardiovasc Risk 1996; 3:352–357.
42. Jialal I, Fuller CJ, Huet BA. The effect of alpha-tocopherol supplementation on LDL oxidation. A dose–response study. Arterioscler Thromb Vasc Biol 1995; 15:190–198.
43. Jialal I, Vega GL, Grundy SM. Physiologic levels of ascorbate inhibit the oxidative modification of low density lipoprotein. Atherosclerosis 1990; 82:185–191.
44. Jialal I, Fuller CJ. Effect of vitamin E, vitamin C and beta-carotene on LDL oxidation and atherosclerosis. Can J Cardiol 1995; 11:97G–103G.
45. Weber C, Erl W, Weber K, Weber PC. Increased adhesiveness of isolated monocytes to endothelium is prevented by vitamin C intake in smokers. Circulation 1996; 93:1488–1492.
46. Washko PW, Wang Y, Levine M. Ascorbic acid recycling in human neutrophils. J Biol Chem 1993; 268:15531–15535.
47. Mukhopadhyay CK, Chatterjee IB. Free metal ion-independent oxidative damage of collagen. Protection by ascorbic acid. J Biol Chem 1994; 269:30200–30205.
48. Stampfer MJ, Hennekens CH, Manson JE, Colditz GA, Rosner B, Willett WC. Vitamin E consumption and the risk of coronary disease in women. N Engl J Med 1993; 328:1444–1449.
49. Rimm EB, Stampfer MJ, Ascherio A, Giovannucci E, Colditz GA, Willett WC. Vitamin E consumption and the risk of coronary heart disease in man. N Engl J Med 1993; 328:1450–1456.
50. Gey KF. Cardiovascular disease and vitamins. Concurrent correction of "suboptimal" plasma antioxidant levels may, as important part of "optimal" nutrition, help to prevent early stages of cardiovascular disease and cancer, respectively. Bibl Nutr Dieta 1995; 52:75–91.
51. Rathbone BJ, Johnson AW, Wyatt JI, Kelleher J, Heatley RV, Losowsky MS. Ascorbic acid: a factor concentrated in human gastric juice. Clin Sci 1989; 76:237–241.
52. Correa P. Human gastric carcinogenesis: a multistep and multifactorial process—First American Cancer Society Award Lecture on Cancer Epidemiology and Prevention. Cancer Res 1992; 52:6735–6740.

53. Sobala GM, Schorah CJ, Pignatelli B, Crabtree JE, Martin IG, Scott N, Quirke P. High gastric juice ascorbic acid concentrations in members of a gastric cancer family. Carcinogenesis 1993; 14:291–292.
54. Sobala GM, Schorah CJ, Shires S, Lynch DA, Gallacher B, Dixon MF, Axon AT. Effect of eradication of *Helicobacter pylori* on gastric juice ascorbic acid concentrations. Gut 1993; 34:1038–1041.
55. Byers T, Guerrero N. Epidemiologic evidence for vitamin C and vitamin E in cancer prevention. Am J Clin Nutr 1995; 62:1385S–1392S.
56. Davidsson L, Walczyk T, Morris A, Hurrell RF. Influence of ascorbic acid on iron absorption from an iron-fortified, chocolate-flavored milk drink in Jamaican children. Am J Clin Nutr 1998; 67:873–877.
57. Hunt JR, Mullen LM, Lykken GI, Gallagher SK, Nielsen FH. Ascorbic acid: effect on ongoing iron absorption and status in iron-depleted young women. Am J Clin Nutr 1990; 51:649–655.
58. Stack T, Aggett PJ, Aitken E, Lloyd DJ. Routine L-ascorbic acid supplementation does not alter iron, copper, and zinc balance in low-birth-weight infants fed a cows'-milk formula. J Pediatr Gatroenterol Nutr 1990; 10:351–356.
59. Harju E, Lindberg H. Ascorbic acid does not augment the restoration effect of iron treatment for empty iron stores in patients after gastrointestinal surgery. Am Surg 1986; 52:463–466.
60. Rhode BM, Shustik C, Christou NV, MacLean LD. Iron absorption and therapy after gastric bypass. Obes Surg 1999; 9:17–21.
61. Hunt JR, Gallagher SK, Johnson LK. Effect of ascorbic acid on apparent iron absorption by women with low iron stores. Am J Clin Nutr 1994; 59:1381–1385.
62. Hornig D. Distribution of ascorbic acid, metabolites and analogues in man and animals. Ann NY Acad Sci 1975; 258:103–118.
63. Rebec GV, Pierce RC. A vitamin as neuromodulator: ascorbate release into the extracellular fluid of the brain regulates dopaminergic and glutamatergic transmission. Prog Neurobiol 1994; 43:537–565.
64. Keith MO, Pelletier O. Ascorbic acid concentrations in leukocytes and selected organs of guinea pigs in response to increasing ascorbic acid intake. Am J Clin Nutr 1974; 27:368–372.
65. Hornig D, Weber F, Wiss O. Tissue distribution of labelled material in vitamin C-deficient guinea pigs after intravenous injection of $(1-^{14}C)$ ascorbic acid or $(1-^{14}C)$ dehydroascorbic acid. Int J Vitam Nutr Res 1972; 42:511–523.
66. Chinoy NJ. Ascorbic acid levels in mammalian tissues and its metabolic significance. Comp Biochem Physiol A 1972; 42:945–952.
67. Horning D, Gallo–Torres HE, Weiser H. Tissue distribution of labelled ascorbic acid in normal and hypophysectomized rats. Int J Vitam Nutr Res 1972; 42:487–496.
68. Wang Y, Russo TA, Kwon O, Chanock S, Rumsey SC, Levine M. Ascorbate recycling in human neutrophils: induction by bacteria. Proc Natl Acad Sci USA 1977; 94:13816–13819.
69. Daruwala R, Song J, Koh WS, Rumsey SC, Levine M. Cloning and functional characterization of the human sodium-dependent vitamin C transporters hSVCT1 and hSVCT2. FEBS Lett 1999; 460:480–484.
70. Tsukaguchi H, Tokui T, Mackenzie B, Berger UV, Chen XZ, Wang Y, Brubaker RF, Hediger MA. A family of mammalian Na^+-dependent L-ascorbic acid transporters. Nature 1999; 399:70–75.
71. Wang Y, Mackenzie B, Tsukaguchi H, Weremowicz S, Morton CC, Hediger MA. Human vitamin C (L-ascorbic acid) transporter SVCT1. Biochem Biophys Res Commun 2000; 267:488–494.
72. Stratakis CA, Taymans S, Daruwala R, Song J, Levine M. Mapping of the human genes (SLCA23A2 and SLCA23A1) coding for vitamin C transporters 1 and 2 (SVCT1 and SVCT2), to 5q23 and 20p12, respectively. J Med Genet 2000; 37:E20.
73. Vera JC, Rivas CI, Fischbarg J, Golde DW. Mammalian facilitative hexose transporters mediate the transport of dehydroascorbic acid. Nature 1993; 364:79–82.
74. Rumsey SC, Kwon O, Xu GW, Burant CF, Simpson I, Levine M. Glucose transporter isoforms GLUT1 and GLUT3 transport dehydroascorbic acid. J Biol Chem 1997; 272:18982–18989.
75. Rumsey SC, Daruwala R, Al-Hasani H, Zarnowski M, Simpson IA, Levine M. Dehydroascorbic acid transport by GLUT4 in *Xenopus* oocytes and isolated rat adipocytes. J Biol Chem 1997; 272:18982–18989.
76. Welch RW, Wang Y, Crossman A Jr, Park JB, Kirk KL, Levine M. Accumulation of vitamin C (ascorbate) and its oxidized metabolite dehydroascorbic acid occurs by separate mechanisms. J Biol Chem 1995; 270:12584–12592.

77. Padh H, Aleo JJ. Ascorbic acid transport by 3T6 fibroblasts. Regulation by and purification of human serum complement factor. J Biol Chem 1989; 264:6065–6069.
78. Dixon SJ, Wilson JX. Adaptive regulation of ascorbate transport in osteoblastic cells. J Bone Miner Res 1992; 7:675–681.
79. Agus DB, Gambhir SS, Pardridge WM, Spielholz C, Baselga J, Vera JC, Golde DW. Vitamin C crosses the blood–brain barrier in the oxidized form through the glucose transporters. J Clin Invest 1997; 100:2842–2848.
80. Agus DB, Vera JC, Golde DW. Stromal cell oxidation: a mechanism by which tumors obtain vitamin C. Cancer Res 1999; 59:4555–4558.
81. Dhariwal KR, Shirvan M, Levine M. Ascorbic acid regeneration in chromaffin granules. In situ kinetics. J Biol Chem 1991; 266:5384–5387.
82. Levine M, Wang Y, Rumsey SC. Analysis of ascorbic acid and dehydroascorbic acid in biological samples. Methods Enzymol 1999; 299:65–76.
83. Rumsey SC, Wang Y, Levine M. Ascorbic acid and dehydroascorbic acid analyses in biological samples. In: Song WO, Beecher GR, eds. Modern Analytical Methodologies on Fat and Water Soluble Vitamins. New York: John Wiley & Sons, 2001 (in press).
84. Dhariwal KR, Hartzell WO, Levine M. Ascorbic acid and dehydroascorbic acid measurements in human plasma and serum. Am J Clin Nutr 1991; 54:712–716.
85. Hegsted DM. Truly quantitative dietary studies have stringent requirements. Am J Clin Nutr 1997; 66:1477–1479.
86. Baker EM, Hodges RE, Hood J, Sauberlich HE, March SC. Metabolism of ascorbic-1-^{14}C acid in experimental human scurvy. Am J Clin Nutr 1969; 22:549–558.
87. Hodges RE, Hood J, Canham JE, Sauberlich HE, Baker EM. Clinical manifestations of ascorbic acid deficiency in man. Am J Clin Nutr 1971; 24:432–443.
88. Bake EM, Hodges RE, Hood J, Sauberlich HE, March SC, Canham JE. Metabolism of ^{14}C- and ^{3}H-labeled L-ascorbic acid in human scurvy. Am J Clin Nutr 1971; 24:444–454.
89. Hodges RE. What's new about scurvy? Am J Clin Nutr 1971; 24:383–384.
90. Block G, Mangels AR, Patterson BH, Levander OA, Norkus EP, Taylor PR. Body weight and prior depletion affect plasma ascorbate levels attained on identical vitamin C intake: a controlled-diet study. J Am Coll Nutr 1999; 18:628–637.
91. Leggott PJ, Robertson PB, Rothman DL, Murray PA, Jacob RA. The effect of controlled ascorbic acid depletion and supplementation on periodontal health. J Periodontol 1986; 57:480–485.
92. Leggott PJ, Robertson PB, Rothman DL, Murray PA, Jacob RA. Response of lingual ascorbic acid test and salivary ascorbate levels to changes in ascorbic acid intake. J Dent Res 1986; 65:131–134.
93. Holloway DE, Hutton SW, Peterson FJ, Duane WC. Lack of effect of subclinical ascorbic acid deficiency upon antipyrine metabolism in man. Am J Clin Nutr 1982; 35:917–924.
94. Blanchard J, Conrad KA, Watson RR, Garry PJ, Crawley JD. Comparison of plasma, mononuclear and polymorphonuclear leucocyte vitamin C levels in young and elderly women during depletion and supplementation. Eur J Clin Nutr 1989; 43:97–106.
95. Leggott PJ, Robertson PB, Jacob RA, Zambon JJ, Walsh M, Armitage GC. Effects of ascorbic acid depletion and supplementation on periodontal health and subgingival microflora in humans. J Dent Res 1991; 70:1531–1536.
96. Blanchard J. Depletion and repletion kinetics of vitamin C in humans. J Nutr 1991; 121:170–176.
97. Mangels AR, Block G, Frey CM, Patterson BH, Taylor PR, Norkus EP, Levander OA. The bioavailability to humans of ascorbic acid from oranges, orange juice and cooked broccoli is similar to that of synthetic ascorbic acid. J Nutr 1993; 123:1054–1061.
98. Washko P, Rotrosen D, Levine M. Ascorbic acid transport and accumulation in human neutrophils. J Biol Chem 1989; 264:18996–19002.
99. Bergsten P, Amitai G, Kehrl J, Dhariwal KR, Klein HG, Levine M. Millimolar concentrations of ascorbic acid in purified human mononuclear leukocytes. Depletion and reaccumulation. J Biol Chem 1990; 265:2584–2587.
100. King J, Wang Y, Welch RW, Dhariwal KR, Conry–Cantilena C, Levine M. Use of a new vitamin C-deficient diet in a depletion/repletion clinical trial. Am J Clin Nutr 1997; 65:1434–1440.
101. Piotrovskij VK, Kallay Z, Gajdos M, Gerykova M, Trnovec T. The use of a nonlinear absorption model in the study of ascorbic acid bioavailability in man. Biopharm Drug Dispos 1993; 14:429–442.
102. Gregory JFD. Ascorbic acid bioavailability in foods and supplements. Nutr Rev 1993; 51:301–303.

103. Sacharin R, Taylor T, Chasseaud LF. Blood levels and bioavailability of ascorbic acid after administration of a sustained-release formulation to humans. Int J Vitam Nutr Res 1977; 47:68–74.
104. Vinson JA, Bose P. Comparative bioavailability to humans of ascorbic acid alone or in a citrus extract. Am J Clin Nutr 1988; 48:601–604.
105. Graumlich JF, Ludden TM, Conry–Cantilena C, Cantilena LR Jr, Wang Y, Levine M. Pharmacokinetic model of ascorbic acid in healthy male volunteers during depletion and repletion. Pharm Res 1997; 14:1133–1139.
106. Washko P, Levine M. Inhibition of ascorbic acid transport in human neutrophils by glucose. J Biol Chem 1992; 267:23568–23574.
107. Park JB, Levine M. Intracellular accumulation of ascorbic acid is inhibited by flavonoids via blocking of dehydroascorbic acid and ascorbic acid uptakes in HL-60, U937 and Jurkat cells. J Nutr 2000; 130:1297–1302.
108. Clydesdale FM, Ho CT, Lee CY, Mondy NI, Shewfelt RL. The effects of postharvest treatment and chemical interactions on the bioavailability of ascorbic acid, thiamin, vitamin A, carotenoids, and minerals. Crit Rev Food Sci Nutr 1991; 30:599–638.
109. Mayersohn M. Vitamin C bioavailability. J Nutr Sci Vitaminol (Tokyo) 1992; Spec:446–449.
110. Kallner A, Hartmann D, Hornig D. Steady-state turnover and body pool of ascorbic acid in man. Am J Clin Nutr 1979; 32:530–539.
111. Kallner A, Hartmann D, Hornig D. On the absorption of ascorbic acid in man. Int J Vitam Nutr Res 1977; 47:383–388.
112. Mitch WE, Johnson MW, Kirshenbaum JM, Lopez RE. Effect of large oral doses of ascorbic acid on uric acid excretion by normal subjects. Clin Pharmacol Ther 1981; 29:318–321.
113. Wagner ES, Lindley B, Coffin RD. High-performance liquid chromatographic determination of ascorbic acid in urine: effect on urinary excretion profiles after oral and intravenous administration of vitamin C. J Chromatogr 1979; 163:225–229.
114. Blanchard J, Conrad KA, Garry PJ. Effects of age and intake on vitamin C disposition in females. Eur J Clin Nutr 1990; 44:447–460.
115. Tomson CR, Channon SM, Parkinson IS, McArdle P, Qureshi M, Ward MK, Laker MF. Correction of subclinical ascorbate deficiency in patients receiving dialysis: effects on plasma oxalate, serum cholesterol, and capillary fragility. Clin Chim Acta 1989; 180:255–264.
116. Balcke P, Schmidt P, Zazgornik J, Kopsa H, Haubenstock A. Ascorbic acid aggravates secondary hyperoxalemia in patients on chronic hemodialysis. Ann Intern Med 1984; 101:344–345.
117. Ono K. Secondary hyperoxalemia caused by vitamin C supplementation in regular hemodialysis patients. Clin Nephrol 1986; 26:239–243.
118. Ono K. The effect of vitamin C supplementation and withdrawal on the mortality and morbidity of regular hemodialysis patients. Clin Nephrol 1989; 31:31–34.
119. Pru C, Eaton J, Kjellstrand C. Vitamin C intoxication and hyperoxalemia in chronic hemodialysis patients. Nephron 1985; 39:112–116.
120. Rolton HA, McConnell KM, Modi KS, Macdougall AI. The effect of vitamin C intake on plasma oxalate in patients on regular haemodialysis. Nephrol Dial Transplant 1991; 6:440–443.
121. Allman MA, Truswell AS, Tiller DJ, Stewart PM, Yau DF, Horvath JS, Duggin GG. Vitamin supplementation of patients receiving haemodialysis. Med J Aust 1989; 150:130–133.
122. Sullivan JF, Eisenstein AB. Ascorbic acid depletion during hemodialysis. JAMA 1972; 220:1697–1699.
123. Sullivan JF, Eisenstein AB. Ascorbic acid depletion in patients undergoing chronic hemodialysis. Am J Clin Nutr 1970; 23:1339–1346.
124. Bohm V, Tiroke K, Schneider S, Sperschneider H, Stein G, Bitsch R. Vitamin C status of patients with chronic renal failure, dialysis patients and patients after renal transplantation. Int J Vitam Nutr Res 1997; 67:262–266.
125. Papastephanidis C, Agroyannis B, Tzanatos–Exarchou H, Orthopoulos B, Koutsicos D, Frangos–Plemenos M, Kallitsis M, Yatzidis H. Re-evaluation of ascorbic acid deficiency in hemodialysed patients. Int J Artif Organs 1987; 10:163–165.
126. Wang S, Eide TC, Sogn EM, Berg KJ, Sund RB. Plasma ascorbic acid in patients undergoing chronic haemodialysis. Eur J Clin Pharmacol 1999; 55:527–532.
127. Shah GM, Ross EA, Sabo A, Pichon M, Bhagavan H, Reynolds RD. Ascorbic acid supplements in patients receiving chronic peritoneal dialysis. Am J Kidney Dis 1991; 18:84–90.
128. Johnston CS. Recommendations for vitamin C intake. JAMA 1999; 282:2118; discussion 2119.

129. Koplan JP, Annest JL, Layde PM, Rubin GL. Nutrient intake and supplementation in the United States (NHANES II). Am J Public Health 1986; 76:287–289.
130. Patterson BH, Block G, Rosenberger WF, Pee D, Kahle LL. Fruit and vegetables in the American diet: data from the NHANES II survey. Am J Public Health 1990; 80:1443–1449.
131. Simon JA, Schreiber GB, Crawford PB, Frederick MM, Sabry ZI. Dietary vitamin C and serum lipids in black and white girls. Epidemiology 1993; 4:537–542.
132. Basch CE, Zybert P, Shea S. 5-A-DAY: dietary behavior and the fruit and vegetable intake of Latino children. Am J Public Health 1994; 84:814–818.
133. Murphy SP, Rose D, Hudes M, Viteri FE. Demographic and economic factors associated with dietary quality for adults in the 1987–88 Nationwide Food Consumption Survey. J Am Diet Assoc 1992; 92:1352–1357.
134. Food and Nutrition Board; Panel on Dietary Antioxidants and Related Compounds. Dietary Reference Intakes for Vitamin C, Vitamin E, Selenium and Beta Carotene, and other Carotenoids. Washington DC: National Academy Press, 2000:95–185.
135. Levine M, Rumsey SC, Daruwala R, Park JB, Wang Y. Criteria and recommendations for vitamin C intake. JAMA 1999; 281:1415–1423.
136. Washko PW, Welch RW, Dhariwal KR, Wang Y, Levine M. Ascorbic acid and dehydroascorbic acid analyses in biological samples. Anal Biochem 1992; 204:1–14.
137. Dyer DL, Kanai Y, Hediger MA, Rubin SA, Said HM. Expression of a rabbit renal ascorbic acid transporter in *Xenopus laevis* oocytes. Am J Physiol 1994; 267:C301–306.
138. Park JB, Levine M. Purification, cloning and expression of dehydroascorbic acid-reducing activity from human neutrophils: identification as glutaredoxin. Biochem J 1996; 315:931–938.

8
Vitamin C and Cardiovascular Diseases

Anitra C. Carr and Balz Frei
Linus Pauling Institute, Oregon State University, Corvallis, Oregon

I. INTRODUCTION
A. Vitamin C Is a Potent Water-Soluble Antioxidant

Vitamin C (ascorbate) is an essential micronutrient required for normal metabolic functioning of the body (1). Humans, and other primates, have lost the ability to synthesize vitamin C owing to a mutation in the gene coding for L-gulono-γ-lactone oxidase, an enzyme required for the biosynthesis of vitamin C via the glucuronic acid pathway (2). As a result, humans have to obtain vitamin C through the diet; the vitamin is especially plentiful in fresh fruit and vegetables (3). A lack of vitamin C in the diet causes the deficiency disease scurvy (4). Vitamin C is a cosubstrate for various biosynthetic enzymes, including the hydroxylases and oxygenases involved in the synthesis of collagen, carnitine, and catecholamines (5,6). The role of vitamin C is to reduce the active center metal ion of these enzymes (5,6), and the ability to maintain metal ions in the reduced state is related to the redox potential of vitamin C (7).

Vitamin C is also an important water-soluble antioxidant in biological fluids (8,9). It readily scavenges reactive oxygen, nitrogen, and chlorine species, thereby effectively protecting other substrates from oxidative damage. The reactive species scavenged by vitamin C include superoxide and aqueous peroxyl radicals, singlet oxygen, ozone, peroxynitrite, nitrogen dioxide, and hypochlorous acid (Table 1) (7). In addition to scavenging these reactive species, vitamin C can regenerate other small-molecule antioxidants, such as α-tocopherol, glutathione (GSH), urate, and β-carotene, from their respective radical species (see Table 1) (7). Interaction of vitamin C with the α-tocopheroxyl radical to regenerate α-tocopherol moves radicals from the lipid phase into the aqueous phase and, thereby, prevents tocopherol-mediated peroxidation in lipoproteins (19). Although vitamin C acts as a coantioxidant for α-tocopherol in isolated lipoproteins and cells (20,21), it is uncertain whether vitamin C recycles, or rather spares, α-tocopherol in vivo (22–25). In contrast, vitamin C spares GSH under conditions of increased oxidative stress in vivo (26).

Vitamin C is an effective antioxidant for several reasons. First, both ascorbate and the ascorbyl radical, the latter formed by one electron oxidation of ascorbate (Fig. 1), have low

Table 1 Vitamin C Scavenges Reactive Oxygen, Nitrogen, and Chlorine Species and Regenerates Antioxidant Radicals to Their Parent Compound

Chemical species scavenged by vitamin C	Ref.
Reactive oxygen species	
Alkoxyl radicals (RO$^{\cdot}$)	10
Hydroxyl radical ($^{\cdot}$OH)	10
Ozone (O_3)	11
Peroxyl radicals ($RO_2^{\cdot}$)	10
Singlet oxygen ($^1O_2$)	12
Superoxide anion/hydroperoxyl radical ($O_2^{\cdot-}$/$HO_2^{\cdot}$)	10
Reactive nitrogen species	
Dinitrogen trioxide/dinitrogen tetroxide (N_2O_3/N_2O_4)	13
Nitrogen dioxide ($NO_2^{\cdot}$)	14
Nitroxide (NO)	15
Peroxynitrite/peroxynitrous acid ($ONOO^-$/ONOOH)	16
Reactive chlorine species	
Chloramines (RNHCl)	17
Hypochlorous acid (HOCl)	17
Antioxidant-derived radicals	
β-Carotene radical cation (β-$C^{\cdot+}$)	18
Thiyl/sulfonyl radicals ($RS^{\cdot}$/$RSO^{\cdot}$)	10
α-Tocopheroxyl radical (α-$TO^{\cdot}$)	10
Urate radical ($UH^{\cdot-}$)	10

reduction potentials (27); hence, they can react with most other biologically relevant radicals and oxidants (several of which are listed in Table 1). For this reason, vitamin C has been said to be "at the bottom of the pecking order" and "to act as the terminal water-soluble small molecule antioxidant" in biological systems (27). Second, the ascorbyl radical has a low reactivity because of resonance stabilization of the unpaired electron, and readily dismutates to ascorbate and dehydroascorbic acid (DHA) (10). In addition, ascorbate can be regenerated from both the ascorbyl radical and DHA by enzyme-dependent and enzyme-independent pathways. The ascorbyl radical is reduced by an NADH-dependent semidehydroascorbate reductase (28) and the NADPH-dependent selenoenzyme thioredoxin reductase (29). DHA can be reduced back to ascorbate nonenzymatically by GSH (28), as well as by thioredoxin reductase (30) and the GSH-dependent enzyme glutaredoxin (31).

B. Oxidative Processes Are Involved in Cardiovascular Diseases

Oxidative processes have been strongly implicated in atherosclerosis, myocardial infarction, and stroke (32). The oxidative modification hypothesis of atherosclerosis is currently the most widely accepted model of atherogenesis. Low-density lipoprotein (LDL), the major carrier of cholesterol and lipids in the blood (33), infiltrates into the intima of lesion-prone arterial sites where it is oxidized over time by oxidants generated by local vascular cells or enzymes (34) to a form that exhibits atherogenic properties (Table 2). Minimally oxidized LDL is able to activate endothelial cells to express surface adhesion molecules, primarily vascular cell adhesion molecule-1 (VCAM-1) and intercellular adhesion molecule-1 (ICAM-1), as well as monocyte chemotactic protein-1 (MCP-1), which cause circulating monocytes to adhere

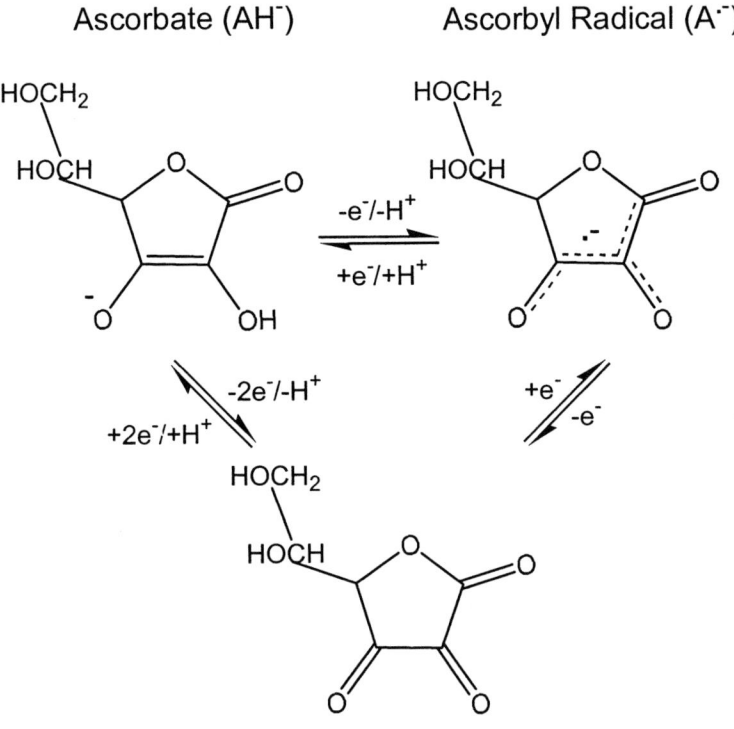

Figure 1 Ascorbate (AH$^-$) is oxidized to the ascorbyl radical (A$^{\cdot-}$) and then to dehydroascorbic acid (DHA) by one-electron oxidants (e.g., superoxide or nitrogen dioxide radicals), or directly to DHA by two-electron oxidants (e.g., hypochlorous acid or chloramines). DHA rapidly hydrolyzes to diketogulonic acid and other products, or is reduced back to AH$^-$ by chemical or enzymatic systems utilizing GSH or NAD(P)H. A$^{\cdot-}$ spontaneously dismutates to AH$^-$ and DHA or is reduced back to AH$^-$ by chemical or enzymatic systems.

Table 2 Oxidatively Modified Low-Density Lipoprotein (LDL) Has Potentially Atherogenic Properties Toward Vascular Cells

Potentially atherogenic properties of oxidatively modified LDL	Ref.
Chemotaxis of leukocytes and smooth muscle cells	35, 36
Cytotoxicity	37–39
Induction of monocyte chemotactic protein-1, granulocyte and macrophage colony-stimulating factors and cell adhesion molecules in vascular cells	40–42
Inhibition of endothelium-derived nitric oxide synthesis and biological activity	43, 44
Inhibition of macrophage migration	35
Recognition by macrophage scavenger receptors	45, 46
Stimulation of leukocyte adhesion to the endothelium	42, 47
Stimulation of smooth muscle cell growth	48

to the endothelium and migrate into the artery wall (35,40,42). The monocytes subsequently differentiate into macrophages in response to macrophage colony-stimulating factor (M-CSF), the expression of which by vascular cells is also enhanced by modified LDL (41). The oxidized LDL further inhibits the egress of macrophages from the artery wall, where the cells recognize and readily take up the oxidized LDL through a scavenger receptor-mediated process (45,46). Unlike the normal apolipoprotein (apo)B/E LDL receptor that recognizes native LDL, the scavenger receptors on macrophages that recognize modified LDL are not tightly regulated and, as a result, the macrophages are converted into foam cells, a component of fatty streaks and the hallmark of atherosclerosis.

Endothelium-derived nitric oxide (EDNO) is a pivotal molecule in the regulation of vascular tone by the stimulation of vascular smooth muscle cell relaxation and concomitant vasodilation (49,50). In addition to causing vasodilation, EDNO exerts several other potent antiatherogenic effects, including inhibition of leukocyte–endothelial interactions, smooth-muscle cell proliferation, and platelet aggregation (49,50). Endothelial vasodilator dysfunction has been observed in patients with coronary artery disease or associated risk factors, such as hypercholesterolemia, hyperhomocysteinemia, essential hypertension, diabetes mellitus, smoking, and aging (51–53). Most of these conditions are associated with increased oxidative stress, particularly increased production of superoxide radicals, which can directly inactivate EDNO (54,55). In addition, oxidized LDL can inhibit the synthesis or release of EDNO by endothelial cells, or can attenuate its biological activity (44,56) (Fig. 2).

It is still uncertain which factors are responsible for the oxidation of LDL in vivo. LDL can be oxidized into a potentially atherogenic form in vitro through metal ion-dependent oxidation of its lipid component, with subsequent modification of apolipoprotein (apo)B-100 by reactive aldehyde products of lipid peroxidation, particularly malondialdehyde (MDA) and 4-hydroxynonenal (HNE) (57). However, whether catalytic metal ions are available in the early lesion in vivo remains a matter of debate (58). Several metal ion-independent mechanisms have been proposed, primarily enzymatic, including 15-lipoxygenase and myeloperoxidase (59,60).

There are several lines of evidence that point to the formation and existence of oxidized LDL in vivo. Antibodies to aldehyde-modified LDL recognize epitopes in human atheroscle-

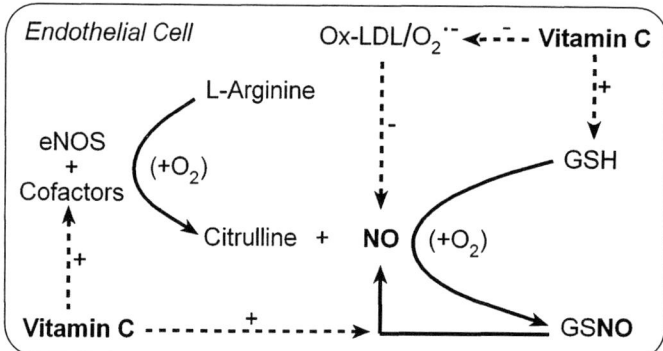

Figure 2 Vitamin C preserves the bioavailability of nitric oxide (NO) by several mechanisms: Vitamin C scavenges superoxide ($O_2^{\cdot-}$) and prevents the formation of oxidized LDL (Ox-LDL), which otherwise would decrease the bioavailability of NO. Vitamin C spares intracellular thiols (e.g., GSH), which stabilize NO through the formation of S-nitrosothiols (e.g., GSNO). In addition, vitamin C is involved in the release of NO from S-nitrosothiols, and preserves cofactors of endothelial NO synthase (eNOS) (e.g., tetrahydrobiopterin). Solid arrows indicate reactions, and dashed arrows effects.

rotic plaques (61), and LDL extracted from these lesions reacts with antibodies to oxidized LDL and exhibits characteristics identical with those of in vitro-oxidized LDL. Aldehyde-modified LDL has also been detected in plasma, as have been autoantibodies to oxidized LDL (32). Antibodies to hypochlorous acid-modified protein have detected epitopes in lesions, suggesting an alternative or additional mechanism of LDL oxidation involving myeloperoxidase (62). Furthermore, F_2-isoprostanes, which are specific lipid peroxidation biomarkers formed from nonenzymatic, radical-mediated oxidation of arachidonyl-containing lipids (63), have been detected at elevated levels in human atherosclerotic lesions (64,65), as have other oxidized lipids (66). Increased levels of F_2-isoprostanes have also been detected in plasma of patients with coronary risk factors, such as diabetics, hypercholesterolemia, or smoking (67,68). Indirect evidence that oxidative processes are involved in cardiovascular diseases has come from studies showing that antioxidant supplements, such as vitamin C, can decrease markers of in vivo lipid peroxidation (see Sec. II.B) (69) and can reverse endothelial dysfunction in patients with coronary artery disease or coronary risk factors (see Sec. IV.B) (70). In addition, numerous epidemiological studies have indicated that dietary antioxidants reduce the incidence of and mortality from cardiovascular diseases in humans (see Sec. V) (71).

II. LIPID PEROXIDATION

A. Vitamin C Inhibits In Vitro Lipid Peroxidation

Numerous studies have been carried out to investigate how vitamin C affects lipid oxidation in isolated LDL and whole plasma exposed to different oxidants. Vitamin C, either added to or present as a "contaminant" in LDL preparations, inhibited the accumulation of thiobarbituric acid-reactive substances (TBARS), lipid hydroperoxides, and F_2-isoprostanes when LDL was exposed to aqueous peroxyl radicals (20,72–74), peroxynitrite (75), or activated neutrophils (74,76). Vitamin C also inhibited the formation of lipid chlorohydrins in LDL exposed to myeloperoxidase-derived hypochlorous acid (77). Several studies have shown that endogenous vitamin C in plasma protects against lipid hydroperoxide and F_2 isoprostane formation induced by aqueous peroxyl radicals (8,72,78), peroxynitrite (75), cigarette smoke (79,80), or activated neutrophils (78). These latter findings are not surprising because vitamin C is such an efficient scavenger of reactive oxygen, nitrogen, and chlorine species present in cigarette smoke or produced by activated phagocytes.

What perhaps is surprising is the effect of vitamin C addition on lipoprotein oxidation in the presence of redox-active transition metal ions. Iron-dependent oxidation of LDL requires the presence of a reducing agent, such as superoxide or low molecular weight thiols (81–83). Vitamin C can also reduce iron and thereby enhance the production of hydroxyl or lipid alkoxyl radicals (LO·) by reaction of the reduced metal ions with, respectively, hydrogen peroxide or lipid hydroperoxides (LOOH) (see following reactions 1–3). Vitamin C, however, paradoxically inhibits hemin- or myoglobin-dependent oxidation of LDL (84,85), rather than enhancing oxidation, as would be expected from Fenton chemistry (see Reactions 1–3). Two studies, however, showed mixed results with ferritin-mediated LDL oxidation and cell-free LDL oxidation in Hams F-10 medium, which contains redox-active transition metal ions: depending on the concentrations of vitamin C used, pro- or antioxidant effects were observed (86,87). This observation has been previously suggested to be due to the effect of different concentrations of vitamin C on the ratio of Fe^{2+} to Fe^{3+} (88). Endothelial cells and macrophages are able to oxidize LDL in the presence of Ham's F-10 medium; however, addition of vitamin C strongly inhibited cell-mediated LDL oxidation (87,89–91). In addition, endogenous and exogenous vitamin C inhibits, rather than promotes, the formation of lipid hydroperoxides in iron-overloaded human plasma (92).

$$AH^- + Fe^{3+} \rightarrow A^{\cdot -} + Fe^{2+} + H^+ \quad (1)$$

$$H_2O_2 + Fe^{2+} \rightarrow {}^{\cdot}OH + {}^-OH + Fe^{3+} \quad (2)$$

$$LOOH + Fe^{2+} \rightarrow LO^{\cdot} + {}^-OH + Fe^{3+} \quad (3)$$

In contrast with iron, which requires the presence of a reducing agent, copper alone can induce lipid peroxidation in LDL, which is due to binding and reduction of copper ions by LDL itself (81,82). However, in the presence of vitamin C, copper-induced LDL oxidation is strongly inhibited (84,89,93–96). This activity is likely due to side-specific oxidation of histidine residues and subsequent loss of bound copper from the LDL particle (97,98). Interestingly, vitamin C, in the presence of copper ions, also eliminates preformed lipid hydroperoxides (84), although the mechanism is not presently known. In contrast, studies by Stait and Leake (90,91) showed that vitamin C can stimulate copper-induced lipid peroxidation if the LDL is already (mildly) oxidized. Another recent paper (99) has confirmed these findings by showing that vitamin C can act as a pro- or antioxidant toward LDL depending on when it is added to the copper- and LDL-containing incubation. Finally, when vitamin C is added to human serum supplemented with copper, antioxidant, rather than pro-oxidant, effects were observed (100), similar to the findings with iron-supplemented plasma (92).

B. Vitamin C Inhibits In Vivo Lipid Peroxidation

Several studies have been carried out in humans to determine the effects of vitamin C supplementation (500–2000 mg/day) on in vivo lipid peroxidation (Table 3). Smokers are under enhanced oxidative stress, as evidenced by reduced plasma levels of vitamin C (113) and increased levels of circulating lipid oxidation products, such as F_2-isoprostanes (68,101). Smoking is also a major risk factor for cardiovascular diseases (114,115). In one study, urinary levels of the F_2-isoprostane, 8-epiPGF$_{2\alpha}$, in five heavy smokers were decreased by one-third following supplementation with 2000 mg/day of vitamin C for only 5 days. However, another recent study, in which coronary artery disease patients were supplemented with 500 mg/day of vitamin C for 30 days, showed no change in plasma 8-epiPGF$_{2\alpha}$ levels (102). Plasma levels of TBARS have been used as a marker of lipid oxidation in several studies of smokers (104,106,107). Of these, one reported a reduction (107), one no change (106), and the third an increase (104) in plasma TBARS levels following vitamin C supplementation.

Of the vitamin C intervention studies carried out with healthy individuals or nonsmokers (25,108–110), two reported a significant reduction in plasma MDA levels following supplementation with vitamin C (25,108). These investigators also reported reduced plasma levels of allantoin, an oxidation product of urate (108), and increased levels of vitamin E and GSH in red blood cells (25). A trial in which nonsmokers were supplemented with 6000 mg/day of vitamin C (109) showed a nonsignificant trend toward reduced plasma levels of MDA and HNE. Another study (110), however, found no change in urinary TBARS following supplementation with vitamin C.

Several studies have also investigated the effect of vitamin C supplementation on ex vivo LDL oxidizability. The oxidizability, or susceptibility to oxidation, of isolated LDL is determined by measuring the lag time and propagation rate of lipid peroxidation in LDL exposed to copper ions or other oxidants, and is dependent on the antioxidant content and lipid composition of the lipoprotein (33,116). In smokers, two studies showed no effect of vitamin C supplementation on ex vivo copper-stimulated LDL oxidation (103,104), whereas a third study found a

Table 3 Effects of Vitamin C Supplementation on In Vivo and Ex Vivo Biomarkers of Lipid Oxidation

Study system	Challenge	Effects of vitamin C	Ref.
Urine	(Smokers), none	↓ 8-*epi*-PGF$_{2\alpha}$	101
Plasma	(CAD patients), none	X 8-*epi*-PGF$_{2\alpha}$	102
LDL	(Smokers), ex vivo copper	X CD	103
Plasma, LDL	(Smokers), none	↑ MDA	104
	ex vivo copper, hemin/H$_2$O$_2$	X CD	
LDL	(Smokers), ex vivo copper	↓ TBARS, CD	105
Serum	(Smokers), none	X TBARS	106
Plasma, LDL	Smoking	↓ TBARS	107
Plasma	None	↓ MDA	108
Plasma	None	↓ MDA/HNE (ns)	109
Urine	None	X TBARS	110
Plasma, LDL	None	↓ MDA	25
	Ex vivo copper	X TBARS, CD	
LDL	Ex vivo copper	↓ CD	111
LDL	Ex vivo copper	↓ TBARS	112

↑, increased damage; ↓, decreased damage; X, no change; CAD, coronary artery disease; CD, conjugated dienes; HNE, 4-hydroxynonenal; LDL, low-density lipoprotein; MDA, malondialdehyde; ns, not significant; TBARS, thiobarbituric acid-reactive substances.

decreased oxidizability of LDL (105). In healthy individuals or nonsmokers two studies have reported decreased ex vivo LDL oxidation following vitamin C supplementation (111,112), whereas another showed no change (25).

The ex vivo LDL oxidation studies are difficult to rationalize, however, because vitamin C, being a water-soluble molecule, is removed from LDL during isolation from plasma. Therefore, no change in ex vivo LDL oxidation would be expected, as was observed in three of the foregoing ex vivo studies (25,103,104). The observed decrease in LDL oxidation following vitamin C supplementation in the other studies (105,111,112) may be explained by "contamination" of the LDL preparation with vitamin C, which has been observed previously (74), or possibly by sparing, or regeneration, of LDL-associated vitamin E by vitamin C (111).

III. CELLULAR MECHANISMS

A. Vitamin C Attenuates Cellular Oxidant Production

Low-density lipoprotein can be oxidatively modified by several different cell types, including neutrophils, monocytes, macrophages, and endothelial cells (32). Vitamin C protects against neutrophil-mediated oxidation of LDL (74,76), presumably by scavenging reactive oxygen and chlorine species generated by the cells following stimulation of the respiratory burst. An alternative mechanism of vitamin C may involve decreasing the production of oxidants at the cellular level. Stimulation of the respiratory burst of neutrophils results in oxidation of 30–40% of the intracellular vitamin C to dehydroascorbic acid (117), and supplementation of subjects with vitamins C and E decreases production of oxidants by subsequently isolated neutrophils (118). Loading of human vascular endothelial cells with vitamin C decreases cellular levels of hydrogen peroxide and inhibits modification of LDL by these cells (87). Furthermore, vitamin C may act indirectly by sparing intracellular glutathione (26), the latter of which has been implicated in decreased oxidation of LDL by macrophages (119).

B. Vitamin C Reduces Cellular Adhesion

Adhesion of leukocytes to the endothelium is an important initiating step in atherogenesis (32). Monocytes isolated from smokers exhibit increased adhesion to endothelial cells compared with cells isolated from nonsmokers (120,121). Supplementation of smokers with 2000 mg/day of vitamin C for 10 days elevated plasma levels of vitamin C almost twofold and significantly reduced monocyte adhesion to endothelial cells (120). In another study, however, supplementation of smokers with 2000 mg of vitamin C 2 hours before collection of serum had no effect on ex vivo monocyte–endothelial cell adhesion, despite a more than threefold increase in serum vitamin C levels (121). Supplementation may have been too short, however, to affect intracellular vitamin C levels. Interestingly, supplementation with 7000 mg of L-arginine, the physiological substrate for nitric oxide (NO) synthase, significantly reduced monocyte–endothelial cell adhesion (121), suggesting the involvement of NO in decreased adhesion (see Sec. IV.A). Nevertheless, several in vivo animal studies suggest an important role for vitamin C in inhibiting leukocyte–endothelial cell interactions induced by cigarette smoke (122,123) or oxidized LDL (124).

IV. ENDOTHELIUM-DEPENDENT VASODILATION

A. Vitamin C Increases In Vitro Endothelium-Derived Nitric Oxide

Vitamin C may be able to increase the bioavailability of EDNO by increasing its synthesis or decreasing the levels of superoxide and oxidized LDL, both of which react with and inactivate NO (see Fig. 2). Vitamin C also spares intracellular thiols, which, in turn, can stabilize EDNO through the formation of biologically active S-nitrosothiols (125). In addition, reducing agents such as vitamin C have been implicated in the rapid release of NO from S-nitrosothiols (126–128). Recent in vitro studies have shown that vitamin C (0.1–10 mM) reverses the impairment of vasodilation of isolated arterial segments and aortic rings exposed to oxidized LDL (129) or to the superoxide-generating enzyme xanthine oxidase (130,131). Although relatively high concentrations of vitamin C (10 mM) are required to effectively inhibit the reaction of NO with superoxide (131), these concentrations are potentially achievable in extracellular fluids, such as plasma, by vitamin C infusion or in the cytoplasm by active cellular uptake of vitamin C. Heller and co-workers (132) recently showed that vitamin C (0.1–100 μM) increases the production of both citrulline, the byproduct of NO synthesis (see Fig. 2), and cyclic GMP, a marker of NO bioactivity, by cultured human vascular cells (132). The authors implicated modulation by vitamin C of the availability or affinity of tetrahydrobiopterin, an essential cofactor of NOS, as a possible mechanism for the observed increase in EDNO synthesis and activity.

B. Vitamin C Preserves Endothelium-Dependent Vasodilation

Patients with, or at risk for, cardiovascular diseases exhibit impaired endothelium-dependent vasodilation (51–53). Numerous clinical trials have been published over the past few years consistently demonstrating beneficial effects of vitamin C supplementation on endothelium-dependent vasodilation in humans. Increased agonist-induced and flow-mediated vasodilation were observed in patients with coronary spastic angina (133) and chronic heart failure (134,135) following intra-arterial infusion of vitamin C (10–25 mg/min). Oral supplementation with vitamin C (a single dose of 2000 or 500 mg/day for 4 weeks) also increased flow-mediated vasodilation in coronary artery disease patients (102,136) (Fig. 3). Individuals with coronary risk factors, such as hypertension (137–139), hypercholesterolemia (139,140), diabetes (141,142), hyperhomocysteinemia (143,144), and smoking (145,146), also show improved vasodilation following supplementation with vitamin C. Motoyama and co-workers (145) found a positive correlation between serum levels of vitamin C and endothelium-dependent vasodilation. Two

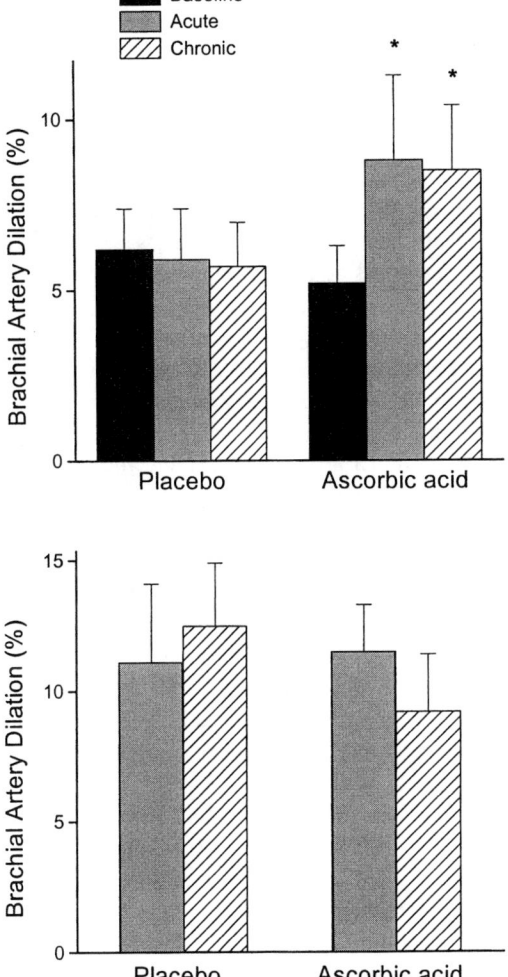

Figure 3 The effects of short-term and long-term ascorbic acid administration on flow- or nitroglycerin-mediated vasodilation in coronary artery disease patients: Subjects with flow-mediated dilation less than 10% underwent brachial ultrasound examination at baseline (black bars), 2 h after a single 2000-mg–oral dose of ascorbic acid (gray bars), and following 1 month of oral 500-mg/day supplementation (hatched bars). Both short-term and long-term ascorbic acid therapy had significant effects on flow-mediated dilation (*$p = 0.002$ by repeated measures ANOVA) (upper panel), but not on nitroglycerin-mediated dilation (lower panel). Data are presented as mean ± SEM and are derived from 17 subjects treated with ascorbic acid and 16 subjects treated with placebo. (From Ref. 102.)

of the studies assessing vasodilation (133,145) also showed reduced levels of TBARS following vitamin C administration, although a third (102) found no change in biomarkers of lipid and protein oxidation. Finally, in all of the foregoing in vivo studies (102,133–136), vitamin C supplementation had no effect on endothelium-independent vasodilation by nitroglycerin or sodium nitroprusside, indicating that vitamin C is acting by improving the synthesis of ENDO, rather than the responsiveness of the smooth-muscle cells to NO.

V. EPIDEMIOLOGICAL STUDIES

A. Vitamin C Intake Is Associated with a Reduced Risk of Cardiovascular Diseases

Many epidemiological studies and a limited number of clinical trials have indicated that dietary intake of, or supplementation with, antioxidant vitamins is associated with a reduction in the incidence of cardiovascular disease morbidity and mortality (22,147,148). Over the last 15 years, several prospective cohort studies have been published on the association between vitamin C intake and the risk of cardiovascular diseases (22,114,147–149). However, observed associations between vitamin C intake, or plasma levels, and cardiovascular disease risk do not prove cause–effect relations and may be limited by numerous confounding factors, which have been discussed previously (150,151).

Several prospective cohort studies have reported a reduced cardiovascular or cerebrovascular disease risk of 25–50% with moderate intake of vitamin C, between 45 and 113 mg/day (152–155). Other studies found similar reductions in the risk of cardiovascular diseases, but with considerably higher intakes of vitamin C (300–400 mg/day) (156–158). Kritchevsky et al. (159) measured carotid artery wall thickness as a measure of atherosclerosis and found a significant reduction in this endpoint in people older than 55 years who consumed amounts of vitamin C greater than 982 mg/day, compared with those consuming less than 88 mg/day.

Interestingly, several epidemiological studies have indicated no association of vitamin C intake, or regular supplementation, with the risk of cardiovascular or cerebrovascular diseases (160–164). Kushi et al. (161) and Rimm et al. (160), in two large epidemiological studies, reported no additional risk reduction for coronary heart disease with vitamin C intakes of about 200 and 400 mg/day, respectively, compared with intakes of about 90 mg/day. One intervention trial found no reduction of stroke or hypertension in a population of Chinese men and women supplemented with 120 mg/day of vitamin C and 30 μg/day of molybdenum for 5 years (164).

The lack of a protective effect of vitamin C supplementation (161,162,164) or dietary vitamin C intakes greater than about 100 mg/day (152,160,161) in several of the foregoing studies is likely explained by the fact that an intake of 100 mg/day of vitamin C results in tissue saturation (165). Thus, increasing vitamin C intakes over this amount may have only a small or no additional effect on tissue levels and, hence, on disease risk. Thus, the evidence from the foregoing prospective cohort studies suggests that vitamin C reduces the risk of cardiovascular diseases, although probably little or no additional benefit can be derived from vitamin C intakes greater than about 100 mg/day.

B. Vitamin C Status Is Associated with a Reduced Risk of Cardiovascular Diseases

Several investigators studying cardiovascular disease and stroke have measured plasma levels of vitamin C, which is a considerably more accurate and reliable measure of body vitamin C status than dietary intake estimated from questionnaires. Several studies observed a reduced risk of 30–60% with moderate plasma levels of vitamin C, between 11 and 57 μmol/L (153,166–170). Interestingly, patients suffering from coronary artery disease, myocardial infarction and angina pectoris have significantly lower plasma levels of vitamin C than controls or survivors (168,169,171,172). Other studies have found similar reductions in the risk of cardiovascular diseases with higher plasma levels of vitamin C (67–153 μmol/L) (158). A large study by Simon et al. (173) that comprised 6624 men and women enrolled in the Second National Health and Nutrition Examination Study (NHANES II), showed 26 and 27% risk reductions for stroke and coronary heart disease, respectively, with saturating serum vitamin C levels of 63–153 μmol/L, compared with low to marginal levels of 6–23 μmol/L. In a subsequent study (NHANES III) (174), analysis of the relative prevalence of coronary heart disease and stroke among individuals who also reported alcohol consumption showed a 52 and a 54% decrease in angina and stroke, respectively, with serum vitamin C levels of 57–170 μmol/L compared with less than 23 μmol/L.

In a recent comprehensive review article (22), Gey proposed that plasma vitamin C levels of 50 μmol/L or more provide optimum benefit for cardiovascular diseases (22), and this number seems to be in good agreement with the majority of the studies discussed here. Most interestingly, a plasma vitamin C level of 50 μmol/L is achieved by a dietary intake of approximately 100 mg/day of vitamin C (165), in good agreement with the foregoing suggested protective intake level of about 100 mg/day derived from diet-based prospective cohort studies, as well as the level required for tissue saturation (165). In the foregoing cited studies reporting an inverse association between plasma vitamin C levels and angina pectoris (168) and coronary heart disease (169), the association was substantially reduced after adjustment for smoking. This finding is to be expected given the known effect of smoking on plasma vitamin C levels (113), and suggests that smoking may increase cardiovascular disease risk, in part, by lowering vitamin C status.

VI. SUMMARY

Cardiovascular diseases are the leading cause of morbidity and mortality in the United States and other westernized populations, and are responsible for nearly 1 million deaths every year in the United States alone (57). Major risk factors associated with cardiovascular diseases are hypercholesterolemia, hyperhomocysteinemia, essential hypertension, diabetes mellitus, smoking, and aging, most of which are associated with increased oxidative stress, particularly increased production of superoxide radicals (51–53). Considerable evidence has also accumulated implicating lipid peroxidation and oxidative modification of LDL in atherosclerotic lesion development (32,175). As such, the role of antioxidants in these chronic conditions is of clinical relevance.

Many biochemical, clinical, and epidemiological studies have indicated that vitamin C may be of benefit in cardiovascular disease prevention and treatment. Vitamin C acts as an efficient scavenger of aqueous radicals and oxidants, thereby protecting other biomolecules from oxidative damage. In addition, vitamin C can spare, or recycle, vitamin E and GSH, two other physiologically important antioxidants. In vitro studies have shown that endogenous and added vitamin C effectively protect plasma and isolated LDL against lipid peroxidation under many different types of oxidizing conditions, including metal ion-independent and ion-dependent processes. Incubation of vitamin C with vascular cells or leukocytes decreases their oxidant production and adhesive properties, both of which are important early steps in LDL oxidation, arterial monocyte recruitment, and atherosclerotic lesion development. Vascular cells incubated with vitamin C also show increased synthesis of NO, a pivotal molecule in the regulation of vascular homeostasis.

Numerous studies in humans indicate that vitamin C supplementation protects against in vivo oxidation of lipids, particularly in individuals exposed to enhanced oxidative stress, such as smokers. In addition, many clinical studies have consistently shown beneficial effects of vitamin C treatment on endothelium-dependent vasodilation in patients with cardiovascular disease or coronary risk factors. Finally, numerous epidemiological studies strongly suggest that increased vitamin C intake or status lowers the incidence of and mortality from cardiovascular diseases.

ACKNOWLEDGMENTS

The authors are supported by grants from the U. S. National Institutes of Health (HL-56170 to B. F.) and the American Heart Association (9920420Z to A. C.).

REFERENCES

1. Jaffe GM. Vitamin C. In: Machlin L, ed. Handbook of Vitamins. New York: Marcel Dekker, 1984:199–244.
2. Woodall AA, Ames BN. Diet and oxidative damage to DNA: the importance of ascorbate as an antioxidant. In: Packer L, Fuchs J, eds. Vitamin C in Health and Disease. New York: Marcel Dekker, 1997:193–203.
3. Bendich A. Vitamin C safety in humans. In: Packer L, Fuchs J, eds. Vitamin C in Health and Disease. New York: Marcel Dekker, 1997:367–379.
4. Levine M. New concepts in the biology and biochemistry of ascorbic acid. N Engl J Med 1986; 314:892–902.
5. Burri BJ, Jacob RA. Human metabolism and the requirement for vitamin C. In: Packer L, Fuchs J, eds. Vitamin C in Health and Disease. New York: Marcel Dekker, 1997:341–366.
6. Tsao CS. An overview of ascorbic acid chemistry and biochemistry. In: Packer L, Fuchs J, eds. Vitamin C in Health and Disease. New York: Marcel Dekker, 1997:25–58.
7. Halliwell B. Vitamin C: antioxidant or pro-oxidant in vivo? Free Radic Res 1996; 25:439–454.
8. Frei B, England L, Ames BN. Ascorbate is an outstanding antioxidant in human blood plasma. Proc Natl Acad Sci USA 1989; 86:6377–6381.
9. Frei B, Stocker R, England L, Ames BN. Ascorbate: the most effective antioxidant in human blood plasma. Adv Exp Med Biol 1990; 264:155–163.
10. Buettner GR, Jurkiewicz BA. Catalytic metals, ascorbate and free radicals: combinations to avoid. Radiat Res 1996; 145:532–541.
11. Menzel DB. Oxidation of biologically active reducing substances by ozone. Arch Environ Health 1971; 23:149–153.
12. Chou PT, Khan AU. L-Ascorbic acid quenching of singlet delta molecular oxygen in aqueous media: generalized antioxidant property of vitamin C. Biochem Biophys Res Commun 1983; 115:932–937.
13. Licht WR, Tannenbaum SR, Deen WM. Use of ascorbic acid to inhibit nitrosation: kinetic and mass transfer considerations for an in vitro system. Carcinogenesis 1988; 9:365–372.
14. Cooney RV, Ross PD, Bartolini GL. N-Nitrosation and N-nitration of morpholine by nitrogen dioxide: inhibition by ascorbate, glutathione and α-tocopherol. Cancer Lett 1986; 32:83–90.
15. Kveder M, Pifat G, Pecar S, Schara M, Ramos P, Esterbauer H. Nitroxide reduction with ascorbic acid in spin labeled human plasma LDL and VLDL. Chem Phys Lipids 1997; 85:1–12.
16. Bartlett D, Church DF, Bounds PL, Koppenol WH. The kinetics of the oxidation of L-ascorbic acid by peroxynitrite. Free Radic Biol Med 1995; 18:85–92.
17. Chesney JA, Mahoney JR, Eaton JW. A spectrophotometric assay for chlorine-containing compounds. Anal Biochem 1991; 196:262–266.
18. Edge R, Truscott TG. Prooxidant and antioxidant reaction mechanisms of carotene and radical interactions with vitamins E and C. Nutrition 1997; 13:992–994.

19. Neuzil J, Thomas SR, Stocker R. Requirement for, promotion, or inhibition by α-tocopherol of radical-induced initiation of plasma lipoprotein lipid peroxidation. Free Radic Biol Med 1997; 22:57–71.
20. Bowry VW, Mohr D, Cleary J, Stocker R. Prevention of tocopherol-mediated peroxidation in ubiquinol-10-free human low density lipoprotein. J Biol Chem 1995; 270:5756–5763.
21. May JM, Qu ZC, Mendiratta S. Protection and recycling of alpha-tocopherol in human erythrocytes by intracellular ascorbic acid. Arch Biochem Biophys 1998; 349:281–289.
22. Gey KF. Vitamins E plus C and interacting conutrients required for optimal health. Biofactors 1998; 7:113–174.
23. Jacob RA, Kutnink MA, Csallany AS, Daroszewska M, Burton GW. Vitamin C nutriture has little short-term effect on vitamin E concentrations in healthy women. J Nutr 1996; 126:2268–2277.
24. Burton GW, Wronska U, Stone L, Foster DO, Ingold KU. Biokinetics of dietary RRR-α-tocopherol in the male guinea pig at three dietary levels of vitamin C and two levels of vitamin E. Evidence that vitamin C does not "spare" vitamin E in vivo. Lipids 1990; 25:199–210.
25. Wen Y, Cooke T, Feely J. The effect of pharmacological supplementation with vitamin C on low-density lipoprotein oxidation. Br J Clin Pharmacol 1997; 44:94–97.
26. Meister A. Glutathione–ascorbic acid antioxidant system in animals. J Biol Chem 1994; 269:9397–9400.
27. Buettner GR. The pecking order of free radicals and antioxidants: lipid peroxidation, α-tocopherol, and ascorbate. Arch Biochem Biophys 1993; 300:535–543.
28. Wells WW, Jung C. Regeneration of vitamin C. In: Packer L, Fuchs J, eds. Vitamin C in Health and Disease. New York: Marcel Dekker, 1997:109–121.
29. May JM, Cobb CE, Mendiratta S, Hill KE, Burk RF. Reduction of the ascorbyl free radical to ascorbate by thioredoxin reductase. J Biol Chem 1998; 273:23039–23045.
30. May JM, Mendiratta S, Hill KE, Burk RF. Reduction of dehydroascorbate to ascorbate by the selenoenzyme thioredoxin reductase. J Biol Chem 1997; 272:22607–22610.
31. Park JB, Levine M. Purification, cloning and expression of dehydroascorbic acid-reducing activity from human neutrophils: identification as glutaredoxin. Biochem J 1996; 315:931–938.
32. Frei B. Vitamin C as an antiatherogen: mechanisms of action. In: Packer L, Fuchs J, eds. Vitamin C in Health and Disease. New York: Marcel Dekker, 1997:163–182.
33. Esterbauer H, Gebicki J, Puhl H, Jurgens G. The role of lipid peroxidation and antioxidants in oxidative modification of LDL. Free Radic Biol Med 1992; 13:341–390.
34. Heinecke JW. Cellular mechanisms for the oxidative modification of lipoproteins: implications for atherogenesis. Coron Artery Dis 1994; 5:205–210.
35. Quinn MT, Parthasarathy S, Fong LG, Steinberg D. Oxidatively modified low density lipoproteins: a potential role in recruitment and retention of monocyte/macrophages during atherogenesis. Proc Natl Acad Sci USA 1987; 84:2995–2998.
36. Quinn MT, Parthasarathy S, Steinberg D. Lysophosphatidylcholine: a chemotactic factor for human monocytes and its potential role in atherogenesis. Proc Natl Acad Sci USA 1988; 85:2805–2809.
37. Cathcart MK, Morel DW, Chisolm GM. Monocytes and neutrophils oxidize low density lipoprotein making it cytotoxic. J Leukoc Biol 1985; 38:341–350.
38. Hughes H, Mathews B, Lenz ML, Guyton JR. Cytotoxicity of oxidized LDL to porcine aortic smooth muscle cells is associated with the oxysterols 7-ketocholesterol and 7-hydroxycholesterol. Arterioscler Thromb 1994; 14:1177–1185.
39. Coffey MD, Cole RA, Colles SM, Chisolm GM. In vitro cell injury by oxidized low density lipoprotein involves lipid hydroperoxide-induced formation of alkoxyl, lipid, and peroxyl radicals. J Clin Invest 1995; 96:1866–1873.
40. Navab M, Imes SS, Hama SY, et al. Monocyte transmigration induced by modification of low density lipoprotein in cocultures of human aortic wall cells is due to induction of monocyte chemotactic protein 1 synthesis and is abolished by high density lipoprotein. J Clin Invest 1991; 88:2039–2046.
41. Rajavashisth TB, Andalibi A, Territo MC, et al. Induction of endothelial cell expression of granulocyte and macrophage colony-stimulating factors by modified low-density lipoproteins. Nature 1990; 344:254–257.
42. Berliner JA, Territo MC, Sevanian A, et al. Minimally modified low density lipoprotein stimulates monocyte endothelial interactions. J Clin Invest 1990; 85:1260–1266.

43. Murohara T, Kugiyama K, Ohgushi M, Sugiyama S, Ohta Y, Yasue H. LPC in oxidized LDL elicits vasocontraction and inhibits endothelium-dependent relaxation. Am J Physiol 1994; 267:H2441–H2449.
44. Chin JH, Azhar S, Hoffman BB. Inactivation of endothelial derived relaxing factor by oxidized lipoproteins. J Clin Invest 1992; 89:10–18.
45. Henriksen T, Mahoney EM, Steinberg D. Enhanced macrophage degradation of low density lipoprotein previously incubated with cultured endothelial cells: recognition by receptors for acetylated low density lipoproteins. Proc Natl Acad Sci USA 1981; 78:6499–6503.
46. Suits AG, Chait A, Aviram M, Heinecke JW. Phagocytosis of aggregated lipoprotein by macrophages: low density lipoprotein receptor-dependent foam-cell formation. Proc Natl Acad Sci USA 1989; 86:2713–2717.
47. Frostegard J, Haegerstrand A, Gidlund M, Nilsson J. Biologically modified LDL increases the adhesive properties of endothelial cells. Atherosclerosis 1991; 90:119–126.
48. Heery JM, Kozak M, Stafforini DM, et al. Oxidatively modified LDL contains phospholipids with platelet-activating factor-like activity and stimulates the growth of smooth muscle cells. J Clin Invest 1995; 96:2322–2330.
49. Furchgott RF. The discovery of endothelium-derived relaxing factor and its importance in the identification of nitric oxide. JAMA 1996; 276:1186–1188.
50. Loscalzo J, Welch G. Nitric oxide and its role in the cardiovascular system. Prog Cardiovasc Dis 1995; 38:87–104.
51. Keaney JF, Vita JA. Atherosclerosis, oxidative stress, and antioxidant protection in endothelium-derived relaxing factor action. Prog Cardiovasc Dis 1995; 38:129–154.
52. Lyons D. Impairment and restoration of nitric oxide-dependent vasodilation in cardiovascular disease. Int J Cardiol 1997; 62(suppl 2):S101–S109.
53. Taddei S, Virdis A, Ghiadoni L, Salvetti A. Endothelial dysfunction in hypertension: fact or fancy? J Cardiovasc Pharmacol 1998; 32(suppl 3):S41–S47.
54. Gryglewski RJ, Palmer RM, Moncada S. Superoxide anion is involved in the breakdown of endothelium-derived vascular relaxing factor. Nature 1986; 320:454–456.
55. Rubanyi GM, Vanhoutte PM. Superoxide anions and hyperoxia inactivate endothelium-derived relaxing factor. Am J Physiol 1986; 250:H822–H827.
56. Simon BC, Cunningham LD, Cohen RA. Oxidized low density lipoproteins cause contraction and inhibit endothelium-dependent relaxation in the pig coronary artery. J Clin Invest 1990; 86:75–79.
57. Keaney JF, Frei B. Antioxidant protection of low-density lipoprotein and its role in the prevention of atherosclerotic vascular disease. In: Frei B, ed. Natural Antioxidants in Human Health and Disease. San Diego: Academic Press, 1994:303–351.
58. Bucala R. Lipid and lipoprotein oxidation: basic mechanisms and unresolved questions in vivo. Redox Rep 1996; 2:291–307.
59. Heinecke JW. Oxidants and antioxidants in the pathogenesis of atherosclerosis: implications for the oxidized low density lipoprotein hypothesis. Atherosclerosis 1998; 141:1–5.
60. Chisolm GM, Hazen SL, Fox PL, Cathcart MK. The oxidation of lipoproteins by monocytes–macrophages. Biochemical and biological mechanisms. J Biol Chem 1999; 274:25959–25962.
61. Ylä-Herttuala S, Palinski W, Rosenfeld ME, et al. Evidence for the presence of oxidatively modified low density lipoprotein in atherosclerotic lesions of rabbit and man. J Clin Invest 1989; 84:1086–1095.
62. Hazell LJ, Arnold L, Flowers D, Waeg G, Malle E, Stocker R. Presence of hypochlorite-modified proteins in human atherosclerotic lesions. J Clin Invest 1996; 97:1535–1544.
63. de Zwart LL, Meerman JHN, Commandeur JNM, Vermeulen NPE. Biomarkers of free radical damage: applications in experimental animals and in humans. Free Radic Biol Med 1999; 26:202–226.
64. Gniwotta C, Morrow JD, Roberts LJ, Kuhn H. Prostaglandin F_2-like compounds, F_2-isoprostanes, are present in increased amounts in human atherosclerotic lesions. Arterioscler Thromb Vasc Biol 1997; 17:3236–3241.
65. Pratico D, Luliano L, Mauriello A, et al. Localization of distinct F_2-isoprostanes in human atherosclerotic lesions. J Clin Invest 1997; 100:2028–2034.
66. Suarna C, Dean RT, Southwell-Keeley PT, Moore DE, Stocker R. Separation and characterization of cholesterol oxo- and hydroxy-linoleate isolated from human atherosclerotic plaque. Free Radic Res 1997; 27:397–408.

67. Davi G, Alessandrini P, Mezzetti A, et al. In vivo formation of 8-*epi*-prostaglandin $F_{2\alpha}$ is increased in hypercholesterolemia. Arterioscler Thromb Vasc Biol 1997; 17:3230–3235.
68. Morrow JD, Frei B, Longmire AW, et al. Increase in circulating products of lipid peroxidation (F_2-isoprostanes) in smokers. N Engl J Med 1995; 332:1198–1203.
69. Carr AC, Frei B. Does vitamin C act as a pro-oxidant under physiological conditions? FASEB J 1999; 13:1007–1024.
70. Carr AC, Frei B. The role of natural antioxidants in preserving the biological activity of endothelium-derived nitric oxide. Free Radic Biol Med 2000; 28:1806–1814.
71. Carr AC, Frei B. Toward a new recommended dietary allowance for vitamin C based on antioxidant and health effects in humans. Am J Clin Nutr 1999; 69:1086–1107.
72. Lynch SM, Morrow JD, Roberts LJ, Frei B. Formation of non–cyclooxygenase-derived prostanoids (F_2-isoprostanes) in plasma and low density lipoprotein exposed to oxidative stress in vitro. J Clin Invest 1994; 93:998–1004.
73. Ma YS, Stone WL, LeClair IO. The effects of vitamin C and urate on the oxidation kinetics of human low-density lipoprotein. Proc Soc Exp Biol Med 1994; 206:53–59.
74. Stocker R, Bowry VW, Frei B. Ubiquinol-10 protects human low density lipoprotein more efficiently against lipid peroxidation than does α-tocopherol. Proc Natl Acad Sci USA 1991; 88:1646–1650.
75. Thomas SR, Davies MJ, Stocker R. Oxidation and antioxidation of human low-density lipoprotein and plasma exposed to 3-morpholinosydnonimine and reagent peroxynitrite. Chem Res Toxicol 1998; 11:484–494.
76. Scaccini C, Jialal I. LDL modification by activated polymorphonuclear leukocytes: a cellular model of mild oxidative stress. Free Radic Biol Med 1994; 16:49–55.
77. Heinecke JW, Li W, Mueller DM, Bohrer A, Turk J. Cholesterol chlorohydrin synthesis by the myeloperoxidase–hydrogen peroxide–chloride system: potential markers for lipoproteins oxidatively damaged by phagocytes. Biochemistry 1994; 33:10127–10136.
78. Frei B, Stocker R, Ames BN. Antioxidant defenses and lipid peroxidation in human blood plasma. Proc Natl Acad Sci USA 1988; 85:9748–9752.
79. Cross CE, O'Neill CA, Reznick AZ, et al. Cigarette smoke oxidation of human plasma constituents. Ann NY Acad Sci 1993; 686:72–89.
80. Frei B, Forte TM, Ames BN, Cross CE. Gas phase oxidants of cigarette smoke induce lipid peroxidation and changes in lipoprotein properties in human blood plasma: protective effects of ascorbic acid. Biochem J 1991; 277:133–138.
81. Lynch SM, Frei B. Mechanisms of copper and iron-dependent oxidative modification of human low density lipoprotein. J Lipid Res 1993; 34:1745–1753.
82. Lynch SM, Frei B. Reduction of copper, but not iron, by human low density lipoprotein (LDL). J Biol Chem 1995; 270:5158–5163.
83. Lynch SM, Frei B. Physiological thiol compounds exert pro- and anti-oxidant effects, respectively, on iron- and copper-mediated oxidation of human low-density lipoprotein. Biochim Biophys Acta 1997; 1345:215–221.
84. Retsky KL, Frei B. Vitamin C prevents metal ion-dependent initiation and propagation of lipid peroxidation in human low-density lipoprotein. Biochim Biophys Acta 1995; 1257:279–287.
85. Vieira O, Laranjinha J, Madeira V, Almeida L. Cholesterol ester hydroperoxide formation in myoglobin-catalyzed low density lipoprotein oxidation: concerted antioxidant activity of caffeic acid and *p*-coumaric acids with ascorbate. Biochem Pharmacol 1998; 55:333–340.
86. Dai L, Winyard PG, Zhang Z, Blake DR, Morris CJ. Ascorbic acid promotes low density lipoprotein oxidation in the presence of ferritin. Biochim Biophys Acta 1996; 1304:223–228.
87. Martin A, Frei B. Both intracellular and extracellular vitamin C inhibit atherogenic modification of LDL by human vascular endothelial cells. Arterioscler Thromb Vasc Biol 1997; 17:1583–1590.
88. Miller DM, Aust SD. Studies of ascorbate-dependent, iron-catalyzed lipid peroxidation. Arch Biochem Biophys 1989; 271:113–119.
89. Jialal I, Grundy SM. Preservation of the endogenous antioxidants in low density lipoprotein by ascorbate but not probucol during oxidative modification. J Clin Invest 1991; 87:597–601.
90. Stait SE, Leake DS. The effects of ascorbate and dehydroascorbate on the oxidation of low-density lipoprotein. Biochem J 1996; 320:373–381.
91. Stait SE, Leake DS. Ascorbic acid can either increase or decrease low density lipoprotein modification. FEBS Lett 1994; 341:263–267.

92. Berger TM, Polidori MC, Dabbagh A, et al Antioxidant activity of vitamin C in iron-overloaded human plasma. J Biol Chem 1997; 272:15656–15660.
93. Retsky KL, Freeman MW, Frei B. Ascorbic acid oxidation product(s) protect human low density lipoprotein against atherogenic modification: anti- rather than prooxidant activity of vitamin C in the presence of transition metal ions. J Biol Chem 1993; 268:1304–1309.
94. Jialal I, Vega GL, Grundy SM. Physiologic levels of ascorbate inhibit the oxidative modification of low density lipoprotein. Atherosclerosis 1990; 82:185–191.
95. Ortwerth BJ, Linetsky M, Olesen PR. Ascorbic acid glycation of lens proteins produces UVA sensitizers similar to those in human lens. Photochem Photobiol 1995; 62:454–462.
96. Mathiesen L, Wang S, Halvorsen B, Malterud KE, Sund RB. Inhibition of lipid peroxidation in low-density lipoprotein by the flavonoid myrigalone B and ascorbic acid. Biochem Pharmacol 1996; 51:1719–1725.
97. Chen K, Frei B. The effect of histidine modification on copper-dependent lipid peroxidation in human low-density lipoprotein. Redox Rep 1997; 3:175–181.
98. Retsky KL, Chen K, Zeind J, Frei B. Inhibition of copper-induced LDL oxidation by vitamin C is associated with decreased copper-binding to LDL and 2-oxo-histidine formation. Free Radic Biol Med 1999; 26:90–98.
99. Otero P, Viana M, Herrera E, Bonet B. Antioxidant and prooxidant effects of ascorbic acid, dehydroascorbic acid and flavonoids on LDL submitted to different degrees of oxidation. Free Radic Res 1997; 27:619–626.
100. Dasgupta A, Zdunek T. In vitro lipid peroxidation of human serum catalyzed by cupric ion: antioxidant rather than prooxidant role of ascorbate. Life Sci 1992; 50:875–882.
101. Reilly M, Delanty N, Lawson JA, Fitzgerald GA. Modulation of oxidant stress in vivo in chronic cigarette smokers. Circulation 1996; 94:19–25.
102. Gokce N, Keaney JF, Frei B, et al. Long-term ascorbic acid administration reverses endothelial vasomotor dysfunction in patients with coronary artery disease. Circulation 1999; 99:3234–3240.
103. Samman S, Brown AJ, Beltran C, Singh S. The effect of ascorbic acid on plasma lipids and oxidisability of LDL in male smokers. Eur J Clin Nutr 1997; 51:472–477.
104. Nyyssonen K, Poulsen HE, Hayn M, et al. Effect of supplementation of smoking men with plain or slow-release ascorbic acid on lipoprotein oxidation. Eur J Clin Nutr 1997; 51:154–163.
105. Fuller CJ, Grundy SM, Norkus EP, Jialal I. Effect of ascorbate supplementation on low density lipoprotein oxidation in smokers. Atherosclerosis 1996; 119:139–150.
106. Mulholland CW, Strain JJ, Trinick TR. Serum antioxidant potential, and lipoprotein oxidation in female smokers following vitamin C supplementation. Int J Food Sci Nutr 1996; 47:227–231.
107. Harats D, Ben–Naim M, Dabach Y, et al. Effect of vitamin C and E supplementation on susceptibility of plasma lipoproteins to peroxidation induced by acute smoking. Atherosclerosis 1990; 85:47–54.
108. Naidoo D, Lux O. The effect of vitamin C and E supplementation on lipid and urate oxidation products in plasma. Nutr Res 1998; 18:953–961.
109. Anderson D, Phillips BJ, Yu T, Edwards AJ, Ayesh R, Butterworth KR. The effects of vitamin C supplementation on biomarkers of oxygen radical generated damage in human volunteers with "low" or "high" cholesterol levels. Environ Mol Mutagen 1997; 30:161–174.
110. Cadenas S, Rojas C, Mendez J, Herrero A, Barja G. Vitamin E decreases urine lipid peroxidation products in young healthy human volunteers under normal conditions. Pharmacol Toxicol 1996; 79:247–253.
111. Harats D, Chevion S, Nahir M, Norman Y, Sagee O, Berry EM. Citrus fruit supplementation reduces lipoprotein oxidation in young men ingesting a diet high in saturated fat: presumptive evidence for an interaction between vitamins C and E in vivo. Am J Clin Nutr 1998; 67:240–245.
112. Rifici VA, Khachadurian AK. Dietary supplementation with vitamins C and E inhibits in vitro oxidation of lipoproteins. J Am Coll Nutr 1993; 12:631–637.
113. Lykkesfeldt J, Loft S, Nielsen JB, Poulsen HE. Ascorbic acid dehydroascorbic acid as biomarkers of oxidative stress caused by smoking. Am J Clin Nutr 1997; 65:959–963.
114. Lynch SM, Gaziano JM, Frei B. Ascorbic acid and atherosclerotic cardiovascular disease. In: Harris JR, ed. Ascorbic Acid: Biochemistry and Biomedical Cell Biology. New York: Plenum Press, 1996:331–367.
115. Simon JA. Vitamin C and cardiovascular disease: a review. J Am Coll Nutr 1992; 11:107–125.

116. Frei B, Gaziano JM. Content of antioxidants, preformed lipid hydroperoxides, and cholesterol as predictors of the susceptibility of human LDL to metal ion-dependent and -independent oxidation. J Lipid Res 1993; 34:2135–2145.
117. Winterbourn CC, Vissers MCM. Changes in ascorbate levels on stimulation of human neutrophils. Biochim Biophys Acta 1983; 763:175–179.
118. Herbaczynska–Cedro K, Wartanowicz M, Panczenko–Kresowska B, Cedro K, Klosiewicz–Wasek B, Wasek W. Inhibitory effect of vitamins C and E on the oxygen free radical production in human polymorphonuclear leucocytes. Eur J Clin Invest 1994; 24:316–319.
119. Rosenblat M, Aviram M. Macrophage glutathione content and glutathione peroxidase activity are inversely related to cell-mediated oxidation of LDL: in vitro and in vivo studies. Free Radic Biol Med 1998; 24:305–317.
120. Weber C, Wolfgang E, Weber K, Weber PC. Increased adhesiveness of isolated monocytes to endothelium is prevented by vitamin C intake in smokers. Circulation 1996; 93:1488–1492.
121. Adams MR, Jessup W, Celermajer DS. Cigarette smoking is associated with increased human monocyte adhesion to endothelial cells: reversibility with oral L-arginine but not vitamin C. J Am Coll Cardiol 1997; 29:491–497.
122. Lehr H, Frei B, Arfors K. Vitamin C prevents cigarette smoke-induced leukocyte aggregation and adhesion to endothelium in vivo. Proc Natl Acad Sci 1994; 91:7688–7692.
123. Lehr HA, Weyrich AS, Saetzler RK, et al. Vitamin C blocks inflammatory platelet-activating factor mimetics created by cigarette smoking. J Clin Invest 1997; 99:2358–2364.
124. Lehr H, Frei B, Olofsson M, Carew TE, Arfors K. Protection from oxidized LDL-induced leukocyte adhesion to microvascular and macrovascular endothelium in vivo by vitamin C but not by vitamin E. Circulation 1995; 91:1525–1532.
125. Stamler JS, Singel DJ, Loscalzo J. Biochemistry of nitric oxide and its redox-activated forms. Science 1992; 258:1898–1902.
126. Scorza G, Pietraforte D, Minetti M. Role of ascorbate and protein thiols in the release of nitric oxide from S-nitroso-albumin and S-nitroso-glutathione in human plasma. Free Radic Biol Med 1997; 22:633–642.
127. Kashiba–Iwatsuki M, Yamaguchi M, Inoue M. Role of ascorbic acid in the metabolism of S-nitroso-glutathione. FEBS Lett 1996; 389:149–152.
128. Kashiba–Iwatsuki M, Kitoh K, Kasahara E, et al. Ascorbic acid and reducing agents regulate the fates and functions of S-nitrosothiols. J Biochem (Tokyo) 1997; 122:1208–1214.
129. Fontana L, McNeill KL, Ritter JM, Chowienczyk PJ. Effects of vitamin C and of a cell permeable superoxide dismutase mimetic on acute lipoprotein induced endothelial dysfunction in rabbit aortic rings. Br J Pharmacol 1999; 126:730–734.
130. Dudgeon S, Benson DP, MacKenzie A, Paisley–Zyszkiewicz K, Martin W. Recovery by ascorbate by impaired nitric oxide-dependent relaxation resulting from oxidant stress in rat aorta. Br J Pharmacol 1998; 125:782–786.
131. Jackson TS, Xu A, Vita JA, Keaney JF. Ascorbate prevents the interaction of superoxide and nitric oxide only at very high physiological concentrations. Circ Res 1998; 83:916–922.
132. Heller R, Munscher–Paulig F, Grabner R, Till U. L-Ascorbic acid potentiates nitric oxide synthesis in endothelial cells. J Biol Chem 1999; 274:8254–8260.
133. Kugiyama K, Motoyama T, Hirashima O, et al. Vitamin C attenuates abnormal vasomotor reactivity in spasm coronary arteries in patients with coronary spastic angina. J Am Coll Cardiol 1998; 32:103–109.
134. Ito K, Akita H, Kanazawa K, et al. Comparison of effects of ascorbic acid on endothelium-dependent vasodilation in patients with chronic congestive heart failure secondary to idiopathic dilated cardiomyopathy versus patients with effort angina pectoris secondary to coronary artery disease. Am J Cardiol 1998; 82:762–767.
135. Hornig B, Arakawa N, Kohler C, Drexler H. Vitamin C improves endothelial function of conduit arteries in patients with chronic heart failure. Circulation 1998; 97:363–368.
136. Levine GL, Frei B, Koulouris SN, Gerhard MD, Keaney JF, Vita JA. Ascorbic acid reverses endothelial vasomotor dysfunction in patients with coronary artery disease. Circulation 1996; 93:1107–1113.
137. Taddei S, Virdis A, Ghiadoni L, Magagna A, Salvetti A. Vitamin C improves endothelium-dependent vasodilation by restoring nitric oxide activity in essential hypertension. Circulation 1998; 97:2222–2229.

138. Solzbach U, Hornig B, Jeserich M, Just H. Vitamin C improves endothelial dysfunction of epicardial coronary arteries in hypertensive patients. Circulation 1997; 96:1513–1519.
139. Jeserich M, Schindler T, Olschewski M, Unmussig M, Just H, Solzbach U. Vitamin C improves endothelial function of epicardial coronary arteries in patients with hypercholesterolaemia or essential hypertension-assessed by cold pressor testing. Eur Heart J 1999; 20:1676–1680.
140. Ting HH, Timimi FK, Haley EA, Roddy M, Ganz P, Creager MA. Vitamin C improves endothelium-dependent vasodilation in forearm resistance vessels of humans with hypercholesterolemia. Circulation 1997; 95:2617–2622.
141. Timimi FK, Ting HH, Haley EA, Roddy M, Ganz P, Creager MA. Vitamin C improves endothelium-dependent vasodilation in patients with insulin-dependent diabetes mellitus. J Am Coll Cardiol 1998; 31:552–557.
142. Ting HH, Timimi FK, Boles KS, Creager SJ, Ganz P, Creager MA. Vitamin C improves endothelium-dependent vasodilation in patients with non–insulin-dependent diabetes mellitus. J Clin Invest 1996; 97:22–28.
143. Chambers JC, McGregor A, Jean–Marie J, Obeid OA, Kooner JS. Demonstration of rapid onset vascular endothelial dysfunction after hyperhomocysteinemia: an effect reversible with vitamin C therapy. Circulation 1999; 99:1156–1160.
144. Kanani PM, Sinkey CA, Browning RL, Allaman M, Knapp HR, Haynes WG. Role of oxidant stress in endothelial dysfunction produced by experimental hyperhomocyst(e)inemia in humans. Circulation 1999; 100:1161–1168.
145. Motoyama T, Kawano H, Kugiyama K, et al. Endothelium-dependent vasodilation in the brachial artery is impaired in smokers: effect of vitamin C. Am J Physiol 1997; 273:H1644–H1650.
146. Heitzer T, Just H, Munzel T. Antioxidant vitamin C improves endothelial dysfunction in chronic smokers. Circulation 1996; 94:6–9.
147. Weber P, Bendich A, Schalch W. Vitamin C and human health—a review of recent data relevant to human requirements. Int J Vitam Nutr Res 1996; 66:19–30.
148. Enstrom JE. Vitamin C in prospective epidemiological studies. In: Packer L, Fuchs J, eds. Vitamin C in Health and Disease. New York: Marcel Dekker, 1997:381–398.
149. Jha P, Flather M, Lonn E, Farkouh M, Yusuf S. The antioxidant vitamins and cardiovascular disease: a critical review of epidemiologic and clinical trial data. Ann Intern Med 1995; 123:860–872.
150. Fontham ETH. Vitamin C, vitamin C-rich foods, and cancer: epidemiologic studies. In: Frei B, ed. Natural Antioxidants in Human Health and Disease. San Diego: Academic Press, 1994:157–197.
151. Gaziano JM, Manson JE, Hennekens CH. Natural antioxidants and cardiovascular disease: observational epidemiological studies and randomized trials. In: Frei B, ed. Natural Antioxidants in Human Health and Disease. San Diego: Academic Press, 1994:387–409.
152. Knekt P, Reunanen A, Jarvinen R, Seppanen R, Heliovaara M, Aromaa A. Antioxidant vitamin intake and coronary mortality in a longitudinal population study. Am J Epidemiol 1994; 139:1180–1189.
153. Gale CR, Martyn CN, Winter PD, Cooper C. Vitamin C and risk of death from stroke and coronary heart disease in cohort of elderly people. Br Med J 1995; 310:1563–1566.
154. Pandey DK, Shekelle R, Selwyn BJ, Tangney C, Stamler J. Dietary vitamin C and β-carotene and risk of death in middle-aged men. Am J Epidemiol 1995; 142:1269–1278.
155. Fehily AM, Yarnell JWG, Sweetnam PM, Elwood PC. Diet and incident ischaemic heart disease: the Caerphilly Study. Br J Nutr 1993; 69:303–314.
156. Enstrom JE, Kanim LE, Klein MA. Vitamin C intake and mortality among a sample of the United States population. Epidemiology 1992; 3:194–202.
157. Enstrom JE. Counterpoint—vitamin C and mortality. Nutr Today 1993; 28:28–32.
158. Sahyoun NR, Jacques PF, Russell RM. Carotenoids, vitamins C and E, and mortality in an elderly population. Am J Epidemiol 1996; 144:501–511.
159. Kritchevsky SB, Shimakawa T, Tell GS, et al. Dietary antioxidants and carotid artery wall thickness. Circulation 1995; 92:2142–2150.
160. Rimm EB, Stampfer MJ, Asherio A, Giovannucci E, Colditz GA, Willett WC. Vitamin E consumption and the risk of coronary heart disease in men. N Engl J Med 1993; 328:1450–1456.
161. Kushi LH, Folsom AR, Prineas RJ, Mink PJ, Wu Y, Bostick RM. Dietary antioxidant vitamins and death from coronary heart disease in postmenopausal women. N Engl J Med 1996; 334:1156–1162.
162. Losonczy KG, Harris TB, Havlik RJ. Vitamin E and vitamin C supplement use and risk of all cause and coronary heart disease mortality in older persons: the established populations for epidemiologic studies of the elderly. Am J Clin Nutr 1996; 64:190–196.

163. Ascherio A, Rimm EB, Hernan MA, et al. Relation of consumption of vitamin E, vitamin C, and carotenoids to risk for stroke among men in the United States. Ann Intern Med 1999; 130:963–970.
164. Mark SD, Wang W, Fraumeni JF, et al. Do nutritional supplements lower the risk of stroke or hypertension? Epidemiology 1998; 9:9–15.
165. Levine M, Conry–Cantilena C, Wang Y, et al. Vitamin C pharmacokinetics in healthy volunteers: evidence for a recommended dietary allowance. Proc Natl Acad Sci USA 1996; 93:3704–3709.
166. Eichholzer M, Stahelin HB, Gey KF. Inverse correlation between essential antioxidants in plasma and subsequent risk to develop cancer, ischemic heart disease and stroke respectively: 12-year follow-up of the Prospective Basel Study. EXS 1992; 62:398–410.
167. Gey KF, Stahelin HB, Eichholzer M. Poor plasma status of carotene and vitamin C is associated with higher mortality from ischemic heart disease and stroke: Basel Prospective Study. Clin Invest 1993; 71:3–6.
168. Riemersma RA, Wood DA, Macintyre CCA, Elton RA, Gey KF, Oliver MF. Risk of angina pectoris and plasma concentrations of vitamins A, C, and E and carotene. Lancet 1991; 337:1–5.
169. Singh RB, Ghosh S, Niaz MA, et al. Dietary intake, plasma levels of antioxidant vitamins, and oxidative stress in relation to coronary artery disease in elderly subjects. Am J Cardiol 1995; 76; 1233–1238.
170. Nyyssonen K, Parviainen MT, Salonen R, Tuomilehto J, Salonen JT. Vitamin C deficiency and risk of myocardial infarction: prospective population study of men from eastern Finland. Br Med J 1997; 314:634–638.
171. Vita JA, Keaney JF, Raby KE, et al. Low plasma ascorbic acid independently predicts the presence of an unstable coronary syndrome. J Am Coll Cardiol 1998; 31:980–986.
172. Halevy D, Thiery J, Nagel D, et al. Increased oxidation of LDL in patients with coronary artery disease is independent from dietary vitamins E and C. Arterioscler Thromb Vasc Biol 1997; 17:1432–1437.
173. Simon JA, Hudes ES, Browner WS. Serum ascorbic acid and cardiovascular disease prevalence in U. S. adults. Epidemiology 1998; 9:316–321.
174. Simon JA, Hudes ES. Serum ascorbic acid and cardiovascular disease prevalence in U. S. adults: the Third National Health and Nutrition Examination Survey (NHANES III). Ann Epidemiol 1999; 9:358–365.
175. Steinbrecher UP, Zhang H, Lougheed M. Role of oxidatively modified LDL in atherosclerosis. Free Radic Biol Med 1990; 9:155–168.

9
Epidemiological and Clinical Aspects of Ascorbate and Cancer

James E. Enstrom
School of Public Health, University of California, Los Angeles, California

I. INTRODUCTION

Vitamin C (ascorbic acid or ascorbate) is an antioxidant that has received a great deal of attention in recent years relative to prevention and treatment of cancer (1–11), including use of vitamin C supplements (12–16). The human body is under constant attack by reactive oxygen molecules (free radicals and singlet oxygen) that are formed as a natural consequence of normal biochemical activity. Reactive oxygen can damage the body in many ways by altering membrane structure and function. The hypothesis that free radicals may be involved in carcinogenesis is primarily based on observations that many carcinogens are free radicals, are the product of free radical reactions, are converted to free radicals in vivo, or stimulate the production of free radicals. Also, free radicals may be important in tumor initiation or promotion.

Because this damage can be life-threatening, the human body has evolved with antioxidant defense mechanisms to protect against free radical oxidation. Many antioxidants inhibit carcinogenesis in a variety of animal models, and antioxidant molecules may retard atherogenesis by interfering with this oxidation process. These defenses include small molecules, such as vitamin C, that act as antioxidants or scavengers of reactive oxygen species. However, because our antioxidant defense systems are not completely efficient, it has been proposed that increasing the intake of dietary antioxidants, such as vitamin C, may be important in diminishing the cumulative effects of oxidative damage over the long human life span. Vitamin C is the major water-soluble antioxidant.

Epidemiological studies of the relation between vitamin C and cancer or other diseases consist of two types: observational studies and intervention trials. Observational studies examine the association between antioxidant nutrient intake and disease incidence or between blood or tissue levels of vitamin C and disease. However, these observational studies must be interpreted cautiously, because the effects observed may result from factors correlated with vitamin C intake, rather than from vitamin C itself. Thus, supporting data from intervention studies are important for causal inference. Randomized, controlled intervention trials, unlike the observational studies, generally are not subject to bias or confounding. However, these trials are extraordinarily expensive, difficult to conduct, and relatively short in duration.

There are over 100 epidemiological studies that have examined some aspect of the relation between vitamin C and disease. Most of these are case–control studies of cancer patients compared with appropriately matched control subjects without cancer. Most of these case–control studies were reviewed in 1991 by Block (1) and in 1995 by Byers and Guerrero (5). The majority of studies show an inverse relation between vitamin C intake and risk of cancer, when examined on a site-by-site basis. Many of these studies have focused on tobacco-related cancers, such as oral cavity, esophagus, and lung cancer. The observational studies have failed to find any consistent adverse effects associated with increased vitamin C intake. In addition, data from in vitro and animal carcinogenesis studies have supported this association.

The focus of this chapter is on prospective epidemiological studies that are generally methodologically superior to case–control studies because they obtain information about vitamin C intake and other characteristics before cancer or other diseases develop and are less subject to selection bias. This review includes all known prospective epidemiological studies that involve vitamin C intake or an index of vitamin C intake, most of which have been published during the 1990s. Included are findings that come from published papers, book chapters, and dissertations, although there are essentially no significant findings in dissertations that are not already published. Several prospective studies with results based solely on general fruit/vegetable intake or on vitamin supplement intake are not included since these studies involve incomplete measures of vitamin C intake. This chapter updates our previous review (7) and focuses more on cancer.

II. METHODS

We present the essential characteristics of 20 prospective studies that measured vitamin C intake in the diet or in blood samples and had cancer mortality or incidence as an outcome (17–52). Vitamin C intake in all 20 cohorts was determined based on the consumption of fruits and other foods containing vitamin C or supplements containing vitamin C in the 20 cohorts; blood samples—plasma ascorbic acid—were measured in four cohorts (20,45,51,52). The studies are described in chronological order by the first publication for each cohort. For the ten cohorts with multiple publications, the publications are grouped together chronologically.

Table 1 describes the study population, number of subjects, geographic location, age range, follow-up period, health status, and type of data collected for the 20 cancer-related population cohorts (17–52). Several small cohorts measuring vitamin C intake that were followed for all-cause mortality only are described in our previous review (8).

Table 2 describes the results of those studies that give all-cause mortality for males, females, or both sexes. The number of years of follow-up, the high and low vitamin C intake groups, and the controlled variables are presented along with the total number of deaths, relative risk (RR) of high-intake group versus low-intake group, and 95% confidence interval (CI) or statistical significance level (p value) for the relative risk.

Table 3 describes the results of these same studies in which results are presented for mortality or incidence from all cancer for males, females, or both sexes. The mortality or incidence results for specific cancer sites are given in the following tables: Table 4 for lung cancer, Table 5 for breast cancer, and Table 6 for stomach, colorectal, and prostate cancer.

Table 7 compares the Block (1) and Byers and Guerrero (5) reviews of case–control studies with the prospective results in this review.

Table 1 Description of Populations for Prospective Vitamin C Studies: Mortality and Incidence

Author (yr)	Population description	Ages at entry	Start	End	Initial health	Type of study
Bjelke (1982)	13,785 males and 2,928 females; random sample of Norwegian men and their family members	≥35	1967	1978	Average	Mailed dietary questionnaire
Kvale (1983)	10,602 males		1967	1978		
Long-de (1985)	~350,000 white males from 25 states enrolled by ACS (Cancer Prevention Study I)	40–74	1960	1970	No history of cancer; not sick at entry	Mailed lifestyle and dietary questionnaire
Enstrom (1986)	1,369 males and 1,654 females; representative sample of residents of Alameda County, CA	16+	1974	1983	Noninstitutionalized	Lifestyle and dietary interview
Gey (1987)	2,975 male employees of the three major Swiss pharmaceutical companies in Basel (Basel Study)	ave 51	1971–73	1980	Apparently healthy	Exam with blood samples
Stahelin (1991)	2,975 males		1971–73	1985		
Eichholzer (1996)	2,975 males		1971–73	1990		
Kromhout (1987)	878 middle-aged males randomly sampled from Zutphen, Netherlands (Zutphen Study)	40–59	1960	1985	Average	Lifestyle and dietary interview of subjects and wives
Ocke (1997)	561 males	52–71	1971	1990	No history of cancer	
Heilbrun (1989)	8,006 Japanese men residing on Oahu, HI	45–67	1965–68	1985	Cancer-free	Clinical exam and dietary history
Knekt (1991)	4,538 males; participants in Finnish multiphasic Mobile Clinic Health Examination Survey	20–69	1967–72	1986	Cancer-free	Dietary history interview and health exam
Jarvinen (1997)	4,697 females	15+	1967–72	1991		

(continued)

Table 1 (Continued)

Author (yr)	Population description	Ages at entry	Start	End	Initial health	Type of study
Chow (1992)	17,818 white males; Lutheran Brotherhood Insurance Society policy holders from 9 states	35+	1966	1986	Already insured	Mailed lifestyle and dietary questionnaire
Enstrom (1992)	4,479 males and 6,869 females; national sample (NHANES I Epidemiologic Follow-up Study)	25–74	1971–74	1982–84	Average	Lifestyle and dietary interview and exam with blood samples
Enstrom (1994)	4,479 males and 6,869 females		1971–74	1987	Average	
Enstrom (1999)	4,479 males and 6,869 females		1971–74	1992	Average	
Yong (1997)	3,968 males and 6,100 females		1971–74	1992	Average, good dietary data	
Graham (1992)	18,586 postmenopausal females in New York State selected from DMV file (New York State Cohort)	>50	1980	1987	Cancer-free	Mailed dietary questionnaire
Bandera (1997)	27,544 males and 20,456 females	~40–80	1980	1987		Mailed dietary questionnaire: nested case–control analysis
Shibata (1992)	~4,277 males and ~7,300 females; elderly residents of Leisure World, Laguna Hills, CA	> 50 ave 74	1981–85	1989	Cancer-free, 1st year follow-up excluded	Mailed dietary questionnaire
Hunter (1993)	87,494 female registered nurses from 11 large states (Nurses Health Study)	34–59	1980	1988	Cancer-free	Mailed dietary questionnaire
Zhang (1999)	83,234 females	33–60	1980	1994		Mailed dietary questionnaire

Study	Cohort	Age	Baseline	Follow-up	Health status	Assessment
Rohan (1993)	56,837 females enrolled in multicenter Canadian National Breast Screening Study (NBSS)	40–59	1982	1987	Cancer-free	Lifestyle and dietary questionnaire: nested case–control analysis
Pandey (1995)	1,556 male employees of Western Electric Company in Chicago, IL (Western Electric Study)	40–55	1958–59	1983	No history of CHD, cancer, or other serious illness	Lifestyle and dietary interview and numerous exams
Daviglus (1996)	1,899 males		1957–58	1989	No history of cancer	
Bostick (1993)	35,216 females recruited from a random DMV sample in Iowa	55–69	1986	1990	No history of cancer	Mailed dietary questionnaire
Zheng (1995)	34,691 females		1986	1992		
Kushi (1996)	34,387 females		1986	1992		
Zheng (1998)	34,702 females		1986	1993		
Kushi (1999)	34,702 females		1986	1993		
Hertog (1996)	2,112 males recruited from all residents of Caerphilly, South Wales, UK (Caerphilly Study)	45–69	1979–83	~1995	Average	Baseline and follow-up exams with lifestyle and dietary questionnaire
Sahyoun (1996)	254 males and 471 females; noninstitutionalized recruited from MA community groups	60–101	1981–84	1992	Free of terminal disease and severe disorders	Physical, medical, dietary and biochemical exam
Verhoeven (1997)	62,573 females in Netherlands Cohort Study	55–69	1986	1990	Average	Mailed dietary questionnaire: nested case–control analysis
Botterweck (2000) Loria (2000)	58,279 males and 62,573 females 3,347 males and 3,724 females; national sample (NHANES II Mortality Follow-up Study)	30–75	1976–80	1992	No history of CHD, stroke, or cancer	Lifestyle and dietary interview and exam with blood samples
Khaw (2001)	8,860 males and 10,636 females; general practices sample in Norfolk, UK (EPIC study)	45–79	1993–97	1999	No history of CHD, stroke, or cancer	Lifestyle and dietary questionnaire and exam with blood sample

Table 2 Results for Prospective Vitamin C Studies: All-Cause Mortality

Author (yr)	Low vitamin C group (L)	High vitamin C group (H)	Control variables	Years of FU	Males Total deaths	Males RR (H vs L)	Males CI of RR	Females Total deaths	Females RR (H vs L)	Females CI of RR	Both sexes Total deaths	Both sexes RR (H vs L)	Both sexes CI of RR
Enstrom (1986)	VC < 250 mg/d	VC ≥ 250 mg/d	Age	10	134	0.95	0.61–1.42	130	1.03	0.68–1.51	264	0.97	0.67–1.38
Enstrom (1992)	VC < 50 mg/d	VC ≥ 50 mg/d and reg supps	Age	5	473	0.52	0.35–0.73	276	0.77	0.53–1.06	749	0.66	0.53–0.82
Enstrom (1992)	VC < 50 mg/d	VC ≥ 50 mg/d and reg supps	Age, 10 confounders	5	473	0.61	0.43–0.86				749	0.68	0.52–0.89
Enstrom (1992)	VC < 50 mg/d	VC ≥ 50 mg/d and reg supps	Age	Ave 10	1069	0.59	0.47–0.72	740	0.90	0.74–1.09	1809	0.74	0.64–0.85
Enstrom (1992)	VC < 50 mg/d	VC ≥ 50 mg/d and reg supps	Age, 10 confounders	Ave 10	1069	0.78	0.62–0.97				1809	0.86	0.73–1.02
Enstrom (1994)	VC < 50 mg/d	VC ≥ 50 mg/d and reg supps	Age	Ave 14	1595	0.63	0.53–0.74	1242	0.86	0.73–1.00	2837	0.76	0.68–0.85
Enstrom (1994)	VC < 50 mg/d	VC ≥ 50 mg/d and reg supps	Age, 10 confounders	Ave 14	1595	0.80	0.67–0.96				2837	0.88	0.82–0.99
Enstrom (1999)	VC < 50 mg/d	VC ≥ 50 mg/d and reg supps	Age	Ave 19	2132	0.67	0.57–0.77	1876	0.86	0.76–0.98	4008	0.79	0.72–0.87
Enstrom (1999)	VC < 50 mg/d	VC ≥ 50 mg/d and reg supps	Age, 10 confounders	Ave 19	1883	0.90	0.78–1.04	1652	1.01	0.88–1.17	3535	0.95	0.85–1.05
Enstrom (1999)	VC < 20 mg/d	VC ≥ 50 mg/d	Age	Ave 19	2132	0.78	0.70–0.87	1876	0.90	0.76–1.00	4008	0.83	0.77–0.90
Enstrom (1999)	VC < 20 mg/d	VC ≥ 50 mg/d	Age, 10 confounders	Ave 19	1883	0.90	0.78–1.04	1652	1.01	0.89–1.14	3535	0.97	0.89–1.06
Pandey (1995)	VC = 21–82 mg/d	VC = 113–393 mg/d	Age, 11 confounders	Ave 24	667	0.73	0.58–0.91						
Sahyoun (1996)	VC < 90 mg/d	VC > 388 mg/d	Age, sex	Ave 10							217	0.53	0.33–0.84
Sahyoun (1996)	VC < 90 mg/d	VC > 388 mg/d	Age, sex, 3 confounders	Ave 10							217	0.55	0.34–0.88
Sahyoun (1996)	PAA < 0.91 mg/dL	PAA > 1.56 mg/dL	Age, sex, 3 confounders	Ave 10								0.56	0.34–0.91
Loria (2000)	PAA < 0.5 mg/dL	PAA > 1.3 mg/dL	Age	Ave 14	242	0.52	0.41–0.67	127	0.68	0.51–0.92	369	~0.57	$p < 0.05$
Loria (2000)	PAA < 0.5 mg/dL	PAA > 1.3 mg/dL	Age, 8 confounders	Ave 14	242	0.64	0.49–0.83	127	0.84	0.60–1.16	369	~0.70	$p < 0.05$
Khaw (2001)	PAA ≲ 0.5 mg/dL	PAA ≳ 1.4 mg/dL	Age	Ave 4	309	0.48	0.33–0.70	187	0.50	0.32–0.81	496	~0.49	$p < 0.05$
Khaw (2001)	PAA ≲ 0.5 mg/dL	PAA ≳ 1.4 mg/dL	Age, 6 confounders	Ave 4	309	~0.50	$p < 0.05$	187	~0.57	$p < 0.05$	496	~0.52	$p < 0.05$

VC, vitamin C intake in mg/day; reg supps, daily use of vitamin C and/or multivitamin supplements; PAA, plasma ascorbic acid (1.0 mg/dL = 0.568 mmol/dL = 56.8 μmol/L)

Table 3 Results for Prospective Vitamin C Studies: All-Cancer Mortality and Incidence

Author (yr)	Low vitamin C group (L)	High vitamin C group (H)	Control variables	Years of FU	Males Total deaths*	Males RR (H vs L)	Males CI of RR	Females Total deaths*	Females RR (H vs L)	Females CI of RR	Both sexes Total deaths*	Both sexes RR (H vs L)	Both sexes CI of RR
Enstrom (1986)	VC < 250 mg/d	VC ≥ 250 mg/d	Age	10	33	0.80	$p > 0.05$	35	1.21	$p > 0.05$	68	1.01	$p > 0.05$
Gey (1987)	PAA < 0.4 mg/dL	PAA > 0.4 mg/dL	Age, smoking	7	102	0.72	$p > 0.05$						
Stahelin (1991)	PAA < 0.4 mg/dL	PAA > 0.4 mg/dL	Age, smoking, lipids	12	204	0.83	0.57–1.19						
Eichholzer (1996)	PAA < 0.4 mg/dL	PAA > 0.4 mg/dL	Age, smoking, lipids	17	290	0.81	0.59–1.12						
Kromhout (1987)	VC < 63 mg/d	VC = 83–103 mg/d	Age, smoking	25	155	<1.00	$p > 0.05$						
Enstrom (1992)	VC < 50 mg/d	VC ≥ 50 mg/d and reg supps	Age	Ave 10	228	0.79	0.51–1.18	169	0.93	0.60–1.40	397	0.85	0.63–1.14
Enstrom (1994)	VC < 50 mg/d	VC ≥ 50 mg/d and reg supps	Age	Ave 14	346	0.69	0.47–0.97	269	0.92	0.65–1.27	615	0.78	0.60–0.98
Shibata (1992)	VC < 145 mg/d	VC > 210 mg/d	Age, smoking	Ave 7	645[a]	0.90	0.74–1.09	690[a]	0.76	0.63–0.91	1335[a]	~0.82	$p < 0.05$
Shibata (1992)	VC = no supps	VC = median 500 mg/d supps	Age, smoking	Ave 7	642[a]	0.94	0.80–1.10	683[a]	0.93	0.80–1.09	1325[a]	~0.93	$p > 0.05$
Pandey (1995)	VC = 21–82 mg/d	VC = 113–393 mg/d	Age, 11 confounders	Ave 24	155	0.61	0.40–0.94						
Sahyoun (1996)	VC < 90 mg/d	VC > 388 mg/d	Age, sex, 2 confounders	Ave 10							57	0.94	0.36–2.44
Sahyoun (1996)	PAA < 0.91 mg/dL	PAA > 1.56 mg/dL	Age, sex, 3 confounders	Ave 10							57	0.68	0.25–1.83
Loria (2000)	PAA < 0.5 mg/dL	PAA > 1.3 mg/dL	Age	Ave 14	73	0.49	0.31–0.76	34	0.83	0.51–1.35	107	~0.56	$p < 0.05$
Loria (2000)	PAA < 0.5 mg/dL	PAA > 1.3 mg/dL	Age, 8 confounders	Ave 14	73	0.62	0.39–0.99	34	0.94	0.53–1.67	107	~0.70	$p < 0.05$
Khaw (2001)	PAA ≳ 0.5 mg/dL	PAA ≳ 1.4 mg/dL	Age	Ave 4	116	0.47	0.27–0.88	84	0.73	0.38–1.40	200	~0.55	$p < 0.05$
Khaw (2001)	PAA ≳ 0.5 mg/dL	PAA ≳ 1.4 mg/dL	Age, 6 confounders	Ave 4	116	~0.43	$p < 0.05$	84	~0.83	$p > 0.05$	200	~0.54	$p < 0.05$

[a] Cancer deaths in all studies except for cancer incidence in Shibata (1992).

Table 4 Results for Prospective Vitamin C Studies: Lung Cancer Mortality and Incidence

Author (yr)	Low vitamin C group (L)	High vitamin C group (H)	Control variables	Sex	Years of FU	Total sample	Outcome[a] D or I	Total events	RR (H vs. L)	CI of RR
Kvale (1983)	VC index < 15	VC index > 29	Age, smoking, region, residence	Males	11.5	10,602	I	72	0.88	p > 0.05
Long-de (1985)	FFJ = 0–2 d/wk	FFJ = 5–7 d/wk	Age	Males	10	~350,000	D	2,952	0.57	p < 0.05
Long-de (1985)	FFJ = 0–2 d/wk and no pills	FFJ = 5–7 d/wk and pills	Age	Males	10	~350,000	D	2,952	0.61	p < 0.05
Kromhout (1987)	VC < 63 mg/d	VC = 83–103 mg/d	Age, smoking	Males	25	878	D	63	0.36	0.18–0.75
Ocke (1997)	VC < 80 mg/d	VC > 102 mg/d	Age, smoking, energy	Males	19	561	I	54	0.46	0.24–0.88
Knekt (1991)	VC = lowest quintile	VC = highest quintile	Age, smoking (combined result)	Males	18	4,538	I	117	~0.8	p > 0.05
Shibata (1992)	VC < 145 mg/d	VC ≥ 210 mg/d	Age, smoking	Males	Ave 7	~4,277	I	94	1.11	0.68–1.81
Shibata (1992)	VC < 155 mg/d	VC ≥ 225 mg/d	Age, smoking	Females	Ave 7	~7,300	I	70	0.56	0.31–1.02
Chow (1992)	VC = lowest quintile	VC = highest quintile	Age, smoking, industry	Males	20	17,818	D	219	0.80	0.5–1.2
Enstrom (1994)	VC < 50 mg/d	VC ≥ 50 mg/d and reg supps	Age	Males	Ave 14	4,479	D	95	0.59	0.2–1.3
Enstrom (1994)	VC < 50 mg/d	VC ≥ 50 mg/d and reg supps	Age	Females	Ave 14	6,869	D	35	0.57	0.1–2.0
Yong (1997)	VC < 23 mg/d	VC > 113 mg/d	Age, sex	Both sexes	19	11,068	I	248	0.53	0.37–0.76
Yong (1997)	VC < 23 mg/d	VC > 113 mg/d	Age, sex, smoking, 7 confounders	Both sexes	19	11,068	I	248	0.66	0.45–0.96
Eichholzer (1996)	PAA < 0.4 mg/dL	PAA > 0.4 mg/dL	Age, smoking, lipids	Males	17	2,974	D	87	0.55	0.26–1.16
Hertog (1996)	VC < 38 mg/d	VC > 63 mg/d	Age	Males	14	2,112	D	51	1.30	p > 0.05
Hertog (1996)	VC < 38 mg/d	VC > 63 mg/d	Age, smoking, 5 confounders	Males	14	2,112	D	51	2.00	0.8–4.9
Bandera (1997)	VC = low tertile	VC = high tertile	Age, education	Males	7	27,554	I (nccs)[b]	395	0.63	0.53–0.88
Bandera (1997)	VC = low tertile	VC = high tertile	Age, education	Females	7	20,456	I (nccs)[b]	130	0.88	0.57–1.37

[a] Outcome events are mortality (D) or incidence (I).
[b] Analyzed as a nested case-control study (nccs).
FFJ, fruit or fruit juice.

Table 5 Results for Prospective Vitamin C Studies: Breast Cancer Mortality and Incidence

Author (yr)	Low vitamin C group (L)	High vitamin C group (H)	Control variables	Sex	Years of FU	Total sample	Outcome D or I	Total events	RR (H vs. L)	CI of RR
Graham (1992)	VC = 0–34 mg/d	VC = 79–498 mg/d	Age, education	Females	7	18,586	I	344	0.81	0.59–1.12
Shibata (1992)	VC < 155 mg/d	VC ≥ 225 mg/d	Age, smoking	Females	Ave 7	~7,300	I	219	0.86	0.63–1.18
Shibata (1992)	VC = no supps	VC = median 500 mg/d supps	Age, smoking	Females	Ave 7	~7,300	I	102	0.67	0.45–0.99
Rohan (1993)	VC < 101 mg/d	VC > 220 mg/d	Age	Females	6	56,837	I (nccs)	519	0.84	0.61–1.16
Rohan (1993)	VC < 101 mg/d	VC > 220 mg/d	Age, 7 confounders	Females	6	56,837	I (nccs)	519	0.88	0.62–1.26
Rohan (1993)	VC = no supps	VC > 250 mg/d supps	Age	Females	6	56,837	I (nccs)	519	1.37	1.01–1.87
Enstrom (1994)	VC < 50 mg/d	VC ≥ 50 mg/d and reg supps	Age	Females	Ave 14	6,869	D	61	1.34	0.6–2.5
Kushi (1996)	VC < 112 mg/d	VC ≥ 392 mg/d	Age	Females	7	34,387	I	879	0.88	0.71–1.09
Kushi (1996)	VC < 112 mg/d	VC ≥ 392 mg/d	Age, 11 confounders	Females	7	34,387	I	879	0.88	0.70–1.11
Jarvinen (1997)	VC = low tertile	VC = high tertile	Age, body mass	Females	25	4,697	I	88	0.80	$p > 0.05$
Verhoeven (1997)	VC = med 59 mg/d	VC = med 165 mg/d	Age, energy	Females	4.3	62,573	I (nccs)	650	0.77	0.55–1.08
Zhang (1999)	VC = med 70 mg/d (food only)	VC = med 205 mg/d	Age, 10–12 confounders	Females (comb)	~14	83,234	I	2,697	1.04	0.8–1.2
Zhang (1999)	VC = med 83 mg/d (food and supps)	VC = med 710 mg/d	Age, 10–12 confounders	Females (comb)	~14	83,234	I	2,697	1.00	0.8–1.2

Table 6 Results for Prospective Vitamin C Studies: Other Cancer Sites Mortality and Incidence

Author (yr)	Low vitamin C group (L)	High vitamin C group (H)	Control variables	Cancer site	Sex	Years of FU	Total sample	Outcome D or I	Total events	RR (H vs. L)	CI of RR
Bjelke (1982)	VC index < 15	VC index > 22	Age, sex, region, urbanization	Stomach	Both sexes	12	16,713	I	116	0.60	0.4–0.9
Enstrom (1994)	VC < 50 mg/d	VC ≥ 50 mg/d and reg supps	Age	Esophagus and stomach	Both sexes (combined)	Ave 14	11,348	D	39	0.20	0.0–0.8
Zheng (1995)	VC < 145 mg/d	VC > 262 mg/d	Age, smoking	Stomach	Females	7	34,691	I	33	0.50	0.2–1.3
Eichholzer (1996)	PAA < 0.4 mg/dL	PAA > 0.4 mg/dL	Age, smoking	Stomach	Males	17	2,974	D	28	1.41	0.31–6.25
Botterweck (2000)	Median 55 mg/d	Median 135 mg/d	Age, sex, smoking, educ, disease his	Stomach	Both sexes (combined)	6	120,852	I	282	0.70	0.5–1.0
Heilbrun (1989)	VC < 37 mg/d	VC ≥ 160 mg/d	Age	Colon	Males	Ave 18	8,006	I (nccs)	113	0.53	0.4–0.7
Heilbrun (1989)	VC < 37 mg/d	VC ≥ 160 mg/d	Age, alcohol	Rectum	Males	Ave 18	8,006	I (nccs)	65	1.25	0.9–1.6
Shibata (1992)	VC < 145 mg/d	VC ≥ 210 mg/d	Age, smoking	Colon	Males	Ave 7	~4,277	I	97	1.15	0.70–1.88
Shibata (1992)	VC < 155 mg/d	VC ≥ 225 mg/d	Age, smoking	Colon	Females	Ave 7	~7,300	I	105	0.61	0.38–0.99
Bostick (1993)	Total VC < 112 mg/d	Total VC > 392 mg/d		Colon	Females	5	41,837	I	212	0.70	0.45–1.07
Bostick (1993)	Total VC < 112 mg/d	Total VC > 392 mg/d	Age, calories, diet, height	Colon	Females	5	41,837	I	212	1.23	0.75–2.02
Enstrom (1994)	VC < 50 mg/d	VC ≥ 50 mg/d and reg supps	Age	Colon and rectum	Both sexes (combined)	Ave 14	11,348	D	76	0.87	0.4–1.8
Eichholzer (1996)	PAA < 0.4 mg/dL	PAA > 0.4 mg/dL	Age, smoking	Colon	Males	17	2,974	D	22	0.58	0.36–3.23
Hertog (1996)	VC < 38 mg/d	VC > 63 mg/d	Age, smoking, 5 confounders	Digestive system	Males	14	2,112	D	46	0.50	0.2–1.2
Zheng (1998)	VC < 145	VC > 262	Age, smoking	Rectum	Females	8	34,702	I	144	0.84	0.56–1.26
Shibata (1992)	VC < 145 mg/d	VC ≥ 210 mg/d	Age, smoking	Prostate	Males	Ave 7	~4,277	I	208	0.96	0.68–1.35
Enstrom (1994)	VC < 50 mg/d	VC ≥ 50 mg/d and reg supps	Age	Prostate	Males	Ave 14	4,479	D	49	0.91	0.3–2.0
Daviglus (1996)	VC < 75 mg/d	VC > 121 mg/d	Age, smoking	Prostate	Males	30	1,899	I	132	1.27	0.75–2.14
Eichholzer (1996)	PAA < 0.4 mg/dL	PAA > 0.4 mg/dL	Age, smoking	Prostate	Males	17	2,974	D	29	0.97	0.35–3.06

Table 7 Comparison of Case–Control and Prospective Vitamin C Studies: Major Cancer Sites

Cancer site	ICD9	1991 Block review (1) (40 case–control and 4 prospective studies)			1995 Byers review (5) (40 case–control and 9 prospective studies)			2001 Enstrom review (20 prospective cohorts)				Number of unanalyzed cohorts
		Number of studies			Number of studies			Number of cohorts with results				
		RR < 1.0 with $p < 0.05$	Total	RR median	All with RR < 1.0	Total	RR range	RR < 1.0 with $p < 0.05$	All with RR < 1.0	Total	RR range	
Stomach	151	7	7	0.5	9	9	0.4–0.8	2	4	5	0.2–1.4	14
Colorectal	153–154	8	14	0.8	12	15	0.4–1.3	0	7	7	0.5–0.9	12
Lung	162	5	10	0.6	9	11	0.6–1.1	4	9	10	0.4–2.0	9
Breast	174	5	9	0.7	7	10	0.3–1.4	0	6	8	0.8–1.3	4
Prostate	185	0	4	1.2	1	4	0.9–2.3	0	3	4	0.9–1.3	12
All sites	140–208							4	8	9	0.6–1.0	11

Table 8 describes the study population, cancer site, number of subjects, and number of cancer cases or deaths for the 9 cohorts with results for all cancer sites and the 11 cohorts with results for one or more cancer sites, but not for all cancer sites.

Table 9 describes the population, age range, follow-up period, initial health status, and type of study (randomized, controlled trial or patient survival) for the intervention studies that assessed the influence of vitamin C intake on subsequent cancer mortality, incidence, or survival (53–68).

Table 10 describes the results of those intervention studies in Table 9. The placebo and intervention groups are described in terms of level of vitamin C intake (diet or supplements), number of subjects, and number of deaths or other outcomes. Also presented are the characteristics controlled for, years of follow-up, relative risk of intervention versus placebo, and 95% confidence interval or statistical p value.

III. RESULTS

There have been six cohorts analyzed for both death from all causes and death from all cancer. Table 2 shows the relative risk (RR) for all-cause mortality. Each relative risk is based on comparing persons with the highest and lowest vitamin C intake, generally values close to the recommended dietary allowance (RDA). The 16 RRs for males from five cohorts range between 0.48 and 0.95: all 16 are less than 1.00 and 13 are significantly less than 1.0 ($p < 0.05$). The 12 RRs for females from four cohorts range between 0.58 and 1.03: 9 are less than 1.0 and 4 are significantly less than 1.0. The 18 RRs for both sexes from six cohorts range between 0.49 and 0.97: 22 are less than 1.0 and 18 are significantly less. Of the RRs that control for confounding variables, 6 of 8 for males, 1 of 4 for females, and 6 of 9 for both sexes are significantly less than 1.00.

Table 3 shows the RRs for mortality or incidence from all cancer sites by sex: 32 of 34 RRs are less than 1.0, but only 12 are significantly less than 1.0. Table 4 shows the mortality or incidence RRs for lung cancer: 15 of 18 are less than 1.0 and 7 are significantly less. These ratios are more consistently less than 1.0 than those for any other cancer site. Table 5 shows the RRs for breast cancer: 9 of 13 are less than 1.0, but only 1 is significantly less. Table 6 shows the RRs for stomach, colorectal, and prostate cancer: 11 of 14 are less than 1.0, but only 3 are significantly less. Some RRs that are less than 1.00 do not control for confounding variables.

Table 7 compares the results of the case–control studies in the reviews by Block (1) and Byers and Guerrero (5) with the results from the prospective cohorts in Tables 3–6. For stomach, colorectal, lung, breast, and prostate cancer, most of the RRs from case–control studies are less than 1.0. Of the studies in the Byers review, $38/49 = 78\%$ of the RRs are less than 1.0; of the studies in the Block review, $25/44 = 57\%$ of the RRs are significantly ($p < 0.05$) less than 1.0. Of the results in Tables 4–6 for individual cancer sites, $29/34 = 85\%$ of the RRs are less than 1.0, but only $6/34 = 18\%$ are significantly ($p < 0.05$) less than 1.0. Thus, the vast majority of both case–control and cohort studies indicate a beneficial effect for increased vitamin C intake. Also, except for breast cancer, most of the cohort studies have not been analyzed for outcomes of specific cancer sites, a point worthy of further discussion.

Table 8 shows the analysis status of the prospective studies. The total number of subjects in the 20 cohorts are shown, along with the actual or estimated number of total cancer events (deaths or cases) available with existing follow-up. If not published, the total number of available cancer events is estimated for each cohort from the published site-specific results. Of the 20 cohorts, no results for all cancer sites have been published for 11 cohorts, including

Table 8 Results for Every Prospective Vitamin C Cohort: Actual and Estimated Events for All Cancer

Author (most appropriate references)	Outcome D or I	Cancer site	Males Total sample	Males Cancer events	Females Total sample	Females Cancer events	Both sexes Cancer site	Both sexes Total sample	Both sexes Cancer events
			Actual		Actual			Actual	
Cohorts with results for all cancer									
Enstrom (1986)	D	All	1,369	33	1,654	35	All	3,023	68
Gey (1987), Eichholzer (1996)	D	All	2,975	290			All	2,975	290
Kromhout (1987)	D	All	878	155			All	878	155
Enstrom (1992), Enstrom (1994)	D	All	4,479	346	6,869	269	All	11,348	615
Shibata (1992)	I	All	~4,277	645	7,300	690	All	11,577	1335
Pandey (1995)	D	All	1,556	155			All	1,556	155
Sahyoun (1996)	D	All	254	~20	471	~37	All	725	57
Loria (2000)	D	All	3,347	73	3,724	34	All	7,071	107
Khaw (2001)	D	All	8,860	116	10,636	84	All	19,496	200
Total (9 cohorts)			27,995	1,833	30,654	1,149	All	58,649	2,982
Percent of grand total				5.5%		10.4%			7.3%
			Actual		Actual			Estimated	
Cohorts without results for all cancer									
Bjelke (1982)	I	Stomach	13,785	~97	2,928	~19	All	16,713	1,000
Long-de (1985)	D	Lung	~350,000	2,952			All	~350,000	12,000
Heilbrun (1989)	I	Colon	8,006	113			All	8,006	1,100
Knekt (1991)	I	Lung	4,538	117			All	9,235	900
Jarvinen (1997)	I	Breast			4,697	88			
Chow (1992)	D	Lung	17,818	219			All	17,818	1,100
Graham (1992), Bandera (1997)	I	Lung	27,554	395	20,456	130	All	48,010	2,100
Rohan (1993)	I	Breast			56,837	519	All	56,837	1,800
Bostick (1993), Zheng (1998)	I	Rectum			34,702	144	All	34,702	3,000
Hertog (1996)	D	Lung	2,112	51			All	2,112	300
Verhoeven (1997), Botterweck (2000)	I	Stomach	58,279	219	62,573	63	All	120,852	2,500
Zhang (1999)	I	Breast			83,234	2,697	All	83,234	9,000
Total (11 cohorts)			482,092		265,427			747,519	34,800
Grand total (20 cohorts, 9 with and 11 without results for all cancer)			510,087		296,081			806,168	37,782

Table 9 Description of Populations for Intervention Studies Involving Vitamin C and Cancer

Author (yr)	Population description	Ages at entry	Start	End	Initial health	Type of study
Cameron (1976)	52 males and 48 females; terminal patients with cancer of 20 sites from Vale of Leven Hospital, Scotland	32–93	1971	1975	Terminal cancer	Patients compared with matched historical controls
Cameron (1978)	53 males and 47 females; terminal patients with cancer of 16 sites from Vale of Leven Hospital, Scotland	38–93	1971	1978	Terminal cancer	Patients compared with matched historical controls
Creagan (1979)	76 males and 47 females; terminal cancer patients from Mayo Clinic in Rochester, MN	Mean ~65	1978	1978	Terminal cancer	Randomized controlled trial
Moertel (1985)	57 males and 43 females; terminal colorectal cancer patients from Mayo Clinic in Rochester, MN	Mean ~65	1982	1984	Terminal cancer	Randomized controlled trial
McKeown (1988)	90 males and 47 females; Canadian patients with at least one sporatic adenomatous polyp removed	Mean 58	1979	1986	Prior adenomatous polyp	Randomized secondary prevention trial
DeCosse (1989)	15 males and 23 females; colectomy patients from New York hospital with familial adenomatous polypsis	Mean 33	1984	1988	Prior adenomatous polyps and colectomy	Randomized secondary prevention trial
Blot (1993)	~6,600 males and ~8,140 females out of 29,584 adults from four Linxian communes in China	40–69	1986	1991	No debilitating diseases or prior cancer	Randomized primary prevention trial

Study	Subjects	Age	Start	End	Condition	Type
Rohan (1993)	412 female breast cancer patients in Adelaide, Australia	20–74	1982	1989	Confirmed cancer diagnosis	Observational survival study
Roncucci (1993)	94 males and 54 females; Italian patients with at least one colorectal adenoma removed	Mean 59	1985	1990	Prior adenomatous polyp	Randomized secondary prevention trial
Greenberg (1994)	317 males and 75 females; patients from six U.S. cities with at least one colorectal adenoma removed	Mean 61	1984	1992	Good health, no colorectal cancer	Randomized secondary prevention trial
Ingram (1994)	103 female breast cancer patients from Perth, Australia		1985	1992	Cancer diagnosis	Observational survival study
Jain (1994)	678 female breast cancer patients from National Breast Screening Study in Canada	40–59	1982	1992	Confirmed cancer diagnosis	Observational survival study
Lamm (1994)	54 males and 11 females; transitional cell bladder cancer patients from West Virginia	Mean 67	1985	1992	Confirmed cancer diagnosis	Randomized controlled trial
de Lorgeril (1998)	~545 males and ~60 females; survivors of a first acute MI recruited from coronary care unit in Lyon, France	Mean 54	~1990	~1994	Survived first acute myocardial infarction	Randomized secondary prevention trial
Hercberg (1998)	5,056 males and 7,679 females; general population recruits from multimedia campaign in France	35–60	1994	2002	Healthy, cooperative	Randomized, blinded primary prevention trial
Christen (2000)	~15,000 male physicians recruited through American Medical Association (Physician Health Study II)	55–89	2000	2005	Healthy, cooperative	Randomized, blinded primary prevention trial

Table 10 Results for Intervention Studies Involving Vitamin C and Cancer

	Placebo group (P)			Intervention group (I)							
Author (yr)	Vitamin C intake	Sample	Outcome events[a]	Vitamin C intake	Sample	Outcome events[a]	Control variables	Sex	Years of FU	RR (I vs. P)	CI of RR
Cancer patient survival											
Cameron (1976)	0 mg	1000	880	10 g	100	47	Sex, age, site, tumor status	Both sexes	0.27	0.53	$p < 0.01$
Cameron (1978)	0 mg	1000	~900	10 g	100	~36	Sex, age, site, tumor status	Both sexes	0.27	~0.40	$p < 0.01$
Rohan (1993)	< 71 mg/d	80	30	> 234 mg/d	84	23	Age, energy, risk factor	Females	5.5	0.74	0.42–1.30
Ingram (1994)	Low tertile	34	11	High tertile	34	3	Age, energy, smoking, weight	Females	6	0.25	$p < 0.05$
Jain (1994)	< 111 mg/d	~168	~29	> 210 mg/d	~168	~13		Females	~5	0.43	0.21–0.86
Cancer patient trials											
Creagan (1979)	0 mg	63	56	10 g	60	54	Sex, age, site, tumor status	Both sexes	0.50	1.01	$p > 0.05$
Moertel (1985)	0 mg	49	24	10 g	51	25	Sex, age, prior radiation treatment	Both sexes	1	0.96	$p > 0.05$
Lamm (1994)	RDA supps	30	24[b]	2000 mg VC and other supps	35	14[b]	Sex, age, diet, tumor history	Both sexes	Ave 3.75	0.45	$p = 0.0014$
Polyp patient trials											
McKeown (1988)	0 mg	67	34[c]	400 mg VC and 400 mg VE	70	29[c]	Sex, age, tobacco, diet, polyp history	Both sexes	2	0.86	0.51–1.45
DeCosse (1989)	0 mg	22	1.05[d]	4000 mg VC and 400 mg VE	16	0.92[d]	Sex, age, polyp history	Both sexes	4	0.88	$p > 0.05$
Roncucci (1993)	0 mg	78	28[c]	1000 mg VC and VA and VE	70	4[c]	Sex, age, polyp history	Both sexes	3	0.16	$p < 0.05$
Greenberg (1994)	0 mg	187	64[c]	1000 mg VC and 400 mg VE	205	79[c]	Sex, age, diet, adenoma history	Both sexes	1	1.08	0.91–1.29
Acute MI patient trial											
de Lorgeril (1998)	112 mg/d in Medit. diet	302	14	132 mg/d in prudent diet	303	24	Sex, age, health status	Both sexes	4	0.44	0.21–0.94
General population trial											
Blot (1993)	0 mg	~3,700	107	120 mg + 30 μg Mo	~11,100	312	Sex, age, tobacco, cancer history	Both sexes	5.25	1.06	0.92–1.21

[a]Outcome events are deaths unless otherwise indicated.
[b]Tumor recurrence.
[c]Polyp (adenoma) recurrence.
[d]Polyp ratio after treatment (average of 16 visits).

the 6 largest cohorts. As a result, only about 7% of the total number of subjects and about 8% of the total number of cancer events have been analyzed. In addition, there are several other existing cohorts not shown in Tables 1 and 8 that have not been analyzed at all relative to vitamin C and cancer, reducing the percentage of analyzed data even further. If all the available cancer data were analyzed and published, these new results would greatly refine the relation of vitamin C intake with cancer.

Table 10 shows the results for intervention studies involving vitamin C and cancer. Two groups of terminal cancer patients given 10 g of vitamin C survived significantly longer than matched historical controls. In three groups of breast cancer patients, there was an increased survival rate among those with the highest vitamin C intake. There have been two small randomized controlled trials of terminal cancer patients (median survival of 7 weeks) and neither of these showed any benefit from 10 g of vitamin C supplements. However, one small trial of bladder cancer patients showed a significant benefit for 2 g of vitamin C. A randomized trial of bladder cancer patients showed that a multivitamin that included vitamin C reduced tumor recurrence significantly. In general, the potential rate of vitamin C in the treatment of human cancer has not been fully investigated.

Several intervention trials have examined the effect of vitamin C supplementation on the recurrence of colorectal polyps, considered a precursor to colorectal cancer. Only one of the four largest randomized trials has demonstrated efficacy for vitamin C in reducing polyp recurrence. One intervention trial among acute MI patients showed a Mediterranean-type diet with vitamin C intake of about 130 mg/day resulted in a lower cancer death rate. One large community intervention trial in China showed no mortality benefit for vitamin C supplements of 120 mg/day.

IV. CONCLUSIONS

A large majority of epidemiological studies show a decrease in risk of cancer mortality or incidence with an increase of vitamin C intake, particularly for levels of vitamin C intake close to the current U. S. RDA of 60 mg/day (69). The inverse relation is strongest for males, next strongest for both sexes combined, and weakest for females. However, several studies show no significant relation after controlling for confounding variables, and others do not properly control for confounding variables. Indices of varying quality have been used, and they have usually been based on dietary sources alone. There does not appear to be a relation with vitamin C supplement intake per se, but only a few studies have examined use of supplements (13). Most studies have dealt with only one cancer site at a time, without regard for the influence of vitamin C on all cancer or overall health. The vast majority of available prospective data remain unanalyzed.

Several studies show that cancer patients with increased vitamin C intake have longer survival, but only one of three randomized patient trials show a benefit for supplemental vitamin C. One general population trial showed no benefit. However, there have been so few trials involving vitamin C that the results thus far should not be overinterpreted. The trials may apply only to populations with similar baseline nutritional status and risk factors and to the specific intervention used. The nutrient intervention may have been given too late in the disease process, may have been given for an inadequate duration, or may have been given to an already well-nourished population.

Although the specific mechanism by which vitamin C may be causally related to cancer has not yet been clearly established, there is substantial epidemiological evidence that increased vitamin C intake is associated with reduced cancer risk. Because of this epidemiological evidence and other supporting evidence (10,11), the RDA has been to be increased to 90 mg/day for males and 75 mg/day for females (70–71). This relation can be substantially refined by complete analysis of available prospective cohort data. Additional well-designed trials are required to measure the influence of specific vitamin C interventions. It is important to further examine the promising role of vitamin C in reducing cancer risk, because it is a risk factor that can be easily changed and one for which even a small benefit can have a large influence on the population.

ACKNOWLEDGMENTS

This review has been supported in part by the Wallace Genetic Foundation. The author thanks Ted Luppen for technical assistance.

REFERENCES

1. Block G. Vitamin C and cancer prevention: the epidemiologic evidence. Am J Clin Nutr 1991; 53:270S–282S.
2. Dorgan JF, Schatzkin A. Antioxidant micronutrients in cancer prevention. Hematol Oncol Clin North Am 1991; 5:43–68.
3. Byers T, Perry G. Dietary carotenes, vitamin C, and vitamin E as protective antioxidants in human cancers. Annu Rev Nutr 1992; 12:139–159.
4. Manson JE, Jonas MA, Hunter DJ. Prospective cohort studies of vitamins and cancer. In: Bray GA, Ryan DH, eds. Vitamins and Cancer Prevention. Baton Rouge: Louisiana State University Press, 1993:87–109.
5. Byers T, Guerrero N. Epidemiologic evidence for vitamin C and vitamin E in cancer prevention. Am J Clin Nutr 1995; 62(6 suppl):1385S–1392S.
6. Mayne ST. Antioxidant nutrients and cancer incidence and mortality: an epidemiologic perspective. Adv Pharmacol 1997; 38:657–675.
7. Enstrom JE. Vitamin C in prospective epidemiologic studies. In: Packer L, Fuchs J, eds. Vitamin C in Health and Disease. New York: Marcel Dekker, 1997:381–398.
8. Lee IM. Antioxidant vitamins in the prevention of cancer. Proc Assoc Am Physicians 1999; 111:10–15.
9. Byers T. What can randomized controlled trials tell us about nutrition and cancer prevention? CA Cancer J Clin 1999; 49:353–361.
10. Carr AC, Frei B. Toward a new recommended dietary allowance for vitamin C based on antioxidant and health effects in humans. Am J Clin Nutr 1999; 69:1086–1107.
11. Levine M, Rumsey SC, Daruwala R, Park JB, Wang Y. Criteria and recommendations for vitamin C intake. JAMA 1999; 281:1415–1423.
12. Bendich A, Langseth L. The health effects of vitamin C supplementation: a review. J Am Coll Nutr 1995; 14:124–136.
13. Patterson RE, White E, Kristal AR, Neuhouser ML, Potter JD. Vitamin supplements and cancer risk: the epidemiological evidence. Cancer Causes Control 1997; 8:786–802.
14. Kaegi E. Unconventional therapies for cancer: 5. Vitamins A, C and E. The Task Force on Alternative Therapies of the Canadian Breast Cancer Research Initiative. Can Med Assoc J 1998; 158:1483–1488.
15. Head KA. Ascorbic acid in the prevention and treament of cancer. Altern Med Rev 1998; 3:175–186.
16. Prasad KN, Kumar A, Kochupillai V, Cole WC. High doses of multiple antioxidant vitamins: essential ingredients in improving the efficacy of standard cancer therapy. J Am Coll Nutr 1999; 18:13–25.
17. Bjelke E. The recession of stomach cancer: selected aspects. In: Magnus K, ed. Trends in Cancer Incidence. Washington, DC: Hemisphere, 1982:162–181.
18. Kvale G, Bjelke E, Gart JJ. Dietary habits and lung cancer risk. Int J Cancer 1983; 31:397–405.
19. Long-de W, Hammond EC. Lung cancer, fruit, green salad and vitamin pills. Chin Med J 1985; 98:206–210.

20. Enstrom JE, Kanim LE, Breslow L. The relationship between vitamin C intake, general health practices, and mortality in Alameda County, California. Am J Public Health 1986; 76:1124–1130.
21. Gey KF, Brubacher GB, Staehelin HB. Plasma levels of antioxidant vitamins in relation to ischemic heart disease and cancer. Am J Clin Nutr 1987; 45:1368–1377.
22. Stahelin HB, Gey KF, Eichholzer M, Ludin E, Bernasconi F, Thurneysen J, Brubacher G. Plasma antioxidant vitamins and subsequent cancer mortality in the 12-year follow-up of the prospective Basel Study. Am J Epidemiol 1991; 133:766–775.
23. Eichholzer M, Stahelin HB, Gey KF, Ludin E, Bernasconi F. Prediction of male cancer mortality by plasma levels of interacting vitamins: 17 year follow-up of the prospective Basel Study. Int J Cancer 1996; 66:145–150.
24. Kromhout D. Essential micronutrients in relation to carcinogenesis. Am J Clin Nutr 1987; 45:1361–1367.
25. Ocke MC, Bueno-de-Mesquita HB, Feskens EJ, van Staveren WA, Kromhout D. Repeated measurements of vegetables, fruits, beta-carotene, and vitamins C and E in relation to lung cancer. The Zutphen Study. Am J Epidemiol 1997; 145:358–365.
26. Heilbrun LK, Nomura A, Hankin JH, Stemmermann GN. Diet and colorectal cancer with special reference to fiber intake. Int J Cancer 1989; 44:1–6.
27. Knekt P, Jarvinen R, Seppanen R, Rissanen A, Aromaa A, Heinonen OP, Albanes D, Heinonen M, Pukkala E, Teppo L. Dietary antioxidants and the risk of lung cancer. Am J Epidemiol 1991; 134:471–479.
28. Jarvinen R, Knekt P, Seppanen R, Teppo L. Diet and breast cancer risk in a cohort of Finnish women. Cancer Lett 1997; 114:251–253.
29. Chow WH, Schuman LM, McLaughlin JK, Bjelke E, Gridley G, Wacholder S, Chien HT, Blot WJ. A cohort study of tobacco use, diet, occupation, and lung cancer mortality. Cancer Causes Control 1992; 3:247–254.
30. Enstrom JE, Kanim LE, Klein MA. Vitamin C intake and mortality among a sample of the United States population. Epidemiology 1992; 3:194–202.
31. Enstrom JE. Vitamin C intake and mortality among a sample of the United States population: new results. In: Packer L, Cadenas E, eds. Biological Oxidants and Antioxidants. Germany: Hippokrates Verlag, 1994:229–241.
32. Enstrom JE. Antioxidants and mortality among a national sample. Technology 1999; 6:131–139.
33. Yong LC, Brown CC, Schatzkin A, Dresser CM, Slesinski MJ, Cox CS, Taylor PR. Intake of vitamins E, C, and A and risk of lung cancer. The NHANES I epidemiologic followup study. First National Health and Nutrition Examination Survey. Am J Epidemiol 1997; 146:231–243.
34. Graham S, Zielezny M, Marshall J, Priore R, Freudenheim J, Brasure J, Haughey B, Nasca P, Zdeb M. Diet in the epidemiology of postmenopausal breast cancer in the New York State cohort. Am J Epidemiol 1992; 136:1327–1337.
35. Bandera EV, Freudenheim JL, Marshall JR, Zielezny M, Priore RL, Brasure J, Baptiste M, Graham S. Diet and alcohol consumption and lung cancer risk in the New York State Cohort (United States). Cancer Causes Control 1997; 8:828–840.
36. Shibata A, Paganini–Hill A, Ross RK, Henderson BE. Intake of vegetables, fruits, beta-carotene, vitamin C and vitamin supplements and cancer incidence among the elderly: a prospective study. Br J Cancer 1992; 66:673–679.
37. Hunter DJ, Manson JE, Colditz GA, Stampfer MJ, Rosner B, Hennekens CH, Speizer FE, Willett WC. A prospective study of the intake of vitamin C, E, and A and the risk of breast cancer. N Engl J Med 1993; 329:234–240.
38. Zhang S, Hunter DJ, Forman MR, Rosner BA, Speizer FE, Colditz GA, Manson JE, Hankinson SE, Willett WC. Dietary carotenoids and vitamins A, C, and E and risk of breast cancer. J Natl Cancer Inst 1999; 91:547–556.
39. Rohan TE, Howe GR, Friedenreich CM, Jain M, Miller AB. Dietary fiber, vitamins A, C, and E, and risk of breast cancer: a cohort study. Cancer Causes Control 1993; 4:29–37.
40. Pandey D, Shekelle R, Tangney C, Stamler J. Dietary vitamin C and beta carotene and risk of death in middle-aged men: the Western Electric Study. Am J Epidemiol 1995; 142:1269–1278.
41. Daviglus ML, Dyer AR, Persky V, Chavez N, Drum M, Goldberg J, Liu K, Morris DK, Shekelle RB, Stamler J. Dietary beta-carotene, vitamin C, and risk of prostate cancer: results from the Western Electric Study. Epidemiology 1996; 7:472–477.

42. Bostick RM, Potter JD, McKenzie DR, Sellers TA, Kushi LH, Steinmetz KA, Folsom AR. Reduced risk of colon cancer with high intake of vitamin E: the Iowa Women's Health Study. Cancer Res 1993; 53:4230–4237.
43. Zheng W, Sellers TA, Doyle TJ, Kushi LH, Potter JD, Folsom AR. Retinol, antioxidant vitamins, and cancers of the upper digestive tract in a prospective cohort study of postmenopausal women. Am J Epidemiol 1995; 142:955–960.
44. Kushi LH, Fee RM, Sellers TA, Zheng W, Folsom AR. Intake of vitamins A, C, and E and postmenopausal breast cancer. The Iowa Women's Health Study. Am J Epidemiol 1996; 144:165–174.
45. Zheng W, Anderson KE, Kushi LH, Sellers TA, Greenstein J, Hong CP, Cerhan JR, Bostick RM, Folsom AR. A prospective cohort study of intake of calcium, vitamin D, and other micronutrients in relation to incidence of rectal cancer among postmenopausal women. Cancer Epidemiol Biomarkers Prev 1998; 7:221–225.
46. Kushi LH, Mink PJ, Folsom AR, Anderson KE, Zheng W, Lazovich D, Sellers TA. Prospective study of diet and ovarian cancer. Am J Epidemiol 1999; 149:21–31.
47. Hertog MG, Bueno-de-Mesquita HB, Fehily AM, Sweetnam PM, Elwood PC, Kromhout D. Fruit and vegetable consumption and cancer mortality in the Caerphilly Study. Cancer Epidemiol Biomarkers Prev 1996; 5:673–677.
48. Sahyoun NR, Jacques PF, Russell RM. Carotenoids, vitamins C and E, and mortality in the elderly population. Am J Epidemiol 1996; 144:501–511.
49. Verhoeven DT, Assen N, Goldbohm RA, Dorant E, van'tVeer P, Sturmans E, Hermus RJ, van den Brandt PA. Vitamins C and E, retinol, beta-carotene and dietary fibre in relation to breast cancer risk: a prospective cohort study. Br J Cancer 1997; 75:149–155.
50. Botterweck AAM, van den Brandt P, Goldbohm RA. Vitamins, carotenoids, dietary fiber, and the risk of gastric carcinoma. Cancer 2000; 88:737–748.
51. Loria CM, Klag MJ, Caulfield LE, Whelton PK. Vitamin C status and mortality in US adults. Am J Clin Nutr 2000; 72:139–145.
52. Khaw KT, Bingham S, Welch A, Luben R, Wareham N, Oakes S, Day N. Relation between plasma ascorbic acid and mortality in men and women in EPIC-Norfolk prospective study. Lancet 2001; 357:657–663.
53. Cameron E, Pauling L. Supplemental ascorbate in the supportive treatment of cancer: prolongation of survival time in terminal human cancer. Proc Natl Acad Sci USA 1976; 73:3685–3689.
54. Cameron E, Pauling L. Supplemental ascorbate in the supportive treatment of cancer: reevaluation of prolongation of survival time in terminal human cancer. Proc Natl Acad Sci USA 1978; 75:4538–4542.
55. Creagan ET, Moertel CG, O'Fallon JR, Schutt AJ, O'Connell MJ, Rubin J, Frytak S. Failure of high-dose vitamin C (ascorbic acid) therapy to benefit patients with advanced cancer: a controlled trial. N Engl J Med 1979; 301:687–690.
56. Moertel CG, Fleming TR, Creagen ET, Rubin J, O'Connell MJ, Ames MM. High-dose vitamin C versus placebo in the treatment of patients with advanced cancer who have had no prior chemotherapy: a randomized double-blind comparison. N Engl J Med 1985; 312:137–141.
57. McKeown-Eyssen G, Holloway C, Jazmaji V, Bright-See E, Dion P, Bruce WR. A randomized trial of vitamins C and E in the prevention of recurrence of colorectal polyps. Cancer Res 1988; 48:4701–4705.
58. DeCosse JJ, Miller HH, Lesser ML. Effect of wheat fiber and vitamin C and E on rectal polyps in patients with familial adenomatous polyposis. J Natl Cancer Inst 1989; 81:1290–1297.
59. Blot WJ, Li JY, Taylor PR, Guo W, Dawsey S, Wang GQ, Yang CS, Zheng SF, Gail M, Li GY, Yu Y, Liu BQ, Tangrea J, Sun YH, Liu F, Fraumeni JF Jr, Zhang YH, Li B. Nutrition intervention trials in Linxian, China: supplementation with specific vitamin/mineral combinations, cancer incidence, and disease-specific mortality in the general population. J Natl Cancer Inst 1993; 85:1483–1492.
60. Rohan TE, Hiller JE, McMichael AJ. Dietary factors and survival from breast cancer. Nutr Cancer 1993; 20:167–177.
61. Roncucci L, DiDonato P, Carati L, Ferrari A, Perini M, Bertoni G, Bedogni G, Paris B, Svanoni F, Girola M, Ponz de Leon M. Antioxidant vitamins or lactulose for the prevention of the recurrence of colorectal adenomas. Dis Colon Rectum 1993; 36:227–234.
62. Greenberg ER, Baron JA, Tosteson TD, Freeman DH Jr, Beck GJ, Bond JH, Colacchio TA, Coller JA, Frankl HD, Haile RW, Mandel JS, Nierenberg DW, Rothstein R, Snover DC, Stevens MM,

Summers RW, van Stolk RU, the Polyp Prevention Study Group. A clinical trial of antioxidant vitamins to prevent colorectal adenoma. N Engl J Med 1994; 331:141–147.
63. Ingram D. Diet and subsequent survival in women with breast cancer. Br J Cancer 1994; 69:592–595.
64. Jain M, Miller AB, To T. Premorbid diet and the prognosis of women with breast cancer. J Natl Cancer Inst 1994; 86:1390–1397.
65. Lamm DJ, Riggs DR, Shriver JS, vanGilder PF, Rach JF, DeHaven JI. Megadose vitamins in bladder cancer: a double-blind clinical trial. J Urol 1994; 151:21–26.
66. De Lorgeril M, Salen P, Martin J–L, Monjaud I, Boucher P, Mamelle N. Mediterranean dietary pattern in a randomized trial: prolonged survival and possible reduced cancer rate. Arch Intern Med 1998; 158:1181–1187.
67. Hercberg S, Preziosi P, Briancon S, Galan P, Triol I, Malvy D, Roussel A–M, Favier A. A primary prevention trial using nutritional doses of antioxidant vitamins and minerals in cardiovascular diseases and cancers in a general population: the SU.VI.MAX study—design, methods, and participant characteristics. Controlled Clin Trials 1998; 19:336–351.
68. Christen WG, Gaziano JM, Hennekens CH. Design of Physicians' Health Study II—a randomized trial of beta-carotene, vitamin E and C, and multivitamins, in prevention of cancer, cardiovascular disease, and eye disease, and review of results of completed trials. Ann Epidemiol 2000; 10:125–134.
69. Food and Nutrition Board, Institute of Medicine. Recommended Dietary Allowances. Washington, DC: National Academy Press, 1989.
70. Food and Nutrition Board, Institute of Medicine. Dietary reference intakes. Washington, DC: National Academy Press, 1998.
71. Food and Nutrition Board, Institute of Medicine. Recommended Dietary Allowances. Washington, DC: National Academy Press, 2000.

10
Carotenoids: Linking Chemistry, Absorption, and Metabolism to Potential Roles in Human Health and Disease

Denise M. Deming, Thomas W.-M. Boileau, Kasey H. Heintz, Christine A. Atkinson, and John W. Erdman, Jr.
University of Illinois, Urbana, Illinois

I. INTRODUCTION

In the past few decades, dietary carotenoids have been implicated in biological processes that may have physiological relevance to human health and chronic disease. Some of the biological actions of carotenoids include antioxidant activity, intercellular communication, cell differentiation, immunoenhancement, and inhibition of mutagenesis and transformation. A variety of hypotheses concerning the potential role of carotenoids in health and disease arose from the effects of carotenoids observed in model systems in vitro and animal studies in vivo. Numerous epidemiological studies have also supported an inverse association between dietary intake or blood levels of carotenoids and risk of some chronic diseases. One of the most dramatic and consistent epidemiological observations from these studies was the inverse association between intake of fruits and vegetables high in β-carotene and lung cancer, which stimulated subsequent human intervention trials in high-risk groups of asbestos workers and smokers. The unexpected negative results that emerged from these trials brought into question the mechanisms of action of β-carotene and other carotenoids and their role in health and disease prevention.

This disparity is not a total surprise as carotenoid-containing foods also possess numerous other potential bioreactive components. Carotenoids are a large group of compounds (Fig. 1) with various structural features and biological actions. Classes of carotenoids, as well as their structural and geometric isomers, are absorbed and metabolized differentially by the body and among species of animals. As a result, carotenoids may compete or act synergistically with each other, or with other protective components in foods. Such diversity among carotenoids makes it extremely difficult to uncover a mechanism of action for a single carotenoid in vivo and relate it to a potential role in disease.

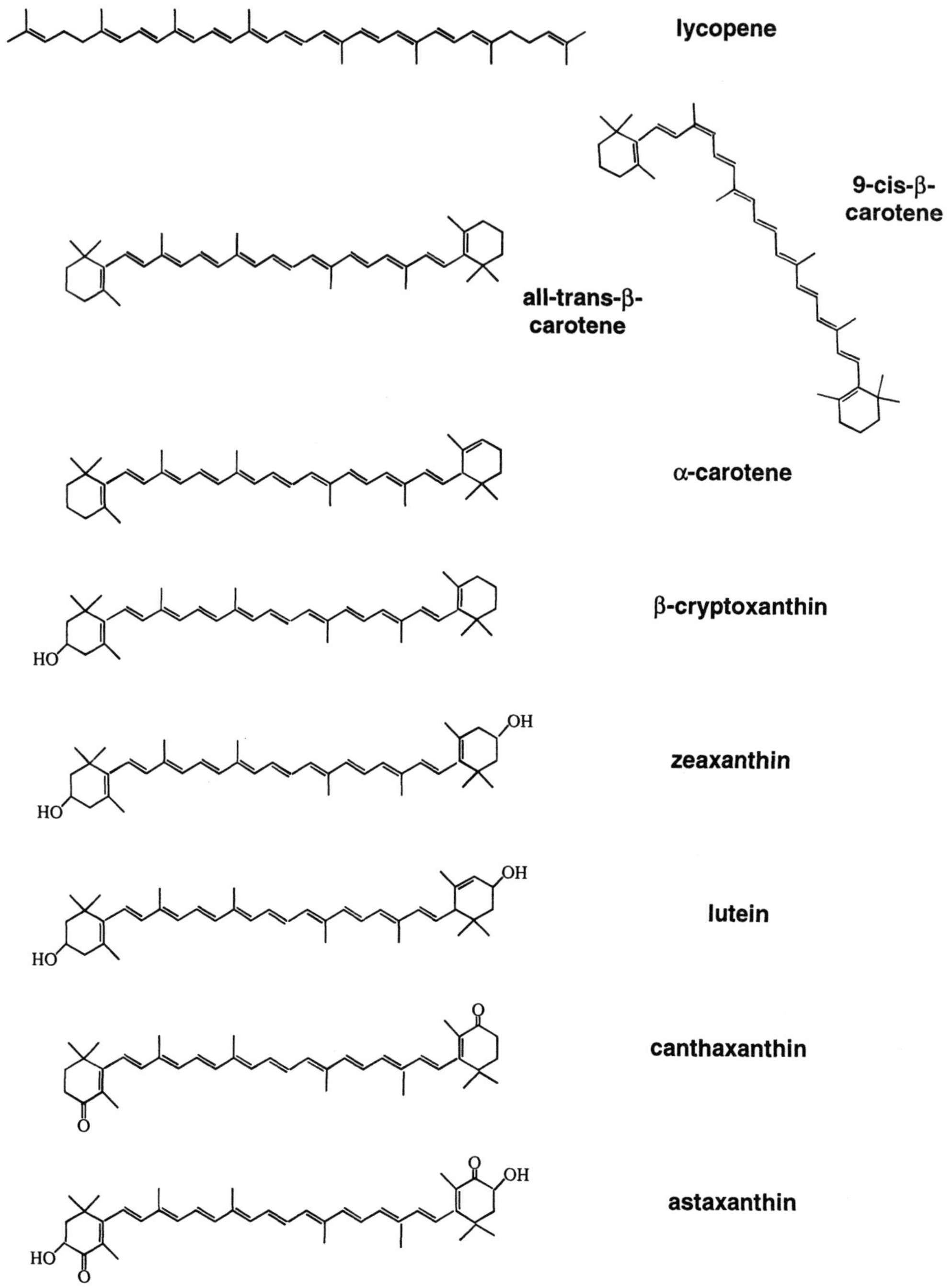

Figure 1 Structures of common carotenoids.

This chapter will examine and discuss the link between the chemistry, absorption, and metabolism of carotenoids as they relate to their potential role in human health and disease. First, the chemistry of carotenoids will be presented in relation to structure and observed biological actions. Carotenoid absorption, transport, and metabolism will then be described in relation to their structural features and properties. A final discussion will link associations of specific carotenoids with their potential roles in human health and disease.

II. CHEMISTRY OF CAROTENOIDS RELATED TO BIOLOGICAL EFFECTS

Olson (1) and Krinsky (2) have eloquently categorized and described the biological effects of carotenoids in terms of *functions, actions,* and *associations*. The only universally accepted biological function of carotenoids related to human health is the role of a select few carotenoids as precursors of vitamin A. An example of a biological action, which may or may not have physiological significance, is the ability of some carotenoids to enhance intercellular gap junction communication, in vitro. Finally, a biological association is exemplified by the strong inverse relation between consumption of fruits and vegetables rich in carotenoids and risk of several chronic diseases, such as cancer, heart disease, and age-related macular degeneration.

The purported biological functions, actions, and associations of carotenoids appear to be influenced by their chemical structure and physicochemical properties. An unsubstituted β-ionone ring, part of the chemical structure of β-carotene, α-carotene, and β-cryptoxanthin, provides these carotenoids with the capacity to be metabolized to vitamin A in mammals (3,4). A ring-structure in non-provitamin A carotenoids has also been linked to the induction of gap junction proteins. The distinctive, conjugated double-bond system of carotenoids is responsible for their antioxidant properties in vitro, which have been suggested to provide protection against oxidative stress associated with a variety of chronic diseases. However, the antioxidant activity of carotenoids is not clearly linked to disease mechanisms, in vivo.

There are obvious gaps in knowledge that separate the functions, actions, and associations of carotenoids. The chemistry and properties of carotenoids can provide a foundation for unraveling their potential biological actions. The following section will describe carotenoid structure and properties and relate them to these potential actions.

A. Chemical Structure of Carotenoids

1. Basic Molecular Features

More than 600 different carotenoids have been identified in nature, and remarkably, they all have common molecular features. The basic molecular structure of most carotenoids consists of a polyisoprenoid, C_{40} carbon chain with a series of conjugated, double bonds located in the central portion of the molecule (see Fig. 1). This distinctive feature permits effective delocalization of electrons along the entire length of the polyene chain, and provides carotenoids not only with their definitive molecular shape, but also their pigmentation, light-harvesting potential during photosynthesis, and chemical reactivity.

Another structural feature of most carotenoid molecules is the presence of cyclic end groups, discussed in greater detail elsewhere (5). Lycopene is an "open chain" or acyclic polyene, whereas β-carotene is dicyclic with β-ionone rings at both ends of the molecule. Lycopene and β-carotene are also examples of carotenoids exhibiting internal molecular symmetry in which one half of the molecule is identical with the other half. The significance of lycopene cleavage at this point of symmetry is unclear, but central cleavage of β-carotene has the potential of producing two molecules of retinol, resulting in the assignment of the highest vitamin A value to β-carotene compared with any other provitamin A carotenoids. Lycopene, β-carotene, and α-carotene belong to the class of carotenoids known as carotenes. Carotenoids such as β-cryptoxanthin, lutein, and zeaxanthin have oxygenated end groups and are classified as xanthophylls.

The parent carotenoid molecule can be further modified by alterations in the double-bond structure and by addition of oxygenated side groups. Apocarotenoids and norcarotenoids are examples of carotenoids that have lost carbon atoms from the ends or within the polyene chain, respectively, either by oxidative or biological cleavage. Hydroxylated carotenoids are often present in nature as glycosides or esterified to long-chain fatty acids, making them more hydrophobic (1).

2. Geometric Isomers and Structural Conformation

In principle, carotenoids can adopt a tremendous number of different configurations and conformations because of the possibility of isomerism and rotation around their carbon–carbon double and single bonds, respectively. Interconversion of geometric forms of carotenoids occurs when they are exposed to light and thermal energy, or when they undergo chemical reactions. However, carotenoids will stereochemically rearrange and ultimately exist in a form with the preferred, lowest state of energy. Carotenoids are most stable when their polyene chains are in a linear, all-*trans*-conformation because the double bonds are in a plane and steric hindrance is at a minimum (6). *cis*-Isomers of carotenoids are thermodynamically less stable than *trans*-isomers because of the closer proximity between hydrogen atoms or methyl groups resulting from the *cis* double bond. However, steric hindrance can also play a critical role in stabilizing ring-chain conformations associated with carotenoids having cyclic end groups (7).

Cyclic end groups have been associated with specific biological actions of carotenoids, such as stimulation of intercellular gap junctional communication. Stahl et al. (8) reported that β-carotene and canthaxanthin—carotenoids containing six-membered rings—are quite active in the induction of gap junction communication in murine fibroblasts. In addition to β-carotene and canthaxanthin, Zhang et al. (9) reported an up-regulation of connexin43 gene expression in C3H/10T1/2 cells by lutein and lycopene. Because lycopene is an acyclic carotenoid, it may be that cyclic end groups are not related to gap junction communication. However, Khachick and co-workers have proposed a possible alternative antioxidant mechanism of action for lycopene (10) that could result in the formation of an oxidative, five-membered cyclic, metabolite of lycopene, which has been identified in human serum (11). This compound, 2,6-cyclolycopene-1,5-diol (Fig. 2) may be the biologically active component that up-regulates connexin43 gene expression in C3H/10T1/2 cells. However, it is not clear whether lycopene, itself, or the oxidation products of lycopene are most active in up-regulation of gap junction cellular communication. Notably, Zhang and co-workers reported that the positive effects of carotenoids on up-regulating the gap junctional cellular communication appears to be unrelated to their antioxidant properties, because carotenoids increased levels of connexin43 mRNA and protein, whereas the antioxidants methyl-bixin and α-tocopherol were inactive (12).

Interest in the potential biological actions of *cis*-isomers of carotenoids has been further stimulated by the evidence that isomers of retinoids clearly have specific biological effects (13,14), which may also be true for isomers of carotenoids. Hanusch and co-workers (15) demonstrated that the all-*trans*- and 13-*cis*-isomers of 4-oxoretinoic acid—decomposition products of canthaxanthin (Fig. 3)—are efficient inducers of gap junctional communication in C3H/10T1/2 murine fibroblasts, specifically by enhanced expression of connexin43 mRNA. Interestingly, although Zhang et al. (9) demonstrated similar effects for the parent molecule,

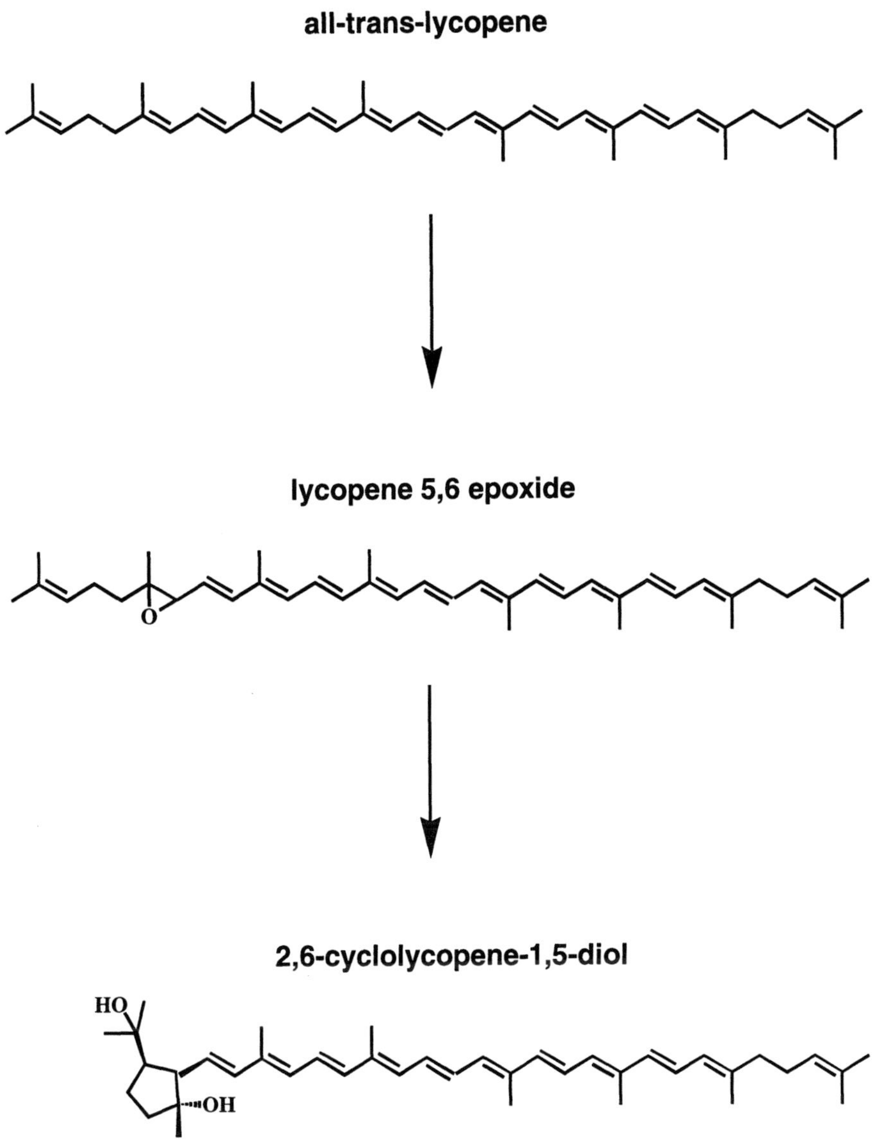

all-trans-lycopene

lycopene 5,6 epoxide

2,6-cyclolycopene-1,5-diol

Figure 2 Potential mechanism for formation of 2,6-cyclolycopene-1,5-diol, an oxidative metabolite of lycopene. (From Refs. 10, 11.)

canthaxanthin, they also reported that canthaxanthin did not induce the retinoic acid receptor β (RARβ). Further study is required to determine whether RARβ is induced by the all-*trans*- and 13-*cis*-isomers of 4-oxoretinoic acid. Stahl and Seis (16) have recently reviewed the effects of structurally different carotenoids and retinoids on the gap junctional communication pathway.

Retinoids play an essential role in vertebrate growth, embryonic development, vision, immune response, and reproduction. In particular, retinoids are well known for their ability to induce cellular differentiation, thereby reducing the ability of many cells to proliferate. Conversion of β-carotene to retinoic acid is one potential pathway (Fig. 4) by which carotenoids

all-trans canthaxanthin

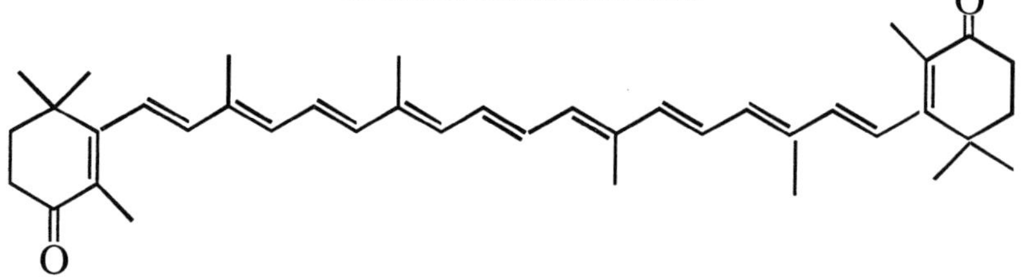

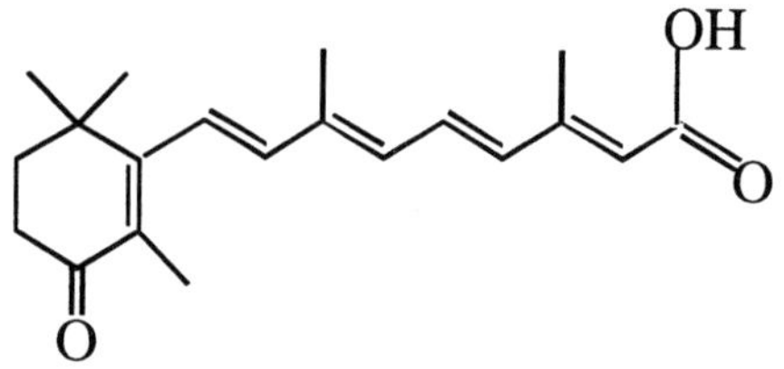

all-trans-4-oxo-retinoic acid

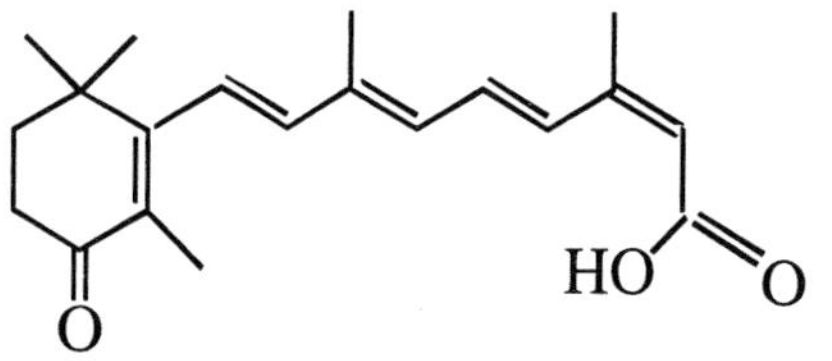

13-cis-oxo-retinoic acid

Figure 3 Structures of all-*trans*-canthaxanthin and all-*trans*- and 13-*cis*-isomers of 4-oxoretinoic acid, oxidation products of canthaxanthin. (From Ref. 15.)

may provide protection from carcinogenesis and other diseases. In addition, there is evidence to suggest that the effect may differ with different isomeric forms of β-carotene. All-*trans*- and 9-*cis*-retinoic acids are active retinoids in the regulation of expression of retinoid responsive genes. Both are physiological ligands for two classes of ligand-dependent transcription factors (i.e., all-*trans*-retinoic acid for retinoic acid receptors (RAR) and 9-*cis*-retinoic acid for retinoid X receptors (RXR). In fact, 9-*cis*-β-carotene has been demonstrated to be a precursor of 9-*cis*-retinoic acid in vitro (17,18) and in vivo (19). Moreover, 9-*cis*-retinoic acid is the only known retinoid ligand for RXR (20,21). Retinoic acid-mediated gene expression occurs following the formation of RAR–RXR heterodimers that interact with specific retinoic acid response elements (RARE) in the promoter region of different genes. Thus, the biological actions of β-carotene, such as canthaxanthin and lycopene, could be partly due to the formation of active metabolites and not the intact parent molecule.

B. Carotenoid Properties

1. Light Absorption

Carotenoids have relatively low excited energy states during light absorption because of the delocalization of electrons along the conjugated double-bond chain of the molecule. As a result the transition from the ground state to a higher excited state allows carotenoids to strongly absorb light in the visible region and, consequently, emit intensely colored yellow, orange, and red hues. Although the absorption maxima and the shapes of the absorption spectra are tools

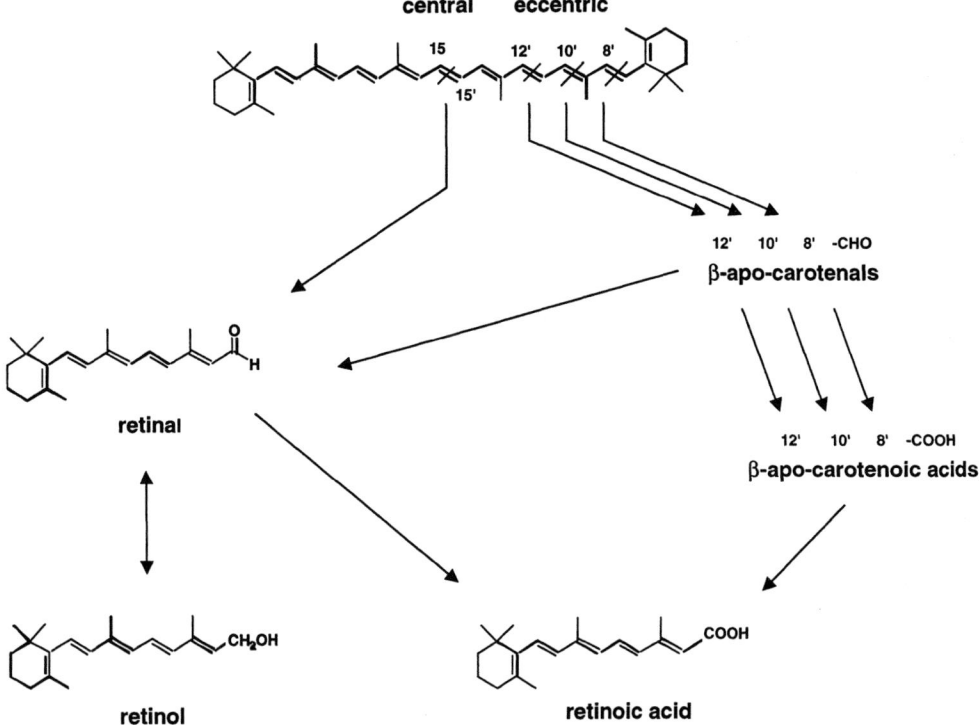

Figure 4 Possible central and eccentric cleavage pathways of all-*trans*-β-carotene.

used in the structural characterization of carotenoids, light absorption properties of a carotenoid are dependent on the medium. Notably, the absorption spectrum of a carotenoid in an organic solvent may differ significantly from that of a carotenoid in vivo, which may be affected by interactions of carotenoids with proteins and lipids (22). α-Crustacyanin, an astaxanthin–protein complex found in lobster, shifts the light absorption spectrum of astaxanthin toward the red, resulting in the natural blue pigment of this carotenoprotein (7). Interestingly, Rao et al. (4) have suggested that the formation of a stable, carotenoprotein complex may protect the carotenoid from degradation, thereby providing the system with enhanced antioxidant protection against oxidative damage.

2. Antioxidant Activity

The antioxidant activity of carotenoids is largely due to the extended system of conjugated double bonds, a structural feature that allows carotenoids to quench or inactivate some excited molecules. Thus, carotenoids can be efficient quenchers of singlet oxygen species and can directly scavenge free radicals (2,23), which has been one driving force for the interest in carotenoids as potential disease modulators. The system of conjugated double bonds, characteristic of carotenoids, can also be associated with pro-oxidant activity under certain conditions (24). β-Carotene exhibits free radical scavenging behavior at the low oxygen partial pressures found under physiological conditions, but at high oxygen pressures, β-carotene exhibits a pro-oxidant effect, particularly at relatively high concentrations. Palozza (25) has critically reviewed the evidence supporting the pro-oxidant activity of carotenoids and the possible biological consequences associated with human disease.

Free radical reactions in biological systems are not always harmful. In fact, many normal biological processes in vivo depend on free radicals (26). Oxidative stress associated with disease states results from an imbalance between pro-oxidants and antioxidants, in favor of the pro-oxidants (27). Thus, the antioxidant or pro-oxidant activity of carotenoids can create beneficial or harmful results in biological systems depending on the redox potential of the molecules and their environment.

The ability to easily transcend excited states of energy, to accept excitation energy from other moieties, such as chlorophyll or O_2, and to dissipate this energy harmlessly, allows some carotenoids to be efficient photosensitizers. In fact, the most characterized function of carotenoids in biological systems is their ability to harvest light during photosynthesis in plants and protect cells from photosensitization (28). In humans, β-carotene has also been reported to protect against photosensitivity in diseases such as erythropoietic protoporphyria, a condition in which free porphyrins accumulate, thereby sensitizing the skin to light and thus leading to the formation of singlet oxygen (29). Interestingly, photosensitization is effective only for carotenoids containing at least eight conjugated double bonds (5,30), and the molecules must be held in close proximity and in a specific orientation with other molecules, such as protein, for efficient energy transfer to occur (31).

The relation between the structure of carotenoids and their ability to act as chain-breaking, free radical scavengers has been demonstrated in vitro. Studies suggest that opening the β-ionone ring, adding chemical groups to the β-ionone ring, or replacing the β-ionone ring with other functional groups can modify the antioxidant capacity. Di Mascio and co-workers (32) compared the structures of carotenoids with their quenching ability using chemiluminescence intensity. They reported the following rank order of antioxidant activities: lycopene > β-carotene > lutein, suggesting that quenching properties of carotenoids are influenced not only by the length of the conjugated double-bond system, but also by the functional end groups. Similar conclusions were suggested by Miller and co-workers (33) after assessing the antioxidant activities of carotenes and xanthophylls by measuring the extent of their abilities to scavenge the ABTS radical cation. Overall, this group reported that the carotenes with 11 conjugated double bonds were more active ABTS radical quenchers than xanthophylls, with the exception of β-cryptoxanthin. Siems and co-workers (34) also reported a faster rate of breakdown for carotenes than for xanthophylls following exposure to various radical-initiated autooxidation conditions, suggesting that the slower degradation of the xanthophylls may be linked to tissue-specific accumulation in the human retina.

Woodall et al. (35) have suggested that different antioxidant reactivities of carotenoids cannot be attributed solely to differences in electron distribution along the polyene chain of the chromophore. The introduction of a *cis*-bond into the polyene chain of a carotenoid may also affect the antioxidant potency of carotenoids (36). Levin and Mokady (37) compared the in vitro peroxyl–radical-scavenging abilities of all-*trans*-β-carotene with that of 9-*cis*-β-carotene by measuring degradation of each in the presence of methyl linoleate. Their results showed higher degradation and thus greater antioxidant potency for 9-*cis*-β-carotene than all-*trans*-β-carotene. They explained the isomeric difference to be an effect of the steric hindrance and thus higher reactivity of the *cis*-bond compared with that of the *trans*-bond. Even though many carotenoids exert antioxidant activity under specific conditions in vitro, their in vivo relevance to disease is unknown and speculative (38). The presence of a conjugated keto group on the β-ionone ring also increases the efficiency of the peroxyl–radical-trapping ability of carotenoids. Terao (39) demonstrated that canthaxanthin and astaxanthin had superior ability to inhibit the formation of hydroperoxides in an in vitro radical-initiated system of methyl linoleate compared with β-carotene and zeaxanthin.

3. Biological Systems

Although the physical and chemical properties of free carotenoids are well-characterized in simple organic solvents and in vitro model systems, it is unclear how these properties are expressed in complex biological environments, in vivo. Selective orientation of carotenoids in biological systems, such as micelles, lipoproteins, and membranes, is most likely similar to other lipid molecules and is based on polarity, length, and structure of the carotenoid molecule (1,5,40,41). The use of in vitro, lipid emulsion models have supported the selective orientation of carotenoids into biological systems. Borel and co-workers (42) proposed that the polarity of specific carotenoids may directly affect their solubilization into triacylglycerol-phospholipid emulsion particles. β-Carotene, a nonpolar carotene, migrates to the triacylglycerol-rich core of the particle, whereas zeaxanthin, a more polar xanthophyll, orients at the surface monolayer along with phospholipids and fatty acids. Boileau and co-workers (43) also suggested that the geometry of the carotenoid molecule may influence orientation of carotenoids into bile acid micelles. This group reported greater incorporation of *cis*-lycopene than *trans*-lycopene into in vitro, bile acid micelles suggesting that the shorter length of the *cis*-isomer compared with that of the all-*trans*-isomer of a carotenoid may enhance solubilization into biological systems.

The tendency of carotenoids to aggregate or crystallize may or may not interfere with their ability to participate in biological actions. Hydrocarbon carotenoids, such as β-carotene and lycopene, may form small clathrate complexes with bile acids (44). However, *cis*-isomers of carotenoids are less likely to crystallize than their all-*trans*-counterpart (5).

4. Membranes

Carotenoids are one of many possible dietary components that can influence membrane characteristics such as fluidity, stability, and susceptibility to oxidative damage (45). Because carotenoids are essentially hydrophobic molecules, they are thought to orient in close proximity to lipids within membranes of living cells. The use of model systems, such as phospholipid liposome monolayers and bilayers, have shown that the properties of membranes are influenced by carotenoid localization which, in turn, may influence membrane integrity and biological functioning. Hydrophobic carotenes, such as lycopene and β-carotene, tend to be solubilized in the core parallel to the membrane surface. Solubilization of β-carotene and lycopene in the core of membranes could be related to their proposed ability to act as photosensitizers in the skin, or to maintenance of membrane fluidity, which may enhance the ability of lymphocytes to respond to challenges on the immune system (46).

The presence of polar functional groups on carotenoid molecules dramatically influences their orientation within membranes (47). Xanthophylls most likely orient toward the surface of membranes where they can expose their polar moieties to the aqueous environment, and where associations with proteins may be enhanced. Consequently, dioxycarotenoids—xanthophylls with two polar end groups—can orient themselves in a position perpendicular to the membrane surface. Indeed, this membrane orientation has been demonstrated for lutein and zeaxanthin. Woodall and co-workers (35) suggested that strong interactions between the polar end groups on zeaxanthin with the polar head groups on membrane phospholipids hold the carotenoid molecule in a fixed position spanning the membrane. Moreover, Gruszecki and co-workers (48) recently reported that the orientation of lutein in lipid membranes formed with egg yolk lecithin was different from that of zeaxanthin, in spite of their similar molecular structure. Using specific pigment antisera, spectrophotometry, and monomolecular layering techniques, they demonstrated that zeaxanthin adopted an orientation perpendicular to the membrane, whereas lutein was distributed within the hydrophobic phase of the membrane in two different pools, one oriented parallel and the other perpendicular to the membrane (48). This same group later demonstrated that lutein and zeaxanthin were equally protective against initial UV-induced oxidative damage to lipid membranes, but zeaxanthin appeared to be a better photoprotector than lutein during prolonged UV exposure (49). The differential organization of lutein and zeaxanthin in membranes and their protective efficacy against oxidative damage may be related to their proposed role in reducing photooxidative stress in the human macula.

Stability and properties of membranes may be affected by positioning of carotenoid molecules. In general, studies using model systems suggest that carotenoids will affect the thickness, fluidity, strength, and ultimately the permeability of the membrane (47,50,51). For example, membrane fluidity is enhanced by solubilization of carotenes within the membrane core parallel to the surface. In contrast, the rigidity and mechanical strength of a membrane may increase when dioxycarotenoids are anchored perpendicular to the membrane (52), suggesting that polar carotenoids increase the stability of lipid bilayers. The orientation of carotenoid–glucoside esters, similar to that of dihydroxylated carotenoids, may also enhance membrane stability (53). Interestingly, Wisniewska and Subczynski (50) reported that incorporation of polar carotenoids into phospholipid bilayers significantly increases the hydrophobicity of the membrane interior, while increasing membrane permeability in the polar headgroup region.

In vitro studies using liposomes have provided some insight into the relation between carotenoid orientation and reactivity in lipid bilayers. Kennedy and Liebler (54,55) have demonstrated that β-carotene prevented peroxidation of soybean phosphatidylcholine (PC) liposomes, resulting in the formation of β-carotene epoxides. β-Carotene regenerates α-tocopherol from the α-tocopheroxy radical in liver microsomes, suggesting a synergistic effect of β-carotene with other antioxidants (25). Although xanthophylls (i.e., canthaxanthin, zeaxanthin, and astaxanthin) also have the ability to act as antioxidants during the peroxidation of PC liposomes, their chain-breaking activity was much less than that of α-tocopherol (56). Moreover, Stahl and co-workers (8) have reported that mixtures of carotenoids were more effective than single compounds in protecting multilamellar liposomes against oxidative damage, and that the superior protection of mixtures, especially the synergistic effect of lycopene and lutein, may be related to different physicochemical properties or the specific positioning of carotenoids in membranes.

III. CAROTENOID ABSORPTION AND METABOLISM

The absorption and metabolism of carotenoids is an ambiguous process and many questions about the mechanisms of carotenoid passage through the body remain unanswered. Nonetheless, studies conducted over the last 10–15 years have greatly improved the understanding of the pathway of absorption and metabolism of carotenoids and are summarized in numerous reviews (3,40,41,57–62). The following discussion will specifically highlight the provocative research that links structural features and properties of carotenoids with their absorption and metabolism.

A. Release from the Food Matrix

The release of carotenoids from the food matrix is the first step in the absorptive process (Fig. 5), and is considered to be an important determinant of the bioavailability of carotenoids (63). It is widely accepted that (1) carotenoids from commercial preparations, such as water-miscible beadlets, or from oil preparations or emulsions are more bioavailable than carotenoids from fruits and vegetables (64,65); and (2) carotenoids are less available from raw than from

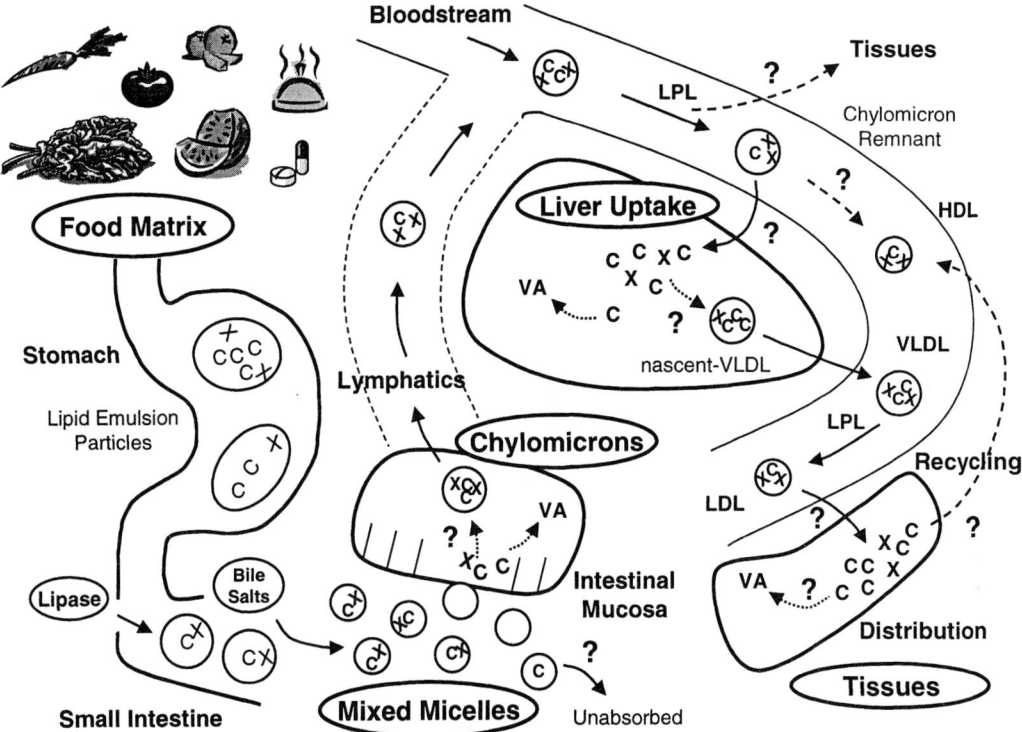

Figure 5 Pathway of absorption and metabolism of carotenoids: C, carotenes; X, xanthophylls; VA, vitamin A; LPL, lipoprotein lipase; VLDL, very low-density lipoproteins; LDL, low-density lipoproteins; HDL, high-density lipoproteins. (From Ref. 41.)

processed fruits and vegetables (66). In addition, studies using β-carotene support a hypothesis that carotenoids are about three times more available from fruits than from vegetables (67). The differences in the intact cell matrix (68) and intracellular localization of carotenoid molecules in fruits and vegetables may partially account for differences in their release from the matrix of these foods and thus their bioavailability (62). Two recent studies appear to suggest that because of its polar properties, the hydroxycarotenoid lutein may be less affected by disruption of the cell wall matrix of spinach than the more hydrophobic carotene, β-carotene, and thus may be more bioavailable (63,69).

Various food-processing techniques have the potential to further enhance carotenoid bioavailability (70). Mechanical homogenization and controlled-heat treatment are particularly effective in enhancing bioavailability of β-carotene from carrots and spinach (66) and lycopene from tomatoes (71), especially with the addition of fat during processing (72). Fat provides a lipophilic environment in which hydrophobic carotenoids will migrate and subsequently deliver a more bioavailable form of carotenoid from the food product. Because the linear, all-*trans*-configuration of carotenoids is particularly stable, it is not surprising that most carotenoids occur in nature in this form, which incidentally is the predominant form found in foods (73).

Although heat treatment may improve bioavailability of carotenoids from fruits and vegetables by rupturing cell wall matrices, it also promotes formation of *cis*-isomers of carotenoids. β-Carotene *cis*-isomers are found in significant quantities in processed foods (74–77). Canning of fresh sweet potatoes, carrots, and tomatoes, vegetables with negligible amounts of *cis*-β-carotene isomers, increased total levels of *cis*-isomers of β-carotene, in particular the 9-*cis* and 13-*cis*, to approximately 25, 27, and 48%, respectively (78). Interestingly, heat treatment of tomato paste in the presence of oil results in higher *cis*-isomerization of lycopene than in the absence of oil (79), and *cis*–*trans*-isomers of lycopene were found only in the oil phase, suggesting that the extent of isomerization of lycopene may be dependent on the extent of transfer of lycopene from matrix of the tomato paste into the oil phase (70). Enhancement of transfer of carotenes into oil droplets has also been reported by conditions of low pH, suggesting an explanation for why carotene absorption in vivo is depressed by conditions of low gastric acidity (80).

Overall, the extent of *cis*-isomerization depends on the duration and temperature of heat treatment used in specific processing techniques (81–83). Exposure to excessive heat treatment causes extensive *cis*-isomerization and oxidation of carotenoids, resulting in structural changes that may decrease the vitamin A activity of the food (84,85) and perhaps alter other biological properties of carotenoids. There is evidence that *cis*-isomers of carotenoids from processed foods and supplements are indeed absorbed or metabolized differently by the body (43,66,86–89), details of which will be discussed in the next two sections.

B. Absorption and Transport

The uptake of carotenoids into intestinal mucosal cells is aided by the formation of bile acid micelles in the lumen of the small intestine (see Fig. 5), and it is thought to occur by passive diffusion (44,90). The extent of carotenoid solubilization into micelles may be affected by polarity (42), geometry (43), or both, of the carotenoid molecule, as well as micellar fatty acid composition and saturation (90).

The intramucosal processing of carotenoids is one of the least understood areas of carotenoid absorption. Once uptake is complete, some of the absorbed β-carotene and other provitamin A carotenoids, such as α-carotene and β-cryptoxanthin, can be oxidatively cleaved to retinol (i.e., vitamin A) by a specific enzyme, β-carotene 15,15′-dioxygenase (91,92). An in vitro assay has been developed (17,93,94) to assess the influence of various treatments on the cleavage activity of this enzyme (95–99). Both central and eccentric cleavage pathways of all-*trans*-β-carotene (see Fig. 4) can produce retinol and retinoic acid. Notably, central cleavage produces retinal, whereas eccentric cleavage predominantly produces β-apocarotenals and retinoic acid (100,101). Products from both cleavage mechanisms have been identified in homogenates of small-intestinal mucosa of animals and humans using the in vitro assay (93,100–103). The existence of two cleavage pathways may be due to the presence of two different enzymes in the intestinal mucosa that convert β-carotene to retinal and retinol or to retinal and retinoic acid (104). In addition, it has also been proposed that central cleavage may take place when retinol is needed, and when retinoic acid is needed, eccentric cleavage occurs (104). The inability to purify β-carotene 15,15′-dioxygenase remains an obstacle and the mechanisms of β-carotene oxidative cleavage are a subject of ongoing research.

Although most of the absorbed β-carotene is thought to be converted to vitamin A, a small portion is transported as the intact molecule. Whether carotenoids are transported intracellularly by specific proteins, or whether they migrate in lipid droplets, remains to be elucidated (105). Carotenoids are esterified with palmitic acid and packaged in chylomicrons before export from the mucosal cell by the mesenteric lymph system into the blood. As with micelle formation, it appears that polarity of a carotenoid may be an important determinant of the efficiency of carotenoid incorporation into chylomicrons and subsequent transport in the lymph and blood. If during the digestive process, a less lipophilic xanthophyll, such as lutein, resides closer to the surface of lipid micelles, the likelihood of intestinal uptake might be greatly enhanced compared with that of a more lipophilic carotene, such as β-carotene, that resides in the triacylglycerol core of the micelle. Studies in animals and humans support this hypothesis. Gartner and coworkers (106) reported preferential increase in lutein and zeaxanthin compared with β-carotene in human chylomicrons, suggesting that the presence of hydroxyl moieties may indeed enhance uptake and transport within the enterocyte and packaging into chylomicrons. In agreement with Gartner et al., O'Neill and Thurnham (107) reported the appearance of the xanthophyll, lutein, in human chylomicrons before the carotenes, β-carotene and lycopene, following a dose of all three carotenoids. Similar preferential uptake has also been demonstrated in the preruminant calf (108). In addition, competition between xanthophylls and carotenes for uptake and transport may also be reflected by their appearance in chylomicrons or serum (109–111).

Geometry of the carotenoid may be another important factor influencing uptake and transport of carotenoids in the lymph and blood. Boileau and co-workers (43) reported a study using the lymph-cannulated ferret to support their hypothesis, discussed earlier, which stated that the shorter length of a *cis*-isomer of a carotenoid compared with that of the *trans*-isomer may enhance its solubility in biological systems. In this study, ferrets were fed an oral dose of lycopene and *cis–trans*-lycopene isomers in stomach contents, small intestinal contents, mucosal cells, lymph, and several tissues were quantified by high-performance liquid chromatography (HPLC). *cis*-Lycopene isomers were no different among the dose, stomach contents, and small intestinal contents (9–17%). However, *cis*-lycopene isomers increased to 59% in intestinal mucosal cells and to 72% in lymph collections, suggesting than *cis*-lycopene isomers are preferentially absorbed over all-*trans*-lycopene. These results are consistent with results demonstrating greater incorporation of *cis*-lycopene than *trans*-lycopene into in vitro, bile acid micelles reported by the same group.

Intestinal absorption and transport of β-carotene isomers is less clear than that of lycopene isomers. The ingestion of *cis*-isomers of β-carotene from foods and supplements is significant; however, their metabolic fate is poorly understood. Several human studies suggest that there may be a discrimination in absorption and transport among β-carotene isomers, in particular the 9-*cis* (88,112). Elevated concentrations of all-*trans*-β-carotene in human plasma or serum have been reported in response to dietary or supplemental intake, but initial low blood concentrations of 9-*cis*-β-carotene were not increased even following high dose of this isomer (89,113,114). Interestingly, increased proportions of *cis*-isomers of β-carotene in thermally processed vegetables did not negate the enhancement of total and all-*trans*-β-carotene in plasma of humans compared with that of the raw counterparts (66). A similar preferential accumulation of all-*trans*-β-carotene compared with 9-*cis*-β-carotene has also been reported in human chylomicrons (115).

Despite the low serum and chylomicron concentrations in human and animals following a dose of 9-*cis*-β-carotene, relatively high levels of this isomer are present in tissues. In fact, it has been estimated that 9-*cis*-β-carotene may account for up to 25% of the total β-carotene in human liver (87,89). A substantial accumulation of 9-*cis*-β-carotene has also been reported in the livers of chicks (116), rats (117), and ferrets (118) after supplementation with 9-*cis*-β-carotene. However, 9-*cis*-β-carotene appears to be less efficient compared with all-*trans*-β-carotene as a precursor of retinol. The vitamin A activity of 9-*cis*-β-carotene in rats has been estimated to be only 57% that of all-*trans*-β-carotene using a storage bioassay of liver retinyl ester (85). Overall, these studies suggest that 9-*cis*-β-carotene could (1) be inefficiently absorbed or rapidly converted to vitamin A in the intestinal mucosa; (2) be absorbed and more rapidly taken up into tissues than other β-carotene isomers; or (3) undergo isomerization in tissues.

Isomerization of 9-*cis*-β-carotene to the all-*trans*-isomer in the intestinal mucosa has been postulated to partially explain the negligible amounts of 9-*cis*-β-carotene in the blood and could regulate the supply of the 9-*cis*-retinoid precursor to tissues. In one study using isotopically labeled β-carotene, You et al. (86) reported an estimated isomerization of 9-*cis*-β-carotene to all-*trans*-β-carotene of 54% in human small intestinal mucosa at physiological doses. Because the isomerization of 9-*cis*- to all-*trans* β-carotene is not a thermodynamically favorable reaction (119), it has been suggested that a tissue isomerase that converts 9-*cis*-β-carotene to the all-*trans*-isomer must be present (86,120). In contrast with You et al., Hebuterne et al. (19) reported similar absorption of 9-*cis*- and all-*trans*-β-carotene in ferrets following intestinal perfusion with either isomer. Although total retinoic acid levels in portal blood, liver, and intestine were similar for both β-carotene isomers, 9-*cis*-retinoic acid represented only half the total retinoic acid formed when 9-*cis*-β-carotene was perfused (19). If extensive *cis–trans*-isomerization of 9-*cis*-β-carotene in intestinal mucosa is indeed a regulatory mechanism to control levels of retinoic acid in vivo, other factors may be more important than the proportions of β-carotene isomers in the diet in determining the distribution of β-carotene isomers or their retinoid conversion metabolites in body pools (66).

Carotenoids are transported in the serum by lipoproteins, and distribution in individual classes of lipoproteins is not homogeneous. Low-density lipoproteins (LDL) are the main carriers of hydrophobic carotenes, such as β-carotene and lycopene in human blood (121–124), whereas high-density lipoproteins (HDL) are carriers of the more polar xanthophylls (125,126). This distribution appears to suggest greater exchange of xanthophylls, which may localize on the surface among lipoproteins, than carotenes, which probably migrate to the core (127,128). Until recently, it was thought that xanthophyll esters, such as from β-cryptoxanthin, were cleaved before absorption and uptake (129). However, lutein esters were recently identified in human serum following supplementation of a mixture of lutein esters (i.e., lutein monopalmitate and lutein diesters) (130). Because lutein esters are more hydrophobic than free lutein, their distribution in lipoproteins and, thus, their transfer among lipoproteins and tissue uptake may be affected.

Patterns of serum carotenoids reflect absorption of a wide variety of carotenoids in the diet. The most prevalent serum carotenoids include β-carotene, lycopene, lutein, and in lower levels, α-carotene, zeaxanthin, and cryptoxanthin (11). Structural and geometric isomers of carotenes and xanthophylls have been identified in human blood (87,131–133). *cis*-Isomers of lycopene are more commonly found in serum than are β-carotene isomers. Stahl and co-workers (87) reported that *cis*-isomers of lycopene were at least 50% of total serum lycopene, whereas *cis*-isomers of β-carotene, primarily 13-*cis*- and 15-*cis*-, were present at only 5% of the all-*trans*-isomer. As mentioned previously, 9-*cis*-β-carotene is present in tissues, but in insignificant amounts in serum.

Other less-studied dietary carotenoids have recently been identified in human blood. The absorption of *cis*-isomers of astaxanthin, xanthophylls present in marine seafood, was recently reported in humans for the first time (134). Maximum plasma concentrations of astaxanthin isomers were observed 6 h following a meal containing a defined mixture (Carophyll Pink, Hoffmann LaRoche) of all-*trans*-, 9-*cis*-, and 13-*cis*-isomers of astaxanthin (1:2:1 ratio, respectively) (134). Similar to lycopene *cis*-isomers, the presence of *cis*-isomers of astaxanthin in human plasma may suggest preferential tissue uptake and biological activity. However, further study is required to determine tissue distribution of these carotenoids and potential mechanisms of action in humans.

Even though epoxy-carotenoids are abundant in fruits and vegetables (73), little is known about their absorption and metabolism. Barua (135) identified epoxy-β-carotenes in human plasma following orally administered dietary or synthetic epoxy-β-carotenes. In light of the demonstration of the high activity of 5,6-epoxy-β-carotene in induction of human leukemic NB4 cell differentiation (136), it was hypothesized that epoxy-β-carotenes or their potential conversion metabolites, epoxyretinoids, may have biological actions that affect physiological and disease states in vivo (135). The knowledge that epoxy-β-carotenes are indeed absorbed is significant. Tomato-based food products are major sources of lycopene 5,6-epoxides (73) and are proposed intermediates in the formation of oxidative metabolites of lycopene, one of which is biologically active in up-regulating gap junction proteins in vitro (12). However, lycopene epoxides have not yet been identified in human plasma.

Oxidative metabolites of carotenoids have been identified in human serum, suggesting an antioxidant role of carotenoids in vivo. Khachik and co-workers (11) have recently identified 34 carotenoids, including 13 geometric isomers and 8 metabolites in serum and breast milk of lactating women. Among the metabolites were oxidative products of lycopene and lutein–zeaxanthin and additional dehydration products of lutein, presumably formed under acidic conditions similar to those found in the stomach (11). This same group further proposed that the oxidative metabolites of lutein and zeaxanthin can occur from four types of reactions involving the end groups of these carotenoids (10). It has been suggested that presence of these oxidative metabolites in serum may be an indication that carotenoids are quenching peroxides and other free radical species, thereby protecting cells from oxidative damage (10). However, little is known about the sites and mechanisms of formation of these metabolites.

C. Tissue Accumulation and Metabolism

Once in the blood, carotenoids are passively taken up into various tissues following degradation of lipoproteins by lipoprotein lipase (LPL; see Fig. 5). Chylomicron remnants are cleared from the blood in the liver by the chylomicron receptor. Carotenoids accumulate in the liver, but regulation of their storage is poorly understood. Recently, Rao and co-workers (4) purified a cellular carotenoid-binding protein (CCBP) from ferret liver, which had a high degree of specificity toward carotenoids with at least one β-ionone ring, but not toward other carotenoids. This group proposed that CCBP may play a role in storage, transport, and metabolism of provitamin A carotenoids, as well as act as a natural substrate for metabolic reactions involving these carotenoids (4). Carotenoids may exit the liver into the blood following incorporation into very low-density lipoproteins (VLDL). Subsequent uptake of carotenoids into tissues from VLDL, and especially LDL, is thought to occur through the LDL receptor because the tissues with the highest levels of carotenoids (e.g., liver, adrenal glands, testes) tend to have high LDL receptor activity (128,137,138).

Carotenoids are present in many tissues in humans, including liver, adipose, pancreas, kidney, lung, adrenal, spleen, heart, thyroid, testes, ovary (87,139), and eye (140–142). Total quantitative levels of carotenoids are highest in liver and adipose tissue, the main storage sites for carotenoids (128). Concentrations of carotenoids (i.e., per gram of tissue basis) are highest in the liver, adrenal, and reproductive tissues. As is true for serum, β-carotene, lycopene, lutein, α-carotene, zeaxanthin, and cryptoxanthin are the main tissue carotenoids (137,139). In addition, the geometrical isomers of lycopene and β-carotene found in serum are also found in tissues (87). Some tissues exhibit specific patterns of carotenoid accumulation, suggesting that certain carotenoids may exert a biological effect in one tissue over another. For example, whereas lycopene is predominantly found in the all-*trans*-form in foods, at least 13 isomeric forms of lycopene have been found in the prostate (143), the biological significance of which will be discussed in greater detail in the last section of this chapter.

The extent to which plasma and serum concentrations of carotenoids reflect those of organs may or may not be important to biological actions of carotenoids. The differences in quantities and ratios of carotenoids in human blood could be attributed to dietary intake or to specific mechanisms of absorption and utilization of these compounds (131). It has been proposed that the uneven but wide distribution of most dietary carotenoids in tissues may indicate an active biological role of these compounds (137). A new hypothesis suggests that reduced tissues levels of β-carotene, in particular, may actually reflect the effect of disease, rather than the cause (144). Because of its high susceptibility to oxidation and other chemical transformation, β-carotene may simply be an indicator of cellular insult (144). This thinking is supported by some studies associating low tissue levels of β-carotene with disease (145,146) or compromised health (147,148), and further studies demonstrating the same relation even when β-carotene intake was no different between case and control groups (149). However, it is possible that some potential biological actions of β-carotenes may be exerted through their conversion to retinoids and subsequent gene regulation, which may differ with isomeric form of β-carotene.

IV. POTENTIAL ROLE IN HUMAN HEALTH AND DISEASE PREVENTION

This section outlines specific health- and disease-related areas of carotenoid research that have been the subject of recent interest and debate. Each subject area is supported by varying degrees of evidence associating dietary or supplemental carotenoid intake with tissue-specific carotenoid accumulation or biological effects in humans, animal models, or cell culture. The focus of this section will be to link the structural features, physical and chemical properties, biological actions, and epidemiological associations of carotenoids with their potential role in human health and disease.

A. β-Carotene and Lung Cancer

Almost 20 years ago Peto et al. (150) proposed that β-carotene may reduce the risk of certain types of cancer. Since then, a compelling amount of epidemiological evidence has suggested a role for fruits and vegetables, rich in β-carotene, in the prevention of lung carcinogenesis (151). Smoking, a strong risk factor for lung cancer, increases oxidative damage in lung tissue, which theoretically, could at least partially be reversed by dietary antioxidants. β-Carotene is both a chain-breaking antioxidant (24) and a quencher of singlet oxygen (32). Because it accumulates in human lung tissue (139), investigators speculated that β-carotene, the most widely distributed carotenoid in fruits and vegetables, may be the protective factor. These observations formed the basis for two large-scale intervention trials in smokers, the Alpha Tocopherol, β-Carotene Cancer Prevention Study (ATBC) (145) and the Carotenoid and Retinol Efficacy Trial (CARET) (152), designed to test the efficacy of β-carotene (and vitamin A in CARET) supplements in preventing lung cancer in smokers. Surprisingly, both studies resulted in an increase in lung cancer incidence in the β-carotene-supplemented group.

In the years since these two trials, investigators have considered several hypotheses explaining the results of these trials. One possible mechanism, as mentioned previously, may be attributed to the chain-breaking antioxidant properties of β-carotene, which occur only at low oxygen pressures. At high oxygen pressures, as would be encountered in the lung, β-carotene may act as a pro-oxidant. In a recent study using smoke-exposed ferrets, Wang and co-workers (153) demonstrated that incubating β-carotene with lung postnuclear fractions from smoke-exposed ferrets resulted in a three-fold greater increase in apocarotenal formation (i.e., oxidative metabolites of β-carotene) than equivalent fractions from unexposed ferrets. Additionally, lung tissue from the β-carotene-fed ferrets exposed to smoke had reduced concentrations of retinoic acid and a downregulation of the retinoic acid receptor β (RARβ). The authors suggest that the higher apocarotenal formation, decreased lung retinoic acid, and a down-regulation of RARβ in smoke-exposed ferrets may interfere with normal retinoid signaling in the lung of smokers that might enhance the lung cancer process. They proposed that apocarotenoids induce cytochrome P450 enzymes that destroy retinoic acid and also up-regulate activator protein-1.

Others have suggested that the results of the human intervention trial may have been skewed by intake of ethanol (154), which may have affected the metabolism of retinoic acid, a metabolite of β-carotene. Ethanol increases oxidative stress (155). Retinoids have the ability to induce cell differentiation in vitro (156) and thus may reduce the ability of many cell types to proliferate. Alcohol intake increases lung retinol concentration in lung tissues of rats fed β-carotene (157). It is postulated that increased lung retinol may also lead to increased lung retinoids and interfere with normal retinoid signaling, a mechanism similar to that postulated for tobacco smoke. Upon further assessment, the investigators from both the ATBC and CARET trials have shown that alcohol may indeed exacerbate the negative effects of β-carotene on lung cancer in smokers. In the ATBC trial, participants with an alcohol intake of greater than 11 g of alcohol per day was associated with higher lung cancer incidence than in participants with lower alcohol intakes (158). Similarly, in the CARET trial, participants in the highest quartile of alcohol intake (i.e., > 30 g alcohol per day) had increased risk for lung cancer (152). Overall it appears that β-carotene metabolism and its antioxidant–pro-oxidant equilibrium may be altered in smokers and be further exacerbated in smokers who also consume alcohol.

B. Lycopene, β-Carotene, and Prostate Cancer

Epidemiological studies have shown that high intakes of tomatoes and tomato products (159,160) as well as high blood levels of lycopene (161) are associated with a decreased risk for prostate cancer. Lycopene is the predominant carotenoid in tomatoes and tomato products and is also a potent scavenger of singlet oxygen in vitro (32). Additionally, lycopene is found in the human prostate as all-*trans*-lycopene and a variety of *cis*-isomers (143). Approximately 79–88% of the lycopene in the human prostate is in the *cis*-form although only 9–21% of lycopene in tomatoes and tomato-based foods is present as *cis*-isomers, suggesting preferential absorption or selective tissue uptake of *cis*-lycopene over all-*trans*-lycopene. The biological significance of *cis*-lycopene isomers remains to be elucidated. However, studies comparing the antioxidant capabilities of *cis*- and *trans*-β-carotene have suggested that *cis*-carotenoid isomers may be more efficient antioxidants (36,37). This suggestion may be significant, in light of the presence of oxidation products of lycopene in human serum (11) that up-regulate gap junction proteins in vitro (12), but the potential enzymes and pathways of formation of these products require further study. The role of lycopene in prostate carcinogenesis has been limited by both gaps in the understanding of lycopene uptake, absorption, and metabolism in humans and animal models as well a lack of relevant models of prostate carcinogenesis. McCormick and co-workers (162) have recently used a model of chemically induced prostate carcinogenesis to study the effects of retinoids on tumor incidence in rats (162–164). This model may prove useful for studying the effects of lycopene and other dietary components on earlier stages of prostate carcinogenesis.

Lycopene-feeding studies in rodents commonly used in cancer trials have shown that tissue lycopene concentrations, similar to those of humans, are achievable. Williams et al. (165) reported tumor lycopene levels and *cis–trans*-lycopene profiles similar to humans in nude mice implanted with androgen-responsive LNCap human prostate cells that were fed diets containing 6.0 g/kg lycopene as tomato oleoresin. Boileau and co-workers (166) have recently found, that in rats, serum, liver, and prostate lycopene plateaus between 0.05 and 0.5 g/kg dietary lycopene incorporated into diets as commercially available lycopene beadlets. Interestingly, as dietary lycopene levels increased, so did the percentage of lycopene as *cis*-isomers in tissues and serums. Furthermore, castrated rats accumulated 2.5-fold more liver lycopene than intact controls or castrated rats implanted with testosterone suggesting that androgens may influence liver lycopene metabolism. Addition of testosterone back to the castrated rats decreased liver lycopene to concentrations that were no different from those of intact control rats. This effect was independent of serum insulin-like growth factor-I (IGF-I). The finding that lycopene metabolism and tissue distribution may be affected by testosterone indicates that androgens and lycopene should be evaluated together in both animal and human studies designed to evaluate the chemopreventive efficacy of carotenoids. In addition, some investigators have hypothesized that androgens increase oxidation in the prostate (167). If this is true, an equilibrium may exist between the protective effects of prostate antioxidants, such as lycopene, other carotenoids, vitamin E, and selenium, and promoting effects of androgens and other hormones on antioxidant turnover and development of prostate cancer.

No clear associations between supplemental β-carotene and prostate cancer incidence have been made in the ATBC, CARET trials, or Physicians' Health Study (PHS). However, a recent reexamination of the PHS data has shown that men with the lowest baseline levels of β-carotene had decreased risk for prostate cancer with β-carotene supplementation. In that study, Cook and co-workers (168) reported that prostate cancer risk was decreased by 32% in men who initially had the lowest serum β-carotene and were subsequently given β-carotene supplements.

In vitro findings do support a role for β-carotene in prostate carcinogenesis. Williams and co-workers (169) have recently shown that β-carotene inhibits growth of three human prostate cancer cell lines in vitro. Additionally, this group has shown that β-carotene undergoes intracellular conversion to retinol by prostate cancer cells, suggesting the ability of cancer cells to locally convert β-carotene to retinol, bypassing normal regulation of tissue retinol uptake.

C. Lutein and Zeaxanthin and the Eye

By 2050, the U. S. Census Bureau estimates that more than 80 million Americans will be over the age of 65 (170), and as the population ages, a sharp increase in the incidence of diseases of the eye is expected. Age-related macular degeneration (AMD) is currently the leading cause of blindness in persons older than age 65 in the United States. Age-related cataractogenesis (ARC) is also common in older adults, affecting 55–85% of people older than 75 years of age (171,172). Although both AMD and ARC are multifactorial diseases, a strong body of scientific evidence supports a protective role for lutein and zeaxanthin in the prevention of age-related diseases of the eye (173,174). High intakes of leafy green vegetables—rich sources of lutein and zeaxanthin—have been associated with reduced risk of cataracts (175) and macular degeneration (176). Furthermore, lutein and zeaxanthin are the main carotenoids present in the human macula (140,177) and the only carotenoids present in the human lens (142,178,179). Two hypotheses have emerged to explain the protective action of these xanthophylls (180). Over the course of a lifetime, the eye is exposed to the damaging effects of light and oxygen. Lutein and zeaxanthin absorb blue light and may act as filters to protect photoreceptors of the eye and retinal pigment epithelium from damage. In addition, their antioxidant activity may limit the creation of reactive species that may attack lipids, carbohydrates, and DNA.

AMD is characterized by atrophy of photoreceptors and the retinal pigment epithelium in the macular region of the retina (181). An ongoing subject of debate over the last few years has revolved around the role of the macular carotenoids in the etiology of AMD. Dietary supplementation with lutein can increase macular pigment density (182). However, to date, no intervention trials have been carried out to test for a direct relation between increased lutein and zeaxanthin intake and decreased incidence of ADM. The macula lutea is so named because of its yellow color caused by the presence of lutein and zeaxanthin, and several of their stereo- and geometric isomers that selectively accumulate in this tissue of the eye (141). The ratio of zeaxanthin to lutein in the macular region of the retina varies with the distance from the center of the fovea, the central part of the macula that is thought to be rich in photoreceptors and be responsible for visual acuity (141,183). Khachik and co-workers (184) have identified oxidation products of lutein and zeaxanthin in human and monkey retinas, suggesting that these carotenoids may be acting as antioxidants to protect the macula from short-wavelength light. Lutein and zeaxanthin have recently been associated with the rods and cones, respectively (i.e., photoreceptors) in the human eye (185), and potential xanthophyll-binding proteins in the human macula have tentatively been identified (186). The perpendicular orientation of lutein and zeaxanthin in membranes has the potential to enhance interactions of their polar groups with proteins (35), thereby anchoring these carotenoids in a fixed position spanning the membrane (52). In addition, it has been suggested that when bound to proteins, carotenoids are less prone to degradation and are more effective antioxidants than free carotenoids and thus are able to protect the system from oxidative damage (4).

ARC is characterized by loss of lens transparency. Opacity of the lens is related to the precipitation of damaged proteins that may accumulate with age from normal metabolic pathways (187). However, oxidation, osmotic stress, and chemical adduct formation are thought to play a major role in the modulation of lens protein (188) and in lipid peroxidation within the lens epithelium (189). Thus, it is hypothesized that intake of dietary antioxidants may block these processes (190). Data on localization of lutein and zeaxanthin in the human lens is scarce. However, one study (179) supports a protective role of lutein–zeaxanthin, α-tocopherol, and retinol in the epithelium and cortex of the human lens. This group reported that concentrations of lutein–zeaxanthin, α-tocopherol, and retinol in younger, more metabolically active tissue (epithelial and cortex layers) of human lenses were 3-, 1.8-, and 1.3-fold higher, respectively, than that in older, less metabolically active tissue (nuclear layer). Another study (191) suggests that macular lutein and zeaxanthin concentrations may be a marker for lutein and zeaxanthin in the lens. This group observed a significant inverse relationship ($p < 0.0001$) between macular pigment density and lens density in women. The biological actions of lutein and zeaxanthin in the lens appear to parallel those of the human macula. However, an explanation of the intricate patterns of selective uptake and distribution of xanthophylls into the human retina and lens remain to be elucidated.

D. Carotenoids and Skin

In the 1960s Mathews–Roth and co-workers (192) were able to demonstrate a protective effect of β-carotene in erythropoietic protoporphyria, a photosensitivity disease resulting in itching and burning of the skin on exposure to visible light. It was hypothesized that β-carotene acts to prevent diseases of photosensitivity by quenching light-activated species and thereby preventing cellular damage, which accounts for the symptoms of these diseases. Since then, ongoing research, investigating the potential role of carotenoids in UV-induced skin damage, has been driven by the wide use of β-carotene supplements as sun protectants.

UV-irradiation of the skin leads to acute sunburn reactions and erythema (premature aging of the skin), and is associated with an increased risk for skin cancer (193). These detrimental effects are thought to be associated with the UV-light induced formation of reactive oxygen species that are capable of damaging cellular lipids, proteins, and DNA. Since carotenoids are efficient scavengers of singlet oxygen and peroxyl radicals (23), they are speculated to provide the skin with protection from acute and chronic exposure to UV light. In particular, the positioning of hydrophobic carotenes, such as β-carotene and lycopene, in the core of membranes parallel to the surface may enhance protection through various layers of the skin and aid in retention of membrane fluidity and biological functioning.

Several studies have demonstrated increased levels of β-carotene in the skin after single (194,195) and multiple doses (196–198). Prince and Frisoli (194) found that a single 51-mg dose of β-carotene increased serum β-carotene by 2.5-fold after 40 h, but an increase in skin β-carotene concentrations as measured by skin remittance spectroscopy were delayed by as much as 14 days. Ribaya–Mercado and co-workers (195) reported a similar magnitude of increase in serum β-carotene following a 120-mg oral dose of β-carotene after 1 day. The subsequent increase in skin β-carotene also occurred in a shorter time period (5 days postdose), as measured by HPLC of skin biopsies. Interestingly, a single exposure of skin to UV light 6 days following this 120-mg oral dose of β-carotene resulted in no decrease in skin β-carotene concentration, but a significant decrease in skin lycopene, suggesting that skin lycopene may be preferentially destroyed over β-carotene.

Little data are available on the distribution of β-carotene in skin from various locations on the body. In one study in which 24 mg/day of β-carotene was supplemented for 12 weeks, Stahl and co-workers (197) observed an increase in β-carotene levels in serum, which paralleled that observed in skin and correlated with levels in skin from the forehead and palm of the hand. Notably, 2 weeks after the end of supplementation, β-carotene concentration in all areas of the skin decreased. This same research group also demonstrated the presence of xanthophyll esters in skin (199) and, more recently, the protective effects of a supplement containing a mixture of carotenoids alone and in combination with a vitamin E supplement against erythema in humans (200). After 8 weeks of supplementation, skin damage from an application of a blue-light solar simulator to the dorsal region of the back was significantly diminished ($p < 0.01$), and the suppression was greater with the combination of carotenoids and vitamin E than with carotenoids alone. These data support their earlier work in which they reported superior antioxidant protection with mixtures of carotenoids than single carotenoids in multilamellar liposomes in vitro (8) and that a synergistic effect may be related to different physicochemical properties or to the specific positioning of compound in membranes.

The inhibitory effects of β-carotene on cyclooxygenase and lipoxygenase pathways are also being investigated as a potential mechanism of action in skin protection. In a study using ^{14}C-labeled-arachidonic acid and ^{14}C-labeled-arachidonic acid and ^{14}C-labeled-linoleic acid, Bar-Natan and co-workers (201) observed a significant decrease in major metabolites of both substrates in human skin homogenates following exposure to low concentrations of β-carotene (0.3 mM). Similar results were observed by Lomnitski et al. (202) using skin homogenates of rats. In a subsequent study by this group, significant increases in lipoxygenase activity in rat skin following exposure to UVA irradiation were prevented for 4 h by topical pretreatment of skin with β-carotene (202) suggesting that β-carotene applied to the skin surface may provide mild protection from sunburn.

E. Carotenoids and Cardiovascular Disease

Cardiovascular disease (CVD) remains the major cause of mortality in developed countries. Although conclusive evidence has not been elucidated for a role of carotenoids in CVD, several epidemiological studies have investigated the relation between carotenoid intake and CVD risk. Inverse associations between serum β-carotene and CVD, for example, have been reported in numerous studies, such as in The Lipid Research Clinics Coronary Primary Prevention Trial and Follow-Up Study, in which 1899 men were followed for 13 years (203). Carotenoids are found in lipoproteins and accumulate in atherosclerotic plaques (194). As previously mentioned, the series of conjugated double bonds characteristic to the structure of carotenoids enables them to quench singlet oxygen and to terminate lipid peroxidation. That carotenoids can function as antioxidants in vitro and are transported in lipoproteins led to the hypothesis that carotenoids may act in the process of atherosclerosis by preventing oxidation, specifically of LDL.

The role of carotenoids in the prevention of CVD has been reviewed recently (204), with variable results between in vitro and in vivo studies. In addition, several prospective epidemiological studies, case–control, cross-sectional, and clinical studies report variable results, some of which are summarized here. In 1992, Princen et al. (205) reported that β-carotene did not protect LDL from lipid peroxidation in vitro. Similarly, Gaziano et al. (206) demonstrated that supplementation with β-carotene in vitro or in vivo did not enhance the protection of LDL against metal ion-dependent and ion-independent oxidation. In one human study, when β-carotene was supplemented at 60 mg/day for 3 months, β-carotene plus vitamin E (VE) (1600 mg/day) for an additional 3 months, and then β-carotene plus VE and vitamin C (2 g/day) for another 3 months, levels of β-carotene in LDL increased nearly 20-fold, but LDL susceptibility to oxidation did not change (207). β-Carotene supplementation was also studied in an intervention trial using a subgroup of Finnish men from the Alpha Tocopherol, β-Carotene Cancer Prevention Study (ATBC), who had experienced a previous myocardial infarction (208). Although a significant difference in the number of major coronary events was not observed between the β-carotene–supplemented group and the placebo group, there were more deaths from coronary heart disease reported in the group receiving β-carotene supplements. In addition, the supplemented group had an 11% increase in ischemic heart disease mortality and a 20% increase in stroke mortality (208). Another intervention study in Lixian, China, showed that supplementation with β-carotene alone or in combination with vitamin E or selenium did not reduce the risk of CVD in this malnourished population (209). Furthermore, in a group of 34,486 Iowa women, it was reported that fatal coronary heart disease was not associated with carotenoid intake (210).

Several human studies have found positive associations between carotenoid intake and reduced risk of CVD. In a large prospective study of 2974 middle-aged men in Switzerland, an increased risk of death from coronary heart disease (CHD) was observed among those in the lowest quartile of plasma carotene levels (211). The Atherosclerosis Risk in Communities Study involving 12,773 participants, aged 45–64 years, reported that those in the highest quintile of carotenoid consumption had a lower prevalence of plaques (women, 25.4%; men, 36%) than those in the lowest quintile of carotenoid consumption (women, 29.3%; men, 39.8%) (212). It was suggested that carotenoids of other plant-derived compounds may play a role in preventing arterial plaque formation (212).

Supplementary to these results, are various case–control and cohort studies that reported a decrease in risk of CHD with intake of carotenoids. In the United States, Blot and co-workers (209) conducted two studies, one cohort with 87,245 healthy women, and the other with 39,910 men. Women and men in the highest quintile of β-carotene intake had a 22% lower risk of CHD and a 25% lower risk of suffering a CHD event, respectively, than did those in the lowest quintile (209). However, Lee et al. (213) reported no overall benefits of β-carotene supplementation on incidence of CVD in women in the Nurses' Health Study. An additional case–control study, referred to as the European Community Multicenter Study on Antioxidants, Myocardial Infarction, and Breast Cancer (EURAMIC) Study (214) investigated the incidence of myocardial infarction (MI) in relation to levels of carotenoids in adipose. β-Carotene and α-carotene did not show associations with MI; however, lycopene with an odds ratio of 0.52 for the contrast of the 10th and the 90th percentiles remained independently protective against incidence of MI (214). It was concluded that lycopene, or other bioactive components found in a similar common food source (e.g., tomato products) may contribute to the protective effect of vegetable consumption on risk of MI (214). Subsequently, Argarwal and co-workers (215) reported a significant decrease in serum lipid peroxidation and LDL oxidation in 19 human subjects following supplementation with tomato juice, spaghetti sauce, or the oleoresin fraction of tomatoes for 1 week.

F. Carotenoids and Immune Response

Interest in the study of carotenoids and the immune response was sparked in the 1930s when Green and Mellanby (216) reported that vitamin A-deficient rats fed β-carotene did not develop infections. Thus, the role of carotenoids in modulating host defense systems was originally thought to be due to their provitamin A activity. Conditions that suppress immune function, such as low vitamin A status, increase the risk of infectious diseases and have been associated with increased cancer risk in animals and human (217,218). Environmental factors, such as cigarette smoking, UV-light exposure, and viral infection, as well as the aging process, are also associated with loss of cell-mediated immune response followed by a concomitant increase in infections and cancer incidence (46).

Several protective functions of immune cells are thought to depend on the fluidity of cell membranes (46). Thus, loss of membrane fluidity resulting from lipid peroxidation is directly related to the ability of lymphocytes to respond to challenges to the immune system (219). As mentioned previously, specific positioning of carotenoids in membranes may affect their thickness, fluidity, strength, and permeability (47,50,51); thus, carotenoids may aid in maintaining cell function. In addition to membrane fluidity, carotenoids may regulate immune function by managing various separate or interrelated cell events (220), including induction of heat-shock proteins (221), enhancement of gap junction communication (9), and inhibition of arachidonic acid oxidation (222), which is related to the free radical scavenging properties of carotenoids.

Whereas most of the work on carotenoids and immune response has focused on β-carotene, the influence of various carotenoids on immunoenhancement has been investigated in recent years. α-Carotene in addition to carotenoids, such as astaxanthin, canthaxanthin, lutein, and lycopene, have received attention. Although studies on immunomodulation with non–provitamin A carotenoids are limited, evidence shows that both provitamin A and non–provitamin A carotenoids enhance many aspects of immune function. Studies with various carotenoids have demonstrated significant immunomodulating actions relative to humoral immune responses to T-dependent antigens. Jyonouchi et al. (223) reported an enhancement of antibody production by lutein, astaxanthin, and β-carotene in response to T-dependent antigens in vitro and in vivo. In a subsequent study by the same group, astaxanthin increased human immunoglobin production in response to T-dependent stimuli (224).

Some studies report positive effects of carotenoids on lymphocyte proliferation in animals and humans. Cigarette smoke can impose free radical burden on lymphocytes. However, supplemental β-carotene (20 mg/day), administered to healthy male smokers for 14 weeks, enhanced proliferation of lymphocytes (225). A similar enhancement of T- and B-lymphocyte proliferation was observed in rats fed diets containing 0.2% β-carotene or canthaxanthin for up to 66 weeks (226). In contrast, Kramer and Burri (227) reported that a low-dose β-carotene supplement had no effect on suppressed mitogenic proliferative responsiveness of human blood lymphocytes, but was corrected with supplementation of a carotenoid complex containing α-carotene, β-carotene, β-cryptoxanthin, lutein, zeaxanthin, and lycopene. These observations are supported by the work of Stahl et al. (8) who demonstrated superior protection of carotenoid mixtures, especially lycopene and lutein, in protecting multilamellar liposomes against oxidative damage in vitro. Thus, although most studies have focused on the influence of β-carotene, the influence of other carotenoids in addition to and other than β-carotene has been established.

Mixed results have been reported in studies investigating the effects of β-carotene on various immunological parameters in elderly populations. T-helper cells, natural killer (NK) cells, and various cytokines were increased in a dose–response relation with β-carotene supplementation in elderly individuals (228). Santos et al. (229) also observed an enhancement of NK cell activity in elderly men, participating in the Physicians' Health Study (PHS), who had been supplemented with 50 mg β-carotene every other day for 10–12 years compared with those taking placebo. However, in subsequent short-term and long-term studies, this same research group reported no effects of β-carotene supplementation on several immunological parameters, including lymphocyte proliferation, production of interleukin-2 (IL-2), production of prostaglandin E_2 (PGE_2), and immunological cell profiles (230). The overall conclusion was that β-carotene supplementation did not have an enhancing or suppressive effect on T-cell–mediated immunity of healthy elderly (230).

Recent research investigating the protective role of carotenoids in UV-induced skin damage, is described elsewhere in this chapter. However, earlier studies have linked the immunosuppressive effects of UV-light exposure with increased development of skin and other tumors (231). Supplemental intakes of canthaxanthin and retinol reduced the growth of experimentally implanted tumors in mice exposed to UV irradiation (232). In addition, β-carotene supplementation to young adult men before exposure to UV light prevented suppression of delayed-type hypersensitivity responses (DTH), a clinical index of cell-mediated immune response (233).

V. CONCLUSION

Our objective for this chapter was to investigate the link between the chemistry, absorption, and metabolism of carotenoids and their potential role in human health and disease. The evidence supporting an association between intake of carotenoid-rich fruits and vegetables and reduced risk of some chronic diseases, as well as the biological effects of carotenoids in model systems is promising. However, research still has not been able to confirm that carotenoids are a principal factor in reduced risk of disease associated with elevated intakes of carotenoid-rich fruits and vegetables, or that carotenoids, through their biological actions, can affect specific disease states.

The pathways of carotenoid absorption and metabolism can be explained with knowledge of the many chemical and structural properties of these molecules. However, the link with the selective patterns of carotenoid uptake into tissues, as well as the significance of tissue levels and subsequent metabolism is less clear. The presence or absence of various dietary carotenoids, their geometric isomers, and their oxidative metabolites in human blood and tissues suggest that specific carotenoids may exhibit different degrees of biological activity, depending on their environment in vivo (10). Although the antioxidant activity exhibited by carotenoids in vitro is one mechanism related to their potential role as modulators of health and disease, they may exert biological actions by several other mechanisms. These include (1) production of retinoids, (2) enhancement of cellular communication, (3) stimulation of cell differentiation, (4) stimulation of phase I enzyme (detoxification enzymes) activity, (5) enhancement of anti-inflammatory or immune-related properties, and (6) inhibition of mutagenesis and transformation.

It has been proposed that the observed effects of a specific carotenoid on cells or tissues may be the result of specific properties of that carotenoid, and it only remains to associate a chemical property with the specific biological action (234). In contrast, low tissue levels of β-carotene, in particular, may simply be an indicator or marker of cellular insult rather than a causal effect of disease (144). We must keep in mind, however, that some biological actions attributed to β-carotene may reflect conversion to retinoids and subsequent gene regulation. Low levels of β-carotene metabolites may exert substantial and highly controlled physiological effects, many that have yet to be elucidated. In addition, explorations of the interactions of carotenoids with each other and with other potentially bioactive components in foods are just beginning.

REFERENCES

1. Olson JA. Carotenoids. In: Shils ME, Olson JA, Shike M, Ross AC, eds. Modern Nutrition in Health and Disease. Baltimore: Williams & Wilkins, 1999:525–541.
2. Krinsky NI. Actions of carotenoids in biological systems. Annu Rev Nutr 1993; 13:561–587.
3. Wang X–D. Review: absorption and metabolism of β-carotene. J Am Coll Nutr 1994; 13:314–325.
4. Rao MN, Ghosh P, Lakshaman MR. Purification and partial characterization of a cellular carotenoid-binding protein from ferret liver. J Biol Chem 1997; 272:24455–24460.
5. Britton G. Structure and properties of carotenoids in relation to function. FASEB J 1995; 9:1551–1558.
6. Stahl W, Seis H. Separation of geometrical isomers of β-carotene and lycopene. Methods Enzymol 1994; 234:388–400.
7. Britton G, Weesie RJ, Askin D, Warburton J, Gallardo–Guerro L, Jansen FJ, Groot HJMD, Lugtenburg J, Cornard JP, Merlin JC. Carotenoid blues: structural studies on carotenoproteins. Pure Appl Chem 1997; 69:2075–2084.
8. Stahl W, Nicolai S, Briviba K, Hanusch M. Biological activities of natural and synthetic carotenoids: induction of gap junctional communication and singlet oxygen quenching. Carcinogenesis 1997; 18:89–92.
9. Zhang L–X, Cooney RV, Bertram JS. Carotenoids up-regulate connexin43 expression independent of their provitamin A or antioxidant properties. Cancer Res 1992; 52:5707–5712.
10. Khachik F, Beecher GR, Smith JC Jr. Lutein, lycopene, and their oxidative metabolites in chemoprevention of cancer. J Cell Biochem 1995; 22:236–146.
11. Khachik F, Spangler CJ, Smith JC Jr. Identification, quantification, and relative concentrations of carotenoids and their metabolites in human milk and serum. Anal Chem 1997; 69:1873–1881.
12. Zhang L–X, Cooney RV, Bertram JS. Carotenoids up-regulate connexin43 expression independent of their provitamin A or antioxidant properties. Cancer Res 1992; 52:5707–5712.
13. Achkar C, Derguini F, Blumberg B, Langston A, Levin AA, Speck J, Evans RM, Bolando J Jr, Nakanishi K, Buck J, Gudas LJ. 4-Oxoretinol, a new natural ligand and transactivator of the retinoic acid receptors. Proc Natl Acad Sci USA 1996; 93:4879–4884.
14. Pijnappel W, Hendriks H, Folkers G. The retinoid ligand 4-oxoretinoic acid is a highly active modulator of positional specification. Nature 1993; 366:340–344.
15. Hanusch M, Stahl W, Schulz WA, Sies H. Induction of gap junctional communication by 4-oxoretinoic acid generated from its precursor canthaxantin. Arch Biochem Biophys 1995; 317:423–428.
16. Stahl W, Sies H. The role of carotenoids in gap junctional communication. Int J Vitam Nutr Res 1998; 68:354–359.
17. Nagao A, Olson JA. Enzymatic formation of 9-*cis*, 13-*cis*, and all *trans* retinals from isomers of β-carotene. FASEB J 1994; 8:968–973.
18. Wang X–D, Krinsky NI, Benotti PN, Russell RM. Biosynthesis of 9-*cis*-retinoic acid from 9-*cis*-β-carotene in human intestinal mucosa in vitro. Arch Biochem Biophys 1994; 313:150–155.
19. Hebuterne X, Wang X–D, Johnson E, Krinsky NI, Russell RM. Intestinal absorption and metabolism of 9-*cis* β-carotene in vivo: biosynthesis of 9-*cis* retinoic acid. J Lipid Res 1995; 36:1264–1273.
20. Levin AA, Sturzenbecker LJ, Kazmer S, Bosakowski T, Huselton C, Allenby G, Speck J, Kratzeisen C, Rosenberger M, Lovey A, Grippo JF. 9-*cis*-Retinoic acid stereoisomer binds and activates the nuclear receptor RXRα. Nature 1992; 355:359–361.
21. Heyman RA, Mangelsdorf DJ, Dyck JA, Stein RB, Eichele G, Evans RM, Thalle C. 9-*cis* Retinoic acid is a high affinity ligand for the retinoid X receptor. Cell 1992; 68:397–406.
22. Britton G. UV/visible spectroscopy. In: Britton G, Liaaen–Jensen S, Pfander H, eds. Carotenoids. Basel: Birkhauser Verlag, 1995:13–62.

23. Sies H, Stahl W. Vitamins E and C, β-carotene, and other carotenoids as antioxidants. Am J Clin Nutr 1995; 62:1315S–1321S.
24. Burton GW, Ingold KU. β-Carotene: an unusual type of lipid antioxidant. Science 1984; 224:569–573.
25. Palozza P, Krinsky NI. β-Carotene and α-tocopherol are synergistic antioxidants. Arch Biochem Biophys 1992; 297:184–187.
26. Diplock AT. Antioxidant nutrients and disease prevention: an overview. Am J Clin Nutr 1991; 53:189S–193S.
27. Bast A, Haenen GRMM, van den Berg R, van den Berg H. Antioxidant effects of carotenoids. Int J Vitam Nutr Res 1998; 68:399–403.
28. Demmig–Adams B, Gilmore AM, Adams WW. In vivo functions of carotenoids in higher plants. FASEB J 1996; 10:403–412.
29. Mathews–Roth MM. β-Carotene: clinical aspects. In: Spiller GA, Scala J, eds. Current Topics in Nutrition and Disease. New York: Alan R Liss, 1989:17–38.
30. Hirayama O, Nakamura K, Hamada S, Kobayasi Y. Singlet oxygen quenching ability of naturally occurring carotenoids. Lipids 1994; 29:149–150.
31. Frank HA, Cogdell RJ. The photochemistry and function of carotenoids in photosynthesis. In: Young A, Britton G, eds. Carotenoids in Photosynthesis. London: Chapman & Hall, 1993:252–326.
32. Di Mascio P, Kaiser S, Sies H. Lycopene as the most efficient biological carotenoid singlet oxygen quencher. Arch Biochem Biophys 1989; 274:532–538.
33. Miller NJ, Sampson J, Candeias LP, Bramley PM, Rice–Evans CA. Antioxidant activities of carotenes and xanthophylls. FEBS Lett 1996; 384:240–242.
34. Siems WG, Sommerburg O, Kuijk FJV. Lycopene and β-carotene decompose more rapidly than lutein and zeaxanthin upon exposure to various prooxidants in vitro. Biofactors 1999; 10:105–113.
35. Woodall AA, Britton G, Jackson MJ. Carotenoids and protection of phospholipids in solution or in liposomes against oxidation by peroxyl radicals: relationship between carotenoid structure and protective ability. Biochim Biophys Acta 1997; 1336:575–586.
36. Levin G, Yeshurun M, Mokady S. In vivo antiperoxidative effect of 9-cis-β-carotene compared with that of the all-trans isomer. Nutr Cancer 1997; 27:293–297.
37. Levin G, Mokady S. Antioxidant activity 9-cis compared to all-trans β-carotene in vitro. Free Radic Biol Med 1994; 17:77–82.
38. Halliwell B. Free radicals, antioxidants, and human disease: curiosity, cause or consequence? Lancet 1994; 244:721–724.
39. Terao J. Antioxidant activity of β-carotene-related carotenoids in solution. Lipids 1989; 24:659–661.
40. Parker RS, Swanson JE, You C–S, Edwards AJ, Huang T. Bioavailability of carotenoids in human subjects. Proc Nutr Soc 1999; 58:1–8.
41. Deming DM, Erdman JW Jr. Mammalian carotenoid absorption and metabolism. Pure Appl Chem 1999; 71(12):2213–2223.
42. Borel P, Grolier P, Armand M, Partier A, Lafone H, Lairon D, Azais–Braesco V. Carotenoids in biological emulsions: solubility, surface to core distribution, and release from lipid droplets. J Lipid Res 1996; 37:250–261.
43. Boileau AC, Merchen NR, Wasson K, Atkinson CA, Erdman JW Jr. cis-Lycopene is more bioavailable than trans-lycopene in vitro and also in vivo in the lymph cannulated ferret. J Nutr 1999; 129:1176–1181.
44. El-Gorab MI, Underwood BA, Loerch JD. The roles of bile salts in the uptake of β-carotene and retinol by rat everted gut sacs. Biochim Biophys Acta 1975; 401:265–277.
45. Wiseman H. Dietary influences on membrane function: importance in protection against oxidative damage and disease. Nutr Biochem 1996; 7:2–15.
46. Bendich A. Antioxidants, immune response, and animal function. J Dairy Sci 1993; 76:2789–2794.
47. Gruszecki WI, Sielewiesiuk J. Orientation of xanthophylls in phosphatidyl choline multilayers. Biochim Biophys Acta 1990; 1023:405–412.
48. Gruszecki WI, Sujak A, Strzalka K, Radunz A, Schmis GH. Organization of xanthophyll–lipid membranes studied by means of specific pigment antisera, spectrophotometry and monomolecular layer technique: lutein versus zeaxanthin. Z Naturforsch 1999; 54:517–525.

49. Sujak A, Gabrielska J, Grudzinski W, Borc R, Mazurek P, Gruszecki WI. Lutein and zeaxanthin as protectors of lipid membranes against oxidative damage: the structural aspects. Arch Biochem Bioiphys 1999; 37:301–307.
50. Wisniewska A, Subczynski WK. Effects of polar lipids on the shape of the hydrophobic barrier of phospholipid bilayers. Biochim Biophys Acta 1998; 1368:235–246.
51. Subcznyski WK, Markowska E, Sielewiesiuk J. Effect of polar carotenoids on the oxygenated diffusion–concentration product in lipid bilayers: an ESR spin label study. Biochim Biophys Acta 1991; 1068:68–72.
52. Lazrak T, Milton A, Wolf G, Albrecht AM, Mieche M, Ourisson G, Nakatani Y. Comparison of the effects of inserted C_{40} and C_{50} terminally dihydroxylated carotenoids on the mechanical properties of various phospholipid vesicles. Biochim Biophys Acta 1987; 903:132–141.
53. Hara M, Yuan H, Yang Q, Hoshino T, Yokoyama A, Miyake J. Stabilization of liposomal membranes by thermozeaxanthins: carotenoid–glucoside esters. Biochim Biophys Acta 1999; 1461: 147–154.
54. Kennedy TA, Liebler DC. Peroxyl radical scavenging by β-carotene in lipid bilayers. Effect of oxygen partial pressure. J Biol Chem 1992; 267:4658–4663.
55. Kennedy TA, Liebler DC. Peroxyl radical oxidation of β-carotene: formation of beta-carotene. Chem Res Toxicol 1991; 4:290–295.
56. Lim BP, Nagao A, Terao J, Tanaka K, Suzuki T, Takama K. Antioxidant activity of xanthophylls on peroxyl radical-mediated phospholipid peroxidation. Biochim Biophys Acta 1992; 1126:178–184.
57. Olson JA. Absorption, transport, and metabolism of carotenoids in humans. Pure Appl Chem 1994; 66:1011–1016.
58. Furr HC, Clark RM. Intestinal absorption and tissue distribution of carotenoids. Nutr Biochem 1997; 8:364–377.
59. Castenmiller JJM, West CE. Bioavailability and bioconversion of carotenoids. Nutr Rev 1998; 18: 19–38.
60. Boileau TWM, Moore AC, Erdman JW Jr. Carotenoids and vitamin A. In: Papas AM, ed. Antioxidant Status, Diet, Nutrition, and Health. Boca Raton, FL: CRC Press, 1999:133–158.
61. Silveira ER, Moreno FS. Natural retinoids and β-carotene: from food to their actions on gene expression. J Nutr Biochem 1998; 9:446–456.
62. van het Hof KH, West CE, Westrate JA, Hautvast JGAJ. Dietary factors that affect the bioavailability of carotenoids. J Nutr 2000; 130:503–506.
63. Castenmiller JJM, West CE, Linssen JPH, van het Hof KH, Voragen AGJ. The food matrix of spinach is a limiting factor in determining the bioavailability of β-carotene and to a lesser extent of lutein in humans. J Nutr 1999; 129:349–355.
64. Brown ED, Micozzi MS, Craft NE, Bieri JG, Beecher G, Edwards BK, Rose A, Taylor PR, Smith JC Jr. Plasma carotenoids in normal men after a single ingestion of vegetables or purified β-carotene. Am J Clin Nutr 1989; 49:1258–1265.
65. Micozzi MS, Brown ED, Edwards BK, Bieri JG, Taylor PR, Khachik F, Beecher GR, Smith JC Jr. Plasma carotenoid response to chronic intake of selected foods and β-carotene supplements in men. Am J Clin Nutr 1992; 55:1120–1125.
66. Rock CL, Lovalvo JL, Emenhiser C, Ruffin MT, Flatt SW, Schwartz SJ. Bioavailability of β-carotene is lower in raw than in processed carrots and spinach. J Nutr 1998; 128:913–916.
67. de Pee S, West CE, Permaesih D, Martuti S, Muuhilal, Hautvast JG. Orange fruit is more effective than are dark-green, leafy vegetables in increasing serum concentrations of retinol and β-carotene in school children in Indonesia. Am J Clin Nutr 1998; 68:1058–1067.
68. van het Hof KH, Boer BCJ, Tijburg LBM, Lucius BRHM, Zijp I, West CE, Hautvast JGAJ, Westrate JA. Carotenoid bioavailability in humans from tomatoes processed in different ways. Comparison of carotenoid response in triglyceride-rich lipoprotein fraction of plasma after a single consumption of tomato products and plasma in four days. J Nutr 2000; 130:1189–1196.
69. van het Hof KH, Tijburg LBM, Pietrzik K, Westrate JA. Bioavailability of carotenoids and folate from different vegetables. Effect of disruption of the vegetable matrix. Br J Nutr 1999; 82:203–212.
70. van het Hof KH, Gartner C, West CE, Tijburg LBM. Potential of vegetable processing to increase the delivery of carotenoids to man. Int J Vitam Nutr Res 1998; 68:366–370.
71. Stahl W, Sies H. Uptake of lycopene and its geometrical isomers is greater from heat-processed than from unprocessed tomato juice in humans. J Nutr 1992; 122:2161–2166.

72. Gartner C, Stahl W, Sies H. Lycopene is more bioavailable from tomato paste than from fresh tomatoes. Am J Clin Nutr 1997; 66:116–122.
73. Khachik F, Goli MB, Beecher GR, Holden J, Lusby WR, Tenorio MD, Barrera MR. Effect of food preparation on qualitative and quantitative distribution of major carotenoid constituents of tomatoes and several green vegetables. J Agric Food Chem 1992; 40:390–398.
74. Schwartz SJ. Chromatographic analysis of cis/trans carotenoid isomers. J Chromatogr 1992; 624:235–252.
75. Khachik F, Beecher GR, Lusby WR. Separation, identification, and quantification of the major carotenoids in extract of apricots, peaches, cantaloupe, and pink grapefruit by liquid chromatography. J Agric Food Chem 1989; 37:1465–1473.
76. Panalaks T, Murray TK. The effect of processing on the content of carotene isomers in vegetables and peaches. J Inst Can Technol Alimen 1970; 3:145–151.
77. Lessin WJ, Catigani CL, Schwartz SJ. Quantification of cis–trans isomers of provitamin A carotenoids in fresh and processed fruits and vegetables. J Agric Food Chem 1997; 45:3728–3732.
78. Chandler LA, Schwartz SJ. HPLC separation of cis–trans carotene isomers in fresh and processed fruits and vegetables. J Food Sci 1987; 52:669–672.
79. Schierle J, Bretzel W, Buhler I, Faccin N, Hess D, Steiner K, Schuep W. Content and isomeric ratio of lycopene in food and plasma. Food Chem 1997; 59:459–465.
80. Rich GT, Fillery–Travis A, Parker ML. Low pH enhances the transfer of carotene from carrot juice to olive oil. Lipids 1998; 33:985–992.
81. Williams AW, Erdman JW Jr. Effects of food processing techniques on the content and bioavailability of vitamins: a focus on carotenoids. In: Micronutrient Interactions: Impact on Child Health and Nutrition. Washington, DC: ILSI Press, 1998:43–49.
82. Shi J. Lycopene in tomatoes: chemical and physical properties affected by food processing. Crit Rev Food Sci Nutr 2000; 40:1–42.
83. Desobry SA, Netto FM, Labuza TP. Preservation of β-carotene from carrots. Crit Rev Food Sci Nutr 1998; 38:381–396.
84. Jonsson L. Thermal degradation of carotenes and influence on their physiological functions. In: Friedman, M, ed. Nutritional and Toxicological Consequences of Food Processing. New York: Plenum Press, 1991:75–82.
85. Sweeney JP, Marsh AC. Effect of processing on provitamin A in vegetables. J Am Diet Assoc 1971; 59:238–243.
86. You C–S, Parker RS, Goodman KJ, Swanson JE, Corso TN. Evidence of cis–trans isomerization of 9-cis-β-carotene during absorption in humans. Am J Clin Nutr 1996; 64:177–183.
87. Stahl W, Schwarz W, Sundquist AR, Sies H. cis–trans Isomers of lycopene and β-carotene in human serum and tissues. Arch Biochem Biophys 1992; 294:173–177.
88. Stahl W, Sies H. Geometrical isomers of β-carotene and lycopene: in vivo studies with humans. In: Livrea MA, Vidali G, eds. Retinoids: From Basic Science to Clinical Applications. Basel: Birkhäuser Verlag, 1994:29–34.
89. Stahl W, Schwartz W, Sies H. Human serum concentrations of all-trans β- and α-carotene but not 9-cis β-carotene increase upon ingestion of a natural isomer mixture obtained from *Dunaliella salina* (Betatene). J Nutr 1993; 123:847–851.
90. Hollander D, Paul E, Ruble J. β-Carotene intestinal absorption: bile, fatty acid, pH, and flow rate effects on transport. Am J Physiol 1978; 235:E686–E691.
91. Olson JA, Hayaishi O. The enzymatic cleavage of β-carotene into vitamin A by soluble enzymes of rat liver and intestine. Proc Natl Acad Sci USA 1965; 54:1364–1369.
92. Olson JA. Provitamin A function of carotenoids: the conversion of β-carotene into vitamin A. J Nutr 1989; 119:105–108.
93. Olson JA. The conversion of radioactive β-carotene into vitamin A by rat small intestine in vivo. J Biol Chem 1961; 236:349–356.
94. During A, Nagao A, Hoshino C, Terao J. Assay of β-carotene 15,15'-dioxygenase activity by reverse-phase high-pressure liquid chromatography. Anal Biochem 1996; 241:199–205.
95. Grolier P, Duszka C, Borel P, Alexandre–Gouabau M, Azais–Baesco V. In vitro and in vivo inhibition of β-carotene dioxygenase activity by canthaxanthin in rat intestine. Arch Biochem Biophys 1997; 348:233–238.
96. van Vliet T, Schaik FV, Berg HVD. β-Carotene metabolism: the enzymatic cleavage to retinal. Voeding 1992; 53:186–190.

97. van Vliet T, van Schaik F, Schreurs WHP, van den Berg H. In vitro measurement of β-carotene cleavage activity: methodological considerations and the effect of other carotenoids on β-carotene cleavage. Int J Vitam Nutr Res 1996; 66:77–85.
98. van Vliet T, van Vlissingen MF, van Schaik F, van den Berg H. β-Carotene absorption and cleavage in rats is affected by the vitamin A concentration of the diet. J Nutr 1996; 126:499–508.
99. During A, Nagao A, Terao A. β-Carotene 15,15′-dioxygenase activity and cellular retinol-binding protein type II are enhanced by dietary unsaturated triacylglycerols in rat intestine. J Nutr 1998; 128:1614–1619.
100. Wang X–D, Krinsky NI, Tang G, Russell RM. Retinoic acid can be produced from eccentric cleavage of β-carotene in human intestinal mucosa. Arch Biochem Biophys 1992; 293:298–304.
101. Napoli JL, Race KR. Biogenesis of retinoic acid from β-carotene. J Biol Chem 1988; 263:17372–17377.
102. Sharma RV, Mathur SN, Ganguly J. Studies on the relative biopotencies and intestinal absorption of different apo-β-carotenoids in rats and chickens. Biochem J 1976; 158:377–383.
103. Wang X–D, Tang G–W, Fox JG, Krinsky NI, Russell RM. Enzymatic conversion of β-carotene into β-apocarotenals and retinoids by human, monkey, ferret, and rat tissues. Arch Biochem Biophys 1991; 285:8–16.
104. Wolf G. The enzymatic cleavage of β-carotene: still controversial. Nutr Rev 1995; 53:134–137.
105. Gugger ET, Erdman JW Jr. Intracellular β-carotene transport in bovine liver and intestine is not mediated by cytosolic proteins. J Nutr 1996; 126:1470–1474.
106. Gartner C, Stahl W, Sies H. Preferential increase in chylomicron levels of the xanthophylls lutein and zeaxanthin compared to β-carotene in the human. Int J Vitam Nutr Res 1996; 66:119–125.
107. O'Neill ME, Thurnham DI. Intestinal absorption of β-carotene, lycopene and lutein in men and women following a standard meal: response curves in the triacylglycerol-rich lipoprotein fraction. Br J Nutr 1998; 79:149–159.
108. Bierer TL, Merchen NR, Erdman JW Jr. Comparative absorption and transport of five common carotenoids in preruminant calves. J Nutr 1995; 125:1569–1577.
109. Kostic D, White WS, Olson JA. Intestinal absorption, serum clearance, and interactions between lutein and β-carotene when administered to human adults in separate and combined oral doses. Am J Clin Nutr 1995; 62:604–610.
110. van den Berg H, van Vliet T. Effect of simultaneous, single oral doses of β-carotene with lutein or lycopene on the β-carotene and retinyl ester responses in the triacylglycerol-rich lipoprotein fraction of men. Am J Clin Nutr 1998; 68:82–89.
111. van den Berg H. Carotenoid interactions. Nutr Rev 1999; 57:1–10.
112. Gaziano JM, Johnson EJ, Russell RM, Manson JE, Stampfer MJ, Ridker PM, Frei B, Hennekens CH, Krinsky NI. Discrimination in absorption or transport of β-carotene isomers after oral supplementation with either all-*trans*- or 9-*cis*-β-carotene. Am J Clin Nutr 1995; 61:1248–1252.
113. Jensen CD, Howes TW, Spiller GA, Thomas SP, Whittam JH, Scala J. Observations on the effects of ingesting *cis*- and *trans*-β-carotene isomers on human serum concentrations. Nutr Rep Int 1987; 35:413–422.
114. Johnson EJ, Krinsky NI, Russell RM. Serum response of all-*trans* and 9-*cis* isomers of β-carotene in humans. J Am Coll Nutr 1996; 15:620–624.
115. Stahl W, Schwarz W, Laar JV, Sies H. All-*trans* β-carotene preferentially accumulates in human chylomicrons and very low density lipoproteins compared with the 9-*cis* geometrical isomer. J Nutr 1995; 125:2128–2133.
116. Ben-Amotz A, Shoshana M, Edelstein S, Avron M. Bioavailability of a natural isomer mixture as compared with synthetic all-*trans* β-carotene in rats and chicks. J Nutr 1989; 119:1013–1019.
117. Weiser HG, Riss G, Biesalski HK. Uptake and metabolism of β-carotene isomers in rats. In: Canfield LM, Krinsky NI, Olson JA, eds. Carotenoids in Human Health. New York: New York Academy of Sciences, 1993; 223–225.
118. Erdman JW Jr, Thatcher AJ, Hofmann NE, Lederman JD, Block SS, Lee CM, Mokady S. All-*trans* β-carotene is absorbed preferentially to 9-*cis* β-carotene, but the latter accumulates in the tissues of domestic ferrets (*Mustela purotius furo*). J Nutr 1998; 128:2009–2013.
119. Doering WE, Sotiriou–Leventis C, Roth WR. Thermal interconversions among 15-*cis*, 13-*cis*, and all-*trans*-β-carotene: kinetics, Arrhenius parameters, thermochemistry, and potential relevance to anticarcinogenicity of all-*trans*-β-carotene. J Am Chem Soc 1995; 117:2747–2757.

120. Stahl W, Schwarz W, Sies H. Human serum concentrations of all-*trans* β-carotene and α-carotene but not 9-*cis* β-carotene increase upon ingestion of a natural isomer mixture obtained from *Dunaliella salina* (Betatene). J Nutr 1993; 123:847–851.
121. Bjornson LK, Kayden HJ, Miller E, Moshell AN. The transport of α-tocopherol and β-carotene in human blood. J Lipid Res 1976; 17:343–352.
122. Johnson EJ, Russell RM. Distribution of orally administered β-carotene among lipoproteins in healthy men. Am J Clin Nutr 1992; 56:128–135.
123. Traber MG, Diamond DR, Lane JC, Brody RI, Kayden JH. β-Carotene transport in human lipoproteins. Comparisons with α-tocopherol. Lipids 1994; 29:665–669.
124. Pateau I, Khachik F, Brown ED, Beecher GR, Kramer TR, Chittans J, Clevidence BA. Chronic ingestion of lycopene-rich tomato juice or lycopene supplements significantly increases plasma concentrations of lycopene and related tomato carotenoids in humans. Am J Clin Nutr 1998; 68: 1187–1195.
125. Clevidence BA, Bieri JG. Association of carotenoids with human plasma lipoproteins. In: Abelson J, Simon MI, eds. Methods in Enzymology. San Diego: Academic Press, 1993:33–46.
126. Reddy PP, Clevidence BA, Berlin E, Taylor PR, Bieri JG, Smith JC. Plasma carotenoid content and vitamin E profile of lipoprotein fractions of men fed a controlled typical U. S. diet. FASEB J 1989; 3:A955.
127. Romanchik JE, Morel DW, Harrison EH. Distributions of carotenoids and alpha-tocopherol among lipoproteins do not change when human plasma is incubated in vitro. J Nutr 1995; 125:2610–2617.
128. Parker RS. Absorption, metabolism, and transport of carotenoids. FASEB J 1996; 10:542–551.
129. Wingerath T, Stahl W, Sies H. β-Cryptoxanthin selectively increases in human chylomicrons upon ingestion of tangerine concentrate rich in β-cryptoxanthin esters. Arch Biochem Biophys 1995; 324:385–390.
130. Granado F, Olmedilla B, Gil–Martinez E, Blanco I. Lutein esters in serum after lutein supplementation in human subjects. Br J Nutr 1998; 80:445–449.
131. Krinsky NI, Russett MD, Handelman GJ, Snodderly DM. Structural and geometrical isomers of carotenoids in human plasma. J Nutr 1991; 120:1654–1662.
132. Rushin WG, Catignani GL, Schwartz SJ. Determination of β-carotene and its *cis* isomers in serum. Clin Chem 1990; 36:1986–1989.
133. Khachik F, Englert G, Daitch CE, Beecher GR, Tonucci LH, Lusby WR. Isolation and structural elucidation of the geometrical isomers of lutein and zeaxanthin in extracts from human plasma. J Chromatogr 1992; 582:153–566.
134. Bjerkeng OM, Liaaen–Jensen S. Humans administered a single meal with astaxanthin. 12th International Carotenoid Symposium, Cairns, Australia, July 19–23, 1999.
135. Barua AB. Intestinal absorption of epoxy-β-carotenes by humans. Biochem J 1999; 339:359–362.
136. Duitsman PK, Becker B, Barua AB, Olson JA. Effects of epoxycarotenoids, β-carotene, and retinoic acid on the differentiation and viability of the leukemia cell line NB4 in vitro. Int J Vitam Nutr Res 1999; 69:303–308.
137. Kaplan LA, Lau JM, Stein EA. Carotenoid composition, concentrations, and relationships in various human organs. Clin Physiol Biochem 1990; 8:1–10.
138. Erdman JW Jr, Fahey GC Jr, White CB. Effects of purified dietary fiber sources on β-carotene utilization by the chick. J Nutr 1986; 116:2415–2423.
139. Schmitz HH, Poor CL, Wellman RB, Erdman JW Jr. Concentrations of selected carotenoids and vitamin A in human liver, kidney and lung tissue. J Nutr 1991; 121:1613-1621.
140. Bone RA, Landrum JT, Fernandez L, Tarsis SL. Analysis of the macular pigment by HPLC: retinal distribution and age study. Inv Ophthalmol Vis Sci 1988; 29:843–849.
141. Bone R, Landrum JT, Friedes LM, Gomez CM, Kilburn MD, Menendez E, Vidal I, Wang W. Distribution of lutein and zeaxanthin stereoisomers in the human retina. Exp Eye Res 1997; 64: 211–218.
142. Yeum K–J, Taylor A, Tang G, Russell RM. Measurement of carotenoids, retinoids, and tocopherols in human lenses. Inv Ophthalmol Vis Sci 1995; 36:2756–2761.
143. Clinton SK, Emenhiser C, Schwartz SJ, Bostwick DG, Williams AW, Moore BJ, John W, Erdman J. *cis–trans* Lycopene isomers, carotenoids, and retinol in the human prostate. Cancer Epidemiol Biomarkers Prev 1996; 5:823–833.
144. Jandacek RJ. The canary in the cell: a sentinal role for β-carotene. J Nutr 2000; 130:648–651.

145. The alpha-Tocopherol β-Carotene Cancer Prevention Study Group. The effect of vitamin E and β-carotene on the incidence of lung cancer and other cancers in male smokers. N Engl J Med 1994; 330:1029–1035.
146. Levy Y, Bartha P, Ben-Amotz A, Brook JG, Danker G, Lin S, Hammerman H. Plasma antioxidants and lipid peroxidation in acute myocardial infarction and thrombolysis. J Am Coll Nutr 1998; 7:337–341.
147. Benton D, Haller J, Fordy J. The vitamin status of young British adults. Int J Vitam Nutr Res 1997; 67:34–40.
148. Stich HF, Hornby AP, Dunn BP. β-Carotene levels in exfoliated mucosa cells of population groups at low and elevated risk for oral cancer. Int J Cancer 1986; 37:389–393.
149. Zhang S, Tang G, Russell RM, Mayzel KA, Stampfer MJ, Willet WC, Hunter DJ. Measurements of retinoids and carotenoids in breast adipose tissue and a comparison of concentrations in breast cancer cases and control subjects. Am J Clin Nutr 1997; 66:626–632.
150. Peto R, Doll R, Buckley JD, Sporn MB. Can dietary β-carotene materially reduce human cancer rates? Nature 1981; 290:201–208.
151. Block G, Patterson B, Subar A. Fruit, vegetable, and cancer prevention: a review of the epidemiological evidence. Nutr Cancer 1992; 18:1–29.
152. Omenn GS, Goodman GE, Thornquist MD. Effects of a combination of β-carotene and vitamin A on lung cancer and cardiovascular disease. N Engl J Med 1996; 334:1150–1155.
153. Wang X-D, Liu C, Bronson RT, Smith DE, Krinsky NI, Russell RM. Retinoid signaling and activator protein-1 expression in ferrets given β-carotene supplements and exposed to tobacco smoke. J Natl Cancer Inst 1999; 91:60–66.
154. CARIG. β-Carotene and the carotenoids: beyond the intervention trials. Nutr Rev 1996; 54:185–188.
155. Leo MA, Aleynik SI, Aleynik MK, Liebler CS. β-Carotene beadlets potentiate hepatotoxicity of alcohol. Am J Clin Nutr 1997; 66:1461–1469.
156. Strickland S, Mahdavi V. The induction of differentiation in teratocarcinomic stem cells by retinoic acid. Cell 1978; 15:393–403.
157. Grummer MA, Erdman JW Jr. Effect of chronic alcohol consumption and moderate or high fat diet upon tissue distribution of vitamin A or β-carotene. Nutr Res 1986; 6:61–73.
158. Albanes D, Heinonen O, Taylor P, Virtamo J, Edwards B, Rautalahti M, Hartman AM, Palmgren J, Freedman LS, Haapakoski J, Barrett MJ, Pietinen P, Malila N, Tala E, Liippo K, Salomaa P, Huttunen JK. α-Tocopherol and β-carotene supplements and lung cancer incidence in The alpha-Tocopherol, β-Carotene Cancer Prevention Study: effects of baseline characteristics. J Natl Cancer Inst 1996; 88:1560–1570.
159. Giovannucci E, Ascherio A, Rimm EB, Stampfer MJ, Colditz GA, Willett WC. Intake of carotenoids and retinol in relation to risk of prostate cancer. J Natl Cancer Inst 1995; 87:1767–1776.
160. Mills PK, Beeson L, Phillips RL, Fraser GE. Cohort study of diet, lifestyle, and prostate cancer in Adventist men. Cancer 1989; 64:598–604.
161. Gann PH, Ma J, Giovannucci E, Willet W, Sacks FM, Hennekens CH, Stampfer MJ. Lower prostate cancer risk in men with elevated plasma lycopene levels: results of a prospective analysis. Cancer Res 1999; 59:1225–1230.
162. McCormick DL, Rao KVN, Steele VE, Lubert RA, Kelloff GJ, Bosland MC. Chemoprevention of rat prostate carcinogenesis by 9-*cis* retinoic acid. Cancer Res 1999; 59:521–524.
163. Rao KVN, Johnson WD, Bosland MC, Lubert RA, Steele VE, Kelloff GJ, McCormick DL. Chemoprevention of rat prostate carcinogenesis by early and delayed administration of dehydroepiandrosterone. Cancer Res 1999; 59:3084–3089.
164. McCormick DL, Rao KVN, Dooley L, Steele VE, Lubet RA, Kelloff GJ, Bosland MC. Influence of *N*-methyl-*N*-nitrosourea, testosterone, and *N*-(4-hydroxyphenyl)-all-*trans*-retinamide on prostate cancer induction in Wistar Unilever rats. Cancer Res 1998; 58:3282–3288.
165. Williams AW, Boileau TWM, Zhou JR, Clinton SK, Erdman JW Jr. β-Carotene modulates human prostate cancer cell growth in vitro and evidence for conversion of β-carotene to retinol. J Nutr 2000; 130:728–732.
166. Boileau TWM, Clinton SK, Erdman JW Jr. Lycopene tissue accumulation and isomer patterns are determined by dietary lycopene concentration and androgen status in male F344 rats. J Nutr 2000; 130:1613–1618.

167. Ripple MO, Henry WF, Rago RP, Wilding G. Prooxidant–antioxidant shift induced by androgen treatment of human prostate carcinoma cells. J Natl Cancer Inst 1997; 89:40–48.
168. Cook NR, Stampfer MJ, Ma J, Manson JE, Sacks FM, Buring J, Hennekens CE. β-Carotene supplementation of low baseline levels and decreased risk of total prostate cancer. Cancer 1999; 86:1783–1792.
169. Williams AW, Boileau TWM, Clinton SK, Erdman JW Jr. β-Carotene stability and uptake by prostate cancer cells is dependent upon delivery vehicle. Nutr Cancer 2000; 36(2):185–190.
170. Census U. S., Bot. Statistical Brief: Sixty Plus in the United States. U. S. Dept of Commerce, Economics and Statistics Administration, 1995.
171. Klein BEK, Klein R, Linton KLP. Prevalence of age-related lens opacities in a population. The Beaver Dam Study. Ophthalmology 1992; 99:546–552.
172. Sperduto RD, Hiller R. The prevalence of nuclear, cortical, and posterior subcapsular lens opacities in a general population sample. Ophthalmology 1984; 91:815–818.
173. Brown L, Rimm EB, Seddon JM, Giovannucci EL, Chasan–Taber L, Spiegelman D, Willet WC, Hankinson SE. A prospective study of carotenoid intake and risk of cataract extraction in U. S. men. Am J Clin Nutr 1999; 70:517–524.
174. Chasan–Traber L, Willet WC, Seddon JM, Stampfer MJ, Rosner B, Colditz GA, Speizer FE, Hankinson SE. A prospective study of carotenoid and vitamin A intakes and risk of cataract extraction in U. S. women. Am J Clin Nutr 1999; 70:509–516.
175. Jacques PF, Chylack LTJ. Epidemiologic evidence of a role for the antioxidant vitamins and carotenoids in cataract prevention. Am J Clin Nutr 1991; 53:352S–355S.
176. Seddon JM, Ajani UA, Sperduto RD, Hiller R, Blair N, Burton TC, Farber MD, Gragoudas ES, Haller J, Miller DT, Yannuzzi LA, Willet W, The Eye Disease Case–Control Study Group. Dietary carotenoids, vitamins A, C, and E, and advanced age-related macular degeneration. JAMA 1994; 9272:1413–1420.
177. Handelman GJ, Dratz EA, Collin C, van Kujik FJGM. Carotenoids in the human macula and whole retina. Invest Ophthalmol Vis Sci 1988; 29:850–855.
178. Bates CJ, Chen S, Macdonald A, Holden R. Quantitation of vitamin E and a carotenoid pigment in cataractous human lenses, and the effect of a dietary supplement. Int J Vitam Nutr Res 1996; 66:316–321.
179. Yeum K–J, Shang FM, Schalch WM, Russell RM, Taylor A. Fat-soluble nutrient concentrations in different layers of the human cataractous lens. Curr Eye Res 1999; 19:502–505.
180. Schalch W. Carotenoids in the retina—a review of their possible role in preventing or limiting damage caused by light and oxygen. In: Emerit I, Chance B, eds. Free Radicals and Aging. Basel: Birkäuser Verlag, 1992.280–298.
181. Pratt S. Dietary prevention of age-related macular degeneration. J Am Optom Assoc 1999; 70: 39–47.
182. Hammond BRJ, Johnson EJ, Russell RM, Krinsky NI, Yeum K–J, Edwards RB, Snoddderly DM. Dietary modification of human macular pigment density. Invest Ophthalmol Vis Sci 1997; 38: 1795–1801.
183. Bone RA, Landrum JT, Tarsis SL. Preliminary identification of the human macular pigment. Vis Res 1985; 25:1531–1535.
184. Khachik F, Bernstein PS, Garland DL. Identification of lutein and zeaxanthin oxidation products in human and monkey retinas. Invest Ophthalmol Vis Sci 1997; 38:1802–1811.
185. Sommerburg O, Siems WG, Hurst JS, Lewis JW, Kliger DS, van Kuijk FJGM. Lutein and zeaxanthin are associated with photoreceptors in the human retina. Curr Eye Res 1999; 19:491–495.
186. Bernstein PS, Balashov NA, Tsong ED, Rando RR. Retinal tubulin binds macular carotenoids. Invest Ophthalmol Vis Sci 1997; 38:167–175.
187. Taylor A. Cataract: relationship between nutrition and oxidation. J Am Coll Nutr 1993; 12:138–146.
188. Bunce GE, Kinoshita J, Horowitz J. Nutritional factors in cataract. Annu Rev Nutr 1990; 10: 233–254.
189. Bhuyan KC, Bhuyan DK. Molecular mechanism of cataractogenesis: III. Toxic metabolites of oxygen as initiators of lipid peroxidation. Curr Eye Res 1984; 3:67–81.
190. Jacques PF, Taylor A. Micronutrients and age-related cataracts. In: Bendich A, Butterworth CE Jr, eds. Micronutrients. In Health and Disease Prevention. New York: Marcel Dekker, 1991:359–379.
191. Hammond BR, Wooten BR. Density of the human crystalline lens is related to the macular pigment carotenoids, lutein and zeaxanthin. Optom Vis Sci 1997; 74:499–504.

192. Mathews–Roth MM. Carotenoids in erythropoietic protoporphyria and other photosensitivity diseases. Ann NY Acad Sci 1993; 691:127–138.
193. Taylor CR, Stern RS, Leyden JJ, Gilchrest BA. Photoaging, photodamage, and photoprotection. J Am Acad Dermatol 1990; 22:1–15.
194. Prince MR, Frisoli JK. β-Carotene accumulation in serum and skin. Am J Clin Nutr 1993; 57:175–181.
195. Ribaya–Maercado JD, Garmyn M, Gilchrest BA, Russel RM. Skin lycopene is destroyed preferentially over β-carotene during ultraviolet irradiation in humans. J Nutr 1995; 125:1854–1859.
196. Biesalski HK, Hemmes C, Hopfenmuller W, Schmid C, Gollnick HP. Effects of controlled exposure of sunlight on plasma and skin levels of β-carotene. Free Radic Res 1996; 24:215–224.
197. Stahl W, Heinrich U, Jungmann H, von Laar J, Schietzel M, Seis H, Tronnier H. Increased dermal carotenoid levels by noninvasive reflection spectrophotometry correlate with serum levels in women ingesting Betatene. J Nutr 1998; 128:903–907.
198. Garmyn M, Ribaya–Mercado JD, Russel RM, Bhawan J, Gilchrest BA. Effect of β-carotene supplementation on the human sunburn reaction. Exp Dermatol 1995; 4:104–111.
199. Wingerath T, Seis H, Stahl W. Xanthophyll esters in human skin. Arch Biochem Biophys 1998; 355:271–274.
200. Stahl W, Heinrich U, Jungmann H, Sies H, Tronnier H. Carotenoids and carotenoids plus vitamin E protect against ultraviolet-light induced erythema in humans. Am J Clin Nutr 2000; 71:795–798.
201. Bar-Natan R, Lomnitski L, Sofer Y, Segman S, Neeman I, Grossman S. Interaction between β-carotene and lipoxygenase in human skin. Int J Biochem Cell Biol 1996; 28:935–941.
202. Lomnitski L, Grossman S, Bergman M, Sofer Y, Sklan D. In vitro and in vivo effects of β-carotene on rat epidermal lipoxygenases. Int J Vitam Nutr Res 1997; 67:407–414.
203. Morris DL, Kritchevsky SB, Davis CE. Serum carotenoids and coronary heart disease: The Lipid Research Clinics Coronary Primary Prevention Trial and Follow-Up Study. JAMA 1994; 2272:1439–1441.
204. Cooper DA, Eldridge AL, Peters JC. Dietary carotenoids and certain cancers, heart disease, and age-related macular degeneration: a review of recent research. Nutr Rev 1999; 57:201–214.
205. Princen HMG, van Poppel G, Vogelezang C, Buytenhek R, Kok FJ. Supplementation with vitamin E but not β-carotene in vivo protects low density lipoprotein from lipid peroxidation in vitro: effect of cigarette smoking. Arterioscler Thromb 1992; 12:554–562.
206. Gaziano JM, Hatta A, Flynn M, Johnson EJ, Krinsky NI, Ridker PM, Hennekens CH, Frei B. Supplementation with β-carotene in vivo and in vitro does not inhibit low density lipoprotein oxidation. Atherosclerosis 1995; 112:187–195.
207. Reaven PD, Khouw A, Beltz WF, Parthasarathy S, Witztum JL. Effect of dietary antioxidant combinations in humans: protection of LDL by vitamin E, but not by β-carotene. Arterioscler Thromb 1993; 13:590–600.
208. Rapola JM, Vortamo J, Ripatti S, Huttunen JK, Albanes D, Taylor PR, Heinonen OP. Randomized trial of alpha-tocopherol and β-carotene supplements on incidence of major coronary events in men with previous myocardial infarction. Lancet 1997; 349:1717–1720.
209. Blot WJ, Li J–Y, Taylor PR, Guo W, Dawsey S, Wang G–Q, Yang CS, Zheng S–F, Gail M, Li G–Y, Yu Y, Liu B–Q, Tangrea J, Sun Y–H, Liu F, Fraumeni JF Jr, Zhang Y–H, Li B. Nutrition intervention trials in Linxian, China: supplementation with specific vitamin/mineral combinations, cancer incidence, and disease-specific mortality in the general population. J Natl Cancer Inst 1993; 85:1483–1492.
210. Kushi LH, Folsom AR, Prineas RJ, Mink PJ, Wu Y, Bostick RM. Dietary antioxidant vitamins and death from coronary heart disease in postmenopausal women. N Engl J Med 1996; 334:1156–1162.
211. Gey FK, Stahelin HB, Eichholzer M. Poor plasma status of carotene and vitamin C is associated with higher mortality from ischemic heart disease and stroke: Basel Prospective Study. Clin Invest 1993; 71:3–6.
212. Kritchevsky SB, Tell GS, Shimakawa T, Dennis B, Li R, Kohlmeier L, Steere E, Heiss G. Provitamin A carotenoid intake and carotid artery plaques: the Atherosclerosis Risk in Communities Study. Am J Clin Nutr 1998; 68:726–733.
213. Lee IM, Cook NR, Manson JE, Buring JE, Hennekens CH. β-Carotene supplementation and incidence of cancer and cardiovascular disease: the Women's Health Study. J Natl Cancer Inst 1999; 91:2102–2106.

214. Kohlmeier L, Kark JD, Gomez–Garcia E, Martin BC, Stech SE, Kardinaal AF, Ringstad J, Thamm M, Massev V, Riemersma R, Martin–Moreno JM, Huttunen JK, Kolkand FJ. Lycopene and myocardial infarction. Am J Epidemiol 1997; 146:618–626.
215. Argarwal S, Rao V. Tomato lycopene and low density lipoprotein oxidation: a human dietary intervention study. Lipids 1998; 33:981–984.
216. Green HN, Mellanby E. Carotene and vitamin A: the anti-infective action of carotene. Br J Exp Pathol 1930; 11:81–89.
217. Karter DL, Karter AJ, Yarrish R, Patterson C, Kass PH, Nord J, Kislak JW. Vitamin A deficiency in non-vitamin supplemented patients with AIDS: a cross-sectional study. J Acquir Immune Defic Syndr 1995; 8:199–203.
218. Hennekens CH, Mayrent SL, Willet W. Vitamin A, carotenoids, and retinoids. Cancer 1986; 58: 1827–1841.
219. Bendich A. Antioxidant vitamins and immune response. In: Chandra RK, ed. Nutrition and Immunology. New York: Alan R. Liss, 1988:125–147.
220. Chew BP. Role of carotenoids in the immune response. J Dairy Sci 1993; 76:2804–2811.
221. Schwartz JL, Singh RJ, Teicher B, Wright JE, Trites DH, Shklar G. Induction of a 70-kD protein associated with the selective cytotoxicity of the β-carotene in human epidermal carcinoma. Biochim Biophys Commun 1990; 169:941–946.
222. Halevy O, Sklan D. Inhibition of arachadonic acid oxidation by β-carotene, retinol, and α-tocopherol. Biochim Biophys Acta 1987; 918:304–307.
223. Jyonouchi H, Zang L, Gross M, Tomita Y. Immunomodulating actions of carotenoids: enhancement of in vivo and in vitro antibody production to T-dependent antigens. Nutr Cancer 1994; 21:47–58.
224. Jyonouchi H, Sun S, Gross M. Effect of carotenoids on in vitro immunoglobulin production by human peripheral blood mononuclear cells: astaxanthin, a carotenoid without vitamin A activity, enhances in vitro response to a T-dependent stimulant antigen. Nutr Cancer 1995; 23:171–183.
225. Van Poppel G, Spanhaak G, Ockhuizen T. Effect of β-carotene on immunological indexes in healthy male smokers. Am J Clin Nutr 1993; 57:402–407.
226. Bendich A, Shapiro SS. Effect of β-carotene and canthaxanthin on the immune responses of the rat. J Nutr 1986; 116:2254–2262.
227. Kramer TR, Burri BJ. Modulated mitogenic proliferative responsiveness of lymphocytes in whole-blood cultures after a low-carotene diet and mixed-carotenoid supplementation in women. Am J Clin Nutr 1997; 65:871–875.
228. Watson R, Prabhala R, Plezia P, Alberts D. Effect of β-carotene on lymphocyte sub-populations in elderly humans: evidence for a dose–response relationship. Am J Clin Nutr 1991, 53:90–94.
229. Santos MS, Meydani SN, Leka L, Wu D, Fotouhi N, Meydani M, Hennekens CH, Gaziano JM. Natural killer cell activity in elderly men is enhanced by β-carotene supplementation. Am J Clin Nutr 1996; 64:772–777.
230. Santos MS, Leka LS, Ribay–Mercado JD, Russell RM, Maydani M, Hennekens CH, Gaziano JM, Meydani SN. Short- and long-term β-carotene supplementation do not influence T-cell mediated immunity in healthy elderly persons. Am J Clin Nutr 1997; 66:917–924.
231. Punnonen K, Autio P, Kiistala U. In-vivo effects of solar-simulated ultraviolet irradiation on antioxidant enzymes and lipid peroxidation in human epidermis. Br J Dermatol 1991; 125:18.
232. Gensler HL. Reduction of immunosuppression in UV-irradiated mice by dietary retinyl palmitate plus canthaxanthin. Carcinogenesis 1989; 10;203–207.
233. Fuller CJ, Faulkner H, Bendich A, Parker RS, Roe DA. Effect of β-carotene supplementation on photosuppression of delayed-type hypersensitivity in normal young men. Am J Clin Nutr 1992; 56:684–690.
234. Krinsky NI. Cellular aspects of carotenoid actions. In: Cadenas E, Packer L, eds. Handbook of Antioxidants. New York: Marcel Dekker, 1996:315–336.

11
Antioxidant Effects of Carotenoids: Implication in Photoprotection in Humans

Wilhelm Stahl and Helmut Sies
Heinrich-Heine-Universität, Düsseldorf, Germany

I. INTRODUCTION

The sun provides energy necessary for life on earth, and its electromagnetic spectrum covers γ- and x-ray, ultraviolet (UV) and visible light, as well as infrared (IR) and microwave radiation. Relative to photooxidative stress and diseases related to sun exposure, UV and visible radiation play a particularly important role. This includes the spectrum from 280 to 750 nm, that comprises UVB (280–315 nm), UVA (315–380 nm), and visible light (380–750 nm). Most of the UV light is absorbed by the ozone layer of the atmosphere, and less than 4% of the UVB intensity reaches the surface of earth. However, the thickness of the shielding ozone layer is decreasing; therefore, exposure to UV light increases. UV light is directly damaging to living organisms by inducing chemical reactions with relevant biomolecules. Visible light drives photosynthesis, which is essential for converting radiation energy. However, visible light may also cause damage resulting from physicochemical processes, reactive oxygen species being formed in light-exposed tissues. The modification of biologically important molecules in photooxidative reactions has been associated with pathological processes in the development of several diseases of light-exposed tissue, including cataract, age-related macular degeneration, skin cancer, skin aging, or skin erythema formation. There is increasing evidence that dietary antioxidants such as carotenoids, tocopherols, or ascorbate protect against photooxidative reactions.

II. CAROTENOIDS: ANTIOXIDANT FUNCTION

Carotenoids are a class of structurally related compounds found in plants, algae, and several lower organisms (1). Because of the presence of an extended system of conjugated double bonds the carotenoids are deeply colored in yellow, orange, or red (Fig. 1). The absorption maxima depend on the number of conjugated double bonds ranging from 400 to 500 nm. The major sources for carotenoids in the human diet are fruits and vegetables, containing

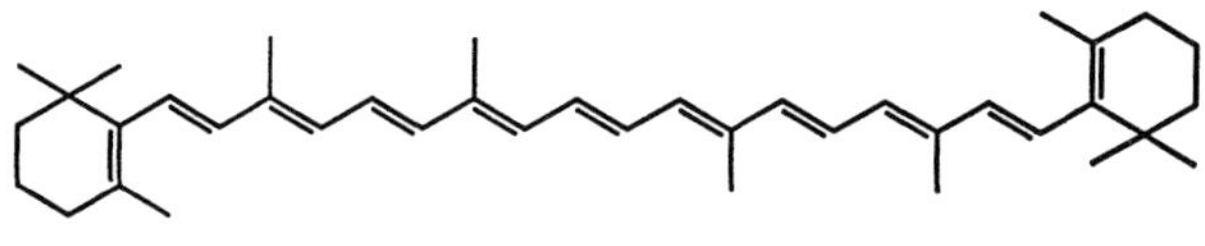

β-Carotene

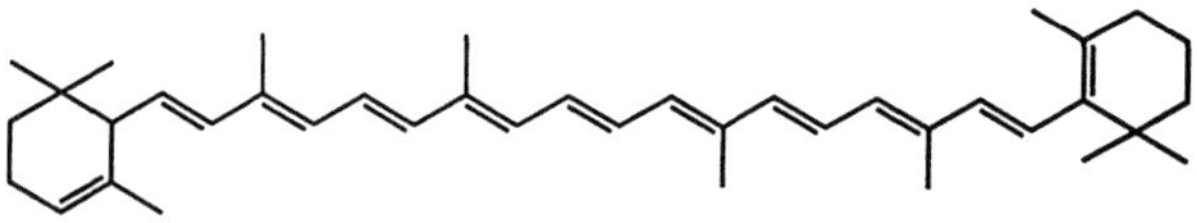

α-Carotene

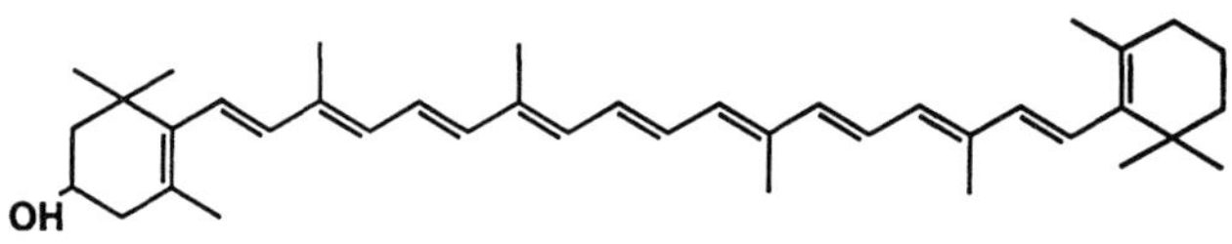

β-Cryptoxanthin

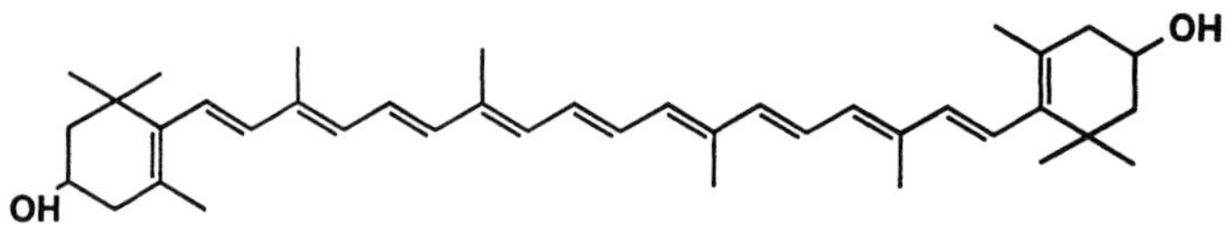

Zeaxanthin

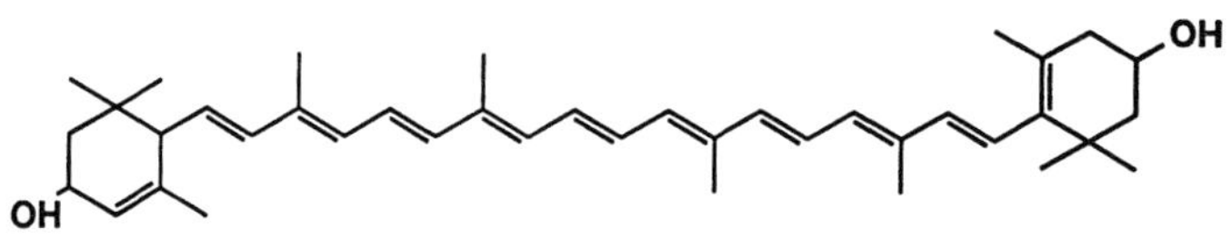

Lutein

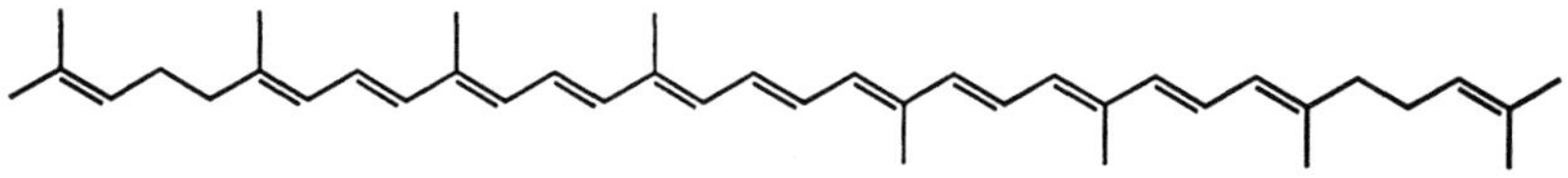

Lycopene

Figure 1 Chemical structures of carotenoids.

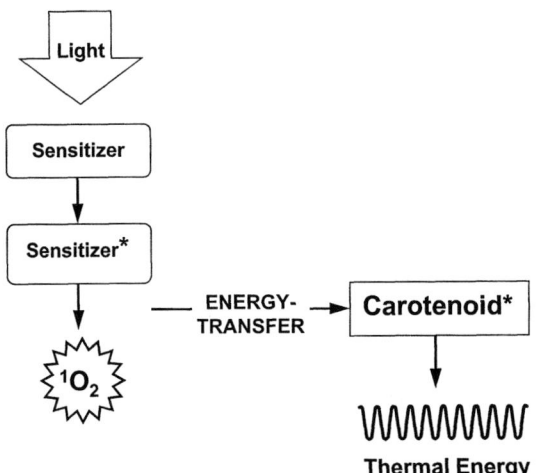

Figure 2 Formation of singlet oxygen by irradiation in the presence of a sensitizer—quenching of singlet oxygen by carotenoids.

α-carotene, β-carotene, lycopene, lutein, zeaxanthin, and β-cryptoxanthin (2,3). Carotenoids are efficient scavengers of reactive oxygen species, especially singlet molecular oxygen and peroxyl radicals. Furthermore, they are capable of quenching excited triplet states, which is an important property for their photoprotective effects in plants.

Singlet molecular oxygen ($^1O_2$) is the electronically excited form of oxygen, formed in biological systems by type II photosensitization reactions (Fig. 2); for example, in light-exposed tissue (4,5). $^1O_2$ can interact with target molecules either by transferring its excitation energy or by chemical reaction. Preferential targets for chemical reactions are double bonds; for example, in polyunsaturated fatty acids or in guanine bases in DNA (6–10).

Carotenoids scavenge singlet oxygen by physical or chemical quenching (11–13). Physical quenching involves the transfer of excitation energy from $^1O_2$ to the carotenoid, resulting in ground-state oxygen and an excited triplet-state carotenoid (see Fig. 2). The energy is dissipated between the excited carotenoid and the surrounding solvent to yield a nonreactive ground-state carotenoid and thermal energy. In the process of physical quenching the carotenoid remains intact, so that it can undergo further cycles of singlet oxygen quenching. The rate constants for the reaction of carotenoids with singlet oxygen are in the range of 10^9 M^{-1} s^{-1} (14,15). Chemical quenching contributes less than 0.05% to the overall quenching of $^1O_2$ by carotenoids. However, this process, known as photobleaching, is responsible for the final decomposition of carotenoids.

Carotenoids efficiently scavenge peroxyl radicals, especially at low oxygen tension (16–19). In this process the carotenoid reacts chemically with the radical. Carotenoids act synergistically in this process with tocopherol (20); mixtures of carotenoids are more effective than single compounds (21).

III. AGE-RELATED MACULAR DEGENERATION

Oxidative damage and antioxidant protection in ocular tissues is of increasing interest, as the organ is highly susceptible to damage by sunlight and reactive oxygen species (22). The present chapter will focus on photooxidative damage of the lens and the macula lutea and the implication of carotenoids in protection. The macula lutea ("yellow spot") is part of the retina, and it is the area of maximal visual acuity, dedicated to high-resolution tasks and detailed color discrimination (23,24). The visual axis meets the retina at the fovea centralis. Lutein and zeaxanthin are the pigments responsible for coloration of this tissue (25–27). These carotenoids are so-called xanthophylls or oxocarotenoids and carry two functional hydroxyl groups. Other important carotenoids, such as lycopene, α-carotene, or β-carotene, which are present in the blood and in most human tissues (28), are not found in the macula lutea.

Age-related macular degeneration (AMD) is a major cause for irreversible blindness among the elderly in the Western world and it affects about 20% of the population older than the age of 65 years (23,29). Several risk factors for AMD have been identified and include advanced age; light skin and eye color; high exposure to sunlight; and low dietary intake and low serum levels of xanthophylls (30–32); a genetic disposition has been suggested (33). The disease develops gradually over many years and occurs in two major forms: dry AMD, characterized by atrophic pigment epithelium and the presence of drusen; and wet AMD, characterized by neovascularization (29).

Only limited information is now available on the biochemical mechanisms involved in the development of the disease. Epidemiological studies, in vivo and in vitro data, as well as analyses of the risk factors suggest that photooxidative damage plays an important role in the pathobiochemistry of AMD (23,24,34,35).

In the presence of appropriate sensitizers singlet molecular oxygen may be formed in light-exposed tissues, which further reacts to yield other reactive oxygen species capable of damaging proteins, lipids, and DNA (5,36). Drusen, which are characteristic of dry AMD, are rich in lipids, and it has been supposed that they form when lipofuscin accumulates in the retinal pigment epithelium (23). Lipofuscin is an indigestible, fluorescent product of lipid oxidation including some oxidation products of vitamin A (35). Excessive blue light may increase its formation. In vitro studies demonstrate that lipofuscin acts as a photosensitizer (37). After photoactivation of lipofuscin granules, singlet oxygen and other reactive oxygen species, including superoxide anion, hydrogen peroxide, or lipid hydroperoxides, are generated. The action spectrum of singlet oxygen formation indicates that this process is strongly wavelength-dependent, and its efficiency decreased with increasing wavelength by a factor of ten, comparing 420 and 520 nm (38). The quantum yield of singlet oxygen increased with increasing concentration of oxygen. A possible mechanism of singlet oxygen formation was studied with laser flash photolysis (38). A triplet intermediate with a broad absorption spectrum peaking at near 440 nm was identified; it was quenched by β-carotene with concomitant formation of a β-carotene triplet state. These results indicate the potential role of lipofuscin in blue light-induced damage to the retina pigment epithelium related to the formation singlet molecular oxygen. However, other sensitizers may also be involved in such processes (35). Most carotenoids are efficient antioxidants, quenching singlet oxygen and trapping peroxyl radicals (36), and lycopene is the most efficient singlet oxygen quencher of the natural carotenoids (39). The rate constants for the reaction of lutein and zeaxanthin with singlet oxygen are in the range of 10^9 M^{-1} s^{-1} (39,40). Both these compounds may also act as blue-light filters with the absorption maxima being at near 450 nm, with extinction coefficients of more than 120,000 M^{-1} cm^{-1} (41).

Epidemiological data support the concept that the macular pigment has a protective role. In the multicenter Eye Disease Case–Control Study (42) a high dietary intake of carotenoids was associated with a diminished risk for AMD; a strong epidemiological association was found for lutein and zeaxanthin. Among the different carotenoid sources, the strongest correlation between intake and diminished risk was found for spinach, a vegetable rich in lutein. Short-term positive effects on the visual function of AMD patients were observed after increased consumption of spinach (43). In comparison with controls unaffected by AMD, lower serum levels of lutein and zeaxanthin were found in patients suffering from AMD (44,45). It should be noted that data are still conflicting, and some smaller studies did not report correlations between lutein and zeaxanthin serum levels and the risk for AMD (24). Protective effects have also been reported for other carotenoids, including β-carotene and lycopene (45). However, these compounds do not occur in the macula lutea. Other antioxidant vitamins, such as ascorbate or tocopherol, appear to be of minor importance in the protection from AMD (31,46).

Lutein serum levels can be increased after supplementation or dietary modification (23,47). After ingestion of 30 mg/day of lutein for 3 weeks, serum levels of about 1.7 nmol/mL were measured, an increase from about 0.1 nmol/mL at baseline. This was accompanied by an increase in the optical density of the macular pigment, as determined by heterochromatic flicker photometry.

It is unknown why lutein and zeaxanthin are selected as macular pigments, although other carotenoids are available in the organism. There is also no explanation for the different topographical distribution of these carotenoids in the macula. Lutein dominates over zeaxanthin in human serum and tissues, but the latter is found enriched in the center of the macula lutea (23,24). The ratio of lutein/zeaxanthin increases in outer segments of the tissue. Specific membrane-stabilizing effects of zeaxanthin may be the reason. In contrast to β-carotene, lutein, and zeaxanthin are specifically oriented perpendicular to the plane of the membrane owing to the interaction of their hydroxyl groups with hydrophilic segments of the membrane (48,49).

meso-Zeaxanthin ($3R,3'S$-zeaxanthin), an optical isomer of the natural $3R,3'R$-form, is found in high amounts in the center of the macula, which is unusual because this compound does not occur in dietary sources, serum, or other tissues (23). The $3R,3'S$-zeaxanthin might be formed in enzymatic, chemical, or photochemical reactions in the center of the macula.

Summing up, there is increasing evidence that the carotenoids lutein and zeaxanthin are involved in the protection of the macula lutea, preventing macular degeneration. However, final proof requires appropriate intervention studies.

IV. CATARACT

Cataract is an age-related eye disease and one of the major causes of impaired vision worldwide. The oxidation of lens proteins is thought to play an important role in the development and progression of cataractous lesions (50). Most likely, reactive oxygen species generated in photochemical reactions within the lens are the damaging agents. Because the turnover of lens proteins is slow with a half-life of decades, altered proteins may accumulate, aggregate, and finally precipitate in opacities. Additionally, reactive oxygen species are capable of modifying repair enzymes important for elimination of dysfunctional proteins and thus accelerate cataractogenesis (50).

There is increasing evidence that dietary and endogenous antioxidants provide protection against oxidative modification of proteins and are involved in the maintenance of lens function. Primary defense to protect from oxidative insult consist of low molecular weight antioxidants, such as ascorbate, tocopherol, glutathione, and carotenoids; the major antioxidant enzymes superoxide dismutase, catalase, and glutathione peroxidase contribute to protection. Several epidemiological studies on the relation between antioxidant nutrients and cataract risk revealed a lower risk for individuals with a high intake or blood level of vitamin C, vitamin E, vitamin A, and carotenoids (50). The most convincing data have been presented for vitamin C. Long-term supplementation with vitamin C over a period of more than 10 years was associated with a 77% lower prevalence of early lens opacities (51) and also with a lower incidence of cataract extraction (52). Lens vitamin C levels are significantly decreased with cataract severity (53).

Inconsistent findings have been reported for the lipophilic antioxidants. Plasma tocopherol levels were inversely associated with nuclear opacities as reported in the Baltimore Longitudinal Study on Aging and the Lens Opacities Case–Control Study (54–56); no significant correlation was found in the Italian–American Cataract Study and the India–U.S. Case–Control Study (57,58). Data on the effects of carotenoids in cataract prevention are conflicting. Individuals with high carotenoid plasma levels had a diminished prevalence of cataract, compared with persons with low carotenoid levels (59), but no association between carotenoid intake and cataract incidence could be demonstrated. Serum carotenoid and tocopherol levels and their relation to cataractous lesions was studied in a sample of 400 adults from the Beaver Dam Eye Study (60). Here, only serum tocopherol was inversely related to cataract. A marginal inverse association was found for lutein and cryptoxanthin. However, data from another study showed that the dietary intake of lutein and zeaxanthin is associated with a lower risk for cataract extraction; no significant effects were found for other carotenoids or vitamin A (61). In an intervention trial (ATBC Study), supplementation with either β-carotene or α-tocopherol had no effect on the incidence of cataract among male smokers (62). Carotenoid levels in the lens are quite low. In contrast to vitamin C, which is concentrated in this tissue against a steep concentration gradient, carotenoids appear to play a minor role in the antioxidant defense system of the lens.

V. SKIN PROTECTION

Skin is a large and complex organ consisting of distinct layers: stratum corneum, epidermis, and dermis. Its primary physiological function is that of a barrier protecting against mechanical force, contaminants, pathogenic microorganisms, or radiation ranging from UV to IR. Extensive exposure to sunlight affects the skin and may result in skin damage (63). Acute effects include erythema and photosensitivity reactions; long-term consequences are carcinogenesis and photoaging. In addition to irradiation the skin is continuously exposed to oxygen. The presence of both factors is required for photochemical reactions, yielding reactive oxygen species (64). Photooxidative stress is thought to be involved in the pathogenesis of several skin diseases. UV light is a major component of the solar spectrum and produces reactive oxygen species by interaction with cellular chromophores. Singlet molecular oxygen and hydrogen peroxide are suggested to be the most important reactive oxygen species formed on UV exposure. Further reactive oxygen species can be generated by iron-catalyzed reactions, including the highly reactive hydroxyl radical; iron may be released from cellular stores by UV light (65). UV light induces damage typical for reactive oxygen species, such as protein modification, lipid peroxidation, or DNA damage, resulting in the formation of thymine dimers or 8-oxo-7,8-dihydrodeoxyguanosine (66,67).

In the presence of suitable sensitizers, visible light also induces photochemical reactions. An example for that is the inherited disease erythropoietic protoporphyria (EPP) (68,69). EPP is characterized by elevated levels of protoporphyrin, an efficient sensitizer molecule, and sensitivity to visible light in the range of 380–560 nm. The patients experience burning sensation followed by erythema formation. It has been suggested that $^1O_2$ or excited triplet intermediates, or both, are responsible for the symptoms, which are ameliorated by high doses of β-carotene.

Ultraviolet light affects signal transduction and ultimately gene expression in exposed tissues (70). These effects overlap with signaling pathways responsive to reactive oxygen species, as it has been demonstrated for the activation of the transcription factors NF-κB or AP-1 (71).

The skin is equipped with several antioxidant defense systems and contains carotenoids, ascorbate, glutathione, tocopherols, ubiquinone, as well as several antioxidant enzymes, such as glutathione peroxidase or superoxide dismutase. It is thought that these enzymes contribute to the protection of skin against photooxidative damage, although further evidence from clinical trials is needed to confirm this suggestion (72,73). Antioxidants are depleted after UV irradiation and oxidative damage is observed (74).

The levels of carotenoids in skin are different in different areas (75). When using reflection spectroscopy, higher basal values were measured in skin of the forehead, palm of the hand, and dorsal skin; lower levels were found in skin of the arm and the back of the hand. After treatment, increases in carotenoid skin levels are found in all areas. In facial skin, the mean β-carotene values of about 0.1–0.3 nmol/g wet tissue have been measured by means of HPLC (76); lutein and α-carotene concentrations were lower. Small amounts of xanthophyll esters are detectable in skin tissues (77). Higher levels at about 1.5 nmol/g wet tissue are found when subcutaneous fat is included in sample analyses (78).

Several in vitro and animal studies have shown protective effects of β-carotene and other carotenoids on skin cancer, whereas other studies provided no evidence for protection. The results of epidemiological studies showed no diminished risk for skin cancer associated with dietary intake or blood levels of β-carotene. No diminished risk for basal- or squamous-cell skin cancer after supplementation with β-carotene for up to 5 years was determined in a clinical trial (79). Data on intervention studies with other carotenoids are not available.

β-Carotene is often supplemented before sun exposure to prevent sunburn reactions. The protective effects are thought to be related to the antioxidant properties of the carotenoid, because photooxidative damage is considered to be involved in the pathobiochemistry of erythema formation. The data obtained in different studies on this topic are conflicting. Gollnick et al. (80) found that the development of erythema induced by natural sunlight was lower under supplementation with β-carotene; treatment was with 30 mg of β-carotene per day for 10 weeks. A slight but statistically significant protective effect of oral supplementation with β-carotene on the prevention of erythema was also reported by Mathews–Roth and co-workers (81). In this study high doses of 180 mg/day of β-carotene were applied for a period of 10 weeks. Volunteers were exposed to natural sunlight for up to 2 h and the protective effects were attributed to an increase in the minimal erythema dose after treatment. In another study, carotenoid supplementation (25 mg/day of carotenoids) was given over 12 weeks (82). Erythema was induced by illumination with a blue-light solar simulator. In this study, erythema formation on dorsal skin was significantly diminished from week 8 on.

However, no effects were reported in a study for which 90 mg/day of β-carotene were applied for 3 weeks (83). Treatment with β-carotene provided no clinically or histologically detectable protection when skin was irradiated with 3 MED to provoke a sunburn reaction. The authors concluded that β-carotene supplementation is unlikely to modify the severity of cutaneous photodamage. No protection against erythema formation was also found (84) when the volunteers received 150 mg/day of oral carotenoids over 4 weeks.

Because of differences in the study design for doses, duration of treatment, or UV exposure, it is difficult to compare these studies directly. However, it is interesting that in the studies in which protective effects were found, treatment with carotenoids was for at least 10 weeks, whereas only a 3- to 4-week treatment design was applied in the studies that showed no effects.

VI. CONCLUSION

Carotenoids are efficient scavengers of reactive oxygen species, and there is increasing evidence that these natural polyenes play a role in the protection against photooxidative damage. Data are most promising for the preventive effects of oral treatment with carotenoids on erythema formation. More research is necessary to provide insight in the very important relation that probably exists between lutein and zeaxanthin intake and the protection against age-related macular degeneration.

ACKNOWLEDGMENTS

Our studies were supported by the VERUM Foundation, Munich, and by the European Community (FAIR CT 97-3100). H.S. is a Fellow of the National Foundation for Cancer Research (NFCR) Bethesda, MD.

REFERENCES

1. Olson JA, Krinsky NI. Introduction: the colorful fascinating world of the carotenoids: important physiologic modulators. FASEB J 1995; 9:1547–1550.
2. Olmedilla B, Granado F, Blanco I, Rojas–Hidalgo E. Seasonal and sex-related variations in six serum carotenoids, retinol, and α-tocopherol. Am J Clin Nutr 1994; 60:106–110.
3. Khachik F, Spangler CJ, Smith JC, Canfield LM, Steck A, Pfander H. Identification, quantification, and relative concentrations of carotenoids and their metabolites in human milk and serum. Anal Chem 1997; 69:1873–1881.
4. Kanofsky JR. Singlet oxygen production in biological systems. Chem Biol Interact 1989; 70:1–28.
5. Kanofsky JR. Singlet oxygen in biological systems: a comparison of biochemical and photochemical mechanisms for singlet oxygen generation. In: Tarr M, Samson F, eds. Oxygen Free Radicals in Tissue Damage. Boston: Birkhäuser, 1993:77–92.
6. Halliwell B, Gutteridge JMC. Free Radicals in Biology and Medicine. Oxford: Clarendon, 1989.
7. Piette J. Mutagenic and genotoxic properties of singlet oxygen. J Photochem Photobiol B Biol 1990; 4:335–339.
8. Briviba K, Klotz LO, Sies H. Toxic and signaling effects of photochemically or chemically generated singlet oxygen in biological systems. Biol Chem 1997; 378:1259–1265.
9. Sies H, Menck CFM. Singlet oxygen induced DNA damage. Mutat Res 1992; 275:367–375.
10. Sies H. Biochemistry of oxidative stress. Angew Chem Int Ed Engl 1986; 25:1058–1071.
11. Edge R, McGarvey DJ, Truscott TG. The carotenoids as antioxidants—a review. J Photochem Photobiol B Biol 1997; 41:189–200.
12. Stahl W, Sies H. Physical quenching of singlet oxygen and cis–trans isomerization of carotenoids. Ann NY Acad Sci 1993; 691:10–19.
13. Foote CS, Denny RW. Chemistry of singlet oxygen. VII. Quenching by β-carotene. J Am Chem Soc 1968; 90:6233–6235.
14. Baltschun D, Beutner S, Briviba K, Martin H–D, Paust J, Peters M, Röver S, Sies H, Stahl W, Steigel A, Stenhorst F. Singlet oxygen quenching abilities of carotenoids. Liebigs Ann 1997; 1887–1893.
15. Fukuzawa K, Inokami Y, Tokumura A, Terao J, Suzuki A. Rate constants for quenching singlet oxygen and activities for inhibiting lipid peroxidation of carotenoids and α-tocopherol in liposomes. Lipids 1998; 33:751–756.
16. Burton GW, Ingold KU. β-Carotene: an unusual type of lipid antioxidant. Science 1984; 224:569–573.
17. Kennedy TA, Liebler DC. Peroxyl radical scavenging by β-carotene in lipid bilayers. J Biol Chem 1992; 267:4658–4663.
18. Palozza P, Krinsky NI. Antioxidant effects of carotenoids in vivo and in vitro: an overview. Methods Enzymol 1992; 213:403–420.
19. Rice–Evans CA, Sampson J, Bramley PM, Holloway DE. Why do we expect carotenoids to be antioxidants in vivo? Free Radic Res 1997; 26:381–398.

20. Palozza P, Moualla S, Krinsky NI. Effects of β-carotene and α-tocopherol on radical-initiated peroxidation of microsomes. Free Radic Biol Med 1992; 13:127–136.
21. Stahl W, Junghans A, de Boer B, Driomina E, Briviba K, Sies H. Carotenoid mixtures protect multilamellar liposomes against oxidative damage: synergistic effects of lycopene and lutein. FEBS Lett 1998; 427:305–308.
22. Rose RC, Picher SP, Bode AM. Ocular oxidants and antioxidant protection. Proc Soc Exp Biol Med 1998; 217:397–407.
23. Landrum JT, Bone RA, Kilburn MD. The macular pigment: a possible role in protection from age-related macular degeneration. Adv Pharmacol 1997; 38:537–556.
24. Schalch W, Dayhaw–Barker P, Barker FM. The carotenoids of the human retina. In: Taylor A, ed. Nutritional and Environmental Influences on the Eye. Boca Raton, FL: CRC Press, 1999:215–250.
25. Snodderly DM, Brown PK, Delori FC, Auran JD. The macular pigment. I. Absorbance spectra, localization, and discrimination from other yellow pigments in primate retinas. Invest Ophthalmol Vis Sci 1984; 25:660–673.
26. Bone RA, Landrum JT, Tarsis SL. Preliminary identification of the human macular pigment. Vis Res 1985; 11:1531–1535.
27. Handelman GJ, Dratz EA, Reay CC, van Kuijk FJGM. Carotenoids in the human macula and whole retina. Invest Ophthalmol Vis Sci 1988; 29:850–855.
28. Stahl W, Schwarz W, Sundquist AR, Sies H. cis–trans Isomers of lycopene and β-carotene in human serum and tissues. Arch Biochem Biophys 1992; 294:173–177.
29. Hyman L. Epidemiology of AMD. In: Hampton GR, Nelsen PT, eds. Age-Related Macular Degeneration: Principles and Practice. New York: Raven Press, 1992:1–35.
30. Sandberg MA, Gaudio AR, Miller S, Weiner A. Iris pigmentation and extent of disease in patients with neovascular age-related macular degeneration. Invest Ophthalmol Vis Sci 1994; 353:2734–2740.
31. Christen WG, Ajani UA, Glynn RJ, Manson JE, Schaumberg DA, Chew EC, Buring JE, Hennekens CH. Prospective cohort study of antioxidant vitamin supplement use and the risk of age-related maculopathy. Am J Epidemiol 1999; 149:476–484.
32. Seddon JM, Willett WC, Speizer FE, Hankinson SE. A prospective study of cigarette smoking and age-related macular degeneration in women. JAMA 1996; 276:1141–1146.
33. Allikmets R, Shroyer NF, Singh N, Seddon JM, Lewis RA, Bernstein PS, Pfeiffer A, Zabriskie NA, Li Y, Hutchinson A, Dean M, Lupski JR, Leppert M. Mutation of the Stargardt disease gene (ABCR) in age-related macular degeneration. Science 1997; 277:1805–1807.
34. Schalch W. Carotenoids in the retina—a review of their possible role in preventing or limiting damage caused by light and oxygen. In: Emerit I, Chance B, eds. Free Radicals and Aging. Basel: Birkhäuser Verlag, 1992:280–298.
35. Snodderly DM. Evidence for protection against age-related macular degeneration by carotenoids and antioxidant vitamins. Am J Clin Nutr 1995; 62:1448S–1461S.
36. Sies H, Stahl W. Vitamins E and C, β-carotene, and other carotenoids as antioxidants. Am J Clin Nutr 1995; 62:1315S–1321S.
37. Rozanowska M, Jarvis–Evans J, Korytowski W, Boulton ME, Burke JM, Sarna T. Blue light-induced reactivity of retinal age pigment. In vitro generation of oxygen-reactive species. J Biol Chem 1995; 270:18825–18830.
38. Rozanowska M, Wessels J, Boulton M, Burke JM, Rodgers MA, Truscott TG, Sarna T. Blue light-induced singlet oxygen generation by retinal lipofuscin in non-polar media. Free Radic Biol Med 1998; 24:1107–1112.
39. Di Mascio P, Kaiser S, Sies H. Lycopene as the most efficient biological carotenoid singlet oxygen quencher. Arch Biochem Biophys 1989; 274:532–538.
40. Conn PF, Schalch W, Truscott TG. The singlet oxygen carotenoid interaction. J Photochem Photobiol B Biol 1991; 11:41–47.
41. Britton G, Liaaen–Jensen S, Pfander H. Carotenoids. Vol. 1B: Spectroscopy. Basel: Birkhäuser Verlag, 1995:57–61.
42. Seddon JM, Ajani UA, Sperduto RD, Hiller R, Blair N, Burton TC, Farber MD, Gragoudas ES, Haller J, Miller DT, Yannuuzzi LA, Willett WC. Dietary carotenoids, vitamins A, C, and E, and advanced age-related macular degeneration. JAMA 1994; 272:1413–1420.
43. Richer S. Part II: ARMD-pilot (case series) environmental intervention data. J Am Optom Assoc 1999; 70:24–36.

44. Eye Disease Case–Control Study Group. Antioxidant status and neovascular age-related macular degeneration. Arch Ophthalmol 1993; 111:104–109.
45. Mares–Perlman JA, Brady WE, Klein R, Klein BEK, Bowen P, Stacewicz–Sapuntzakis M, Palta M. Serum antioxidants and age-related macular degeneration in a population-based case–control study. Arch Ophthalmol 1995; 113:1518–1523.
46. Smith W, Mitchell P, Rochester C. Serum beta carotene, alpha tocopherol, and age-related maculopathy: the Blue Mountains Eye Study. Am J Ophthalmol 1997; 124:838–840.
47. Hammond BR, Johnson EJ, Russell RM, Krinsky NI, Yeum K–J, Edwards RB, Snodderly DM. Dietary modification of human macular pigment density. Invest Ophthalmol Vis Sci 1997; 38:1795–1801.
48. Gabrielska J, Gruszecki WI. Zeaxanthin (dihydroxy-β-carotene) but not β-carotene rigidifies lipid membranes: a H-NMR study of carotenoid–egg phosphatidylcholine liposomes. Biochim Biophys Acta 1996; 1285:167–174.
49. Gruszecki WI, Sielewiesiuk J. Orientation of xanthophylls in phosphatidylcholine multilayers. Biochim Biophys Acta 1990; 1023:405–412.
50. Taylor A, Nowell T. Oxidative stress and antioxidant function in relation to risk for cataract. Adv Pharmacol 1997; 38:516–536.
51. Jacques PF, Taylor A, Hankinson SE, Willett WC, Mahnken B, Lee Y, Vaid K, Lahav M. Long-term vitamin C supplement use and prevalence of early age-related lens opacities. Am J Clin Nutr 1997; 66:911–916.
52. Hankinson SE, Stampfer MJ, Seddon JM, Colditz GA, Rosner B, Speizer FE, Willett WC. Nutrient intake and cataract extraction in women: a prospective study. Br Med J 1992; 305:335–339.
53. Tessier F, Moreaux V, Birlouez–Aragon I, Junes P, Mondon H. Decrease in vitamin C concentration in human lenses during cataract progression. Int J Vitam Nutr Res 1998; 68:309–315.
54. Vitale S, West S, Hallfrisch J, Alston C, Wan F, Moorman C, Muller D, Singh V, Taylor HR. Plasma antioxidants and risk of cortical and nuclear cataract. Epidemiology 1993; 4:195–203.
55. Leske MC, Chylack LT, He Q, Wu S–Y, Schoenfeld E, Friend J, Wolfe J. Antioxidant vitamins and nuclear opacities. Ophthalmology 1998; 105:831–836.
56. Leske MC, Wu S–Y, Hyman L, Sperduto R, Underwood B, Chylack LT, Milton RC, Srivastava S, Ansari N. Biochemical factors in the lens opacities. Case–control study. The Lens Opacities Case–Control Study Group. Arch Ophthalmol 1995; 113:1113–1119.
57. The Italien–American Cataract Study Group. Risk factors for age-related cortical, nuclear, and posterior subcapsular cataracts. Am J Epidemiol 1991; 133:541–553.
58. Mohan M, Sperduto RD, Angra SK, Milton RC, Mathur RL, Underwood BA, Jaffery N, Pandya CB, Chhabra VK, Vajpayee RB, Kalra VK, Sharma YR. India–US case–control study of age-related cataracts. India–US Case–Control Study Group. Arch Ophthalmol 1989; 107:670–676.
59. Jacques PF, Chylack LT. Epidemiologic evidence of a role for the antioxidant vitamins and carotenoids in cataract prevention. Am J Clin Nutr 1991; 53:352S–355S.
60. Lyle BL, Mares–Perlman JA, Klein BEK, Klein R, Palta M, Bowen PE, Greger JL. Serum carotenoids and tocopherols and incidence of age-related nuclear cataract. Am J Clin Nutr 1999; 69:272–277.
61. Chasan–Taber L, Willett WC, Seddon JM, Stampfer MJ, Rosner B, Colditz GA, Speizer FE, Hankinson SE. A prospective study of carotenoid and vitamin A intakes and risk of cataract extraction in US women. Am J Clin Nutr 1999; 70:509–516.
62. Teikari JM, Rautalahti M, Haukka J, Järvinen P, Hartman AM, Virtamo J, Albanes D, Heinonen O. Incidence of cataract operation in Finnish male smokers unaffected by α-tocopherol or β-carotene supplements. J Epidemiol Community Health 1998; 52:468–472.
63. Taylor CR, Stern RS, Leyden JJ, Gilchrest BA. Photoaging, photodamage and photoprotection. J Am Acad Dermatol 1990; 22:1–15.
64. Darr D, Fridovich I. Free radicals in cutaneous biology. J Invest Dermatol 1994; 102:671–675.
65. Pourzand C, Watkin RD, Brown JE, Tyrrell RM. Ultraviolet A radiation induces immediate release of iron in human primary skin fibroblasts: the role of ferritin. Proc Natl Acad Sci USA 1999; 96:6751–6756.
66. Thiele J, Hsieh S, Briviba K, Sies H. Presence of a physiological keratin oxidation gradient in human forehead stratum corneum. J Invest Dermatol 1999; 112:778.
67. Ahmed NU, Ueda M, Nikaido O, Osawa T, Ichihashi M. High levels of 8-hydroxy-2'-deoxyguanosine appear in normal human epidermis after a single dose of ultraviolet radiation. Br J Dermatol 1999; 140:226–231.

68. Mathews–Roth MM, Pathak MA, Fitzpatrick TB, Harber LC, Kass EH. β-Carotene as an oral protective agent in erythropoietic protoporphyria. JAMA 1974; 228:1004–1008.
69. Fritsch C, Bolsen K, Ruzicka T, Goerz G. Congenital erythropoietic porphyria. J Am Acad Dermatol 1997; 36:594–610.
70. Scharffetter–Kochanek K. Photoaging of the connective tissue of skin: its prevention and therapy. Adv Pharmacol 1997; 38:639–655.
71. Sen CK, Packer L. Antioxidant and redox regulation of gene transcription. FASEB J 1996; 10:709–720.
72. Steenvorden DPT, Beijersbergen van Henegouwen GMJ. The use of endogenous antioxidants to improve photoprotection. J Photochem Photobiol B Biol 1997; 41:1–10.
73. Fuchs J. Potentials and limitations of the natural antioxidants *RRR*-alpha-tocopherol, L-ascorbic acid and β-carotene in cutaneous photoprotection. Free Radic Biol Med 1998; 25:848–873.
74. Podda M, Traber MG, Weber C, Yan L–J, Packer L. UV-irradiation depletes antioxidants and causes oxidative damage in a model of human skin. Free Radic Biol Med 1998; 24:55–65.
75. Stahl W, Heinrich U, Jungmann H, von Laar J, Schietzel M, Sies H, Tronnier H. Increased dermal carotenoid levels assessed by noninvasive reflection spectrophotometry correlate with serum levels in women ingesting Betatene. J Nutr 1998; 128:903–907.
76. Peng Y–M, Peng Y–S, Lin Y. A nonsaponification method for the determination of carotenoids, retinoids, and tocopherols in solid human tissues. Cancer Epidemiol Biomarker Prev 1993; 2:139–144.
77. Wingerath T, Sies H, Stahl W. Xanthophyll esters in human skin. Arch Biochem Biophys 1998; 355:271–274.
78. Ribaya–Mercado JD, Garmyn M, Gilchrest BA, Russell RM. Skin lycopene is destroyed preferentially over β-carotene during ultraviolet irradiation in humans. J Nutr 1995; 125:1854–1859.
79. Baron JA, Bertram JS, Britton G, Buiatti E, De Flora S, Feron VJ, Gerber M, Greenberg ER, Kavlock RJ, Knekt P, Malone W, Mayne ST, Nishino H, Olson JA, Pfander H, Stahl W, Thurnham DI, Virtamo J, Ziegler RG. IARC Handbooks of Cancer Prevention: Carotenoids. Vol 2. Lyon: IARC, 1998.
80. Gollnick HPM, Hopfenmüller W, Hemmes C, Chun SC, Schmid C, Sundermeier K, Biesalski HK. Systemic beta carotene plus topical UV-sunscreen are an optimal protection against harmful effects of natural UV-sunlight: results of the Berlin–Eilath study. Eur J Dermatol 1996; 6:200–205.
81. Mathews–Roth MM, Pathak MA, Parrish JA, Fitzpatrick TB, Kass EH, Toda K, Clemens W. A clinical trial of the effects of oral beta-carotene on the responses of human skin to solar radiation. J Invest Dermatol 1972; 59:349–353.
82. Stahl W, Heinrich U, Jungmann H, Sies H, Tronnier H. Carotenoids and carotenoids plus vitamin E protect against ultraviolet light-induced erythema in humans. Am J Clin Nutr 2000; 71:795–798.
83. Garmyn M, Ribaya–Mercado JD, Russell RM, Bhawan J, Gilchrest BA. Effect of beta-carotene supplementation on the human sunburn reaction. Exp Dermatol 1995; 4:104–111.
84. Wolf C, Steiner A, Hönigsmann H. Do oral carotenoids protect human skin against ultraviolet erythema, psoralen phototoxicity, and ultraviolet-induced DNA damage? J Invest Dermatol 1988; 90:55–57.

12

Oxidative Breakdown of Carotenoids and Biological Effects of Their Metabolites

Werner G. Siems
Herzog–Julius Hospital, Bad Harzburg, Germany

Olaf Sommerburg
University Children's Hospital, Ulm, Germany

Frederik J. G. M. van Kuijk
University of Texas Medical Branch, Galveston, Texas

I. INTRODUCTION

Chemical and biological properties of carotenoids are described in several reviews (1–5). It is known that about 600 distinct compounds are identified as naturally occurring carotenoids (6). They include cyclic hydrocarbon carotenoids (carotenes), acyclic hydrocarbon carotenoids (lycopene), and oxygenated hydrocarbon carotenoids (xanthophylls). The distribution of each carotenoid is quite different in the tissues and organs of humans (7–9). Major carotenoids in the human plasma are lutein, zeaxanthin, β-cryptoxanthin, lycopene, α-carotene, and β-carotene (10). The necessity of carotenoids for normal visual function referring to their provitamin A activity has long been known. However, also the role of a carotenoid itself in eye tissue, namely in the retina, has been intensively studied. It was demonstrated that the two polar substances, lutein and zeaxanthin, are the major carotenoids in the eye (11). They are concentrated throughout the whole retina; however, their highest concentration is at the locus of sharpest vision, the macula, forming the macular pigment. Handelman et al. (11) showed the carotenoid concentration in the macula to be fivefold higher compared with the peripheral retina. Lutein is the major carotenoid in the peripheral retina, whereas zeaxanthin becomes more and more dominant approaching the foveal center.

There are different suggestions for the biological functions of carotenoids in the eye tissues. Already 50 years ago it was suggested that the macular pigment is selectively able to absorb blue light. Later carotenoids have been proposed to be potent antioxidants, protecting membrane lipids from peroxidation (9,12). Carotenoids are effective singlet oxygen ($^1O_2$) quenchers

(13–18). DiMascio et al. (18) suggested that $^1O_2$-quenching capacities of lycopene, β-carotene, and tocopherols are of comparable magnitudes in plasma when the concentration difference is taken into account (18,19). Thus, the molar $^1O_2$-quenching capacity of lycopene and β-carotene is even higher than that of vitamin E (18,19). Lycopene was characterized as the most efficient biological carotenoid singlet oxygen quencher. However, the peroxyl radical trapping reactions of β-carotene were also intensively investigated (20,21).

In our studies, the first step of investigations on major carotenoids of human plasma and tissues was to expose them to radical-initiated autoxidation conditions in vitro. Different free radical-generating sources were selected for measurement of degradation rates of lutein, zeaxanthin, lycopene, and β-carotene: azobisisobutyronitrile (AIBN) as source of a peroxyl radical initiator; the so-called bleaching procedure using the action of hypochloric acid (NaOCl); UV light in presence of rose bengal as singlet oxygen generator; and natural sunlight.

In the second step of investigation the inhibition of Na^+,K^+-ATPase by carotenoid oxidative breakdown products was checked as an indicator of the biological activity of those metabolites.

II. ANTIOXIDANT ACTION OF CAROTENOIDS IS CONNECTED WITH THEIR FREE-RADICAL-INITIATED BREAKDOWN

β-Carotene and other carotenoids have excellent antioxidant activity, which under some conditions is higher than the antioxidant action of α-tocopherol (19). The $^1O_2$-quenching rate constants for carotenoids are at about 10^{10} M^{-1} s^{-1} much higher than those of tocopherols (16,22). The impressive antioxidant effects of β-carotene were first pointed out by Burton and Ingold (12). These authors have suggested that β-carotene serves as a chain-breaking antioxidant by trapping chain-propagating peroxyl radicals under low oxygen partial pressure (12). Carotenoids can act as chain-breaking antioxidants in solutions (23), membranes (12), and subcellular organelles (24). Carotenoids are important components of the well-organized defense system of human plasma against oxidative damages, especially against oxidative modification of plasma low-density lipoprotein (LDL) (25).

The antioxidant action of carotenoids is essentially connected with their free radical-initiated breakdown and with the formation of carotenoid breakdown products (CBP). Therefore, the understanding of the antioxidative effects of carotenoids includes a knowledge about the kinetics of their breakdown and, consequently, also the analysis of CBP and their biological effects. The free radical-initiated breakdown of different carotenoids was studied by several groups, and different methods were described to observe the degradation of these substances. For many years, the oxidative breakdown of β-carotene was monitored simply by following its bleaching; that is, the loss of the major absorption peak at 450 nm (26). An important physiological and pathophysiologically relevant source for the destruction of carotenoids is ultraviolet (UV) light exposure. UV light exposure of the eye has been associated with cataract formation and retinal degeneration (27). One mechanism that is thought to play an important role involves the generation of oxygen radicals. Under experimental conditions in vitro, the generation of free radicals in UV light exposure can be increased by the addition of natural and artificial compounds, such as rose bengal. Under those conditions the formation of singlet oxygen was demonstrated.

El-Tinay and Chichester (28) and later Handelman et al. (29) used radical initiators such as AIBN to accelerate the formation of oxidation products of β-carotene. This compound breaks down thermally to a radical species that rapidly reacts with oxygen to form a peroxyl radical. Mortensen and colleagues compared the radical-scavenging activity of different carotenoids and postulated an antioxidant hierarchy (30–32). These authors determined the comparative mechanisms and relative rates of nitrogen dioxide, thiyl, and sulfonyl radical scavenging by the carotenoids lycopene, lutein, zeaxanthin, astaxanthin, and canthaxanthin by pulse radiolysis (31). Furthermore, they studied the interaction between carotenoids and tocopherols by real-time detection following laser flash photolysis of transient carotenoid radical cations and tocopheroxyl radicals formed in chloroform (30,32).

In their studies on the kinetics of carotenoid breakdown Ojima et al. (22) compared the consumption of different carotenoids in photosensitized oxidation of human plasma and plasma LDL. In that paper the authors compared the behavior of endogenous carotenoids in $^1O_2$ generation systems with methylene blue or 12-(pyrene)dodecanoid acid (P-12) as water-soluble and lipid-soluble photosensitizers, respectively. They found, that in P-12-sensitized photooxidation of human plasma and LDL, the breakdown rate of xanthophylls (zeaxanthin and lutein) was slower than that of lycopene and carotenes. Thus, the polar carotenoids are less reactive with $^1O_2$ generated within lipid phase, in contrast to nonpolar carotenoids, lycopene and carotenes. In the presence of methylene blue almost equal consumption rates of those carotenoids during photoirradiation of LDL were observed. In methylene blue experiments in plasma the xanthophylls decreased even faster than lycopene and β-carotene. From those findings the authors concluded, that the antioxidant activity of individual carotenoids is influenced by the site of $^1O_2$ generation (22).

The chemical reactions between the different free radical species and the carotenoids essentially result in the formation of breakdown products. If those products possess reactive functional groups, they may exert biological effects. In such a case it is important to know which metabolites are formed and which biological effects they can exert.

Handelman et al. characterized some products formed during the autoxidation of β-carotene (29). Kennedy and Liebler demonstrated the formation of β-carotene epoxides (20), and recently, Liebler and McClure identified carotenoid–radical adducts (33). It has been estimated that each carotenoid molecule can quench 1000 $^1O_2$ molecules before they react chemically and form products (4). Many of these products have been characterized and consist of carbonyls and epoxides (4,34). Obviously, different radical sources can modify the pattern and the rate of carotenoid degradation. Under some conditions the highest degradation rate was for lycopene, under other radical-initiating conditions, for β-carotene. In our study the lycopene-breakdown overwhelmed the β-carotene breakdown in presence of AIBN. These results might be explained by comparing the chemical formulas of both compounds. For the lycopene structure the possibility of formation of peroxyl groups is higher than for β-carotene, in which the lateral ring structure reduces the number of double bonds.

III. COMPARISON OF DIFFERENT METHODS FOR THE ANALYSIS OF CAROTENOID BREAKDOWN

The breakdown of carotenoid mixtures from lutein, zeaxanthin, lycopene, and β-carotene was monitored and compared under different conditions.

Bleaching can destroy high amounts of carotenoids within short time periods. Figure 1 shows the degradation of lutein, zeaxanthin, lycopene, and β-carotene under conditions of bleaching mediated by 1 mM hypochlorite. Within 3 min between 500 and 750 nmol/L of the single carotenoid compounds were destroyed using initial concentrations of 1 μM of each carotenoid. The highest degradation rates were found for lycopene and β-carotene. The degradation of lycopene is twice as fast as the degradation of lutein and zeaxanthin.

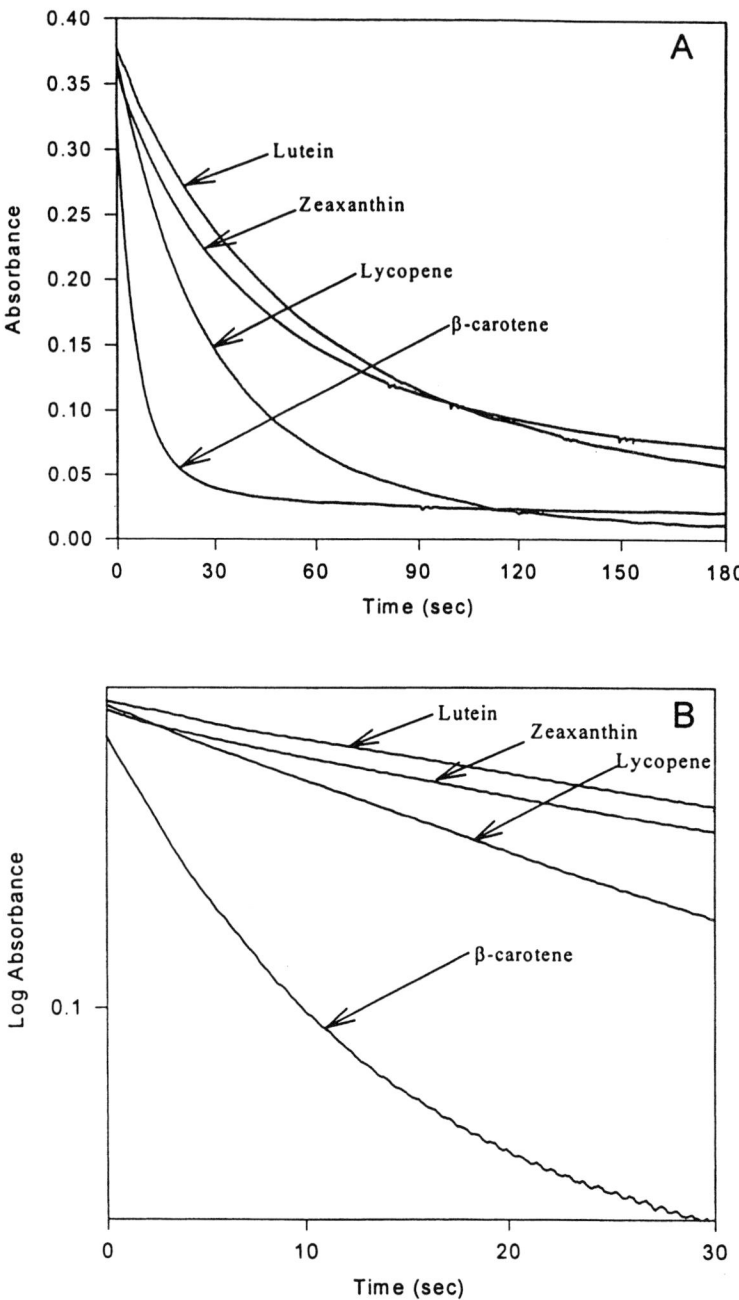

Figure 1 Loss of different carotenoids during bleaching in a NaOCl-containing solution (final NaOCl concentration 1 mM). The initial concentration of each of the carotenoids (lutein, zeaxanthin, lycopene, and β-carotene) was 1 μM. Data are shown with linear (A) and logarithmic (B) ordinate axis. The figure shows the continuous spectrophotometric monitoring at 450 nm of the breakdown of a single carotenoid compound in a cuvette. In parallel, measurement of carotenoid breakdown in carotenoid mixtures was carried out (data not shown here). In one experiment aliquots were taken for extraction and carotenoid analysis by HPLC at defined time points.

Figure 2A shows the rapid degradation of carotenoid concentrations from equimolar 1 μM mixtures under conditions of UV light exposure in presence of rose bengal. Within the first 2 min 30% of lutein, 40% of zeaxanthin, 55% of lycopene, and 85% of β-carotene were degraded.

Table 1 shows the carotenoid breakdown from UV light exposure in presence of rose bengal for the different initial concentrations of carotenoids (1 μM, 250 nM, and 50 nM). The lower the initial concentration of carotenoids, the lower are the remaining levels as a percentage of initial concentration after defined time periods of UV light irradiation in presence of rose bengal. Starting with 50-nM levels, after 15 min the β-carotene level is zero (not detectable). At the same time point, about 5 nM of lutein and zeaxanthin, and about 3 nM of lycopene are still present in the irradiated solution. Figure 2B shows the breakdown of carotenoid mixtures (1 μM each) during natural sunlight exposure. During sunlight exposure the most rapid breakdown rate was measured for lycopene, followed by β-carotene. At the end of sunlight experiments (36 h of irradiation) the remaining levels of lycopene and β-carotene (about 0.15 μM) were significantly different from remaining levels of lutein and zeaxanthin (about 0.30 μM).

The same sequence of carotenoid degradation rates as under natural sunlight irradiation was also found during carotenoid autoxidation in presence of AIBN. Table 2 shows the degradation of carotenoids at 1 μM each in presence of 5 mM AIBN. Within 30 min of incubation 50% of lycopene and 35% of β-carotene autoxidized, but only 20% of lutein and zeaxanthin did, respectively. Under all the experimental conditions that we used, the breakdown rates for lycopene and β-carotene were higher than those for lutein and zeaxanthin.

IV. POSSIBLE CONSEQUENCES OF THE UNEQUAL LIGHT-INDUCED CAROTENOID BREAKDOWN FOR RETINAL CAROTENOID PATTERN

Lutein and zeaxanthin are the dominant carotenoids in the peripheral retina and in the macular region, respectively (11,37). Sommerburg et al. investigated the localization of carotenoids in the different parts of the human eye and demonstrated that lutein and zeaxanthin are associated with the photoreceptors in human retina (38). Lycopene and β-carotene are not found in the retina, although retinal tissue should be supplied with all compounds by the blood stream. Thus, the question arises: Why are lycopene and β-carotene lacking in human and animal retinas in contrast to xanthophylls which are highly concentrated in the same tissue?

The superficial slices of the skin and the tissues of the eye are the only sites of the organism that are continuously exposed to photoirradiation. Photooxidation of unsaturated lipid proceeds at least partially by $^1O_2$ oxygenation. Probably, the skin and the eye are the only organs with significant generation of $^1O_2$ under physiological conditions. At least, the retina underlies accelerated generation of reactive oxygen species including peroxyl radicals and singlet oxygen during all periods of light exposure. After photoirradiation β-carotene and other antioxidants are consumed in skin and blood plasma (39). Ribaya–Mercado et al. (40) measured rapid β-carotene and lycopene decreases in plasma and skin during ultraviolet irradiation in humans, with a preference of lycopene degradation in exposed skin areas.

We follow the suggestion (22) that the antioxidant activity of carotenoids in photosensitized oxidation depends on the site of $^1O_2$ generation. Furthermore, we investigated the autoxidation of carotenoids themselves under both natural and artificial conditions with increased formation of reactive oxygen species. In those autoxidation experiments the breakdown of lycopene and β-carotene was higher than the breakdown of xanthophylls. What does that mean for carotenoid pattern of the retina? Lycopene and β-carotene, which are highly concentrated in the retinal

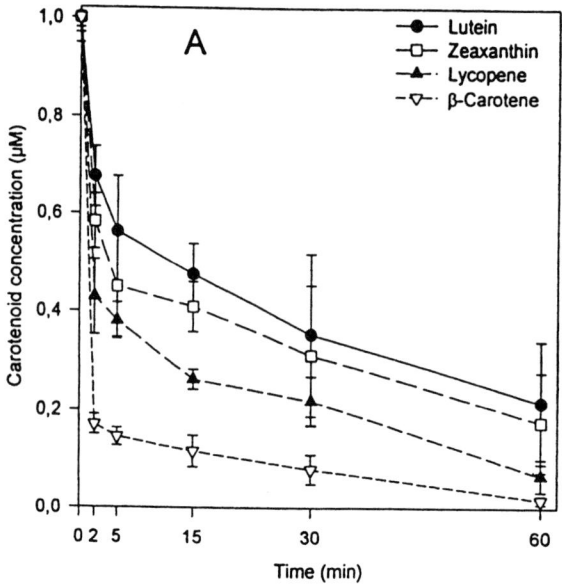

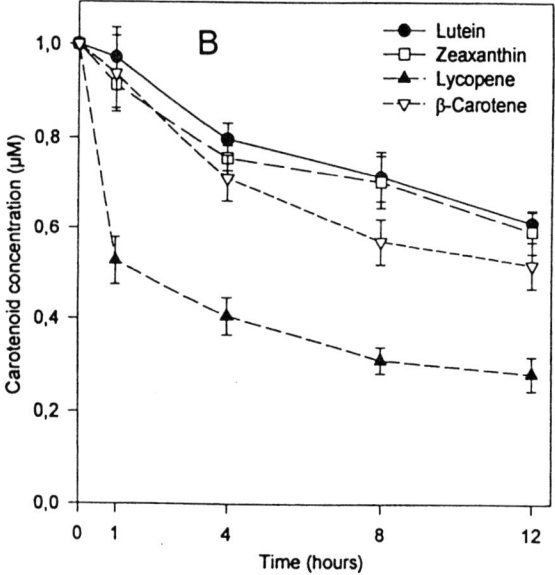

Figure 2 Time course of the carotenoid loss (A) during UV irradiation in presence of rose bengal and (B) during sunlight exposure. Initial concentration of carotenoids was 1 μM each; $n = 10$ (UV irradiation); $n = 6$ (sunlight exposure). Experimental details: rose bengal concentration was 125 μg/mL; carotenoid mixtures were photoirradiated by fluorescent lamp (light intensity 8000 lux) at 22°C. The sunlight exposure was started at 9 AM, ended at 6 PM; during the night the samples were kept in the dark in the freezer at −20°C until the next day when the exposure was continued in the same manner. The procedure was repeated for 4 days, thus experiments ended finally after 36 h of sunlight exposure. Closed scintillation vials were used in both experiments for irradiation of the solutions of the carotenoid mixture (1-mL solution in 5-mL vials). At defined time points aliquots were taken for extraction and carotenoid analysis by HPLC: details of the extraction procedure and the HPLC analysis are given elsewhere (36).

Table 1 Loss of Carotenoids in a Mixture of Lutein, Zeaxanthin, Lycopene, and β-Carotene[a]

	Lutein	Zeaxanthin	Lycopene	β-Carotene
1 μM	0.48 ± 0.15	0.41 ± 0.12	0.26 ± 0.02	0.12 ± 0.05
0.25 μM	0.085 ± 0.007	0.078 ± 0.018	0.052 ± 0.017	0.033 ± 0.010
0.05 μM	0.005 ± 0.001	0.004 ± 0.001	0.003 ± 0.002	nd

[a]During 15 min of UV irradiation in presence of rose bengal ($n = 10$). Values are given as mean ± SD (remaining amounts) in μM; nd, not detectable. [The extraction procedure and the HPLC analysis of carotenoids were described in Ref. 36.]
Source: Ref. 35.

arterial system, are rapidly lost in this tissue. The first reason for that is suggested to be the high autoxidation rate of lycopene and β-carotene during photoirradiation processes. As a second mechanism leading to the almost complete lack of both nonpolar compounds (in analogy to Ref. 22), the dominance of hydrophobic $^1O_2$ generators in the retina could be postulated.

Nevertheless, a final proof of the theory on the unusual carotenoid pattern in the human macula is lacking.

V. DO CAROTENOIDS EXERT PRO-OXIDATIVE OR OTHER SIDE EFFECTS?

There are some findings on prooxidative actions of carotenoids. Burton and Ingold first presented evidence that β-carotene can act as a pro-oxidant during radical-initiated lipid peroxidation, although this was observed only at 100% oxygen (12,41). Truscott presented a theoretical basis for the antioxidant and pro-oxidant effects of β-carotene under low and high oxygen tensions (42). Krinsky (4) summarized the reports on prooxidant effects at different oxygen tensions and concluded that the pro-oxidant effect is seen at 100% oxygen, but not under ambient conditions (21%). Up to now there is no evidence for a pro-oxidant effect at the physiological level or at tissue levels, where oxygen tension is about 1–2%. Thus, in his opinion, it seems to be very little support of the concept that β-carotene acts as a pro-oxidant in the body (4).

Further discussion and thinking on biological effects, signal functions, and possibly partial toxicity is derived from unexpected results in some clinical supplementation trials. In general, intake of carotenoids is supposed to lead to beneficial clinical effects. Antioxidant functions

Table 2 Carotenoid Breakdown[a] in Presence of 5 mM AIBN

	Lutein	Zeaxanthin	Lycopene	β-Carotene
After 2 min	0.94 ± 0.05	0.96 ± 0.06	0.86 ± 0.04	0.90 ± 0.06
After 15 min	0.85 ± 0.03	0.85 ± 0.04	0.62 ± 0.10	0.79 ± 0.28
After 30 min	0.81 ± 0.02	0.80 ± 0.04	0.52 ± 0.21	0.61 ± 0.06

[a]The initial concentration of each carotenoid was 1 μM, values are given as mean ± SD (remaining amounts) in μM, $n = 4$. [Extraction and HPLC measurement of carotenoids were described in Ref. 36.]
Source: Ref. 35.

of carotenoids are associated with reduction of DNA damage, malignant transformation, and other parameters of cell damage in vitro. In epidemiological studies, carotenoid intake was associated with decreased incidence of certain types of cancer and degenerative diseases, such as Alzheimer's disease, atherosclerosis, coronary heart disease, cataract, and age-related macular degeneration (ARMD) (17,42,43). These associations were originated from excellent observational studies, which have quite consistently indicated that diets containing fruits and vegetables enriched in carotenoids have a significant risk reduction for chronic diseases. However, in a few interventional studies, high-dose supplementation of β-carotene did not result in clinical improvement, and in men who were heavy smokers, even an increased mortality caused by lung cancer was found (44–46). The conclusion that major public health benefits could be achieved by increasing consumption of carotenoid-rich fruits and vegetables still appears to stand. However, the pharmacological supplementation of β-carotene to prevent cardiovascular disease and lung cancer, particularly in smokers, should no longer be recommended (45).

In an attempt to understand the phenomenon of partial toxicity seen during supplementation of β-carotene in smokers, Krinsky et al. (47) exposed ferrets fed high doses of β-carotene to cigarette smoke. Interestingly, they observed unexpected changes in the lung nuclear receptors and histology. These changes were attributed to oxidative metabolites of β-carotene, rather than to the intact carotenoid precursor (47). This could perhaps explain how these compounds, lacking specific-binding proteins or nuclear receptors, can exert such profound biological effects. The author reported that these oxidative metabolites modulated the activity of protein kinase C, a major player in cell signaling. Krinsky's summarizing statement was that biological properties of the carotenoids may be much more related to the products of carotenoid interaction under oxidant stress (e.g., breakdown products such as apocarotenals and retinoids) (4,47).

Many of the carotenoid breakdown products were identified as aldehydes (48), and aldehydes, even at low cellular levels, may react rapidly with sulfhydryl groups, lysyl residues, and histidine residues. The interrelations of other endogenous aldehydic compounds, such as the end product of lipid peroxidation 4-hydroxynonenal (HNE) with enzymes and other proteins were intensively studied (49–55). If a bulk of carotenoid breakdown products has aldehydic groups one should expect biological reactions of those compounds that are similar to the effects of HNE. Previously, we reported the irreversible inhibition of Na^+,K^+-ATPase by HNE (53). The IC_{50} value for this reaction was calculated 120 μM (53). Now we measured the effect of oxidative carotenoid breakdown products on Na^+,K^+-ATPase activity and compared the results with those of HNE and related aldehydes. Additionally, restoration of enzyme activity was evaluated in the presence of hydroxylamine (HA) and β-mercaptoethanol (BME).

VI. INHIBITION OF Na^+,K^+-ATPase ACTIVITY BY CAROTENOID BREAKDOWN PRODUCTS AS INDICATOR OF THEIR BIOLOGICAL ACTIVITY

The regulation of Na^+,K^+-ATPase activity, including its phosphorylation by protein kinases (56,57) and subunit interactions (55,59), has been extensively studied. Furthermore, pharmacological effects especially those related to the activity of cardiac glycosides, such as digoxin (see exogenous inhibitors of Na^+,K^+-transporting ATPase 3.6.1.37 listed in Ref. 60) have been described. There are also endogenous inhibitors of Na^+,K^+-ATPase, and endogenous digitalis-like factors have been partially isolated and characterized from mammalian organs (61–63).

Several studies have reported inactivation of Na^+,K^+-ATPase by agents that react with either lysine or cysteine residues (53,64–69). Kim and Akera reported that oxygen free radicals caused ischemia–reperfusion injury to cardiac Na^+,K^+-ATPase (70). They showed a partial inactivation of ATPase during lipid peroxidation following ischemia–reperfusion injury, which could be reduced by antioxidants (70). The kinetic parameters of Na^+,K^+-ATPase are modified by free radicals in vitro and in vivo (71,72). Oxygen free radicals directly attack the ATP-binding site of the cardiac Na^+,K^+-ATPase (73).

The results of our investigation now show that this enzyme is inhibited by another group of endogenous aldehydes, those derived from oxidative breakdown of carotenoids. In our experiments CBP potently inhibited Na^+,K^+-ATPase activity. Furthermore, the inhibition was much more effective than that of 4-HNE and related aldehydic compounds. Table 3 shows the inhibition of Na^+,K^+-ATPase activity by carotenoid oxidation products (CBP, β-apo-10′-carotenal, and retinal) and by HNE at 10-μM concentration of those compounds (48). Figure 3A shows the inhibition of Na^+,K^+-ATPase activity by CBP and related compounds. For comparison the inhibition of HNE and related compounds nonanal (NA), and trans-2,3-nonenal (NE) on the enzyme activity is shown in Figure 3B. Figure 3A shows that the inhibition of Na^+,K^+-ATPase activity by CBP, apo-10, and retinal (0.1–10 M) is concentration-dependent. Similarly, a concentration-responsive inhibition for HNE, NE, and NA (1–100 M) is shown in Figure 3B. The slopes for both curves are similar except for the concentration range at which equivalent inhibition is obtained. The IC_{50} values for the ATPase inhibition were obtained from these curves. The IC_{50} for CBP is 11 μM, which is one-tenth the value for HNE. Thus, CBPs are more potent as inhibitors of Na^+,K^+-ATPase than HNE. Additionally, GC separations of CBP without derivatization and after formation of ethyloxime derivatives were carried out. From comparison of the chromatograms it was concluded that several of the CBP are aldehydes that were converted to ethyloxime derivatives. The enzyme activity once inhibited by CBP could only be partially recovered by means of hydroxylamine and β-mercaptoethanol. The BME was more effective than HA. An almost complete restoration of enzyme activity resulted after addition of HA to the samples that were incubated with β-apo-10′-carotenal or retinal, but for these compounds, the addition of BME did not increase enzyme activity.

Table 3 Inhibition of Na^+,K^+-ATPase by Carotenoid Oxidative Breakdown Products (CBP) and 4-Hydroxynonenal

Compound	ATP splitting	% of control	n
CBP	291 ± 27	52.4 ± 4.8	20
Apo-10	461 ± 44	83.0 ± 7.9	20
Retinal	403 ± 7	72.5 ± 1.2	12
4-HNE	445 ± 18	89.0 ± 3.2	8

Values expressed as nmol/mg protein/min for ATP splitting and as percentage of control. The rate of ATP splitting in the control was 556±33 ($n = 49$). The initial concentrations used were 10 μM for all compounds. CBPs were used in a concentration corresponding to an equivalent of oxidation products of 10 μM β-carotene. [For details of CBP formation and of measurement of enzyme activity, see method section in Refs. 48, 53.]
Source: Ref. 48.

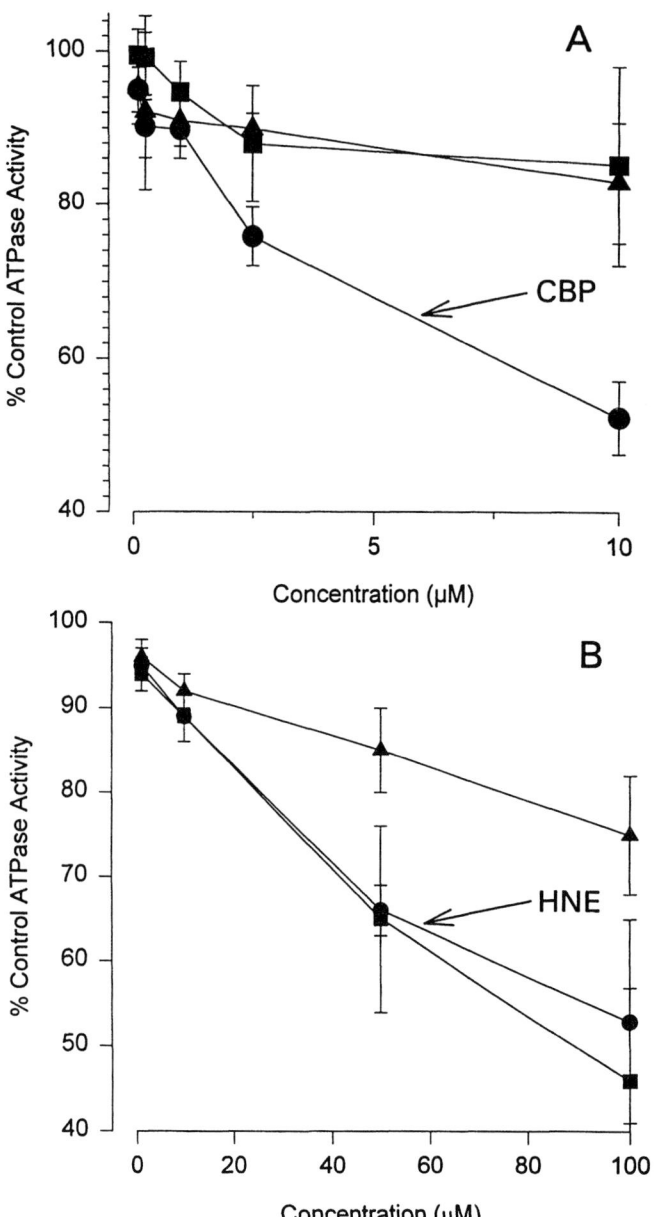

Figure 3 Inhibition of Na^+,K^+-ATPase activity by aldehydes: (A) by oxidized carotenoids and related compounds, (B) by 4-HNE and related aldehydes: symbols: Fig. 3A. ●, CBP; ▲, APO-10; ■, β-carotene; Fig. 3B: ●, 4-HNE; ▲, NA; ■, NE. The CBP concentrations are given as concentrations of nondegraded β-carotene equivalents. The methodological approach for the measurement of enzyme activity is given elsewhere (53).

VII. TOXICITY OF OXIDATIVE METABOLITES OF CAROTENOIDS

Aldehydes derived either from PUFA oxidation or carotenoid breakdown are much more stable than the initial reactive oxygen species and can act as both autocrine and paracrine agents at the intra- and extracellular levels, attacking targets close and far from the site of generation. Therefore, they are not only end products of oxidative breakdown processes, but may also act as "second-messengers" for the primary reactive species—free radicals or singlet oxygen—that initiated their formation. We propose that aldehydic breakdown products of carotenoids and lipid peroxidation should be classified together as one group in relation to those biological effects. These endogenous aldehydes are able to interact with proteins, which has been extensively demonstrated for HNE (49–55,74). In our studies, the inhibition Na^+,K^+-ATPase by CBP was shown, and in vitro it was much more toxic than HNE. However, the toxicity of both CBP and HNE in vivo will ultimately depend on the capacity of the metabolic pathways for both products. The metabolic pathways for HNE, including their capacity in different tissues, has been previously elucidated (75–77). However, very little is known about the capacity of CBP metabolic pathways in animal and human tissues.

In our investigations an inhibition of ATPase activity by CBP was shown at concentrations between 0.25 and 1 μM. At 2.5 μM, an inhibition of 25% was observed. We suggest that the inhibitory effect of CBP may be cumulative because of the irreversible binding of these metabolites to the enzyme. Carotenoid levels, especially β-carotene, in blood plasma and in various animal and human tissues are dependent on the carotenoid content of food and may contain higher CBP concentrations than used in our Na^+,K^+-ATPase inhibition studies. We propose that, under conditions of oxidative stress, tissues with high carotenoid levels accumulate aldehydic metabolites that could activate stress-signaling pathways similar to those postulated by Uchida et al. for 4-hydroxy-2-nonenal (78).

VIII. SUMMARY

The antioxidant action of carotenoids essentially is connected with the free radical-initiated breakdown of carotenoids and with the formation of carotenoid breakdown products (CBP). The kinetics of carotenoid breakdown and biological effects of CBP were studied in vitro. In the first step of investigations major carotenoids of human plasma and tissues were exposed to radical-initiated autoxidation conditions. The consumption of lutein and zeaxanthin, the only carotenoids in the retina, and lycopene and β-carotene, the most effective quenchers of singlet oxygen in plasma, were compared.

Under all conditions of free radical-initiated autoxidation of the investigated carotenoids, the breakdown of lycopene and β-carotene was much faster than that of lutein and zeaxanthin. Under influence of UV light in presence of rose bengal by far the highest breakdown rate was found for β-carotene, followed by lycopene. Bleaching of carotenoid mixtures mediated by NaOCl, addition of azobisisobutyronitril (AIBN), and the photoirradiation of carotenoid mixtures by natural sunlight led to the following sequence of breakdown rates: lycopene > β-carotene > zeaxanthin > lutein.

The slow degradation of the xanthophylls zeaxanthin and lutein may explain most of the zeaxanthin and lutein in the retina of humans and other species. In correlation with that, the rapid degradation of β-carotene and lycopene under the influence of natural sunlight and UV light is postulated to be the reason for the almost lack of those two carotenoids in the human retina. Nevertheless, a final proof of that theory is lacking.

In a second step of investigations the inhibition of Na^+,K^+-ATPase by carotenoid oxidative breakdown products was checked as an indicator of the biological activity of those metabolites. For that purpose β-carotene was completely oxidized by hypochlorous acid. To assess biological activity the Na^+,K^+-ATPase activity was assayed in the presence of these oxidation products. Its activity is rapidly inhibited by oxidized carotenoids. This was demonstrated for a mixture of β-carotene oxidative breakdown products, β-apo-10′-carotenal and retinal. Most of the β-carotene oxidation products are aldehydic compounds. The concentration of the mixture of carotenoid oxidation products that inhibited 50% Na^+,K^+-ATPase activity was equivalent to 10 μM nondegraded β-carotene, whereas 4-hydroxy-2-nonenal (HNE), a major product of lipid peroxidation, has a more than tenfold higher IC_{50} value (120 μM). It is concluded that oxidation products of carotenoids are more potent inhibitors of Na^+,K^+-ATPase than HNE. Enzyme activity could be only slightly recovered with hydroxylamine or β-mercaptoethanol. Thus, in vitro binding of carotenoid oxidation products results in strong enzyme inhibition. These data indicate the potential toxicity of oxidative carotenoid metabolites and their activity as key enzyme regulators and signal modulators.

REFERENCES

1. Krinsky NI. The biological properties of carotenoids. Pure Appl Chem 1994; 66:1003–1010.
2. Britton G. Structure and properties of carotenoids in relation to function. FASEB J 1995; 9:1551–1558.
3. Krinsky NI. Carotenoid properties define primary biological actions and metabolism defines secondary biological actions. In: Oezben T, ed. Free Radicals, Oxidative Stress, and Antioxidants: Pathological and Physiological Significance. London: NATO Advanced Study Institute, 1998:323–332.
4. Krinsky NI. The antioxidant and biological properties of the carotenoids. Ann NY Acad Sci 1998; 854:443–447.
5. Palozza P, Krinsky NI. Antioxidant effects of carotenoids in vitro and in vivo: an overview. Methods Enzymol 1992; 213:403–420.
6. Olson JA. Biological actions of carotenoids. J Nutr 1989; 119:94–95.
7. Kaplan LA, Lau JM, Stein EA. Carotenoid compositions and relationship in various human organ. Clin Physiol Biochem 1990; 8:1–10.
8. Stahl W, Schwarz W, Sundquist AR, Sies H. cis–trans-Isomers of lycopene and beta-carotene in human serum and tissues. Arch Biochem Biophys 1992; 294:173–177.
9. Sies H, Stahl W. Vitamins E and C, beta-carotene, and other carotenoids as antioxidants. Am J Clin Nutr 1995; 62:1315S–1321S.
10. Ito I, Ochiai J, Sasaki R, Suzuki S, Kusuhara Y, Morimitsu Y, Otani M, Aoki K. Serum concentrations of carotenoids, retinol, and α-tocopherol in healthy persons determined by high-performance liquid chromatography. Clin Chim Acta 1990; 194:131–144.
11. Handelman GJ, Dratz EA, Reay CC, van Kuijk FJGM. Carotenoids in the human macula and whole retina. Invest Ophthalmol Vis Sci 1988; 29:850–855.
12. Burton GW, Ingold KU. β-Carotene: an unusual type of lipid antioxidant. Science 1984; 224:569–573.
13. Foote CS, Denny RW. Chemistry of singlet oxygen VII. Quenching by β-carotene. J Am Chem Soc 1969; 90:6233–6235.
14. Dalle–Carbonare M, Pathak MA. Skin photosensitizing agent and the role of reactive oxygen species in photoaging. J Photochem Photobiol B 1992; 14:105–124.
15. Boehm F, Haley J, Truscott TG, Schalch W. Cellular bound β-carotene quenches singlet oxygen in man. J Photochem Photobiol B 1993; 21:219–221.
16. Kaiser S, DiMascio P, Murphy ME, Sies H. Physical and chemical scavenging of singlet molecular oxygen by tocopherols. Arch Biochem Biophys 1990; 277:101–108.
17. Sies H, Stahl W, Sundquist AR. Antioxidant functions of vitamin E and C, β-carotene, and other carotenoids. Ann NY Acad Sci 1992; 669:7–20.

18. DiMascio P, Kaiser S, Sies H. Lycopene as the most efficient biological carotenoid singlet oxygen quencher. Arch Biochem Biophys 1989; 274:532–538.
19. Miller NJ, Sampson J, Candeias LP, Bramley PM, Rice–Evans CA. Antioxidant activities of carotenes and xanthophylls. FEBS Lett 1996; 384:240–242.
20. Kennedy TA, Liebler DC. Peroxyl radical oxidation of β-carotene epoxides. Chem Res Toxicol 1991; 4:290–295.
21. Kennedy TA, Liebler DC. Peroxyl radical scavenging by β-carotene in lipid bilayers. J Biol Chem 1992; 267:4658–4663.
22. Ojima F, Sakamoto H, Ischiguro Y, Terao J. Consumption of carotenoids in photosensitized oxidation of human plasma and plasma low-density lipoprotein. Free Radic Biol Med 1993; 15:377–384.
23. Terao J. Antioxidant activity of β-carotene-related carotenoid in solution. Lipids 1989; 24:659–661.
24. Palozza P, Moualla S, Krinsky NI. Effects of β-carotene and α-tocopherol on radical-initiated peroxidation of microsomes. Free Radic Biol Med 1992; 13:127–136.
25. Frei B, Stocker R, Ames BN. Antioxidant defenses and lipid peroxidation in human blood plasma. Proc Natl Acad Sci USA 1988; 85:9748–9752.
26. Ben-Aziz A, Grossman S, Ascarelli I, Budowski P. Carotene-bleaching activities of lipoxygenase and heme proteins as studied by a direct spectrophotometric method. Phytochemistry 1971; 10;1445–1452.
27. van Kuijk FJGM. Effects of ultraviolet light on the eye: role of protective glasses. Environ Health Perspect 1991; 96:177–184.
28. El-Tinay AH, Chichester CO. Oxidation of β-carotene. Site of initial attack. J Org Chem 1970; 35: 2290–2293.
29. Handelman GJ, van Kuijk FJGM, Chatterjee A, Krinsky NI. Characterization of products formed during the autoxidation of beta-carotene. Free Radic Biol Med 1991; 10:427–437.
30. Mortensen A, Skibsted LH. Kinetics of photobleaching of β-carotene in chloroform and formation of transient carotenoid species absorbing in the near infrared. Free Radic Res 1996; 25:355–368.
31. Mortensen A, Skibsted LH, Sampson J, Rice–Evans C, Everett SA. Comparative mehcanisms and rates of free radical scavenging by carotenoid antioxidants. FEBS Lett 1997; 418:91–97.
32. Mortensen A, Skibsted LH. Relative stability of carotenoid radical cations and homologue tocopheroxyl radicals. A real time kinetic study of antioxidant hierarchy. FEBS Lett 1997; 417:261–266.
33. Liebler DC, McClure TD. Antioxidant reactions of β-carotene: identification of carotenoid–radical adducts. Chem Res Toxicol 1996; 9:8–11.
34. Stratton SP, Schaefer WH, Liebler DC. Isolation and identification of singlet oxygen oxidation products of β-carotene. Chem Res Toxicol 1993; 6:542–547.
35. Siems WG, Sommerburg O, van Kuijk FJGM. Lycopene and β-carotene decompose more rapidly than lutein and zeaxanthin upon exposure to various pro-oxidants in vitro. BioFactors 1999; 10: 105–113.
36. Sommerburg O, Zang LY, van Kuijk FJGM. Simultaneous detection of carotenoids and vitamin E in human plasma. J Chromatogr B 1997; 695:209–215.
37. Schalch W. Carotenoids in the retina—a review of their possible role in preventing or limiting damage caused by light and oxygen. In: Emerit I, Chance B, eds. Free Radicals and Aging. Basel: Birkhaeuser Verlag, 1992:280–298.
38. Sommerburg O, Siems WG, Hurst JS, Lewis JW, Kliger DS, van Kuijk FJGM. Lutein and zeaxanthin are associated with photoreceptors in human retina. Curr Eye Res 1999; 19:491–495.
39. Biesalski HK, Hemmes C, Hopfenmueller W, Schmid C, Gollnick HP. Effects of controlled exposure of sunlight on plasma and skin levels of beta-carotene. Free Radic Res 1996; 24:215–224.
40. Ribaya–Mercado JD, Garmyn M, Gilchrest BA, Russell RM. Skin lycopene is destroyed preferentially over β-carotene during ultraviolet irradiation in humans. J Nutr 1995; 125:1854–1859.
41. Burton GW. Antioxidant action of carotenoids. J Nutr 1989; 119:109–111.
42. Liebler DC. Antioxidant reactions of carotenoids. Ann NY Acad Sci 1993; 691:20–31.
43. Seddon JM, Ajani UA, Sperduto RD, Hiller R, Blair N, Burton TC, Farber MD, Gragoudas ES, Haller J, Miller DT, Yannuzzi LA, Willett W. Dietary carotenoids, vitamins A, C, and E, and advanced age-related macular degeneration. JAMA 1994; 272:1413–1420.
44. The alpha-tocopherol, beta-Carotene Cancer Prevention Study Group. The effect of vitamin E and beta carotene on the incidence of lung cancer and other cancers in male smokers. N Engl J Med 1994; 330:1029–1035.
45. Mayne ST. β-Carotene, carotenoids, and disease prevention in humans. FASEB J 1996; 10:690–701.

46. Omaye ST, Krinsky NI, Kagan VE, Mayne ST, Liebler DC, Bidlack WR. β-Carotene: friend or foe? Fundam App Toxicol 1997; 40:163–174.
47. Krinsky NI. Carotenoid metabolites as cell signaling modulators. In: Packer L, Davies KJA, Cadenas E, eds. Oxidants and Antioxidants in Biology, Oxygen Club of California World Congress Abstracts. Santa Barbara: Oxygen Club of California, 1991:1–2.
48. Siems WG, Sommerburg O, Hurst JS, van Kuijk FJGM. Carotenoid oxidative degradation products inhibit Na^+-K^+-ATPase. Free Radic Res 2000; 33:427–435.
49. Uchida K, Stadtman ER. Modification of histidine residues in proteins by reation with 4-hydroxynonenal. Proc Natl Acad Sci USA 1992; 89:4544–4548.
50. Uchida K, Stadtman ER. Selective cleavage of thioether linkage in proteins modified with 4-hydroxynonenal. Proc Natl Acad Sci USA 1992; 89:5611–5615.
51. Szweda LI, Uchida K, Tsai L, Stadtman ER. Inactivation of glucose-6-phosphate dehydrogenase by 4-hydroxynonenal: selective modification of an active-site lysine. J Biol Chem 1993; 268:3342–3347.
52. Uchida K, Stadtman ER. Covalent attachment of 4-hydroxynonenal to glyceraldeyde-3-phosphate dehydrogenase: a possible involvement of intra- and intermolecular cross-linking reaction. J Biol Chem 1993; 268:6388–6393.
53. Siems WG, Hapner SJ, van Kuijk FJGM. 4-Hydroxynonenal inhibits Na^+-K^+-ATPase. Free Radic Biol Med 1996; 20:215–223.
54. Siems WG, Capuozzo E, Verginelli D, Salerno C, Crifo C, Grune T. Inhibition of NADPH oxidase-mediated superoxide radical formation in PMA-stimulated human neutrophils by 4-hydroxynonenal-binding to -SH and -NH_2 groups. Free Radic Res 1997; 27:353–358.
55. Sommerburg O, Ullrich O, Sitte N, von Zglinicki D, Siems W, Grune T. Dose- and wavelength-dependent oxidation of crystallins by UV light-selective recognition and degradation by the 20S proteasome. Free Radic Biol Med 1999; 24:1369–1374.
56. Feschenko MS, Sweadner KJ. Phosphorylation of Na,K-ATPase by protein kinase C at Ser18 occurs in intact cells but does not result in direct inhibition of ATP hydrolysis. J Biol Chem 1997; 272: 17726–17733.
57. Bertorello AM, Aperia A, Walaas SI, Nairn AC, Greengard P. Phosphorylation of the catalytic subunit of Na^+,K^+-ATPase inhibits the activity of the enzyme. Proc Natl Acad Sci USA 1991; 88: 11359–11362.
58. Daly SE, Lane LK, Blostein R. Cytoplasmic regions of the alpha subunit of the sodium pump involved in modulating the Na,K-ATPase reaction. Ann NY Acad Sci 1997; 834:489–497.
59. Colonna T, Kostich M, Hamrick M, Hwang B, Rawn JD, Fambrough DM. Subunit interactions in the sodium pump. Ann NY Acad Sci 1997; 834:498–513.
60. Zollner H. Handbook of Enzyme Inhibitors, Part A. 2nd ed. Basel: VCH, 1993:340–344.
61. Goto A, Yamada K, Yagi N, Yoshioka M, Sugimoto T. Physiology and pharmacology of endogenous digitalis-like factors. Pharmacol Rev 1992; 44:377–399.
62. Zhao N, Lo LC, Berova N, Nakanishi K, Tymiak AA, Ludens JH, Haupert GT, Jr. Na,K-ATPase inhibitors from bovine hypothalamus and human plasma are different from ouabain: nanogram scale CD structural analysis. Biochemistry 1995; 34:9893–9896.
63. Lichtstein D, Gati I, Samuelov S, Berson D, Rozenman Y, Landau L, Deutsch J. Identification of digitalis-like compounds in human cataractous lenses. Eur J Biochem 1993; 216:261–268.
64. Skou JC, Hilberg C. The effect of sulfhydryl-blocking reagents and of urea on the (Na^+/K^+)-activated enzyme system. Biochim Biophys Acta 1965; 110:359–369.
65. Xu K. Any of several lysines can react with 5'-isothiocyanatofluorescein to inactivate sodium and potassium ion activated adenosinetriphosphatase. Biochemistry 1989; 28:5764–5772.
66. Winslow JW. The reaction of sulfhydryl groups of sodium and potassium ion-activated adenosine triphosphatase with N-ethylmaleimide. J Biol Chem 1981; 256:9522–9531.
67. Schoot BM, Schoots AFM, de Pont JJHHM, Schuurmans Stekhoven FMAH, Bonting SL. Studies on (Na^+/K^+) activated ATPase, XLI: Effects of N-ethylmaleimide on overall and partial reactions. Biochim Biophys Acta 1977; 483:181–192.
68. Tobin T, Akera T. Showdomycin, a nucleotide-site directed inhibitor of (Na^+/K^+)-ATPase. Biochim Biophys Acta 1975; 389:126–136.
69. Askari A, Huang W, Henderson GR. Functional and structural modifications induced by mercurials in Na,K-ATPase. In: Skou JC, Noerby JG, eds. Na,K-ATPase: Structure and Kinetics. New York: Academic Press, 1979:205–215.

70. Kim M, Akera T. O_2 free radicals cause of ischemia–reperfusion injury to cardiac Na^+K^+-ATPase. Am J Physiol 1987; 252:252-H257.
71. Kurella E, Kukley M, Tyulina O, Dobrota D, Matejovicova M, Mezesova V, Boldyrev A. Kinetic parameters of Na/K-ATPase modified by free radicals in vitro and in vivo. Ann NY Acad Sci 1997; 834:661–665.
72. Huang WH, Wang YH, Askari A. Na-K-ATPase: inactivation and degradation induced by oxygen radicals. Int J Biochem 1992; 24:621–626.
73. Xu KY, Zweier JL, Becker LC. Oxygen-free radicals directly attack the ATP binding site of the cardiac Na^+,K^+-ATPase. Ann NY Acad Sci 1997; 834:680–683.
74. van Kuijk FJGM. 4-Hydroxynonenal interaction with rhodopsin. Biochem Biophys Res Commun 1997; 230:275–279.
75. Siems WG, Zollner H, Grune T, Esterbauer H. Metabolic fate of 4-hydroxynonenal in hepatocytes: 1,4-dihydroxynonene is not the main product. J Lipid Res 1997; 38:612–622.
76. Siems WG, Pimenov AM, Esterbauer H, Grune T. Metabolism of 4-hydroxynonenal, a cytotoxic lipid peroxidation product, in thymocytes as an effective secondary antioxidative defense mechanism. J Biochem 1998; 123:534–539.
77. Grune T, Siems WG, Zollner H, Esterbauer H. Metabolism of 4-hydroxynonenal, a cytotoxic lipid peroxidation product, in Ehrlich mouse ascites cells at different proliferation stages. Cancer Res 1994; 54:5231–5235.
78. Uchida K, Shiraishi M, Naito Y, Torii Y, Nakamura Y, Osawa T. Activation of stress signaling pathways by the end product of lipid peroxidation: 4-hydroxy-2-nonenal is a potential inducer of intracellular peroxide production. J Biol Chem 1999; 274:2234–2242.

13
Carotenoids in the Nutrition of Infants

Olaf Sommerburg and Michael Leichsenring
University Children's Hospital, Ulm, Germany

Werner G. Siems
Herzog-Julius Hospital, Bad Harzburg, Germany

Kristina Meissner
University Children's Hospital, Würzburg, Germany

I. INTRODUCTION

In the last decades pediatricians learned more about the balance of oxidants and antioxidants in biological systems. As a consequence, the importance of dietary micronutrients with antioxidant function was acknowledged. Today a number of vitamins, such as vitamins A, C, or E, are supplemented regularly in fortified food for infants to prevent vitamin deficiency–related diseases. However, several other biologically active nutrients can be isolated from dietary plants and plants used in herbal medicine (1–3). These micronutrients include carotenoids, flavonoids, and polyphenols. Some of them serve as antioxidants; however, the spectrum of their biological functions is broader then previously thought.

Carotenoids have long been known because some of them play an important role as precursors of vitamin A (4). The role of vitamin A in growing infants has been intensively studied during the last several years. Therefore, until today, many clinicians understand carotenoids in nutrition exclusively as source for that vitamin. Although vitamin A has to be considered as an important nutrient, the knowledge about its biological functions is not the object of this chapter. Thus, we will focus more on the nonvitamin A–related functions of carotenoids and on the dietary supply of these micronutrients for infants.

II. IMPORTANCE OF CAROTENOIDS IN INFANCY

It is widely accepted that carotenoids play a preventive role in age-related diseases, such as cancer, cardiovascular disease, or macular degeneration (4), but still, not much is known about the specific role of these micronutrients in the first years of life. However, for some of these diseases, it is accepted that pathology has already begun in early life; thus, the importance of carotenoids for infants might be assumed. Therefore, we will focus in more detail on possible functions of carotenoids in infancy.

A. Antioxidant Defense

The ability of carotenoids to serve as radical scavenger has long been known (5). Notably, β-carotene and lycopene, as well as the oxycarotenoids zeaxanthin and lutein, exert antioxidant functions in lipid phases by free radical on singlet oxygen ($^1O_2$) quenching (6).

Oxidative stress has been implicated as one of the major pathogenetic factors in prematurity. Disorders of preterm infants, such as retinopathy, intraventricular hemorrhage, bronchopulmonary dysplasia, or necrotizing enterocolitis are associated with accelerated lipid peroxidation (7). Moreover, not only preterm infants suffer increased oxidative stress, term-born infants are also confronted by temporary hypoxic situations during birth. Each kind of oxygen deficiency is associated with accelerated purine degradation, leading to increased formation of superoxide radicals and H_2O_2 by the xanthine oxidase reaction. The cascade of peroxidation reactions of unsaturated fatty acids results in the formation of aldehydic lipid peroxidation (LPO) products. These aldehydes are able to act as "second toxic messengers" of free radicals, leading to cell damage from cytotoxic and genotoxic activity even in nanomolar concentrations (8,9). Schmidt et al. were able to show increased amounts of those aldehydic LPO products in cord blood plasma of term neonates with asphyxia as well as in term infants having an acidosis (umbilical artery pH < 7.20) but no postnatal disturbances of adaptation (10). Oxidative stress might be assumed in all infants with postnatal disturbances of pulmonary adaptation. These infants would suffer either temporary hypoxic conditions or, if treated by respirator, increased amounts of oxygen. Interestingly, Lindeman et al. showed that preterm and term infants have an increased total radical-trapping ability compared with adults (11). However, several studies have shown that levels of lipophilic antioxidants, vitamin E as well as carotenoids, are low in infants after birth (11–17). The only way, for instance, for vitamin E to contribute to the total antioxidant capacity would be an extensive recycling process. Water-soluble antioxidants, such as bilirubin, uric acid, and vitamin C are increased in neonates: They probably guarantee a higher recycling rate of lipid-soluble antioxidants within the first hours of life. However, the trapping capacity of neonates decreases postnatally, mainly owing to the decline of uric acid and vitamin C (14). Bilirubin levels follow a typical biphasic course and may compensate longer for the loss of antioxidant capacity. Attempts to limit the incidence and severity of oxygen toxicity within the first days of life by prophylactic therapy with vitamin E has produced conflicting results (18). However, within few days, healthy infants show plasma levels of antioxidants, including vitamin E, comparable with those of adults (14,15).

No specific data are yet available about the role of carotenoids in the network of antioxidant defense of infants.

B. Immune System

The immune system of newborn infants is still not fully developed; accordingly, clinicians distinguish between inborn and acquired immunity. In the first weeks of life infants are much less capable of responding to infections because of immunological deficiencies involving complement, polymorphonuclear leukocytes, cytokines, antibody, or cell-mediated immunity. Infections are a frequent and important cause of morbidity and mortality during the infant period. To the best of our knowledge there are no data showing a direct influence of carotenoids on the state of the immune system in infants. However, 10 years ago Bendich had already defined the role of carotenoids in immune response (19). In the last decade more precise information on the role of carotenoids at the molecular level of immunity became available. For example, Jyonouchi et al. could demonstrate in rodent models that astaxanthin, a carotenoid without vitamin A activity, enhances T-dependent humoral immunity in vivo and in vitro (20,21). Moreover, it was also shown that human peripheral blood mononuclear cells produce more IgM, IgG, and IgA in carotenoid-supplemented cultures than in unsupplemented cultures (22). In utero IgM production starts from the 10th to 12th week of gestation. IgG synthesis starts later, but the major amount of IgG found in neonates after birth is acquired by placental transport from the mother. Because synthesis of IgA does not begin until the 30th week of gestation, serum IgA levels after birth are extremely low compared with those of IgM and IgG (23). The findings that carotenoids are able to enhance IgA production against a T-cell-dependent polyclonal stimulant may be of special value. IgA is present mainly in the gastrointestinal and airway mucosa and is believed to have an essential role in the first-line defense mechanisms against pathogen invasion.

Other important implications in regulation of the immune system might be assumed from the property of some carotenoids to inhibit neoplastic transformation (24). Carotenoids also modulate gene expression in human cells (24). Moreover, some carotenoids are able to induce gap junctional communication between cells (25–27), which plays a key role in morphogenesis, cell differentiation, and secretion of hormones (28–30). In 1993, a report of the Cancer in Children and Antioxidant Micronutrients French Study Group showed that the incidence of tumors in children, such as leukemia, lymphoma, bone, and renal tumors, were inversely related to the plasma concentration of β-carotene (31).

The latter findings agree with the results of a study done with ten children with acute lymphoblastic leukemia (ALL) by our group (unpublished data). These children showed lower plasma values of β-carotene, α-carotene, lycopene, and cryptoxanthine than those of healthy children. Moreover, the plasma levels of these carotenoids were further decreasing in these children during chemotherapy. Although this was probably the result of the side effects of chemotherapy (vomiting, diarrhea) it may have an effect on the success of the whole treatment, considering the antioxidant and immunological actions assumed for carotenoids.

C. Development of Visual Function

The development of vision in infants is a long-term process that is not completely finished until birth. Although the optic vesicle is identifiable by the fourth week of gestation, and vascular supply of the retina is nearly complete by the term due date, development of the macular region continues for the first 3–4 years after birth. Photoreceptors differentiate from ganglion cells and represent the outer plexiform layer of the retina. They develop radially from the optic disc and reach the ora serratia at about 29 weeks of gestation (32). With increasing maturity of the photoreceptors, an increasing concentration of interstitial retinol-binding protein can be found in the retina. Vitamin A has a special implication for the function of the photoreceptors and much is already known about the importance of this vitamin for the development of neuronal and ocular tissues (33,34). However, the only carotenoids found in measurable amounts in eye tissues are lutein and zeaxanthin, which do not have a provitamin A function (35–37). These oxycarotenoids are distributed throughout the neuronal retina (36,37), and it is proposed that their major fraction is concentrated in the plasma membrane of the rod outer segments (38). A linear relation between the regional ratio of lutein and zeaxanthin and the regional ratio of rods and cones was shown (39). Thus, zeaxanthin is dominant in the foveal center, whereas lutein is more abundant farther out in the periphery (37,39). Both carotenoids are proposed to serve as an optical filter, by absorbing blue light and reducing chromatic aberration, and as antioxidants. Interestingly, several authors report that the macular pigment is absent in infants younger than 6 months and propose that lutein and zeaxanthin gradually accumulate with time from dietary sources (39,40). Because visual function, especially of the macular region, is still developing during the first months of human life, and these carotenoids are assumed to protect neuronal eye structures, one can assume that lutein and zeaxanthin should be considered as important micronutrients in infancy.

Cognitive development of infants is suggested to be highly related to the quality of vision (41–43). It remains to be investigated whether a delayed accumulation of lutein and zeaxanthin in children who do not have a sufficient supply of these oxycarotenoids also leads to delayed development of visual function and, consequently, to a delay in cognitive development. Over several years, long-chain polyunsaturated fatty acids (LCP) have been discussed as important for the development of neuronal and eye tissues (44–47). As a consequence, LCP are now regularly added as supplements in formula preparation for infants. For almost 15 years it has been known that lutein and zeaxanthin are present in the retina. Furthermore, their function in visual acuity is well known, and their absence was acknowledged to be one of the major pathogenetic factors of age-related macular degeneration. However, despite this knowledge of the nature of the macular pigment, the question of supplementation of lutein and zeaxanthin to infants was not discussed.

III. CAROTENOIDS IN NUTRITION OF NEONATES

Lipid-soluble vitamins, such as vitamin E and carotenoids, are markedly lower in cord blood of neonates in comparison with the serum levels of their mothers (12,13). This is also true for carotenoids (15–17). For α-tocopherol it is generally accepted that plasma concentration is closely associated with plasma lipid levels. Several authors showed that the α-tocopherol/lipid ratio in cord blood is comparable with the maternal ratio (48–51). Because carotenoids in plasma are also transported by lipoproteins, the lower amount of body lipids might be considered as a limiting factor for the storage capacity of neonates. For the investigated carotenoids, cord blood plasma concentrations were reported to be approximately 9–25% that of plasma levels in the mothers (15–17). Oostenbrug et al. found a correlation between cord blood plasma levels and maternal levels of lutein and α- and β-carotene when a ratio was calculated between the absolute carotenoid value and the unsaturation index of plasma phospholipid fatty acids (16). They found no such correlation for lycopene (16).

As oxidative stress is considered to be a key element in the pathology of many disturbances in preterm infants, the question arose whether plasma levels of lipophilic antioxidants are related to gestational age. For vitamin E the data in the literature are conflicting (11,15,52). For β-carotene in 1986, Ostrea et al. reported an almost linear correlation between cord blood plasma levels and gestational age (15). For other carotenoids no data are available in the literature comparing these antioxidants in preterm and term infants. However, in own investigations we did not find differences in plasma levels of β-cryptoxanthin, lycopene, α-, and β-carotene between preterm and term neonates (unpublished data; 53).

Nevertheless, a replenishment of the neonate's carotenoid levels to values comparable with adults can be reached only by diet. For β-carotene Ostrea et al. reported an increase of plasma levels within 5 days in breastfed infants but not in infants fed formula preparation (15). Therefore, a more detailed study of mother's milk and formula preparations for infants was necessary.

A. Mother's Milk

A more complex investigation on the relation between carotenoid concentrations in plasma of infants and feeding was performed by our group (54). In a first step, 24 breast milk samples (6 samples of colostrum and 18 samples of mature breast milk) were analyzed for β-carotene, α-carotene, lycopene, and β-cryptoxanthin. The data show that all four measured carotenoids are present in breast milk. Similar to other nutrients, carotenoid concentrations were significantly higher (by a factor of 3.5–4.5) in colostrum than in mature mother's milk (Table 1). In the light of these findings the rapid postnatal replenishment of β-carotene in breastfed neonates found by Ostrea et al. (15) may be explained.

Khachik et al. performed probably the most comprehensive investigation on qualitative and quantitative analysis of carotenoids in human serum and human breast milk (55). With a highly sophisticated method they were able to detect 34 carotenoids including 13 of their geometric isomers in both serum and corresponding breast milk of three lactating women. Although it is not clear whether all these isomers are necessary for infant's feeding, these results show that all carotenoids obtained from the daily diet are present in breast milk and are available for nutrition. Only recently, it was shown that manipulation of the daily diet by increased amounts of β-carotene resulted in elevated plasma concentrations of this carotenoid and, subsequently, also in higher amounts of β-carotene in the milk of lactating women (56,57).

B. Formula Preparations

The first investigation about the content of carotenoids in formula preparations was performed by Ostrea et al. in 1986, probably after they found that formula-fed infants, in contrast with breastfed, did not show a postnatal replenishment of plasma β-carotene. At this time, neither of the two investigated formula preparations available on the American market (Similac and Enfamil) contained β-carotene (15). More than 1 decade later, a total of eight formula preparations, available on the European market, for preterm (Beba 0 and Humana 0) and term infants (Pre Beba, Pre Aptamil, Pre Aletemil, and Pre Aponti), including two preparations that were considered to be hypoallergenic (Humana HA and Aletemil HA) were investigated for their content of carotenoids (β-carotene, α-carotene, lycopene, and β-cryptoxanthin) and compared with mother's milk (54). The results of this study show that formula preparations today still do not have the profile of the main carotenoids found in mother's milk. However, in contrast to the investigation of Ostrea et al., β-carotene was found at least in four of the eight preparations. Moreover, in three of the investigated preparations contained β-cryptoxanthin. However, four formulas, including the hypoallergenic, did not contain any of the detected carotenoids.

Table 1 Concentrations[a] of Different Carotenoids in Colostrum ($n = 6$) and Mature Breast Milk ($n = 18$)

Carotinoid	Colostrum	Mature breast milk
β-Carotene	254 (176–351)	58 (46–74)
α-Carotene	61 (42–78)	17 (0–26)
Lycopene	121 (104–141)	32 (30–41)
Cryptoxanthin	75 (66–142)	18 (14–27)

[a] Values are given in micrograms per liter (μg/L) as median and interquartile ranges.

Figure 1 compares the contents of carotenoids in the investigated formula preparations with mature breast milk.

C. Influence of the Kind of Feeding on Carotenoids in the Plasma of Infants

In the light of these findings, it is evident that different carotenoid profiles present in mother's milk and the currently available formula preparations also provide a different carotenoid supply to neonates. Therefore, the content of β-carotene, α-carotene, lycopene, and β-cryptoxanthin was investigated in a total of 83 blood samples from different preterm and term-born infants fed breast milk or formula preparations (see foregoing) (54). For statistical analysis the infants were divided into four groups that described their feeding situation: (1) neonates within the first 24 h after birth; (2) breastfed infants (BF); (3) infants fed both breast milk and formula preparations (BF/FF); and (4) formula-fed infants (FF). To exclude the influence of the carotenoid profile after birth obtained from the placenta during pregnancy, samples from formula-fed infants were analyzed only when the babies were older than 14 days. At this point, all of the investigated

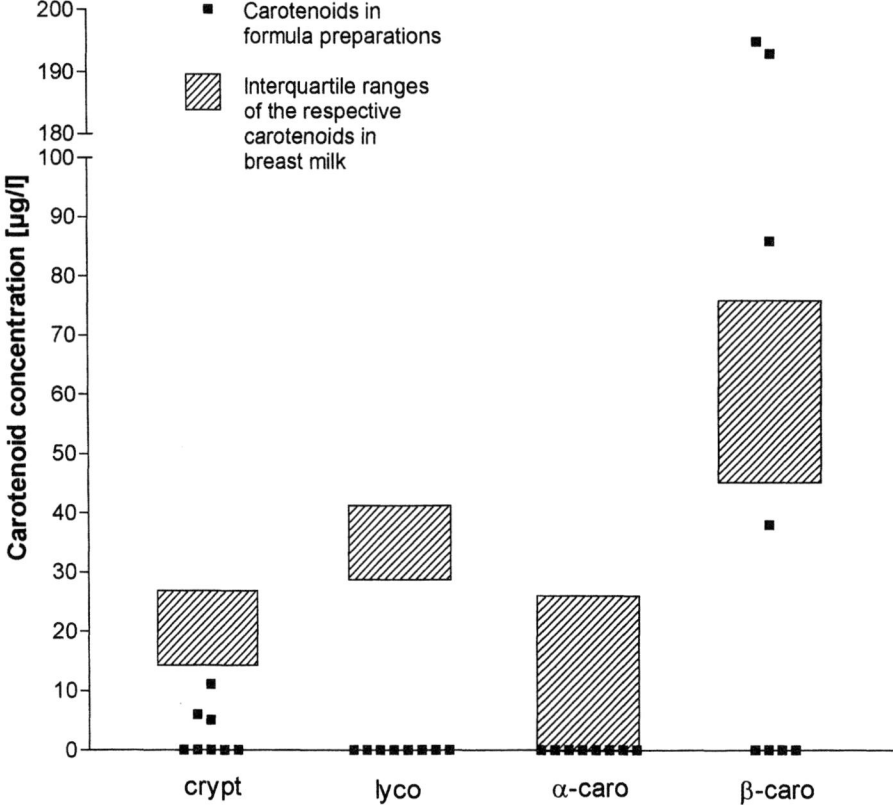

Figure 1 Carotenoid contents in different brands of formula preparation in comparison with mature breast milk. Concentrations of formula preparations are given as single values ($n = 8$) in micrograms per liter (μg/L) as means of three measurements. Values of mature breast milk ($n = 18$) are given in μg/L as interquartile ranges: crypt, cryptoxanthine; lyco, lycopene; α-caro, α-carotene; β-caro, β-carotene. (From Ref. 54.)

infants had normal plasma concentrations of tocopherols (α and γ) and retinol (unpublished data; 53).

Within 24 h after birth (group 1) all four carotenoids could be detected in plasma of the neonates. α-Carotene was not found in only two samples by comparing these results with BF infants (group 2) it could be shown that plasma concentrations of β-carotene, α-carotene, lycopene, and β-cryptoxanthin increased during breast-feeding, although the difference in α-carotene was not statistically significant. In contrast, carotenoid profiles of FF infants (group 4) were completely different from those of neonates after birth and from those of BF infants. Lycopene and α-carotene, which were not found in any of the formula preparations, were also not detectable in the plasma of FF infants older than 2 weeks. Also in BF/FF infants (group 3) lycopene and α-carotene were measured in much lower concentrations than in BF infants. These results clearly demonstrate that carotenoids in infants are consumed and disappear from plasma if not sufficiently supplied by nutrition. Considering lycopene as one of the most potent singlet oxygen scavengers (58,59), this might well affect the antioxidant capacity, compared with breastfed infants in which this carotenoid increased after birth.

β-Carotene was found in four of eight formula preparations. Two of them had levels close to the concentrations measured in mature mother's milk; however, in two others, β-carotene concentrations were about four times as high as in mature breast milk. On an average the group of FF newborns showed significantly lower β-carotene levels than neonates after birth and BF newborns. However, some singlet exclusions were seen, when FF newborns had β-carotene levels up to four times higher than BF infants (Fig. 2). The only explanation for these plasma concentrations is feeding with formula preparations containing very high β-carotene concentrations. However, the discussions about the benefit of a high-dose supplementation of one single carotenoid are not yet finished (60,61). Furthermore, β-carotene is known to exert pro-oxidative activity under certain conditions and some of the breakdown metabolites of that carotenoid have been discussed relative to signal function (62,63).

IV. CAROTENOIDS IN NUTRITION OF OLDER INFANTS AND CHILDREN

It is generally accepted that inclusion of solid food in the diet after 4–6 months of age contributes significantly to the health of the normal infant. Precooked cereals provide a convenient way to feed infants a variety of grains containing iron and vitamin B and having a greater caloric density than milk. Fruits and vegetables contain carotenoids beside many other important ingredients for infants, such as minerals, water-soluble vitamins, and B-complex vitamins. For infants the diet has to be introduced as strained, pureed-cooked, or in the form of fruit and vegetable juices. A greater number of parents in Western countries use commercially prepared preparations in which a wide variety of fruits and vegetables are used. These preparations mixed with mashed fruits and vegetables should provide the required amounts of carotenoids. However, there are no data in the literature in which the amounts of carotenoids in such preparations were evaluated. For infants, formula preparations fed before the introduction of fruit and vegetables in the daily diet seems to be the first opportunity to obtain carotenoids after placental transfer from the mother was no longer available.

Although meat does not contain substantial amounts of carotenoids (64), egg yolk is considered a good source for lutein and zeaxanthin (65). Orange is rich in vitamin C and also contains substantial amounts of oxycarotenoids and cryptoxanthin (65). However, many young infants do not tolerate citrus juices in amounts large enough to supply an adequate vitamin intake. Two of the most used vegetables in commercially fortified preparations for infant

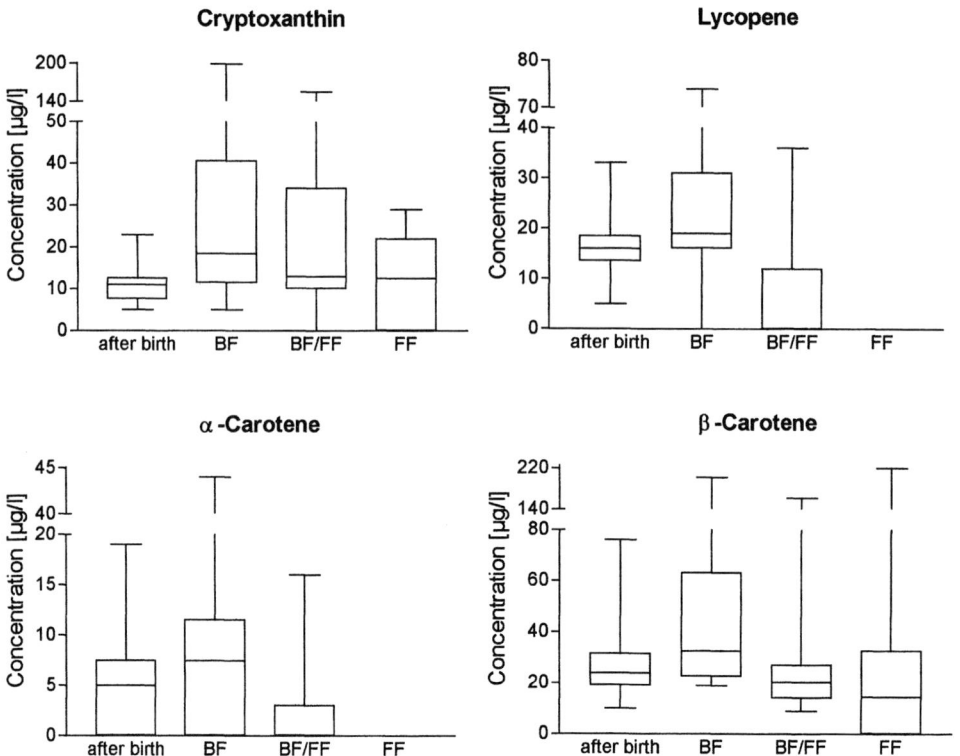

Figure 2 Plasma carotenoid concentrations of neonates after birth ($n = 23$), breastfed infants (BF; $n = 18$), formula fed infants (FF; $n = 20$), and infants fed both breast milk and formula preparations (BF/FF; $n = 22$). Values are given in micrograms per liter (μg/L) as median, interquartile ranges, minimum, and maximum. (From Ref. 54.)

are carrots and spinach. They provide mainly β-carotene and lutein, respectively. For older children it is recommended that they eat five servings of fruit and vegetables per day. Reviews of the literature databases are available providing information for physicians and nutritional physiologists about quantity and qualitative composition of carotenoids in different fruits and vegetables (66). Because supplementation of single carotenoids failed in interventional studies (67,68) more information about food consumption and recommendations to change eating behavior from nutrition physiologists and physicians are required to reach a decrease in the incidence of cancer and cardiovascular diseases. However, the failure of supplementation of a single carotenoid does not necessarily mean that the supplementation of a carotenoid mixture adapted to extracts from fruits and vegetables might not be effective.

A. Carotenoid Supplements in Infancy?

In several diseases, low levels of plasma carotenoids are observed in children (69–72). The most drastic decrease in all antioxidants is seen in malnourished children. Becker et al. did not find any substantial amounts of carotenoids in plasma of Nigerian children with kwashiorkor and marasmus (69). Rankins et al. reported comparable results from children from Senegal (70). One can expect that the lack of carotenoids may contribute to the well-documented impairment of immune response in these children. However, to the best of our knowledge no trials were reported in the literature in which malnourished children received antioxidant supplementation with carotenoids for improvement of their situation.

A huge problem in Africa, but also to some extent in Western countries, is the infection of children with human immunodeficiency virus (HIV). Omene et al. reported decreased β-carotene levels in children suffering from the acquired immune deficiency syndrome (AIDS) (71). It is generally accepted that disturbances in the regulation of the T-helper cells play a fundamental role in the pathology of AIDS. According to the results of Jyonouchi et al. (22), who showed carotenoids to be important regulators of T cells, one may raise the question of whether correction or carotenoid levels in plasma of HIV patients may have a positive effect on their immune system and further in the history of their disease.

In reviewing the literature, there is only one promising attempt to add carotenoid supplementation to the treatment regimen of a pediatric disease. Children who have cystic fibrosis show markedly decreased levels of several carotenoids in their plasma (72–74), mainly owing to the malabsorption of fat and lipophilic substances, which is typical for that disease. Some of these children were also deficient in retinol, leading to impaired nocturnal vision (75). In several trials, promising results were achieved when physicians added supplementation of β-carotene to the treatment of patients with cystic fibrosis. It was shown by several authors that levels of β-carotene could be effectively reestablished to normal ranges by β-carotene supplementation (76–78). Some investigators also recorded a reduction of LPO parameters in the patients receiving β-carotene (77,79,80). However, because of the malabsorption of lipophilic substances in these patients, large doses of β-carotene (60 mg twice a day) were necessary to improve LPO (76). In the study of Huet et al. (75), even an improvement of the nocturnal vision was found in some of his patients. Unfortunately, despite these promising results, no prospective studies with a greater number of patients were conducted to prove the assumed positive effects in children with cystic fibrosis. Consequently, supplementation of β-carotene did not reach significance in the treatment regimen of that disease. However, considering that the whole profile of carotenoids is depleted in cystic fibrosis patients (72), it has to be questioned whether supplementation of a multiple carotenoid mixture might be more effective.

In conclusion, carotenoids are a unique group of substances that exert different functions. According to the results of the intensive investigations of the last few years, it should be recognized that supplementation of one single carotenoid cannot replace the functions of the other substances. In the future, mixtures made from different carotenoid sources or representing the carotenoid profile normally present in plasma of healthy volunteers should be used for supplementation and enrichment of fortified food. Furthermore, we have to consider a large discrepancy between the knowledge about carotenoid action in vitro and the knowledge about carotenoid function in children in vivo.

REFERENCES

1. Khachik F, Beecher GR, Goli MB, Lusby WR. Separation and quantitation of carotenoids in foods. Methods Enzymol 1992; 213:347–359.
2. Packer L, Rimbach G, Virgili F. Antioxidant activity and biologic properties of a procyanidin-rich extract from pine (*Pinus maritima*) bark, pycnogenol. Free Radic Biol Med 1999; 27:704–724.
3. Luper S. A review of plants used in the treatment of liver disease: part 1. Altern Med Rev 1998; 3:410–421.
4. Krinsky NI. Actions of carotenoids in biological systems. Annu Rev Nutr 1993; 13:561–587.
5. Krinsky NI. Antioxidant functions of carotenoids. Free Radic Biol Med 1989; 7:617–635.
6. Sies H, Stahl W, Sundquist AR. Antioxidant functions of vitamins. Vitamins E and C, beta-carotene, and other carotenoids. Ann NY Acad Sci 1992; 669:7–20.

7. Sullivan JL. Iron, plasma antioxidants, and the "oxygen radical disease of prematurity." Am J Dis Child 1988; 142:1341–1344.
8. Esterbauer H, Schaur RJ, Zollner H. Chemistry and biochemistry of 4-hydroxynonenal, malonaldehyde and related aldehydes. Free Radic Biol Med 1991; 11:81–128.
9. Cadenas E, Muller A, Brigelius R, Esterbauer H, Sies H. Effects of 4-hydroxynonenal on isolated hepatocytes. Studies on chemiluminescence response, alkane production and glutathione status. Biochem J 1983; 214:479–487.
10. Schmidt H, Grune T, Muller R, Siems WG, Wauer RR. Increased levels of lipid peroxidation products malondialdehyde and 4-hydroxynonenal after perinatal hypoxia. Pediatr Res 1996; 40:15–20.
11. Lindeman JH, van-Zoeren GD, Schrijver J, Speek AJ, Poorthuis BJ, Berger HM. The total free radical trapping ability of cord blood plasma in preterm and term babies. Pediatr Res 1989; 26:20–24.
12. Leonard PJ, Doyle E, Harrington W. Levels of vitamin E in the plasma of newborn infants and of the mothers. Am J Clin Nutr 1972; 25:480–484.
13. Mino M, Nishino H. Fetal and maternal relationship in serum vitamin E level. J Nutr Sci Vitaminol (Tokyo) 1973; 19:475–482.
14. van-Zoeren GD, Lindeman JH, Houdkamp E, Brand R, Schrijver J, Berger HM. Postnatal changes in plasma chain-breaking antioxidants in healthy preterm infants fed formula and/or human milk. Am J Clin Nutr 1994; 60:900–906.
15. Ostrea EM J, Balun JE, Winkler R, Porter T. Influence of breast-feeding on the restoration of the low serum concentration of vitamin E and beta-carotene in the newborn infant. Am J Obstet Gynecol 1986; 154:1014–1017.
16. Oostenbrug GS, Mensink RP, Al MD, van Houwelingen A, Hornstra G. Maternal and neonatal plasma antioxidant levels in normal pregnancy, and the relationship with fatty acid unsaturation. Br J Nutr 1998; 80:67–73.
17. Kiely M, Cogan PF, Kearney PJ, Morrissey PA. Concentrations of tocopherols and carotenoids in maternal and cord blood plasma. Eur J Clin Nutr 1999; 53:711–715.
18. Karp WB, Robertson AF. Vitamin E in neonatology. Adv Pediatr 1986; 33:127–147.
19. Bendich A. Carotenoids and the immune response. J Nutr 1989; 119:112–115.
20. Jyonouchi H, Hill RJ, Tomita Y, Good RA. Studies of immunomodulating actions of carotenoids. I. Effects of beta-carotene and astaxanthin on murine lymphocyte functions and cell surface marker expression in in vitro culture system. Nutr Cancer 1991; 16:93–105.
21. Jyonouchi H, Zhang L, Tomita Y. Studies of immunomodulating actions of carotenoids. II. Astaxanthin enhances in vitro antibody production to T-dependent antigens without facilitating polyclonal B-cell activation. Nutr Cancer 1993; 19:269–280.
22. Jyonouchi H, Sun S, Gross M. Effect of carotenoids on in vitro immunoglobulin production by human peripheral blood mononuclear cells: astaxanthin, a carotenoid without vitamin A activity, enhances in vitro immunoglobulin production in response to a T-dependent stimulant and antigen. Nutr Cancer 1995; 23:171–183.
23. Gitlin D, Biasucci A. Development of γG, γA, γM, β1C/β1A, C1-esterase inhibitor, ceruloplasmin, transferrin, hemopexin, haptoglobin, fibrinogen, plasminogen, α1-antitrypsin, orosomucoid, β-lipoprotein, α_2-macroglobulin and prealbumin in human conceptus. J Clin Invest 1969; 48:1433–1446.
24. Bertram JS, Bortkiewicz H. Dietary carotenoids inhibit neoplastic transformation and modulate gene expression in mouse and human cells. Am J Clin Nutr 1995; 62:1327S–1336S.
25. Stahl W, Hanusch M, Sies H. 4-Oxo-retinoic acid is generated from its precursor canthaxanthin and enhances gap junctional communication in 10T1/2 cells. Adv Exp med Biol 387:121–128.
26. Stahl W, Nicolai S, Briviba K, Hanusch M, Broszeit G, Peters M, Martin HD, Sies H. Biological activities of natural and synthetic carotenoids: induction of gap junctional communication and singlet oxygen quenching. Carcinogenesis 1997; 18:89–92.
27. Zhang LX, Acevedo P, Guo H, Bertram JS. Upregulation of gap junctional communication and connexin43 gene expression by carotenoids in human dermal fibroblasts but not in human keratinocytes. Mol Carcinog 1995; 12:50–58.
28. Yamasaki H, Krutovskikh V, Mesnil M, Columbano A, Tsuda H, Ito N. Gap junctional intercellular communication and cell proliferation during rat liver carcinogenesis. Environ Health Perspect 1993; 101(suppl 5):191–197.

29. Dahl E, Winterhager E, Traub O, Willecke K. Expression of gap junction genes, connexin40 and connexin43, during fetal mouse development. Anat Embryol (Berl) 1995; 191:267–278.
30. Allen F, Tickle C, Warner A. The role of gap junctions in patterning of the chick limb bud. Development 1990; 108:623–634.
31. Malvy DJ, Burtschy B, Arnaud J, Sommelet D, Leverger G, Dostalova L, Drucker J, Amedee MO. Serum beta-carotene and antioxidant micronutrients in children with cancer. The "Cancer in Children and Antioxidant Micronutrients" French Study Group. Int J Epidemiol 1993; 22:761–771.
32. Kretzer FL, Hittner HM. Initiating events in the development of retinopathy of prematurity. In: Silverman WA, Flynn JT, eds. Retinopathy of Prematurity. New York: Blackwell Scientific, 1985:121–152.
33. Maden M, Holder N. Retinoic acid and development of the central nervous system. Bioessays 1992; 14:431–438.
34. Pirie A. Vitamin A deficiency and child blindness in the developing world. Proc Nutr Soc 1983; 42:53–64.
35. Yeum KJ, Taylor A, Tang G, Russell RM. Measurement of carotenoids, retinoids, and tocopherols in human lenses. Invest Ophthalmol Vis Sci 1995; 36:2756–2761.
36. Bone RA, Landrum JT, Friedes LM, Gomez CM, Kilburn MD, Menendez E, Vidal I, Wang W. Distribution of lutein and zeaxanthin stereoisomers in the human retina. Exp Eye Res 1997; 64:211–218.
37. Handelman GJ, Dratz EA, Reay CC, van Kuijk FJGM. Carotenoids in the human macula and whole retina. Invest Ophthalmol Vis Sci 1988; 29:850–855.
38. Sommerburg O, Siems WG, Hurst JS, Lewis JW, Kliger DS, van Kuijk FJGM. Lutein and zeaxanthin are associated with photoreceptors in the human retina. Curr Eye Res 1999; 19:491–495.
39. Bone RA, Landrum JT, Fernandez L, Tarsis SL. Analysis of the macular pigment by HPLC: retinal distribution and age study. Invest Ophthalmol Vis Sci 1988; 29:843–849.
40. Nussbaum JJ, Pruett RC, Delori FC. Historic perspectives. Macular yellow pigment. The first 200 years. Retina 1981; 1:296–310.
41. Kulp MT, Schmidt PP. Visual predictors of reading performance in kindergarten and first grade children. Optom Vis Sci 1996; 73:255–262.
42. Golding J, Rogers IS, Emmett PM. Association between breast feeding, child development and behaviour. Early Hum Dev 1997; 49(suppl):S175–S184.
43. Cass HD, Sonksen PM, McConachie HR. Developmental setback in severe visual impairment. Arch Dis Child 1994; 70:192–196.
44. Birch EE, Birch DG, Hoffman DR, Uauy R. Dietary essential fatty acid supply and visual acuity development. Invest Ophthalmol Vis Sci 1992; 33:3242–3253.
45. Carlson SE, Werkman SH, Peeples JM, Wilson WM. Long-chain fatty acids and early visual and cognitive development of preterm infants. Eur J Clin Nutr 1994; 48(suppl 2):S27–S30.
46. Carlson SE, Ford AJ, Werkman SH, Peeples JM, Koo WW. Visual acuity and fatty acid status of term infants fed human milk and formulas with and without docosahexaenoate and arachidonate from egg yolk lecithin. Pediatr Res 1996; 39:882–888.
47. Uauy R, Birch E, Birch D, Peirano P. Visual and brain function measurements in studies of n-3 fatty acid requirements of infants. [Published erratum appears in J Pediatr 1992 Aug;121(2):329.] J Pediatr 1992; 120:S168–S180.
48. Dison PJ, Lockitch G, Halstead AC, Pendray MR, Macnab A, Wittmann BK. Influence of maternal factors on cord and neonatal plasma micronutrient levels. Am J Perinatol 1993; 10:30–35.
49. Jain SK, Wise R, Bocchini JJJ. Vitamin E and vitamin E–quinone levels in red blood cells and plasma of newborn infants and their mothers. J Am Coll Nutr 1996; 15:44–48.
50. Lughetti L, Maggi E, Volta C, Palladini G, Bellomo G, Bernasconi S. Neonatal and maternal levels of lipid-soluble antioxidants. Acta Biomed Ateneo Parmense 1997; 68(suppl 1):81–83.
51. Kiely M, Cogan P, Kearney PJ, Morrissey PA. Relationship between smoking, dietary intakes and plasma levels of vitamin E and beta-carotene in matched maternal–cord pairs. Int J Vitam Nutr Res 1999; 69:262–267.
52. Huertas JR, Palomino N, Ochoa JJ, Quiles JL, Ramirez TM, Battino M, Robles R, Mataix J. Lipid peroxidation and antioxidants in erythrocyte membranes of full-term and preterm newborns. Biofactors 1998; 8:133–137.
53. Meissner K. Die Rolle der Carotinoide bei Früh- und Neugeborenen. MD dissertation, University of Heidelberg, Germany, 1999.

54. Sommerburg O, Meissner K, Nelle M, Lenhartz H, Leichsenring M. Carotenoid supply in breast-fed and formula-fed neonates. Eur J Pediatr 2000; 159(1–2):105–113.
55. Khachik F, Spangler CJ, Smith JJ, Canfield LM, Steck A, Pfander H. Identification, quantification, and relative concentrations of carotenoids and their metabolites in human milk and serum. Anal Chem 1997; 69:1873–1881.
56. Johnson EJ, Qin J, Krinsky NI, Russell RM. beta-Carotene isomers in human serum, breast milk and buccal mucosa cells after continuous oral doses of all-*trans* and 9-*cis* beta-carotene. J Nutr 1997; 127:1993–1999.
57. Canfield LM, Giuliano AR, Neilson EM, Blashil BM, Graver EJ, Yap HH. Kinetics of the response of milk and serum beta-carotene to daily beta-carotene supplementation in healthy, lactating women. Am J Clin Nutr 1998; 67:276–283.
58. Di Mascio P, Devasagayam TP, Kaiser S, Sies H. Carotenoids, tocopherols and thiols as biological singlet molecular oxygen quenchers. Biochem Soc Trans 1990; 18:1054–1056.
59. Wagner JR, Motchnik PA, Stocker R, Sies H, Ames BN. The oxidation of blood plasma and low density lipoprotein components by chemically generated singlet oxygen. J Biol Chem 1993; 268:18502–18506.
60. Omaye ST, Krinsky NI, Kagan VE, Mayne ST, Liebler DC, Bidlack WR. beta-Carotene: friend or foe? Fundam Appl Toxicol 1997; 40:163–174.
61. Halliwell B. Establishing the significance and optimal intake of dietary antioxidants: the biomarker concept. Nutr Rev 1999; 57:104–113.
62. Krinsky NI. Carotenoid metabolites as cell signaling modulators. OCC 1999 World Congress—Oxidants and Antioxidants in Biology, March 3–6, 1999: abstr 6.
63. Siems WG, Sommerburg O, van Kuijk FJGM. Discrepancy between majority of lutein and zeaxanthin and lack of lycopene and beta-carotene in human retina is due to different radical-initiated breakdown rates of carotenoids. Biofactors 1999; 10:105–113.
64. Chug–Ahuja JK, Holden JM, Forman MR, Mangels AR, Beecher GR, Lanza E. The development and application of a carotenoid database for fruits, vegetables, and selected multicomponent foods. J Am Diet Assoc 1993; 93:318–323.
65. Sommerburg O, Keunen JE, Bird AC, van Kuijk FJGM. Fruits and vegetables that are sources for lutein and zeaxanthin: the macular pigment in human eyes. Br J Ophthalmol 1998; 82:907–910.
66. Mangels AR, Holden JM, Beecher GR, Forman MR, Lanza E. Carotenoid content of fruits and vegetables: an evaluation of analytic data. [Published erratum in J Am Diet Assoc 1993 May;93(5):527.] J Am Diet Assoc 1993; 93:284–296.
67. Blumberg J, Block G. The Alpha-Tocopherol, Beta-Carotene Cancer Prevention Study in Finland. Nutr Rev 1994; 52:242–245.
68. Smigel K. beta Carotene fails to prevent cancer in two major studies; CARET intervention stopped. J Natl Cancer Inst 1996; 88:145.
69. Becker K, Botticher D, Leichsenring M. Antioxidant vitamins in malnourished Nigerian children. Int J Vitam Nutr Res 1994; 64:306–310.
70. Rankins J, Green NR, Tremper W, Stacewitcz–Sapuntzakis M, Bowen P, Ndiaye M. Undernutrition and vitamin A deficiency in the Department of Linguere, Louga Region of Senegal. [Published erratum in Am J Clin Nutr 1993 Sept;58(3):453.] Am J Clin Nutr 1993; 58:91–97.
71. Omene JA, Easington CR, Glew RH, Prosper M, Ledlie S. Serum beta-carotene deficiency in HIV-infected children. J Natl Med Assoc 1996; 88:789–793.
72. Homnick DN, Cox JH, Deloof MJ, Ringer TV. Carotenoid levels in normal children and in children with cystic fibrosis. J Pediatr 1993; 122:703–707.
73. Benabdeslam H, Abidi H, Garcia I, Bellon G, Gilly R, Revol A. Lipid peroxidation and antioxidant defenses in cystic fibrosis patients. Clin Chem Lab Med 1999; 37:511–516.
74. Portal BC, Richard MJ, Faure HS, Hadjian AJ, Favier AE. Altered antioxidant status and increased lipid peroxidation in children with cystic fibrosis. Am J Clin Nutr 1995; 61:843–847.
75. Huet F, Semama D, Maingueneau C, Charavel A, Nivelon JL. Vitamin A deficiency and nocturnal vision in teenagers with cystic fibrosis. Eur J Pediatr 1997; 156:949–951.
76. Homnick DN, Spillers CR, Cox SR, Cox JH, Yelton LA, Deloof MJ, Oliver LK, Ringer TV. Single- and multiple-dose-response relationships of beta-carotene in cystic fibrosis. J Pediatr 1995; 127:491–494.
77. Rust P, Eichler I, Renner S, Elmadfa I. Effects of long-term oral beta-carotene supplementation on lipid peroxidation in patients with cystic fibrosis. Int J Vitam Nutr Res 1998; 68:83–87.

78. Winklhofer–Roob BM, van't Hof MA, Shmerling DH. Response to oral beta-carotene supplementation in patients with cystic fibrosis: a 16-month follow-up study. [Published erratum appears in Acta Paediatr 1996 Jan;85(1):124.] Acta Paediatr 1995; 84:1132–1136.
79. Lepage G, Champagne J, Ronco N, Lamarre A, Osberg I, Sokol RJ, Roy CC. Supplementation with carotenoids corrects increased lipid peroxidation in children with cystic fibrosis. [Published erratum appears in Am J Clin Nutr 1997 Feb;65(2):578.] Am J Clin Nutr 1996; 64:87–93.
80. Winklhofer–Roob BM, Puhl H, Khoschsorur G, van't Hof MA, Esterbauer H, Shmerling DH. Enhanced resistance to oxidation of low density lipoproteins and decreased lipid peroxide formation during beta-carotene supplementation in cystic fibrosis. Free Radic Biol Med 1995; 18:849–859.

14

Human Studies on Bioavailability and Serum Response of Carotenoids

Elizabeth J. Johnson
Jean Mayer USDA Human Nutrition Research Center on Aging at Tufts University, Boston, Massachusetts

I. INTRODUCTION

Carotenoids are a family of compounds comprising over 600 fat-soluble pigments; however, only about 24 are found in human plasma and tissues. The two subclasses of carotenoids are the oxygenated xanthophylls and the hydrocarbon carotenes. Evidence is emerging to indicate that these plant pigments may have a role in reducing the risk of certain diseases. For example, lycopene has been suggested to be a factor in the prevention of prostate cancer, and lutein has been implicated to play a role in reducing the risk of age-related macular degeneration. Also, some carotenoids are precursor to vitamin A (e.g., β-carotene, α-carotene, β-cryptoxanthin) and are the major sources of dietary vitamin A in many parts of the world. For these reasons, there is growing need for information on the factors involved in the bioavailability of carotenoids.

The bioavailability of a carotenoid is considered to be the fraction of ingested carotenoids utilized for normal physiological functions or storage (1). Published information on carotenoid bioavailability is still largely based on serum or plasma levels after ingestion. Currently, more sophisticated methods are being developed to provide more accurate assessments of carotenoid bioavailability. Regardless of the method of choice, the bioavailability of a carotenoid involves the processes of intestinal absorption, transport, and distribution to tissues.

All measures of bioavailability are estimates. Much of the research has focused on β-carotene. The reasons for this are (1) β-carotene is a carotenoid of high provitamin A activity, (2) it is a major carotenoid in foods and human tissues, and (3) there is a mass commercial production of β-carotene, thus making it widely available for study. However, with the emerging data to suggest a role of other carotenoids in health and disease, studies are being conducted to examine the bioavailability of the other major carotenoids found in diet and human serum and tissues.

II. ABSORPTION AND METABOLISM OF CAROTENOIDS

Carotenoids, being fat soluble, follow the same intestinal absorption path as dietary fat. Release from the food matrix and dissolution in the lipid phase appears to be important initial steps in the absorption process. Carotenoids are thought to be absorbed in the small intestinal mucosa by a passive, diffusion process. Fatty acid esters of xanthophylls are cleaved in the lumen of the small intestine before uptake by the mucosa. Carotenoids are taken up by the mucosa of the small intestine and packaged into triacylglycerol-rich chylomicrons. β-Carotene and other provitamin A carotenoids are partly converted to vitamin A, primarily retinyl esters, in the intestinal mucosa, and both carotenoids and retinyl esters are incorporated into chylomicrons and secreted into lymph for transport to the liver. A more comprehensive review of carotenoid absorption can be found elsewhere in Chapter 10.

In fasting serum, hydrocarbon carotenes are found primarily in low-density lipoprotein (LDL), whereas xanthophylls (containing one or more polar functional groups) are more evenly distributed between LDL and high-density lipoprotein (HDL) (2). The carotenes, being lipophilic, are located in the core of a lipoprotein, which may explain why they do not transfer between lipoproteins at an appreciable rate (3). Because the xanthophylls are more polar, they are probably located on the surface of lipoproteins, and are likely to undergo more rapid surface transfer, resulting in the observed apparent equilibration between LDL and HDL.

III. METHODS TO MEASURE BIOAVAILABILITY

A. Serum Concentrations After Carotenoid Ingestion

The method of concentration–time curves for carotenoids in serum or plasma has been widely used as a measure of carotenoid bioavailability. In this method quantitated amounts of carotenoids are ingested and the changes in serum concentration at various time intervals after ingestion are determined. The advances in high-performance liquid chromatography (HPLC) techniques have permitted quantitation of individual carotenoids and their isomers in serum at low concentrations. Relative differences in absorption are determined by comparing the serum carotenoid concentrations with baseline values at various postingestion intervals. With this method, comparisons of relative bioavailabilities can be made among carotenoids, formulations (purified sources vs. food; food processing vs. unprocessed), or persons. In such serum response curves, bioavailability is taken to be synonymous with absorption and used to reflect carotenoid entering the serum following ingestion.

Serum response curves are carried out using either single or multiple doses. The single-dose method attempts to measure carotenoid entering the body in chylomicrons during the absorption period following a single dose. Therefore, a rise in serum concentrations followed by a fall is generally measured. In longer-term multiple dose trials, serum carotenoid concentrations reach a constant elevated level after prolonged intake.

The use of serum response curves is limited by several factors. First, the serum response to a single oral dose of a carotenoid can be highly variable. This has been observed for β-carotene and lycopene (4) and lutein (5). Also, because of the rapid rate of chylomicron catabolism and hepatic uptake of chylomicron remnants (half-life 10–15 min), even in the postprandial state chylomicron-association carotenoids represent a small proportion of total serum carotenoids. Furthermore, regardless of the times at which the measurements are taken, the concentration of carotenoid in the serum represents a balance among intestinal absorption, breakdown, tissue uptake, and release from body stores. These factors limit the possibility of measuring absolute bioavailabilities. Consequently, relatively large doses, usually exceeding the typical daily intake by at least fivefold are needed to observe a significant increase in concentration over baseline levels. The question arises of whether results from pharmacological doses represent the situation with physiological doses. It is likely that large doses saturate transport and metabolic processes, thereby making interpretation of results difficult. This is supported by the observation that the plasma area under the concentration–time curve (AUC) in studies that used β-carotene as the test carotenoid, were not proportional to the carotenoid dose (6,7).

With a provitamin A carotenoid, the metabolism of a portion of the test dose to retinyl esters during intestinal absorption may further complicate the interpretation of results. This would not occur for xanthophylls. However, xanthophylls may undergo rapid exchange among lipoproteins. This could substantially influence the quantification of serum carotenoids concentration–time curves.

Although serum carotenoid concentrations–time curves have their limitations, they are still widely used because methods can provide an estimate on relative bioavailabilities with relatively simple procedures.

B. Lipoprotein Concentrations After Carotenoid Ingestion

The concentration of β-carotene in triglyceride-rich lipoprotein (TRL) fractions (mixtures of chylomicrons and very low-density lipoproteins; VLDL) have been used to estimate between-person and within-person variability in β-carotene absorption and intestinal conversion to retinyl esters (8). Advantages of this method over the serum response curve method are (1) accounting for intestinal conversion to retinyl esters, (2) allowing the use of smaller test dose, and (3) improving the discrimination of newly absorbed carotenoids from endogenous pools (mainly LDL). Because this method separates lipoproteins using density gradients, a major disadvantage is that the intestinal-derived chylomicrons are not separated from the liver-derived VLDL. Consequently, there is overlap between the density range of chylomicrons and that of VLDL in the $d < 1.006$ fraction. The proportion of the remnant pool that is recovered will be dependent on separation parameters (e.g., gradient density, period of centrifugation, and speed). Indeed, different parameters have been used with this technique (9–11). Although the TRL carotenoid concentration–time curves are considered to be a better estimate of bioavailability than that of serum response curves, it also measures relative, rather than absolute, bioavailabilities.

It is possible that different centrifugation methods will result in differing recoveries. None of the published data using this method have assessed the recovery of chylomicrons in the collected fraction. This limits the ability to estimate absolute absorption efficiency, because a low recovery will result in an underestimation of absorption efficiency. It is likely that differences in reported AUC data using this method [e.g., that of van Vliet et al. (8) and O'Neill et al. (11)] are due to different recovery of chylomicrons.

As observed with serum response curves, data from TRL are typically highly variable (8,10), especially among subjects, even though treatment conditions are usually standardized. This may be due to carotenoid absorption among subjects being highly variable. It may also be a result of differences in the kinetics of chylomicron secretion and clearance (hepatic remnant uptake) among individuals, given that, at any moment in time, the serum chylomicron remnant population will reflect the concentration of carotenoid in the secreted particle, the rate of serum input, and the rate of hepatic remnant uptake. It is highly likely that different individuals have different kinetics of chylomicron input or removal; such differences have not yet been taken into account. Such variability can limit the ability to determine differences in bioavailabilities among individuals or treatments. Nonetheless, the TRL curves have been useful to obtain relative bioavailabilities, such as lycopene from raw versus heated tomato products (see later discussion) (9).

The use of TRL carotenoid concentration versus time for the estimate of the bioavailability of xanthophylls may present additional problems. These carotenoids, which possess polar functional groups, are susceptible to rapid surface transfer to LDL or HDL, such as that that occurs for other polar lipid constituents, such as cholesterol, phospholipid, and tocopherols. Furthermore, the use of this method in determining the bioavailability of carotenoids from foods may be limited because food matrices are slowly digested and would yield slow rates of carotenoid absorption. A slow rate would result in broad concentration–time curves, which would make the measure of AUC difficult, inaccurate, or impossible.

C. Balance Techniques (Oral–Fecal or Gastrointestinal Lavage)

Comparison of the amount of a substance consumed with its fecal excretion has been a method used for the estimation of absorption. The basis of the balance method is the quantitative measurement of all intake (input) and excretion (output) of the carotenoid over a specific period of time. No urinary excretion of either free, or conjugated carotenoids has been found, and there is negligible loss with exfoliation from skin. Therefore, balance studies involve the estimation of carotenoid intake for a period of days, and the collection and analysis of all fecal output for carotenoids for the same time period. Output is subtracted from input, and divided by the number of days of the balance period, to obtain the quantity of carotenoid apparently absorbed.

For carotenoids, the balance method has the major disadvantage of an inability to account for carotenoid degradation in the upper (chemical oxidation) or lower (microbial degradation or alteration) regions of the gastrointestinal tract. In an attempt to overcome this, Bowen et al. (12) have modified the traditional oral–fecal balance approach to include gastrointestinal lavage (washout) after allowing a defined period of digestion and absorption. This method involves a preparatory gastrointestinal lavage using a polyethylene glycol–electrolyte solution. Subjects then consume a standardized test meal containing a known amount of carotenoid. After a 24-h period, a second lavage is performed. Fecal output is collected from the test meal through the postmeal lavage and analyzed for carotenoids. The difference between ingested carotenoid and that recovered in fecal effluent is interpreted to represent efficiency of absorption. The advantage of this approach is that it controls the residence time of nonabsorbed carotenoid in the lower gut, thereby possibly limiting microfloral degradation or modification. This would permit a more precise estimation of the amounts of carotenoids retained in the gastrointestinal tract that would be available for absorption. However, the duration of the allowed absorption period is currently arbitrary, and the quantitative extent to which microfloral metabolism is limited is unknown.

The gastrointestinal lavage method requires further evaluation and confirmation, and it may have limited use in bioavailability studies. However, this technique may prove useful when used, along with specific stable isotopes of individual carotenoids, to assess isotope dilution from endogenous carotenoids in an effort to determine true absorption.

D. Stable Isotope Applications

The development of stable isotope-labeled carotenoids has made possible the ability to clearly discriminate between dosed and endogenous carotenoids. Isotopic labeling has also made it possible to use doses sufficiently low to avoid influencing endogenous pools. Stable isotopes eliminates the risks associated with radioactive isotopes. To date, the published research on isotopic applications to determine carotenoid bioavailability have been with β-carotene. In one study, chemically synthesized, octadeuterated β-carotene and conventional mass spectrometry (MS) were employed (13), and in another, biosynthetic, ^{13}C-labeled β-carotene and combustion-isotope ratio mass spectrometry were used (14). An added advantage to isotopic labeling is that it permits an assessment of the extent of intestinal conversion to vitamin A, and for subsequent empirical or compartmental modeling to estimate absolute absorption and postabsorptive metabolism (15).

In this method, single doses of deuterated or ^{13}C-enriched β-carotene are administered to subjects under standardized conditions, following a brief period of dietary intervention to clear the upper gastrointestinal tract of carotenoids and vitamin A. Serial blood samples are drawn at baseline and frequently over the first 16 h, then less frequently if postabsorption data are needed. Because the absorption (chylomicron) peak typically occurs at 4–5 h after dosing, frequent sampling (at least hourly) is needed during this period to obtain an accurate AUC of kinetic parameters concerning absorption and intestinal metabolism. Because the dosed carotenoid is labeled, isolation of chylomicrons is not required. With both conventional and isotope ratio–MS approaches, extensive fraction purification is required, making these methods labor-intensive and costly, which limits the size of sample groups.

Bioavailability of carotenoid from different formulations can potentially be compared simultaneously using different isotopomers of the same carotenoid, varying either in number of deuterium atoms or in ^{13}C enrichment and monitoring of the appropriate masses. In this way, direct comparisons can be made under identical dosing conditions, avoiding the need for separate tests and washout periods for each formulation.

IV. FACTORS RELATED TO THE BIOAVAILABILITY OF CAROTENOIDS

A. Carotenoid Type

Xanthophylls, such as lutein and zeaxanthin, are lipophilic molecules, but are more polar than carotenes, such as β-carotene and lycopene. Therefore, xanthophylls may be more easily incorporated into the outer portions of lipid micelles within the gastrointestinal tract and may be more easily taken up by enterocyte membranes and, eventually, chylomicrons, presumably increasing the bioavailability. This idea is supported by the work of van het Hof et al. (16) in which over a period of 4 weeks, healthy young men and women (mean age: 22 years) consumed controlled diets high (490 g/day) or low (130 g/day) in vegetables. The low-vegetable diet was provided with and without a supplement of highly bioavailable β-carotene (6 mg/day) and lutein (9 mg/day). In this study, the bioavailability of carotenoid was measured using the change in plasma concentrations. Comparison of the plasma results for the high-vegetable diet with the low-vegetable diet plus the supplemental carotenoids found a substantial difference between the relative bioavailabilities of β-carotene (14%) and lutein (67%).

A difference in bioavailability between β-carotene and lutein was also found in a recent prospective study (17) in which seven healthy adult women and men modified their usual daily diets by adding 60 g/day of spinach for 15 weeks, providing 10.8 mg/day of lutein and 5 mg/day of β-carotene. Lutein concentrations in serum significantly increased twofold from baseline values after 4 weeks of spinach feeding. The serum lutein concentrations remained higher than baseline throughout the 15-week–supplementation period. Despite the daily consumption of at least 5 mg β-carotene contained in the spinach, the mean serum concentrations of β-carotene did not change throughout the entire study. These findings may reflect the differences between a relatively hydrophilic xanthophyll and a lipophilic carotene. Given that this study was conducted with a food source rather than pure supplements, they may also reflect a difference in the location of the carotenoid in the food matrix (i.e., the pigment–protein complexes of cell chloroplasts versus the crystalline form in chromoplasts).

B. Food Matrix

Studies that examine the effect of food matrix on carotenoid bioavailability compare responses between a pure supplement and an equivalent carotenoid dose found in a food source. Several investigators have found that β-carotene dissolved in oil is absorbed more readily than β-carotene from foods (18–20). Presumably, this is because a pure form of β-carotene does not need to release from a food matrix for intestinal absorption. In several human studies, the serum response of β-carotene from foods varied, when compared with the response from β-carotene supplements. In raw carrots, the bioavailability has been reported to range from 17 to 26% (21–23), in mixed vegetables from 7 to 14% (16,24), and in spinach the bioavailability was measured to vary between 5 and 10% (25). The low bioavailability of β-carotene in spinach may be due to its entrapment and complexing to proteins in chloroplasts and within cell structures. In carrots, β-carotene exists as crystals, up to 1000 μm in length, which may explain the relatively higher bioavailability.

The large difference in bioavailability between a pure source and a food source of a carotenoid may not be true for all carotenoids. van het Hof et al. found that the relative bioavailability of lutein from a high-vegetable diet was 67% (16), and others found that the serum lutein response, as measured by the 24-h AUC, from a lutein supplement was no different from an equal amount of lutein contained in cooked spinach (5). The reason for the discrepancy between β-carotene and lutein bioavailability from foods could lie in where the particular carotenoid is located within the plant cell matrix, or it could reflect the difference between a xanthophyll and a carotene. Xanthophylls, being more water-soluble than lipophilic carotenes, may be positioned differently within the lipoproteins, which may cause them to be absorbed, transported, and cleared differently from those of hydrocarbons. Different serum responses for xanthophylls and carotenes have been reported in preruminant calves (26).

C. Food Processing

Studies examining the effect of food processing on carotenoid bioavailability compare responses among a raw, whole food and food that has been heat-treated or mechanically homogenized. Cooking and mechanical homogenization increases the bioavailability of carotenoids (27). The mechanism by which this occurs is most likely the disruption of the food matrix to release the carotenoid from the matrix and from protein complexes (28). For example, in a 4-week–feeding study, the plasma response of β-carotene was approximately three times greater in spinach and carrots that were pureed and thermally processed than it was when these vegetables were consumed in raw, large pieces (29).

Similar to the effect on β-carotene bioavailability, heating tomato was associated with an increase in lycopene absorption when compared with the serum response for unprocessed tomato juice (30). Also, the lycopene bioavailability (as measured by TRL response curves) was greater from a single dose of tomato paste than it was from an equal lycopene dose from fresh tomatoes (9). Interestingly, these studies support the findings of Giovannucci et al. that the association between consumption of various tomato products and the risk of prostate cancer depends on the bioavailability of lycopene (31). That is, there is an association with the consumption of tomato paste, not with consumption of minimally processed tomato juice.

The improved effect on bioavailability by processing may not occur for xanthophylls. In a study designed to examine the carotenoid bioavailability in various preparations of spinach, subjects received, over a 3-week period, a control diet, a control diet supplemented with carotenoids, or one of four spinach products: whole-leaf spinach, minced spinach, enzymatically liquefied spinach, and liquefied spinach to which dietary fiber was added (25). Consumption of spinach was observed to significantly increase serum concentrations of β-carotene and lutein; however, serum β-carotene responses differed significantly between the whole-leaf and liquefied spinach groups and between the minced and liquefied groups, whereas the serum lutein response did not differ among spinach groups.

D. Amount of Carotenoids

At low doses, the efficiency of β-carotene absorption from the diet is higher than that with higher doses (21,32); this is also true for lycopene (30). Absorption of carotenoids appears to be linear at dosages up to 20–30 mg, but becomes limited at higher levels because of factors, such as solubility (33).

E. Interactions with Other Carotenoids

Human studies on carotenoid interactions have been recently reviewed by van den Berg (34). These studies have demonstrated interactions among carotenoids, largely through the use of serum response data.

Kostic et al. (35) examine plasma responses after a single oral dose of β-carotene and lutein, both alone and after an equimolar mixture (0.5 μmol/kg body weight for each), and found that when combined in the same dose, β-carotene significantly reduced the serum AUC values for lutein to 53–61% of control values, whereas lutein reduced the AUC value for β-carotene in five subjects, but enhanced it in three subjects. The effects of lutein on the AUC for β-carotene were inversely related to the AUC for β-carotene alone. These investigations concluded that β-carotene and lutein interact with each other; however, individual responses were highly varied.

Combined doses of β-carotene and canthaxanthin (25 mg each) resulted in a plasma canthaxanthin response significantly lower than after treatment with canthaxanthin alone, but this was not true for the β-carotene response (36). Similarly, Paetau et al. recently reported that ingestion of a 25-mg–each dose of β-carotene and canthaxanthin reduced plasma canthaxanthin response, but not that of β-carotene (37). Similar to the results reported by Kostic et al. using lutein and β-carotene, this study found an enhanced β-carotene plasma response after combined dosage with canthaxanthin in subjects with the lowest plasma AUCs for β-carotene.

Van den Berg and van Vliet (10) studied the relative bioavailability of β-carotene with lutein and lycopene using the TRL response curve method. The carotenoid and retinyl palmitate responses in the TRL fraction, after a separate 15-mg–β-carotene dose, were compared with those after a combined dose of 15 mg β-carotene (suspension in palm oil) plus 15 mg lycopene (as a 5% tomato oleoresin) or with 15 mg lutein (xanthophyll concentrate from marigold). Combined dosage with lutein decreased the AUC of β-carotene and retinyl palmitate in the TRL fraction by 66 and 74%, respectively, compared with the response for β-carotene alone. A combined dosage with lycopene had no significant effect of β-carotene and retinyl palmitate response. β-Carotene cleavage, as estimated by the ratio between the AUC for retinyl esters and the AUC for β-carotene, was not significantly affected by combined dosing with lutein or with lycopene.

A single-dose study was conducted in healthy men to investigate serum β-carotene and lycopene responses after ingestion of individual and combined doses of β-carotene and lycopene (4). After ingestion of the combined dose, the serum β-carotene response, as measured by AUC, was no different from that for the β-carotene dose alone. However, the lycopene response after the combined dose was significantly enhanced. These investigators suggested that the finding of an improved lycopene absorption when administered with β-carotene was due to some components in the β-carotene suspension that enhanced the solubilization of crystalline lycopene, thereby providing a better serum response. This effect would be a physicochemical one; however, it would be dependent on the nature of the preparations of administered carotenoids, but not of biological events in the gastrointestinal tract. These results are in contrast to the observation of Prince et al. (38), who suggested that high-dose β-carotene supplementation (300 mg/day for 21 days added to a self-selected diet) resulted in a decrease in serum lycopene concentrations, which they attributed to a possible competition in absorption. The differing results may be due to the differences in dose size and duration of supplementation.

The foregoing studies were designed to specifically examine interactions among carotenoids. Further information can be gained from the results of intervention studies in which the changes in serum concentrations or carotenoids were not the main objectives, but nonetheless, were considered important to the study design.

In a short-term study with β-carotene (12 or 30 mg/day for 6 weeks) both β- and α-carotene plasma concentrations increased with supplementation, a small, but significant, decrease in serum lutein concentration was seen (20). Pappalardo et al. also measured a small, significant increase in serum α-carotene concentration after β-carotene supplementation (30 mg/day for 43 days) (39). These results could thus be due to the presence of trace amounts of α-carotene in the supplement, as seen in the study conducted by Mayne et al., in which a β-carotene dose of 50 mg/day for 5 years resulted in a twofold increase in plasma concentrations of α-carotene (40). Prince et al. (38) reported a strong decrease in serum lycopene levels after high-dose β-carotene supplementation (300 mg/day for 21 days), whereas another high-dose supplementation study, using 100 mg/day for 6 days, found a decrease in the lycopene content in LDL, the major carrier of carotenes in the circulation (41). In contrast, others found no effect of β-carotene supplementation (90 mg/day for 3 weeks) on serum carotenoid levels in healthy older women (42).

In the α-tocopherol and β-carotene (ATBC) trial in male smokers (43), when compared with the placebo, treatment with 20 mg β-carotene daily for 6.7 years, resulted in a small, but significant, decrease in the average serum lutein concentration. In the Australian polyp prevention study (44), a dose of 20 mg/day of β-carotene for 24 months resulted in a significant increase in serum lycopene and α-carotene, whereas the placebo-supplemented group had no such changes. However, in another polyp prevention study in the United States, there was no effect of supplementation with β-carotene (25 mg/day for 4 years) on the serum concentrations of carotenoids, other than β-carotene (45). Similarly, the Physicians Health Study reported that β-carotene supplementation (50 mg every-other day for 12 years) did not change plasma concentrations of other carotenoids (46).

Carotenoids may interact with each other at any point during the absorption and metabolic processes. In the intestinal lumen, carotenoids may compete for uptake in mixed micelles, or may enhance the solubilization of a carotenoid to improve micellular uptake. In the intestinal mucosa a carotenoid may inhibit or enhance the provitamin A cleavage enzyme. Carotenoids may also compete for uptake in chylomicrons. In the circulation, there may be exchange among plasma lipoproteins for carotenoids, which may be affected by the type and amount of carotenoid present. Finally, there may be inhibition or enhancement of tissue uptake or release by carotenoids. The specifics of at which points carotenoids interact have not been fully investigated.

F. Isomeric Form

β-Carotene can exist in food and human tissues as several different geometric isomers, including the all-*trans*-, 9-*cis*-, 13-*cis*-, and 15-*cis*-isomers (47). The major β-carotene isomer in human serum is all-*trans*-β-carotene, with small or negligible amounts of 13-*cis*- and 9-*cis*-β-carotene (48–50). However, there are considerable amounts of 9-*cis*- and 13-*cis*-β-carotene present in human tissue (49).

Data examining the serum response to a single large oral dose of either all-*trans*-β-carotene or 9-*cis*-β-carotene in men indicated that the all-*trans*-isomer attains a far greater postprandial concentration, but that the 9-*cis*-isomer reaches peak levels sooner (41,51). In an attempt to determine if these serum response differences were due to differences in tissue uptake, the concentration of β-carotene isomers in human serum, breast milk, and buccal mucosa cells after continuous oral doses of β-carotene isomers were examined in healthy lactating women (52). The changes milk and buccal mucosa cells of all-*trans*- and 9-*cis*-β-carotene followed a pattern similar to that for serum. The investigators concluded that the differences in the serum response curve of all-*trans*-β-carotene and 9-*cis*-β-carotene are not due to differences in tissue uptake, but may reflect a selective intestinal absorption of the all-*trans*-isomer.

Isomers of lycopene have been detected in human plasma and tissues (30,48,53,54). In one report it was observed that processed tomato juice contained a small amount of 9-*cis*-lycopene in addition to the predominant all-*trans*-isomer (30). Relative to their concentrations in tomato juice, the serum response to 9-*cis*-lycopene was significantly more than that of all-*trans* lycopene, suggesting that the *cis*-isomers are better absorbed that the all-*trans*-form, although in vivo isomerization would be another explanation.

Little research has been conducted on the bioavailability of isomers of other carotenoids. It is reasonable to assume that, as with β-carotene and lycopene, bioavailability would vary among the *trans*- and *cis*-forms. The importance of this to human health and disease remains to be determined.

G. Interactions with Other Food Components

1. Dietary Fat

The absorption and bioconversion of β-carotene is significantly reduced when the intake of dietary fat is low (55). Also, when β-carotene is given in the absence of fat no detectable change in serum β-carotene occurs (7). Dimitrov et al. (56) showed that dietary fat (63–69 g from breakfast and lunch plus an unreported quantity for the self-selected evening meal) increases the plasma response to β-carotene supplements, although the quantity of fat required for optimal absorption of vegetable carotenoids is thought to be small (57). In general, there is no dose–response relation between dietary fat intake and serum response to dietary carotenoids, but there is some increase in serum β-carotene response to a high-fat diet (56,58,59). The serum response to dietary β-carotene is related to the serum response to dietary triglyceride (6). After a single 120-mg dose of β-carotene the β-carotene response in chylomicrons was lower after ingestion of a meal composed of triglycerides from C-8 and C-10 rather than C-16 and C-18 fatty acids (60). This may be explained by the observation that the solubility of β-carotene decreased with increased chain length in triglyceride fatty acids (33).

2. Dietary Fiber

In a study to examine the effect of dietary fiber on serum carotene values, the increase in plasma β-carotene concentration after ingestion of β-carotene in a capsule was significantly reduced (42%) by pectin (61). Also, dietary fiber, being a part of the food matrix, may entrap carotenoids to result in a decreased bioavailability. Another effect of dietary fiber on carotenoid metabolism may be due to an interaction with bile acids, resulting in increased fecal excretion of bile acids; therefore, in decreased absorption of fats and fat-soluble substances, such as carotenoids.

V. SUMMARY

The bioavailability of carotenoids is considered to be the amount of ingested carotenoids that is used for normal physiological functions and storage. Therefore, any factor that affects intestinal absorption will affect bioavailability. There are several methods to measure bioavailability, each with advantages and disadvantages that are mostly related to accuracy, time, and cost. The simplest and most widely used method to assess carotenoid bioavailability is the serum response of carotenoid concentration after single or multiple doses of carotenoid. In general, carotenoid bioavailability is considered to be highly varied among individuals. Factors that affect the bioavailability of carotenoids include vehicle type (supplement vs. food; processed vs. unprocessed food) or dietary factors (amount and type of carotenoid(s), fat, or fiber). To date, most information on carotenoid bioavailability has come through studies with β-carotene. However, with the emergence of the possible protective effects of other carotenoids (e.g., lutein and lycopene), there is a growing need for information on the factors involved in the bioavailability of other carotenoids.

REFERENCES

1. Jackson MJ. The assessment of bioavailability of micronutrients: introduction. Eur J Clin Nutr 1997; 51(suppl):S1–S2.
2. Clevidence BA, Bieri JG. Association of carotenoids with human plasma lipoproteins. Methods Enzymol 1993; 214:3–17.
3. Massey JB. Kinetics of transfer of α-tocopherol between model and native plasma lipoproteins. Biochim Biophys Acta 1984; 793:387–392.
4. Johnson EJ, Qin J, Krinsky NI, Russell RM. Ingestion by men of a combined dose of β-carotene and lycopene does not affect the absorption of β-carotene but improves that of lycopene. J Nutr 1997; 127:1833–1837.
5. Johnson EJ, Krinsky NI, Russell RM. Serum response of lutein in humans after ingestion of a lutein supplement or spinach. (in preparation).
6. Henderson CT, Mobarahan S, Powen P, Stacewicz–Sapuntzakis M, Langenberg P, Kioni R, Lucchesi D, Sugarman S. Normal serum response to oral beta-carotene in humans. J Am Coll Nutr 1989; 8:625–635.
7. Prince MR, Frisoli JK. beta-Carotene accumulation in serum and skin. Am J Clin Nutr 1993; 57:175–181.
8. van Vliet T, Schreurs WHP, van den Berg H. Intestinal β-carotene absorption and cleavage in men: response of β-carotene and retinyl esters in the triacylglyceride-rich lipoprotein fraction after a single oral dose of β-carotene. Am J Clin Nutr 1995; 62:110–116.
9. Gartner C, Stahl W, Sies H. Lycopene is more bioavailable from tomato paste than from fresh tomatoes. Am J Clin Nutr 1997; 66:116–122.
10. van den Berg H, van Vliet T. Effect of simultaneous, single oral doses of β-carotene and retinyl ester responses in the triacylglycerol-rich lipoprotein fraction of men. Am J Clin Nutr 1998; 68:82–89.
11. O'Neill ME, Thurham DI. Intestinal absorption of β-carotene, lycopene, and lutein in men and women following a standard meal: response curves in the triacylglycerol-rich lipoprotein fraction. Br J Nutr 1998; 79:149–159.
12. Bowen PE, Mobarhan S, Smith JC. Absorption of carotenoids in humans. Methods Enzymol 1993; 214:3–17.

13. Dueker SR, Jones AD, Smith GM, Clifford AJ. Stable isotope methods for the study of β-carotene-d8 metabolism in humans utilizing tandem mass spectrometry and high performance liquid chromatography. Anal Chem 1994; 66:4177–4185.
14. Parker RS, Swanson JE, Marmor B, Goodman KJ, Spielman AB, Brenna JT, Viereck SM, Canfield WK. Study of β-carotene metabolism in humans using ^{13}C-β-carotene and high precision isotope ratio mass spectrometry. Ann NY Acad Sci 1993; 691:86–95.
15. Novotny JA, Dueker SR, Zech LA, Clifford AJ. Compartmental analysis of the dynamics of β-carotene metabolism in an adult volunteer. J Lipid Res 1995; 36:1825–1838.
16. van het Hof KH, Brouwer IA, West CE, Haddeman E, Steegers-Theunissen RPM, van Dusseldorp M, Weststrate JA, Eskes TKAB, Hautvast JGAJ. Bioavailability of lutein from vegetables is 5 times higher than that of β-carotene. Am J Clin Nutr 1999; 70:261–268.
17. Johnson EJ, Hammond BR, Yeum KJ, Qin J, Wang XD, Castaneda C, Snodderly DM, Russell RM. Relation among serum and tissue concentrations of lutein and zeaxanthin and macular pigment density. Am J Clin Nutr 2000; 71:1555–1562.
18. Rao CN, Rao BSN. Absorption of dietary carotenes in human subjects. Am J Clin Nutr 1970; 23:105–109.
19. WHO Technical Report Series 362. Requirements of vitamin A, thiamine, riboflavin and niacin. FAO Nutr Meet Rep Ser 1967; 41:74–76.
20. Micozzi MS, Brown ED, Edwards BK, Bieri JG, Taylor PR, Khachik F, Beecher GR, Smith JC Jr. Plasma carotenoid response to chronic intake of selected foods and β-carotene supplements in men. Am J Clin Nutr 1992; 55:1120–1125.
21. Brown ED, Micozzi MS, Craft NE, et al. Plasma carotenoids in normal men after a single ingestion of vegetables or purified β-carotene. Am J Clin Nutr 1989; 49:1258–1265.
22. Bulux J, Quan de Serrano J, Guiliano A, Perez R, Lopez CY. Plasma response of children to short-term chronic β-carotene supplementation. Am J Clin Nutr 1994; 59:1369–1375.
23. Torronen R, Lehmusaho M, Hakkinen S, Hanninen O, Mykkanen H. Serum β-carotene response to supplementation with raw carrots, carrot juice or purified β-carotene in healthy non-smoking women. Nutr Res 1996; 16:565–575.
24. De Pee S, West CE, Muhilal, Karyadi D, Hautvast JGAJ. Lack of improvement in vitamin A status with increased consumption of dark-green leafy vegetables. Lancet 1995; 346:75–81.
25. Castenmiller JJ, West CE, Linssen JP, van het Hof KH, Voragen AG. The food matrix of spinach is a limiting factor in determining the bioavailability of beta-carotene and to a lesser extent of lutein in humans. J Nutr 1999; 129:349–355.
26. Bierer TL, Merchen NR, Erdman JW Jr. Comparative absorption and transport of five common carotenoids in preruminant calves. J Nutr 1995; 125:1569–1577.
27. van het Hof KH, Gartner C, West CE, Tijburg LBM. Potential of vegetable processing to increase the delivery of carotenoids to man. Int J Vit Res 1998; 68:366–370.
28. Britton G. Structure and properties of carotenoids in relation to function. FASEB J 1995; 9:1551–1558.
29. Rock CL, Lovalvo JL, Emenhiser C, Ruffin MT, Flatt SW, Schwartz SJ. Bioavailability of β-carotene is lower in raw than in processed carrots and spinach in women. J Nutr 1998; 128:913–916.
30. Stahl W, Sies H. Uptake of lycopene and its geometrical isomers is greater from heat-processed than from unprocessed tomato juice in humans. J Nutr 1992; 122:2161–2166.
31. Giovannucci E, Ascherio A, Rimm EB, Stampfer MJ, Colditz GA, Willett WC. Intake of carotenoids and retinol in relation to risk of prostate cancer. J Natl Cancer Inst 1995; 87:1767–1776.
32. Erdman J. The physiology chemistry of carotenes in man. Clin Nutr 1988; 7:101–106.
33. Borel P, Grolier P, Armand M, Partier A, Lafont H, Lairon D, Azais-Braesco V. Carotenoids in biological emulsions: solubility, surface-to-core distribution, and release from lipid droplets. J Lipid Res 1996; 37:250–261.
34. van den Berg H. Carotenoid interactions. Nutr Rev 1999; 57:1–10.
35. Kostic D, White WS, Olson JA. Intestinal absorption, serum clearance, and interactions between lutein and β-carotene when administered to human adults in separate or combined oral doses. Am J Clin Nutr 1995; 62:604–620.
36. White WS, Stacewicz-Sapuntzakis M, Erdman JW, Bowen PE. Pharmacokinetics of β-carotene and canthaxanthin after ingestion of individual and combined doses by human subjects. J Am Coll Nutr 1994; 13:665–671.

37. Paetau I, Chen H, Goh NMY, White WS. Interactions in the postprandial appearance of β-carotene and canthaxanthin in plasma triacylglycerol-rich lipoproteins in humans. Am J Clin Nutr 1997; 66:1133–1143.
38. Prince MR, Frisoli JK, Goetschkes MM, Stringham JM, LaMuraglia GM. Rapid serum carotene loading with high-dose beta-carotene: clinical implications. J Cardiovasc Pharmacol 1991; 17:343–347.
39. Pappalardo G, Maiani G, Mobarhan S, Guadalaxara A, Azzini E, Raguzzini A, Sallucci M, Serfini M, Trifero M, Illomei G, Ferro–Luzzi A. Plasma (carotenoids, retinol, α-tocopherol) and tissue (carotenoid) levels after supplementation with β-carotene in subjects with precancerous and cancerous lesions of the sigmoid colon. Eur J Clin Nutr 1997; 51:661–666.
40. Mayne ST, Cartmel B, Silva F, Silva F, Kim CS, Fallon BG, Briskein K, Zheng T, Baum M, Shor–Posner G, Goodwin WJ Jr. Effect of supplemental β-carotene on plasma concentrations of carotenoids, retinol, and tocopherol in humans. Am J Clin Nutr 1998; 68:642–647.
41. Gaziano JM, Johnson EJ, Russell RM, Manson JE, Stampfer MJ, Ridker PM, Frei B, Hennekens CH, Krinsky NI. Discrimination in absorption or transport of β-carotene isomers after oral supplementation with either all-*trans* or 9-*cis* β-carotene. Am J Clin Nutr 1995; 61:1248–1252.
42. Ribaya–Mercado JD, Ordovas JM, Russell RM. Effect of β-carotene supplementation on the concentrations and distribution of carotenoids, vitamin E, vitamin A, and cholesterol in plasma lipoprotein and non-lipoprotein fractions in healthy older women. J Am Coll Nutr 1995; 14:614–620.
43. Albanes D, Virtamo J, Taylor PR, Rautalahi M, Pietinen PM, Heinonen OP. Effects of supplemental β-carotene, cigarette smoking, and alcohol consumption on serum carotenoids in the ATBC carotene study. Am J Clin Nutr 1997; 66:366–372.
44. Wahlquist ML, Wattanapenpaiboon N, Macrae FL, Lambert JR, MacLennan R, Hsu–Hage BH. Changes in serum carotenoids in subjects with colorectal adenomas after 24 months of β-carotene supplementation. Am J Clin Nutr 1994; 60:936–943.
45. Nierenberg DW, Dain BJ, Mott LA, Baron JA, Greenberg ER. Effect of 4 years of oral supplementation with β-carotene on serum concentrations of retinol, tocopherol, and five carotenoids. Am J Clin Nutr 1997; 66:315–319.
46. Fotouhi N, Meydani M, Santos MS, et al. Carotenoid and tocopherol concentrations in plasma, peripheral blood mononuclear cells, and red blood cells after long-term β-carotene supplementation in men. Am J Clin Nutr 1996; 63:553–558.
47. Chandler LA, Schwartz SJ. HPLC separation of *cis–trans* carotene isomers in fresh and processed fruits and vegetables. J Food Sci 1987; 52:669–672.
48. Stahl W, Schwarz W, Sundquist AR, Sies H. *cis-trans* Isomers of lycopene and β-carotene in human serum and tissues. Arch Biochem Biophys 1992; 294:173–177.
49. Stahl W, Schwartz W, Sies H. Human serum concentrations of all-*trans* β- and α-carotene but not 9-*cis* β-carotene increase upon ingestion of a natural isomer mixture obtained from *Dunaliella salina* (Betatene). J Nutr 1993; 123:847–851.
50. Tamai H, Murata T, Morinoby T, Manago M, Takenaka H, Hayashi K, Mino M. Bioavailability of β-carotene in a carotenoid preparation derived from *Dunaliella bardawil* in human male adults. In: Canfield LI, Krinsky NI, Olson JA, eds. Carotenoids in Human Health. NY Acad Sci 1993; 691:238–240.
51. Johnson EJ, Krinsky NI, Russell RM. Serum response of all-*trans* and 9-*cis* isomers of β-carotene in humans. J Am Coll Nutr 1996; 15:620–624.
52. Johnson EJ, Qin J, Krinsky NI, Russell RM. β-Carotene isomers in human serum, breast milk and buccal mucosa cells after continuous oral doses of all-*trans* and 9-*cis* β-carotene. J Nutr 1997; 127:1993–1997.
53. Schmitz HH, Poor CL, Wellman RB, Erdman JW Jr. Concentrations of selected carotenoids and vitamin A in human liver, kidney, and lung tissue. J Nutr 1992; 121:1613–1621.
54. Krinsky NI, Russett MD, Handelman GJ, Snodderly DM. Structural and geometrical isomers of carotenoids in human plasma. J Nutr 1990; 120:1654–1662.
55. Jialal I, Norkus EP, Cristol L, Grundy SM. β-Carotene inhibits the oxidative modification of low-density-lipoprotein. Biochim Biophys Acta 1991; 1089:134–138.
56. Dimitrov NV, Meyer C, Ullrey DE, Chenworth W, Michelakis A, Malone W, Boone C, Fink G. Bioavailability of β-carotene in humans. Am J Clin Nutr 1988; 48:298–304.
57. Jayarajan P, Reddy V, Mohanram M. Effect of dietary fat on absorption of β-carotene from green leafy vegetables. J Med Ind Res 1980; 71:53–56.

58. Nierenberg DW, Stukel TA, Baron JA, Dain BJ, Greenberg ER (Skin Cancer Prevention Study Group). Determinants of increase in plasma concentration of β-carotene after chronic oral supplementation. Am J Clin Nutr 1991; 53:1443–1449.
59. Shiau A, Morbaran S, Stacewicz–Sapuntzakis M, et al. Assessment of the intestinal retention of β-carotene in humans. J Am Coll Nutr 1994; 13:369–375.
60. Borel P, Tyssandier V, Mekki N, Grolier P, Rochette Y, Alexandre–Gouabau MC, Lairon D, Azais–Braesco V. Chylomicron beta-carotene and retinyl palmitate responses are dramatically diminished when men ingest beta-carotene with medium-chain rather than long-chain triglycerides. J Nutr 1998; 128:1361–1367.
61. Rock CL, Swendseid ME. Plasma β-carotene response in humans after meals supplemented with dietary pectin. Am J Clin Nutr 1992; 55:96–99.

15
Caffeic Acid and Related Antioxidant Compounds: Biochemical and Cellular Effects

João Laranjinha
University of Coimbra, Coimbra, Portugal

I. INTRODUCTION

The hydroxycinnamic acids are phenylpropanoid plant metabolites, chemically and biologically related, that are commonly found in plant-derived foodstuff (1). Among them, caffeic acid, its quinic ester derivative, chlorogenic acid, as well as its precursor, *p*-coumaric acid, are the phenolic acids most widely distributed in plant tissues. In addition to other functions, they take part in the biosynthesis of the more complex and more studied class of phenolic compounds, the flavonoids (2,3). Evidence concerning the antioxidant and anticarcinogenic properties of these phenolic acids originates from epidemiological studies (4–6), that inversely associate fruit and vegetable intake with the incidence of coronary heart disease and cancer, and are supported by biological and biochemical data.

A considerable amount of experimental data on the antioxidant activity of hydroxycinnamates, in particular caffeic acid, is available, and reviews with emphasis on structure–antioxidant activity relations have been recently forwarded (7). It is not the purpose of this chapter to review exhaustively all the available information concerning the chemistry, biochemistry, and biology of phenolic acids, instead we critically discuss selected topics relevant for the evaluation of the potential role of caffeic acid in human physiology.

The formation of reactive oxygen and nitrogen species is a feature of many degenerative diseases, such as atherosclerosis. The lipid peroxidation of low-density lipoproteins (LDL) is a critical initial event in atherogenesis. This is connected with the consensus that the oxidation of LDL occurs predominantly in arterial intima in microdomains sequestered from plasmatic antioxidants (8) ensued by the formation of the earliest atherosclerotic lesion, the fatty streak, under a structurally intact layer of endothelial cells (9). Consequently, there has been a great interest in understanding the involvement of free radicals in LDL oxidation and the mechanisms by which antioxidants may inhibit such processes. In particular, the concerted activity of antioxidant compounds, which is more relevant in a biological milieu, requires additional progress in its understanding. This review primarily focuses on the general antioxidant activity of caffeic acid (and derivatives), grounded in its physicochemical properties (kinetic, thermodynamic, and solubility parameters), and how this phenolic compound undergoes redox cycles with vitamins E and C enhancing the protection of isolated human LDL against oxidation. Pro-oxidant activities and bioavailability are also discussed. Finally, we refer to recent advances made in understanding the molecular action of caffeic acid at the cellular level by interfering with the toxic-signaling pathways related to atherogenesis through mechanisms that are not necessarily related to antioxidant activity.

II. PHYSICOCHEMICAL PROPERTIES

A. Structures

Hydroxycinnamic acids are phenolic compounds that derive biosynthetically from phenylalanine and play a central role in phenolic metabolism in plants (1,2) (Fig. 1). They also contribute to the structure of the plants as components of cell walls and are biosynthetic precursors of flavonoids (2). Usually, these phenolic acids occur in plants as esters or combined with sugars, organic acids, and lipids, apparently in dynamic interconversion with an intracellular pool of the free acids (10). Because of their almost universal distribution, phenolic acids are an integral part of the human diet; they have been found in fruits, vegetables, flowers, nuts, seeds, and in plant-derived products, such as wine, tea, coffee, and olive oil (11,12). Caffeic acid, its quinic ester derivative—chlorogenic acid—as well as its precursor—*p*-coumaric—are among the phenolic acids most widely distributed in plant tissues. Chlorogenic acid can be considered

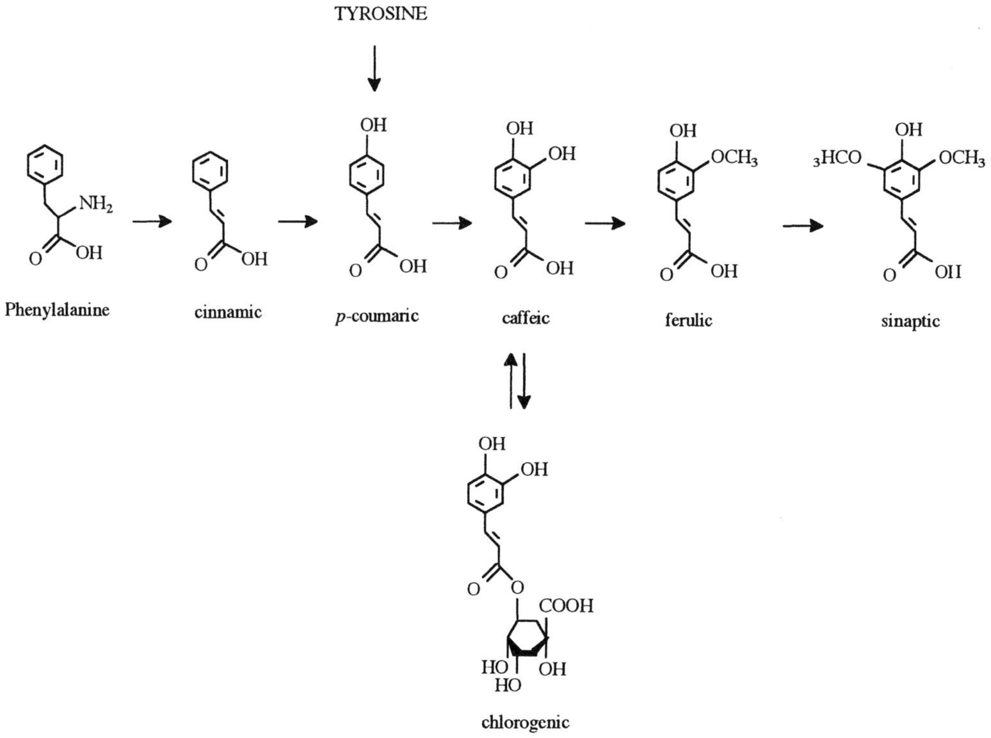

Figure 1 Structures and biosynthetic relation of hydroxycinnamates.

a storage form of caffeic acid because the transferase that couples quinic acid to caffeic moiety during the biosynthesis of chlorogenic acid is reversible (13,14). The hydroxycinnamates occur in nature in the more stable *trans*-configuration (see Fig. 1), but isomerization to the *cis*-configuration gradually occurs on exposure to ultraviolet (UV) and visible light (15).

B. Scavenging Rate Constants

Despite the closure structural relation among hydroxycinnamates, replacement of one of the OH groups in the *o*-dihydroxy structure of caffeic and chlorogenic acids by an OCH_3 group (as in ferulic acid) or by an H atom (as in *p*-coumaric acid), strongly affects physicochemical behavior and, therefore, antioxidant activities. The same applies if the lateral double bond becomes saturated (as in the dehydro derivatives) or replaced by a COOH group (as in hydroxybenzoic acids; e.g., protocatechuic acid). On the contrary, the esterification of caffeic acid with quinic acid producing chlorogenic acid, is likely to have a minor influence on the physicochemical parameters that support the antioxidant activities. These considerations can be rationalized on the basis of the work of Wolf Bors et al. with more complex polyphenols.

Bors et al. (16), on the basis of the reaction rate constants of flavonoids with several radicals and the stability of flavonoid-derived radicals, established the most relevant structural principles for effective radical scavenging by flavonoids; namely, an *o*-dihydroxy (catechol) structure in conjugation with a lateral double bond and an oxo function. Additional OH groups are considered much less reactive and acquire importance only for high concentrations of the phenols. Among the hydroxycinnamates, caffeic acid retains the structural features that maximize radical-scavenging activity in flavonoids, which is predictive of higher rate constants toward several types of oxidant species, as shown in Table 1 (17–23,37,64). It could be argued that caffeic acid is the "active site" of flavonoids for radical scavenging (in particular flavones and flavonols). The *o*-dihydroxy group is typically the radical target site, which after

Table 1 Scavenging Properties of Caffeic Acid (or Its Ester Derivative, Chlorogenic Acid)

Oxidant	Product/rate constant	Ref.
ROO·	$1.5 \times 10^7 \, M^{-1}s^{-1}$	17[a]
$O_2^{·-}$	$0.96 \times 10^6 \, M^{-1}s^{-1}$	18[b]
OH·	$3.24 \times 10^9 \, M^{-1}s^{-1}$	18[b]
ONOO$^-$	Quinone	
	(for chlorogenic $1.6 \times 10^5 \, M^{-1}s^{-1}$)	37, 18[b]
·NO$_2$	$8.6 \times 10^8 \, M^{-1}s^{-1}$	19[b]
MbFe^{IV}=O	MbFe^{III}	
	Semiquinone radical	23[c], 64
N$_2$O$_3$	$8.6 \times 10^9 \, M^{-1}s^{-1}$	21[d]
HOCl	*o*-Quinone of chlorogenic	22
$^1O_2$	$5.1 \times 10^6 \, M^{-1}s^{-1}$	20[e]

[a] Kinetic chemiluminescence in chlorobenzene at 50°C and peroxyl radical derived from diphenyl methane.
[b] Pulse radiolysis.
[c] MbFe^{IV}=O, ferrylmyoglobin; MbFe^{III}, metmyoglobin.
[d] Competition spectrophotometric assay.
[e] Time-resolved infrared phosphorescence in acetonitrile.

one-electron oxidation produces a phenoxyl radical (*o*-semiquinone). Accordingly, the caffeic acid-derived *o*-semiquinone radical has been observed by electron paramagnetic resonance (EPR) after reaction of the phenolic acid with several oxidants, including peroxynitrite and ferrylmyoglobin (23). Even so, a recent study on the scavenging activity of caffeic acid derivatives against 1,1-diphenyl-2-picrylhydrazyl (DPPH) radical indicated that a saturated lateral group in the aromatic ring had a slightly higher inhibitory activity when compared with an unsaturated group (24).

Data on radical-scavenging properties of flavonoids is far more abundant than for these more simple phenols (25). In view of the structural relations between hydroxycinnamates and flavonoids, one would be tempted to predict that, generally, the phenolic acids exhibit similar radical-scavenging activity compared with the flavonoids (particularly flavones and flavonols). However, this is not necessarily so, as inferred from Table 1. Although the rate constant for the reaction with peroxyl radicals is comparable with those of flavonoids exhibiting a catechol structure, such as quercetin and fisetin, the rate constant for the reactions of $O_2^{\cdot-}$ with caffeic and chlorogenic acid are two or three orders of magnitude higher than those of $O_2^{\cdot-}$ with flavonoids (26). Apparently, these are the highest rates yet reported for the reactions of phenolic antioxidants with $O_2^{\cdot-}$, and this is a meaningful observation. Superoxide anion itself is not a very reactive radical; it can oxidize (4Fe–4S) clusters of enzymes, such as aconitase, and it can also oxidize catecholamines and related compounds, but it is unable to initiate the free radical oxidation of polyunsaturated lipids and DNA (27). However, one may consider $O_2^{\cdot-}$ as a precursor of more damaging oxidants by mechanisms that include (1) production of hydroxyl radical by the Haber–Weiss reaction; (2) oxidation of (4Fe–4S) clusters followed by release of Fe^{2+} and Fenton chemistry; (3) protonation to the more reactive conjugate acid ($HO_2^{\cdot}$, $pK_a = 4.8$); and (4) formation of $ONOO^-$ by the rapid interaction of superoxide and nitric oxide (28) [$K = 6.7 \times 10^9$ $M^{-1}s^{-1}$ (29)].

Peroxynitrite has acquired biological relevance as a potential oxidant and nitrating agent in vivo, inducing lipid peroxidation (30,31), and modification of amino acids, proteins, (32,31), and DNA (33). The rate constant for the reaction of $ONOO^-$ and chlorogenic acid (presumably the rate constant for caffeic acid is similar) is orders of magnitude higher as compared with those for the reactions of $ONOO^-$ with ascorbate and glutathione (34,35). Apparently, peroxynitrite, reacts with the hydroxycinnamates through nitration or addition according to the OH pattern; the reaction with monophenols, such as *p*-coumaric acid, involves nitration, whereas the reaction with catechols, including caffeic and chlorogenic acids, is likely to involve preferentially two consecutive electron transfer steps, producing intermediary *o*-semiquinone radicals (Laranjinha J, unpublished observations) and quinones (36,37). However, in view of the high concentrations of hemeproteins and CO_2/HCO_3^- in vivo and the rate constants (38,39) of their reactions with peroxynitrite (on the order of 10^4 $M^{-1}s^{-1}$) it is unlikely that the catecholic cinnamic acids play a significant role in direct reactions with peroxynitrite in vivo.

Nevertheless, under particular experimental conditions in vitro, caffeic acid behaves as a strong antioxidant in peroxynitrite-mediated damage; namely, (1) inhibition of peroxynitrite-induced oxidation of dopamine (40); (2) inhibitory effects against peroxynitrite-mediated nitration of tyrosine residues in proteins (41); and (3) prevention of the damage to LDL evaluated in terms of the formation of carbonyl groups, as well as the oxidation of tryptophan and thiols groups in the apoB protein (Dinis T, personal communication).

C. Antioxidant Radical Decay

It has been emphasized (16,42) that, in addition to the rate constants with different types of radicals, other kinetic parameters, such as the stability of the antioxidant-derived radical as

Table 2 One-Electron Reduction Potentials at pH7 for Hydroxycinnamate Radicals

Compound	E_7/mV	Ref.
Caffeic acid	534–540	20, 26, 195
Chlorogenic acid	550	20
p-Coumaric acid	590	20
Ferulic acid	595	20

well as stoichiometry, should be taken into account to evaluate the antioxidant potential of a particular compound. That is to say, the antioxidant must efficiently eliminate the oxidant, but the radical of the antioxidant must be harmless toward the target to be protected. The structure of hydroxycinnamates, exhibiting the conjugated double bond with the phenol ring, enables an extensive electron delocalization, a prerequisite condition for radical stabilization because a "safe" decay of the antioxidant-derived radical by reaction with another radical, by disproportionation or reaction with another antioxidant, becomes more feasible. This concept can be inferred from studies comparing the antioxidant activities of caffeic and chlorogenic acids with that of the hydroxybenzoic acid derivative, protocatechuic acid, devoid of the conjugated double bond. In an experimental system consisting of LDL challenged with AAPH-derived peroxyl radicals (43), the hydroxycinnamates exhibited higher stoichiometric numbers and reactivity with peroxyl radicals, as compared with the hydroxybenzoic acid, thereby more efficiently protecting LDL from lipid peroxidation. Moreover, UV spectral data on the decay of the phenolic compounds showed that for protocatechuic acid, intermediates accumulate during the reaction with peroxyl radicals, whereas spectral patterns for caffeic and chlorogenic revealed the appearance of well-defined isosbestic points as the reaction proceeds, suggesting the presence of only two species in solution, the catechol and the corresponding o-quinone.

D. Redox Potentials

The redox potentials of phenolic compounds, which are important to assess the thermodynamic feasibility of reactions, are very sensitive to structural modifications in the aromatic ring (44). Accordingly, the structural features that determine radical-scavenging efficiency also control the redox potential. This notion can be verified by comparing the redox potentials for the family of hydroxycinnamates (Table 2); the catechol group in conjugation with a side double bond provides the compound with lower redox potentials.

III. MECHANISMS OF ANTIOXIDANT ACTIVITY

On the basis of the radical-scavenging properties discussed in the foregoing, and given the general rule that free radical scavengers must react spontaneously and very rapidly with the most frequently encountered free radicals, it can be anticipated that caffeic acid and related hydroxycinnamates inhibit radical-mediated process at several levels:

1. Preventing initiating process through scavenging of ·OH, ONOO⁻, and ferrylmyoglobin through reactions involving electron transfer and possible by chelating transition metals.
2. Breaking peroxidative chain reactions by stabilizing peroxyl radicals in the form of peroxides through H atom donation.
3. Regenerating α-tocopherol by reducing α-tocopheroxyl radical.

These concepts have been extensively illustrated in lipid systems, inasmuch as the antioxidant potential of hydroxycinnamates has been particularly studied in connection with lipid peroxidation.

This section surveys the mechanistic aspects of antioxidant activity of caffeic and related phenolic acids and also discusses structure–activity relations and pro-oxidant activities. Particular emphasis is given to recent advances made in the understanding of concerted antioxidant activity of caffeic acid with ascorbate and α-tocopherol in relation to the protection of LDL against oxidation.

A. Radical Scavenging

In 1976, Sharma (45) showed that caffeic acid was a potent inhibitor of in vitro lipid peroxidation of rat brain homogenates. Subsequent studies in solution have demonstrated its ability to scavenge hydroxyl (46) and peroxyl radicals, thus protecting linoleic acid (47) and methyl linoleate (48,49) from oxidation. Observations in cellular and lipoprotein systems further focused the interest in these compounds as potentially useful biological antioxidants: (1) inhibitory effects on hydroperoxide-initiated chemiluminescence of mouse liver homogenates were described (50); (2) Liu et al. (51) showed that caffeic acid exerted a protective action against peroxidative damage to liver microsomes induced by Fe^{2+}/cysteine or vitamin C–NADPH, to hepatocytes challenged with CCl_4 and to erythrocytes incubated with H_2O_2 or MDA; (3) chain-breaking-type activities for caffeic and chlorogenic acids were observed in LDL challenged with AAPH-derived peroxyl radicals (52), exhibiting stoichiometric values toward peroxyl radicals greater than those of α-tocopherol (43). These observations have been reproduced and further extended to several lipid systems under several oxidant conditions. Examples include studies of lipid oxidation in lipoproteins challenged with reactive high oxidation states of myoglobin (53,54), such as ferrylmyoglobin (55); studies in copper-dependent LDL oxidation in solution (56,57), or in in vitro oxidation model for heart disease (58); studies in peroxyl radical-induced oxidation of erythrocytes and of linoleic acid-containing sodium dodecyl sulfate (SDS) micelles as well as erythrocytes incubated with AAPH (59,60); studies of lipid peroxidation in rat liver microsomes and mitochondria challenged with CCL_4 and ascorbate/Fe^{2+} (61). Antioxidant activities toward DNA and proteins, although less studied, have also been reported (62,63).

Attempts have been made to establish structure–activity relations. Generally, conclusions agree with the previously mentioned structural criteria established by Bors et al. (16) for radical scavenging, suggesting that this is an important mechanism underlying antioxidant activities: a catechol group confers higher antioxidant capacity compared with monophenols (e.g., caffeic vs. p-coumaric acid), and a double bond conjugated with the catechol ring has a great effect in stabilizing the antioxidant-derived radical, thus enhancing antioxidant activity (7). These notions are supported by, among others, experiments demonstrating (1) higher scavenging activity toward aqueous peroxyl radicals (43) and higher TEAC values (trolox equivalent antioxidant capacity) (7) of caffeic acid as compared with protocatechuic acid, a hydroxybenzoic acid derivative displaying a catechol structure, but devoid of a conjugated double bond with the phenolic ring; (2) higher efficiency of caffeic acid (or chlorogenic) when compared with its biosynthetic monophenolic precursor, p-coumaric acid, or to ferulic acid, a methoxylated derivative in a phenolic OH group, to reduce ferrylmyoglobin to metmyoglobin (64) and to scavenge peroxyl radicals, thereby protecting LDL against oxidation (53,54,58); (3) stronger inhibitory activity of caffeic acid than that of p-coumaric and protocatechuic on hemolysis and lipid peroxidation of erythrocytes challenged with H_2O_2 (65). Additional substituents in the catechol ring may affect the overall antioxidant activity and two concepts are usually forwarded to explain differences among the phenolic metabolites: the electron-donating character of the substituents in the phenol ring (66,67,194) favors scavenging, and internal hydrogen bonding involving phenolic OH groups decrease reactivity with peroxyl radicals. Accordingly, ferulic acid, a phenolic compound containing an electron-donating methoxy group is more efficient than the monophenol p-coumaric acid in inhibiting peroxidation of linoleic acid micelles (65) and protecting LDL from oxidation by ferrylmyoglobin (54). Electron-donating ability to the hypervalent iron in ferrylmyoglobin follows the order caffeic > chlorogenic > ferulic > p-coumaric and further supports the aforementioned concepts (64).

B. Metal Interaction (Anti- and Pro-Oxidant Activities)

Chelation of transition metals, species that produce radicals through the monovalent reduction of hydroperoxides, could be envisaged as an operative mechanism of prevention of radical-mediated oxidations. For example, caffeic acid is more efficient in inhibiting Cu^{2+}-catalyzed than peroxyl radical-initiated LDL oxidation (56), and chlorogenic acid inhibited the iron-induced lipid peroxidation of bovine liver microsomes (68). Generally, phenols exhibit a chelating activity of iron either in the form of Fe^{3+} (69) or Fe^{2+} (70), and those having a catechol structure (including caffeic acid and flavonoids containing a catechol group in the B-ring) reduce Fe^{3+} to Fe^{2+} in a pH-dependent way (decreasing from pH 5.5 to pH 7.0) (71). Therefore, the metal chelating and reducing abilities of catechols, maintaining metals in a reduced catalytic active form, may, on the other hand, support pro-oxidant activities through Fenton catalysis (reductive cleavage of hydroperoxides). An illustrative example is given by the acceleration of TBARS formation upon caffeic acid addition to LDL seeded with peroxides during incubation with Cu^{2+} (72); similar effects were observed for other reductants such as ascorbate (73) and catechins (74). The ability of phenolics to maintain metals in a redox-active form may be of biological relevance in the later stages of atherosclerosis, because advanced human atherosclerotic lesions contain available iron and copper ions (75).

Caffeic acid also stimulates DNA and deoxyribose degradation in the presence of bleomycin and EDTA (71), effects that are ascribed to the capacity of phenols to reduce the rather inactive bleomycin–Fe^{3+} and EDTA–Fe^{3+} complexes (76,77). These effects are strictly dependent on the presence of EDTA and bleomycin and, therefore, the assays are important because bleomycin and EDTA are used in food and pharmaceutical industry (78), but they are difficult to extrapolate to in vivo conditions. Moreover, two observations oppose the putative biological relevance of those reactions: first, human albumin protects DNA and deoxyribose from the pro-oxidant action of plant phenols in those systems (79). Second, the pro-oxidant effects were observed for concentrations one order of magnitude higher compared with the concentrations at which phenolics effectively inhibit lipid peroxidation.

The observation that o-diphenols, including caffeic acid, reduce and release iron from ferritin, at a rate directly related to the reducing power of the compounds (80,81), is also of interest in the context of pro-oxidation, because such a reaction would increase the availability of catalytic metals. This could, in principle, support a ferritin-dependent lipid peroxidation as observed for other phenolic compounds, such as 6-hydroxydopamine (82). This view is, again, particularly relevant in the context of atherosclerosis when considering the reported synergistic association of ferritin and LDL-cholesterol with cardiovascular disease (83) and the role of oxidized LDL in atherogenesis (see later discussion).

In connection with chelating ability of phenolics, two other concepts are worth mentioning. On one hand, it was recently reported that caffeic acid decreases zinc (but not copper) absorption in rats (84), an observation that points to the potential effects of caffeic acid in mineral nutrition. On the other hand, reduction of ferric iron to the ferrous form in the active center of enzymes supports the inhibition of several enzymatic activities by caffeic acid. In view of the facile redox interaction of hydroxycinnamates with ferrylmyoglobin (64), a hemeprotein exhibiting a peroxidase-like activity (55), peroxidases and other heme proteins are obvious candidates. Of particular interest is the reductive inactivation of lipoxygenases (85–88), enzymes that catalyze dioxygenation of specific polyunsaturated fatty acids to hydroperoxides during leukotriene biosynthesis. Because of the role of leukotrienes in inflammation, regulation of lipoxygenase activity may be of pharmacological interest in the prevention of vascular disease (89). Likewise, and considering the aging-associated up-regulation of neuronal 5-lipoxygenase expression, caffeic acid may have a role in neuroprotection (90).

C. Redox Cycling

1. LDL Oxidation and Atherosclerosis

Strong evidence suggests that oxidized LDL critically contributes to the initiation of atherogenesis and that lipid peroxidation plays a key role in its development (8,9,91). Therefore, the inhibition of lipid peroxidation in LDL by exogenous and endogenous antioxidants has become a matter of major interest in order to develop a method for atherosclerosis prevention (92); antioxidants are potential antiatherogenic compounds. Several agents are competent in vitro inducers of LDL oxidation, including cells (93–95), Cu^{2+} (92), lipoxygenase (96), peroxidases (97), peroxynitrite (98), higher oxidation states of myoglobin (54,99), hemin (100), and azo-initiators (101).

Caffeic acid and related compounds, including hydroxycinnamates and the hydroxybenzoic derivative, protocatechuic acid, exhibit antioxidant activities under most of the aforementioned oxidant conditions (43,52–54,56–58). However, although much work has been done with the individual compounds, the potential dynamic interactions among antioxidants are still unclear, and are more relevant in a biological milieu.

Mechanistically, the synergistic interaction of phenolics with major antioxidants, such as vitamins E and C, is of great relevance for its antioxidative functions. The reported studies on the synergistic interaction of hydroxycinnamates involve reactions with α-tocopherol and ascorbate in connection with the inhibition of LDL lipid peroxidation.

α-Tocopherol is quantitatively the major endogenous antioxidant in human LDL (102), reacting either with the initiating radical or breaking the radical chain of lipid peroxidation on reaction with chain-carrying lipid peroxyl radical. Generally, in either of the situations, it produces the α-tocopheroxyl radical. Tocopheroxyl radicals have a very low rate constant value for the reversible dimerization (i.e., 10^2 $M^{-1}s^{-1}$) (103). So, they are stable and decay slowly. Bowry and Stocker (104) have shown that, under particular conditions, the α-tocopheroxyl radical may itself react with unsaturated lipids, acting as a chain-transfer compound, rather than acting as a chain-breaking antioxidant. This mechanism of LDL oxidation was described as the "tocopherol-mediated lipid peroxidation" and increases with the reduction of the reactivity of the radical oxidants and radical flux to which LDL is exposed (105). The fluxes and types of radical oxidants to which LDL becomes exposed in the subendothelial space of arteries are not known. However, as pointed out by Stocker (106), atherosclerosis is a chronic disease implying that if LDL oxidation theory applies, there must be a low tonus of LDL oxidation in vivo. Therefore, an efficient prevention of LDL oxidation requires the export of the radical character from the lipoprotein to the aqueous medium. An operative mechanism is the rapid elimination (reduction) of α-tocopheroxyl radical by an amphiphilic "coantioxidant," maintaining α-tocopherol in a high steady-state concentration in the lipoprotein particles and a "safe" reaction decay for the coantioxidant radical. Ascorbate is the best known example of such a coantioxidant. Ascorbate rapidly reduces α-tocopherol radicals to tocopherol (107–109) in membranes (110–112) and lipoproteins (113,114). Tocopherol is located at or near the membrane surface (115) and the efficiency of radical scavenging decreases as the radical goes deeper into the interior of the membranes (116). Therefore, the particular localization of α-tocopherol at the membrane surface and ascorbate in water phase facilitates the interaction between the two antioxidants at the interface between the membrane or lipoprotein and water. This makes possible the export of radical character from lipid to water. In this way, unpaired electrons are channeled from reactive free radicals to ascorbate. The ascorbate free radical, semidehydroascorbate is, in turn, eliminated by disproportionation or by reductase activities. This is the mechanistic basis for synergistic protection of LDL against oxidation.

2. Reactions of Caffeic Acid and α-Tocopherol

Similarly to ascorbate, caffeic acid inhibits lipid peroxidation synergistically with α-tocopherol in LDL challenged with ferrylmyoglobin (117). In this system, LDL became depleted of α-tocopherol and the peroxidative chain propagated after tocopherol consumption. Caffeic acid prevented α-tocopherol consumption when added either before or during the depletion reaction, partially restoring α-tocopherol levels. These findings, as well as the chain-breaking activity exhibited by caffeic acid when added during the propagation chain of LDL lipid peroxidation (43), led us to suggest the reduction of α-tocopherol radical to tocopherol by the phenolic acid as a mechanism contributing to the antioxidant activity of caffeic acid. In accordance with this mechanistic interpretation, Nardini et al. (118) observed that lipoproteins from caffeic acid-fed rats were markedly resistant to oxidative modification and that caffeic acid dietary supplementation resulted in a statistically significant increase of α-tocopherol both in plasma and lipoproteins. Additionally, Stocker et al. (106,119) have reported the ability of caffeic acid to quench the α-tocopheroxyl radical in micelles, and they have proposed a one-electron transfer reaction as the underlying mechanism.

The ability to reduce α-tocopherol radical cannot be extended to the hydroxycinnamate family because the biosynthetic precursor of caffeic acid, p-coumaric acid, accelerates the rate of α-tocopherol consumption in LDL challenged with ferrylmyoglobin when added either before or during the ongoing reaction (117). This effect of p-coumaric acid was interpreted in terms of the stability of hydroxycinnamate-derived phenoxyl radicals and is sustained by the higher reduction potential of p-coumaric radical as compared with that of the caffeic radical (20) (i.e., conversely to caffeic acid o-semiquinone radical, p-coumaric acid phenoxyl radical, was able to oxidize α-tocopherol). This conclusion is in agreement with the observation that sterically unprotected phenoxyl radical is highly reactive toward tocopherol, inducing H abstraction in nonpolar medium with rate constants three orders of magnitude higher than the H abstraction from α-tocopherol by peroxyl radicals (120).

3. Reactions of Caffeic Acid and Ascorbate

The ability of caffeic acid to interact with ascorbate and provide synergistic protection to LDL has also been scrutinized (121). A combination of caffeic acid with ascorbate synergistically increased the lag times required for linoleate hydroperoxide and 7-ketocholesterol formation as well as for cholesteryl linoleate consumption, major oxidation products and unsaturated lipid in LDL, respectively. Given that caffeic acid was a better antioxidant than ascorbate in the system used, the potential recycling of phenoxyl radical from caffeic acid by ascorbate as a reaction contributing to the increased protection of LDL against oxidation was discussed (23). Such an interaction would provide a constant resupply of caffeic acid and would limit the decay of caffeic radical by a second-order reaction. In view, of the lower reduction potential of ascorbate radical as compared with caffeic radical, this reaction is likely to occur (see following section). In fact, the redox interaction of ascorbate with hydroxycinnamates may be a common reaction in higher plants; ascorbate and hydroxycinnamates colocalize in plant cellular compartments, such as the vacuoles, at millimolar concentrations. In plants, ascorbate inhibits peroxidase-dependent univalent oxidation of caffeic acid and, for soluble peroxidases, the reduction of caffeic radical by ascorbate has been proposed as part of the mechanism (122). Moreover, the redox couple of caffeic with ascorbate has been proposed as the basis for a very effective mechanism of detoxification in plants: the facile electron donation to peroxidases by caffeic acid and the subsequent reduction of caffeic radicals by ascorbate can efficiently reduce H_2O_2 without any accumulation of oxidized phenolic products (123,124). It may be envisaged, however, that in systems where ascorbate is the more important antioxidant, the recycling of caffeic radical by ascorbate can result in pro-oxidant effects.

4. *Reactions of Caffeic Acid, Ascorbate, and α-Tocopherol*

Further studies on the dynamic interactions of caffeic acid with α-tocopherol and ascorbate provided evidence for a sequence entailing transfer of the radical character required to accomplish optimal synergistic protection of LDL against oxidation (23). Figure 2 shows a continuous-flow EPR measurement of a mixture of α-tocopherol-containing SDS micelles oxidized with ferrylmyoglobin and the effect of sequential introduction of caffeic and ascorbate into the medium. Although the independent recycling of α-tocopherol by ascorbate can occur,

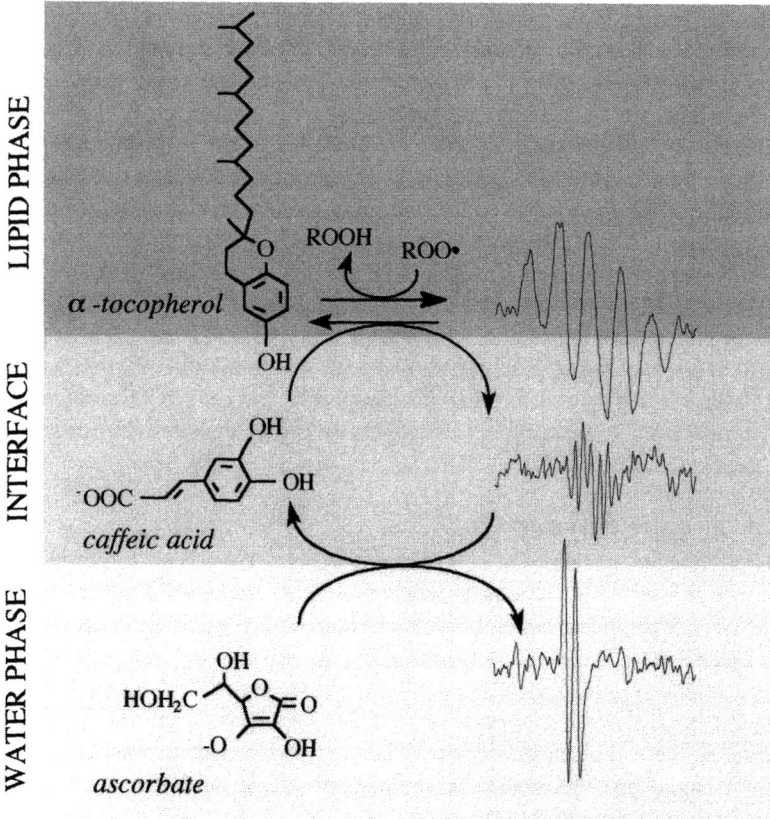

Figure 2 Continuous-flow EPR measurements (see text and Ref. 23 for details).

the results indicate that the radical character can be sequentially transferred from the lipoprotein particle to the aqueous medium through the one-electron reduction of tocopheroxyl radical by caffeic acid and, in turn, of caffeic radical by ascorbate. Under these conditions it was observed that α-tocopherol, caffeic acid, and ascorbate acted synergistically to afford optimal protection of LDL against oxidation (Fig. 3). Moreover, caffeic acid worked more efficiently as a coantioxidant with α-tocopherol than did ascorbate. These experimental findings suggest that in addition to reduction potential and decay kinetics of antioxidant-derived radicals, the solubility (localization) of antioxidant is relevant for the antioxidant activity of caffeic acid (see Fig. 2). These points require further discussion:

The reported one-electron reduction potential of caffeic o-semiquinone radical ($E7 = 0.54$ V) at pH 7 is slightly higher than $E7 = 0.48$ V for trolox phenoxyl radical (the water-soluble analogue of vitamin E assumed to have identical reduction potential) (125). Therefore, if the figures can apply, the reduction of tocopheroxyl radical by caffeic acid is not thermodynamically feasible. However, the reaction can be kinetically pulled, overcoming the thermodynamic constraints, considering that the concentration of caffeic acid is far more than that of tocopheroxyl radical.

Ascorbate, the terminal electron donor in the free radical-scavenging chain (126), has the lowest reduction potential (0.28 V), implying that the reduction of caffeic acid radical to the parent compound by ascorbate is thermodynamically feasible. Conceivably, EPR evidence for the interaction of ascorbate with hydroxycinnamates supports the regeneration of caffeic (23) and chlorogenic (124) acids from their corresponding radicals by ascorbate. However, similar to the interaction of flavonoids with ascorbate (44), a redox equilibrium involving several

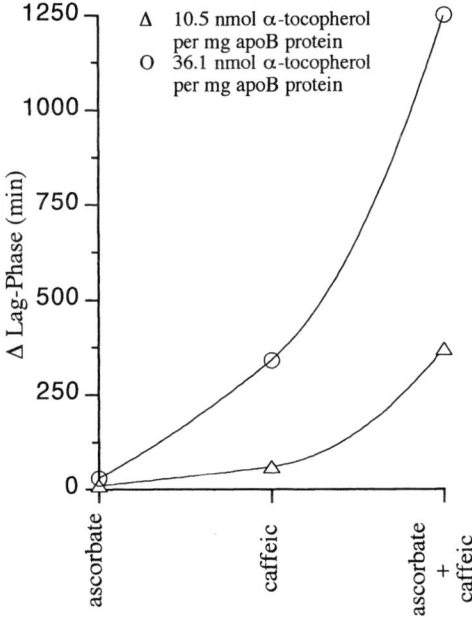

Figure 3 Concerted effects of α-tocopherol, caffeic acid, and ascorbate in the inhibition of LDL oxidation by ferrylmyoglobin. Differences in the length of lag phases of conjugated dienes' formation in the presence of antioxidants from those in the absence, in two populations of LDL (normal and α-tocopherol-enriched) obtained from the same plasma sample (see details in Ref. 23).

reactions can be established between hydroxycinnamates and ascorbate (23,127). In addition, it has also been reported that quinone formed from caffeic acid by peroxidase-dependent reaction is reduced to the original compound by ascorbate (123).

The physical accessibility of the reductant to the tocopheroxyl radical is critical in determining the synergistic antioxidant activity in LDL and membrane systems (116,128,129). The greater effect of caffeic acid over ascorbate to synergistically inhibit LDL oxidation (see Fig. 3) appears attributable to its physical characteristics. Conversely to ascorbate, caffeic acid is relatively poorly soluble in water. This property would allow the caffeic acid to gain easier access to the lipoprotein particle, facilitating the repair of the lipophilic tocopheroxyl radical and, on the other hand, to prevent the initial attack on LDL by free radicals generated in the water phase.

That the solubility properties of flavonoids facilitate their localization at water–lipid interfaces and, in turn, influence their antioxidant activities, is a concept that has been observed in liposomal membranes (130–132). Concerning the hydroxycinnamates, and caffeic acid in particular, much indirect evidence emphasizes the amphiphilic properties that support the localization of caffeic at the interface of LDL and membrane systems. First, Tyson et al. (133), running two-phase partition experiments to assess the ionophoretic ability of Fe^{3+} chelators, showed that caffeic acid was effective in transferring Fe^{3+} from an aqueous phase to an organic hydrophobic phase. Second, Foti et al. (60) studied the antioxidant activity of flavonoids, coumarins, and cinnamic acids in a micellar system, in correlation with the partition coefficient of the compounds in octanol–water mixtures at 50°C and observed that caffeic acid exhibited a partition coefficient lower than flavonols, such as quercetin, but higher than glycosilated flavanones, such as naringin and hesperidin. Third, although caffeic acid displays one of the highest reactivities toward peroxyl radicals (see Table 1), only a moderate capability to quench peroxyl radicals inside SDS micelles of methyl linoleate was observed (60). The analysis of data in this later system requires the consideration that the repulsion exerted by the negative charges of SDS makes difficult the access of caffeic monoanions to the interior of micelles, but the results also suggest that the high antioxidant activity of caffeic acid in lipoproteins (23; see Fig. 3) may be largely related to the reduction of α-tocopheroxyl radical at the LDL interface, rather than directly intercept any secondary lipid peroxyl radicals. Fourth, lipoprotein-bound antioxidant activity was shown for chlorogenic acid using an in vitro oxidation model for heart disease (134). Fifth, Carbonneau et al. (135) suggested a location for caffeic acid and other wine phenolic compounds at the lipoprotein surface based on the loss of antioxidant effects against LDL oxidation after extensive dialysis.

Obviously, in addition to a nonspecific interaction with the phospholipid monolayer, the binding of caffeic acid to apoB protein in the LDL particle, cannot be disregarded. Abu-Amsha et al. (57) found that caffeic acid spared α-tocopherol in LDL challenged with copper and that the presence of caffeic acid alters the binding of copper to the apoB protein, thus suggesting an interaction of the phenolic compound with the apoprotein. This is not surprising, for binding of caffeic acid to proteins, such as albumin, in vitro has already been shown (136,137). In the structure of phenolic acids, aromatic rings, and carbon–hydrogen skeletons of lateral chains provide binding sites of a hydrophobic nature to interact with proteins. Also, if one takes into account the capacity of phenolics to establish ionic and H-bonding, it may be suggested that phenolic acids have the ability to interact with a wide range of proteins.

If we consider that copper binding to apoB protein is a prerequisite for LDL oxidation (138), the modification of binding sites for copper in LDL may be viewed as a new antioxidant mechanism for caffeic acid that is reminiscent of that observed for ascorbate (73,139). In fact, the incubation of LDL with the potential pro-oxidant mixture consisting of ascorbate and copper

IV. BIOAVAILABILITY AND PHARMACOKINETICS

is not followed by lipoprotein oxidation, an effect partially ascribed to the ascorbate-induced modification of copper-binding sites, most notably His, in the lipoprotein particle (140).

An important question remaining to be unequivocally answered relates to the bioavailability and metabolism of the hydroxycinnamates in humans (141). Implicitly, information about the human toxicology of hydroxycinnamates is scarce. Given the ubiquitous distribution of these phenolic acids in plant-derived foodstuff, it is conceivable that they are ingested by humans in high amounts and, therefore, a consistent toxic risk is not expected to take place. A recent work in a Bavarian subpopulation described an average phenolic acid intake of 222 mg/day and the dominating phenol was identified as caffeic acid (206 mg/day) (142).

The information on the absorption, distribution, and excretion of phenolic acids is limited, but from available preliminary data in animals and humans some broad indications can be retrieved:

1. After oral ingestion, hydroxycinnamates can reach human plasma in a concentration-dependent manner, although the levels detected are very low in relation to the amounts ingested.

Dietary supplementation studies with fruit, green tea, and red wine in humans have suggested the uptake of hydroxycinnamates. Bourne et al. (143) identified free ferulic, caffeic, and p-coumaric acids in human urine after high levels of fruit intake. Maiani et al. (144) were able to detect caffeic acid in human plasma and, in spite of the chromatographically impure fraction contaminated with caffeine, the results indicate a plasma concentration peak of caffeic acid 1–2 h after tea ingestion in the high nanomolar to micromolar range. A significant increase in plasma caffeic acid was also observed after consumption of red wine, although, no immediate effect on ex vivo LDL oxidizability was found (145). Studies in animals further support bioavailability of hydroxycinnamates. When added to the diet, caffeic acid has been recovered in substantial concentrations (low micromolar range) in rat (118) and rabbit plasma (146). Yet, a pharmacokinetic study of caffeic acid in isolated perfused rat liver indicated that metabolic rates of individual compounds are affected by accompanying substances; caffeic acid was clearly better metabolized when given alone than when applied in crude plant extracts (147). Finally, evidence for the existence of mechanisms of transport across the intestinal epithelium was provided by the description of a Na^+-dependent saturable transport of cinnamic acid across the brush-border membrane of rat jejunum (148,149).

2. After ingestion, the phenolic compounds are partially recovered as derivatives, after methylation and conjugation with sulfate and glucuronic acid (150); a notion that has already been clearly documented for the flavonoid quercetin (151).

Biotransformation studies of caffeic acid by means of the isolated perfused rat liver point in this direction (152). Though 93.3% of caffeic acid dose appeared unchanged after one liver passage, several products of caffeic acid oxidation, including methylation products, ferulic and isoferulic acid, and a cyclization product, esculetin, were found in the perfusion medium. It is important to recognize that this work raises the notion of "antioxidant phenolic interconversion"; the metabolism of caffeic acid in vivo may originate phenolic products that still exhibit antioxidant activity. The conversion of caffeic to ferulic acid is a prime example: oral administration of caffeic acid to humans caused the urinary appearance of O-methylated phenolic acids, including ferulic acid and its conjugates (153).

Although endothelial cells in the gastrointestinal tract as well as liver cells are likely to be involved in the metabolism of the phenolic compounds, intestinal microflora of humans and experimental animals also plays an important role in the metabolism of caffeic acid (153–155).

Peppercorn and Goldman (154) have shown that germ-free rats were able to excrete only caffeic and ferulic acids in urine when caffeic was given in the diet. However, when the germ-free rats were selectively infected with bacteria characteristic of the gastrointestinal tract, the feeding of caffeic acid led to the urinary excretion of dehydroxylated and decarboxylated metabolites of caffeic acid. Nevertheless, the physiological significance of these processes requires the evaluation of the different regions of the gut where absorption and microflora metabolization may occur; for example, if absorption of hydroxycinnamates preferentially takes place in the jejunum (156), metabolization by microflora in the colon may be bypassed.

In connection with the concept of phenolic interconversion just discussed, one should also consider the potential formation of phenolic acids through the metabolization of more complex polyphenols by processes that may include scission of the flavonoid structure by intestinal microflora or mammal enzymatic activities. A recent study shows that after oral administration of rosmarinic acid to rats, caffeic, ferulic, and coumaric acids, as well as their sulfate derivatives, were found in the urine (157). Microflora in the gastrointestinal tract of mammals are also capable of releasing phenolic acids from carbohydrate complexes (158).

Despite increased water solubility achieved through glucuronidation, studies in rats suggest that renal excretion is not the main route of elimination of the hydroxycinnamates, ferulic and chlorogenic acids (150). In fact, glucuronides as well as sulfates of caffeic acid could be determined in the bile in isolated perfused rat liver models (152). On the other hand, pharmacokinetic studies of caffeic acid after intravenous administration in rabbits (159) indicated that more than 50% of unchanged caffeic acid was excreted in urine.

Curiously, it was claimed that dehydrocaffeic acid is a contaminant in human plasma for the electrochemical determination of catecholamines, particularly in persons who intake more than 3 cups of coffee a day, a beverage known to contain high amounts of caffeic acid (160).

3. Evidence on the in vivo antioxidant effects of caffeic acid (or metabolites) indirectly supports its bioavailability.

Oral administration of caffeic and chlorogenic acids inhibited the elevation of serum lipid peroxides, as well as liver peroxides, in rats fed peroxidized oil (161), treated with CCl_4 or irradiated with ^{60}Co (162). Dietary supplementation of caffeic acid increased plasma and LDL α-tocopherol in rats as compared with controls given no phenolic acid (118). Another study reported the prevention of paraquat-induced oxidative stress, as followed by measuring the activities of superoxide dismutase (SOD), catalase, and GSH peroxidase activities, in the liver of rats supplemented with chlorogenic acid in the diet (163).

V. CELLULAR EFFECTS

A. Modulation of Cell Signaling

Novel findings are being reported in connection with direct effects of caffeic acid at the cellular level that are not necessarily related to antioxidant activities. Studies related to the role of LDL in atherogenesis are of particular interest and are discussed in the following.

Oxidized LDL is cytotoxic to cultured cells (164,165), and cell death by apoptosis in human cultured endothelial cells through a calcium-dependent mechanism has been observed (166). Hydroxycinnamic acids, most notably caffeic acid, exhibited a potent cytoprotective effect of cultured endothelial cells against oxidized LDL, blocking concomitantly the intracellular Ca^{2+} peak and the apoptotic process (167). In addition to an "indirect" cytoprotective effect of caffeic acid related to the inhibition of LDL oxidation (antioxidant effect), the same study presented evidence for a "direct" protective effect of endothelial cells against apoptosis induced by oxidized LDL, independently of the inhibition of LDL oxidation. Specifically, LDL particles were preoxidized by UV or treatment with ferrylmyoglobin, in the absence of the phenolic compound and, after oxidation, were added to the cultured medium simultaneously with caffeic acid. Nevertheless, the "indirect" cytoprotective effect supported by the antioxidant activity of caffeic acid was significantly higher than the "direct" effect.

The ability of caffeic acid to interfere with the intracellular signaling cascade triggered by oxidized LDL was explored by the same authors. Several studies indicate that oxidized LDL interferes with signaling pathways involving, among others (168–174), the epithelial growth factor receptor (EGFR) (175), a transmembrane receptor apparently implicated in cell proliferation or differentiation. Salvayre et al. (personal communication) demonstrated that caffeic acid inhibited the activation of EGFR induced by oxidized LDL by multiple mechanisms, ranging from inhibition of intracellular oxidative stress, assessed in terms of 6-carboxy-$2',7'$-dichlorodihydrofluorescein oxidation, to the competitive inhibition of the EGFR kinase activity.

Further evidence supporting a potential involvement of caffeic acid in the modulation of cellular functions was recently forwarded by Scaccini et al. who have observed that the phenolic acid inhibited the activities of phosphorylase kinase, protein kinase C, and protein kinase A in vitro by noncompetitive mechanisms (176).

The competence of caffeic acid to exert an antioxidant action and to modulate a response to an oxidative challenge inside the cell has also been observed in cellular cultures of human monocytes (U937) incubated with t-butyl hydroperoxide (tBOOH) (177). Under the experimental conditions used this study, caffeic acid was incorporated into cells without any cytotoxic effect up to a concentration of 100 μM in the culture medium. Cells preincubated with caffeic acid were more resistant to cell death induced by tBOOH treatment, its proliferative capacity was maintained at higher levels, and the loss of cellular glutathione was slowed down, when compared with the control cells not preincubated with caffeic acid.

On the other hand, caffeic acid alone or in combination with copper (but not iron) ions was claimed to induce apoptosis in human promyelocytic leukemic HL-60 cells (178), effects that could be decreased by α-tocopherol previously incorporated in the cells (179). In summary, a complex picture is emerging that includes several targets for the action of caffeic acid at the cellular level. Relative to the inhibition of the deregulation of cell signaling triggered by oxidized LDL, several levels of caffeic acid intervention can be considered that may operate complementary: namely, (1) quenching of free radicals outside the cells; (2) modulating toxic-signaling pathways evoked by oxidized LDL through mechanisms that are not necessarily related to its antioxidant activity; (3) reducing intracellular oxidative stress.

B. Mutagenicity

In contrast to the beneficial effects of antioxidant and protective activities, caffeic acid acts as a mutagen in several test systems (180). These activities are likely to result from pro-oxidant effects. Usually, mutagenicity tests require the presence of transition metals (181) and redox cycling of phenolics, with the consequent production free radical-dependent damage. However, in this discussion, it is relevant to consider that caffeic acid is a very efficient scavenger of radicals, including $O_2^{\cdot -}$, as discussed earlier; therefore, the overall reaction, depending on available phenol and competition reactions, could be the annihilation of reactive oxygen species.

The ability of phenolic compounds to bind DNA has also been suggested in connection with their mutagenicity effects (182). A dose-dependent mutagenicity effect may also be of significance, and this is suggested by the observations that at a very high brief dietary dose

(183,184) or a low (0.04–0.8%) long-term dose (185) of caffeic acid promoted forestomach carcinogenesis in rats.

On the contrary, phenolic acids have been strong inhibitors of carcinogenesis at the initiation and promotion stages (180,186) induced by different compounds (187–189). These effects are reflected by the capacity of caffeic acid to (1) prevent cancer in skin, tongue, liver, lung, and esophagus of rats (190,191), as well as by the inhibition of nitrosamine formation in vivo (192); (2) induce phase II drug-metabolizing enzymes in rat liver, including glutathione S-transferases and quinone reductase (193).

VI. CONCLUDING REMARKS

Caffeic acid and related compounds exert several actions in a biological setting. These actions are linked to antioxidant and, eventually, to pro-oxidant activities, but new effects at the cellular level also point to actions not necessarily related to antioxidation.

Despite the pro-oxidant and mutagenic activities found under particular conditions, its antioxidant activity, particularly at the initial stages of oxidative stress, is strongly supported by data obtained both in vitro and in vivo. In this regard, bioavailability and metabolism are largely unknown and require further development. Nevertheless, the potential use of caffeic acid and hydroxycinnamates in the development of pharmaceutical products cannot be disregarded in the design of antioxidants for prevention of disorders related to lipid oxidation.

Pathogenic cell signaling triggered by oxidized LDL, leading to cellular dysfunction, is critically involved in atherogenesis. The modulation effects of caffeic acid on these cascades beyond its antioxidant activity, indicates new trends in the biological activity of the dietary phenolic compounds related to the prevention of atherosclerosis, which requires further studies.

The potential for caffeic acid to behave as an effective antioxidant in lipid systems, such as the LDL, appears to be dictated by thermodynamic and kinetic parameters and by location of the phenol at the lipid–water interface.

Overall, physicochemical data and novel findings at the cellular level and on the concerted activity with vitamins E and C, point to the biological intervention of caffeic acid at several levels and including several targets:

1. Extracellular activities related to the quenching of several types of free radicals, thus inhibiting cellular and LDL damage.
2. Interface phenomena, encompassing antioxidant activities, that include the modification of binding sites for transition metals in LDL and, also, the regeneration of α-tocopherol in the lipoprotein particles.
3. Intracellular effects by modulating toxic-signaling pathways evoked by oxidized LDL through mechanisms that are largely unknown, but are not necessarily related to its antioxidant activity and by reducing intracellular oxidative stress.
4. In addition to specific actions in the framework of oxidative stress, broad and unspecific biological actions of these compounds can be envisaged supported by interaction with enzymes either unspecifically or specifically through reduction of metals in the active center.

ACKNOWLEDGMENTS

Supported by Programa PRAXIS XXI, Fundação para a Ciência e Tecnologia (grants PRAXIS/PCNA/BIA/160/96 and PRAXIS/P/BIA/1395/1998), Portugal.

REFERENCES

1. Abu-Amsha R, Croft KD, Puddey IB, Proudfoot JM, Beilin LJ. Phenolic content of various beverages determines the extent of inhibition of human serum and low density lipoprotein oxidation in vitro: identification and mechanism of action of some cinnamic acid derivatives from red wine. Clin Sci 1996; 91:449–458.
2. Heller W, Forkmann G. Biosynthesis of flavonoids. In: Harborne J, ed. The Flavonoids: Advances in Research Since 1986. London: Chapman & Hall, 1993:499–535.
3. Stafford HA. The metabolism of aromatic compounds. Annu Rev Plant Physiol 1974; 25:459–486.
4. Hertog M, Feskens E, Hollman P, et al. Dietary antioxidant flavonoids and risk of coronary heart disease: the Zutphen Elderly Study. Lancet 1993; 342:1007–1011.
5. Knekt P, Jarvinen R, Reunamen A, Maatela J. Flavonoid intake and coronary mortality in Finland: a cohort study. Br Med J 1996; 312:478–481.
6. Hollman P, Hertog M, Katan M. Role of dietary flavonoids in protection against cancer and coronary heart disease. Biochem Soc Trans 1996; 24:785–789.
7. Rice-Evans CA, Miller NJ, Paganga G. Structure–antioxidant activity relationships of flavonoids and phenolic acids. [Published erratum appears in Free Radic Biol Med 1996; 21(3):417.] Free Radic Biol Med 1996; 20:933–956.
8. Witzum J. The oxidation hypothesis of atherosclerosis. Lancet 1994; 344:793–795.
9. Steinberg D. A critical look at the evidence for the oxidation of LDL in atherogenesis. Atherosclerosis 1997; 131(suppl):S5–S7.
10. Wallace G, Fry SC. Phenolic components of the plant cell wall. Int Rev Cytol 1994; 151:229–267.
11. Herrmann K. Occurrence and content of hydroxycinnamic and hydroxybenzoic acid compounds in foods. Crit Rev Food Sci Nutr 1989; 28:315–347.
12. Shahidi F, Naczk M. Food Phenolics: Sources, Chemistry, Effects, Applications. Lancaster, PA: Technomic, 1995.
13. Rhodes M, Wooltorton L. The enzymic conversion of hydroxycinnamic acids to p-coumarylquinic and chlorogenic acids in tomato fruits. Phytochemistry 1976; 15:947–951.
14. Ulbrich B, Zenk M. Partial purification and properties of hydroxycinnamoyl-CoA: quinate hydroxycinnamoyl transferase from higher plants. Phytochemistry 1979; 18:929–933.
15. Kahnt G. Phytochemistry 1967; 6:755–758.
16. Bors W, Heller W, Mitchel C, Saran M. Flavonoids as antioxidants: determination of radical-scavenging efficiencies. Methods Enzymol 1990; 186:343–355.
17. Belyakov V, Roginsky V, Bors W. Rate constants for the reaction of peroxyl free radical with flavonoids and related compounds as determined by the kinetic chemiluminescence method. J Chem Soc Perkin Trans 1995; 2:2319–2326.
18. Kono Y, Kobayashi K, Tagawa S, et al. Antioxidant activity of polyphenolics in diets. Rate constants of reactions of chlorogenic acid and caffeic acid with reactive species of oxygen and nitrogen. Biochim Biophys Acta 1997; 1335:335–342.
19. Zhouen Z, Side Y, Weizhen L, et al. Mechanism of reaction of nitrogen dioxide radical with hydroxycinnamic acid derivatives: a pulse radiolysis study. Free Radic Res 1998; 29:13–16.
20. Foley S, Navaratnam S, McGarvey D, et al. Singlet oxygen quenching and the redox properties of hydroxycinnamic acids. Free Radic Biol Med 1999; 26:1202–1208.
21. Kono Y, Shibata H, Kodama Y, Sawa Y. The suppression of the N-nitrosating reaction by chlorogenic acid. Biochem J 1995; 312:947–953.
22. Kono Y, Shibata H, Kodama Y, et al. Chlorogenic acid as a natural scavenger for hypochlorous acid. Biochem Biophys Res Commun 1995; 217:972–978.
23. Laranjinha J, Cadenas E. Redox cycles of caffeic acid, α-tocopherol, and ascorbate: implications for protection of low-density lipoproteins against oxidation. IUBMB Life 1999; 48:1–9.
24. Chen CP, Yokozawa T, Chung HY. Inhibitory effect of caffeic acid analogues isolated from *Salviae miltiorrhizae* Radix against 1,1-diphenyl-2-picrylhydrazyl radical. Exp Toxicol Pathol 1999; 51:59–63.
25. Bors W, Heller W, Michel C, Stettmaier K. Flavonoids and polyphenols: chemistry and biology. In: Cadenas E, Packer L, eds. Handbook of Antioxidants. New York: Marcel Dekker, 1996:409–466.
26. Jovanovic SV, Steenken S, Tosic M, et al. Flavonoids as antioxidants. J Am Chem Soc 1994; 116:4846–4851.
27. Fridovich I. Superoxide anion radical ($O_2^{\cdot-}$), superoxide dismutases and related matters. J Biol Chem 1997; 279:18515–18517.

28. Beckman J, Beckman T, Chen J, et al. Apparent hydroxyl radical production by peroxynitrite: implications for endothelial injury from nitric oxide and superoxide. Proc Natl Acad Sci USA 1990; 87:1620–1624.
29. Huie R, Padmaja S. The reaction of NO with superoxide. Free Radic Res Commun 1993; 18:195–199.
30. Radi R, Beckman J, Bush K, Freeman B. Peroxynitrite-induced membrane lipid peroxidation: the cytotoxic potential of superoxide and nitric oxide. Arch Biochem Biophys 1991; 288:481–487.
31. Squadrito GL, Pryor WA. The formation of peroxynitrite in vivo from nitric oxide and superoxide. Chem Biol Interact 1995; 96:203–206.
32. Ischiropoulos H, Zhu L, Chen J, et al. Peroxynitrite mediated tyrosine nitration catalyzed by superoxide dismutase. Arch Biochem Biophys 1992; 298:431–437.
33. Salgo MG, Bermudez E, Squadrito GL, Pryor WA. Peroxynitrite causes DNA damage and oxidation of thiols in rat thymocytes [corrected]. [Published erratum appears in Arch Biochem Biophys 1995 Dec 1; 324(1):200.] Arch Biochem Biophys 1995; 322:500–505.
34. Bartlett D, Church D, Bounds P, Koppenol W. The kinetics of the oxidation of L-ascorbic acid by peroxynitrite. Free Radic Biol Med 1995; 18:85–92.
35. Lee. Bioorg Med Chem Lett 1997; 118:2913–2918.
36. Pannala A, Razaq R, Halliwell B, et al. Inhibition of peroxynitrite dependent tyrosine nitration by hydroxycinnamates: nitration or electron donation. Free Radic Biol Med 1998; 24:594–606.
37. Kerry N, Rice–Evans C. Peroxynitrite oxidises catechols to *o*-quinones. FEBS Lett 1998; 437:167–171.
38. Denicola A, Freeman B, Trujillo M, Radi R. Peroxynitrite reaction with carbon dioxide/bicarbonate: kinetics and influence on peroxynitrite-mediated oxidations. Arch Biochem Biophys 1996; 333:49–58.
39. Alayash A, Ryan B, Cashon R. Peroxynitrite-mediated heme oxidation and protein modification of native and chemically modified hemoglobins. Arch Biochem Biophys 1998; 349:65–73.
40. Kerry N, Rice–Evans C. Inhibition of peroxynitrite-mediated oxidation of dopamine by flavonoid and phenolic antioxidants and their structural relationships. J Neurochem 1999; 73:247–253.
41. Niwa T, Doi U, Kato Y, Osawa T. Inhibitory mechanism of sinapinic acid against peroxynitrite-mediated tyrosine nitration of protein in vitro. FEBS Lett 1999; 459:43–46.
42. Cadenas E. Mechanisms of antioxidant action. In: Ozben T, ed. Mechanisms of Antioxidant Action. New York: Plenum Press, 1998:237–251.
43. Laranjinha J, Almeida L, Madeira V. Reactivity of dietary phenolic acids with peroxyl radicals: antioxidant activity upon low density lipoprotein peroxidation. Biochem Pharmacol 1994; 48:487–494.
44. Bors W, Michel C, Schikora S. Interaction of flavonoids with ascorbate and determination of their univalent redox potentials: a pulse radiolysis study. Free Radic Biol Med 1995; 19:45–52.
45. Sharma O. Antioxidant activity of curcumin and related compounds. Biochem Pharmacol 1976; 25:1811–1812.
46. Iwahashi H, Ishii T, Sugata R, Kido R. The effects of caffeic acid and its related catechols on hydroxyl radical formation by 3-hydroxyanthranilic acid, ferric chloride and hydrogen peroxide. Arch Biochem Biophys 1990; 276:242–247.
47. Chimi H, Cillard J, Cillard P, Rahmani M. Peroxyl and hydroxyl radical scavenging activity of some natural phenolic antioxidants. J Am Oil Chem Soc 1991; 68:307–312.
48. Terao J, Karasawa H, Arai H, et al. Peroxyl radical scavenging activity of caffeic acid and its related phenolic compounds in solution. Biosci Biotechnol Biochem 1993; 57:1204–1205.
49. Cuvelier M, Richard H, Berset C. Comparison of the antioxidative activity of some acid-phenols: structure–activity relationship. Biosci Biotechnol Biochem 1992; 56:324–325.
50. Fraga C, Martino V, Ferraro G, et al. Flavonoids as antioxidants evaluated by in vitro and in situ liver chemiluminescence. Biochem Pharmacol 1987; 36:717–720.
51. Liu G, Zhang T, Wang B, Wang Y. Protective action of seven natural phenolic compounds against peroxidative damage to biomembranes. Biochem Pharmacol 1992; 43:147–152.
52. Laranjinha J, Almeida L, Madeira V. Lipid peroxidation and its inhibition in low density lipoproteins: quenching of *cis*-parinaric acid fluorescence. Arch Biochem Biophys 1992; 297:147–154.
53. Castelluccio C, Paganga G, Melikian N, et al. Antioxidant potential of intermediates in phenylpropanoid metabolism in higher plants. FEBS Lett 1995; 368:188–192.
54. Laranjinha J, Vieira O, Almeida L, Madeira V. Inhibition of metmyoglobin/H_2O_2-dependent low density lipoprotein lipid peroxidation by naturally occurring phenolic acids. Biochem Pharmacol 1996; 51:395–402.

55. Giulivi C, Cadenas E. Ferrylmyoglobin: formation and chemical reactivity toward electron-donating compounds. Methods Enzymol 1994; 233:189–202.
56. Nardini M, D'Aquino M, Tomassi G, et al. Inhibition of human low-density lipoprotein oxidation by caffeic acid and other hydroxycinnamic acid derivatives. Free Radic Biol Med 1995; 19:541–552.
57. Abu-Amsha R, Croft K, Puddey I, et al. Phenolic content of various beverages determines the extent of inhibition of human serum and low density lipoprotein oxidation in vitro: identification and mechanism of action of some cinnamic acid derivatives from red wine. Clin Sci 1996; 91:449–458.
58. Vinson J, Dabbagh Y, Serry M, Jang J. Plant flavonoids, especially tea flavonols, are powerful antioxidants using an in vitro oxidation model for heart disease. J Agric Food Chem 1995; 43:2800–2802.
59. Kitagawa S, Sugiyama Y, Sakuma T. Inhibitory effects of catechol derivatives on hydrophilic free radical initiator-induced hemolysis and their interaction with hemoglobin. Chem Pharm Bull 1996; 44:881–884.
60. Foti M, Piattelli M, Baratta M, Ruberto G. Flavonoids, coumarins and cinamic acids as antioxidants in a micellar system. Structure–activity relationship. J Agric Food Chem 1996; 44:497–501.
61. Uchida M, Nakajin S, Toyoshima S, Shinoda M. Antioxidative effect of sesamol and related compounds on lipid peroxidation. Biol Pharm Bull 1996; 19:623–626.
62. Grace S, Salgo M, Pryor W. Scavenging of peroxynitrite by a phenolic/peroxidase system prevents oxidative damage to DNA. FEBS Lett 1998; 426:24–28.
63. Shibata H, Sakamoto Y, Oka M, Kono Y. Natural antioxidant, chlorogenic acid, protects against DNA breakage caused by monochloramine. Biosci Biotechnol Biochem 1999; 63:1295–1297.
64. Laranjinha J, Almeida L, Madeira V. Reduction of ferrylmyoglobin by dietary phenolic acid derivatives of cinnamic acid. Free Radic Biol Med 1995; 19:329–337.
65. Ohnishi M, Morishita H, Iwahashi T, et al. Inhibitory effects of chlorogenic acids on linoleic acid peroxidation and haemolysis. Phytochemistry 1994; 36:579–583.
66. Scott G. Antioxidants. Bull Chem Soc Jpn 1988; 61:165–170.
67. Burton GW, Doba T, Gabe EJ, et al. Autoxidation of biological molecules. 4. Maximizing the antioxidant activity of phenols. J Am Chem Soc 1985; 107:7053–7065.
68. Kono Y, Kashine S, Yoneyama T, et al. Iron chelation by chlorogenic acid as a natural antioxidant. Biosci Biotechnol Biochem 1998; 62:22–27.
69. Afanes'ev I, Dorozhko A, Brodskii A, et al. Chelating and free radical scavenging mechanisms of inhibitory action of rutin and quercetin in lipid peroxidation. Biochem Pharmacol 1989; 38:1763–1769.
70. van Acker SA, van den Berg DJ, Tromp MN, et al. Structural aspects of antioxidant activity of flavonoids. Free Radic Biol Med 1996; 20:331–342.
71. Moran J, Klucas R, Grayer RJ, et al. Complexes of iron with phenolic compounds from soybean nodules and other legume tissues: prooxidant and antioxidant properties. Free Radic Biol Med 1997; 22:861–870.
72. Yamanaka N, Oda O, Nagao S. Prooxidant activity of caffeic acid, dietary nonflavonoid phenolic acid, on Cu^{2+}-induced low density lipoprotein oxidation. FEBS Lett 1997; 405:186–190.
73. Stait SE, Leake DS. Ascorbic acid can either increase or decrease low density lipoprotein modification. FEBS Lett 1994; 341:263–267.
74. Yamanaka N, Oda O, Nagao S. Green tea catechins such as (−)-epicatechin and (−)-epigallocatechin accelerate Cu^{2+}-induced low density lipoprotein oxidation in propagation phase. FEBS Lett 1997; 401:230–234.
75. Smith C, Mitchinson MJ, Aruoma OI, Halliwell B. Stimulation of lipid peroxidation and hydroxyl-radical generation by the contents of human atherosclerotic lesions. Biochem J 1992; 286:901–905.
76. Evans P, Halliwell B. Measurement of iron and copper in biological systems: bleomycin and copper-phenanthroline assays. Methods Enzymol 1994; 233:82–92.
77. Aruoma O, Murcia A, Butler J, Halliwell B. Evaluation of the antioxidant and prooxidant actions of gallic and its derivatives. J Agric Food Chem 1993; 41:1880–1885.
78. Aruoma O. Pro-oxidant activities: an important consideration for food additives and/or nutrient components. In: Aruoma O, Halliwell B, eds. Free Radicals and Food Additives. London: Taylor & Francis, 1991:173–194.
79. Smith C, Halliwell B, Aruoma O. Protection by albumin against the pro-oxidant actions of phenolic dietary components. Food Chem Toxicol 1992; 30:483–489.

80. Boyer R, Clark H, LaRoche A. Reduction and release of ferritin iron by plant phenolics. J Inorg Biochem 1988; 32:171–181.
81. Kadir F, Al-Massad F. Haem binding to horse spleen ferritin and its effect on the rate of iron release. Biochem J 1992; 282:867–870.
82. Monteiro H, Winterbourn C. 6-Hydroxydopamine releases iron from ferritin and promotes ferritin-dependent lipid peroxidation. Biochem Pharmacol 1989; 38:4177–4182.
83. Kiechl S, Willeit J, Egger G, et al. Body iron stores and the risk of carotid atherosclerosis: prospective results from the Bruneck study. Circulation 1997; 96:3300–3307.
84. Coudray C, Bousset C, Tressol J, et al. Short-term ingestion of chlorogenic or caffeic acids decreases zinc but not copper absorption in rats, utilization of stable isotopes and inductively-coupled plasma mass spectrometry technique. Br J Nutr 1998; 80:575–584.
85. Koshihara Y, Neichi T, Murota S, et al. Caffeic acid is a selective inhibitor for leukotriene biosynthesis. Biochim Biophys Acta 1984; 792:92–97.
86. Kemal C, Louis–Flamberg P, Krupinski–Olsen R, Shorter A. Reductive inactivation of soybean lipoxygenase 1 by catechols: a possible mechanism for regulation of lipoxygenase activity. Biochemistry 1987; 26:7064–7072.
87. Bakovic M, Dunford H. Oxidation kinetics of caffeic acid by prostaglandin H synthase: potential role in regulation of prostaglandin biosynthesis. Prostaglandins Leukot Essent Fatty Acids 1994; 51:337–345.
88. de la Puerta R, Ruiz Gutierrez V, Hoult J. Inhibition of leukocyte 5-lipoxygenase by phenolics from virgin olive oil. Biochem Pharmacol 1999; 57:445–449.
89. Cornicelli J, Trivedi B. 15-Lipoxygenase and its inhibition: a novel therapeutic target for vascular disease. Curr Pharm Des 1999; 5:11–20.
90. Uz T, Pesold C, Longone P, Manev H. Aging-associated up-regulation of neuronal 5-lipoxygenase expression: putative role in neuronal vulnerability. FASEB J 1998; 12:439–449.
91. Steinberg D, Parthasarathy S, Carew TE, et al. Beyond cholesterol. Modifications of low-density lipoprotein that increase its atherogenicity. N Engl J Med 1989; 320:915–924.
92. Esterbauer H, Gebicki J, Puhl H, Jurgens G. The role of lipid peroxidation and antioxidants in oxidative modification of LDL. Free Radic Biol Med 1992; 13:341–390.
93. Steinbrecher UP, Parthasarathy S, Leake DS, et al. Modification of low density lipoprotein by endothelial cells involves lipid peroxidation and degradation of low density lipoprotein phospholipids. Proc Natl Acad Sci USA 1984; 81:3883–3887.
94. Morel D, DiCorleto P, Chisolm G. Endothelial and smooth muscle cells alter low density lipoprotein in vitro by free radical oxidation. Arteriosclerosis 1984; 4:357–364.
95. Aviram M. Modified forms of low density lipoprotein and atherosclerosis. Atherosclerosis 1993; 98:1–9.
96. Parthasarathy S, Wieland E, Steinberg D. A role for endothelial cell lipoxigenase in the oxidative modification of low density lipoprotein. Proc Natl Acad Sci USA 1989; 86:1046–1050.
97. Wieland E, Parthasarathy S, Steinberg D. Peroxidase-dependent metal-independent oxidation of low density lipoprotein in vitro: a model for in vivo oxidation? Proc Natl Acad Sci USA 1993; 90:5929–5933.
98. Darley–Usmar V, Hogg N, O'Leary N, et al. The simultaneous generation of superoxide and nitric oxide can initiate lipid peroxidation in human low density lipoprotein. Free Radic Res Commun 1992; 17:9–20.
99. Dee G, Rice–Evans C, Obeisekera S, et al. The modulation of ferryl myoglobin formation and its oxidative effects on low density lipoproteins by nitric oxide. FEBS Lett 1991; 294:38–42.
100. Balla G, Jacob H, Eaton J, et al. Hemin: a possible physiological mediator of low density lipoprotein oxidation and endothelial injury. Arterioscler Thromb 1991; 11:1700–1711.
101. Sato K, Niki E, Shimasaki H. Free radical-mediated chain oxidation of low density lipoprotein and its synergistic inhibition by vitamin E and vitamin C. Arch Biochem Biophys 1990; 279:402–405.
102. Esterbauer H, Jurgens G, Quehenberger O, Koller E. Autoxidation of human low density lipoprotein: loss of polyunsaturated fatty acids and vitamin E and generation of aldehydes. J Lipid Res 1987; 28:495–509.
103. Lucarini M, Pedulli G, Cipollone M. Bond dissociation enthalpy of α-tocopherol and other phenolic antioxidants. J Org Chem 1984; 59:5063–5070.
104. Bowry V, Stocker R. Tocopherol-mediated peroxidation. The pro-oxidant effect of vitamin E on the radical-initiated oxidation of human low-density lipoprotein. J Am Chem Soc 1993; 115:6029–6040.

105. Upston J, Terentis A, Stocker R. Tocopherol-mediated peroxidation of lipoproteins: implications for vitamin E as a potential antiatherogenic supplement. FASEB J 1999; 13:977–994.
106. Stocker R, Bowry V. Tocopherol-mediated peroxidation of lipoprotein lipids and its inhibition by co-antioxidants. In: Cadenas E, Packer L, eds. Handbook of Antioxidants. New York: Marcel Dekker, 1996:27–41.
107. Packer J, Slater T, Wilson R. Direct observation of a free radical interaction between vitamin E and vitamin C. Nature 1979; 278:737–739.
108. Niki E, Tsuchiya J, Tanimura R, Kamyia Y. Regeneration of vitamin E from α-chromanoxyl radical by glutathione and vitamin C. Chem Lett 1982; 789–792.
109. Mukai K, Nishimura M, Kikuchi S. Stopped-flow investigation of the reaction of vitamin C with tocopheroxyl radical in aqueous Triton X-100 micellar solutions. The structure–activity relationship of the regeneration reaction of tocopherol by vitamin C. J Biol Chem 1991; 266:274–278.
110. Scarpa M, Rigo A, Maiorino M, et al. Formation of α-tocopherol by ascorbate during peroxidation of phosphatidyl choline liposomes. Biochim Biophys Acta 1984; 801:215–219.
111. Niki E, Kawakami A, Yamamoto Y, Kamiya Y. Oxidation of lipids. VIII. Synergistic inhibition of oxidation of phosphatidylcholine liposome in aqueous dispersion by vitamin E and C. Bull Chem Soc Jpn 1985; 58:1971–1975.
112. Doba T, Burton G, Ingold K. Antioxidant activity of vitamin C. The effect of vitamin C either alone or in the presence of vitamin E or a water-soluble analogue upon the peroxidation of aqueous multilamellar phospholipid liposomes. Biochim Biophys Acta 1985; 835:298–303.
113. Kagan V, Serbinova E, Forte T, et al. Recycling of vitamin E in human low density lipoproteins. J Lipid Res 1992; 33:385–397.
114. Kalyanaraman B, Darley-Usmar V, Wood J, et al. Synergistic interaction between the probucol phenoxyl radical and ascorbic acid in inhibiting the oxidation of low density lipoprotein. J Biol Chem 1992; 267:6789–6795.
115. Gomez-Fernandez J, Villalain J, Aranda F, et al. Localization of α-tocopherol in membranes. Ann NY Acad Sci 1989; 570:109–120.
116. Takahashi M, Tsuchiya J, Niki E. Scavenging of radicals by vitamin E in the membranes as studied by spin labeling. J Am Chem Soc 1989; 111:6350–6353.
117. Laranjinha J, Vieira O, Madeira V, Almeida L. Two related phenolic antioxidants with opposite effects on vitamin E content in low density lipoproteins oxidized by ferrylmyoglobin: consumption vs regeneration. Arch Biochem Biophys 1995; 323:373–381.
118. Nardini M, Natella F, Gentili V, et al. Effect of caffeic acid dietary supplementation on the antioxidant defense system in rat: an in vivo study. Arch Biochem Biophys 1997; 342:157–160.
119. Witting PK, Westerlund C, Stocker R. A rapid and simple screening test for potential inhibitors of tocopherol-mediated peroxidation of LDL lipids. J Lipid Res 1996; 37:853–867.
120. Foti M, Ingold K, Lusztyk J. The surprising high reactivity of phenoxyl radicals. J Am Chem Soc 1994; 116:9440–9447.
121. Vieira O, Laranjinha J, Madeira V, Almeida L. Cholesteryl ester hydroperoxide formation in myoglobin-catalyzed low density lipoprotein oxidation: concerted antioxidant activity of caffeic and p-coumaric acids with ascorbate. Biochem Pharmacol 1998; 55:33–340.
122. Takahama U. Regulation of peroxidase-dependent oxidation of phenolics by ascorbic acid: different effects of ascorbic acid on the oxidation of conyferyl alcohol by the apoplastic soluble and cell wall-bound peroxidases. Plant Cell Physiol 1993; 34:809–817.
123. Takahama U, Oniki T. Regulation of peroxidase-dependent oxidation of phenolics in the apoplast of spinach leaves by ascorbate. Plant Cell Physiol 1992; 33:379–387.
124. Yamasaki H, Grace SC. EPR detection of phytophenoxyl radicals stabilized by zinc ions: evidence for the redox coupling of plant phenolics with ascorbate in the H_2O_2-peroxidase system. FEBS Lett 1998; 422:377–380.
125. Stenken S, Neta P. One-electron redox potentials of phenols. Hydroxy- and aminophenols and related compounds of biological interest. J Phys Chem 1982; 86:3661–3667.
126. Buettner G, Jurkiewicz B. Chemistry and biochemistry of ascorbic acid. In: Cadenas E, Packer L, eds. Handbook of Antioxidants. New York: Marcel Dekker, 1996: 91–115.
127. Satoh K, Sakagami H. Ascorbyl radical scavenging of polyphenols. Anticancer Res 1996; 16:2885–2890.
128. Niki E. Antioxidants in relation to lipid peroxidation. Chem Phys Lipids 1987; 44:227–253.
129. Thomas CE, McLean LR, Parker RA, Ohlweiler DF. Ascorbate and phenolic antioxidant interactions in prevention of liposomal oxidation. Lipids 1992; 27:543–550.

130. Ratty A, Sunamoto J, Das N. Interaction of flavonoids with 1,1-diphenyl-2-piryl-hyfrazil free radical, liposomal membranes and soybean lipoxygenase-1. Biochem Pharmacol 1988; 37:989–995.
131. Saija A, Scalese M, Lanza M, et al. Flavonoids as antioxidant agents: importance of their interaction with biomembranes. Free Radic Biol Med 1995; 19:481–486.
132. Terao J, Piskula M. Flavonoids as inhibitors of lipid peroxidation in membranes. In: Rice–Evans C, Packer L, eds. Flavonoids in Health and Disease. New York: Marcel Dekker, 1998:277–293.
133. Tyson CA, LeValley SE, Chan R, et al. Biological evaluation of some ionophore–polymeric chelator combinations for reducing iron overload. J Pharmacol Exp Ther 1984; 228:676–681.
134. Vinson J, Jang J, Dabbagh Y, et al. Plant polyphenols exhibit lipoprotein-bound antioxidant activity using and in vitro oxidation model for heart disease. J Agric Food Chem 1995; 43:2798–2799.
135. Carbonneau M, Leger C, Monnier L, et al. Supplementation with wine phenolic compounds increases the antioxidant capacity of plasma and vitamin E of low-density lipoprotein without changing the lipoprotein Cu(2+)-oxidizability: possible explanation by phenolic location. Eur J Clin Nutr 1997; 51:682–690.
136. Adzet T, Camarasa J, Escubedo E, Merlos M. In vitro study of caffeic acid–bovine serum albumin interaction. Eur J Drug Metab Pharmacokinet 1988; 13:11–14.
137. Muralidhara B, Prakash V. Interaction of 3′-O-caffeoyl D-quinic acid with human serum albumin. Int J Pept Protein Res 1995; 46:1–8.
138. Kuzuya M, Yamada K, Hayashi T, et al. Role of lipoprotein–copper complex in copper catalyzed-peroxidation of low-density lipoprotein. Biochim Biophys Acta 1992; 1123:334–341.
139. Retsky KL, Freeman MW, Frei B. Ascorbic acid oxidation product(s) protect human low density lipoprotein against atherogenic modification. Anti- rather than prooxidant activity of vitamin C in the presence of transition metal ions. J Biol Chem 1993; 268:1304–1309.
140. Retsky KL, Chen K, Zeind J, Frei B. Inhibition of copper-induced LDL oxidation by vitamin C is associated with decreased copper-binding to LDL and 2-oxohistidine formation. Free Radic Biol Med 1999; 26:90–98.
141. Jacobson E, Newmark H, Baptista J, Bruce W. A preliminary investigation of the metabolism of dietary phenolics in humans. Nutr Rep Int 1983; 28:1409–1417.
142. Radtke J, Linseisen J, Wolfram G. Phenolic acid intake of adults in a Bavarian subgroup of the national food consumption survey. Z Ernahrungswiss 1998; 37:190–197.
143. Bourne L, Rice–Evans C. Urinary detection of hydroxycinnamates and flavonoids in humans after high dietary intake of fruit. Free Radic Res 1998; 28:429–438.
144. Maiani G, Serafini M, Salucci M, et al. Application of a new high-performance liquid chromatographic method for measuring selected polyphenols in human plasma. J Chromatogr B Biomed Sci Appl 1997; 692:311–317.
145. Caccetta R, Croft K, Beilin L, Puddey I. Ingestion of red wine significantly increases plasma phenolic acid concentrations but does not acutely affect ex vivo lipoprotein oxidizability. Am J Clin Nutr 2000; 71:67–74.
146. Uang YS, Kang FL, Hsu KY. Determination of caffeic acid in rabbit plasma by high-performance liquid chromatography. J Chromatogr B Biomed Appl 1995; 673:43–49.
147. Wojciechowski H, Gumbinger HG, Vahlensieck U, et al. Analysis of the components of *Lycopus europaeus* L. in body fluids during metabolism studies. Comparison of capillary electrophoresis and high-performance liquid chromatography. J Chromatogr A 1995; 717:261–270.
148. Wolffram S, Weber T, Grenacher B, Scharrer E. A Na(+)-dependent mechanism is involved in mucosal uptake of cinnamic acid across the jejunal brush border in rats. J Nutr 1995; 125:1300–1308.
149. Ader P, Grenacher B, Langguth P, et al. Cinnamate uptake by rat small intestine: transport kinetics and transepithelial transfer. Exp Physiol 1996; 81:943–955.
150. Choudhury R, Srai S, Debnam E, Rice–Evans C. Urinary excretion of hydroxycinnamates and flavonoids after oral and intravenous administration. Free Radic Biol Med 1999; 27:278–286.
151. Manach C, Morand C, Crespy V, et al. Quercetin is recovered in human plasma as conjugated derivatives which retain antioxidant properties. FEBS Lett 1998; 426:331–336.
152. Gumbinger H, Vahlensieck U, Winterhoff H. Metabolism of caffeic acid in the isolated perfused rat liver. Planta Med 1993; 59:491–493.
153. Dayman J, Jepson J. The metabolism of caffeic acid in humans: the dehydroxylating action of intestinal bacteria. Biochem J 1969; 113:111.

154. Peppercorn M, Goldman P. Caffeic acid metabolism by gnotobiotic rats and their intestinal bacteria. Proc Natl Acad Sci USA 1972; 69:1413–1415.
155. Booth A, Williams R. Dehydroxylation of caffeic acid by rat and rabbit caecal contents and sheep rumen liquor. Nature 1963; 198:684–685.
156. Rice–Evans C. Why do we expect flavonoids to be antioxidants in vivo? SFRR Winter Meeting. Bio-flavonoids and Polyphenols in Health and Disease. Dinard, France 1999: book of abstracts p 1.
157. Nakazawa T, Ohsawa K. Metabolism of rosmarinic acid in rats. J Nat Prod 1998; 61:993–996.
158. Goldin B, Lichtenstein A, Sherwood L, Gorbach S. Nutritional and metabolic roles of intestinal flora. In: Shils M, Olson J, Shike M, eds. Modern Nutrition in Health and Disease. Philadelphia: Lea & Febiger, 1994:569–682.
159. Uang YS, Hsu KY. A dose-dependent pharmacokinetic study on caffeic acid in rabbits after intravenous administration. Biopharmacol Drug Dispos 1997; 18:727–736.
160. Goldstein D, Stull R, Markey S, et al. Dihydrocaffeic acid: a common contaminant in the liquid chromatographic–electrochemical measurement of plasma catecholamines in man. J Chromatogr 1984; 311:148–153.
161. Kimura Y, Okuda H, Okuda T, et al. Studies on the activities of tannins and related compounds from medicinal plants and drugs. VII. Effects of extracts of leaves of *Artemesia* species, and caffeic acid and chlorogenic acid on lipid metabolic injury in rats fed peroxidized oil. Chem Pharm Bull 1985; 33:2028–2034.
162. Zhou J, Ashoori F, Susuki S, et al. Protective effect of chlorogenic acid on lipid peroxidation induced in the liver of rats by carbon tetrachloride or ^{60}Co-irradiation. J Clin Biochem Nutr 1993; 15:119–125.
163. Tsuchiya T, Suzuki O, Igarashi K. Protective effects of chlorogenic acid on paraquat-induced oxidative stress in rats. Biosci Biotechnol Biochem 1996; 60:765–768.
164. Henricksen T, Evensen S, Carlander B. Injury to human endothelial cells in culture induced by LDL. Scand J Clin Lab Invest 1979; 39:361–368.
165. Hessler J, Robertson AJ, Chisolm G. LDL-induced cytotoxicity and its inhibition by HDL in human vascular smooth muscle and endothelial cells in culture. Atherosclerosis 1979; 32:213–229.
166. Escargueil–Blanc I, Meilhac O, Pieraggi M, et al. Oxidized LDLs induce massive apoptosis of cultured human endothelial cells through a calcium-dependent pathway. Prevention by aurintricarboxylic acid. Thromb Vasc Biol 1997; 17:331–339.
167. Vieira O, Escargueil–Blanc I, Meilhac O, et al. Effect of dietary phenolic compounds on apoptosis of human cultured endothelial cells induced by oxidized LDL. Br J Pharmacol 1998; 123:565–573.
168. Escargueil–Blanc I, Salvayre R, Negre–Salvayre A. Necrosis and apoptosis induced by oxidized low density lipoproteins occur through two calcium-dependent pathways in lymphoblastoid cells. FASEB J 1994; 8:1075–1080.
169. Parhami F, Fang ZT, Yang B, et al. Stimulation of Gs and inhibition of Gi protein functions by minimally oxidized LDL. Arterioscler Thromb Vasc Biol 1995; 15:2019–2024.
170. Natarajan V, Scribner WM, Hart CM, Parthasarathy S. Oxidized low density lipoprotein-mediated activation of phospholipase D in smooth muscle cells: a possible role in cell proliferation and atherogenesis. J Lipid Res 1995; 36:2005–2016.
171. Claus R, Fyrnys B, Deigner H, Wolf G. Oxidized low-density lipoprotein stimulates protein kinase C (PKC) and induces expression of PKC-isotypes via prostaglandin-H-synthase in P388D1 macrophage-like cells. Biochemistry 1996; 35:4911–4922.
172. Auge N, Escargueil–Blanc I, Lajoie–Mazenc I, et al. Potential role for ceramide in mitogen-activated protein kinase activation and proliferation of vascular smooth muscle cells induced by oxidized low density lipoprotein. J Biol Chem 1998; 273:12893–12900.
173. Deigner H, Claus R. Stimulation of mitogen activated protein kinase by LDL and oxLDL in human U-937 macrophage-like cells. FEBS Lett 1996; 385:149–153.
174. Nagy L, Tontonoz P, Alvarez J, et al. Oxidized LDL regulates macrophage gene expression through ligand activation of PPARgamma. Cell 1998; 93:229–240.
175. Suc I, Meilhac O, Lajoie Mazenc I, et al. Activation of EGF receptor by oxidized LDL. FASEB J 1998; 12:665–671.
176. Nardini M, Scaccini C, Packer L, Virgili F. In vitro inhibition of the activity of phosphorylase kinase, protein kinase C and protein kinase A by caffeic acid and a procyanidin-rich pine bark (*Pinus maritima*) extract. Biochim Biophys Acta 2000; 24974:1–7.

177. Nardini M, Pisu P, Gentili V, et al. Effect of caffeic acid on *tert*-butyl hydroperoxide-induced oxidative stress in U937. Free Radic Biol Med 1998; 25:1098–1105.
178. Satoh K, Kadofuku T, Sakagami H. Copper, but not iron, enhances apoptosis-inducing activity of antioxidants. Anticancer Res 1997; 17:2487–2490.
179. Sakagami H, Satoh K, Makino Y, et al. Effect of α-tocopherol on cytotoxicity induced by UV irradiation and antioxidants. Anticancer Res 1997; 17:2079–2082.
180. Stich HF. The beneficial and hazardous effects of simple phenolic compounds. Mutat Res 1991; 259:307–324.
181. Li Y, Trush M. Reactive oxygen-dependent DNA damage resulting from the oxidation of phenolic compounds by a copper–redox cycle mechanism. Cancer Res 1994; 54:1895s–1898s.
182. Solimani R, Bayon F, Domini I, et al. Flavonoid-DNA interaction studied with flow linear dichroism technique. J Agric Food Chem 1995; 43:876–882.
183. Hirose M, Kawabe M, Shibata M, et al. Influence of caffeic acid and other *o*-dihydroxybenzene derivatives on *N*-methyl-*N'*-nitro-*N*-nitrosoguanidine-initiated rat forestomach carcinogenesis. Carcinogenesis 1992; 13:1825–1828.
184. Lutz U, Lugli S, Bitsch A, et al. Dose response for the stimulation of cell division by caffeic acid in forestomach and kidney of the male F344 rat. Fundam Appl Toxicol 1997; 39:131–137.
185. Hirose M, Takesada Y, Tanaka H, et al. Carcinogenicity of antioxidants BHA, caffeic acid, sesamol, 4-methoxyphenol and catechol at low doses, either alone or in combination, and modulation of their effects in a rat medium-term multi-organ carcinogenesis model. Carcinogenesis 1998; 19:207–212.
186. Kaul A, Khanduja K. Polyphenols inhibit promotional phase of tumorigenesis: relevance of superoxide radicals. Nutr Cancer 1998; 32:81–85.
187. Wood AW, Sayer JM, Newmark HL, et al. Mechanism of the inhibition of mutagenicity of a benzo[*a*]pyrene 7,8-diol 9,10-epoxide by riboflavin 5'-phosphate. Proc Natl Acad Sci USA 1982; 79:5122–5126.
188. Wood AW, Huang MT, Chang RL, et al. Inhibition of the mutagenicity of bay-region diol epoxides of polycyclic aromatic hydrocarbons by naturally occurring plant phenols: exceptional activity of ellagic acid. Proc Natl Acad Sci USA 1982; 79:5513–5517.
189. Stich HF. Teas and tea components as inhibitors of carcinogen formation in model systems and man. Prev Med 1992; 21:377–384.
190. Tanaka T, Kojima T, Kawamori T, et al. Inhibition of 4-nitroquinoline-1-oxide-induced rat tongue carcinogenesis by the naturally occurring plant phenolics caffeic, ellagic, chlorogenic and ferulic acids. Carcinogenesis 1993; 14:1321–1325.
191. Hagiwara A, Kokubo Y, Takesada Y, et al. Inhibitory effects of phenolic compounds on development of naturally occurring preneoplastic hepatocytic foci in long-term feeding studies using male F344 rats. Teratogenesis Carcinog Mutagen 1996; 16:317–325.
192. Kuenzig W, Chau J, Norkus E, et al. Caffeic and ferulic acid as blockers of nitrosamine formation. Carcinogenesis 1984; 5:309–313.
193. Manson MM, Ball HW, Barret MC, et al. Mechanism of action of dietary chemoprotective agents in rat liver: induction of phase I and II drug metabolizing enzymes and aflatoxin B1 metabolism. Carcinogenesis 1997; 18:1729–1738.
194. Jovanovic SV, Tosic M, Simic MG. Use of the Hammett correlation and $\sigma+$ for calculation of one-electron redox potentials of antioxidants. J Phys Chem 1991; 95:10824–10827.
195. Lien EJ, Ren S, Bui HH, Wang R. Quantitative structure–activity relationship of phenolic antioxidants. Free Radic Biol Med 1999; 26:285–294.

16
Polyphenols and Flavonoids Protect LDL Against Atherogenic Modifications

Bianca Fuhrman and Michael Aviram
Rambam Medical Center, Haifa, Israel

I. OXIDATIVE STRESS AND ATHEROSCLEROSIS

Atherosclerosis is the leading cause of morbidity and mortality among people with a Western world lifestyle. The early atherosclerotic lesion is characterized by foam cells derived from cholesterol-loaded macrophages (1,2). Most of the accumulated cholesterol in foam cells originates from plasma low-density lipoprotein (LDL), which is internalized into the cells by the LDL receptor. However, native LDL does not induce cellular cholesterol accumulation, because the LDL receptor activity is down-regulated by the cellular cholesterol content (3,4). LDL has to undergo some modifications, such as aggregation or oxidation, to be taken up by macrophages at an enhanced rate by the macrophage scavenger receptors pathway, which is not subjected to down-regulation by increased cellular cholesterol (5–7). The underlying mechanisms leading to the formation of atherosclerotic lesion are complicated and represent the outcome of multiple interactive processes. Several mechanisms for atherogenesis have evolved, all based on the fact that plasma LDL lipids give rise to the development of the atherosclerotic lesion (8,9).

Atherosclerosis is also related to inflammatory conditions that are initiated by lipoprotein invasion into the artery wall (10). Elevated plasma levels of LDL, a major risk factor for cardiovascular disease, is associated with increased adherence of circulating monocytes to arterial endothelial cells, and to increased rate of LDL entry into the intima.

When LDL particles are entrapped in the artery, they can undergo progressive oxidation followed by a rapid internalization by the macrophage scavenger receptors, leading to foam cells formation. The atherogenicity of LDL in the arterial wall depends on the content of LDL, which is focally retained in the intima.

The "response to retention" hypothesis of atherosclerosis supports subendothelial retention of atherogenic lipoproteins as the central pathological process in atherogenesis (11–13). This theory points to the retention of LDL as a prerequisite step to oxidative modification of the lipoprotein. Lipoprotein retention in the artery wall was suggested to be more important as a risk factor for atherosclerosis than the rate of LDL transport into the artery wall (14,15). Retention of LDL in the intima involves its binding to arterial proteoglycans, and the association of LDL with such proteoglycans depends on structural properties of the LDL, such as its size and density (11,15,16).

Proteoglycan-bound LDL forms aggregates (17), and aggregated LDL is avidly taken up by macrophages, as well as by smooth-muscle cells (18), leading to foam cell formation (19–21). Retention and aggregation of LDL in the arterial wall are key events in atherogenesis, and aggregated LDL exists in atherosclerotic lesion (22). In vitro, LDL aggregation can be induced by phospholipase C, by sphingomyelinase (SMase), or by vortexing (23,24).

Aggregation of LDL stimulates its uptake by macrophages independently of the LDL receptor pathway, thus converting macrophages into foam cells (25).

Recently, it was demonstrated that extensive oxidation of LDL leads to its aggregation (26–28). On the other hand, adherence of LDL to arterial proteoglycans increases the susceptibility of LDL to oxidation (17,29). The oxidative modification hypothesis of atherosclerosis proposes that LDL oxidation (rather than its retention) plays the pivotal role in early atherogenesis (30–38). This hypothesis is supported by evidence that LDL oxidation occurs in vivo (35,39) and contributes to the clinical manifestation of atherosclerosis. Oxidized LDL (Ox-LDL) is more atherogenic than native LDL. In contrast to the cellular uptake of native LDL by the LDL receptor pathway, the uptake of Ox-LDL by the scavenger–receptor pathway promotes cholesterol accumulation and foam cell formation (5,7,38,40). In addition, Ox-LDL atherogenicity is related to recruitment of monocytes to the intima (41), stimulation of monocyte adhesion to the endothelium (42), and cytotoxicity toward arterial cells (43,44). The process of LDL oxidation appears to occur within the artery wall and all major cells of the artery wall, including endothelial cells, smooth-muscle cells, and monocyte-derived macrophages can oxidize LDL (45–48). Macrophage-mediated oxidation of LDL is a key event in early atherosclerosis and requires the binding of LDL to the macrophage LDL receptor (48). The interaction of LDL with macrophages under oxidative stress activates cellular oxygenases, which can then produce reactive oxygen species (ROS) capable of oxidizing LDL (49,50).

Under oxidative stress not only LDL and the other plasma lipoproteins are oxidized, but in cells lipid peroxidation takes place, including arterial macrophages (51). "Oxidized macrophages" can easily oxidize LDL (52). LDL oxidation by arterial cells is facilitated by cellular oxygenases-dependent mechanisms, as well as by some nonenzymatic pathways. Studies in cell culture identified several enzyme systems that could play a role in cell-mediated LDL oxidation, including NADPH oxidase (49), 15-lipoxygenase (53), cytochrome P450 (54), and myeloperoxidase (55,56). Cell-mediated oxidation of LDL depends on the presence of transition metal ions. On the other hand, in vitro oxidation of LDL can also be achieved in a cell-free system, by transition metal ions. Figure 1 depicts major processes associated with LDL atherogenic modifications (oxidation, aggregation) in the arterial wall that lead to macrophage foam cell formation.

Several lines of evidence support the in vivo existence of Ox-LDL (57); LDL from patients with atherosclerosis is more prone to oxidation than LDL from healthy subjects (58–61). LDL from the atherosclerotic apolipoprotein E (apoE)-deficient (E^0) mice is also more prone to oxidation than LDL from control mice (62). Antibodies against epitopes on Ox-LDL have been positively related to the progression of atherosclerosis (30), and LDL isolated from atherosclerotic lesions of humans or E^0 mice is oxidized and aggregated (22). The oxidation rate of LDL is reduced by dietary intervention of antioxidants. Clinical studies investigated the antioxidative effects of antioxidant supplementation to humans on LDL oxidation ex vivo (63,64). Dietary supplementation of β-carotene to healthy subjects resulted in some inhibitory effect on the

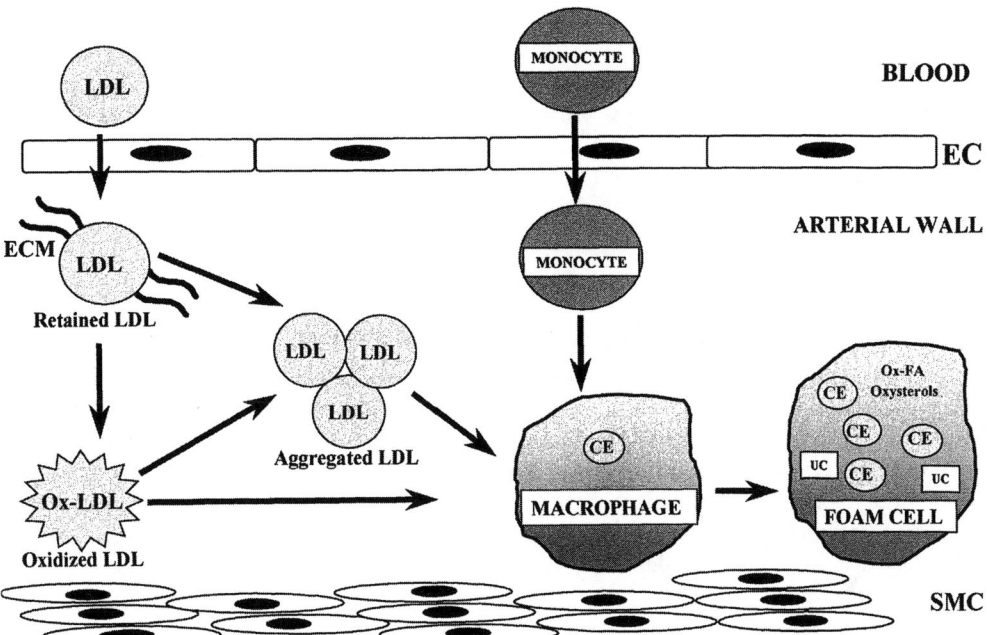

Figure 1 Atherogenic modifications of LDL lead to macrophage foam cell formation: LDL retention by extracellular matrix (ECM) components renders the lipoprotein more susceptible to aggregation and to oxidation. Oxidized LDL (Ox-LDL) formation leads to LDL aggregation (Agg-LDL). Both Agg-LDL and Ox-LDL are extensively taken up by macrophages, leading to cellular cholesterol accumulation and foam cell formation. CE, cholesteryl ester; UC, unesterified cholesterol; Ox-FA, oxidized fatty acids; EC, endothelial cells; SMC, smooth-muscle cells.

susceptibility of LDL to oxidative modification (65–67) in some, but not all, studied subjects. The combination of carotenoids with vitamin E demonstrated a synergistic inhibitory effect on LDL oxidation (67).

Vitamin E supplementation (400 IU/day for 8 weeks) retarded LDL oxidation (68), and supplementation of healthy smokers with vitamin C (ascorbic acid, 1000 mg/day for 4 weeks) resulted in increased plasma ascorbate and reduced LDL susceptibility to oxidation (69). In animal models, the foregoing antioxidants also decreased the atherosclerotic lesion size. Administration of probucol, a lipid-soluble cholesterol-lowering drug with potent antioxidant properties, to Watanabe hereditary hyperlipidemic (WHHL) rabbits, inhibited the formation of atherosclerotic lesions, independently of its cholesterol-lowering properties and was associated with increased resistance of LDL to oxidation (70). Supplementation of vitamin E to the atherosclerotic apolipoprotein E-deficient mice (25 μg/day per mouse for 3 months) inhibited LDL oxidation by 40% and the atherosclerotic lesion area by 35% (28). Dietary supplementation of selenium (1 μg/day per mouse for 6 months) to these mice increased the reduced glutathione (GSH) content and glutathione peroxidase (GPx) activity in the mice peritoneal macrophages by 36 and 30%, respectively. This effect was associated with a 46% reduction in cell-mediated oxidation of LDL, and a 30% reduction in development of atherosclerotic lesions (71). Feeding New Zealand White rabbits a diet containing the antioxidant N,N'-diphenyl-1,4-phenylenediamine (DPPD) 1%, for 10 weeks, resulted in increased resistance of the rabbits' lipoproteins to oxidation in comparison with control lipoproteins, and also substantially reduced the development of atherosclerosis in these mice (72). Feeding the all-*trans*-isomer of β-carotene to cholesterol-fed rabbits attenuated the extent of their atherosclerosis by a mechanism that may not involve only oxidative stress (73). Consumption of another class of antioxidants, the flavonoids, substantially inhibited LDL oxidation and could be related to a reduction in the risk for cardiovascular disease (74,75). Indeed, it was demonstrated that flavonoid intake can be attributed to differences in mortality from coronary heart disease across populations, and dietary consumption of flavonoids was inversely related to morbidity and mortality from coronary heart disease (76).

II. POLYPHENOLS AND FLAVONOIDS

A. Structure, Classification, and Biological Effects

Polyphenols constitute one of the largest category of phytochemicals, most widely distributed among the plant kingdom, and an integral part of the human diet. Dietary phenolics include phenolic acids, phenolic polymers (commonly known as tannins), and flavonoids (77–79). Phenolic acids form a diverse group that includes hydroxybenzoic and hydroxycinnamic acids. Phenolic polymers are compounds of high molecular weight, such as the condensed tannins.

Flavonoids compose the largest and most-studied group of plant phenols. Over 4000 different flavonoids have now been identified, and their molecular structure consists of an aromatic ring A, condensed to heterocyclic ring C, attached to a second aromatic ring B (Fig. 2). They contain several phenolic hydroxyl groups attached to the aromatic rings, which confer their potent antioxidant activity. Flavonoids are usually found in plants as glycosides, and large compositional differences exist between different types of plants, and even between different parts of the same plant. Flavonoids are grouped into anthocyanins and anthoxantins. Anthocyanins are glycosides of anthocyanidin, and they are the most important group of water-soluble plant pigments, responsible for the red, blue, and purple colors of flowers and fruits. The anthoxantins are colorless or white to yellow, and include flavonols, flavanols, flavones, flavans, and isoflavones.

The flavonols are the most widely distributed flavonoids, and the most common flavonols are quercetin, kaempferol, and myricetin. Quercetin is a principal phenolic constituent of plants, and quantitatively the most important dietary flavonoid, found particularly at high levels in onions, apples, kale, and tea. The dietary flavanols catechin and epicatechin commonly occur in combination with gallic acid as epigallocatechin gallate or epicatechin gallate. They are found in tea and in red wine and also in condensed tannin polymers present in fruits, legumes, and grains. The isoflavones are found almost exclusively in the legume family, particularly in soybeans, where genistein and daidzein are the major isoflavones. Table 1 summarizes the Phenolic Phytochemicals content of some selected foods.

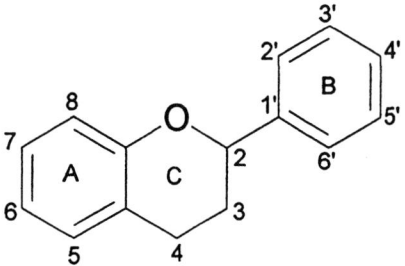

Figure 2 Basic structure of flavonoids.

Table 1 Phenolic Phytochemical Content of Selected Foods

Class and subclass	Representing compounds	Food or beverage	Quantity (mg)[a,b]
Flavonoids			
Flavonols	Quercetin	Olives	550
	Kaempferol	Onions	350
	Myricetin	Kale	320
		Leaf lettuce	310
		Cranberry	250
		Cherry tomato	100
		Broccoli	100
		Apple juice	40
		Green tea	40
		Black tea	20
		Red wine	15
		Grape juice	5
		Grapefruit juice	5
		Orange juice	4
Flavanols	Catechin	Pear	250
	Epicatechin	Red wine	270
		Green tea	180
		White wine	35
		Apple	30
Flavones	Apigenin	Celery	130
	Luteolin	Olives	20
	Chrysin		
Flavanones	Hesperitin	Grapefruit	500
	Hesperidin	Orange	500
	Naringenin		
	Naringin		
Isoflavans	Glabridin	Licorice root	500
Isoflavones	Genistein	Soybean	1500
	Daidzein	Soy nuts	1900

(*continued*)

Table 1 (*Continued*)

Class and subclass	Representing compounds	Food or beverage	Quantity (mg)[a,b]
Phenolic acids and phenolics			
Hydroxycinnamic acids CH=CHCO$_2$CH$_3$	Caffeic acid	Blueberry	2000
	Ferulic acid	Cherry, sweet	800
	Rosmarinic acid	Pear	600
	Carnosic acid	Apple	150
	Gingerol	Orange	100
	Hydroxytyrosol	Grapefruit	40
	Oleuropein	Ginger	
		Olive oil	
Hydroxybenzoic acids CO$_2$H	Ellagic acid	Raspberry	60
	Gallic acid	Strawberry	50
		Grape juice, black	110
		Grape juice, green	
Tannins			
Condensed	Catechin polymers	Red wine	2500
	Epicatechin polymers	White wine	240
		Apple juice	50
		Pomegranate	1200

[a]Quantities given are a total of all phytochemical included in the subclass, and not for individual phytochemicals.
[b]Milligrams per kilogram food, or milligrams per liter juice.

Flavonoids exhibit a wide spectrum of biochemical activities; most, but not all, of them could be related to antioxidant properties. These activities include the following:

1. Inhibition of oxidation processes (radical scavenging and metal ion chelation) (80–84)
2. Inhibition of xanthine oxidase (85)
3. Inhibition of glutathione reductase (86)
4. Inhibition of NADPH oxidase (87)
5. Inhibition of lipoxygenase (88–91)
6. Prevention of cytotoxic effects of oxidized LDL (92)
7. Inhibition of protein kinase C (87,93)
8. Inhibition of cyclic-AMP phosphodiesterase (94)
9. Inhibition of phospholipase A$_2$ (95)
10. Inhibition of calcium-dependent ATPase (96)

B. Antioxidant Activity of Polyphenols and Flavonoids

Polyphenols and flavonoids are powerful antioxidants, and their activity is related to their chemical structures (81–83). Plant polyphenols are multifunctional and can act as reducing agents, as hydrogen atom-donating antioxidants, and as singlet oxygen quenchers. Some polyphenols also act as antioxidants by metal ion chelation properties (97), thereby reducing the metal's capacity to generate free radicals. For a polyphenol to be defined as an antioxidant it must satisfy two basic conditions:

1. When present in low concentration relative to the substrate to be oxidized, it can delay, retard, or prevent auto-oxidation or free radical-mediated oxidation.
2. The resulting radical formed after scavenging must be stable to interrupt the oxidation chain reaction.

Phenolic antioxidants (PPH) inhibit lipid peroxidation by a rapid donation of hydrogen atom to the peroxyl radical (ROO$^\cdot$) resulting in formation of alkyl (aryl) hydroperoxide (ROOH), as illustrated in the following reaction:

$$ROO^\cdot + PPH \rightarrow ROOH + PP^\cdot$$

The polyphenol phenoxyl radical (PP$^\cdot$) produced can be stabilized by further donation of a hydrogen atom and formation of quinones, or by reacting with another radical, including another phenoxyl radical, thereby interrupting the initiation of a new chain reaction.

The free radical-scavenging capability of polyphenols and flavonoids stems from the fact that their reducing potential is lower than that of the alkyl peroxyl radical and the superoxide radical; hence, it results in the free radicals' inactivation. However, under certain conditions, such as high concentrations of phenolic antioxidants, high pH, or the presence of iron ion, phenolic antioxidants can initiate an auto-oxidation process and behave like pro-oxidants, rather than antioxidants (98).

Flavonoids are among the most potent antioxidants owing to their unique structure, which possesses one or more of the following elements:

1. *O*-Dihydroxy structure on ring B, which confers increased stability to the radical form, and participates in electron delocalization
2. Double bond between carbons 2 and 3, which forms a keto group on carbon 4 in the C ring, and increase the electron delocalization of the radical from the B ring
3. Hydroxyl groups in positions 3 and 5 in rings C and A, which are required for a maximal radical-scavenging potential

The antioxidant efficiency of flavonoids is directly related to their degree of hydroxylation and is decreased in the presence of a sugar moiety. Flavonoids are effective scavengers of hydroxyl and peroxyl radicals, and of the superoxide anion (99–102). Some polyphenols act as antioxidants owing to chelation of transition metal ions (92,103), thus inhibiting the Fenton and Haber–Weiss reactions, which are important sources for active oxygen radicals.

III. POLYPHENOLS, FLAVONOIDS, AND LDL ATHEROGENIC MODIFICATIONS

A. Effects of Polyphenols on LDL Oxidation and Aggregation

Aggregation of LDL is an atherogenic modification of the lipoprotein, because aggregated LDL is taken up by macrophages at increased rate, leading to foam cell formation (19–21). There are several lines of evidence implying that LDL aggregation occurs in the arterial wall (22), but little is known about the mechanisms responsible for this modification in vivo. LDL aggregation induced by vortexing is believed to result from interaction between the lipoprotein hydrophobic domains, which are exposed during LDL vortexing (104). Polyphenols, which are multidentate ligands, are able to bind simultaneously to more than one molecule on the lipoprotein surface (105), and thus reduce the susceptibility of LDL to aggregation. Reduced LDL aggregation was demonstrated after dietary consumption of polyphenols, as well as following in vitro enrichment of LDL with polyphenols. Dietary supplementation of licorice, glabridin, gingerol, red wine, quercetin, or catechin (25 μg/day of flavonoids per mouse, for 3 months) to E^0 mice, resulted in a marked decrease in the susceptibility of the mice LDL to aggregation (84).

Furthermore, as oxidation of LDL leads to its aggregation (26–28), inhibition of LDL oxidation by dietary antioxidants, can also lead to inhibition in LDL aggregation. Vitamin E supplementation to E^0 mice resulted in a 40% reduction in LDL oxidation; and in parallel, LDL aggregation was also reduced by 23% (28).

Polyphenols and mainly flavonoids act as potent inhibitors of LDL oxidation by several mechanisms:

1. Scavenging of free radicals
2. Protection of α-tocopherol (vitamin E) and carotenoids in the LDL particle from oxidation
3. Regeneration of vitamin E from oxidized α-tocopherol
4. Chelation of transition metal ions
5. Protection of cells against oxidative damage and, as a result, inhibition of cell-mediated oxidation of LDL
6. Preservation of serum paraoxonase (PON 1) activity and, as a result, hydrolysis of LDL-associated lipid peroxides.

Paraoxonase (PON 1) is an enzyme physically associated in serum with high-density lipoprotein (HDL) (106), and it was recently shown to protect LDL, as well as HDL itself, against oxidation (107). This effect of PON 1 may be relevant to its physiological role in relation to protection against cardiovascular disease (108). Antioxidants preserve PON 1's activity, for they decrease formation of lipid peroxides that can inactivate PON 1 (109).

Flavonoids are quite suitable for protecting cell membranes from free radical-induced oxidation, because they are both lipophilic and hydrophilic. Being partly inside and partly outside of the cell plasma membranes, flavonoids can scavenge free radicals, which are generated within the cells, as well as free radicals that attack the cell from the outside. Indeed, catechins from tea protect erythrocyte membranes and rat liver microsomes from lipid peroxidation (110). Pretreatment of cells with flavanols or flavonols also protected the cells against damage induced by reactive oxygen species (111). The protection of LDL against copper ion or free radical-induced oxidation by flavonoids depends on their structural properties in terms of their response to copper ion (chelation or oxidation), their partitioning between the aqueous and the lipophilic compartments within the LDL particle, and their hydrogen-donating antioxidant properties (112).

The flavanol catechin prevented plasma lipid peroxidation that was induced by azo compounds such as the water-soluble 2,2'-azobis-2-amidinopropane hydrochloride (AAPH), and the lipid-soluble 2,2'-azobis-2,4-dimethylvaleronitrile (AMVN). This antioxidant effect of catechin depends on its plasma concentration, the incubation time, and the physical localization of the generated radicals. As expected from its hydrophilic structure, however, catechin showed a higher antioxidant capacity when the free radical reactions were initiated in the aqueous, rather than the lipid, phase (113). Catechin also inhibits LDL oxidation induced by copper ions, by cultured macrophages, or by vascular endothelial cells (114). Quercetin, rutin, luteolin, and kaempferol also inhibited copper ion-induced LDL oxidation (112), with quercetin, rutin, and luteolin being more effective inhibitors of copper ion-induced LDL oxidation than kaempferol, as they also chelated copper ions. Morin, fisetin, quercetin, and gossypetin inhibited copper ion-induced LDL oxidation, and macrophage-mediated LDL oxidation, with an IC_{50} of 1–2 μM (112). Other flavonoids that inhibited LDL oxidation include the hydroxycinnamic acid-derived phenolic acid; caffeic, ferulic, and p-coumaric acids (115); and the isoflavan glabridin (117,118). Among the different groups of flavonoids, flavonols, flavanols, and the isoflavans are the most potent protectors of LDL against copper ion-induced oxidation. However, although possessing a similar OH group arrangement, the flavonol quercetin was a more potent antioxidant in comparison with the flavanol catechin, owing to the 2–3 double bond and the 4-oxo structure in the quercetin ring C. Similarly, studies on structural aspects of the inhibitory effect of glabridin on LDL oxidation, revealed that the antioxidant effect of glabridin on LDL oxidation resides mainly in the 2'-hydroxyl group of the isoflavan B ring (118). The hydrophobic moiety of the isoflavan was also essential to obtain the inhibitory effect of glabridin on LDL oxidation, and the position of the hydroxyl groups at the B ring significantly affected the ability of glabridin to inhibit LDL oxidation (118).

B. Protection of LDL Against Atherogenic Modifications by Polyphenol-Rich Nutrients

The average daily human intake of flavonoids varies between as low as 25 mg to as high as 1 g (77,78,119–124). Following oral ingestion, some of the ingested flavonoids are absorbed from the gastrointestinal tract, and some of the absorbed flavonoids are metabolized by the gastrointestinal microflora. However, differences in the bioavailability of different flavonoids exist and could be related to chemical structure differences (77,78). The enzymes responsible for intestinal flavonoid metabolism are not supplied by the human intestine, but rather, by gastrointestinal bacteria. One of the first steps in flavonoid absorption is the cleavage of the flavonoid–glycoside bond, followed by a reconjugation in the liver with either sulfate or glucuronate before excretion or further metabolism. The metabolism of flavonoids yields a variety of phenolic compounds, including phenylpropionic acid, phenylacetic acid, and phenyl-γ-valerolactone (78).

Major dietary sources for flavonoids and their effects on LDL atherogenic modifications are presented in the following.

1. Red Wine

The "French paradox" (i.e., low incidence of cardiovascular events in spite of diet high in saturated fat) was attributed to the regular drinking of red wine in southern France (125). Wine has been part of the human culture for over 6000 years, serving dietary and socioreligious functions. In addition to ethanol, red wine contains a range of polyphenols derived from the skin of the grape, with important biological activities (126,127). Red wine contains the flavonols quercetin and myricetin (10–20 mg/L), the flavanols catechin and epigallocatechin (up to 270 mg/L), gallic acid (95 mg/L), condensed tannins (catechin and epicatechin polymers [2500 mg/L]) and polymeric anthocyanidins. The beneficial effect of red wine consumption against the development of atherosclerosis was attributed to the antioxidant activity of its polyphenols. Ingestion of red wine was associated with increased serum antioxidant activity (128). The ex vivo effect of red wine consumption on the propensity of LDL for lipid peroxidation was studied. Administration of 400 mL of red wine to healthy human volunteers for a period of 2 weeks reduced the propensity of the volunteers' LDL to lipid peroxidation (in response to copper ions). This was determined by a 46, 72, and 54% decrement in the content of the lipoprotein-associated aldehydes, lipid peroxides, and conjugated dienes, respectively (129,130). A substantial prolongation of the lag phase required for the initiation of LDL oxidation was also obtained following red wine consumption. The antioxidant effect of dietary red wine against LDL oxidation could be related to the elevation in concentrations of polyphenols in the plasma and in the LDL particle. Thus, some phenolic substances that exist in red wine are absorbed, bind to plasma LDL, and protect the lipoprotein from oxidation (129).

The effect of red wine consumption on the susceptibility of LDL to oxidation was also studied in the postprandial state (131). Five volunteers consumed 300 mL of California red wine, containing 1500 mg/L of total phenolic compounds. LDL isolated from plasma samples taken 1 and 2 h after red wine ingestion was significantly more resistant to copper ion-induced oxidation than LDL obtained before wine consumption, as shown by 50 and 66% inhibition in aldehyde formation, respectively. These results were further confirmed in a study (132) that demonstrated that red wine consumption increased plasma and LDL-associated polyphenols and protected LDL against copper ion-induced oxidation. This was shown by increased lag time and decreased LDL content of lipid peroxides and TBARS (by 34 and 22%, respectively). The effect of the nonalcoholic components of red wine was also studied (133). Dealcoholized red wine did not affect the susceptibility of LDL to copper-induced oxidation. In contrast, a short-term ingestion of purple grape juice reduced LDL susceptibility to oxidation in patients with coronary artery disease (134).

The direct effect of red wine consumption on the development of atherosclerotic lesions was further studied in E^0 mice that were supplemented with 0.5 mL of red wine per day per mouse for 6 weeks (135,136). LDL isolated after red wine consumption, was less susceptible (30–80%) to oxidation induced by either copper ions, by the free radical initiator AAPH, or by J-774 A.1 macrophages in culture, in comparison with LDL isolated from the placebo (alcoholized water)-treated E^0 mice (135,136). The atherosclerotic lesions areas in E^0 mice that consumed red wine, were significantly reduced (by 40%), in comparison with the lesion areas in placebo-treated E^0 mice.

Identification of the active phenolic compounds responsible for the red wine antioxidant properties against LDL oxidation has raised much interest. Phenolic substances in red wine inhibit LDL oxidation in vitro (137). In previous studies, red wine-derived phenolic acids (116,138), resveratrol (139), flavonols (quercetin, myricetin) (115,140,141), catechins (114,142), and the grape extract itself (143,144), all possess antioxidant properties. Confirmation that the active antioxidant components in red wine are phenolic compounds was supported by the finding that ethanol and wine stripped of phenols did not affect LDL oxidation anymore (145). Red wine fractionation revealed major antioxidative potency to monomeric catechins, procyanidins, monomeric anthocyanidins, and phenolic acids (145). The flavonol quercetin and the flavanol catechin (Fig. 3) were tested for antioxidative and antiatherogenic effect, in the atherosclerotic E^0 mice (135). E^0 mice at the age of 4 weeks were supplemented for up to 6 weeks in their drinking water with placebo (1.1% alcohol) or with catechin or quercetin (50 μg/day per mouse). The atherosclerotic lesion area was smaller in the treated mice by 39 or by 46%, respectively, in comparison with E^0 mice that were treated with placebo (Fig. 4A). These results were associated with reduced susceptibility to oxidation (that was induced by different modes, such as copper ions, free radicals generator, or macrophages) of LDL isolated after quercetin, and to a lesser extent after catechin consumption, in comparison with LDL isolated from the placebo group (see Fig. 4B). LDL isolated from E^0 mice that consumed catechin or quercetin for 2 weeks, was also found to be less oxidized (in its basal, not induced, state),

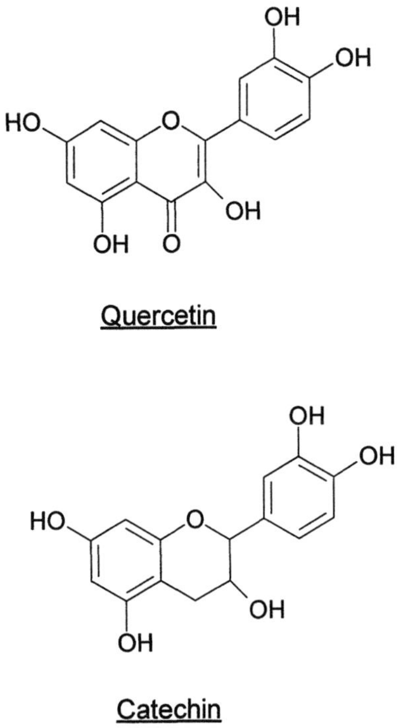

Figure 3 Chemical structure of quercetin and catechin.

in comparison with LDL isolated from E^0 mice that received placebo, as evidenced by 39, or 48% reduced content of LDL-associated lipid peroxides, respectively (135) (see Fig. 4C).

Catechin, quercetin, or red wine consumption affected, besides LDL oxidation, additional atherogenic modifications of LDL; namely, its aggregation. The susceptibility to aggregation of LDL derived from E^0 mice after 6 weeks of dietary consumption of catechin, quercetin, or red wine was decreased in comparison with placebo-treated mice, by 63, 48, or 50%, respectively (see Fig. 4D).

Catechin, quercetin, and red wine consumption also increased serum paroxonase activity by 14, 13, and 75%, respectively, in E^0 mice (135). As paraoxonase protects against lipid peroxidation, the beneficial effect of red wine polyphenols on paraoxonase activity can be considered as an additional antiatherogenic property of red wine.

2. *Licorice*

Glycyrrhiza glabra, the licorice plant, has a history of consumption for more than 3000 years. The licorice roots have long been used as flavoring and sweetening agents. Licorice root has also been used medicinally for a wide range of therapeutics, such as antibacterial, antiviral, anti-inflammatory, antiallergic, and antihepatotoxic. Minor components of licorice, mostly flavonoids from the flavan and chalcon subclasses, possess antioxidative properties. The antioxidative capability of licorice crude extract against LDL oxidation was investigated in vitro and ex vivo (84,146). LDL oxidation induced by copper ions or by AAPH was inhibited by 90% on using as low as 0.3 μg/mL of licorice root extract. Licorice ethanolic extract inhibited LDL oxidation by a mechanism that involves scavenging of free radicals. Evaluation of the protective effect of licorice root extract on the resistance of LDL to ex vivo oxidation was

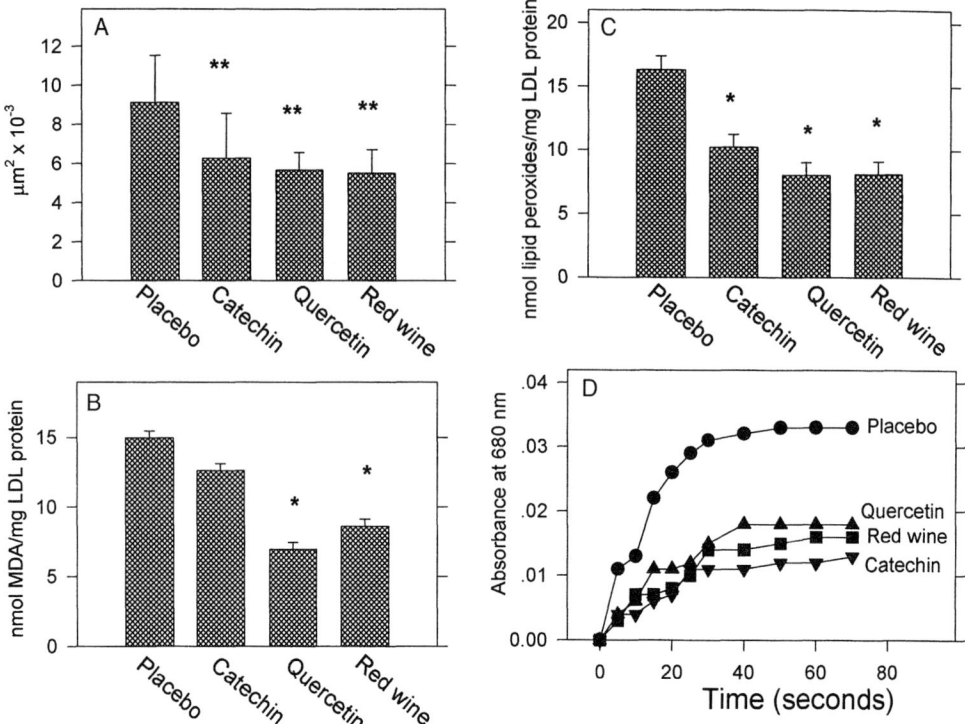

Figure 4 Consumption of red wine or its polyphenols catechin or quercetin by E^0 mice inhibits atherogenic modification of LDL, and decreases the development of atherosclerotic lesions: (A) The aortic arch from E^0 mice that consumed placebo, catechin, quercetin, or red wine was analyzed. Results are expressed as the mean of the lesion area in square micrometers ± SD. $*p < 0.05$ (vs. placebo). (B) LDL was isolated from E^0 mice that consumed placebo, red wine (0.5 mL/day per mouse), catechin, or quercetin (50 μg/day per mouse) for 6 weeks. The susceptibility of LDL to copper ion-induced oxidation was determined following incubation of LDL (100 μL/mL of protein) with 5 μM of $CuSO_4$, and was then measured as TBARS formation. Results are expressed as mean ± SD ($n = 3$); $*p < 0.01$ (vs. placebo). (C) LDL (100 μg/mL of protein) oxidative state (basal, not induced oxidation) was determined as lipid peroxide levels. Results are expressed as mean ± SD ($n = 3$); $*p < 0.01$ (vs. placebo). (D) LDL (100 μg/mL of protein) was subjected to vortex-induced aggregation, and the extent of aggregation was determined by measuring the changes in optical absorbance at 680 nm.

studied in normolipidemic humans and in the atherosclerotic apolipoprotein E-deficient (E^0) mice. LDL, which was isolated from the plasma of ten healthy volunteers after consumption of 100 mg/day of licorice root ethanolic extract for 2 weeks, was more resistant to copper ion-induced oxidation, as well as to AAPH-induced oxidation, by 44 and 36%, respectively, in comparison with LDL isolated before licorice supplementation. Dietary supplementation of licorice (200 μg/day per mouse) to E^0 mice for 6 weeks resulted in an 80% reduction in the susceptibility of their LDL to copper ion-induced oxidation in comparison with LDL isolated from placebo-treated mice (146).

Licorice root contains flavonoids with biological activities, several of which were isolated and purified. Licochalcone B and D, isolated from the roots of *Glycyrrhiza inflata*, inhibit superoxide anion production in the xantine–xantine oxidase system (147), and possess free radical scavenging activity toward the 1,1-diphenyl-2-picrylhydrazyl (DPPH) radical. These phenolic compounds were effective in protecting biological systems against various oxidative processes. They inhibit mitochondrial lipid peroxidation induced by Fe(III)–ADP/NADH, scavenge superoxide anions in microsomes, and protect red blood cells against oxidative hemolysis (147). Other antioxidant constituents that were isolated from licorice were identified as the isoflavans glabridin, hispaglabridin A, hispaglabridin B, 4-O-methyl glabridin, and two chalcones: isoprenylchalcone and isolipuritegenin (117).

Among these compounds, glabridin constituted the major flavonoid in the licorice root extract (500 mg/kg of ethanolic extract) (Fig. 5).

When LDL was incubated with glabridin, the later bound to the LDL particles and, subsequently, protected them from oxidation (118,148). Glabridin inhibited AAPH-induced LDL oxidation in a dose-dependent manner, as shown by the inhibition of cholesteryl linoleate hydroperoxide (CL-OOH) formation, as well as by the inhibition of TBARS and lipid peroxide formation. Addition of glabridin (30 μM) to LDL that was incubated with AAPH or with copper ions also inhibited the formation of oxysterols (7-hydroxycholesterol, 7-ketocholesterol, and 5,5-epoxycholesterol) by 65, 70, and 45%, respectively. Glabridin inhibited the consumption of β-carotene and that of lycopene by 41 and 50%, respectively, after 1 h of LDL oxidation in the presence of AAPH, but failed to protect the major LDL-associated antioxidant, vitamin E, from oxidation (118). Finally, glabridin preserved the arylesterase activity of human serum paraoxonase (PON 1), including its ability to hydrolyze Ox-LDL cholesteryl linoleate hydroperoxides (109).

Administration of glabridin to E^0 mice in their drinking water was followed by analysis of its antioxidative effect against LDL oxidation ex vivo (146). Gas chromatography–mass spectrometry (GC–MS) analysis of the LDL, derived from E^0 mice after consumption of glabridin, revealed that glabridin was absorbed and bound to the LDL particle. Whereas no glabridin could be detected in LDL from control mice, LDL from mice that consumed glabridin (20 μg/day per mouse) contained about 2 nmol of glabridin per milligram LDL protein. LDL derived from E^0 mice after consumption of 20 μg/day of glabridin per mouse for 6 weeks was significantly more resistant than LDL derived from placebo-treated mice, to copper ion-induced oxidation, by 22%. Administration of glabridin (25 μg/day per mouse) to E^0 mice for 3 months also reduced (by 50%) an additional atherogenic modification of LDL (i.e., its susceptibility to aggregation induced by vortexing) (84). Most importantly, inhibition of atherogenic modifications of LDL (oxidation and aggregation) in E^0 mice following glabridin consumption, was associated with a substantial reduction in the development of atherosclerotic lesions (Fig. 6A).

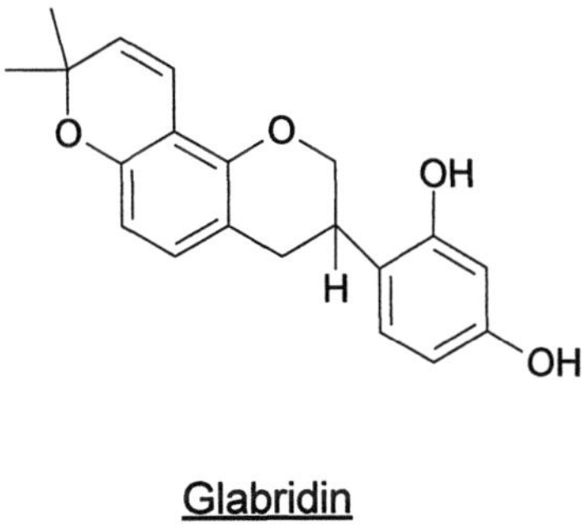

Glabridin

Figure 5 Chemical structure of glabridin.

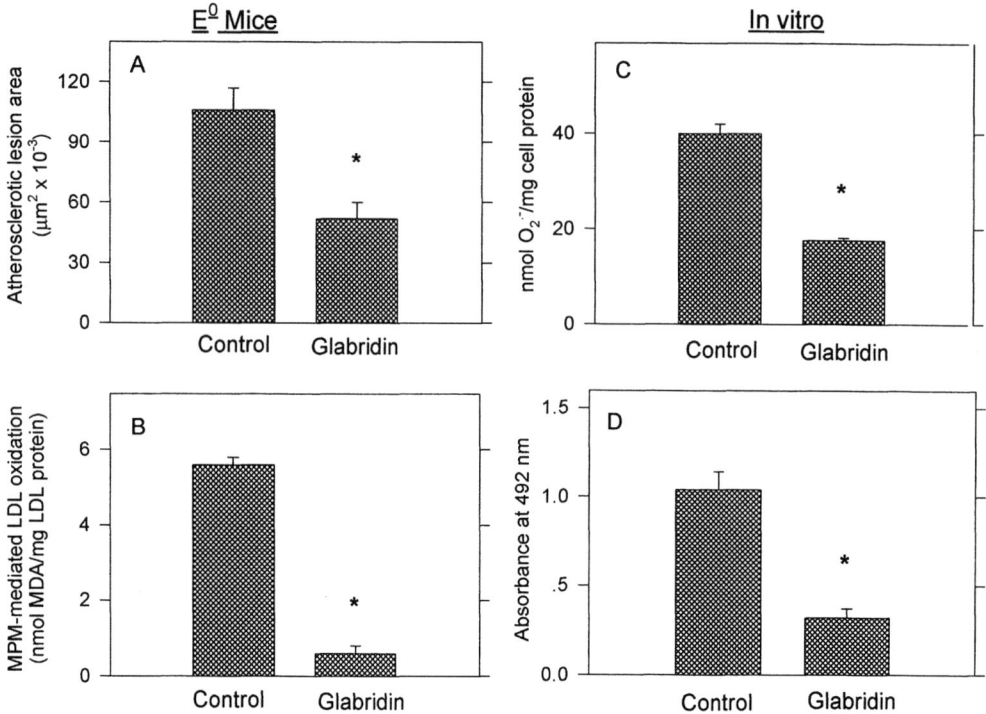

Figure 6 Glabridin inhibits macrophage-mediated oxidation of LDL: (A, B) In vivo studies: E^0 mice were supplemented with placebo (control), or with 20 µg of glabridin per mouse per day, for 6 weeks. (A) Lesion area: the aortic arch derived from E^0 mice that consumed placebo (control) or glabridin was analyzed. Results are expressed as the mean of the lesion area in square micrometers ± SD; *$p < 0.01$ (vs. placebo). (B) Cell-mediated oxidation of LDL: mouse peritoneal macrophages (MPM), harvested from E^0 mice that consumed placebo (control) or glabridin, were incubated with LDL (100 µg/mL of protein) for 6 h under oxidative stress (in the presence of 2 µM $CuSO_4$). The extent of LDL oxidation was measured directly in the medium by the TBARS assays. Results are expressed as mean ± SD ($n = 3$); *$p < 0.01$ (vs. placebo). (C, D) In vitro mechanistic studies: (C) Superoxide anion release: glabridin enrichment of macrophages decreases superoxide anion release in response to PMA. MPM from control mice were incubated with ethanol (0.2%, control) or with 20 µM of glabridin (in 0.2% ethanol) for 2 h at 37°C. Then, the amount of superoxide anion release to the medium in response to 50 ng/mL of PMA was determined. Results are expressed as mean ± SD ($n = 3$). (D) PKC activity: Glabridin inhibits protein kinase C (PKC) in macrophages. Macrophage PKC activity was measured in the cytosolic fraction from macrophages that were enriched with glabridin in comparison with control macrophages. Results are expressed as mean ± SD (= 3).

Glabridin consumption exerts its antioxidative effects also at the cellular level. Enrichment of mouse peritoneal macrophages with glabridin, either in vitro or in vivo (following its consumption by E^0 mice), resulted in 80% inhibition in macrophage-mediated oxidation of LDL, in comparison with control cells (87) (see Fig. 6B). This effect was secondary to the inhibition of the macrophage NADPH oxidase, as reflected by the decrement in superoxide anion release (see Fig. 6C). This latter effect was related to the inhibition of the translocation of the cytosolic component of NADPH oxidase P-47 to the plasma membrane. The foregoing effects of glabridin were associated with the inhibition (by 70%) of macrophage protein kinase C, which is required for P-47 phosphorylation and activation (see Fig. 6D). Thus, glabridin-induced inhibition of P-47 phosphorylation may be the primary event in its inhibitory effect on NADPH oxidase-induced macrophage-mediated oxidation of LDL. All these inhibitory effects of glabridin on the events related to cell-mediated oxidation of LDL required the hydroxyl groups on the isoflavan B ring.

Macrophage foam cell formation during early atherogenesis is determined by the balance between pro-oxidants and antioxidants in arterial cells, as well as in blood lipoproteins (50,149). Because glabridin inhibited oxidative processes both in macrophages and in LDL, these mechanisms may be responsible for the attenuation of atherosclerosis in E^0 mice that consumed glabridin.

3. Soybean

Consumption of diets rich in soy protein has also been claimed to protect against the development of atherosclerosis. The low rates of heart diseases in Japan, in comparison with Western countries, were attributed to the high consumption of soy in Japan. In experimental studies, atherosclerosis was reduced in animals that were fed diets containing soy proteins, compared with those fed diets containing animal proteins (150). In a nonhuman primate study, dietary soybean prevented the development of atherosclerosis in monkeys' aortas (151).

Potential mechanisms for antiatherosclerotic effects of soy include lowering of plasma cholesterol levels, inhibition of cell proliferation, and inhibition of lipoprotein oxidation. These effects could be related to soy proteins or to the isoflavones–genistein, daidzein, or daidzin. Genistein and daidzein (Fig. 7), the major soy isoflavones, occur in nature in their glycosylated or methoxylated derivatives, which are cleaved in the large intestine to yield the free aglycones and additional metabolites. The antioxidant activities of genistein and daidzein were compared with those of their glycosylated or methoxylated derivatives, in a liposomal system, using Fe(II) and Fe(III) metal ions and aqueous-phase, azo-derived peroxyl radicals as the peroxidation initiators (152). Both the parent isoflavonoids and their metabolites were more effective in suppressing metal ion-induced peroxidation than the peroxyl radical-induced perox-

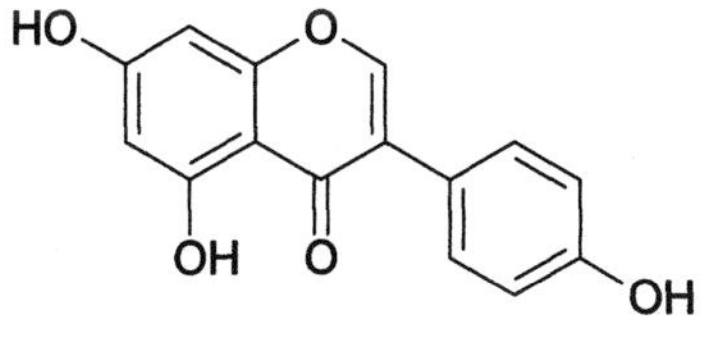

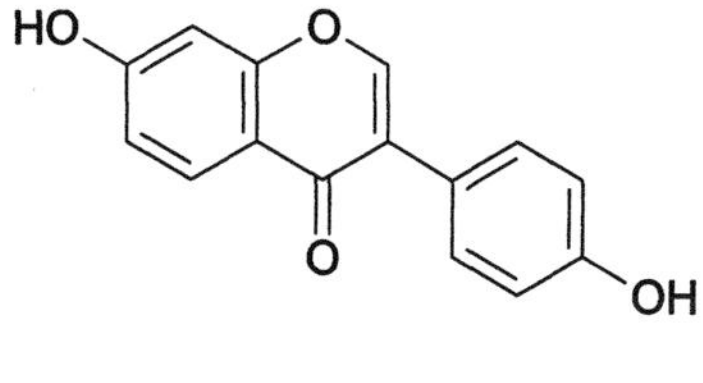

Figure 7 Chemical structure of the phytoestrogens daidzein and genistein.

idation (152). The soybean isoflavone fraction, consisting primarily of genistein, daidzein, and glycetein, also has an hypocholesterolemic effect in both animal and human studies (153). The protective effect of soy isoflavones against atherosclerosis, and their capacity to decrease serum cholesterol levels and lipoprotein oxidation, were studied in control mice (C57BL/6) and in LDL receptor-deficient (LDLr-null) mice (154). For 10 weeks the mice were fed a high fat diet, with isoflavones (IF+, 20.85 g/100 g protein; 0.027 g/100 g genistein; 0.009 g/100 g daidzein) or diet from which the isoflavones were extracted (IF−). The isoflavone-containing diet resulted in a reduction in plasma cholesterol levels, along with an inhibition in the development of atherosclerosis in C57BL/6 mice, but not in LDLr-null mice.

Soy extract containing 40% isoflavones, dose-dependently inhibited copper ion-induced LDL oxidation, with an IC_{50} of about 40 µg/mL, and soy phytoestrogenic isoflavones (genistein, daidzein, daidzin) were shown to possess antioxidant activity (155). Examination of their ability to increase the resistance of LDL to oxidation showed that genistein was the most potent antioxidant among these compounds (155). Analysis of the isoflavones structure–activity relations revealed the importance of the single 4′-hydroxyl group, as well as the 5′,7-dihydroxy structure, in the reactivity of the isoflavones as scavengers of aqueous-phase free radicals.

In human volunteers who were supplemented daily for 2 weeks with 3 soy bars, containing genistein and daidzein (156), the plasma isoflavonoids level markedly increased, but less than 1% of them was associated with the LDL. Subjection of LDL to copper ion-induced oxidation revealed that the lag phase for the initiation of LDL oxidation was prolonged by 20 min in LDL derived after soy intake, in comparison with LDL derived before soy consumption (156). Similarly, it was demonstrated that genistein inhibited copper ion-induced oxidation of LDL, as well as endothelial cell-induced LDL oxidation (157). Finally, genistein effectively protected vascular cells from the cytotoxic damage of oxidized LDL (157). Taken together, all these data support the beneficial action of a soy diet in the prevention of early atherogenic events.

4. Tea

Tea drinking has been associated in epidemiological studies with a decreased risk for cardiovascular disease (120,158–160). The terms green tea and black tea refer to products manufactured from the leaf of the tea plant, *Camellia sinensis*. Green tea is manufactured from fresh leaf and is rich in flavonoids, especially with flavonols from the catechins group, of which epigallocatechin gallate, epicatechin gallate, and epicatechin, account for 30–40% of the green tea solids (161). Black tea manufacture includes an enzymatic step, in which most catechins are converted to complex condensation products, such as the aflavins or thearubigens. Green and black tea also contain small amount of flavonols, such as quercetin.

Absorption studies of tea polyphenols, their effect on LDL oxidation and on atherosclerosis, have shown conflicting results (162). The effect of green or black tea consumption on the resistance of LDL to oxidation was studied in 45 human volunteers who consumed, for 4 weeks, 900 mL (6 cups) of green tea or black tea per day in comparison with mineral water consumption (163). Consumption of tea (green or black) had no effect on the ex vivo resistance of LDL to oxidation. Similar negative results were also demonstrated (164,165). Conversely, in another study (166), ingestion of tea (300 mL after an overnight fast) produced a significant increase of plasma antioxidant capacity, which peaked at 30–50 min after consumption. Similarly (167), ingestion of 400 mL of freshly prepared green tea resulted in a rapid absorption of the tea polyphenols, and it was associated with an increase in plasma total antioxidant state, peaking at 20–40 min after ingestion. Consumption of 750 mL/day of black tea for 4 weeks by 14 healthy volunteers revealed (168) that the lag time for LDL oxidation was significantly prolonged (from 54 to 62 min). The effect of green or black tea on LDL oxidation and atherosclerotic lesion formation was studied in hypercholesterolemic rabbits (169). The results of this study indicated that green tea consumption reduced the atherosclerotic plaque formation, whereas black tea showed no significant effect, although both green and black tea induced a 13 and 15% prolongation in the lag phase of LDL oxidation, respectively (169).

Catechins or theaflavins (25–400 μmol/L) that were added to LDL, dose-dependently inhibited its oxidation (168). Among the catechins, epigallocatechin gallate exerted the most marked effect in prolonging LDL oxidation lag time (168). Furthermore, addition of 1.5 μM of epicatechin and epigallocatechin to a mixture of LDL and copper ion in the initiation phase, inhibited LDL oxidation, whereas higher concentrations were needed (10 μM of epicatechin and 2 μM of epigallocatechin) for the inhibition of the LDL oxidation propagation phase (170).

5. Pomegranate

The pomegranate tree, which is said to have flourished in the Garden of Eden, has been extensively used as a folk medicine in many cultures. Edible parts of pomegranate fruits (about 50% of total fruit weight) comprise 80% juice and 20% seeds. Fresh juice contains 85% moisture, 10% total sugars, 1.5% pectin, ascorbic acid, polyphenols, and flavonoids. Pomegranate seeds are a rich source of crude fibers, pectin, and sugars, and the pomegranate peel contains phenols from the condensed tannins class (171). The dried pomegranate seeds contain the steroidal estrogen estrone (172,173), the isoflavonic phytoestrogens, genistein and daidzein, and the phytoestrogen coumestrol (174).

The content of soluble polyphenols in pomegranate juice varies within the limits of 0.2–1.0%, depending on variety, and includes mainly anthocyanins (such as cyanidin-3-glycoside, cyanidin-3,3-diglycoside, and delphindin-3-glucosid) and anthoxantins [such as catechins, ellagic tannins, and gallic and ellagic acids (171)]. Fermented pomegranate juice and cold-pressed pomegranate seeds, possess antioxidant activity and can reduce prostaglandin and leukotriene formation by inhibition of cyclooxygenases and lipoxygenases (175).

The effect of pomegranate juice on LDL atherogenic modifications, including its oxidation, aggregation, and retention, was studied in vitro and ex vivo in healthy male volunteers and in the atherosclerotic apolipoprotein E-deficient (E^0) mice (176). The in vitro studies demonstrated a significant dose-dependent antioxidant capability of pomegranate juice against LDL oxidation (Fig. 8A). Pomegranate juice also inhibited oxidation of HDL by 22%. The mechanisms for the antioxidative effects of pomegranate juice against LDL oxidation could be related to its capacity to scavenge free radicals. The water-soluble fractions of a pomegranate's inner and outer peels, but not that of the seeds, were even stronger antioxidants against LDL oxidation than the juice (176).

Atherogenicity of LDL is attributed not only to its oxidative modification, but also to its aggregation (26). It was previously shown that LDL oxidation leads to its subsequent aggregation (27,28). The addition of increasing concentrations of pomegranate juice to LDL decreased its susceptibility to aggregation (by vortexing) in a dose-dependent fashion (see Fig. 8B). Pomegranate juice also reduced an additional related modification of LDL: its retention to matrix proteoglycans (as analyzed by LDL binding to chondroitin sulfate).

Extracellular matrix (ECM) proteoglycans (PGs) can bind LDL through their glycosaminoglycan (GAG) moieties, and such interaction leads to entrapment of the LDL particle in the arterial wall, a phenomenon called "LDL retention" (11). Addition of increasing concentrations of pomegranate juice (0–3.5 μmol/L of polyphenols) to LDL (200 μg/mL of lipoprotein protein), induced a substantial dose-dependent reduction in the capacity of LDL to bind chondroitin sulfate (CS; 100 μg/mL). LDL binding to chondroitin sulfate decreased by up to 75% following its incubation with 3.5 μmol/L of pomegranate juice polyphenols (see Fig. 8C).

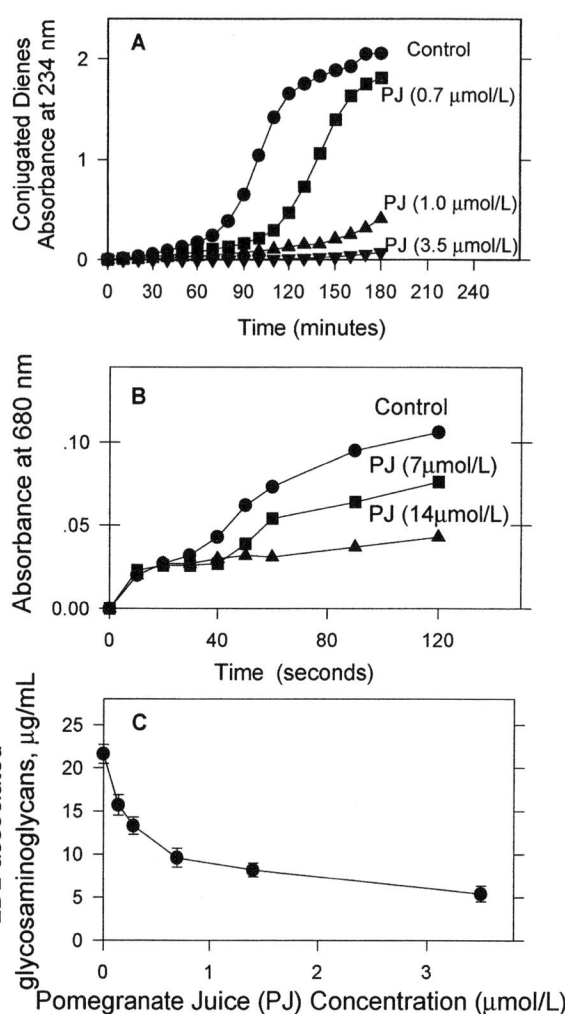

Figure 8 Pomegranate juice inhibits LDL modifications in vitro: (A) LDL oxidation: LDL (100 μg/mL of protein) was incubated without (control) or with increasing concentrations of pomegranate juice (PJ, 0–3.5 μmol/L of polyphenols). LDL oxidation was induced by its incubation with 5 μM of $CuSO_4$, and was measured as conjugated dienes formation that were kinetically monitored at 234 nm. (B) LDL aggregation: LDL (100 μg/mL of protein) was incubated without (control) or with pomegranate juice (PJ, 7 or 24 μmol/L of polyphenols) for 10 min at 25°C. LDL aggregation induced by vortexing was then monitored kinetically at 680 nm. (C) LDL retention: LDL (100 μg/mL of protein) was incubated with increasing concentrations of pomegranate juice (PJ, 0–3.5 μmol/L of polyphenols) for 1 h at 37°C, followed by the addition of chondroitin sulfate (CS; 100 μg/mL), and a further incubation for 30 additional min at 25°C. LDL was then precipitated, and LDL-associated GAG content was analyzed in the precipitate. Results are presented as mean ± SD from three separate experiments.

The antioxidative effect of pomegranate juice dietary consumption was also studied in vivo in humans and in E^0 mice. LDL derived from human healthy volunteers after consumption of pomegranate juice ("wonderful" cultivation, 50 mL/day of pomegranate juice, equivalent to 1.5 mmol/day of total polyphenols), for 2 weeks, was more resistant to copper ion-induced oxidation than LDL obtained before pomegranate juice supplementation (176). This effect was demonstrated by a 43% prolongation of the LDL oxidation lag time (the time required for the initiation of LDL oxidation), after 2 weeks of juice consumption, in comparison with LDL obtained before juice consumption (from 35 ± 6 min before juice consumption to 50 ± 6 min after consumption of pomegranate juice) (Fig. 9A). This latter effect was accompanied by a significant 10% increment in plasma total antioxidant status after 2 weeks of pomegranate juice consumption, in comparison with plasma derived before juice consumption (see Fig. 9B). Finally, pomegranate juice consumption by humans increased the activity of serum paraoxonase (PON 1; which is a HDL-associated esterase that acts as a potent protector against lipid peroxidation) (see Fig. 9C).

Consumption of pomegranate juice by E^0 mice, also has considerable antiatherogenic properties. Pomegranate juice consumption substantially reduced the propensity of E^0 mice-derived LDL to copper ion-induced oxidation (see Fig. 9D).

A reduced capacity of macrophages to oxidize LDL leads to decreased LDL oxidation. Macrophage-mediated oxidation of LDL is considered to be a major event during early atherogenesis, and it is associated with cellular uptake of the modified atherogenic lipoprotein, leading to macrophage cholesterol accumulation and foam cell formation (47,48). Mouse peritoneal macrophages (MPM), which are commonly used as representative of arterial macrophages, were isolated from the peritoneal cavity of control, placebo-treated E^0 mice, as well as from E^0 mice that consumed pomegranate juice (12.5 μL/day per mouse, equivalent to 0.35 μmol of total polyphenols) for 2 months.

Incubation of the MPMs with LDL (100 μg/mL of protein) for 18 h, under oxidative stress (in the presence of 2 μmol/L of $CuSO_4$) revealed that macrophage-mediated oxidation of LDL was inhibited by 90% (see Fig. 9E). The mechanism responsible for this effect was associated with a reduction (by 49%) in superoxide anion release from the macrophages and an elevation in cellular glutathione content by 25% (176). This effect could also be related to reduced levels of macrophage-associated lipid peroxides in MPMs derived after pomegranate juice consumption, in comparison with macrophages isolated from control mice that consumed placebo. Because it was demonstrated that oxidative stress induces macrophage lipid peroxidation (51), and that these oxidized macrophages can oxidatively modify LDL (even in the absence of transition metal ions) (52), inhibition of oxidized macrophages formation by pomegranate juice can possibly result in reduced capacity of the macrophages to oxidize LDL. Finally, and most important, pomegranate juice supplementation to E^0 mice reduced the size of their atherosclerotic lesion and the number of foam cells in the lesion (176), in comparison with control placebo-treated E^0 mice that were supplemented with water (see Fig. 9F).

6. Olive Oil

The Mediterranean diet, rich in fresh fruits and vegetables, is inversely related to the incidence of cardiovascular disease, as shown in the Seven Countries Studies (76,177,178). Olive oil, the dietary fat of choice in the Mediterranean area, in comparison with other vegetable oils, has a peculiar fatty acid composition. The monounsaturated oleic acid (C-18:1, $n = 9$) is the most abundant fatty acid in olive oil (56–84%), whereas the polyunsaturated linoleic acid (C-18:2, $n = 6$), ranges only from 3 to 21%. In addition, olive oil contains a variety of

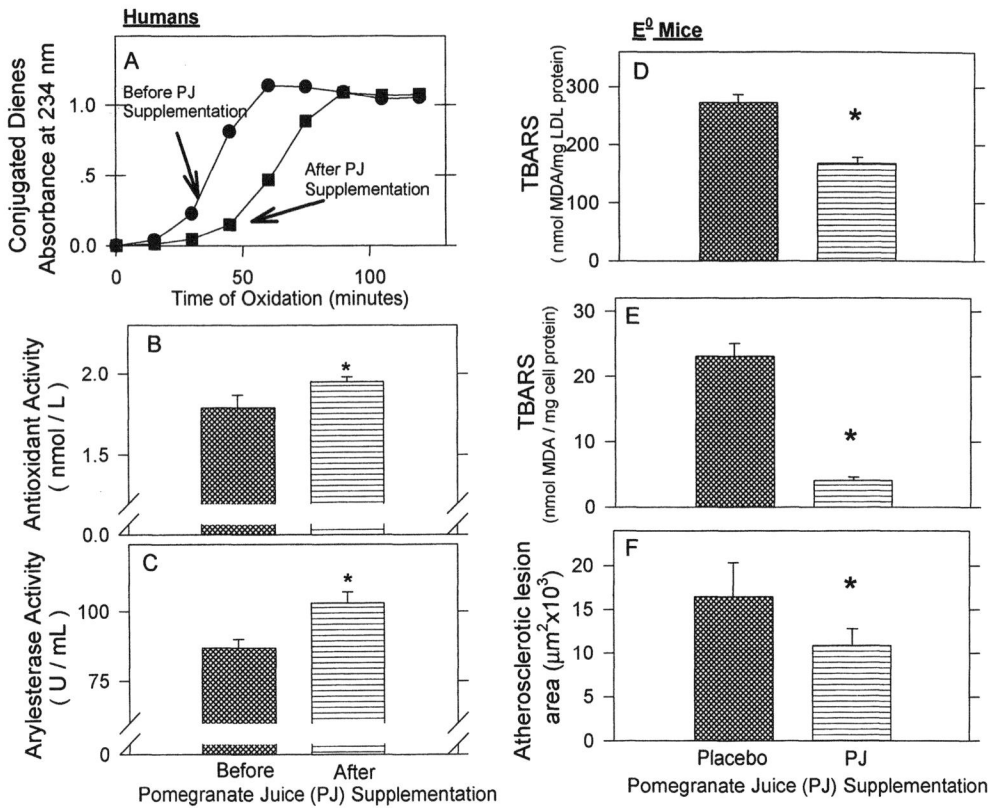

Figure 9 (A,B,C) Pomegranate juice consumption by humans increases the resistance of LDL to oxidation, and increases plasma antioxidant status: (A) LDL oxidation; LDL (100 μg/mL of protein) obtained from healthy human volunteers before or after 2 weeks of pomegranate juice (PJ, 1.5 mmol of total polyphenols) supplementation, was incubated with 5 μM of $CuSO_4$, and the formation of conjugated dienes was kinetically monitored at 234 nm. (B) Plasma antioxidant status: total antioxidant status in plasma obtained before and after pomegranate juice (PJ) supplementation; Results are expressed as mean ± SD ($n = 12$); *$p < 0.01$ (vs. before supplementation). (C) Serum paraoxonase activity: paraoxonase activity was determined in serum obtained before and after pomegranate juice (PJ) consumption, by measuring arylesterase activity. Results are expressed as mean ± SD ($n = 12$); *$p < 0.01$ (after vs. before consumption). (D,E,F) Pomegranate juice consumption by E^0 mice reduces LDL oxidation, along with a reduction in atherosclerotic lesion area. (D) $CuSO_4$-induced LDL oxidation: LDL (100 μg/mL of protein) isolated from E^0 mice that consumed placebo or 12.5 μL of pomegranate juice (PJ; equivalent to 0.35 μmol of total polyphenols) was incubated with 5 μM of $CuSO_4$, and LDL oxidation was measured by the TBARS assay. Results are expressed as mean ± SD of three separate determinations; *$p < 0.01$ (vs. placebo). (E) Cell-mediated LDL oxidation: mouse peritoneal macrophages (MPM) were isolated from the peritoneal fluid of control E^0 mice or from mice that consumed 12.5 μL of pomegranate juice (PJ) per mouse per day, for 2 months. The MPM were incubated for 6 h at 37°C with LDL (100 μg/mL protein) under oxidative stress (in presence of 2 μM of $CuSO_4$). LDL oxidation was measured directly in the medium by the TBARS assay. Results are expressed as mean ± SD ($n = 3$); *$p < 0.01$ (vs. placebo). (F) Lesion size: the aortic arch derived from E^0 mice that consumed placebo or pomegranate juice (PJ; 12.5 μL/mouse per day) for 2 months, was analyzed for lesion size. Results are expressed as the mean of the lesion area in square micrometers; *$p < 0.05$ (vs. placebo).

minor components, including polyphenols (up to 800 mg/kg), which provide the typical taste and aroma of extra virgin olive oil and confer this oil's stability to oxidation (179).

The mechanisms underlying the cardiovascular benefits of the Mediterranean diet may stem from the high content of the monounsaturated oleic acid, as well as from the polyphenols, which are beneficial in reducing LDL atherogenic alterations, including its oxidation (161,179–182). Furthermore, polyphenols in olive oil possess beneficial effects on cellular processes, including inhibition of lipoxygenase (183), production of leukotriene-B_4 (184), and stimulation of nitric oxide (NO) release from macrophages (185).

LDL isolated from Greek subjects who consumed a diet naturally rich in olive oil was significantly less susceptible (by 12%) to oxidation as measured by conjugated diene formation, in comparison with LDL isolated from American subjects who consumed a typical American diet (186). Furthermore, the proinflammatory potential of mildly oxidized LDL derived from Greek subjects measured as LDL promotion of monocyte chemotaxis and adhesion to endothelial cells, was decreased by 42%, in comparison with LDL derived from American subjects. There was an inverse correlation between the LDL oleic acid content and the stimulation of monocyte chemotaxis and adhesion (186).

Consumption of a liquid diet supplemented with oleic acid for 8 weeks by American subjects resulted in an oleic acid-enriched LDL, which subsequently promoted 52% less monocyte chemotaxis and 77% reduced monocyte adhesion, in comparison with linoleate-enriched LDL (186). This study suggested that LDL enriched with oleic acid is less easily converted into the proinflammatory, minimally modified LDL. These results are consistent with another study (187), demonstrating that dietary supplementation of olive oil to healthy human subjects (50 g/day) for 2 weeks, increased the resistance of their LDL to oxidation (187). This was shown by a significant reduction in LDL peroxides, thiobarbituric acid-reactive substances (TBARS), and conjugated dienes content by 73, 28, and 32%, respectively. Furthermore, LDL obtained after olive oil supplementation demonstrated a 61% decreased cellular uptake by macrophages (187). These beneficial effects of olive oil consumption may also be related, in addition to the oleic acid, to the olive oil polyphenols.

Dietary administration of extra virgin olive oil versus refined olive oil, to New Zealand White rabbits (NZW), resulted in increased resistance of their LDL to oxidation only in the group of animals that consumed extra virgin olive oil (188). These results suggest that the beneficial effect of extra virgin olive oil over that of the refined olive oil is probably due to the presence of phenolics, which are lost during the refining process (188). To determine whether the minor polar components of virgin olive oil could have favorable effects on LDL composition and susceptibility to oxidation, ten normolipidemic subjects received different oils in a crossover study (two diet periods of 3 weeks each). They received either virgin olive oil or oleic acid-rich sunflower oil. LDL oxidation, measured as conjugated dienes production, decreased only after the virgin olive oil diet, suggesting a mild antioxidative effect against LDL oxidation for some minor components of virgin olive oil (189).

Some major phenols were extracted and purified from olive oil (179,190,191), and their biological properties have been investigated. Oleuropein and hydroxytyrosol are two major representative phenols in olive oil (Fig. 10). Hydroxytyrosol and oleuropein inhibited, in a dose-related manner the production of LTB_4 by calcium ionophore-stimulated leukocytes (184) through the inhibition of 5-lipoxygenase. Oleuropein also dose-dependently enhanced the release of nitric oxide (NO) from lipopolysaccharide (LPS; endotoxin)-challenged mouse peritoneal macrophages, owing to stimulation of nitric oxide synthase expression (185). NO production during endotoxin challenge, which is accompanied by increased oxidative stress caused by the respiratory burst and cellular production of oxygen free radicals, is believed

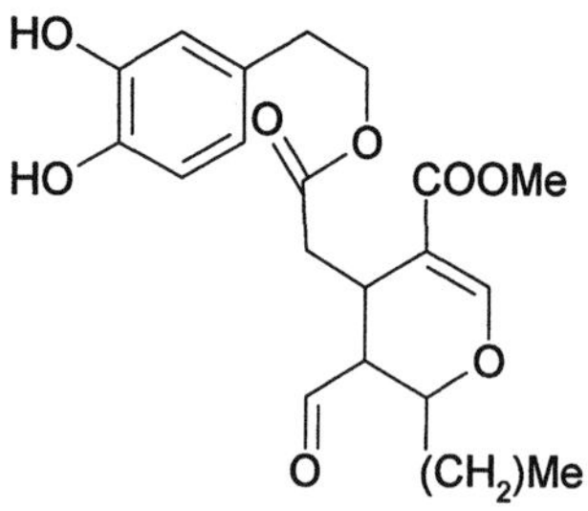

Figure 10 Chemical structure of hydroxytyrosol and oleuropein.

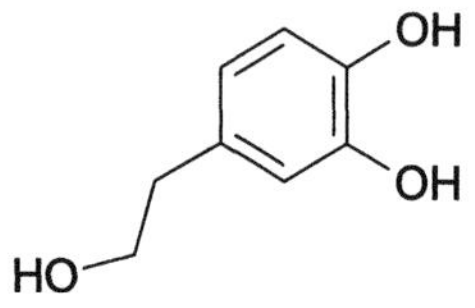

to protect cells against oxidative damage. Reduced cellular oxidative stress can subsequently reduce the capacity of the cells to oxidatively modify LDL. Direct antioxidant activities of oleuropein and hydroxytyrosol against LDL oxidation were demonstrated (190,191). LDL incubation with oleuropein or with hydroxytyrosol resulted in the inhibition of copper ion-induced LDL oxidation. Oleuropein and hydroxytyrosol protection of LDL against oxidation can be related to the potency of these compounds to scavenge free radicals. Both hydroxytyrosol and oleuropein express scavenging capacity for superoxide radical in a cell-free system (based on the generation of urate and superoxide by xanthine/xanthine oxidase) and in a cellular system (based on the production of superoxide by PMA-challenged human neutrophils) (192).

7. Ginger

Ginger (*Zingiber officinale* Roscoe) is one of the world's most known spice, and it has been universally used throughout history for its health benefits. The dried extract of ginger contains monoterpenes and sesquiterpenes. The main antioxidants in ginger are the phenolics, gingerols and shogaols, and some related phenolic ketone derivatives (Fig. 11).

Ginger extract possesses antioxidative characteristics, as it can significantly scavenge superoxide anions and hydroxyl radicals (193–195). Gingerol, at high concentrations, inhibited ascorbate–ferrous-induced lipid peroxidation in rat liver microsomes (195). Gingerol isolated from *Zingiber* inhibits platelet function by the inhibition of thromboxane formation (196), and it also decreases inflammation processes (197). Furthermore, ginger acts as an hypolipidemic agent in cholesterol-fed rabbits (198–200).

The ex vivo effect of a standardized ginger extract on the development of atherosclerosis was studied in E^0 mice, in relation to the resistance of their LDL to oxidation and aggregation (200). Sixty E^0 mice at the age of 6 weeks were divided into three groups, 20 mice in each group, and were supplemented for 10 weeks in their drinking water with placebo (1.1% alcohol), or with ginger extract (25 μg/day or 250 μg/day). Consumption of 250 μg/day of ginger extract reduced atherogenic modifications of LDL, as shown by a 62% decrease in the basal level of

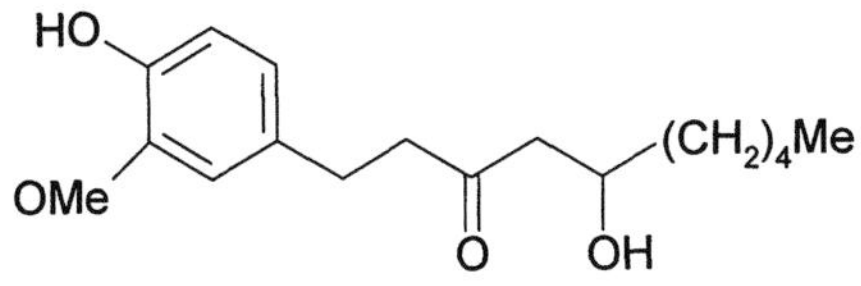

Figure 11 Chemical structure of gingerol and shogaol.

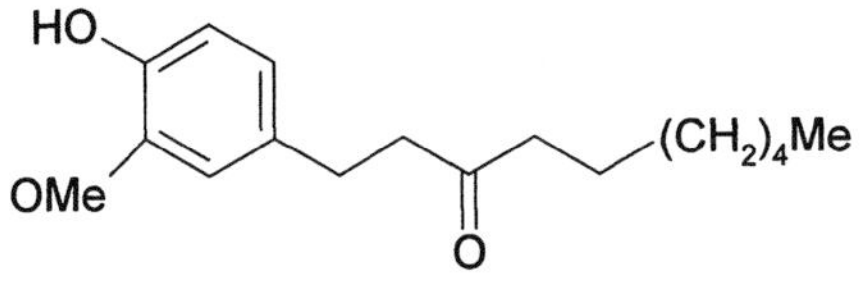

LDL-associated lipid peroxides, and also by a 33% inhibition in LDL aggregation (induced by vortexing). In parallel, the aortic atherosclerotic lesion areas were considerably decreased, by 10 and 44%, in mice that consumed 25 µg/day or 250 µg/day of ginger extract, respectively, in comparison with placebo-treated mice.

Furthermore, consumption of 25 or 250 µg/day of ginger extract by E^0 mice could have reduced LDL oxidation by reducing the capacity of macrophages to oxidize LDL. Indeed, peritoneal macrophages harvested from E^0 mice after consumption of 25 or 250 µg/day of ginger extract, exhibited a significant reduction in their capacity to oxidize LDL (by 45 and 60%, respectively), in comparison with placebo-treated mice (200).

8. Garlic

Garlic is one of the most widely quoted herb with medicinal potentials known in the literature. The therapeutic actions of garlic and its constituents have been widely reported (201,202). Studies suggested that garlic powder manifests direct antiatherogenic action (203–206). The antiatherosclerotic effect of garlic has been attributed to its hypolipidemic activity (201,207), as well as to its antioxidant properties. Garlic possesses antioxidant characteristics that have been demonstrated both in vitro and in vivo (208–211). Garlic extract inhibits copper ion-induced LDL oxidation in a dose-dependent manner, with an IC_{50} of 120 µg/mL (208). Ten healthy volunteers were given 60 mg/day of garlic powder (6 tables of Kwai) for two weeks in a placebo-controlled, randomized, double-blind crossover trial (209). Although serum lipid and lipoprotein levels were not significantly affected in this short study period, the ex vivo susceptibility of apolipoprotein B-containing lipoproteins to oxidation was significantly decreased by 34% (209). The oxidation susceptibility of LDL, derived from patients with coronary artery disease, after garlic consumption (a single dose of 300 mg, or a long-term administration of 300 mg, three times daily for 28 days), was also significantly decreased (210). These antioxidative effects of garlic could be related to its ability to scavenge oxygen free radicals. It was demonstrated (212) that, indeed, garlic extract is a powerful scavenger of the hydroxyl radical (OH·).

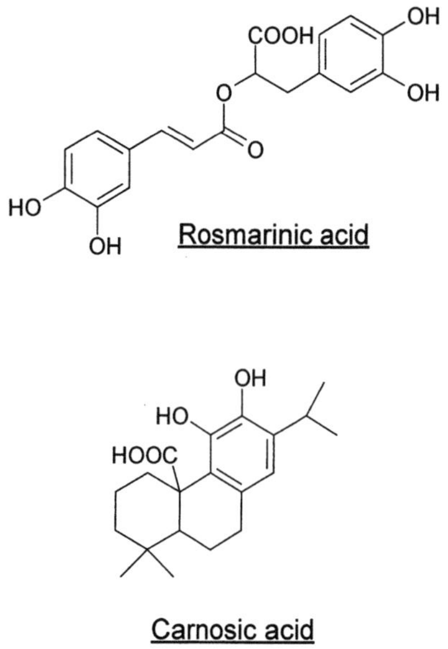

Figure 12 Chemical structure of rosmarinic acid and carnosic acid.

Many compounds with biological activities have been identified and isolated from garlic extract (201,207), including flavonoids, such as kaempferol glycosides (213) and allicin, which can account for protection of LDL from oxidation by the garlic extracts. Allicin is the main biologically active component of garlic clove extracts, and its biological activity is attributed to a thiol–disulfide exchange, as well as to a direct antioxidant activity (214–216).

9. Rosemary

The commonly used spice and flavoring agent rosemary, derived from the leaves of the plant *Rosmarinus officinalis* L, possesses antioxidative properties (217,218). Its most active antioxidant constituents include the phenolics rosmarinic acid and carnosic acid (Fig. 12), which account for 90% of its antioxidant activity (219).

Carnosic acid inhibits superoxide anion production in the xanthine–xanthine oxidase system, thus being effective in protecting biological systems against oxidative damage (220). Carnosic acid also acts as a powerful inhibitor of lipid peroxidation in microsomal and liposomal systems, and scavenges peroxyl radicals and hydrogen peroxides (220). Recently, we have observed that both rosmarinic acid and carnosic acid inhibited LDL oxidation (208). Rosmarinic acid and carnosic acid inhibited copper ion-induced LDL oxidation in a dose-dependent manner, with an IC_{50} of 2 µg/mL and 35 µg/mL for the inhibition of TBARS formation, respectively, and an IC_{50} of 4 and 35 µg/mL for the inhibition of lipid peroxides formation, respectively (208).

IV. SUMMARY

Several dietary polyphenols and flavonoids substantially reduce LDL atherogenic modifications, which lead to foam cell formation. Figure 13 summarizes our current view on the major pathways by which polyphenols protect LDL against atherogenic modifications, and thereby reduce macrophage foam cell formation and the development of advanced atherosclerosis. Polyphenols can protect LDL against atherogenic modifications through two pathways:

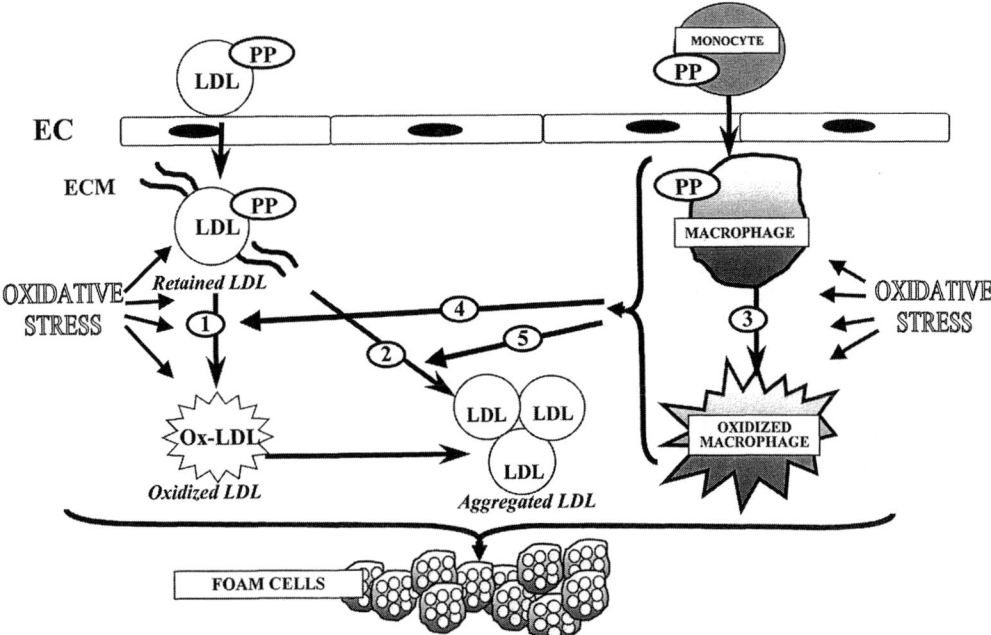

Figure 13 Major pathways by which polyphenols inhibit modified LDL-induced macrophage foam cell formation: Polyphenols (PP) affect LDL directly by their interaction with the lipoprotein and inhibition of LDL retention, LDL oxidation (1) and LDL aggregation (2). Polyphenols can also protect LDL indirectly, by their accumulation in arterial cells and protection of arterial macrophages against oxidative stress (3). This latter effect is associated with inhibition of the formation of oxidized macrophages and the capacity of macrophages to oxidize LDL (4) or to promote LDL aggregation (5).

1. *Direct interaction of the polyphenols with the lipoprotein and protection of LDL against oxidation and aggregation.* LDL enrichment with polyphenols decreases the retention of the lipoprotein to arterial wall extracellular matrix components, reduces LDL oxidation, and inhibits LDL aggregation. Furthermore, polyphenols increase serum paraoxonase activity, resulting in a further protection of the lipoprotein against oxidation.

2. *Protection of LDL against oxidation secondary to polyphenol accumulation in arterial macrophages and, thereby, reducing cell-mediated oxidation of LDL.* Polyphenols accumulate in macrophages, and inhibit the activation of cellular NADPH oxidase by the inhibition of protein kinase C (PKC) activity. This effect results in reduced capacity of the cells to oxidatively modify LDL. Furthermore, enrichment of macrophages with polyphenols inhibits macrophage lipid peroxidation and the formation of oxidized macrophages. Because oxidized macrophages promote LDL oxidation, prevention of oxidized macrophages formation results in decreased LDL oxidation.

All these effects of polyphenols were demonstrated in vitro, as well as in vivo in humans and in the atherosclerotic apolipoprotein E-deficient mice, following dietary supplementation of nutrients rich in diverse polyphenols (221–223). Dietary supplementation of nutrients rich in polyphenols, or of purified polyphenols, to the E^0 atherosclerotic mice resulted, along with the protection of LDL against atherogenic modifications, also in a significant inhibition in the development of atherosclerotic lesions.

REFERENCES

1. Schaffner T, Taylor K, Bartucci EJ, Fischer–Dzoga K, Beenson JH, Glagov S, Wissler R. Arterial foam cells with distinctive immuno-morphologic and histochemical features of macrophages. Am J Pathol 1980; 100:57–80.
2. Gerrity RG. The role of monocytes in atherogenesis. Am J Pathol 1981; 103:181–190.
3. Goldstein JL, Brown MS. Regulation of the mevalonate pathway. Nature 1990; 343:425–430.
4. Brown MS, Goldstein JL. A receptor-mediated pathway for cholesterol homeostasis. Science 1986; 232:34–47.
5. Steinberg D, Parthasarathy S, Carew TE, Khoo JC, Witztum JL. Beyond cholesterol: modifications of low-density lipoprotein that increase its atherogenicity. N Engl J Med 1989; 320:915–924.
6. Aviram M. Modified forms of low density lipoprotein and atherosclerosis. Atherosclerosis 1993; 98:1–9.
7. Aviram M. Beyond cholesterol: modifications of lipoproteins and increased atherogenicity. In: Neri Serneri GG, Gensini GF, Abbate R, Prisco D, eds. Atherosclerosis Inflammation and Thrombosis. Florence, Italy: Scientific Press, 1993:15–36.
8. Berliner JA, Navab M, Fogelman AM, Frank JS, Demer DL, Edwards PA, Watson AD, Lusis AJ. Atherosclerosis: basic mechanisms. Oxidation, inflammation, and genetics. Circulation 1995; 91:2488–2496.
9. Ross R. The pathogenesis of atherosclerosis: a perspective for the 1990s. Nature 1993; 362:801–809.
10. Ross R. Atherosclerosis: an inflammatory disease. N Engl J Med 1999; 340:115–126.
11. Williams KJ, Tabas I. The response-to-retention hypothesis of early atherogenesis. Arterioscler Thromb Vasc Biol 1995; 15:551–561.
12. Williams KJ, Tabas I. The response-to-retention hypothesis of atherogenesis reinforced. Curr Opin Lipidol 1998; 9:471–474.
13. Nordestgaard BG. The vascular endothelial barrier-selective retention of lipoproteins. Curr Opin Lipidol 1996; 7:269–273.
14. Schwenke DC, Carew TE. Initiation of atherosclerotic lesions in cholesterol-fed rabbits I: focal increases in arterial LDL concentrations precede development of fatty streak lesions. Arteriosclerosis 1989; 9:895–907.
15. Schwenke DC, Carew TE. Initiation of atherosclerotic lesions in cholesterol-fed rabbits II: selective retention of LDL vs. selective increase in LDL permeability in susceptible sites of arteries. Arteriosclerosis 1989; 9:908–918.
16. Carmena R, Ascaso JF, Camejo G, Varela G, Hurt–Camejo E, Ordovas JM, Bergstom M, Wallin B. Effect of olive and sunflower oils on low density lipoprotein level, composition, size, oxidation, and interaction with arterial proteoglycans. Atherosclerosis 1996; 125:243–255.
17. Camejo G, Hurt–Camejo E, Olson U, Bonders G. Proteoglycans and lipoproteins in atherosclerosis. Curr Opin Lipidol 1993; 4:385–391.
18. Ismail NA, Alavi MZ, Moore S. Lipoprotein–proteoglycan complexes from injured rabbit aortas accelerate lipoprotein uptake by arterial smooth muscle cells. Atherosclerosis 1994; 105:79–87.
19. Kostner GM, Bihari–Varga M. Is the atherogenicity of Lp(a) caused by its reactivity with proteoglycans? Eur Heart J 1990; 11(suppl E):184–189.
20. Vijayagopal P, Srinivasan SR, Radhakrishnamurthy B, Berenson GS. Lipoprotein–proteoglycan complexes from atherosclerotic lesions promote cholesteryl ester accumulation in human monocyte/macrophages. Arterioscler Thromb 1992; 12:237–249.
21. Hurt E, Bonders G, Camejo G. Interaction of LDL with human arterial proteoglycans stimulates its uptake by human monocyte-derived macrophages. J Lipid Res 1990; 31:443–454.
22. Aviram M, Maor I, Keidar S, Hayek T, Oiknine J, Bar-El Y, Adler Z, Kertzman V, Milo S. Lesioned low density lipoprotein in atherosclerotic apolipoprotein E-deficient transgenic mice and in humans is oxidized and aggregated. Biochem Biophys Res Commun 1995; 216:501–513.
23. Pentikainen MO, Lethonen EM, Kovanen PT. Aggregation and fusion of modified low density lipoprotein. J Lipid Res 1996; 37:2638–2649.
24. Schissel SL, Tweedie–Hardman J, Rapp JH, Graham G, Williams KJ, Tabas I. Rabbit aorta and human atherosclerotic lesion hydrolyze the sphingomyelin of retained low-density lipoprotein. Proposed role for arterial-wall sphingomyelinase in subendothelial retention and aggregation of atherogenic lipoproteins. J Clin Invest 1996; 98:1455–1464.

25. Zhang WY, Gaynor PM, Kruth HS. Aggregated low density lipoprotein induces and enters surface-connected compartments of human monocyte–macrophages. Uptake occurs independently of the low density lipoprotein receptor. J Biol Chem 1997; 272:31700–31706.
26. Hoff HF, O'Neil Y. Lesion-derived low density lipoprotein and oxidized low density lipoprotein share a lability for aggregation, leading to enhanced macrophage degradation. Arterioscler Thromb Vasc Biol 1991; 11:1209–1222.
27. Hoff HF, Whitaker TE, O'Neil Y. Oxidation of low density lipoprotein leads to particle aggregation and altered macrophage recognition. J Biol Chem 1992; 267:602–609.
28. Maor I, Hayek T, Coleman R, Aviram M. Plasma LDL oxidation leads to its aggregation in atherosclerotic apolipoprotein E-deficient mice. Arterioscler Thromb Vasc Biol 1997; 17:2995–3005.
29. Hurt–Camejo E, Camejo G, Rosengren B, Lopez F, Ahlstrom C, Fager G, Bondjers G. Effect of arterial proteoglycan and glycosaminoglycans on low density lipoprotein oxidation and its uptake by human macrophages and arterial smooth muscle cells. Arterioscler Thromb 1992; 12:569–583.
30. Jialal I, Devaraj S. The role of oxidized low density lipoprotein in atherogenesis. J Nutr 1996; 126(suppl):1053S–1057S.
31. Steinberg D. Low density lipoprotein oxidation and its pathobiological significance. J Biol Chem 1997; 272:20963–20966.
32. Berliner JA, Heinecke JW. The role of oxidized lipoproteins in atherosclerosis. Free Radic Biol Med 1996; 20:707–727.
33. Aviram M. Oxidative modification of low density lipoprotein and atherosclerosis. Isr J Med 1995; 31:241–249.
34. Witztum JL, Steinberg D. Role of oxidized low density lipoprotein in atherogenesis. J Clin Invest 1991; 88:1785–1792.
35. Aviram M. Interaction of oxidized low density lipoprotein with macrophages in atherosclerosis and the antiatherogenicity of antioxidants. Eur J Clin Chem Clin Biochem 1996; 34:599–608.
36. Kaplan M, Aviram M. Oxidized low density lipoprotein: Atherogenic and proinflammatory characteristics during macrophage foam cell formation. An inhibitory role for nutritional antioxidants and serum paraoxonase. Clin Chem Lab Med 1999; 37:777–787.
37. Parthasarathy S, Santanam N, Auge N. Oxidized low-density lipoprotein, a two-faced Janus in coronary artery disease? Biochem Pharmacol 1998; 56:279–284.
38. Parthasarathy S, Rankin SM. The role of oxidized LDL in atherogenesis. Prog Lipid Res 1992; 31:127–143.
39. Herttuala SY. Is oxidized low density lipoprotein present in vivo? Curr Opin Lipidol 1998; 9:337–344.
40. Aviram M. The contribution of the macrophage receptor for oxidized LDL to its cellular uptake. Biochem Biophys Res Commun 1991; 179:359–365.
41. Kim JA, Territo MC, Wayner E, Carlos TM, Parhami F, Smith CW, Haberland ME, Fogelman AM, Berliner JA. Partial characterization of leukocyte binding molecules on endothelial cells induced by minimally oxidized LDL. Arterioscler Thromb 1994; 14:427–433.
42. Khan NBV, Parthasarathy S, Alexander RW. Modified LDL and its constituents augment cytokine-activated vascular cell adhesion molecule-1 gene expression in human vascular endothelial cells. J Clin Invest 1995; 95:1262–1270.
43. Rangasamy S, Penn MS, Saidel GM, Chisolm GM. Exogenous oxidized low density lipoprotein injures and alters the barrier function of endothelium in rats in vivo. Circ Res 1997; 80:37–44.
44. Penn MS, Chisolm GM. Oxidized lipoproteins, altered cell function and atherosclerosis. Atherosclerosis 1994; 108(suppl):S21–S29.
45. Witztum JL, Steinberg D. Modification of low density lipoprotein by endothelial cells involves lipid peroxidation and degradation of low density lipoprotein phospholipids. Proc Natl Acad Sci USA 1984; 81:3883–3887.
46. Heinecke JW, Rosen H, Chait A. Iron and copper promote modification of low density lipoprotein by human arterial smooth muscle cells in culture. J Clin Invest 1984; 74:1980–1984.
47. Parthasarathy S, Printz DJ, Boyd D, Joy L, Steinberg D. Macrophage oxidation of low density lipoprotein generates a modified form recognized by the scavenger receptor. Arteriosclerosis 1986; 6:505–510.
48. Aviram M, Rosenblat M. Macrophage mediated oxidation of extracellular low density lipoprotein requires an initial binding of the lipoprotein to its receptor. J Lipid Res 1994; 35:385–398.

49. Aviram M, Rosenblat M, Etzioni A, Levy R. Activation of NADPH oxidase is required for macrophage-mediated oxidation of low density lipoprotein. Metabolism 1996; 45:1069–1079.
50. Aviram M, Fuhrman B. LDL oxidation by arterial wall macrophages depends on the antioxidative status in the lipoprotein and in the cells: role of prooxidants vs. antioxidants. Mol Cell Biochem 1998; 188:149–159.
51. Fuhrman B, Oiknine J, Aviram M. Iron induces lipid peroxidation in cultured macrophages, increases their ability to oxidatively modify LDL and affect their secretory properties. Atherosclerosis 1994; 111:65–78.
52. Fuhrman B, Oiknine J, Keidar S, Kaplan M, Aviram M. Increased uptake of low density lipoprotein (LDL) by oxidized macrophages is the result of enhanced LDL receptor activity and of progressive LDL oxidation. Free Radic Biol Med 1997; 23:34–46.
53. Yla-Herttuala S, Rosenfeld ME, Parthasarathy S, Glass CK, Sigal E, Witztum JL, Steinberg D. Colocalization of 15-lipoxygenase mRNA and protein with epitopes of oxidized low density lipoprotein in macrophage-rich areas of atherosclerotic lesions. Proc Natl Acad Sci USA 1990; 87:6959–6963.
54. Aviram M, Kent UM, Hollenberg PF. Microsomal cytochrome P450 catalyzes the oxidation of low density lipoprotein. Atherosclerosis 1999; 143:253–260.
55. Heinecke JW. Mechanism of oxidative damage of low density lipoprotein in human atherosclerosis. Curr Opin Lipidol 1997; 8:268–274.
56. Heinecke JW. Pathways for oxidation of low density lipoprotein by myeloperoxidase: tyrosyl radical, reactive aldehydes, hypochlorous acid and molecular chlorine. Biofactors 1997; 6:145–155.
57. Yla-Herttuala S, Palinski W, Rosenfeld ME, Pharthasarathy S, Carew TE, Buttler S, Witztum JL, Steinberg D. Evidence for the presence of oxidatively modified low density lipoprotein in atherosclerotic lesions of rabbit and man. J Clin Invest 1989; 84:10867–1095.
58. Lavy A, Brook JG, Dankner G, Ben Amotz A, Aviram M. Enhanced in vitro oxidation of plasma lipoproteins derived from hypercholesterolemic patients. Metabolism 1991; 40:794–799.
59. Keidar S, Kaplan M, Shapira H, Brook JG, Aviram M. Low density lipoprotein isolated from patients with essential hypertension exhibits increased propensity for oxidation and enhanced uptake by macrophages: a possible role for angiotensin II. Atherosclerosis 1994; 104:71–84.
60. Maggi E, Bellazzi R, Gazo A, Secciam T, Bellomo G. Autoantibodies against oxidatively-modified LDL in chronic patients undergoing dialysis. Kidney Int 1994; 46:869–876.
61. Nishigaki I, Hagihara M, Tsunekana H, Maseki M, Yagi K. Lipid peroxide levels of serum lipoprotein fractions of diabetic patients. Biochem Med 1981; 25:373–378.
62. Hayek T, Oiknine J, Brook JG, Aviram M. Increased plasma lipoprotein lipid peroxidation in apo E-deficient mice. Biochem Biophys Res Commun 1994; 201:1567–1574.
63. Keaney JF, Frei B. Antioxidant protection of low-density lipoprotein and its role in the prevention of atherosclerotic vascular disease. In: Frei B, ed. Natural Antioxidants in Human Health and Disease. San Diego, CA: Academic Press, 1994:303–352.
64. Aviram M. Antioxidants in restenosis and atherosclerosis. Curr Interven Cardiol Rep 1999; 1:66–78.
65. Levy Y, Ben-Amotz A, Aivram M. Effect of dietary supplementation of β-carotene to humans on its binding to plasma LDL and on the lipoprotein susceptibility to undergo oxidative modification: comparison of the synthetic all-*trans* isomer with the natural algae β-carotene. J Nutr Environ Med 1995; 5:13–22.
66. Levy Y, Kaplan M, Ben Amotz A, Aviram M. The effect of dietary supplementation of β-carotene on human monocyte–macrophage-mediated oxidation of low density lipoprotein. Isr J Med Sci 1996; 32:473–478.
67. Fuhrman B, Ben-Yaish L, Attias J, Hayek T, Aviram M. Tomato's lycopene and β-carotene inhibit low density lipoprotein oxidation and this effect depends on the lipoprotein vitamin E content. Nutr Metab Cardiovasc Dis 1997; 7:433–443.
68. Jialal I, Fuller CJ, Huet BA. The effect of α-tocopherol supplementation on LDL oxidation a dose–response study. Arterioscler Thromb Vasc Biol 1995; 15:190–198.
69. Fuller CJ, Grundy SM, Norkus EP, Jialal I. Effect of ascorbate supplementation on low density lipoprotein oxidation in smokers. Atherosclerosis 1996; 119:139–150.
70. Kita T, Nagano Y, Yokode M, Ishii K, Kume N, Ooshima A, Yoshida H, Kawai C. Probucol prevents the progression of atherosclerosis in Watanabe heritable hyperlipidemic rabbit, an animal model for familial hypercholesterolemia. Proc Natl Acad Sci USA 1987; 84:5928–5931.

71. Rosenblat M, Aviram M. Macrophage glutathione content and glutathione peroxidase activity are inversely related to cell-mediated oxidation of LDL. Free Radic Biol Med 1997; 24:305–313.
72. Sparrow CP, Doebber TW, Olszewski J, Wu MS, Ventre J, Stevens KA, Cha YS. Low density lipoprotein is protected from oxidation and the progression of atherosclerosis is slowed in cholesterol-fed rabbits by the antioxidant N,N'-diphenyl-phenylenediamine. J Clin Invest 1992; 89:1885–1891.
73. Shaish A, Daugherty A, O'Sullivan F, Schonfeld G, Heineck JW. beta-Carotene inhibits atherosclerosis in hypercholesterolemic rabbits. J Clin Invest 1995; 96:2075–2085.
74. Muldoon MF. Flavonoids and heart disease: evidence of benefit still fragmentary. Br Med J 1996; 312:458–459.
75. Hertog MGL, Feskens EJM, Kromhout D. Antioxidant flavonols and coronary heart disease risk. Lancet 1997; 349:699.
76. Hertog MG, Kromhout D, Aravanis C, et al. Flavonoid intake and long-term risk of coronary heart disease and cancer in the seven countries study. Arch Intern Med 1995; 155:381–386.
77. Bravo L. Polyphenols: chemistry, dietary sources, metabolism, and nutritional significance. Nutr Rev 1998; 56:317–333.
78. Leibovitz BE, Mueller JA. Bioflavonoids and polyphenols: medical application. J Optim Nutr 1993; 2:17–35.
79. King A, Young G. Characteristics and occurrence of phenolic phytochemicals. J Am Diet Assoc 1999; 99:213–218.
80. Catapano AL. Antioxidant effect of flavonoids. Angiology 1997; 48:39–44.
81. Rice–Evans CA, Miller NJ, Bolwell PG, Bramley PM, Pridham JB. The relative antioxidant activities of plant-derived polyphenolic flavonoids. Free Radic Res 1995; 22:375–383.
82. Rice–Evans CA, Miller NJ, Paganga G. Structure–antioxidant activity relationships of flavonoids and phenolic acids. Free Radic Biol Med 1996; 20:933–956.
83. Van Acker SABE, Van-den Berg DJ, Tromp MNJL, Griffioen DH, van Bennekom WP, Van der Vijgh WJF, Bast A. Structural aspects of antioxidants activity of flavonoids. Free Radic Biol Med 1996; 20:331–342.
84. Aviram M, Fuhrman B. Polyphenolic flavonoids inhibit macrophage-mediated oxidation of LDL and attenuate atherogenesis. Atherosclerosis 1998; 137(suppl):S45–S50.
85. Chang WS, Chang YH, Lu FJ, Chiang HC. Inhibitory effects of phenolics on xanthine oxidase. Anticancer Res 1994; 14:501–506.
86. Elliott AJ, Scheiber SA, Thomas C, Pardini RS. Inhibition of glutathione reductase by flavonoids. A structure–activity study. Biochem Pharmacol 1992; 44:1603–1608.
87. Rosenblat M, Belinky P, Vaya J, Levy R, Hayek T, Coleman R, Merchav S, Aviram M. Macrophage enrichment with the isoflavan glabridin inhibits NADPH oxidase-induced cell mediated oxidation of low density lipoprotein. J Biol Chem 1999; 274:13790–13799.
88. Welton A. Effect of flavonoids on arachidonic acid metabolism. In: Plant Flavonoids in Biology and Medicine. Vol 1. New York: Alan R Liss, 1986:231–242.
89. Hsiech R, German B, Kinsella J. Relative inhibitory potencies of flavonoids on 12-lipoxygenase of fish gill. Lipids 1988; 23:322–326.
90. Baumann J, Bruchhausen F, Wurm G. Flavonoids and related compounds as inhibitors of arachidonic acid peroxidation. Prostaglandins 1980; 20:627–639.
91. Luiz da Silva E, Tsushida T, Terao J. Inhibition of mammalian 15-lipoxygenase-dependent lipid peroxidation in low density lipoprotein by quercetin and queretin monoglucosides. Arch Biochem Biophys 1998; 349:313–320.
92. Negre–Salvayre A, Salvayre R. Quercetin prevents the cytotoxicity of oxidized LDL on lymphoid cell lines. Free Radic Biol Med 1992; 12:101–106.
93. Ferriola PC, Cody V, Middleton E Jr. Protein kinase C inhibition by plant flavonoids. Kinetic mechanisms and structure–activity relationships. Biochem Pharmacol 1989; 38:1617–1624.
94. Beretz A, Anton R, Stoclet J. Flavonoid compounds are potent inhibitors of cyclic AMP phosphodiesterase. Experientia 1978; 34:1054–1055.
95. Lindhal M, Tagesson C. Selective inhibition of groups II phospholipase A_2 by quercetin. Inflammation 1993; 17:573–582.
96. Fewtrell C, Gomperts B. Effect of flavone inhibitors of transport ATPases on histamine secretion from rat mast cells. Nature 1997; 265:635–636.
97. Brown JA, Khodr H, Hider RC, Rice–Evans C. Structural dependence of flavonoid interactions with Cu^{2+} ions: implications for their antioxidant properties. Biochem J 1998; 330:1173–1178.

98. Shahidi F, Wanasundara PK. Phenolic antioxidants. Crit Rev Food Sci Nutr 1992; 32:67–103.
99. Bors W, Heller W, Michel C, Saran M. Flavonoids as antioxidants: determination of radical-scavenging efficiencies. Methods Enzymol 1990; 186:343–355.
100. Afanas'ev IB, Dorozhko AI, Brodskii AV, et al. Chelating and free radical scavenging mechanisms of inhibitory action of rutin and quercetin in lipid peroxidation. Biochem Pharmacol 1989; 38:1763–1769.
101. Torel J, Cillard J, Cillard P. Antioxidant activity of flavonoids and reactivity with peroxyl radical. Phytochemistry 1986; 25:91–100.
102. Chen YT, Zheng RL, Jia ZJ, Ju Y. Flavonoids as superoxide scavengers and antioxidants. Free Radic Biol Med 1990; 9:19–21.
103. Morel I, Lescoat G, Cogrel P, et al. Antioxidant and iron-chelating activities of the flavonoids catechin, quercetin and diosmetin on iron-loaded rat hepatocytes cultures. Biochem Pharmacol 1993; 45:13–19.
104. Khoo JC, Miller E, McLoughlin P, Steinberg D. Prevention of low density lipoprotein aggregation by high density lipoprotein or apolipoprotein A-I. J Lipid Res 1990; 31:645–652.
105. Hagerman AE, Butler LG. The specificity of proanthocyanidin–protein interactions. J Biol Chem 1981; 156:4494–4498.
106. Mackness MI, Mackness B, Durrington PN, Fogelman AM, Berliner J, Lusis AJ, Navab M, Shih D, Fonarow GC. Paraoxonase and coronary heart disease. Curr Opin Lipidol 1998; 9:319–324.
107. Aviram M, Rosenblat M, Bisgaier CL, Newton RS, Primo–Parmo SL, La Du BN. Paraoxonase inhibits high density lipoprotein (HDL) oxidation and preserves its functions: a possible peroxidative role for paraoxonase. J Clin Invest 1998; 101:1581–1590.
108. Aviram M. Does paraoxonase play a role in susceptibility to cardiovascular disease? Mol Med Today 1999; 5:381–386.
109. Aviram M, Rosenblat M, Billecke S, Erogul J, Sorenson R, Bisgaier CL, Newton RS, La Du B. Human serum paraoxonase (PON 1) is inactivated by oxidized low density lipoprotein and preserved by antioxidants. Free Radic Biol Med 1999; 26:892–904.
110. Namiki M, Osawa T. Antioxidants/mutagens in foods. Basic Life Sci 1986; 39:131–142.
111. Shimoi K, Masuda S, Furugori M, Esaki S, Kinae N. Radioprotective effect of antioxidative flavonoids in gamma-ray irradiated mice. Carcinogenesis 1994; 15:2669–2672.
112. Brown JA, Khodr H, Hider RC, Rice–Evans C. Structural dependence of flavonoid interactions with Cu^{2+} ions: implications for their antioxidant properties. Biochem J 1998; 330:1173–1178.
113. Lotito SB, Fraga CB. (+)-Catechin prevents human plasma oxidation. Free Radic Biol Med 1998; 24:435–441.
114. Mangiapane H, Thomson J, Salter A, Brown S, Bell GD, White DA. The inhibition of the oxidation of low density lipoprotein by (+)-catechin, a naturally occurring flavonoid. Biochem Pharmacol 1992; 43:445–450.
115. De Whalley CV, Rankin SM, Hoult RS, Jessup W, Leake DS. Flavonoids inhibit the oxidative modification of low density lipoproteins by macrophages. Biochem Pharmacol 1990; 39:1743–1750.
116. Nardini M, D'Aquino M, Tomassi G, Gentili V, Di Felice M, Scaccini C. Inhibition of human low density lipoprotein oxidation by caffeic acid and other hydroxycinnamic acid derivatives. Free Radic Biol Med 1995; 19:541–552.
117. Vaya J, Belinky PA, Aviram M. Antioxidant constituents from licorice roots: isolation, structure elucidation and antioxidative capacity toward LDL oxidation. Free Radic Biol Med 1997; 23:302–313.
118. Belinky PA, Aviram M, Fuhrman B, Rosenblat M, Vaya J. The antioxidative effects of the isoflavan glabridin on endogenous constituents of LDL during is oxidation. Atherosclerosis 1998; 137:49–61.
119. Kuhnau J. The flavonoids: a class of semi-essential food components: their role in human nutrition. World Rev Nutr Diet 1976; 24:117–191.
120. Hertog MGL, Hollman POH, Katan MB, Kromhout D. Intake of potentially anticarcinogenic flavonoids and their determinants in adults in The Netherlands. Nutr Cancer 1993; 20:21–29.
121. Hollman PCH. Bioavailability of flavonoids. Eur J Clin Nutr 1997; 51(suppl 1):S66–S69.
122. Justesen U, Knuthsen P, Leth T. Determination of plant polyphenols in Danish foodstuffs by HPLC–UV and LC–MS detection. Cancer Lett 1997; 114:165–167.
123. Ameer B, Weintraub RA, Johnson JV, Yost RA, Rouseff RL. Flavanone absorption after naringin, hesperidin, and citrus administration. Clin Pharmacol Ther 1996; 60:33–40.

124. de Vries JH, Hollman PC, Meyboom S, Buysman MN, Zock PL, van Staveren WA, Katan MB. Plasma concentrations and urinary excretion of the antioxidant flavonols quercetin and kaempferol as biomarkers for dietary intake. Am J Clin Nutr 1998; 68:60–65.
125. Renaud S, de Lorgeril M. Wine alcohol, platelets and the French paradox for coronary heart disease. Lancet 1992; 339:1523–1526.
126. Soleas GJ, Diamandis EP, Goldberg DM. Wine as a biological fluid: history, production, and role in disease prevention. J Clin Lab Anal 1997; 11:287–313.
127. Hertog MGL, Hollman PCH, van de Putte B. Content of potentially anticarcinogenic flavonoids of tea infusions, wines, and fruit juices. J Agric Food Chem 1993; 41:1242–1246.
128. Whitehead TP, Robinson D, Allaway S, Syms J, Hale A. Effect of red wine ingestion on the antioxidant capacity of serum. Clin Chem 1995; 41:32–35.
129. Fuhrman B, Lavy A, Aviram M. Consumption of red wine with meals reduces the susceptibility of human plasma and LDL to undergo lipid peroxidation. Am J Clin Nutr 1995; 61:549–554.
130. Fuhrman B, Aviram M. White wine reduces LDL susceptibility to oxidation in vitro but not in vivo. Am J Clin Nutr 1996; 63:403–404.
131. Miyagi Y, Miwa K, Inoue H. Inhibition of human low density lipoprotein oxidation by flavonoids in red wine and grape juice. Am J Cardiol 1997; 80:1627–1631.
132. Nigdikar SV, Williams N, Griffin BA, Howard AH. Consumption of red wine polyphenols reduces the susceptibility of low density lipoproteins to oxidation in vivo. Am J Clin Nutr 1998; 68:258–265.
133. de Rijke YB, Demacker PN, Assen NA, Sloots LM, Katan MB, Stalenhoef AF. Red wine consumption does not affect oxidizability of low-density lipoprotein volunteers. Am J Clin Nutr 1996; 63:329–334.
134. Stein JH, Keevil JG, Wiebe DA, Aeschlimann S, Folts JD. Purple grape juice improves endothelial function and reduces the susceptibility of LDL cholesterol to oxidation in patients with coronary artery disease. Circulation 1999; 100:1050–1055.
135. Hayek T, Fuhrman B, Vaya J, Rosenblat M, Belinky P, Coleman R, Elis A, Aviram M. Reduced progression of atherosclerosis in the apolipoprotein E deficient mice following consumption of red wine, or its polyphenols quercetin or catechin, is associated with reduced susceptibility of LDL to oxidation and aggregation. Arterioscler Thromb Vasc Biol 1997; 17:2744–2752.
136. Aviram M, Hayek T, Fuhrman B. Red wine consumption inhibits LDL oxidation and aggregation in humans and in atherosclerotic mice. Biofactors 1997; 6:415–419.
137. Frankel EN, Waterhouse AL, Kinsella JE. Inhibition of oxidation human low density lipoprotein by phenolic substances in red wine. Lancet 1993;341:454–457.
138. Abu-Amsha R, Croft KD, Puddey IB, Proudfoot JM, Beilin LJ. Phenolic content of various beverages determines the extent of inhibition of human serum and low density lipoprotein oxidation in vitro: identification and mechanism of some cinnamic derivatives from red wine. Clin Sci 1996; 91:449–458.
139. Frankel EN, Waterhouse AL, Kinsella JE. Inhibition of human LDL oxidation by resveratrol. Lancet 1993; 341:1103–1104.
140. Manach C, Morand C, Texier O, Favier ML, Agullo G, Demigne C, Regerat F, Remesy C. Quercetin metabolites in plasma of rats fed diets containing rutin or quercetin. J Nutr 1995; 125:1911–1922.
141. Vinson JA, Dabbagh YA, Serry MM, Janj J. Plant flavonoids, especially tea flavonols, are powerful antioxidants using an in vitro model for heart disease. J Agric Food Chem 1995; 45:2800–2802.
142. Salah N, Miller NJ, Paganga G, Tijburg L, Bolwell GP, Rice–Evans C. Polyphenolic flavonols as scavengers of aqueous phase radicals and as chain-breaking antioxidants. Arch Biochem Biophys 1995; 322:339–346.
143. Lanninghamfoster L, Chen C, Chance DS, Loo G. Grape extract inhibits lipid peroxidation of human low density lipoprotein. Biol Pharm Bull 1995; 18:1347–1351.
144. Rao AV, Yatcilla MT. Bioabsorption and in vivo antioxidant properties of grape extract BioVin: a human intervention study. J Med Food 2000; 3:15–22.
145. Kerry NL, Abbey M. Red wine and fractionated phenolic compounds prepared from red wine inhibit low density lipoprotein oxidation in vitro. Atherosclerosis 1997; 135:93–102.
146. Fuhrman B, Buch S, Vaya J, Belinky PA, Coleman R, Hayek T, Aviram M. Licorice extract and its major polyphenol glabridin protect low-density lipoprotein against lipid peroxidation: in vitro and ex vivo studies in humans and in atherosclerotic apolipoprotein E-deficient mice. Am J Clin Nutr 1997; 66:267–275.

147. Haraguchi H, Ishikawa H, Mizutani K, Tamura Y, Kinoshita T. Antioxidative and superoxide scavenging activities of retrochalcones in *Glycyrrhiza inflata*. Bioorg Med Chem 1998; 6:339–347.
148. Belinky PA, Aviram M, Mahmood S, Vaya J. Structural aspects of the inhibitory effect of glabridin on LDL oxidation. Free Radic Biol Med 1998; 24:1419–1429.
149. Aviram M. Macrophage foam cell formation during early atherogenesis is determined by the balance between pro-oxidants and antioxidants in arterial cells and in blood lipoproteins: a need for a dual approach. Antiox Redox Signal 1999; 1:585–594.
150. Anthony MS, Clarkson TB, Williams JK. Effects of soy isoflavones on atherosclerosis: potential mechanisms. Am J Clin Nutr 1998; 68:1390S–1393S.
151. Piliang WG, Djojosoebagio S, Suprayogi A. Soybean hull and its effect on atherosclerosis in non-human primates. Biomed Environ Sci 1996; 9:137–143.
152. Arora A, Nair MG, Strasburg GM. Antioxidant activities of isoflavones and their biological metabolites in a liposomal system. Arch Biochem Biophys 1998; 356:133–141.
153. Lichtenstein AH. Soy protein, isoflavones and cardiovascular disease risk. J Nutr 1998; 128:1589–1592.
154. Kirk EA, Sutherland P, Wang SA, Chait A, LeBoeuf RC. Dietary isoflavones reduce plasma cholesterol and atherosclerosis in C57BL/6 mice but not LDL receptor-deficient mice. J Nutr 1998; 128:954–959.
155. Ruiz–Larrea MB, Mohan AR, Paganga G, Miller NJ, Bolwell GP, Rice–Evans CA. Antioxidant activity of phytoestrogenic isoflavones. Free Radic Res 1997; 26:63–70.
156. Tikkanen MJ, Wahala K, Ojala S, Vihma V, Adlercreutz H. Effect of soybean phytoestrogen intake on low density lipoprotein oxidation resistance. Proc Natl Acad Sci USA 1998; 95:3106–3110.
157. Kapiotis S, Hermann M, Held I, Seelos C, Ehringer H, Gmeiner BM. Genistein, the dietary-derived angiogenesis inhibitor, prevents LDL oxidation and protects endothelial cells from damage by atherogenic LDL. Arterioscler Thromb Vasc Biol 1997; 17:2868–2874.
158. Thelle DS. Coffee, tea and coronary heart disease. Curr Opin Lipidol 1995; 6:25–27.
159. Hertog MG, Feskens EJ, Hollman PC, Katan MB, Kromhout D. Dietary antioxidant flavonoids and risk of coronary heart disease: the Zutphen Elderly Study. Lancet 1993; 342:1007–1011.
160. Stensfold I, Tverdal A, Solvoll K, Foss PO. Tea consumption, relationship to cholesterol, blood pressure and coronary and total mortality. Prev Med 1992; 21:546–553.
161. Graham HN. Green tea composition, consumption and polyphenol chemistry. Prev Med 1992; 21:334–334.
162. Weisburger JH. Tea and health: the underlying mechanisms. Proc Soc Exp Biol Med 1999; 220:271–275.
163. van het Hof KH, de Boer HS, Wiseman SA, Lien N, Westrate JA, Tijburg LB. Consumption of green or black tea does not increase resistance of low density lipoprotein to oxidation in humans. Am J Clin Nutr 1997; 66:1125–1132.
164. McAnlis GT, McEneny J, Pearce J, Young IS. Black tea consumption does not protect low density lipoprotein from oxidative modification. Eur J Clin Nutr 1998; 52:202–206.
165. Princen HM, van Duyvennvoorde W, Buytenhek R, Blonk C, Tijburg LB, Langius JA, Meinders AE, Pijl H. No effect of consumption of green and black tea on plasma lipid and antioxidant levels and on LDL oxidation in smokers. Arterioscler Thromb Vasc Biol 1998; 18:833–841.
166. Serafini M, Ghiselli A, Ferro–Luzzi A. In vivo antioxidant effect of green and black tea in man. Eur J Clin Nutr 1996; 50:28–32.
167. Benzie IFF, Szeto YT, Tomlinson B, Strain JJ. Drinking green tea leads to a rapid increase in plasma antioxidant potential. In: Kumpulainen JT, Salonen JT, eds. Natural Antioxidants and Anticarcinogens in Nutrition, Health and Disease. London: Royal Society of Chemistry, 1999:280–282.
168. Ishikawa T, Suzukawa M, Ito T, Yioshida H, Ayaori M, Nishiwaki M, Yonemura A, Hara Y, Nakamura H. Effect of tea flavonoid supplementation on the susceptibility of low density lipoprotein to oxidative modification. Am J Clin Nutr 1997; 66:261–266.
169. Tijburg LB, Wiseman SA, Meijer GW, Weststrate JA. Effects of green tea, black tea and dietary lipophilic antioxidants on LDL oxidizability and atherosclerosis in hypercholesterolaemic rabbits. Atherosclerosis 1997; 135:37–47.
170. Yamanaka N, Oda O, Nagao S. Green tea catechins such as (−)-epicatechin and (−)-epigallocatechin accelerate Cu^{2+}-induced low density lipoprotein oxidation in propagation phase. FEBS Lett 1997; 20:230–234.

171. Ben Nasr C, Ayed N, Metche M. Quantitative determination of the polyphenolic content of pomegranate peel. Z Lebensm Unters Forsch 1996; 203:374–378.
172. Heftaman E, Bennett ST. Identification of estrone in pomegranate seeds. Phytochemistry 1966; 5:1337–1339.
173. Moneam NMA, El Sharasky AS, Badreldin MM. Oestrogen content of pomegranate seeds. J Chromatogr 1988; 438:438–442.
174. Sharaf A, Nigm SAR. The oestrogenic activity of pomegranate seed oil. J Endocrinol 1964; 29:91–92.
175. Shubert YS, Lansky EP, Neeman I. Antioxidant and eicosanoid enzyme inhibition properties of pomegranate seed oil and fermented juice flavonoids. J Ethnopharmacol 1999; 66:11–17.
176. Aviram M, Dornfeld L, Rosenblat M, Volkova N, Kaplan M, Coleman R, Hayek T, Presser D, Fuhrman B. Pomegranate juice consumption reduces oxidative stress, atherogenic modifications to LDL, and platelet aggregation: studies in humans and in atherosclerotic apolipoprotein E-deficient mice. Am J Clin Nutr 2000; 71:1062–1076.
177. Keys A. Mediterranean diet and public health: personal reflections. Am J Clin Nutr 1995; 61 (6 suppl):1321S–1323S.
178. Fidanza F, Puddu V, Imbimbo AB, Menotti A, Keys A. Coronary heart disease in seven countries. VII. Five-year experience in rural Italy. Circulation 1970; 41(4 suppl):I63–I75.
179. Visioli F, Galli C. Natural antioxidants and prevention of coronary heart disease: a potential role of olive oil and its minor constituents. Nutr Metab Cardiovasc Dis 1995; 5:306–314.
180. Das DK. Naturally occurring flavonoids: structure, chemistry, and high-performance liquid chromatography methods for separation and characterization. Methods Enzymol 1994; 234:410–420.
181. Aruoma OI. Nutrition and health aspects of free radicals and antioxidants. Food Chem Toxicol 1994; 32:671–683.
182. Visioli F, Galli C. The effect of minor constituents of olive oil on cardiovascular disease: new findings. Nutr Rev 1998; 56:142–147.
183. de la Puerta R, Ruiz Gutierrez V, Hoult JR. Inhibition of leukocyte 5-lipoxygenase by phenolics from virgin olive oil. Biochem Pharmacol 1999; 57:445–449.
184. Petroni A, Blasevich M, Papini N, Salami M, Sala A, Galli C. Inhibition of leukocyte leukotriene B4 production by an olive oil-derived phenol identified by mass-spectrometry. Thromb Res 1997; 87:315–322.
185. Visioli F, Bellosta S, Galli C. Oleuropein, the bitter principle of olives, enhances nitric oxide production by mouse macrophages. Life Sci 1998; 62:541–546.
186. Tsimikas S, Philis–Tsimikas A, Alexopoulos S, Sigari F, Lee C, Reaven PD. LDL isolated from Greek subjects on a typical diet or from American subjects on an oleate-supplemented diet induces less monocyte chemotaxis and adhesion when exposed to oxidative stress. Arterioscler Thromb Vasc Biol 1999; 19:122–130.
187. Aviram M, Eias K. Dietary olive oil reduces low-density lipoprotein uptake by macrophages and decreases the susceptibility of the lipoprotein to undergo lipid peroxidation. Ann Nutr Metab 1993; 37:75–84.
188. Wiseman SA, Mathot JN, de Fouw NJ, Tijburg LB. Dietary non-tocopherol antioxidants present in extra virgin olive oil increase the resistance of low density lipoprotein to oxidation in rabbits. Atherosclerosis 1996; 120:15–23.
189. Nicolaiew N, Lemort N, Adorni L, Berra B, Montorfano G, Rapelli S, Cortesi N, Jacotot B. Comparison between extra virgin olive oil and oleic acid rich sunflower oil: effects on postprandial lipemia and LDL susceptibility to oxidation. Ann Nutr Metab 1998; 42:251–260.
190. Visioli F, Bellomo G, Montedoro G, Galli C. Low density lipoprotein oxidation is inhibited in vitro by olive oil constituents. Atherosclerosis 1995; 117:25–32.
191. Visioli F, Galli C. Oleuropein protects low density lipoprotein from oxidation. Life Sci 1994; 55:1965–1971.
192. Visioli F, Bellomo G, Galli C. Free radical-scavenging properties of olive oil polyphenols. Biochem Biophys Res Commun 1998; 247:60–64.
193. Krishnakantha TP, Lokesh BR. Scavenging of superoxide anions by spice principles. Indian J Biochem Biophys 1993; 30:133–134.
194. Cao ZF, Chen ZG, Guo P, Zhang SM, Lian LX, Luo L, Hu WM. Scavenging effects of ginger on superoxide anion and hydroxyl radical. Chung-Kuo Chung Yao Tsa Chih 1993; 18:750–751, 764.
195. Reddy AA, Lokesh BR. Studies on spice principles as antioxidants in the inhibition of lipid peroxidation of rat liver microsomes. Mol Cell Biochem 1992; 111:117–124.

196. Guh JH, Ko FN, Jong TT, Teng CM. Antiplatelet effects of gingerol isolated from *Zingiber officinale*. J Pharm Pharmacol 1995; 47:329–332.
197. Ozaki Y, Kawahara N, Harada M. Anti-inflammatory effect of *Zingiber cassumunar* Roxb. and its active principles. Chem Pharm Bull (Tokyo) 1991; 39:2353–2356.
198. Bhandari U, Sharma JN, Zafar R. The protective action of ethanolic ginger (*Zingiber officinale*) extract in cholesterol fed rabbits. J Ethnopharmacol 1998; 61:167–171.
199. Sharma I, Gusain D, Dixit VP. Hypolipidaemic and antiatherosclerotic effects of *Zingiber officinale* in cholesterol fed rabbits. Phytol Res 1996; 10:517–518.
200. Fuhrman B, Rosenblat M, Hayek T, Coleman R, Aviram M. Ginger extract consumption reduces plasma cholesterol, inhibits LDL oxidation and attenuates development of atherosclerosis in atherosclerotic, apolipoprotein E-deficient mice. J Nutr 2000; 130:1124–1131.
201. Argawal KC. Therapeutic actions of garlic constituents. Med Res Rev 1996; 16:111-124.
202. Nagourney RA. Garlic: medicinal food or nutritious medicine? J Med Food 1998; 1:13–28.
203. Orekhov AN, Tertov VV, Sobenin IA, Pivovarova EM. Direct anti-atherosclerosis-related effects of garlic. Ann Med 1995; 27:63–65.
204. Orekhov AN, Grunwald AJ. Effects of garlic on atherosclerosis. Nutrition 1997; 13:656–663.
205. Berthold HK, Sudhop T. Garlic preparations for prevention of atherosclerosis. Curr Opin Lipidol 1998; 9:565–569.
206. Neil A, Silagy C. Garlic: its cardio-protective properties. Curr Opin Lipidol 1994; 5:6–10.
207. Lawson LD. Bioactive organosulfur compounds of garlic and garlic products. Role in reducing blood lipids. In: Kinghom AD, Balandrin MF, eds. Human Medicinal Agents from Plants. Washington, DC: American Chemical Society Books, 1983:308–330.
208. Fuhrman B, Volkova N, Rosenblat M, Aviram M. Lycopene synergistically inhibits LDL oxidation in combination with vitamin E, glabridin, rosmarinic acid, carnosic acid or garlic. Antiox Redox Signal 2000; 2:491–506.
209. Phelps S, Harris WS. Garlic supplementation and lipoprotein oxidation susceptibility. Lipids 1993; 28:475–477.
210. Orekhov AN, Pivovarova EM, Tertov VV. Garlic powder tablets reduce atherogenicity of low density lipoprotein. A placebo-controlled double-blind study. Nutr Metab Cardiovasc Dis 1996; 6:21–31.
211. Ide N, Nelson AB, Lau BH. Aged garlic extract and its constituents inhibit Cu(2+)-induced oxidative modification of low density lipoprotein. Planta Med 1997; 63:263–264.
212. Prasad K, Laxdal VA, Yu M, Raney BL. Evaluation of hydroxyl radical scavenging property of garlic. Mol Cell Biochem 1996; 154:55–63.
213. Carotenuto A, De Feo V, Fattorusso E, Lanzotti V, Magno S, Cicala C. The flavonoids of *Allium ursinum*. Phytochemistry 1996; 41:531–536.
214. Rabinkov A, Miron T, Konstantinovski L, Wilchek M, Mirelman D, Weiner L. The mode of action of allicin: trapping of radicals and interaction with thiol containing proteins. Biochim Biophys Acta 1998; 1379:233–244.
215. Eilat S, Oestraicher Y, Rabinkov A, et al. Alteration of lipid profile in hyperlipidemic rabbits by allicin, an active constituent of garlic. Coron Artery Dis 1995; 6:985–990.
216. Prasad K, Laxdal VA, Yu M, Raney BL. Antioxidant activity of allicin, an active principle in garlic. Mol Cell Biochem 1995; 148:183–189.
217. Offord EA, Mace K, Ruffieux C, Malnoe A, Pfeifer AMA. Rosemary components inhibit benzo(*a*)pyrene-induced genotoxicity in human bronchial cells. Carcinogenesis 1995; 16:2057–2062.
218. Wu JW, Lee MH, Ho CT, Chang SS. Elucidation of the chemical structures of natural antioxidants isolated from rosemary. J Am Oil Chem Soc 1982; 59:339–345.
219. Aruoma OI, Halliwell B, Aeschbach R, Loligers J. Antioxidant and pro-oxidant properties of active rosemary constituents: carnosol and carnosic acid. Xenobiotica 1992; 22:257–268.
220. Haraguchi H, Saito T, Okamura N, Yagi A. Inhibition of lipid peroxidation and superoxide generation by diterpenoids from *Rosmarinus officinalis*. Planta Med 1995; 61:333–336.
221. Aviram M. Review of human studies on oxidative damage and antioxidant protection related to cardiovascular disease. Free Rad Res 2000; 33:S85–S97.
222. Fuhrman B, Aviram M. Anti-atherogenicity of nutritional antioxidants. IDrugs 2001; 4:82–92.
223. Fuhrman B, Aviram M. Flavonoids protect LDL from oxidation and attenuate atherosclerosis. Curr Opin Lipidol 2001; 12:41–48.

17

Phytoestrogen Content in Foods and Their Role in Cancer

Anna H. Wu and Malcolm C. Pike
University of Southern California, Los Angeles, California

I. DEFINITION OF PHYTOESTROGENS

Very broadly, the term *phytoestrogens* refers to plant-derived compounds that show estrogen-like biological activity. In the last decade, attention has been focused on three classes of phytoestrogen: the isoflavonoids, the coumestans, and the lignan precursors (1–5). The main isoflavones are genistein, daidzein, and glycitein. Coumestrol (the most common coumestan) is not an isoflavone, but shares structural similarity with this compound. Isoflavones and coumestrols are found in relatively few foods. The main dietary sources of isoflavones are soybeans and its food products; staples in the traditional Asian diet (6). Sprouts including mung bean sprouts, soybean sprouts, and alfalfa sprouts are the richest source of coumestrol. These sprouts are not commonly consumed and, generally, in modest quantities, even if consumed (1). On the other hand, the lignan precursors, secoisolariciresinol and matairesinol, are ubiquitous in plant foods. Various food groups (e.g., grains and cereals, oilseeds and nuts, berries, fruits, and vegetables) and beverages (e.g., tea, coffee, and wine) are rich sources of these lignan precursors (7–10). Secoisolariciresinol and matairesinol are converted by bacteria in the intestinal tract to enterolactone and enterodiol, respectively (5).

Intake of foods rich in isoflavones, lignans, or both isoflavones and lignans, has been used to represent phytoestrogen intake in different studies (coumestrols are generally included under isoflavones if they are considered). We believe it is important to study the health effects associated with isoflavones and lignans separately. Our ability to assess intake of these two classes of phytoestrogen differs because isoflavones are found primarily in soybeans, whereas lignans are found in a much larger number of foods. In addition, the population groups with high intake of isoflavones may not have high intake of lignans, and vice versa. The biological activity of these two classes of phytoestrogens may also differ. Accurate food composition data for the specific class of phytoestrogen are essential to study the health effects of isoflavones and lignans. There are now concerted efforts to standardize the analysis and reporting of isoflavones and lignans in foods and to develop databases for these compounds (see following discussion).

A. Isoflavone Content of Foods

High-performance liquid chromatography (HPLC) is the method most often used to determine isoflavone levels in foods (11). In most soyfoods, the proportionate distribution of the three isoflavones, daidzein, genistein, and glycitein is 45, 45, and 10%, respectively (12,13). Each of the three isoflavones may occur in one of four possible forms (the aglycon, the glucoside, the malonylglucoside, and the acetylglucoside). Glucosides and malonylglucosides are the predominant forms (14). Reinli and Block (11) summarized the daidzein and genistein levels reported in plant foods from 22 studies that were published before 1996. The U.S. Department of Agriculture (USDA) and investigators at Iowa State University further developed this isoflavone database; it is now part of the electronic version of the *USDA Handbook No. 8 of Food Composition Data* (15). Thirty-eight peer-reviewed studies [24 were not in the study by Reinli and Block (11)] with relevant information were included and, whenever possible, glycitein values in foods were added to the database. The sum of the three isoflavones comprises the total isoflavone levels in the USDA database (15). To allow comparison among studies, both publications presented isoflavone levels on a wet weight basis by taking the reported values (if available) or by calculating this by assuming a given moisture content for that particular food (11,15). The main sources of isoflavones (in milligrams of isoflavone per gram wet weight) include soybeans (0.6–1.5 mg/g), soy flour (1.3–1.8 mg/g), soy protein isolate and concentrates (aqueous washed; 0.9–1.0 mg/g), and various traditional soyfoods, such as fermented soybeans (natto; 0.6 mg/g), fermented soy paste (miso; 0.4–0.6 mg/g), tempeh (0.4 mg/g), tofu (0.3–0.6 mg/g), and soy milk (0.05–0.12 mg/g) (11,15). There is a growing number of second-generation soyfoods that are made by adding soy ingredients to a variety of foods to replace animal protein, or as an extender. The isoflavone content of second-generation soyfoods, such as soy hot dogs (0.03–0.15 mg/g), soy bacon and hamburgers (0.01–0.12 mg/g), and soy cheese (0.06–0.3 mg/g) tends to be lower and more variable (11–13,15–17). Misclassification is more likely if an average isoflavone value is assigned to the various second-generation soyfoods. The USDA database (15) also included published data on levels of coumestrol, formononetin, and biochanin A (the latter two compounds are precursors of daidzein and genistein, respectively), confirming that alfalfa and clover sprouts are the richest sources of these compounds.

A question of interest is the extent of variability in isoflavone content in the same soyfoods. In a study of soybean varieties grown in the United States and Japan, isoflavone content was influenced largely by crop year, and to a lesser extent, by the variety or the location of crop (14). Differences in processing methods including the variability in moisture factor and the amount of nonsoy ingredients added also influence the isoflavone contents of various fermented and nonfermented Asian soyfoods (12,13,16,17). However, there are no consistent differences in isoflavone levels of commonly consumed traditional soyfoods (i.e., tofu and soymilk) that are produced in different regions of the United States (13), or in different countries (12) [selected soyfoods consumed in Hawaii and Singapore were compared (12)]. Raw and cooked forms of soyfoods also tend to show similar isoflavone values after adjustment of moisture factor (12,13).

Isoflavone levels in many legumes (other than soybeans), sprouts, vegetables, and fruits, are also available. Franke et al. (18) found measurable levels of daidzein and genistein in selected legumes and sprouts, although the levels were low, generally less than 1% of the levels in soybeans (fruits and vegetables were not included in this study). Mazur et al. (9) confirmed these findings in legumes and sprouts and reported no detectable isoflavone levels in some 25 commonly consumed fruits and vegetables (including cruciferous, allium, and other vegetables).

An emerging question is the relative importance of "hidden sources" of isoflavones (19–21). Some processed foods and meat-based mixed dishes may contain varying amounts and various types of soy ingredients (e.g., soy protein, soy flour). It is difficult to accurately assess exposure to these hidden sources of soy isoflavones, as the manufacturers' practice of adding soy ingredients may be brand- and product-specific, and variable over time. These hidden sources of soy intake are unlikely to be very important in epidemiological studies conducted in populations that consume traditional soyfoods, because Asian soyfoods would account for most of the isoflavones consumed. Average daily soyfood intake in Asia varied between 50 and 100 g/day (approximately 15–40 mg/day of isoflavones) in different studies (22–25). However, if an increasing number of products containing soy ingredients become available, and if the consumption of second-generation soyfoods becomes prevalent, then the assessment of isoflavone intake in epidemiological studies may be much more difficult.

B. Lignan Content of Foods

Direct and indirect analytical approaches have been used to determine lignan levels in foods. In the direct method, food samples are hydrolyzed, extracted, purified, and separated, and the lignans are silylated and analyzed using isotope dilution gas chromatography–mass spectrometry (ID–GC–MS–SIM) (9,10). In contrast, the indirect method involves in vitro fermentation with human fecal inoculum, followed by GC–MS analysis of the digesta for mammalian lignan (7,8). Lignan levels are highest in flaxseed; they are at least 20–30 times higher than the next group of foods that are rich in lignan (tea, berries, currants, dried seaweed, and cereal bran) (7–10,20,27). The lignan levels obtained using these two methods are not directly comparable. The direct method measures the lignan precursors (secoisolariciresinol and matairesinol), whereas the indirect method measures the mammalian lignans (enterolactone and enterodiol), resulting, after conversion of the lignan precursors by gut bacteria (27). Moreover, none of the studies actually analyzed the same foods using the two analytical methods and the specific foods that were tested differ in the different studies. In general, lignan levels for most foods for which comparisons could be made were higher when measured using the direct, rather than the indirect approach (20,27). A difference in the efficiency of the two extraction methods that are dependent on the the type of food has been suggested to partly explain the higher values using the in vitro fermentation approach (27).

II. PHYTOESTROGENS AND RISK OF CANCER

Adlercreutz (3), Setchell (5), and Messina and colleagues (6,34) were among the first to suggest that isoflavones and lignans (or foods rich in these compounds) may prevent breast and other hormone-related cancers. Although many investigators have focused on the antiestrogenic properties of various phytoestrogens in possibly preventing hormone-related cancers, there is also increasing evidence that the risk of nonhormone-related cancers may be also lowered. Antioxidant and various antitumor properties, including inhibition of angiogenesis, topoisomerase, and tyrosine kinase, are being vigorously investigated as other mechanisms of action of phytoestrogens (28–33). Thus, high intake of phytoestrogens may reduce the risk of nonhormonally dependent cancers as well as hormonally dependent cancers. In addition, the specific constituents in soybeans (i.e., isoflavones or some other constituents, such as protease inhibitors, phytic acid, saponins, or β-sitosterol) (6,28,35–37) that may confer protection against cancer need to be determined definitively.

A. Isoflavones and Cancer

The cancer sites we have included in this review are breast, endometrium, prostate, colorectum, stomach, and lung (see Sec. III). Results from published, peer reviewed, English-language analytic epidemiological studies that have data on dietary soy intake or urinary excretion of isoflavones on an individual level (isoflavone excretion is used as a marker of soy intake) are summarized in Tables 1–4. The epidemiological studies are presented by cancer site; the studies conducted in Asia are shown first, followed by those conducted outside of Asia. The specific soyfood(s) investigated and the definition of *high* and *low* soy intake are also described. In some studies, soy intake was estimated in terms of grams of soyfood intake per day (22,23,40,49,51,54,58,60). In other studies, the comparison was in terms of the frequency of intake of a specific soyfood (38,39,41–43,46,47,50,52,53,56,57,59). In one study, soy intake was expressed in terms of the milligrams of isoflavones consumed per day (48).

Before presenting the results from the epidemiological studies, it is necessary to discuss the assessment of soy intake in the studies to highlight some of the limitations of this evidence. Because most of these studies were not designed specifically to investigate the role of soyfood, the assessment varied in terms of the specific fermented (i.e., fermented soybean paste or fermented soybeans) and nonfermented soyfoods (i.e., soybeans, tofu, soymilk, and other processed tofu products, such as dried, fried, or pressed tofu) considered. Fermented soybean pastes and processed tofu products are usually used as condiments in cooking, whereas fermented soybeans and nonfermented soyfoods are typically consumed for nourishment (61). In most of the studies conducted among Chinese living in China, Taiwan, Singapore, or elsewhere in Asia, intake of both fermented and nonfermented soyfoods was assessed, and the risk of a particular cancer site was assessed, usually in relation to total soyfood intake. In contrast, some studies conducted in Japan asked only about miso intake (38,44) (a commonly consumed fermented soybean paste among Japanese); this single food represents approximately 25% of the total soy intake in Japan. In other studies (39,41,50,52,59), intake of tofu, representing approximately 45% of the total soy intake in Japan (24,25), was also asked. In almost all the studies conducted among native Japanese or those residing in Hawaii, the risk for a particular cancer site was assessed in relation to intake of miso or tofu separately. The findings associated with miso and tofu intake (if both foods were included) were usually not adjusted for each other (39,41,46,50,52,59), and an index of total soyfoods consumed was seldom calculated in the studies conducted among Japanese. Studies conducted among Asians and non-Asians residing in the United States or other Western countries usually used tofu as a marker of total soy intake (42,43,49), although some studies (54,60) also asked about intake of other soyfoods. The portion size of the soyfood eaten was usually absent in these studies. Because the different soyfoods may be used as a staple (for nourishment) or a condiment, the amount consumed may be particularly important. Thus, there is considerable heterogeneity in the specific soyfoods included and in the level of intake investigated in the different studies. In addition, the role of potential dietary confounders was not considered in most of these studies.

B. Lignans and Cancer

Lignans were first hypothesized to be protective against breast cancer on the basis of reports of higher excretion of enterolactone in women who were vegetarians, compared with omnivores and breast cancer patients (3,62). There is ongoing research to reconcile the differences in lignan levels obtained using the direct and indirect analytical methods (27). In one case–control study, the relation between intake of lignan precursors (secoisolariciresinol and matairesinol) and risk of prostate cancer (48) was investigated. Although one could also examine the relation between lignan-rich foods and risk of cancer, this method is not satisfactory, because lignans are found in many groups of foods (i.e., cereal, grains, legumes, berries or currants, tea, coffee, and alcohol beverage), some of which are also rich in fiber or various micronutrients. Flaxseed (or linseed), the single food that is richest in lignan content, is not typically consumed in the human diet. Thus, unlike the study of isoflavones, which is essentially the study of soyfoods, it is much more difficult to assess intake of lignans through food group analysis. Our discussion on lignans and cancer is limited to the few epidemiological studies with individual dietary data on lignan intake (48) or on urinary enterolactone and enterodiol levels (63).

III. SPECIFIC CANCER SITES

A. Breast Cancer

Table 1 summarizes published case–control and cohort studies with data on soy intake and breast cancer risk; results (if available) are shown separately for pre- and postmenopausal women. The strongest evidence that risk of breast cancer may be reduced in association with soy intake is found in two case–control studies (40,41) conducted in Asia and two other case–control studies conducted in the United States (42,43). A protective effect of soy was observed in both pre- and postmenopausal women in one study (43), but was found only among premenopausal

Table 1 Dietary Soy and Risk of Breast Cancer

Study (ref.), area	Soy food (highest vs. lowest level)	Premenopausal OR (95% CI)	Postmenopausal OR (95% CI)
Studies in Asia			
Cohort studies			
Hirayama 1990 (38), Japan	Miso: daily vs. nondaily	0.85 (0.7–1.1)[a]	
Key 1999 (39), Japan	Tofu: ≥5/wk vs. ≤1/wk	1.07 (0.8–1.5)[b]	
	Miso: ≥5/wk vs. ≤1/wk	0.91 (0.7–1.1)[b]	
Case–control studies			
Lee 1992 (40), Singapore	Soy products: 55+ g/d vs. <20.3 g/d	0.4 (0.2–0.9)[c]	1.1 (0.5–2.3)[c]
Hirose 1995 (41), Japan	Tofu: 3+/wk vs. <3/mo	0.8 (0.6–1.0)[d]	1.0 (0.7–1.3)[d]
	Miso: daily vs. less	1.2 (1.0–1.4)[d]	1.0 (0.8–1.2)[d]
Yuan 1995 (23), China	Soy protein: per 18 g/d		1.0 (0.7–1.4)[e]
Studies outside of Asia			
Case–control studies			
Witte 1997 (42), U.S. and Canada	Tofu: 1 serving/wk	0.5 (0.2–1.1)[f]	NA
Wu 1996 (43), Asian–Americans in California and Hawaii	Tofu dish: 55+/yr vs. <13/yr	0.7 (0.5–1.0)[g]	0.7 (0.4–1.3)[g]

[a] Adjusted for age.
[b] Adjusted for age, calendar period, age at and time of bombing, radiation dose.
[c] Adjusted for age, select menstrual and reproductive factors.
[d] Adjusted for age and year of first visit.
[e] Adjusted for age, energy, and various menstrual and reproductive factors.
[f] Adjusted for age, body mass index, alcohol, energy, and various menstrual and reproductive factors.
[g] Adjusted for age, ethnicity, study area, migration history, and select menstrual and reproductive factors.

women in the other two (40,41). [The study by Witte et al. (42) did not include postmenopausal women]. In contrast, soy intake was not associated with risk of breast cancer in two cohort studies of native Japanese (38,39) and in a large population-based case–control study conducted in Shanghai and Tianjin, China (23). Results were not presented by menopausal status in the two cohort studies (38,39) and were similar for both pre- and postmenopausal women in the case–control study in China (Yuan JM, personal communication).

In addition to the studies on dietary intake of soy, a possible protective role of high urinary excretion of phytoestrogen (as a marker of dietary intake of isoflavones and lignans) was suggested in two small case–control studies. In an Australian study, there was a statistically significant 50% reduction in risk of breast cancer among women whose urinary excretion of equol (a metabolite of daidzen) was in the upper three quartiles (63). However, risk was not significantly associated with urinary levels of daidzen (urinary genistein levels were not measured). This study also investigated the relation between breast cancer risk and urinary excretion of enterolactone, enterediol, and matairesinol. Risk was reduced by some 30 and 60%, respectively, among women whose urinary excretion of enterodiol and enterolactone was in the upper quartile; the finding for enterolactone was statistically significant (63). There was, however, a twofold increased risk associated with the upper three quartiles of matairesinol. The interrelations between these three lignans and the isoflavones were not discussed in this study. In addition, the level of isoflavone excretion was low, even among those in the highest excretion category, and it is unclear whether the effects of lignans and isoflavone were independent of each other.

In a study conducted in China (64), women who had total urinary isoflavone levels (based on daidzein, genistein, and glycitein) in the upper two tertiles showed a statistically nonsignificant 50% reduction in risk of breast cancer, compared with those in the lowest tertile. There was a statistically significant reduction in risk (RR $= 0.14$) for those who displayed high-excretion levels of both isoflavones and phenol (a surrogate marker of fruit and vegetable intake) (64).

Both biomarker studies are limited, in that the urine specimens from breast cancer patients were obtained after their diagnosis and treatment. These results are meaningful only if the intake of foods rich in isoflavone and lignan did not change after cancer diagnosis. Data on intake of soy- or lignan-rich foods were also unavailable in the Australian study and were described only for controls in the Chinese study (26).

B. Endometrial Cancer

In a case–control study of endometrial cancer in Hawaii, Goodman et al. (60) reported a statistically significant 40% reduced risk of endometrial cancer in association with increasing intake of soy. This association was found for intake of tofu, tofu and other soy products, and all legumes combined (i.e., including tofu) after adjustment for total calories and nondietary risk factors. The protective effects of soy (and legumes) were observed in both Asians and nonAsians in this study.

In a case–control study conducted in Shanghai, China, intake of legumes was not associated with risk of endometrial cancer (65). However, it is unclear whether soyfoods were included under "legumes" in this study. Thus, data are currently sparse, and additional studies are needed to determine the role of soybeans in endometrial cancer.

C. Prostate Cancer

The strongest evidence that risk of prostate cancer may be reduced in association with soy (mainly nonfermented soyfoods, such as tofu) intake is found in two cohort (46,47) and two case–control studies conducted in the United States (48,49) (Table 2). In the cohort of Seventh Day Adventists in California, daily intake of soymilk, compared with no intake, was associated with a statistically significant 70% reduction in prostate cancer risk (47). In a cohort of Japanese in Hawaii, high (5+/week) intake of tofu compared with intake once per week or less was also associated with a statistically significant 65% reduction in risk (46). Similarly, a protective effect of nonfermented soyfoods is suggested in a large case–control study conducted among Asian–Americans, African–Americans, and whites in North America (49). Highest quintile of tofu intake (> 39.4 g/day; this is equivalent to 12 mg/day of isoflavones by assuming 0.3 mg of isoflavones per gram of tofu) was associated with a 40% lower risk of prostate cancer (p trend = 0.06). As discussed in the following, the protective effect in this study may be partly due to intake of all legumes, and not specifically to intake of soyfoods. Investigators of a small, hospital-based case–control study conducted among white men in Texas reported a protective effect of soy, based on estimated dietary intake of genistein and daidzein (48).

Table 2 Dietary Soy and Risk of Prostate Cancer

Study (ref.), area	Soy food (highest vs. lowest level of intake)	Odds ratio (95% CI) (lowest level as baseline)
Studies in Asia		
Cohort studies		
Hirayama 1990 (38), Japan	Miso: daily vs. nondaily	1.4 (1.1–1.9)[a]
Case–control studies		
Oishi 1988 (44), Japan	Miso: high vs. < low	1.29 (0.6–2.9)[b]
		0.64 (0.3–1.3)[c]
Lee 1998 (45), China	7 soy foods	Mean soy intake: 71 g/day in cases vs. 84 g/day in controls
Studies outside of Asia		
Cohort studies		
Severson 1989 (46), Japanese in Hawaii	Miso: 5+/wk vs. ≤1/wk	1.24 (0.5–3.0)[a]
	Tofu: 5+/wk vs. ≤1/wk	0.35 (0.1–1.4)[a], p trend = 0.05
Jacobsen 1998 (47), Seventh Day Adventist in California	Soymilk: >1/day vs. never	0.3 (0.1–0.9)[d], p trend = 0.02
Case–control studies		
Strom 1998 (48), Texas	Genistein (0.03 mg/day)[e]	0.71 (0.4–1.3)[f]
	Daidzein (0.02 mg/day)[e]	0.57 (0.3–1.0)[f]
Kolonel (2000) (49) California, Hawaii, and British Columbia, Canada	Tofu: >39.4 g/day vs. none/day	0.62 (0.4–0.9)[g], p trend = 0.06

[a] Adjusted for age.
[b] Subjects with benign prostatic hyperplasia served as controls.
[c] Hospital controls.
[d] Adjusted for age, body mass index, coffee, whole-fat milk, eggs, citrus fruit, and age at first marriage.
[e] Median intake among controls.
[f] Adjusted for age, family history of prostate cancer, alcohol intake, and total caloric intake.
[g] Adjusted for age, education, ethnicity, calories, and saturated fat.

However, the interpretation of this finding is questionable because the intake of isoflavones was extremely low in this population, less than 0.1 mg/day of isoflavones (48), compared with average daily isoflavone intake of 15–40 mg in Asia (24–26). In a case–control study conducted in China, average daily intake of soy (based on seven soyfoods) was lower among prostate cancer cases (71 g/day), compared with population controls (84 g/day) (45).

In contrast, two studies from Japan suggest that the risk of prostate cancer may be increased in association with high intake of miso (38,44); the result was statistically significant in one (38; see Table 2). An increased risk of prostate cancer in association with miso intake was also reported in the cohort study of Japanese men in Hawaii (46). In both studies in Japan, intake of nonfermented soyfoods was unavailable (38,44).

These results suggest that there may be a different effect of fermented and nonfermented soyfoods. Data on intake of both types of soyfoods are needed to sort out this issue. In addition, intake of legumes needs to be considered carefully in studies on soyfoods, as these foods have been associated with a reduced risk of prostate cancer in other cohort (66,67) and case–control (68) studies. It is notable that Mills et al. (67) and Jacobsen et al. (47) studied the same cohort of Seventh Day Adventists. Mills et al. (67) reported a statistically nonsignificant, reduced risk of prostate cancer in association with intake of vegetarian protein products. It is not known whether intake of legume and vegetarian protein was considered in the reported soymilk–prostate cancer association (47).

In the small case–control study mentioned earlier, Strom et al. (48) reported no significant association between risk of prostate cancer and dietary intake of lignan precursors.

D. Colorectal Cancer

Table 3 shows results on soy intake and risk of colon and rectum cancer separately or the two sites combined. In studies conducted in Asia and Hawaii, there is little convincing evidence that intake of fermented soyfoods significantly influence the risk of colon or rectal cancers (38,50,52,53). Of the four studies with data on tofu or soyfoods, excluding miso (50,51,52,54), a statistically significant lower risk of rectal cancer in association with high intake was reported in one study (52). With the exception of one case–control study (54), most of the other studies had relatively modest numbers of colorectal cancers (range was 93–336 cases). The small numbers may have partly contributed to some of the inconsistent subsite-specific results that have been reported (Table 3).

The role of soyfoods was investigated in two studies of colorectal polyps. In a study of adenomas of sigmoid colon in Japan, risk of polyps did not differ between those who consumed miso daily, compared with those who consumed less frequently (69). In a study of polyps conducted in Southern California, risk of polyps was reduced by 45% among those consumed tofu or soybeans at least once a week, compared with nonconsumers; this finding was not statistically significant (70).

E. Stomach Cancer

We recently conducted a metanalysis to examine the relation between fermented and non-fermented soyfoods and risk of stomach cancer, by including some 20 studies of diet and stomach cancer that were conducted in Asia or among Asians living in the United States (71). Our pooled analysis of 14 studies with data on fermented soyfoods yielded a statistically significant 26% increased risk in association with high intake of fermented soyfoods. In contrast, our pooled analysis of 10 studies with data on nonfermented soyfoods found a statistically significant 28% reduced risk in association with high intake of these foods. However, further

Table 3 Intake of Soy Foods and Risk of Colorectal Cancer

Study (Ref.) area	Soy food (highest vs. lowest level of intake)	Odds ratio (95% CI)
Studies in Asia		
Cohort studies		
Hirayama 1990 (38), Japan	Miso: daily vs. nondaily	1.13 (0.97–1.32) [colon][a] 1.04 (0.89–1.21) [rectum]
Case-control studies		
Tajima 1985 (50), Japan	Miso: 1+/d vs. < daily	0.5 [colon][b] 2.0 [rectum]*
	Tofu: 4+/wk vs. <1/wk	1.1 [colon] 1.6 [rectum]
Hu 1991 (51), China	Soyfoods: >27 g/day vs. <4.1 g/day	No association [colorectum, males/females][c] No association [rectum, females] 0.3 (p < 0.05) [rectum, males]
Hoshiyama, 1993 (52), Japan	Miso: 2+/day vs. < daily	1.9 (0.8–4.4) [colon][b] 0.8 (0.4–1.6) [rectum]
	Soybean products: 8+/wk vs. ≤4/wk	0.6 (0.3–1.3) [colon] 0.4 (0.2–0.9)* [rectum]
Studies outside of Asia		
Case–control studies		
Haenszel 1973 (53), Hawaii	Fermented soybeans: above vs. below average intake	1.6 [colorectum][a]
LeMarchand 1997 (54), Hawaii	Tofu: >24.7 g/day vs. none	1.0 [colorectum, males][d] 0.9 [colorectum, females]

[a] Adjusted for age.
[b] Adjusted for age and sex.
[c] Adjustment was not described.
[d] Adjusted for age, family history, alcohol, smoking, physical activity, body mass index, calories and other dietary factors.
*p trend < 0.05.

analyses suggest that fermented and nonfermented soyfoods may be associated with salt and fruit or vegetable intake, respectively. Salt and fruit or vegetable intake are directly associated with stomach cancer risk (72). In most of the studies we reviewed, the possible confounding role of fruit and vegetable intake, salt, and other compounds such as N-nitroso compounds, had not been considered in the analyses on soyfoods. Thus, the role of soyfoods in the etiology of stomach cancer cannot be determined with confidence until the roles of potential confounders, including, in particular, salt, N-nitroso compounds, and fruit and vegetable intake, are more adequately adjusted.

F. Lung Cancer

Intake of soyfoods and risk of lung cancer have been investigated in a Japanese cohort (38) and case–control studies conducted in Japan (59) and among Chinese residing in Hong Kong (55), and several lung cancer high-risk areas in China (56–58) (Table 4). In four studies, there is some suggestion of a reduction in lung cancer risk in association with the highest level of intake

Table 4 Intake of Soy Foods and Risk of Lung Cancer

Study (Ref.) area	Soy food (highest vs. lowest level)	Odds ratio (95% CI)
Cohort studies		
Hirayama 1990 (38), Japan	Soybean paste soup	
	Daily vs. nondaily	1.06 (0.97–1.15)[a]
Case–control studies		
Koo 1988 (55), Hong Kong	Tofu/soy products	
	High vs. low	0.5[b]*
Wu–Williams 1990 (56), Northern China	Soybean products (times/yr)	
	>458 vs. <153	1.0[c]*
Swanson 1992 (57) Yunnan, China	Bean curd	
	>15.9/mo vs. <8/mo	0.44[d], p trend < 0.01
Hu 1997 (58), Northern China	Soybean product	
	>21.9 g/day vs. <5.5 g/day	0.6[e], p trend = 0.10
Wakai 1999 (59), Japan	Miso soup	
	31/day vs. not daily	3.8[f], p trend = .001 (males)
	31/day vs. not daily	4.0, p trend = .04 (females)
	Tofu	
	Almost daily vs. less	0.7, p < 0.10 (males)
	Almost daily vs. less	1.0, p > 0.05 (females)
	Soybeans	
	≥1–2×/wk vs. <1/mo	0.6, p trend = .05 (males)
	≥1–2×/wk vs. <1/mo	1.1, p trend = 0.9 (females)

*p trend > 0.05.
[a] Adjusted for age.
[b] Adjusted for age, number of births, and education.
[c] Adjusted for age, education, smoking, and study area.
[d] Adjusted for age, respondent type, study site, and education.
[e] Adjusted for cigarettes/day, duration of smoking, and family income.
[f] Adjusted for education, smoking, and medical history of lung disease.

of nonfermented soy foods (55,57–59); the result was statistically significant among males in two studies (57,59). However, in two other studies, intake of soybeans (56) and miso (38) was not associated with lung cancer risk, and in a third study, intake of miso was associated with a statistically significant increased risk (59).

IV. SUMMARY

The evidence on the role of soy and the cancer sites discussed in the following is inconclusive. The results tended to differ among studies conducted in Asia and those conducted in the United States, and among studies that asked about intake of fermented (represented mainly by miso intake) or nonfermented soyfoods. The evidence suggests that miso intake is either not associated with cancer risk, or it may be associated with an increased risk of prostate, stomach, and lung cancer. There is insufficient data at this time to determine whether an increased risk associated with miso is real or spurious. It may be that intake of miso is confounded by some other dietary factors (such as dietary salt intake in studies of stomach cancer) or there may be actual harmful effects of fermented soyfoods. On the other hand, the results tend to suggest that high intake of tofu or nonfermented soyfoods may be associated with reduced risks of breast, prostate, endometrium, stomach, and lung cancer. However, it is also uncertain whether these protective effects are real or spurious. A reduced risk may be observed because there are truly protective constituents in these foods. Alternatively, it is also plausible that high intake of tofu is associated with generally high intake of plant foods, and the protection is not specific for soyfoods. Unfortunately, only a few studies considered the major dietary confounders in their analysis of soyfood. In the study by Yuan et al. (23), soyfood intake was not associated with risk of breast cancer before or after adjustment for the other dietary factors (high intake of dietary fiber was associated with significantly lower risk in this study). In the study by Hoshiyama et al. (73), intake of nonfermented soyfoods was associated with a significantly lower risk of stomach cancer, but this finding was largely eliminated when intake of other dietary factors (including vegetables, miso, or salt intake) was considered in the analysis.

More standardized and complete assessment of the major fermented and nonfermented soyfoods is clearly needed in future epidemiological studies. Portion size of soyfood intake may be particularly important, as many of the fermented soyfoods are used as condiments, and the nonfermented soyfoods are eaten for nourishment. Such improved assessment will allow analysis by intake of isoflavone and by specific soyfoods (or group of soyfoods). Information on dose–response relations will also help to further our understanding of the role of this group of foods. Finally, careful consideration of potential dietary and nondietary confounders is needed to sort out the independent effects of fermented and nonfermented soyfoods.

REFERENCES

1. Verdeal K, Ryan DS. Naturally occurring estrogens in plant foodstuffs—a review. J Food Protect 1979; 42:577–583.
2. Setchell KDR, Lawson AM, Mitchell FL, Adlercreutz H, Kirk DN, Axelson M. Lignans in man and in animal species. Nature 1980; 287:740–742.
3. Adlercreutz H, Fotsis T, Heikkinen R, Dwyer JT, Woods M, Goldin BR, Gorbach SL. Excretion of the lignans enterolactone and enterodiol and of equol in omnivorous and vegetarian postmenopausal women and in women with breast cancer. Lancet 1982; 2:1295–1298.
4. Price KR, Fenwick GR. Naturally occurring oestrogens in foods—a review. Food Addit Contam 1985; 2:73–106.
5. Setchell KDR, Adlercreutz H. Mammalian lignans and phytoestrogens recent studies on their formation, metabolism and biological role in health and disease. In: Rowland IR, ed. Role of the Gut Flora in Toxicity and Cancer. San Diego, CA: Academic Press, 1988: pp. 315–345.
6. Messina M, Barnes S. The role of soy products in reducing risk of cancer. J Natl Cancer Inst 1991; 83:541–546.
7. Thompson LU, Robb P, Serraino M, Cheung F. Mammalian lignan production from various foods. Nutr Cancer 1991; 16:43–52.
8. Thompson LU. Experimental studies on lignans and cancer. Bailliere's Clin Endocrinol Metab 1998; 12:691–705.
9. Mazur W. Phytoestrogen content in foods. Bailliere's Clin Endocrinol Metab 1998; 12:729–742.
10. Mazur WM, Duke JA, Wahala K, Rasku S, Adlercreutz H. Isoflavonoids and lignans in legumes: nutritional and health aspects in humans. J Nutr Biochem 1998; 9:193–200.
11. Reinli K, Block G. Phytoestrogen content of foods—a compendium of literature values. Nutr Cancer 1996; 26:123–148.
12. Franke AA, Hankin JH, Yu MC, Maskarinec G, Low SH, Custer LJ. Isoflavone levels in soy foods consumed by multiethnic populations in Singapore and Hawaii. J Agric Food Chem 1999; 47:977–986.
13. Murphy PA, Song TT, Buseman G, Barua K, Beecher GR, Trainer D, Holden J. Isoflavones in retail and institutional soy foods. J Agric Food Chem 1999; 47:2697–2704.

14. Wang HJ, Murphy PA. Isoflavone composition of American and Japanese soybeans in Iowa: effects of variety, crop year, and location. J Agric Food Chem 1996; 42:1674–1677.
15. USDA Handbook No. 8 at http://www.nal.fnic/foodcom/Data/index.html.
16. Wang HJ, Murphy PA. Isoflavone content in commercial soybean foods. J Agric Food Chem 1994; 42:1666–1673.
17. Coward L, Barnes NC, Setchell KDR, Barnes S. Genistein, daidzein, and their β-glycoside conjugates: antitumor isoflavones in soybean foods from American and Asian diets. J Agric Food Chem 1993; 4:1961–1967.
18. Franke AA, Custer LJ, Wang W, Shi CY. Analysis of isoflavonoids and other phenolic agents from foods and from human fluids. Proc Soc Exp Biol Med 1995; 217:263–273.
19. Lampe JW, Gustafson DR, Hutchins AM, Martini MC, Li S, Wahala K, Grandits G, Potter DJ, Slavin JL. Urinary isoflavonoid and lignan excretion on a Western diet: relation to soy, vegetable and fruit intake. Cancer Epidemiol Biomarkers Prev 1999; 8:699–707.
20. Pillow PC, Duphorne CM, Chang S, Contois JH, Strom SS, Spitz MR, Hursting SD. Development of a database for assessing dietary phytoestrogen intake. Nutr Cancer 1999; 33:3–19.
21. Horn-Ross PL, Barnes S, Lee M, Coward L, Mandel JE, Koo J, John EM, Smith M. Assessing phytoestrogen exposure in epidemiologic studies: development of a database (United States). Cancer Causes Control 2000; 11:289–298.
22. Lee HP, Gourley L, Duffy SW, Esteve J, Lee J, Day NE. Dietary effects on breast-cancer risk in Singapore. Lancet 1991; 331:1197–1200.
23. Yuan JM, Wang QS, Ross RK, Henderson BE, Yu MC. Diet and breast cancer in Shanghai and Tianjin, China. Br J Cancer 1995; 71:1353–1358.
24. Nagata C, Takatsuka N, Kurisau Y, Shimizu H. Decreased serum total cholesterol concentration is associated with high intake of soy products in Japanese men and women. J Nutr 1998; 128:209–213.
25. Wakai K, Egami I, Kato K, Kawamura T, Tamakoshi A, Lin Y, Nakayama T, Wada M, Ohno Y. Dietary intake and sources of isoflavones among Japanese. Nutr Cancer 1999; 33:139–145.
26. Chen Z, Zheng W, Custer LJ, Dai Q, Shu XO, Jin F, Franke AA. Usual dietary consumption of soy foods and its correlation with the excretion rate of isoflavonoids in overnight urine samples among Chinese women in Shanghai. Nutr Cancer 1999; 33:82–87.
27. Meagher LP, Beecher GR. Assessment of data on the lignan content of foods. J Food Comp 2000; 13:935–947.
28. Adlercreutz H, Mazur W. Phyto-oestrogens and Western diseases. Ann Med 1997; 29:95–120.
29. Barnes S. Phytoestrogens and breast cancer. Bailliere's Clin Endocrinol Metab 1998; 12:559–579.
30. Thompson LU. Experimental studies on lignans and cancer. Bailliere's Clin Endocrinol Metab 1998; 12:691–705.
31. Bingham SA, Atkinson C, Liggins J, Bluck L, Coward A. Phytoestrogens: where are we now? Br J Nutr 1998; 79:393–406.
32. Messina MJ, Bennick M. Soyfoods, isoflavones and risk of colonic cancer: a review of the in vitro and in vivo data. Bailliere's Clin Endocrinol Metab 1998; 12:707–728.
33. Setchell KDR, Cassidy A. Dietary isoflavones: biological effects and relevance to human health. J Nutr 1999; 129:758S–767S.
34. Messina MJ, Persky V, Setchell KDR, Barnes S. Soy intake and cancer risk: a review of the in vitro and in vivo data. Nutr Cancer 1994; 21:113–131.
35. Kurzer M, Xu X. Dietary phytoestrogens. Annu Rev Nutr 1997; 17:353–381.
36. Fournier DB, Erdman JW Jr, Gordon GB. Soy, its components, and cancer prevention: a review of the in vitro, animal, and human data. Cancer Epidemiol Biomarkers Prev 1998; 7:1055–1065.
37. Kennedy AR. Chemopreventive agents: protease inhibitors. Pharmacol Ther 1998; 78:167–208.
38. Hirayama T. Life-style and mortality. A large-scale census-based cohort study in Japan. In: Wahrendorf J, ed. Contributions to Epidemiology and Biostatistics. Vol. 6. Basel: Karger, 1990.
39. Key TJ, Sharp GB, Appleby PN, Beral V, Goodman MT, Soda M, Mabuchi K. Soya foods and breast cancer risk: a prospective study in Hiroshima and Nagasaki, Japan. Br J Cancer 1999; 81:1248–1256.
40. Lee HP, Gourley L, Duffy SW, Esteve J, Lee J, Day NE. Risk factors for breast cancer by age and menopausal status: a case–control study in Singapore. Cancer Causes Control 1992; 3:313–322.
41. Hirose K, Tajima K, Hamajima N, Inoue M, Takezaki T, Kuroishi T, Yoshida M, Tokudome S. A large-scale, hospital-based case–control study of risk factors of breast cancer according to menopausal status. Jpn J Cancer Res 1995; 86:146–154.

42. Witte JS, Ursin G, Siemiatycki J, Thompson WD, Paganini–Hill A, Haile RW. Diet and premenopausal bilateral breast cancer: a case–control study. Breast Cancer Res Treat 1997; 42:243–251.
43. Wu AH, Ziegler RC, Horn–Ross PL, Nomura AMY, West DW, Kolonel LN, Rosenthal JR, Hoover RN, Pike MC. Tofu and risk of breast cancer in Asian–Americans. Cancer Epidemiol Biomarkers Prev 1996; 5:901–906.
44. Oishi K, Okada K, Yoshida O, Yamaba H, Ohno K, Hayes RB, Schroeder FH. A case–control study of prostatic cancer with reference to dietary habits. Prostate 1988; 12:179–190.
45. Lee MM, Wang RT, Hsing AW, Gu FL, Wang T, Spitz M. Case–control study of diet and prostate cancer in China. Cancer Causes Control 1998; 9:545–552.
46. Severson RK, Nomura AMY, Grove JS, Stemmermann GN. A prospective study of demographics, diet, and prostate cancer among men of Japanese ancestry in Hawaii. Cancer Res 1989; 49:1857–1860.
47. Jacobsen BK, Knutsen SF, Fraser GE. Does high soy milk intake reduce prostate cancer incidence? The Adventist Health Study (United States). Cancer Causes Control 1998; 9:553–557.
48. Strom SS, Yamamura Y, Duphorne CM, Spitz MR, Babaian RJ, Pillow PJ, Hursting SD. Phytoestrogen intake and prostate cancer: a case–control study using a new database. Nutr Cancer 1999; 33:20–25.
49. Kolonel LN, Hankin JH, Whittemore AS, Wu AH, Gallagher RP, Wilkens LR, John ER, Howe GR, Dreon DM, West DW, Paffenbarger RS Jr. Vegetables, fruits, legumes and prostate cancer: a multiethnic case–control study. Cancer Epidemiol Biomarkers Prev 2000; 9:795–804.
50. Tajima K, Tominaga S. Dietary habits and gastro-intestinal cancers: a comparative case–control study of stomach and large intestinal cancers in Nagoya, Japan. Jpn J Cancer Res (Gann) 1985; 76:705–716.
51. Hu J, Liu Y, Yu Y, Zhao T, Liu S, Wang Q. Diet and cancer of the colon and rectum: a case-control study in China. Int J Epidemiol 1991; 20:362–367.
52. Hoshiyama Y, Sekine T, Sasaba T. A case–control study of colorectal cancer and its relation to diet, cigarettes, and alcohol consumption in Saitama Prefecture, Japan. Tohoku J Exp Med 1993; 171:153–165.
53. Haenszel W, Berg JW, Segi M, Kurihara M, Locke FB. Large-bowel cancer in Hawaiian Japanese. J Natl Cancer Inst 1980; 51:1765–1779.
54. Le Marchand L, Hankin JH, Wilkens LR, Kolonel LN, Englyst HN, Lyu LC. Dietary fiber and colorectal cancer risk. Epidemiology 1997; 8:658–665.
55. Koo LC. Dietary habits and lung cancer risk among Chinese females in Hong Kong who never smoked. Nutr Cancer 1988; 11:155–172.
56. Wu–Williams AH, Dai XD, Blot W, Xu ZY, Sun XW, Xiao HP, Stone BJ, Yu SF, Feng YP, Ershow AG, Sun J, Fraumeni JR Jr, Henderson BE. Lung cancer among women in north-east China. Br J Cancer 1990; 62:982–987.
57. Swanson CA, Mao BL, Li JY, Lubin JH, Yao SX, Wang JZ, Cai SK, Hou Y, Luo QS, Blot WJ. Dietary determinants of lung cancer risk: results from a case–control study in Yunnan Province, China. Int J Cancer 1992; 50:876–880.
58. Hu J, Johnson KC, Mayo Y, Xu T, Lin Q, Wang C, Zhao F, Wang G, Chen Y, Yang Y. A case–control study of diet and lung cancer in northeast China. Int J Cancer 1997; 71:924–931.
59. Wakai K, Ohno Y, Genka Y, Ohmine K, Kawamura T, Tamakoshi A, Lin Y, Nakayama T, Aoki K, Fukuma S. Risk modification in lung cancer by a dietary intake of preserved foods and soyfoods: findings from a case–control study in Okinawa, Japan. Lung Cancer 1999; 25:147–169.
60. Goodman MT, Wilkens LR, Hankin JR, Lyu LC, Wu AH, Kolonel LN. Association of soy and fiber consumption with the risk of endometrial cancer. Am J Epidemiol 1997; 146:294–306.
61. Liu K. Oriental soyfoods. In: Ang CYW, Liu K, Huang YW, eds. Asian Foods Science and Technology. Lancaster, PA: Technomic Publishing, 1999.
62. Adlercreutz H, Fotsis T, Bannwart C. Determination of urinary lignans and phytoestrogen metabolites, potential antiestrogens and anticarcinogens, in urine of women on various habitual diets. J Steroid Biochem Mol Biol 1986; 25:791–797.
63. Ingram D, Sanders K, Kolybaba M. Case–control study of phyto-estrogens and breast cancer. Lancet 1997; 350:990–994.
64. Zheng W, Dai Q, Custer LJ, et al. Urinary excretion of isoflavonoids and the risk of breast cancer. Cancer Epidemiol Biomarkers Prev 1999; 8:35–40.

65. Shu XO, Zheng W, Potischman N, et al. A population-based case–control study of dietary factors and endometrial cancer in Shanghai, People's Republic of China. Am J Epidemiol 1993; 137:155–165.
66. Schuurman AG, Goldbohm RA, Dorant E, van den Brandt PA. Vegetable and fruit consumption and prostate cancer risk: a cohort study in The Netherlands. Cancer Epidemiol Biomarkers Prev 1998; 7:673–680.
67. Mills PK, Beeson L, Phillips RL, Fraser GE. Cohort study of diet, lifestyle, and prostate cancer in Adventist Men. Cancer 1989; 64:598–604.
68. Key TJA, Silcocks PB, Davey GK, et al. A case–control study of diet and prostate cancer. Br J Cancer 1997; 76:678–687.
69. Kono S, Imanishi K, Shinchi K, Yanai F. Relationship of diet to small and large adenomas of the sigmoid colon. Jpn J Cancer Res 1993; 84:13–19.
70. Witte JS, Longnecker MP, Bird CL, Lee ER, Frankl HD, Haile RW. Relation of vegetable, fruit, and grain consumption to colorectal adenomatous polyps. Am J Epidemiol 1996; 144:1015–1025.
71. Wu AH, Yang D, Pike MC. Soy foods and risk of stomach cancer—the problem of potential confounders. Cancer Epidemiol Biomarkers Prev 2000; 9:1051–1058.
72. Nomura A. Stomach cancer. In: Schottenfeld D, Fraumeni JF Jr. eds. Cancer Epidemiology and Prevention. New York: Oxford Press, 1996.
73. Hoshiyama Y, Sasaba T. A case–control study of stomach cancer and its relation to diet, cigarettes, and alcohol consumption in Saitama Prefecture, Japan. Cancer Causes Control 1992; 3:441–448.

18

Peroxynitrite Scavenging by Mitochondrial Reductants and Plant Polyphenols

Alberto Boveris, Silvia Alvarez, Silvia Lores Arnaiz, and Laura B. Valdez
School of Pharmacy and Biochemistry, University of Buenos Aires, Buenos Aires, Argentina

I. INTRODUCTION

Peroxynitrite ($ONOO^-$) is an oxidizing and nitrating species produced in vivo both as an intracellular and as an extracellular metabolite in mammals. On the one hand, it is formed in isolated mitochondria (1,2), which indicates the physiological intracellular generation of this species, considering that isolated mitochondria have been recognized as effective sources of nitric oxide (NO) (3) and superoxide anion (O_2^-) (4) under physiological conditions. On the other hand, a series of cell types, such as macrophages (5), neutrophils (6), Kupffer cells (7), and cultured endothelial cells (8) produce $ONOO^-$ vectorially into the extracellular space. In both cases, peroxynitrite is formed in the intracellular and the extracellular spaces through the diffusion-controlled reaction ($k = 1.9 \times 10^{10}$ $M^{-1}s^{-1}$) of NO and O_2^- (9). This free radical termination reaction—both reactants have one unpaired electron in their external orbitals—was proposed 10 years ago by Beckman as the molecular mechanism of ischemic injury (10), and it is now also recognized as the main pathway of intramitochondrial NO utilization (1) and as one of the molecular strategies that are responsible for the cytotoxicity of specialized cells (5–7). At physiological pH, $ONOO^-$ protonates to yield peroxynitrous acid (ONOOH; $pK_a = 6.8$), which rearranges itself to yield nitrate (NO_3^-) or to decompose, producing radical species such as hydroxyl radical ($HO^•$) and nitric dioxide ($NO_2^•$), with a global half-life for $ONOO^-$ of about 1 s (11,12).

Peroxynitrite is a powerful univalent oxidant [$E^{0'}_{ONOO^-/NO_2^•} = 1.40$ V (11,12)] that readily oxidizes the sulfhydryl group of cysteine and glutathione (GSH) (13), the sulfur atom of methionine (14), ascorbate (15), the purine and pirimidine bases of DNA (16), and the reduced forms of nicotinamide nucleotides (NADH and NADPH) (17). It is able to start the lipoperoxidation process in biomembranes and liposomes (18) and in isolated low-density lipoproteins (LDL) (19), likely by the generation of hydroxyl radicals. In addition, $ONOO^-$ sustains nitration reactions, such as the nitration of tyrosine residues in proteins, a process that may alter protein function and interfere with the phosphorylation–dephosphorylation-signaling pathways (2,20,21).

The present chapter is focused on the redox reactions of $ONOO^-$ with intramitochondrial and intracellular reductants, such as NADH, ubiquinol, lipoic acid, GSH, ascorbic acid, and uric acid; and in the reactions of $ONOO^-$ with plant polyphenols such as the flavonoids (+)-catechin, (−)-epicatechin, and myricetin, and the hydroxycinnamates caffeic acid, ferulic acid, and chlorogenic acid. An almost linear relation between the capability of the assayed substances to react with $ONOO^-$ and the inhibition of $ONOO^-$-induced protein nitration is shown. Plant polyphenols are potentially useful antioxidants and anti-inflammatory substances for the vascular space considering that they are bioavailable and, then, that they may reach effective concentrations in plasma and, eventually, in the extracellular fluids. *Ginkgo biloba* and grape seeds extracts, which contain flavonoids among the active compounds, were also tested for $ONOO^-$-scavenging activity.

II. ESTIMATION OF RATE CONSTANTS BY AN INDIRECT METHOD

A. NADH Oxidation by Peroxynitrite

An indirect fluorometric technique was used to estimate the rate constants of the reactions of $ONOO^-$ with NADH and various other reductants. The method is based on a model of simple competition kinetics and on the measurement of product formation, in a system that involves $ONOO^-$ as oxidant, the indicator molecule NADH, and the competitive reductants (22).

The oxidation of NADH by $ONOO^-$ was followed fluorometrically at 37°C in a reaction medium consisting of 100 mM phosphate buffer (pH 7.0), 0.1 mM DTPA, 100 μM NADH, and 100–700 μM $ONOO^-$ using 340 and 463 nm as excitation and emission wavelengths. Exposure of NADH to $ONOO^-$ causes the immediate oxidation, during mixing time, of the reduced pyridine nucleotide, as shown by the decrease of the 463 nm fluorescence emission (Fig. 1). The addition of up to 400 μM $ONOO^-$ produced an almost linear NADH oxidation at a ratio of about 0.25 NAD^+ formed/$ONOO^-$ added. The relatively low oxidation yield is explained by the two-electron donation required to oxidize NADH and by the relatively large contribution of the rearrangement of $ONOO^-$ to yield nitrate [Reactions (1–3)].

The decrease of NADH fluorescence was measured after a constant addition of 200 μM $ONOO^-$ and taken as NAD^+ production in the absence and presence of other reductant scavengers (AH_2), such as mitochondrial reductants and plant polyphenols.

B. Treatment of the Kinetic Data

The treatment of the data was based on the occurrence of the following main and global reactions:

$$ONOO^- + H^+ \rightleftharpoons ONOOH \xrightarrow{ka} NO_3^- + H^+ \tag{1}$$

$$2\ ONOO^- + 2\ H^+ + NADH \xrightarrow{kb} NAD^+ + 2\ NO_2 + 2\ H_2O \tag{2}$$

$$2\ ONOO^- + 2\ H^+ + AH_2 \xrightarrow{kc} A + 2\ NO_2 + 2\ H_2O \tag{3}$$

In alternative oxidation, reactions (2) and (3), where AH_2 means an unspecific reductant, the ratio of the product yield, NAD^+ and A, is proportional to the ratio of each reaction rate, which in each case is the product of each rate constant by the corresponding reductant concentration (23), as given in Eq. (4).

$$\Delta[NAD^+]/\Delta[A] = k_b[NADH]/k_c[AH_2] \tag{4}$$

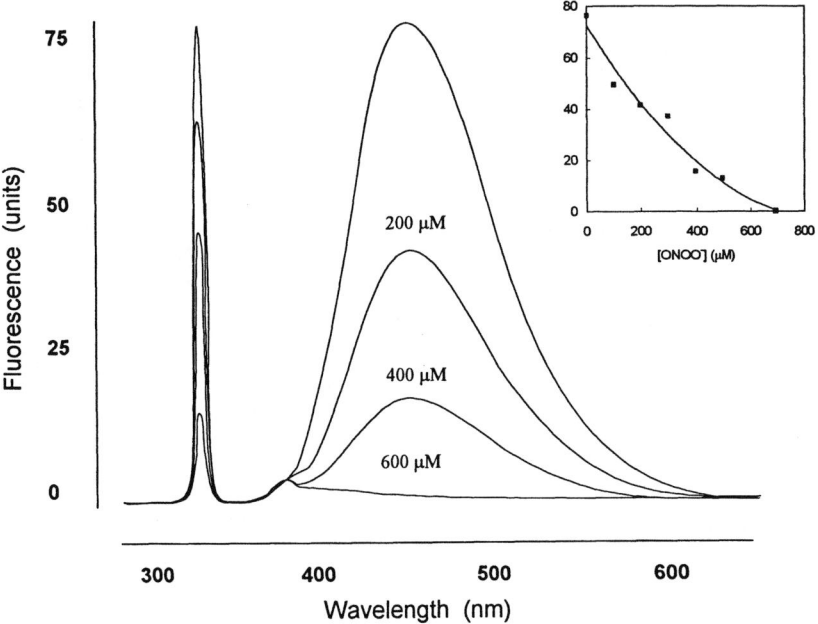

Figure 1 NADH oxidation by peroxynitrite: Changes in NADH fluorescence emission spectrum after addition of 0, 200, 400, or 600 μM ONOO$^-$. Inset: Decrease of NADH fluorescence produced by the addition of 0–700 μM ONOO$^-$.

Moreover, the rate of ONOO$^-$ utilization by alternative reactions (1), (2), and (3) is given by differential Eqs. (5) and (6):

$$-\frac{d[ONOO^-]}{dt} = k_a[ONOO^-] + k_b[NADH][ONOO^-] + k_c[AH_2][ONOO^-] \quad (5)$$

$$-\frac{d[ONOO^-]}{dt} = [ONOO^-](k_a + k_b[NADH] + k_c[AH_2]) \quad (6)$$

Assuming a simple competition oxidation of the detecting molecule (NADH) and a given antioxidant (AH$_2$), the kinetics of alternative reactions (2) and (3) predict that:

$$\frac{\Delta[NADH]_0}{\Delta[NADH]} = 1 + k_c[AH_2]/k_b[NADH] \quad (7)$$

where $\Delta[NADH]_0$ is the fluorescence change observed after ONOO$^-$ addition; $\Delta[NADH]$ is the fluorescence change detected in the presence of ONOO$^-$ and AH$_2$; and k_b and k_c are the apparent second-order rate constants of the reactions of ONOO$^-$ with NADH or AH$_2$ [see reactions (2) and (3)]. The ratio $\Delta[NADH]_0/\Delta[NADH]$ as reductant oxidation, is equivalent to $[NAD^+]_0/[NAD^+]$, where $[NAD^+]_0$ and $[NAD^+]$ are the yields of the oxidized product, NAD$^+$, in the absence and in the presence of scavenger (AH$_2$). Equation (7) can be expressed as:

$$[NAD^+]_0/[NAD^+] = 1 + k_c[AH_2]/k_b[NADH] \quad (8)$$

Thus, plotting the left-hand term of Eq. (8) versus [AH$_2$]/[NADH] will result in a straight line, the slope of which is k_c/k_b and the ordinate intercept is equal to 1.

III. MITOCHONDRIAL REDUCTANTS

A. Determination of Rate Constants

The supplementation of the reaction medium with 0–300 μM ascorbic acid decreased the extent of NADH oxidation by $ONOO^-$ (Fig. 2). The data yielded a straight line, the slope of which, taking as reference $k_c = 569$ M^{-1} s^{-1} for the reaction of ascorbic acid and $ONOO^-$ at 37°C (15), gave a rate constant $k_b = 233$ M^{-1} s^{-1} for the reaction of NADH with $ONOO^-$ (Table 1). Similar experimental procedure and analysis were used with the other reductants: ubiquinol-0 (Q_0H_2, 0–40 μM), glutathione (GSH, 0–150 μM), lipoic acid (LA, 0–250 μM), dihydrolipoic acid (LAH_2, 0–200 μM), uric acid (0–80 μM), and melatonin (0–300 μM). For these reactions, the corresponding rate constants were calculated from the slope of the graphs shown in Figure 3 and from the apparent second-order rate constant for the reaction of NADH and $ONOO^-$ referred to in Table 1. The highest values of the rate constants are those corresponding to the reactions of $ONOO^-$ with Q_0H_2 and ascorbic acid; intermediate values are those for the reactions of $ONOO^-$ and NADH, uric acid, LAH_2, and GSH. The two reductants with –SH groups, GSH, and LAH_2, show about similar rate constants. Melatonin and the oxidized form of lipoic acid showed a poor reactivity; in the latter, it seems that oxidized lipoic acid is able to react with $ONOO^-$ opening the five-atom ring to yield oxidized products. Table 1 also lists the reductant concentrations that inhibited 50% (IC_{50}) the formation of NAD^+, which are inversely related to the rate constants. These concentrations are useful to assess the biological role of the assayed reductants in scavenging $ONOO^-$. Recently, Kirsch

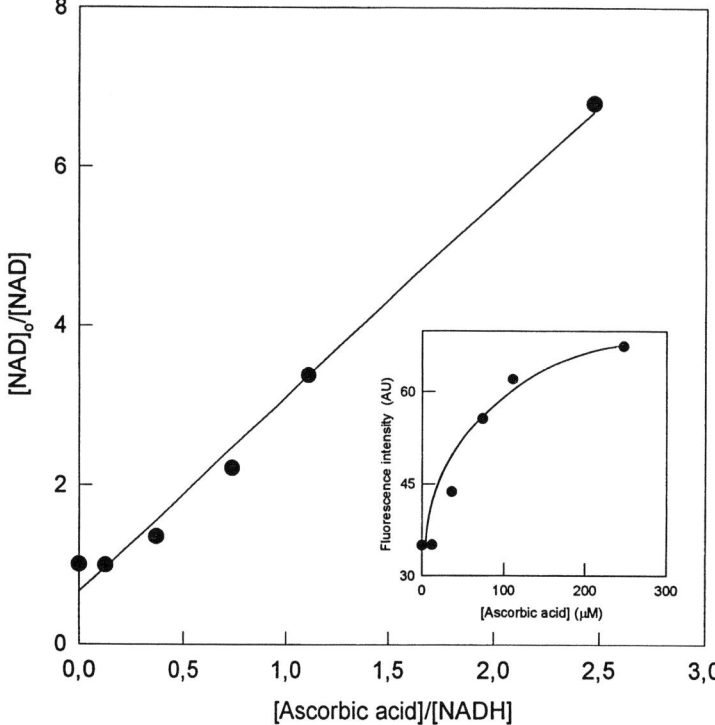

Figure 2 Effect of ascorbic acid on NADH oxidation by peroxynitrite: Plot of $[NAD^+]_0/[NAD^+]$ as a function of [ascorbic acid]/[NADH]. Inset: Inhibition of NAD^+ production by ascorbic acid.

Table 1 Second-Order Rate Constants and IC$_{50}$ of the Reactions of ONOO$^-$ and Reductants

Reductants	k_0/k_b	k (M^{-1} s^{-1})	IC$_{50}$ (μM)
NADH	—	233 ± 27	
Ascorbic acid	2.44 ± 0.28	569[a]	55 ± 6
Ubiquinol-0	2.08 ± 0.23	485 ± 54	48 ± 5
Uric acid	0.89 ± 0.04	207 ± 18	114 ± 11
Glutathione	0.78 ± 0.03	183 ± 12	129 ± 13
Lipoic acid	0.12 ± 0.01	28 ± 1	834 ± 6
Dihydrolipoic acid	0.55 ± 0.17	128 ± 15	211 ± 73
Melatonin	0.19 ± 0.01	43 ± 3	519 ± 21

[a]*Source*: Ref. 15.

and de Groot (17) reported a rate constant of 7.4×10^3 M^{-1} s^{-1} for the reaction of ONOO$^-$ and NADH, also determined by an indirect method and using reduced glutathione as reference. The difference between both values (2.3×10^2 and 7.4×10^3 M^{-1} s^{-1} for the reaction of ONOO$^-$ and NADH reflects mainly the difference in the reference reaction of ONOO$^-$ and GSH [1.8×10^2 (Table 1) and 1.4×10^3 M^{-1} s^{-1} (17)]; in both cases NADH is more reactive (1.3–5.3 times) than GSH toward ONOO$^-$.

In the presence of bicarbonate, ONOO$^-$ readily reacts with CO_2 ($k = 5.8 \times 10^4$ M^{-1} s^{-1} (24–26), forming the adduct ONOOCO$_2^-$. It has been reported that this adduct participates in oxidation and nitration processes (17,20). The effect of CO_2 on NADH oxidation produced by ONOO$^-$ was studied by adding 13 mM NaHCO$_3$ (2.5 mM CO_2 at pH 7.0) and determining the ratios of the apparent rate constants k_c/k_b for the reaction of the formed adduct ONOOCO$_2^-$ with the indicator NADH and with the other competitive reductants, such as ascorbic acid, Q$_0$H$_2$, and GSH (Table 2). The ratios of the apparent reaction constants were in the same magnitude range, both in the presence of CO_2 and in air-equilibrated conditions. It appears that the adduct oxidizes NADH, Q$_0$H$_2$, ascorbic acid, and GSH similarly to ONOO$^-$; and that oxidation occurs directly by the adduct or via homolytic scission, yielding NO$_2^{\bullet}$ and carbonate radical (CO$_3^{\bullet}$) and affording the latter an univalent oxidant similar to HO$^{\bullet}$. These results agree with the reported reactivity of the adduct toward NADH (17).

A rough estimation of the rate constants for the reactions of the adduct ONOOCO$_2^-$ with the assayed reductants can be made by applying the quasi steady-state approach and using 5 ms (200 times less stable than ONOO$^-$) as the $t_{1/2}$ for the spontaneous decomposition of the adduct ($k = 0.69/t_{1/2} = 138$ s^{-1}). At equal rates of adduct production and decomposition (+ d[ONOOCO$_2^-$]/dt = −d[ONOOCO$_2^-$]/dt), at the point of 0.4 mM ONOO$^-$ and at half decomposition of ONOO$^-$ in the experimental conditions of Table 2:

$$+\frac{d[ONOOCO_2^-]}{dt} = k[ONOO^-][CO_2] \qquad (9)$$

$$= 5.8 \times 10^4 \text{ M}^{-1} \text{ s}^{-1} \times 2 \times 10^{-4} \text{ M} \times 2.5 \times 10^{-3} \text{ M}$$

$$= 2.9 \times 10^{-2} \text{ M s}^{-1}$$

$$+\frac{d[ONOOCO_2^-]}{dt} = [ONOOCO_2^-](k_1 + k_2[\text{NADH}]) \qquad (10)$$

where k_1 is the first-order rate constant of the adduct decomposition, and k_2 is the second-order rate constant of the reaction of the adduct and NADH. The rate constants k_1 and k_2 are

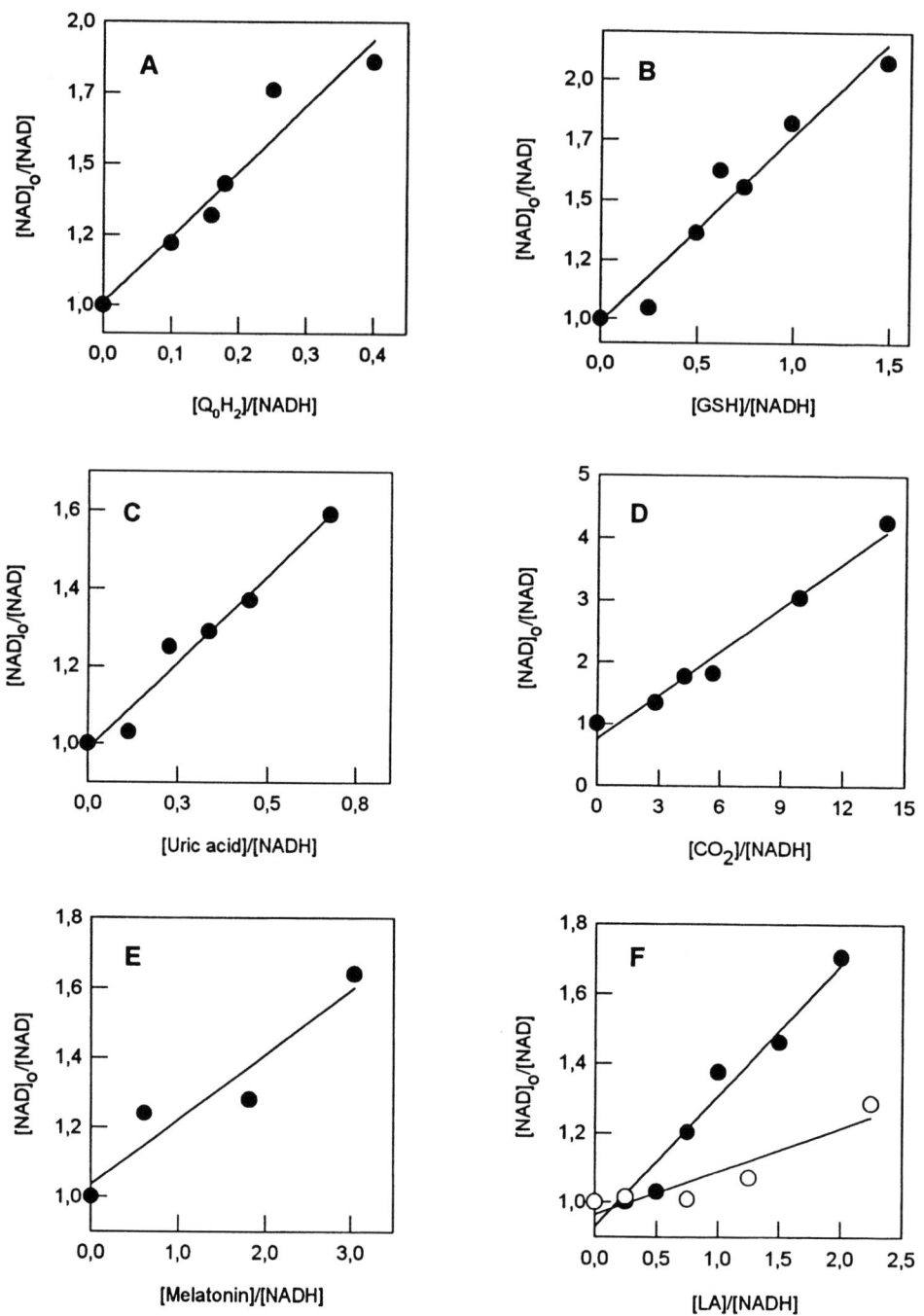

Figure 3 Plot of $[NAD^+]_0/[NAD^+]$ as a function of $[AH_2]/[NADH]$. $[AH_2]$: (A) ubiquinol-0; (B) glutathione; (C) uric acid; (D) carbon dioxide; (E) melatonin; (F) lipoic acid (○); and dihydrolipoic acid (●).

Table 2 Effect of Carbon Dioxide on the NADH Oxidation Produced by ONOO⁻ in the Presence of Ascorbic Acid, Ubiquinol-0, or Glutathione[a]

	Air-equilibrated		CO_2	
	k_0/k_b	IC_{50} (μM)	k_0/k_b	IC_{50} (μM)
Ascorbic acid	2.4 ± 0.3	55 ± 6	2.1 ± 0.4	48 ± 5
Ubiquinol-0	2.1 ± 0.2	48 ± 5	0.57 ± 0.05	178 ± 21
Glutathione	0.78 ± 0.03	129 ± 13	0.14 ± 0.01	735 ± 78

[a] An approximate estimation of the second-order rate constants for the reactions of the adduct $ONOOCO_2^{2-}$ with the assayed reductants yields the following values: with NADH = 1.5×10^6 M^{-1} s^{-1}; with ascorbic acid = 3.2×10^6 M^{-1} s^{-1}; with Q_0H_2 = 8.7×10^5 M^{-1} s^{-1}, and with GSH = 2.1×10^5 M^{-1} s^{-1} (see text).

analogous to k_a and k_b of Eqs. (1) and (2). If we assume an adduct concentration of 100 μM in the quasi steady-state conditions:

$$2.9 \times 10^{-2} \text{ M s}^{-1} = 1 \times 10^{-4} \text{ M} \times (138 \text{ s}^{-1} + k_2 \times 1 \times 10^{-4} \text{ M})$$
$$k_2 = 1.5 \times 10^6 \text{ M}^{-1} \text{ s}^{-1}$$

The following rate constants can be estimated for the reaction of NADH with the adduct by using the ratios of the third column of Table 2: with ascorbic acid = 3.2×10^6 M^{-1} s^{-1}; with Q_0H_2 = 8.7×10^5 M^{-1} s^{-1}; and with GSH = 2.1×10^5 M^{-1} s^{-1}. The biological meaning of adduct formation appears to be the decrease of the intramitochondrial steady-state concentration of ONOO⁻ without markedly changing reductant utilization and oxidized product formation (UQ, NAD⁺, or GSSG), or in other words, without generating another oxidant with different selectivity.

B. Tyrosine Nitration by Peroxynitrite

Mouse liver submitochondrial particles were exposed to a pulse of 200 μM ONOO⁻, in the absence and in the presence of 50–200 μM reductants (ascorbic acid, Q_0H_2, GSH, NADH, uric acid, and melatonin) or 2 mM CO_2. Submitochondrial particles consists mainly of inside out vesicles in which the proteins of the M face of the inner mitochondrial membranes are exposed to the reaction medium and, consequently, afford a model of the exposure of mitochondrial proteins to intramitochondrial ONOO⁻. Protein nitration was evaluated in terms of tyrosine nitration using a specific rabbit polyclonal antibody (gift of Drs. A. Estevez and J. Beckman of the University of South Alabama at Birmingham, AL) and analyzed by Western blot. Effective nitration of proteins was readily observed in the mitochondrial membranes after ONOO⁻ addition (Fig. 4A). Supplementation with CO_2 did not change the nitration level observed when ONOO⁻ was added alone, and no significant protection was obtained when melatonin was used. The other reductants markedly inhibited the tyrosine nitration produced by ONOO⁻ in the following approximate sequence: ascorbic acid > Q_0H_2 = uric acid > NADH = GSH. To estimate the amount of 3-tyrosine nitration, cellulose films were scanned, and the digital image was analyzed with NIH Image 1.62 (by Wayne Rasband, National Institutes of Health, USA). Taken as reference for full nitration was that observed after addition of the ONOO⁻ pulse to submitochondrial particles (see lane 7 in Fig. 4A), and as reference for no nitration was that observed in the absence of ONOO⁻ (see lane 8 in Fig. 4A). The effect is listed in Table 3 as the percentage of tyrosine nitration observed in the presence of 100 μM of each

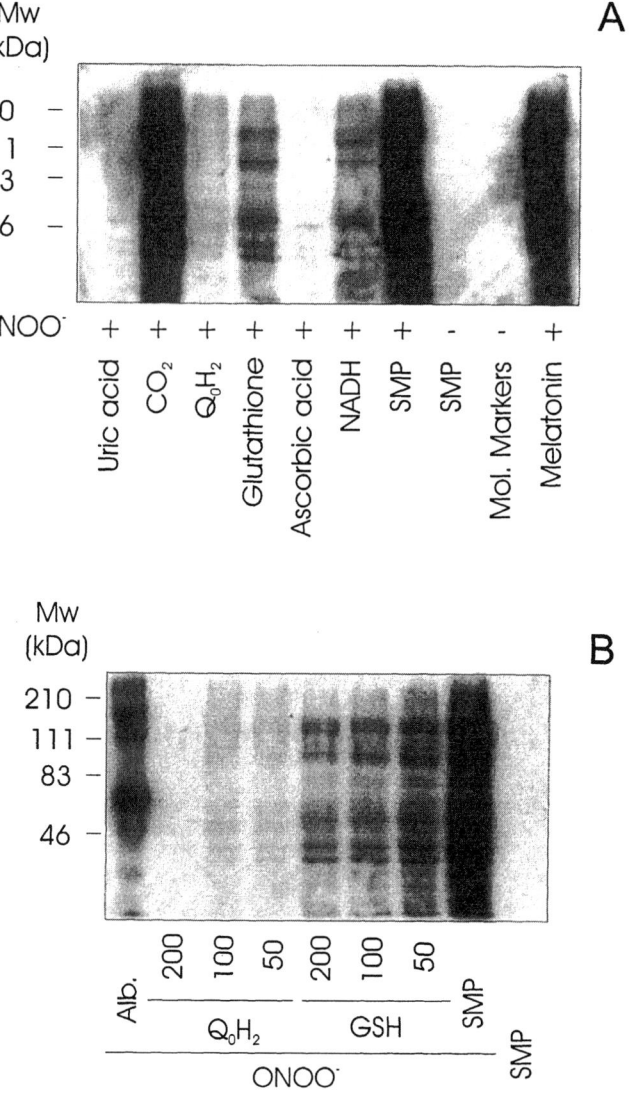

Figure 4 Western blot analysis of 3-nitrotyrosine residues: (A) Effect of 200 μM ONOO$^-$ on mouse liver submitochondrial particles (3 mg/mL) in the absence or presence of 100 μM reductants, except for CO_2 that was 2 mM; (B) the same in the absence or presence of 50–200 μM Q_0H_2 or GSH. The percentages of 3-nitrotyrosine were: 3.8, 2.3, and 0.1% in the presence of 50, 100, and 200 μM Q_0H_2; and 49, 23, and 15% in the presence of 50, 100, and 200 μM GSH.

reductant. Moreover, the effects of different concentrations of Q_0H_2 and of GSH on tyrosine nitration by ONOO$^-$ are shown in Figure 4B; both Q_0H_2 and GSH inhibited tyrosine nitration in a concentration-dependent manner and it can be seen that Q_0H_2 was more effective than GSH in protecting mitochondrial proteins from nitration. The data shown in Figure 4 and in Table 3 can be analyzed in terms of the system ONOO$^-$/submitochondrial particles as a model of the cumulative nitrating effects of the intramitochondrial steady-state concentration of ONOO$^-$, considering that all reactions are linearly proportional to reactant concentration.

Table 3 Effect of Reductants at 100 μM on the Tyrosine Nitration of Mitochondrial Membranes Produced by 200 μM ONOO$^-$

Conditions	Tyrosine nitration (%)
− Peroxynitrite	0
+ Peroxynitrite	100
+ Peroxynitrite + ascorbic acid	0
+ Peroxynitrite + Q$_0$H$_2$	4.5
+ Peroxynitrite + uric acid	4.7
+ Peroxynitrite + NADH	26
+ Peroxynitrite + GSH	26
+ Peroxynitrite + CO$_2$	95
+ Peroxynitrite + melatonin	89

The first point to be considered is that 2 mM CO_2 (at a concentration that is about twice that of the mitochondrial matrix) was unable to prevent protein nitration. The second point is to extrapolate the effects observed at 100 μM of Q_0H_2, NADH, and GSH to their intramitochondrial concentrations. The content of the three reductants in rat liver mitochondria is Q_0H_2, 2.5 nmol/mg protein (27); NADH, 3.8 nmol/mg protein (28); and GSH, 3.0 nmol/mg protein (30), which after considering a mitochondrial matrix value of 6 μL/mg protein (from 35 mg mitochondrial protein per gram of liver and a 0.2 mL of mitochondrial matrix/cm^3 of liver (29) yield an intramitochondrial concentrations of 420 μM Q_0H_2, 640 μM NADH, and 500 μM GSH. As 100 μM Q_0H_2 was able to reduce protein nitration to 4.5%, the intramitochondrial level of 420 μM Q_0H_2 should be able to prevent protein nitration 4.2-fold more effectively (4.5%/4.2), with about 1% of nitration remaining, and an effective protection of 99%. Similarly, intramitochondrial NADH (640 μM) would reduce mitochondrial protein nitration to about 4% (26%/6.4), and intramitochondrial GSH would do so to an extent of about 5% (26%/5). It is then possible to estimate that the combined action of these three intramitochondrial reductants will normally reduce protein nitration to negligible levels and, consequently, to assign an additional and important biological role to ubiquinol, NADH, and GSH; that is, the protection of the matrix proteins from nitration by intramitochondrial ONOO$^-$.

IV. PLANT POLYPHENOLS: FLAVONOIDS AND HYDROXYCINNAMATES

Plant polyphenols constitute a large class of compounds, ubiquitous in plants, containing several phenolic hydroxyl groups that are the chemical basis of their antioxidant activity (31). These polyphenols are reducing agents that function as antioxidants by virtue of the hydrogen-donating properties of their phenolic hydroxyl groups (32,33) as well as by their transition metal-chelating abilities (34,35). The aromatic hydroxyl groups of flavonoids and hydroxycinnamates present an antioxidant pharmacophore comparable with the chroman moiety of tocopherols. Indeed, a high reactivity of flavonoids with radicals such as O_2^- (36), HO$^{\cdot}$ (32), and NO (37) has been reported. In particular, epicatechin, epigallocatechin, and their gallate esters scavenge both aqueous and lipophilic radicals and protect LDL from oxidation by acting as chain-breaking antioxidants (38). In addition, flavonoids are potent scavengers of ONOO$^-$ (39) and red wine exhibits a considerable ONOO$^-$-scavenging activity (37).

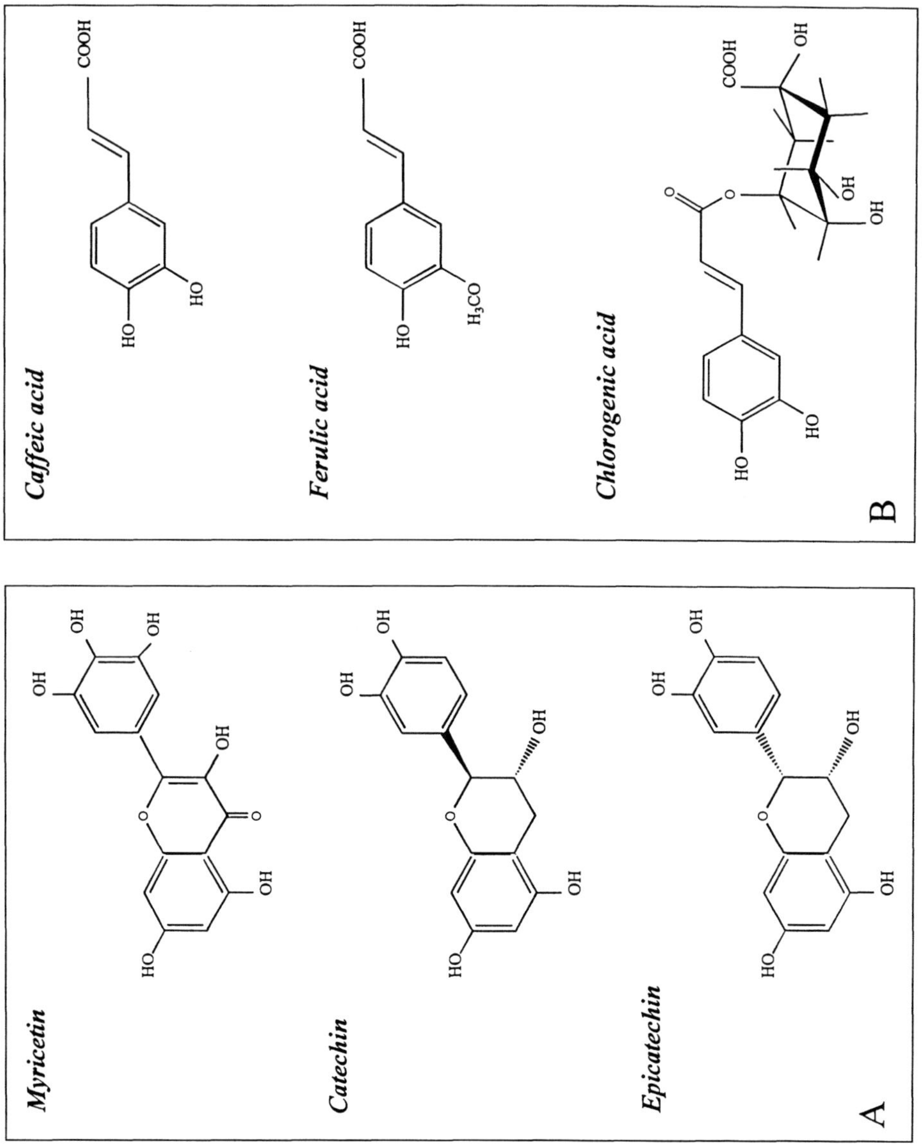

Figure 5 Chemical structures of the assayed (A) polyphenols and (B) hydroxycinnamates.

Hydroxycinnamates or phenylpropanoids are distributed widely in plant tissues, and they are present as dietary phytochemicals at concentrations that are higher than those corresponding to flavonoids (40). These compounds occur in nature in various conjugated forms. It has been reported that hydroxycinnamates exhibit antimicrobial, antiallergic, and anti-inflammatory activities as well as antimutagenic properties (41,42). They possess peroxyl radical-scavenging properties, as measured by their ability to prevent the lipid peroxidation of LDL mediated by heme proteins (32,43). Recently, it has been reported that catechins and hydroxycinnamates can inhibit $ONOO^-$-induced nitration of tyrosine (40).

A. Determination of Rate Constants

The methodology described in Section II.A was used to determine the rate constants of the reactions of $ONOO^-$ with flavonoids and hydroxycinnamates. The chemical structures of these compounds are shown in Figure 5. The corresponding rate constants were calculated from the slope of the corresponding graphs and the second-order rate constant for the reaction of NADH and $ONOO^-$ (Table 4). The highest value of the rate constants was the one corresponding to the reaction of $ONOO^-$ with myricetin; with lower rate constants for the other two flavonoids and the hydroxycinnamates. The concentrations inhibiting 50% NAD^+ formation (IC_{50}) were inversely related and in agreement with the given second-order reaction constants. The $ONOO^-$ scavenging reactivity was markedly higher for myricetin than for the catechins and the hydroxycinnamates.

Ginkgo biloba and grape seed extracts contain a series of flavonoids that are considered responsible for the free radical-scavenging properties of both extracts. When the effect of these two extracts on NADH oxidation by $ONOO^-$ was studied, the estimated half-inhibition concentration, determined from the graphs shown in Figure 6, was lower for *G. biloba* extract than for grape seed extract (see Table 4). Considering that the extracts contain a large number of different substances, it follows that both extracts contain very effective $ONOO^-$ scavengers (see note in Table 4).

Table 4 Second-Order Rate Constants and IC_{50} of the Reactions of $ONOO^-$ with Plant Polyphenols and Hydroxycinnamates

Compounds	Reductants	k_0/k_b	k ($M^{-1}s^{-1}$)	IC_{50} (μM)
Control	NADH	—	233 ± 27	—
	Ascorbic acid	2.44 ± 0.28	569^a	55 ± 6
Flavonoids	Myricetin	2.75 ± 0.10	640 ± 38	35 ± 1
	(+)-Catechin	0.36 ± 0.02	85 ± 6	275 ± 23
	(−)-Epicatechin	0.33 ± 0.02	77 ± 5	313 ± 23
Hydroxycinnamates	Chlorogenic acid	0.61 ± 0.13	142 ± 30	173 ± 36
	Caffeic acid	0.72 ± 0.14	166 ± 32	144 ± 29
	Ferulic acid	0.36 ± 0.02	82 ± 4	507 ± 15
Plant extracts	Grape seed	—	—	118 ± 16^b
	Ginkgo biloba	—	—	85 ± 11^b

[a] *Source*: Ref. 15.
[b] The units are given in $\mu g/mL$, which are roughly comparable to μM, after considering a content of 31% of flavonoids in the extracts and a mean relative mass of 320 Da.

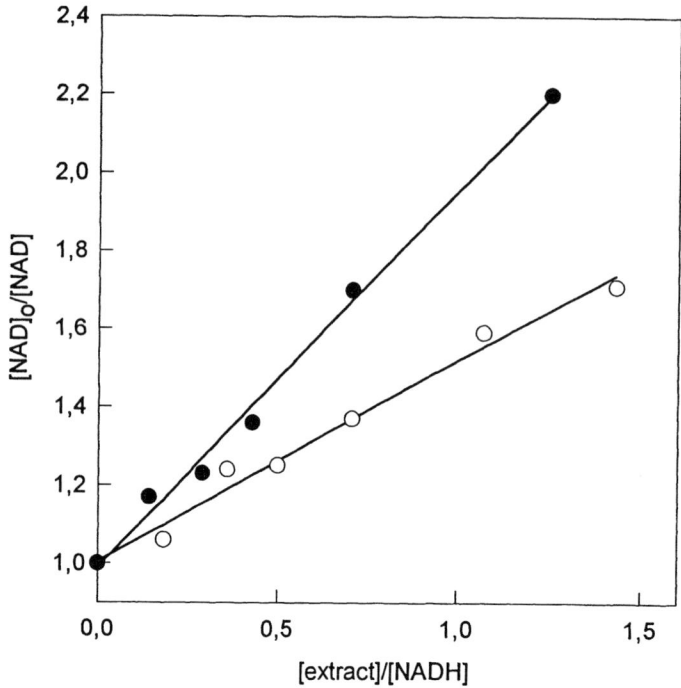

Figure 6 Effect of G. biloba (●) and grape seed extracts (○) on the NADH oxidation produced by peroxynitrite: Plot of $[NAD^+]_0/[NAD^+]$ as a function of [extract]/[NADH].

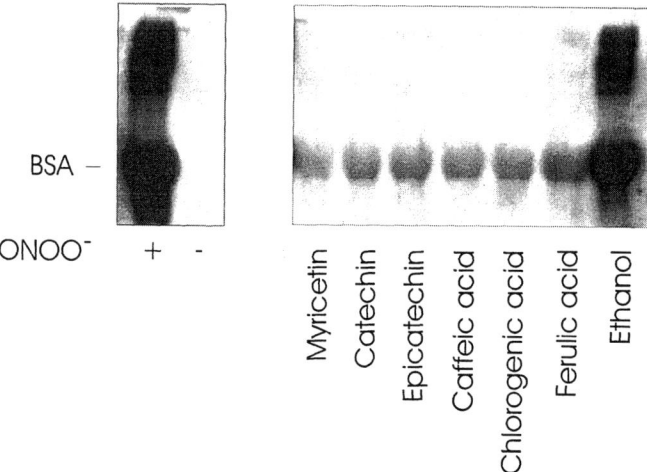

Figure 7 Western blot analysis of 3-nitrotyrosine residues: Effect of 200 μM $ONOO^-$ on bovine serum albumin (2 mg/mL) in the absence or presence of 200 μM polyphenols or hydroxycinnamates. Ethanol, the polyphenol solvent, does not protect albumin from nitration.

Table 5 Effect of Plant Polyphenols and Hydroxycinnamates on the Tyrosine Nitration of Serum Albumin Produced by $ONOO^-$

Conditions	Tyrosine nitration (%)
− Peroxynitrite	0
+ Peroxynitrite	100
+ Peroxynitrite + polyphenols	
+ Myricetin	20
+ (+)-Catechin	23
+ (−)-Epicatechin	24
+ Peroxynitrite + hydroxycinnamates	
+ Caffeic acid	25
+ Chlorogenic acid	27
+ Ferulic acid	35

B. Tyrosine Nitration by Peroxynitrite

Tyrosine nitration of bovine serum albumin (BSA) was used as a model of extracellular protein nitration. Bovine serum albumin (2 mg/mL) was exposed to 200 μM $ONOO^-$, in the absence or presence of 200 μM polyphenols and 3-nitrotyrosine was detected by sodium dodecyl sulfate–polyacrylamide gel electrophoresis (SDS-PAGE) and Western blot analysis (Fig. 7). Supplementation with plant polyphenols was able to inhibit the tyrosine nitration produced by $ONOO^-$ in the following sequence (according to their effect at the same concentrations of 200 μM): myricetin > (+)-catechin = (−)-epicatechin > caffeic acid = chlorogenic acid > ferulic acid.

The amount of 3-nitrotyrosine was quantified, taking as reference for full nitration that observed after $ONOO^-$ addition and for no nitration that observed in the absence of $ONOO^-$ (see Fig. 7, left panel). Flavonoids (myricetin, catechin, and epicatechin) and disubstituted hydroxycinnamates (caffeic acid and chlorogenic acid) decreased tyrosine nitration better than monohydroxycinnamates (ferulic acid) (Table 5). The $ONOO^-$ scavenging effects of flavonoids and hydroxycinnamates observed are in good agreement with the results reported by Rice–Evans et al. (40).

V. CONCLUDING REMARKS

Numerous biomolecules constitute potential targets for $ONOO^-$ in its two chemical actions: as an oxidizing and as a nitrating species. However, only a few molecules are expected to be preferential targets owing to the kinetic conditions (i.e., reaction rates and reactant concentrations). The knowledge of the reaction kinetics of $ONOO^-$ with biomolecules allows not only the prediction of the preferential fates of $ONOO^-$ in biological systems, but also provides information about the use of $ONOO^-$ scavengers in the same systems. Table 6 lists second-order reaction constants for the oxidizing action of $ONOO^-$. As can be observed, a multitude of low molecular mass compounds and proteins are readily oxidized by $ONOO^-$, with rate constants in the range of 10^2–10^6 M^{-1} s^{-1}. Both, monovalent and bivalent reductants are included in Table 6; in the latter, two successive bimolecular reactions are needed to fully oxidize the substrate. For the bivalent reductants, an intermediate radical is formed. The intermediate then, (1) is oxidized by $ONOO^-$ ($Q_0H^{\cdot}$; $NAD^{\cdot+}$, etc.); (2) disproportionates with a similar radical ($Q_0H^{\cdot}$); or (3) dimerizes ($GS^{\cdot}$). A first consideration concerning the rate constants is that they

Table 6 Rate Constants of the Reactions of $ONOO^-$ with Biomolecules and Relevant Compounds at Physiological pH[a]

Compounds	k (M^{-1} s^{-1})	Ref.
Low molecular mass compounds		
Ascorbic acid	2.4×10^{2} [b]	15
	5.7×10^{2} [a]	15
Carbon dioxide	3.0×10^{4} [b]	24
	5.8×10^{4} [c]	26
Cysteine	3.3×10^{3} [b]	44
	5.0×10^{3} [c]	44
Cytochrome c	1.3×10^{4} [b]	45
Ebselen	2.0×10^{6} [b]	46
GSH	6.5×10^{2} [b]	12
	1.4×10^{3} [c]	47
Metalloporphyrins	2.0×10^{6} [b]	47,48
Methionine	1.8×10^{2} [b]	14
Tryptophan	1.0×10^{2} [c]	49
Proteins		
Aconitase	1.4×10^{5} [b]	50
Albumin	5.6×10^{3} [c]	44
Glutathione peroxidase	8.0×10^{6} [b]	51
Hemoglobin	2.5×10^{4} [c]	52
Horseradish peroxidase	7.0×10^{5} [b]	53
Myeloperoxidase	4.8×10^{6} [d]	53
Cu–Zn superoxide dismutase	$10^{3} - 10^{5}$ [c]	54

[a] Reported rate constants were obtained from the literature and are the values (pH-dependent) in the physiological range (pH = 7.2–7.6).
[b] $T = 25°C$.
[c] $T = 37°C$.
[d] $T = 12°C$.

seem to indicate collisional redox reactions with a determined probability of occurrence owing to steric conditions for electron transfer and not a classic free radical reaction involving highly reactive species. However, there is also an understanding that after formation of peroxynitrous acid, this chemical species can (1) rearrange itself to form nitrate [Reaction (1)]; (2) react collisionally with reductants; and (3) dissociate homolitically to form the radicals HO$^{\cdot}$ and NO$_2^{\cdot}$ [Reaction (11)]. An interesting possibility to be considered is that the homolytic scission occurs only in the solvent cage including ONOOH and other reactive molecule [Reaction (12)].

$$ONOOH \rightarrow [HO \cdots NO_2] \rightarrow HO^{\cdot} + NO_2^{\cdot} \qquad (11)$$

$$ONOOH + AH \rightarrow \begin{pmatrix} HO \cdots NO_2 \\ H \cdots A \end{pmatrix} \rightarrow A\text{-}NO_2 + HOH \qquad (12)$$

The almost linear relation found between the suppression of NADH oxidation and $ONOO^-$-mediated protein nitration with the mitochondrial reductants and plant polyphenols (Fig. 8) appears to indicate that the reductants react or interfere with a common intermediate (ONOOH

PEROXYNITRITE SCAVENGING

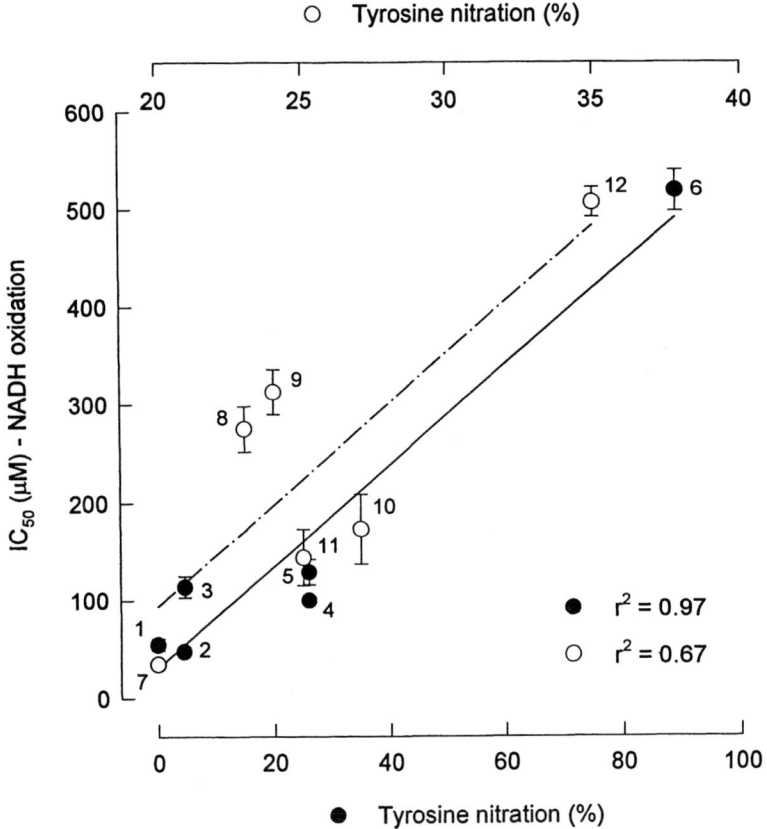

Figure 8 Relations between the inhibition of NADH oxidation, expressed as IC_{50} (μM), and the inhibition of nitration, expressed as percentage of 3-nitrotyrosine: Mitochondrial reductants (●): 1, ascorbic acid; 2, ubiquinol-0; 3, uric acid; 4, NADH; 5, glutathione; 6, melatonin. Polyphenols and hydroxycinnamates (○): 7, myricetin; 8, (+)-catechin; 9, (−)-epicatechin; 10, chlorogenic acid; 11, caffeic acid; 12, ferulic acid.

or HO···NO$_2$), which makes attractive the hypothesis that ONOOH is "activated" in the solvent cage by the coreactant.

The indirect method, based on a fluorometric technique described in this chapter, is sensitive and allows the use of low concentrations of ONOO$^-$ scavengers (0–300 μM) to estimate the reaction rate constants. The assay can be used as an alternative under circumstances in which (1) no direct method or stopped-flow facility is available, (2) pseudo-first-order conditions are not attainable, and (3) high background absorbances are detected.

Peroxynitrite is formed and mediates reactions in both the intracellular and the extracellular spaces. In aerobic cells, ONOO$^-$ is formed in the mitochondrial matrix at rates that are about 1–2% of the rate of oxygen uptake by the organ (1). Figure 9 indicates the intramitochondrial formation of ONOO$^-$ from O$_2^-$ and NO, and of ONOOCO$_2^-$ from CO$_2$ and ONOO$^-$. The scheme also indicates the reaction of both oxidizing species with the matrix reductants NADH, ubiquinol, and reduced glutathione.

In the extracellular environment, ONOO$^-$ is produced by the specialized cells during cytotoxic response (5–7) and by reticuloendothelial cells (8,55,56); O$_2^-$ is produced by the plasma

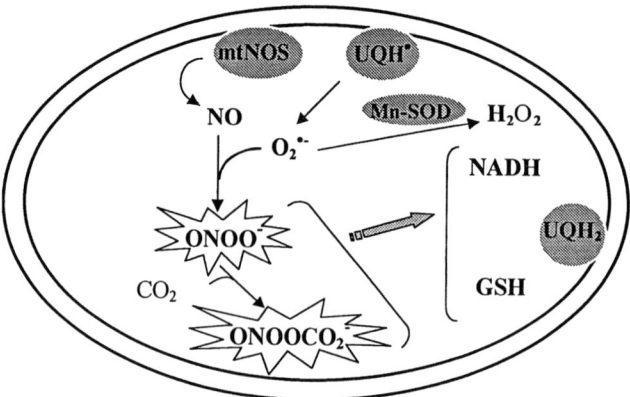

Figure 9 Intramitochondrial metabolism of peroxynitrite.

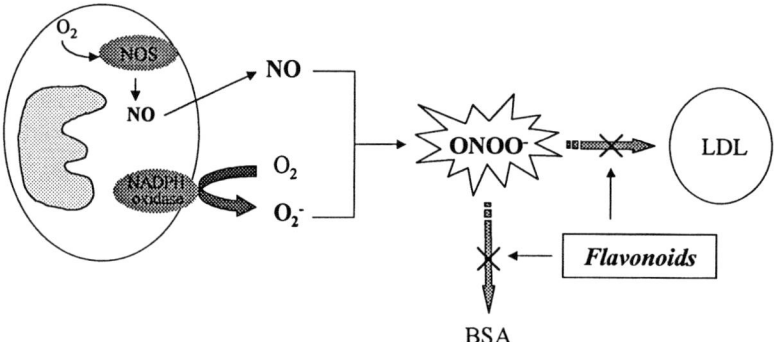

Figure 10 Peroxynitrite produced extracellularly by specialized cells (neutrophils, macrophages, lymphocytes, or others) reaches blood serum albumin and low-density lipoproteins: the oxidation and nitration brought about by peroxynitrite can be prevented by bioavailable flavonoids.

membrane-bound NADPH oxidase (48) and intracellular NO readily diffuses to the extracellular space (48,49) (Fig. 10). Flavonoids are potential useful $ONOO^-$ scavengers because they are bioavailable and reach plasma concentrations in the 0.3 to 3.0-μM range, as flavonoids, glycosides, and conjugates (57–59).

ACKNOWLEDGMENTS

This work was supported by grants PIP 4110/97 from CONICET, PICT 01608 from ANPCYT, and TB11 from the University of Buenos Aires (Argentina).

REFERENCES

1. Poderoso JJ, Lisdero CL, Schöpfer F, Riobó N, Carreras MC, Cadenas E, Boveris A. The regulation of mitochondrial oxygen uptake by redox reactions involving nitric oxide and ubiquinol. J Biol Chem 1999; 274:37709–37716.

2. Boczkowski J, Lisdero CL, Lanone S, Samb A, Carreras MC, Boveris A, Aubier M, Poderoso JJ. Endogenous peroxynitrite mediates mitochondrial dysfunction in rat diaphragm during endotoxemia. FASEB J 1999; 13:1637–1647.
3. Giulivi C, Poderoso JJ, Boveris A. Purification and characterization of a nitric-oxide synthase from rat liver mitochondria. J Biol Chem 1998; 273:11044–11048.
4. Chance B, Sies H, Boveris A. Hydroperoxide metabolism in mammalian organs. Physiol Rev 1979; 59:527–605.
5. Ischiropoulos H, Zhu L, Beckman JS. Peroxynitrite formation from macrophage-derived nitric oxide. Arch Biochem Biophys 1992; 298:446–451.
6. Carreras MC, Pargament GA, Catz SD, Poderoso JJ, Boveris A. Kinetics of nitric oxide and hydrogen peroxide production and formation of peroxynitrite during the respiratory burst of human neutrophils. FEBS Lett 1994; 341:65–68.
7. Wang JF, Komarov P, Sies H, de Groot H. Contribution of nitric oxide synthase to luminol-dependent chemiluminescence generated by phorbol-ester activated Kupffer cells. Biochem J 1991; 279:311–314.
8. Kooy NW, Royall JA. Agonist-induced peroxynitrite production from endothelial cells. Arch Biochem Biophys 1994; 310:352–359.
9. Kissner R, Nauser T, Bugnon P, Lye PG, Koppenol WH. Formation and properties of peroxynitrite as studied by laser flash photolysis, high-pressure stopped-flow technique, and pulse radiolysis. Chem Res Toxicol 1997; 10:1285–1292.
10. Beckman JS. Ischaemic injury mediator. Nature 1990; 345:27–28.
11. Koppenol WH. The basic chemistry of nitrogen monoxide and peroxynitrite. Free Radic Biol Med 1998; 25:385–391.
12. Radi R. Peroxynitrite reactions and diffusion in biology. Chem Res Toxicol 1998; 11:720–721.
13. Radi R, Beckman JS, Bush KM, Freeman BA. Peroxynitrite oxidation of sulfhydryls: the cytotoxic potential of superoxide and nitric oxide. J Biol Chem 1991; 266:4244–4250.
14. Pryor WA, Jin X, Squadrito GL. One- and two-electron oxidations of methionine by peroxynitrite. Proc Natl Acad Sci USA 1994; 91:11173–11177.
15. Bartlett K, Church DF, Bounds PL, Koppenol WH. The kinetics of the oxidation of L-ascorbic acid by peroxynitrite. Free Radic Biol Med 1995; 18:85–92.
16. King PA, Anderson VE, Edwards JO, Gustafson G, Plumb RC, Suggs JW. A stable solid that generates hydroxyl radical upon dissolution in aqueous solution: reactions with proteins and nucleic acid. J Am Chem Soc 1992; 114:5430–5432.
17. Kirsch M, de Groot H. Reaction of peroxynitrite with reduced nicotinamide nucleotides; the formation of hydrogen peroxide. J Biol Chem 1999; 274:24664–24670.
18. Radi R, Beckman JS, Bush KM, Freeman BA. Peroxynitrite-induced membrane lipid peroxidation: the cytotoxic potential of superoxide and nitric oxide. Arch Biochem Biophys 1994; 288:481–487.
19. Darley–Usmar VM, Hogg N, O'Leary VJ, Wilson MT, Moncada S. The simultaneous generation of superoxide and nitric oxide can initiate lipid peroxidation in human low density lipoprotein. Free Radic Res Commun 1992; 17:9–20.
20. Tien M, Berlett BS, Levine RL, Chock PB, Stadtman ER. Peroxynitrite-mediated modification of proteins at physiological carbon dioxide concentration: pH dependence of carbonyl formation, tyrosine nitration and methionine oxidation. Proc Natl Acad Sci USA 1999; 96:7809–7814.
21. Arteel GE, Briviba K, Sies H. Protection against peroxynitrite. FEBS Lett 1999; 445:226–230.
22. Radi R. Kinetic analysis of reactivity of peroxynitrite with biomolecules. Methods Enzymol 1996; 269:354–366.
23. Florence AT, Attwood D, eds. Physicochemical Principles of Pharmacy. Wales, UK: MacMillan Press, Ltd, 1998.
24. Lymar SV, Hurst JK. Rapid reaction between peroxynitrite-ion and carbon dioxide: implications for biological activity. J Am Chem Soc 1995; 117:8867–8868.
25. Bonini MG, Radi R, Ferrer Sueta G, Ferreira ADMC, Augusto O. Direct EPR detection of the carbonate radical anion produced from peroxynitrite and carbon dioxide. J Biol Chem 1999; 274:10802–10806.
26. Denicola A, Freeman BA, Trujillo M, Radi R. Peroxynitrite reaction with carbon dioxide/bicarbonate: kinetics and influence on peroxynitrite mediated oxidations. Arch Biochem Biophys 1996; 333:49–58.
27. Boveris A, Stoppani AOM. Inhibition of electron and energy transfer in mitochondria by 19-nor-ethynyltestosterone acetate. Arch Biochem Biophys 1970; 141:641–655.

28. Chance B, Hess B. Metabolic control mechanisms. I. Electron transfer in the mammalian cells. J Biol Chem 1959; 234:2404–2412.
29. Siliprandi N, Siliprandi A, Bindoli A, Toninello A. Effect of oxidation of glutathione and membrane thiol groups on mitochondrial functions. In: Sies H, Wendel A, eds. Functions of Glutathione in Liver and Kidney. Berlin: Springer-Verlag, 1978:139–147.
30. Costa LE, Boveris A, Koch OR, Taquini AC. Liver and heart mitochondria in rats submitted to chronic hypobaric hypoxia. Am J Physiol 1988; 255:C123–C129.
31. Rice–Evans CA, Miller NJ, Bolwell PG, Bramley PM, Predham JB. The relative antioxidant activities of plant-derived polyphenolic flavonoids. Free Radic Res Commun 1995; 22:375–383.
32. Bors W, Heller W, Michel C, Saran M. Flavonoids as antioxidants: determination of radical-scavenging efficiencies. Methods Enzymol 1990; 186:343–355.
33. Rice–Evans CA, Miller NJ, Paganga G. Structure–antioxidant activity relationships of flavonoids and phenolic acids. Free Radic Biol Med 1996; 20:933–956.
34. Thompson M, Williams CR, Elliot GEP. Stability of flavonoids complexes of copper (II) and flavonoids antioxidant activity. Anal Chim Acta 1976; 85:375–381.
35. Brown JE, Khodr H, Hider RC, Rice–Evans CA. Structural dependence of flavonoid interactions with Cu^{2+} ions: implications for their antioxidant properties. Biochem J 1998; 330:1173–1178.
36. Sichel G, Corsaro C, Scallia M, Di Billio AJ, Bonomo RP. In vitro scavenger activity of some flavonoids and melanins against O_2^-. Free Radic Biol Med 1991; 11:1–7.
37. Haenen GRMM, Bast A. Nitric oxide radical scavenging of flavonoids. Methods Enzymol 1999; 301:490–503.
38. Salah N, Miller NJ, Paganga G, Tijburg L, Bolwell GP, Rice–Evans CA. Polyphenolic flavanols as scavengers of aqueous phase radicals and as chain-breaking antioxidants. Arch Biochem Biophys 1995; 322:339–346.
39. Haenen GRMM, Paquay JBG, Korthouwer REM, Bast A. Peroxynitrite scavenging by flavonoids. Biochem Biophys Res Commun 1997; 236:591–593.
40. Pannala AS, Singh S, Rice–Evans C. Flavonoids as peroxynitrite scavengers in vitro. Methods Enzymol 1999; 300:207–235.
41. Santos AC, Uyemura SA, Lopes JLC, Bazon JN, Mingatto FE, Curti C. Effect of naturally occurring flavonoids on lipid peroxidation and membrane permeability transition in mitochondria. Free Radic Biol Med 1998; 24:1455–1461.
42. Wood AW, Huang MT, Chang RL, Newmark HL, Lehr RE, Yagi H, Sayer JM, Jerina DM, Cooney AH. Inhibition of the mutagenicity of bay-region diol epoxides of polycyclic aromatic hydrocarbons by naturally occurring plant phenols: exceptional activity of ellagic acid. Proc Natl Acad Sci USA 1982; 79:5513–5517.
43. Castelluccio C, Bolwell GP, Gerrish C, Rice–Evans CA. Differential distribution of ferulic acid to the major plasma constituents in relation to its potential as an antioxidant. Biochem J 1996; 316:691–694.
44. Radi R, Beckman JS, Bush KM, Freeman BA. Peroxynitrite oxidation of sulfhydryls: the cytotoxic potential of superoxide and nitric oxide. J Biol Chem 1991; 266:4244–4250.
45. Thomson L, Trujillo M, Telleri R, Radi R. Kinetics of cytochrome c^{2+} oxidation by peroxynitrite: implications for superoxide measurements in nitric oxide-producing biological systems. Arch Biochem Biophys 1995; 319:491–507.
46. Masumoto H, Kissner R, Koppenol WH, Sies H. Kinetic study of the reaction of ebselen with peroxynitrite. FEBS Lett 1996; 398:179–182.
47. Lee JL, Hunt JA, Groves JT. Rapid decomposition of peroxynitrite by manganese porphyrin–antioxidant redox couple. Bioorg Med Chem Lett 1997; 7:2913–2918.
48. Stern MK, Jensen MP, Kramer K. Peroxynitrite decomposition catalysts. J Am Chem Soc 1996; 118:8735–8736.
49. Alvarez B, Rubbo H, Kirk M, Barnes S, Freeman BA, Radi R. Peroxynitrite-dependent tryptophan nitration. Chem Res Toxicol 1996; 9:390–396.
50. Castro L, Rodriguez M, Radi R. Aconitase is readily inactivated by peroxynitrite, but not by its precursor, nitric oxide. J Biol Chem 1994; 269:29409–29415.
51. Briviba K, Kissner R, Koppenol WH, Sies H. Kinetic study of the reaction of glutathione peroxidase with peroxynitrite. Chem Res Toxicol 1998; 11:1398–1401.
52. Alayash AI, Ryan BA, Cashon RE. Peroxynitrite-mediated heme oxidation and protein modification of native and chemically modified hemoglobins. Arch Biochem Biophys 1998; 349:65–73.

53. Floris R, Piersma SR, Yang G, Jones P, Wevwe R. Interaction of myeloperoxidase with peroxynitrite. A comparison with lactoperoxidase, horseradish peroxidase and catalase. Eur J Biochem 1993; 215:767–775.
54. MacMillan–Crow LA, Crow JP, Thompson JA. Peroxynitrite-mediated inactivation of manganese superoxide dismutase involves nitration and oxidation of critical tyrosine residues. Biochemistry 1998; 37:1613–1622.
55. Beckman JS, Ye YZ, Anderson PG, Chen J, Accavitti MA, Tarpey MM, White CR. Extensive nitration of protein tyrosines in human atherosclerosis detected by immunohistochemistry. Biol Chem Hoppe Seyler 1994; 375:81–88.
56. Gabig TG, Babior BM. The superoxide forming oxidase responsible for the respiratory burst in human neutrophils. Properties of the solubilized enzyme. J Biol Chem 1979; 254:9070–9074.
57. Paganga G, Rice–Evans CA. The identification of flavonoids as glycosides in human plasma. FEBS Lett 1997; 401:78–82.
58. Manach C, Morand C, Crespy V, Demigne C, Texier O, Regerat F, Remesy C. Quercetin is recovered in human plasma as conjugated derivatives which retain antioxidant properties. FEBS Lett 1998; 426:331–336.
59. Aziz AA, Edwards CA, Lean ME, Crozier A. Absorption and excretion of conjugated flavonols, including quercetin-$4'$-O-β-glucoside and isorhamnetin-$4'$-O-β-glucoside by human volunteers after the consumption of onions. Free Radic Res 1998; 29:257–269.

19
Antioxidant and Other Properties of Green and Black Tea

Philip J. Rijken, Sheila A. Wiseman, Ute M. Weisgerber, C. A. J. van Mierlo, Paul T. Quinlan, and F. van de Put
Unilever Health Institute, Unilever Research, Vlaardingen, The Netherlands

Douglas A. Balentine and I. Paetau-Robinson
Lipton, Englewood Cliffs, New Jersey

I. GREEN AND BLACK TEA: COMPOSITION, PROCESSING, AND CONSUMPTION

Tea is the second most popular beverage worldwide and a major source of dietary flavonoids. Considerable research effort has been dedicated to unravel the physicochemical and biological properties of tea and tea flavonoids, in particular their antioxidant functionality. The present chapter offers an overview of the state of knowledge in this area and highlights some of the key issues.

A. Green and Black Tea Flavonoid Composition

Green, oolong, and black teas are flavonoid-rich beverages prepared from the processed young leaves of *Camellia sinensis*. Flavonoids are a large family of plant phenolics that are widely distributed in fruits, vegetables, and beverages, such as tea and red wine (Fig. 1 summarizes classification of phenolic phytochemicals and major dietary sources). Flavonoids are chemically classified as dibenzpyrans and pyrones and their derivatives. The core structure consists of a diphenylpropane skeleton (Fig. 2a). The main flavonoids found in fresh tea leaf are the catechins (flavan-3-ols, or flavanols) and the flavonols (see Fig. 2B and C, respectively). These flavonoids typically make up more than 30% of the dry weight of the leaf.

Green tea is produced using thermal processes, such as steaming or dry heating, to inactivate polyphenol oxidases that oxidize catechins to more complex oligomeric flavonoids characteristic of oolong and black teas (Fig. 3 outlines the conversion reactions). The manufacturing process employed determines the types of flavonoids found in tea beverages. Epigallocatechin

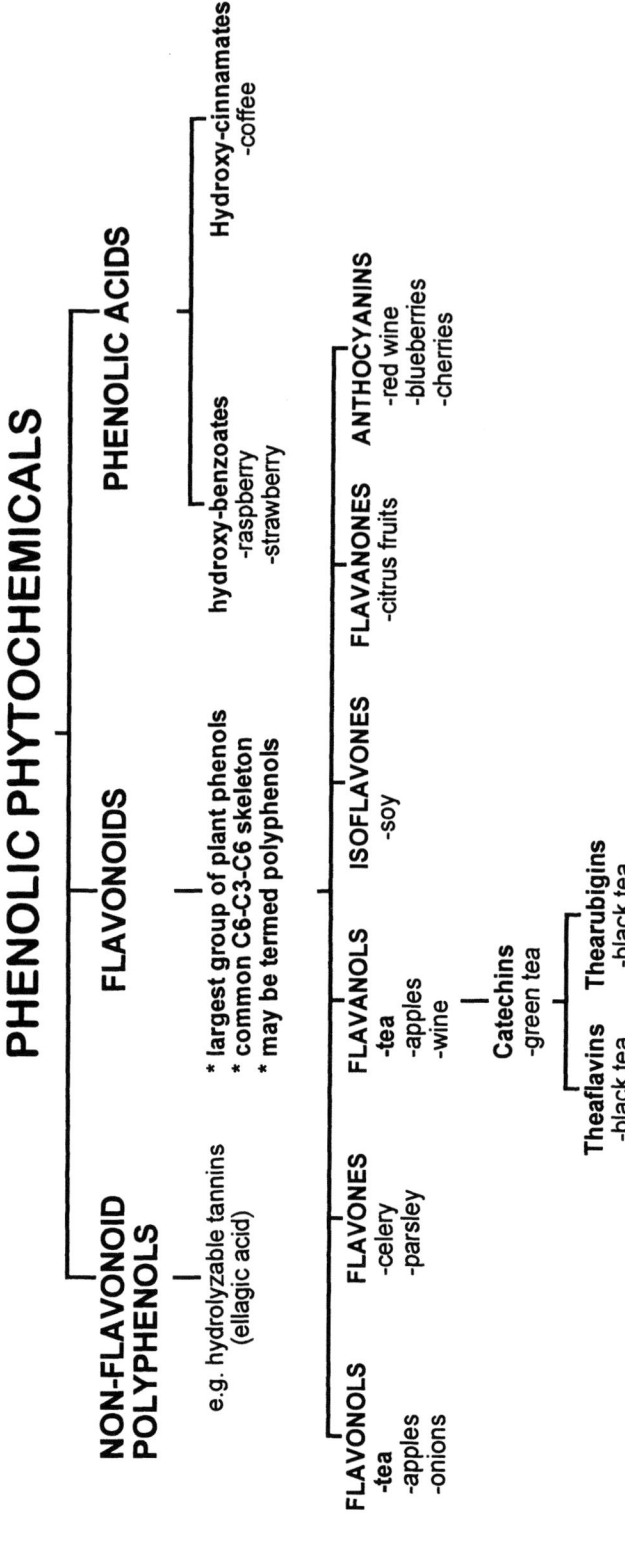

Figure 1 A classification of phenolic phytochemicals and their major dietary sources.

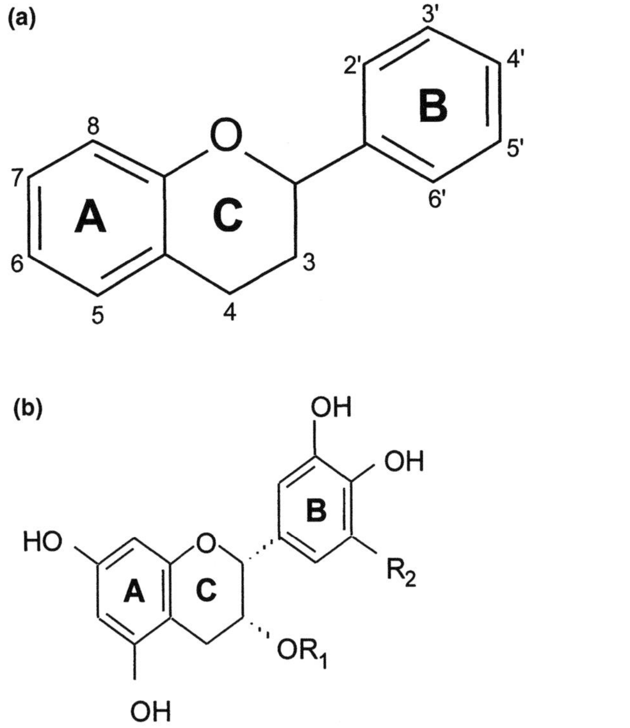

(a)

[Flavonoid diphenylpropane skeleton structure showing rings A, B, C with positions 2'-6' on ring B, 3,4,5 on ring C, and 5-8 on ring A]

(b)

[Flavan-3-ol structure with OH groups and R₁, R₂ substituents]

		R_1	R_2
Epicatechin	EC	H	H
Epicatechin gallate	ECG	Gallate	H
Epigallocatechin	EGC	H	OH
Epigallocatechin gallate	EGCG	Gallate	OH

Figure 2 (a) The flavonoid diphenylpropane skeleton; (b) tea flavanols (flavan-3-ols); (c) tea flavonols; (d) tea theaflavins.

gallate (EGCG) is the most abundant catechin in most green, oolong, and black teas. Some oxidation of the catechins typically occurs during the drying (withering) process and small quantities of a group of flavonoids characteristic of black teas, called theaflavins, can be found in most green teas (see Fig. 2d).

During the manufacture of black tea, the colorless, monomeric catechins are converted to orange-yellow- and red-brown-colored oligomeric flavonoids. Additionally, oxidation of amino acids and lipids results in the generation of numerous volatile flavor compounds. These oxidative changes are reflected in the red-amber color, reduced bitterness, and increased astringency and more complex flavor of black teas (1). Green and oolong tea beverages typically contain 30–130 mg EGCG per cup of tea, and black tea beverages typically contain 0–70 mg EGCG per cup of tea. The flavonols, such as quercetin, kaempferol, myricetin, and their glycosides, are present in much lower concentrations than the catechins and are found in comparable quantities in black, green, and oolong tea beverages (5–15 mg/cup). Flavonol aglycones are found in tea leaf, but are only minor components of tea beverages owing to their poor water solubility (1,2).

(c)

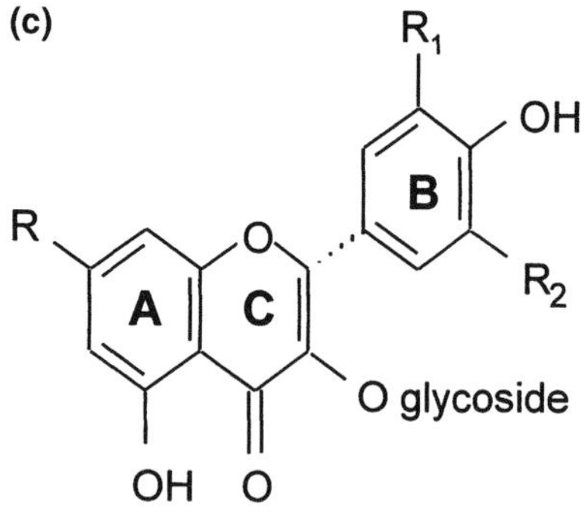

		R_1	R_2
Kaempferol glycoside	KaG	H	H
Quercetin glycoside	QuG	OH	H
Myricetin glycoside	MyG	OH	OH

(d)

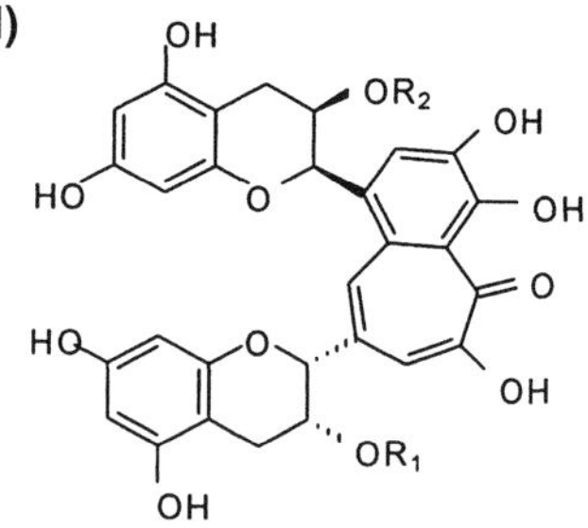

		R_1	R_2
Theaflavin	TF	H	H
Theaflavin 3-gallate	TF-3G	Gallate	H
Theaflavin 3'-gallate	TF-3'G	H	Gallate
Theaflavin di-gallate	TF-DG	Gallate	Gallate

Figure 2 (*Continued*)

Black tea contains several unique classes of flavonoids resulting from the fermentation process, including theaflavins, bisflavonols (theasinensins), theaflavic acid, theaflagallins, and a heterogeneous group of flavonoids called thearubigins. Theaflavins are a well-defined group of benzpyran-substituted benzotropolones that possess a bright red-orange color in solution and impart astringency and brightness to tea beverages (3). Black tea commonly contains four major theaflavins that vary in degree of gallation (see Fig. 2d) and two minor groups called isotheaflavins and neotheaflavins (2,4). The theaflavin content of tea leaf is typically about 2% on a dry weight basis (8–40 mg/cup) as determined by high-performance liquid chromatographic (HPLC) analysis (5). The catechin content of tea leaf is reduced by 85% during fermentation, yet only about 10% can be accounted for in the form of theaflavins and theaflavic acids. The remaining flavonoids form a heterogeneous group of water-soluble products called

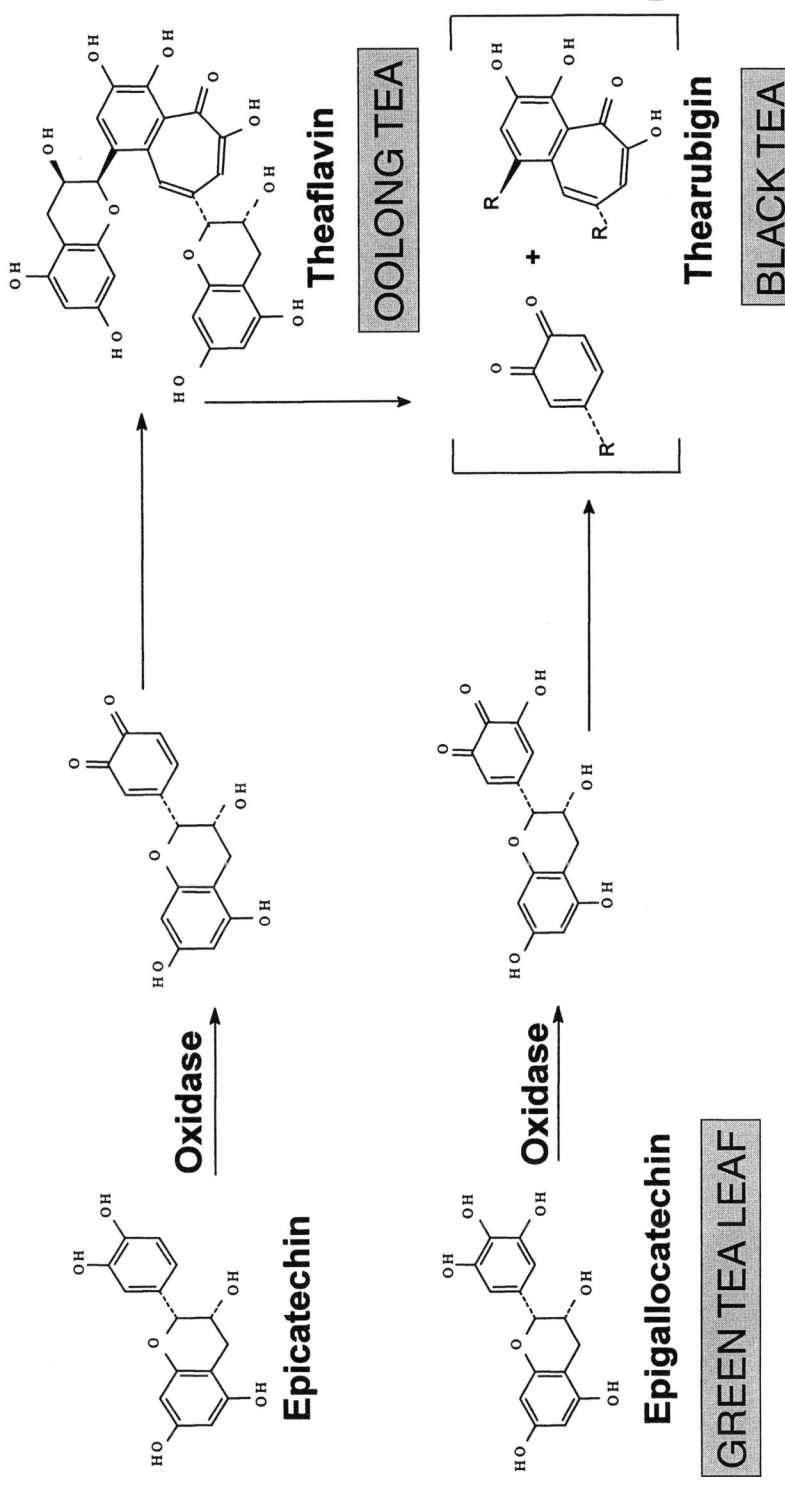

Figure 3 Main conversion reactions during processing of fresh green tea leaf to oolong and black tea.

thearubigins (Fig. 4) that typically comprise 23% of black tea leaf on a dry weight basis (100–200 mg/cup) (1,4). These flavonoid polymers are the brown or black pigments in black tea that provide thickness and astringency to tea beverages. One group of thearubigins are proanthocyanidin polymers, and two other types that have recently been identified are theafulvin (6) and oolongtheanin (7). There are no simple methods to directly determine the thearubigin content of tea beverages.

B. Tea Production and Consumption

Worldwide tea production and consumption is considerable. In 1998 the total world production of tea was 2964 million kilograms of which India, China, Kenya, and Sri Lanka were the major tea-producing countries, with a production of 870, 665, 294, and 281 million kg, respectively (8). Approximately 80% of the world tea harvest is processed to black tea. India has the largest yearly total tea consumption of tea at 632 metric tons, which translates into 660 g per capita. The largest per capita tea consumption is found in Ireland at 2960 g, which approximates to 300 L of tea beverage. The average per capita tea consumption in continental Europe is 300 g and in the United States, it is 330 g, 80% of which is consumed as iced tea.

Flavonoids are not considered to be essential nutrients and do not feature in standard food composition tables, thus studies on dietary flavonoid intakes are relatively few (9). In

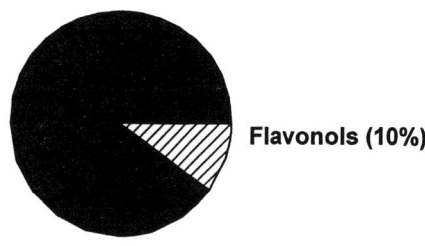

Figure 4 Approximate flavonoid composition of green and black tea.

addition, these reports are incomplete, as they focus only on flavonols and flavones (sources: tea, herbs, vegetables), with little consideration being given to flavanol intake. In populations where tea is consumed, it tends to be the major source of flavonols plus flavones [main sources are tea, herbs, vegetables; e.g., contributing to 48% total intake in a Dutch cohort (10)]. This is significant as the flavonols and flavones constitute only a small proportion (10%) of the total flavonoid complement of tea. Tea beverage, therefore, is a major source of flavonoids in humans.

II. PHYSICOCHEMICAL PROPERTIES OF TEA FLAVONOIDS

Tea flavonoids exhibit typical antioxidant properties, as deduced from a variety of physicochemical and biochemical techniques (11,12). Several groups attached to the diphenylpropane skeleton (see Fig. 2a) and other structural features have been suggested to determine flavonoid antioxidant functionality. The presence of an *ortho*-dihydroxy structure in the B-ring appears key for radical scavenging and transition metal chelation. The function of this catechol group can be further enhanced by features in the central C-ring, promoting electron delocalization and stabilization of the flavonoid aroxyl radical. Its potential relevance is reflected in the values obtained with the Trolox Equivalent Antioxidant Capacity assay (TEAC assay). Table 1 presents a selection of methods frequently used to characterize physicochemical antioxidant properties of flavonoids: TEAC value, redox potential, the ability to inhibit lipid peroxidation in microsomes and in low-density lipoproteins (LDL).

Quercetin has a relatively high TEAC value and is considered to be one of the best flavonoid antioxidants. The structure comprises a catechol moiety in the B-ring and the C-ring contains an unsaturated 2,3-double bond, in conjunction with a 3-hydroxy and a 4-keto group. The importance of the *ortho*-dihydroxy feature in the B-ring can be deduced from kaempferol, which has a structure similar to quercetin, but has only a single hydroxy group

Table 1 Physicochemical Antioxidant Properties of Flavonoids[a]

Flavonoid	TEAC	E_7 (mV)	E_{diff} (mV)[16]	IC$_{50}$ LPO Microsomes (μM)	IC$_{50}$ LPO LDL (μM)
Quercetin	4.7 (12)	330 (14)	110	4.5 (17); 5.2 (18); 9.0 (19)	0.22 (21)
Kaempferol	1.3 (12)	750 (14)	200	47 (18)	1.82 (21)
Rutin	2.4 (12)	600 (14)	230	10 (19); 16 (17); 22 (19)	0.51 (21)
Taxifolin	1.9 (12)	500 (14)			0.34 (21)
Epicatechin	2.5 (12)	570 (14)	190	13 (20); 17 (18)	0.19 (21)
Epigallocatechin	3.8 (12)	420 (14)	90	15 (20)	0.10 (21)
Epicatechin gallate	4.9 (12)		200	3.0 (20)	0.14 (21)
Epigallocatechin gallate	4.9 (12)	430 (14)	140	2.0 (20)	0.08 (21)
Theaflavin	2.9 (13)	510 (15)	160		5.5 (13)
Theaflavin 3-monogallate	4.7 (13)		200		2.8 (13)
Theaflavin 3'-monogallate	4.8 (13)		190		3.4 (13)
Theaflavin 3,3'-digallate	6.2 (13)	540 (15)	190		2.5 (13)

[a] A selection of physicochemical antioxidant properties of the flavonoids, the majority of which are commonly found in tea. Included are TEAC value, "one-electron reduction" potential at pH 7.0 by pulse-radiolysis techniques (E_7); redox potential at pH 6.15 by pulse-voltammetry (E_{diff}); and the efficacy of inhibition transition metal-induced lipid peroxidation (LPO) in microsomes or LDL.
Source: Refs. in parens.

in the B-ring. Apparently, a consequence of this difference is that it exhibits relatively poor antioxidant function. The C-ring features promote electron delocalization. Rutin is glycosylated on the 3-position in the C-ring. Both taxifolin and all tea catechins have a saturated C-ring. The presence of a gallo moiety, rather than a catechol moiety, in the B-ring (epigallocatechin) enhances the radical-scavenging efficiency, which is further boosted when the gallic acid is esterified to the 3-position in the central C-ring (epicatechin gallate, epigallocatechin gallate). Flavonoid biopolymers, such as theaflavins and thearubigins, are commonly present in black tea and also appear to have excellent antioxidant properties (11,12,22).

The "one-electron reduction" or redox potential of flavonoids may be used to predict their electron-donating abilities (14). The redox potential is often inversely related to the flavonoid antioxidant capacity, in particular if galloylated flavonoids (i.e., EGCG, ECG, theaflavin mono- and digallates) are excluded from the analysis ($r = -0.99$). Good correlations were found for the one-electron redox potentials, as determined using pulse radiolysis techniques and differential pulse voltammetry. Galloylation apparently affects the redox potential value, for these flavonoids have, in addition to being efficient antioxidants, relatively high redox potentials (see Table 1). The predicted role of the structural features mentioned was confirmed in microsomal lipid peroxidation studies, and good correlations with redox potential could be identified ($r = 0.91$; see also Refs. 19 and 23). Because transition metals are used in these studies it can be argued that transition metal sequestration, rather than radical scavenging, explains the inhibitory action of flavonoids. This issue was recently addressed by comparing the effects of flavonoids on lipid peroxidation induced by transition metals and by a hydrophilic azo-initiator (19,23). No differences were observed between either system, indicating that radical scavenging, rather than transition metal sequestration, may help explain the mechanism of action of flavonoids.

In more complex models, such as lipid peroxidation in LDL, however, the catechol moiety appears particularly relevant, as kaempferol is a very weak antioxidant (21). The importance of C-ring features as well as galloylation are not convincingly apparent in these studies. Flavonoids behave differently in LDL than in microsomes. It should be kept in mind that lipid peroxidation progresses differently in LDL, as compared with membranes, and LDL contains specific copper-binding sites from which the peroxidation process is thought to be initiated (24,25). Furthermore, antioxidant efficiency is determined by a combination of many properties, including radical scavenging, transition metal sequestration, partitioning, compartmentalization, local availability, and combinations of these. A remarkable deviation from the expected antioxidant efficiency is the poor performance of theaflavins in this system. It has been argued that this is due to their reduced ability to partition in the lipid phase (13,22). Whether this is the most likely explanation remains to be established, because the rutin glycone which is more hydrophilic, is substantially more effective than theaflavins in biochemical assays.

Flavonoids are probably efficient inhibitors of the initiation of the lipid peroxidation process, rather than being effective chain-breaking antioxidants (26,27). Vitamin E (α-tocopherol) is a far superior scavenger of lipid peroxyl radicals than any other flavonoid. Not only the chromanol ring, but also the precise location within the lipophilic environment, are key determinants in this scavenging process (28). Vitamin E is extremely lipophilic when compared with the moderate lipophilicity of flavonoids, as reflected in their calculated partition coefficients (results not shown).

Flavonoids have powerful physicochemical antioxidant properties, in particular when equipped with an *ortho*-dihydroxy function in the B-ring. The data suggest that flavonoids may contribute to the protection of lipids in membranes and LDL predominantly through radical scavenging.

III. TEA FLAVONOID PROPERTIES IN CELL BIOLOGY

A. Biological Availability of Tea Polyphenols

The study of antioxidant functionalities of tea polyphenols in cell culture systems is based on the assumption that these compounds are bioavailable to various human tissues. Indeed, increases in total plasma catechin levels up to 1 μM were observed following consumption of tea by humans (29). In plasma, most flavonoids are found in glucuronidated and sulfated form, the unconjugated molecule usually amounting to less than one-third of the total. The concentrations of individual unconjugated catechins in plasma are submicromolar (30). Consumption of (high-dosed) quercetin supplements leads to a substantial rise in plasma concentration (31,32), showing that transport to the human blood stream occurs. As yet, there are no published data on theaflavin or thearubigin plasma status, or on blood levels of flavonoid degradation products. Nevertheless, it may be concluded that several major tea polyphenols appear rapidly in the human blood circulatory system following ingestion and are, in principle, available as bioactives to humans.

A variety of cell culture studies has been performed to investigate the uptake, fate, functionalities, and mechanism of action of tea polyphenols. Assessment of polyphenol availability to cells in culture is key, because dosage to the cell is evidently intimately linked to function. Only a limited number of studies have addressed this issue. Under in vitro cell culture conditions, quercetin aglycone is taken up by Caco-2 cells, suggesting facile absorption of this compound through the human intestinal epithelium (33). Tea catechins (i.e., EGCG and ECG) are apparently taken up by cells, following a 24-h incubation of Rat-1 fibroblasts (Fig. 5; unpublished observations). Under steady-state conditions, EGCG concentrations rise more than fivefold over the levels of ECG (see Fig. 5), relative to the total amounts offered in the cell

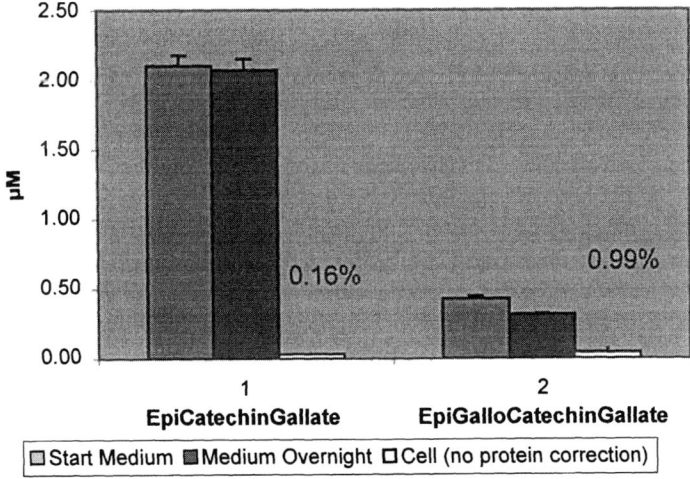

Figure 5 ECG and EGCG concentrations in a Rat-1 fibroblasts: Following a 24-h preincubation with catechins (0.2 μM ECG and 0.4 μM EGCG), cells were washed extensively and catechin levels were determined as described (35) under steady-state conditions. The percentage catechin taken up by cells is indicated relative to the total amount offered in the cell culture medium (percentage of total; $n = 2$). When compared with freshly prepared medium (start medium), no loss of polyphenols in the medium was observed following 24-h exposure to the cell culture (medium overnight). Data were not corrected for protein content, but similar cell numbers were observed in both experiments.

culture medium. Observations such as these provide potential clues to the enhanced antioxidant functionality of EGCG over ECG in experimental systems, and possibly in relation to in vivo bioavailability data (30). Alternatively, degradation of polyphenols may affect the outcome of in vitro studies. Quercetin is rapidly O-methylated in several human cell lines, or degraded with no unchanged compound left after an 8-h incubation (34).

B. Functionalities of Tea Phenolics in Cell Cultures

Cell culture studies have focused on characterization of the biological functionalities of tea catechins, quercetin, and their glycated products. A surprisingly wide range of functionalities of both catechin isomers and quercetin is apparent from the literature (summarised in Table 2). Tea catechins have been demonstrated to inhibit hydroperoxide-dependent toxicity, cell proliferation, cell cycle progression, early gene expression, and to display antimutagenic, antiallergenic, and apoptosis-inducing properties as observed in a variety of cell models. In some cases, catechin's action appears to be indirect (e.g., in linoleic hydroperoxide-induced toxicity through α-tocopherol) (36).

Tea catechins employ different properties, EGCG generally being the most effective agent. EGCG most strongly inhibited histamine release, whereas EC had no effect and moderate inhibition was observed for EGC and ECG. High EGCG effectivity may be attributed to its enhanced antioxidant potential relative to other tea catechins, but may also be related to enhanced availability to the cell.

Quercetin affects a multitude of cell functions, including detoxification enzyme activity, ICAM expression, early proto-oncogene expression, NO production, and signal transduction. This compound can inhibit reactive oxygen species-induced DNA damage and lipid peroxidation, and it displays antiestrogenic properties. In the studies described, the concentration range of polyphenols varied from 1 to 100 μM, and the highest effectivity is found with concentrations higher than 10 μM.

Cell culture studies have indicated that catechins and quercetin are multifunctional molecules that may act through a wide variety of mechanisms in different cell types. These include modulatory effects on gene expression, cell proliferation, and apoptosis, ICAM, and NO-related processes. In addition, antimutagenic, antiallergenic, antiestrogenic properties, as well as various receptor-mediated effects (see also Sec. VI) have been observed. Most studies employed relatively high concentrations of polyphenols, compared with those observed in vivo. Cell studies may reveal more specific functionalities of tea polyphenols, if concentrations that are closer to the levels expected in vivo are employed. The various properties and mechanisms of action of tea polyphenols now listed can be linked to the etiology of a range of conditions and pathologies, including those related to blood vessel function, heart disease, cancer, and immune system function.

IV. FUNCTIONALITIES OF TEA AND TEA FLAVONOIDS IN ANIMAL MODELS

Administration of green or black tea to animal models of oxidative stress and oxidative stress-associated pathologies (e.g., cancer, inflammation, and atherosclerosis), elicits a range of responses that are consistent with the proposal that tea flavonoids or their metabolites are not only bioavailable, but are also active in affecting cellular processes in vivo, by mechanisms that may be related to their antioxidant functionalities.

Table 2 Summary of Functionalities of Catechins and Quercetin in Various Cell Models

Compound	Function[a]	Cell type
Catechin	Protection against linoleic hydroperoxide-induced toxicity by α-tocopherol (36)	Human umbilical vein endothelial cells
EGCG, EGC, ECG	Inhibition of A23187, or 48/80-induced histamine and leukotriene B_4 release, antiallergy (37)	Rat peritoneal exudate cells
EGCG	Preferential growth inhibition, apoptosis induction, and c-*fos*/c-*myc* expression of transformed versus nontransformed cells (38)	WI38 and SV40-transformed WI38 cells, Caco-2 cell line
EGCG	Blocks LPS-induced NO synthase expression and protein levels through down-regulation NF-κB transcription factor (39)	Peritoneal macrophages
Tannin fraction, EGCG, CG, EGC, EC	Inhibition of cell proliferation (40)	Smooth-muscle cells
Green tea catechin extract, EGCG	Growth inhibition and stimulation of apoptosis (41)	Human stomach cancer, KATO III cell line
Green tea extract/ECG	Decrease cell thiol status and cell viability by SH groups (42)	Ehrlich ascites tumor cell line
Catechins, gallates, theaflavins	Review on various antimutagenic and carcinogenic properties, by a multitude of mechanisms (43)	Various
EC, myricetin, quercetin	Differential effects on proliferation, morphology, and detoxification enzyme activity, alter metabolic activation of carcinogens (44)	MCF-7 breast cancer cell line
Quercetin	Inhibition PMA and TNF-α induced ICAM-1 expression by AP-1 and JNK, anti-inflammatory (45)	Human endothelial cells
Quercetin	Inhibition H_2O_2-induced NF-κB binding activity, 8-oxodG and DNA strand breaks (46)	HepG2 cell line
Quercetin	Inhibition LPS-activated NO production possibly by iNOS enzyme expression (47)	LPS-activated RAW 264.7 macrophage cell line
Quercetin	Inhibition estrogen and TGF-induced growth stimulation by antiestrogen action (48)	MCF-7 breast cancer cell line
Flavonols (e.g., quercetin)	Ex vivo protection against H_2O_2-induced DNA damage, independent of plasma antioxidant status (49)	Human (diabetic) lymphocytes
Quercetin	Suppression of growth factor/LPS-induced responses [e.g., cell proliferation, α-actin expression, MAP-kinase activation, TNF-α excretion, NO production (50)]	Rat hepatic stellate and Kupfer cells

(*continued*)

Table 2 (*Continued*)

Compound	Function[a]	Cell type
Quercetin	Cell cycle arrest, blocking of IP3 signaling, synergy with genistein (51)	OVCAR-5 cell line
Quercetin	Hypoxanthine–xanthine oxidase, H_2O_2, 1-chloro-2,4-dinitrobenzene, aminotriazole-induced cell damage by lipid peroxidation, not direct ROS scavenging (52)	Renal tubular epithelial LLC-PK1 cell line

[a]Specific references are in parentheses.

A. Irradiation-Induced Oxidative Stress

Epigallocatechin gallate (EGCG) provided to mice in drinking water for 1 month significantly blocked radiation-induced oxidative damage to hepatic lipids and improved the 30-day survival time after irradiation by 33% (53). In mice, which were gamma-irradiated to induce hydroxyl radical-induced DNA damage in vivo, treatment with flavan-3-ols and flavonols significantly reduced formation of micronuclei in reticulocytes, a marker of DNA damage (54). Exposure of skin to ultraviolet (UV) irradiation can result in either direct or indirect (by reactive oxygen species) damage to DNA and increased risk of skin cancer. Green tea has a marked inhibitory effect on skin tumor size in 7,12-dimethylbenz[a]anthracene (DMBA)-initiated mice treated with UVB (55). Oral administration of 1.25% black tea or green tea, with or without caffeine as the sole source of drinking fluid, also inhibited the formation of UVB-induced tumors in DMBA-initiated SKH-1 mice (56), with black and green teas demonstrating similar inhibitory effects. More recent studies in hairless SKH-1 mice exposed to UVB and UVA+B irradiation, demonstrated that both green and black tea reduced skin tumor formation and suggested that black tea may afford greater protection against UVA+B (solar simulated) irradiation than green tea (57).

B. Diet-Induced Oxidative Stress

Rats fed a high-protein diet (18% [w/w] casein and 0.75% [w/w] adenine) supplemented with either a catechin mixture or EGCG excreted less urinary methylguanidine, an indirect renal marker for hydroxyl radical damage (58). Supplementation of a diet high in polyunsaturated fat (30 energy percent perilla oil) with catechins (1% of diet) reduced the level of oxidative damage, measured as thiobarbituric-reactive substances (TBARS) in rat plasma and erythrocytes, and had a sparing effect on plasma α-tocopherol (59). Ex vivo lipid peroxidation determined in rat liver was reduced following feeding of diets containing 3% (w/w) green or black tea for 50 days (60). Long-term supplementation (19 months) of green tea polyphenols to rat diets significantly reduced the level of plasma TBARS (61).

C. Inflammation

Catechins and quercetin inhibit several aspects related to human neutrophil function in vitro that are considered to be important components of inflammatory reactions, including the release of lysosomal enzymes and the production of free radicals (62). Additionally, the black tea-specific flavonoid, theaflavin-3,3'-digallate, blocks the activation of nuclear factor kappa-B (NF-κB), a necessary transcription factor for inducible (inflammatory) nitric oxide synthase induction

(63). These in vitro anti-inflammatory effects of tea flavonoids have also been demonstrated following tea ingestion in vivo. For example, consumption of green tea polyphenols by SKH-1 hairless mice protects against UVB-induced inflammatory responses (64), and in male BALB/c mice, green tea polyphenols decreased lipopolysaccharide-induced tumor necrosis factor-alpha (TNF-α) production in serum in a dose–response manner and at 0.5 g green tea polyphenols per kilogram bodyweight, serum TNF-α was reduced by 80% compared with the control value (65).

D. Cardiovascular Disease

In studies published to date, tea ingestion in animal models of atherosclerosis does not consistently inhibit the formation of atherosclerotic lesions. In cholesterol-fed rabbits, green or black tea extract supplied in the drinking water at a concentration of 3 g/L did not reduce aortic lesion formation (66). In the same study, vitamin E (200 mg/kg diet) and all-*trans*-β-carotene (20 mg/kg diet) were also ineffective, suggesting that this hypercholesterolemic model may not be sensitive to antiatherosclerotic effects mediated by antioxidants, possibly owing to high levels of β-very low-density lipoprotein (βVLDL) which does not possess a requirement for oxidation before macrophage uptake. A study in homozygous LDL receptor-null mice demonstrated that a dietary antioxidant mixture (0.1% vitamin E, 0.5% β-carotene, and 0.05% vitamin C) inhibited fatty streak formation, whereas black tea (1.25%) provided ad libitum in drinking water had no effect (67). In vitro data suggest that it is more likely that tea flavonoids will exert antithrombotic/antiplatelet effects (68,69), and this is supported by limited data in animals. In a canine thrombosis model, intragastric administration of Earl Grey black tea (10 mL/kg), the equivalent of 3 cups, inhibited platelet activity and prevented experimental coronary thrombosis (70).

E. Carcinogen-Induced Oxidative Stress

The chemical carcinogens 2-nitropropane and 4-(methylnitrosamino)-1-(3-pyridyl)-1-butanone (NNK) induce oxidative damage to DNA. Rats provided green tea infusion or a tea polyphenol isolate, standardized to the same level of EGCG as the green tea, for 2 weeks before exposure to 2-nitropropane had significantly lower levels of hepatic 8-hydroxydeoxyguanosine (8-OHdG) adducts and lipid peroxides (71). In another study, NNK induced 8-OHdG adducts and lung tumors were significantly reduced in mice drinking green tea or EGCG (72). Although these studies indicate that reduction of oxidative DNA damage may be a consequence of tea flavonoid consumption, the compelling anticarcinogenic effects of green and black tea, which have consistently been demonstrated in animal models of carcinogenesis (73,74), may also involve mechanisms unrelated to antioxidant action. Inhibition of angiogenesis (75) and apoptosis (76), as demonstrated for EGCG, are possible alternative anticarcinogenic mechanisms of tea polyphenols. There is now a real requirement for the confirmation of these potential benefits of tea polyphenols at normal consumption levels in humans.

V. FUNCTIONALITIES OF TEA AND TEA FLAVONOIDS IN HUMANS

A. Effect of Green and Black Tea on Plasma Antioxidant Activity in Humans

A growing number of studies have demonstrated that consumption of green and black tea enhances the antioxidant activity (radical-scavenging or ferrous iron-reducing) of human plasma.

One study (77) demonstrated a significant increase in plasma total antioxidant status in human volunteers between 30 and 60 min after consumption of 300 mL of either green or black tea prepared by infusion 2 g of tea leaves with 100 mL water. Consumption of 400 mL green tea prepared from an infusion using 20 g dry tea leaves, resulted in a 4% increase in plasma ferrous iron-reducing ability of plasma (FRAP) 40 min after tea ingestion (78). No increase in FRAP was observed after water intake. In a separate study, ingestion of a single dose of either green or black tea, equivalent to 3 normal cups, significantly increased the plasma FRAP value by 2–3% (79), a result that is in agreement with the findings of Benzie et al. (78). The study by Leenen et al. (79) also demonstrated that addition of milk to tea, which is common practice, particularly in the United Kingdom, India, and Australia, did not significantly negate the observed increase in plasma antioxidant activity following ingestion of tea without milk. These results, from a controlled, crossover study, contrast with those from an earlier report in which addition of milk to tea completely abolished the plasma antioxidant activity response (77), but are consistent with the observation that addition of milk to black tea did not influence the absorption of tea catechins in human volunteers (80). In another short-term study, no significant effect on plasma antioxidant activity was observed in ten healthy subjects after black tea ingestion (81). The lack of significant change in this study could be attributed to the limited power of the study (no control treatment was included and the study comprised only a few subjects) or to differences in the sensitivity of the applied assays.

B. Effect of Tea Flavonoids on Oxidative Damage Markers in Humans

Products of free radical-mediated damage to lipids, protein, and DNA have been identified in biological material, such as plasma, urine, and blood cells, and proposed as "biomarkers" for defining the in vivo protective effects of dietary antioxidants (82). There are currently no consensus "best markers" and little data on their validity in predicting subsequent pathological outcomes are available, although for some markers (e.g., F_2-isoprostanes) this aspect is now being considered. The biomarker approach has been applied in several human intervention trials investigating the biological antioxidant effects of tea and tea flavonoids. In a 4-week intervention study in nonsmokers, consumption of green or black tea (0.9 L/day) had no effect on ex vivo LDL oxidation, plasma levels of malondialdehyde, LPL lipid hydroperoxide levels, or plasma levels of the antioxidant vitamins (83). A similar study in smokers investigated the antioxidant effects of green and black tea consumption (0.9 L/day) and a green tea polyphenol supplement, equivalent to 18 cups/day of green tea (84). Although tea polyphenols strongly inhibited LDL oxidation in vitro, in agreement with the previous trial in nonsmokers, no effects of tea flavonoid ingestion were observed on ex vivo LDL oxidation or plasma levels of antioxidant vitamins. Another study applying the ex vivo approach in whole plasma from healthy volunteers also failed to detect antioxidant effects of black tea (85), although a significantly increased resistance of LDL to oxidation in subjects consuming 750 mL/day of black tea for 4 weeks was shown. Results from ex vivo subjects are, therefore, still inconsistent.

A recent study, has identified biological antioxidant properties of green tea extract (consumption equivalent to 10 cups/day of green tea) in subjects consuming a controlled high linoleic acid diet (87). Green tea extract significantly decreased plasma malondialdehyde concentrations in comparison with placebo treatment. Other putative biomarkers of oxidative stress (i.e., urinary 8-isoprostaglandin $F_{2\alpha}$ and whole blood oxidized glutathione) were not influenced by the tea intervention. Green tea (approximately 1 L/day) reduced urinary malondialdehyde and 8-hydroxydeoxyguanosine concentrations following tea consumption for 1 week (88), and supplementation with green tea catechins significantly reduced plasma phosphatidylcholine hydroperoxide concentrations 60 min after ingestion (89). Tea drinking reduced oxidative damage biomarkers in chronic smokers, such as increased sister chromatid exchange (SCE) and micronucleation in lymphocytes. In a case-controlled study, tea drinking among smokers was associated with a significantly lower level of smoking-induced micronuclei in peripheral blood lymphocytes (90), and smokers who consumed 2–3 cups/day of green tea for 6 months had significantly lower levels of SCE in mitogen-stimulated white blood cells than smokers who consumed 2–3 cups/day of coffee or other beverages (91).

These data indicate that there is evidence for antioxidant functionalities of both green and black tea polyphenols in vivo, but more evidence in humans using validated biomarkers of oxidative damage is certainly required.

C. Effect of Tea Flavonoids on Markers of Cardiovascular Disease in Humans

The effect of black tea consumption on blood lipids has been assessed in several short-term controlled trials. Consumption of 1.8 L/day of black tea for 4 weeks had no effect on total serum cholesterol, LDL, or high-density lipoprotein (HDL) cholesterol or triglyceride levels when compared with water consumption (92). Similar findings were reported when lower amounts (0.75–0.90 L) were consumed for 4 weeks (83,86). Data on green tea and blood lipids in humans are limited, but consumption of 0.9 L/day of green tea for 4 weeks did not significantly change the serum levels of total, LDL, or HDL cholesterol when compared with water (83).

Only a few studies have assessed the effects of tea on markers of thrombosis or hemostasis. Consumption of black tea, 6 mugs/day for 4 weeks, was not associated with altered plasma fibrinogen, tissue plasminogen activator (tPA) or plasminogen activator inhibitor (PAI-1) levels or activities (93), although when the data were reanalyzed according to apolipoprotein E (apoE) genotype, PAI-1 activity was lower in subjects with E2/E3 genotype (94). In a separate study, ingestion of 100 mg/day quercetin-3-glycoside (69) had no significant effects on plasma fibrinogen or PAI-1. Results in genetically heterogeneous populations do not currently suggest that ingestion of tea flavonoids has significant effects on soluble coagulation or fibrinolysis factors in humans. The protective effects of tea ingestion on platelet-mediated thrombus formation, which have been observed in a canine model (70), have yet to be confirmed in humans.

Both green and black tea demonstrate biological effects relative to a wide spectrum of molecular and cellular targets, and a growing body of evidence derived from epidemiological and experimental studies in animals and humans suggests that tea ingestion may be of benefit in various oxidative stress-related pathologies, such as cardiovascular disease, cancer, and inflammation. The composition of green and black tea polyphenols differs considerably, with green tea containing primarily monomeric catechins and black tea containing a high proportion of polymeric flavonoids. However, when green and black tea have been compared at equivalent doses in the same study, similar biological effects have frequently been observed, suggesting common modes of action. This would imply that the polymeric flavonoids found in black tea are bioavailable, and given their molecular weights (700–10,000 Da), it is possible that phenolic scission products of colonic bacterial action on theaflavins and thearubigins are the major absorbed products. Future studies on tea polyphenols need to elucidate the nature of the active forms in vivo, their major molecular or cellular targets, and their mechanisms of action.

VI. COGNITIVE AND MOOD EFFECTS OF BLACK TEA CONSUMPTION

Several components in black tea may affect mood and cognition. Most attention has been focused on the effects of caffeine, present in moderate levels in black tea, and to a lesser extent on the effects of flavonoids, theanine, aroma, and taste.

A. Immediate Effects of Black Tea Consumption and the Role of Caffeine

Caffeine is a mild stimulant of the central nervous system, which increases subjective feelings of energy, alertness, and reaction time on simple tasks, particularly in fatigued subjects (95). Furthermore, it activates the sympathetic nervous system, leading to small increases in blood pressure, changes in regional blood flow, and increases in sweat gland activity (96–98). However, tolerance to the cardiovascular effects of caffeine is thought to develop rapidly, and there is no consistent association between long-term caffeine or tea consumption and blood pressure (99,100).

Levels of caffeine in black tea ($\sim$ 40 mg) are generally less than half that of coffee ($\sim$ 80–160 mg) and a fraction of the level (>200 mg) used in many published studies (101). However, as little as 32 mg caffeine improves vigilance (102). The effects of doses as found in black tea and the interaction with time of day were addressed in a recent study (103). Black tea ingestion associated with rapid increases in alertness and performance, and consumption throughout the day largely prevented the common diurnal pattern of performance decrements over time. A second study showed that high levels of caffeine (four times 150 mg) provided no additional benefit over low levels (four times 37 mg) in the beverage (Hindmarch I, personal communication). Thus, low doses of caffeine can produce pronounced effects on aspects of cognitive performance. Physiological effects on blood pressure, heart rate, and peripheral blood flow are dose-related, with effects observable at about 25–50 mg of caffeine (104).

Caffeine does not appear to be the only factor to contribute to the immediate responses to black tea consumption. In one recent study the effect of black tea, coffee, and water (all with or without caffeine) on autonomic response and mood were monitored in healthy subjects (98). Caffeine augmented many of the physiological responses, and produced positive changes in subjective mood. However, black tea potentiated the increase in skin temperature, compared with coffee and water, indicative of a greater peripheral vasodilatory response plausibly related to the presence of flavonoids in black tea. This acute vasodilatory response may contribute to not only the subjective "warming" effect of drinking tea, but it also indicates tea can influence the microcirculation, with possible implications for cardiovascular function. In this context, it is interesting that flavonoids from a variety of sources have been used in medical practice for over 40 years to treat disorders of peripheral circulation, although their therapeutic value has generally not been evaluated in well-controlled clinical studies (105).

Black tea aroma alone can reliably improve mood in both Asian and United Kingdom consumers (Aspen J, personal communication). This was measured by monitoring the effect of aromas on the physiological "startle response"; the latter is a validated physiological response for monitoring mood state and is modulated by pleasant and unpleasant aromas. There are indications that the bitter–astringent taste of the beverage contributes to an increase in alertness (98,104). Mechanistically, it is possible that these sensory cues can trigger a response in human subjects who have learned to associate these cues with the subsequent physiological effects of the beverage. In conclusion, black tea ingestion can quickly stimulate aspects of mood, cognition, and autonomic nervous system function. These effects may be important drivers of habitual tea consumption in humans.

B. Effects of Other Black Tea Components

Black tea infusion comprises about 30% flavonoids, 7–10% caffeine, 15% carbohydrates, 15% amino acids, and 10% ash, with the rest comprising minor components, including lipids and organic acids. In terms of biological activity, most attention has focused on the flavonoids and, more recently, one of the more unusual amino acids found in tea.

1. Flavonoids

Flavonoids possess potent antioxidant activity, the ability to inhibit various enzyme systems, and can exert a wide range of (receptor-mediated) effects. Relative to the latter, catechins found in black and green tea can inhibit β-adrenergic, opiate, dopamine, and serotonin receptors in vitro (106). There is evidence that cardiovascular β-adrenoreceptor function is not influenced by black tea consumption (6–8 cups/day for 14 days) in humans, but cardiovascular stress responses and lymphocyte β-adrenoreceptor numbers were altered (107). This is suggestive of some effect on receptor-mediated responses, although the mechanisms involved are unclear. Some flavonoids possess a selective and relatively mild affinity for benzodiazepine receptors and a pharmacological profile compatible with a partial agonist action (108). The pharmacological effects of black tea flavonoids have not been thoroughly investigated and, as yet, there is no clear evidence that flavonoids can cross the blood–brain barrier. A more profound understanding of the pharmacokinetics and pharmacodynamics of tea flavonoids and their metabolites is required before more firm conclusions can be drawn about psychological effects in humans.

2. Theanine

Theanine (*N*-ethyl glutamine) is an amino acid present in unusually high levels in tea, tea being virtually the only dietary source. Theanine represents close to 1.3% of the dry weight of green tea (109), although fermentation to black tea can reduce the levels substantially. Theanine has been reported to reduce blood pressure in spontaneously hypertensive rats (110) and to decrease the levels of serotonin and norepinephrine in rat brain (111). These effects are, to some extent, antagonistic to those of caffeine. Levels used have generally been high (1500 mg/kg) and in the absence of well-controlled human studies, it is unclear whether the presence of this compound in tea can exert physiological effects in humans.

C. Chronic Effects on Cognitive Decline

Although dementia and Alzheimer's disease are associated with reduced plasma antioxidant levels, epidemiological evidence for a preventive role of dietary antioxidants is mixed (112,113). The potential role of flavonoids in preventing cognitive decline has not been investigated. A first indication that flavonoids may play a role comes from a double-blind, placebo-controlled study with *Gingko biloba* extract, which stabilized or improved cognitive performance in patients with Alzheimer's or in those who are demented (114). Potentially, the beneficial effects of this extract may be derived from its mixed content of flavonoids, terpenoids, and organic acids, but further work is required to establish a causal relation with flavonoids.

Drinking tea can produce rapid cognitive, mood, and physiological effects in human subjects, resulting from both the biological effects of tea components (caffeine and others) and possibly "learned associations" of the subject acquired through prior experience. A causal relation between tea flavonoids and mood or cognition remains to be established.

VII. EPIDEMIOLOGICAL EVIDENCE ON TEA CONSUMPTION AND THE PREVENTION OF CHRONIC DISEASES

The epidemiological evidence for black tea consumption and its association with cardiovascular disease risk is summarized in this section. In less detail, the state of evidence for a relation between tea and cancer risk is described. Finally, the evidence available on the association between tea consumption and neurodegenerative disease, cataract, and osteoporosis is discussed.

A. Cardiovascular Diseases

Cardiovascular diseases (CVDs) are recognized as multifactorial. The most firmly established risk factors are high blood pressure, smoking, and high blood cholesterol levels. International comparisons indicate that tea consumption could be a modest contributor to the prevention of CVD (115,116). In countries, such as those in the United Kingdom, where both tea intake and heart disease mortality are high, such a modest protective effect might be overwhelmed by the effects of a low consumption of fruit and vegetable, and high rates of smoking. Even a modest effect of tea on heart disease risk would be important from a public health point of view, because tea is, after water, the second most frequently drunk beverage worldwide, and CVD is the most frequent cause of death in adults.

Table 3 summarizes the basic characteristics and results of all case–control and cohort studies that have investigated the association between black tea consumption and risk of myocardial infarction (MI), coronary heart diseases (CHD), mortality, or stroke incidence. A case–control study of the Boston Collaborative Surveillance Program (117) was the first study to show a nonsignificant risk reduction for myocardial infarction of 34% for subjects consuming more than 6 cups/day of tea versus those who did not drink any tea. No adjustment, however, was made for potentially confounding lifestyle and dietary factors. A subsequent, smaller study, comparing male cases of first MI with age-matched controls, found a nonsignificant increased risk with high tea consumption (118). Most known risk factors for CHD were taken into account in a multivariate model, and coffee drinkers were excluded from this analysis. A recent case–control study of the Boston Area Health Study (119) categorized subjects into a relatively narrow range of tea consumption, leaving sufficient statistical power in the highest consumption category. After adjustment for all known risk factors for CHD, including blood LDL/HDL ratio, subjects who drank 1 cup/day or more of black tea had about half the risk of a heart attack compared with those who did not drink tea at all. In support of this finding is the significant trend of a lower risk across tea consumption categories. Also, coffee consumption, although negatively correlated with tea, showed no association with risk of MI in this study, suggesting that the protective effect seen for tea is specific and not likely to be due to confounding. Interestingly, this study provides the suggestion that the mechanism by which tea may exhibit its protection is not by influencing blood lipids, because adjusting for blood lipids did not change the estimated odds ratio.

Prospective studies circumvent the problem of bias largely by evaluating habitual dietary intake in healthy subjects and associate this with diseases occurring many years subsequent to measuring dietary exposure. Several prospective cohort studies have investigated the association between tea intake and subsequent CVD (see Table 3). In a California cohort, tea intake was not related to MI incidence (120), whereas in a Norwegian cohort, drinking more than 1 cup/day of tea reduced the risk of men of dying from CHD by 36%. However, this estimate failed to be statistically significant (121). A long-standing Dutch cohort was able to demonstrate a significantly reduced risk of dying from CHD independent of the major established risk factors (122). This finding was subsequently confirmed for incident stroke by Keli et al. (123).

Table 3 Prospective Cohort Studies Investigating the Association Between Tea Intake and Cardiovascular Disease (CVD)

Ref.	Study, country	Sex, age (yr)	No. of cases/controls	Endpoint	RR	95% CI	Categories of highest versus lowest tea consumption	P for trend
Case–control studies								
Boston Coll, 1972	BCDSP Massachusetts, US	Men and women	276/1104	Nonfatal MI	0.66	0.33–1.30	≥6 versus 0 cups/day	0.2
Rosenberg et al., 1988	Massachusetts, US	Men, 25–54	146/205	First nonfatal MI	1.7	0.6–4.9	≥5 versus 0 cups/day	Not given
Sesso et al., 1999	Boston Area Health Study, US	Men and women, <76 yrs	298/294	First nonfatal MI	0.55	0.32–0.94	≥1 versus 0 cups/day[d]	<0.05

Ref.	Cohort, country	Sex, age (yr)	Length of follow-up (yr)	No events	Endpoint (follow-up)	RR	95% CI	Categories of highest versus lowest tea consumption	P for trend
Cohort studies on black tea									
Klatsky et al., 1990	Kaiser Permanent Hospital Cohort (Oakland + San Francisco), USA	Men and women	5	740	MI incidence	1.11	0.52–2.36	>6 vs. 0 cups/day	Not given
Stensvold et al., 1992	Norway	Men, 35–49[a]	12	141	CHD mortality	0.64	0.38–1.07	>1 vs. <1 cups/day	Not given
Hertog et al., 1993	Zutphen cohort, NL	Men, 65–84	5	43	CHD mortality	0.45	0.22–0.93	>4 vs. ≤2 cups/day[b]	<0.05
Keli et al., 1996	Zutphen cohort, NL	Men, 50–69	15	42	Stroke incidence	0.31	0.12–0.84	≥4.7 vs. <2.6 cups/day[a]	<0.05
Hertog et al., 1997	Caerphilly, Wales	Men, 45–59	14	131	CHD mortality	2.3	1.0–5.1	>8 vs. ≤ 2 cups/day[b]	<0.05
Woodward et al., 1999	Scottish Heart Health Study	Men (46–59)	7.7	402	Fatal	♂1.10	0.51–2.37	≥5 cups vs. 0 cups/day	NS
		Women, 40–59		176	Nonfatal CHD	♀1.06	0.28–4.05		
Yochum et al., 1999	Iowa Women's Health Study	Women, 40–59	10	438	CHD mortality	0.89	0.67–1.17	≥0.7 times vs. 0 times/day	0.4

[a]No analyses were done for women because of few deaths.
[b]1 cup corresponds to 125 mL.
[c]1 cup corresponds to 150 mL.
[d]1 cup corresponds to 237 mL.

The Dutch population provides a wider range of tea consumption than the Norwegian or Californian making it more likely for an association to be identified. On the other hand, in a Welsh population where tea drinking is a universal habit and more than 90% of tea drinkers take milk in their tea, heavy drinkers had the highest risk of death from CHD. Hertog et al. (124) put forward the argument that the addition of milk may lead to binding of milk protein to tea components and thereby prevent their absorption. van het Hof and co-workers (80) have shown in human volunteers that adding milk to black tea does not influence the absorption of quercetin and catechins. They were as yet not able to show the influence on more complex tea polyphenols. However, even if adding milk did prevent the absorption of some of the active compounds in black tea and thereby diminish its potential health benefits, this would not explain an increased risk with increasing tea intake. In the Caerphilly study (124), men with the highest intake of tea tended to be manual workers, they smoked more, consumed less alcohol, and ate more fat. These and other factors were adjusted for in the analysis when studying the association between tea intake and CHD outcome. However, some are adjusted for only in very broad categories, such as smoking (never, ex, or current smoker) and social class (manual or nonmanual workers). It is evident from studies such as the Whitehall study that social class is a very strong predictor for CHD mortality with a 2.3-fold higher CHD mortality in lower-grade civil servants compared with higher-grade ones (125). Hence, the most plausible explanation for a higher mortality in heavy tea drinkers in Wales is residual confounding by imperfectly measured coronary risk factors that cluster with tea intake.

Tea consumption was similarly correlated with socioeconomic status in the Scottish Heart Health Study (126), representing a follow-up of a prevalence study of coronary heart disease in Scotland published in 1993 (127). The elevated risk for coronary morbidity and mortality with increasing tea consumption reported in this study is based on a crude logistic regression analysis that did not account for any of the major risk factors, not even age. According to the earlier paper by Brown et al. (127) on the same study, 21.8% of all subjects were classified as having indications of coronary heart disease at baseline. This is relevant because clinical as well as preclinical symptoms may bring about lifestyle and dietary changes. Tea is generally perceived as "less irritating" than coffee, and cases may therefore revert back to drinking tea. This means that in the analysis cause and effect could be confused. In our table we refer to the most relevant results reported in this study; namely, those for which multiple adjustments were made for other risk factors and in which subjects with CHD at baseline were excluded. Weak, nonsignificant associations in both men and women result from making those appropriate adjustments. The largest women's cohort that studied the association between black tea consumption and death from CHD, found a small, but not significant, reduction in risk with very moderate black tea consumption (128). Multiple adjustments were made for known coronary risk factors.

In a total of ten studies, six showed a reduced risk of MI incidence, CHD mortality, or stroke incidence among regular tea drinkers with varying consumption levels. For three studies, this reduction was statistically significant. Of the remaining studies, one reported an increased risk of borderline significance. Insufficient control for confounding provides the most likely explanation for the discrepancy in results among these studies.

Evidence from epidemiological studies is not conclusive, but that several studies demonstrate lower rates of CHD or stroke in tea drinkers leaves open the possibility of a protective effect of tea against CVD, even at a moderate level of consumption. Confirmation of these findings in countries other than the United States, United Kingdom, and Western Europe is needed.

Epidemiological evidence on the possible role of green tea in the etiology of CVD is scarce. We found two cross-sectional prevalence studies in Japan reporting that subjects who drank green tea regularly were less likely than those not drinking green tea to have a history of stroke or CHD (129,130). Carefully designed case–control studies with newly diagnosed cases and prospective studies are warranted to elucidate the preventive potential of green tea in CVD.

B. Cancer

Evidence from animal models for the effects of tea and tea flavonoids in cancer prevention is strong, and a number of biological mechanisms have been identified by which tea may reduce cancer risk (131). Population-based studies do not provide consistent evidence for tea to play a role in cancer prevention. Case–control studies and cohort studies on black tea were not specifically designed to examine the relation between tea consumption and cancer risk so that often information on type, amount, and strength of tea consumed is very limited or absent. Also, many of the earlier case–control studies published in the 1970s and 1980s have not appropriately adjusted for other known risk factors of specific cancers. Positive associations between tea drinking and cancer risk occur mainly in studies on cancer sites, such as colorectal and bladder cancer, where it is conceivable that preclinical symptoms cause cases to take in more fluid, which leads to biased results. There is a general trend for more recent studies to be of higher quality, where several studies point to the possibility of lowered risk of digestive tract cancers (132,133), prostate cancer (134,135), and pancreatic cancer (132,136,137) among tea drinkers. Prospective studies on bladder cancer (138,139) and breast cancer (140,141) have produced mainly nonsignificant results for tea consumption. Currently, ongoing studies in the United States and Russia use detailed tea questionnaires assessing tea types, amounts consumed, brewing time, and preferred strength of tea (Hakim et al. 2000, in press; Il'yasova, personal communication, 1999). These studies are specifically designed to test the tea and cancer hypothesis and can be expected to generate more convincing evidence for a potential beneficial effect of black tea in cancer prevention. In a recent Japanese study, green tea has significantly decreased the risk of total cancer, with the largest risk reduction seen for lung (RR; 0.36; 0.13–0.96) and colorectal cancer (RR, 0.48; 0.13–1.80) (142). This study was designed with an a priori hypothesis on the role of green tea in cancer prevention.

C. Other Chronic Diseases

The most important adult-onset human *neurodegenerative diseases* are Alzheimer's disease, Parkinson's disease, Huntington's disease, and amyotrophic lateral sclerosis. We were able to identify two small case–control studies on Alzheimer's disease (143,144) and two on Parkinson's disease (145,146), none of which reported results of statistical significance relative to tea consumption. The largest study on Parkinson's disease (342 cases), carried out in Germany, suggested a moderate risk reduction (0.81; CI: 0.41–1.62) in the highest quartile of black tea consumption, compared with non–tea-drinkers (146). As this area of research is in its very early stages, more research is required to determine if there is indeed as association between tea drinking and neurodegenerative diseases.

Cataract is the most important cause of visual impairment worldwide and is related to the precipitation of proteins in the lens with ageing. This process is mediated by oxygen radical activity, and it may be delayed by high intakes of dietary antioxidants. Case–control studies on cataract are hampered by potential misclassification of cases and controls, because more than 50% of people aged 65 years and older have some degree of lens opacity, so that part of the controls are possibly not free of preclinical disease. Nevertheless, two studies showed a reduced risk with increased tea consumption (147), one of which found a statistically significant odds ratio of 0.4 in those drinking 5 cups or more of tea per day (148). However, no adjustment were made beyond age and sex as matching factors. Current evidence is completely insufficient to draw any conclusion on the role of black tea in the development of visual impairment. The pathogenesis of *osteoporosis* is heterogeneous, with genetic, hormonal, nutritional, and other lifestyle factors influencing progression of low bone mass and deterioration of bone tissue. The arising fractures represent a major health care problem. A tendency for decreasing bone mineral density—an effective predictor of fracture risk—with increasing tea consumption was seen in two small cross-sectional studies in women (149,150). Both studies found that caffeine intake may be a determinant of bone density. Two case–control studies in postmenopausal women addressed the relation between tea drinking and fractures. The study by Kreiger et al. (151) including 256 cases of either hip or wrist fracture and more than 500 controls failed to show an association, whereas in the multicenter MEDOS study with more than 2000 cases and almost double as many controls a significant reduction in hip fractures was found with drinking 4 cups/day or more, as compared with drinking no tea at all (152). The authors speculate that a protective effect of tea could be due to the presence of flavonoids with weak estrogen-like activity. More specifically set up investigations with dedicated tea questionnaires are warranted to confirm these results.

Epidemiological evidence supports a moderate protective effect of black tea in cardiovascular disease, but more than 100 studies on tea consumption and cancer risk do not show conclusive results. The role of tea in other chronic conditions has been studied insufficiently to indicate its importance.

VIII. SUMMARY

Antioxidant function of tea flavonoids is apparent from their physicochemical properties and mechanisms of action observed in cell biological studies. Indications for antioxidant effectivity in vivo are observed from a range of studies in animal models for oxidative stress and from human intervention studies. Epidemiological evidence is in line with these observations and indicates a potential role in oxidative–stress-related pathologies and conditions. Multiple mechanisms appear to be associated with potential benefits of tea flavonoid consumption and probably go far beyond radical scavenging and antioxidant functionalities. These may include immunomodulatory effects, effects on processes relevant to carcinogenesis, blood vessel function, heart disease, and possibly estrogen and other receptor-coupled activities. In view of the consistencies of the data available from in vitro and in vivo studies, antioxidant action is likely to contribute to the effects observed, but the relative importance of this particular property of tea polyphenols is as yet difficult to estimate.

REFERENCES

1. Balentine DA. Tea. In: Kirk–Othmer Encyclopedia of Chemical Technology, 4th ed. New York: John Wiley & Sons, 1996:747–768.
2. Harbowy M, Balentine DA. Tea chemistry. Crit Rev Plant Sci 1997; 16:415–480.
3. Obanda M, Owuor PO. Impact of shoot maturity on chlorophyll content, composition of volatile flavour compounds and plain black tea chemical quality parameter of clonal leaf. J Sci Food Agric 1995; 69:529–534.
4. Robertson A. The chemistry and biochemistry of black tea production: the nonvolatiles. In: Wilson KC, Clifford MN, eds. Tea Cultivation to Consumption. London: Chapman & Hall, 1992:553–601.
5. Finger A, Kuhr S, Engelhardt UH. Chromatography of tea constituents. J Chromatogr 1992; 624:293–315.

6. Bailey R, Nursten H, McDowell I. Isolation and analysis of a polymeric thearubigin fraction from tea. J Sci Food Agric 1992; 59:365–375.
7. Hashimoto F, Nonaka G, Nishioka I. Tannins and related compounds. LXXIX. Isolation and structure elucidation of B,B′-linked bisflavanoids, theasinensins D–G and oolong theanin from oolong tea. Chem Pharm Bull 1988; 36:1676–1684.
8. International Tea Committee. Annual Bulletin of Statistics. Colombo, Sri Lanka: Aitken Spence Printing, 1999.
9. Hertog MGL, Hollman PCH, Katan MB. Content of potentially anticarcinogenic flavonoids of 28 vegetables and 9 fruits commonly consumed in the Netherlands. J Agric Food Chem 1992; 40:2379–2383.
10. Hertog MGL, Feskens EJM, Hollman PCH, Katan MB, Kromhout D. Dietary antioxidant flavonoids and risk of coronary heart disease: the Zutphen Elderly Study. Lancet 1993; 342:1007–1011.
11. Bors W, Heller W, Michel C, Stettmaier K. Flavonoids and polyphenols: chemistry and biology. In: Cadenas E, Packer L, eds. Handbook of Antioxidants. New York: Marcel Dekker, 1996:409–465.
12. Rice–Evans CA, Miller NJ, Paganga G. Structure–antioxidant activity relationships of flavonoids and phenolic acids. Free Radic Biol Med 1996; 20:933–956.
13. Miller NJ, Castelluccio C, Tijburg L, Rice–Evans CA. The antioxidant properties of theaflavins and their gallate esters—radical scavengers or metal chelators? FEBS Lett 1996; 392:40–44.
14. Jovanovic SV, Steenken S, Simic M, Hara Y. Antioxidant properties of flavonoids: reduction potentials and electron transfer reactions of flavonoid radicals. In: Rice–Evans CA, Packer L, eds. Flavonoids in Health and Disease. New York: Marcel Dekker, 1998:137–161.
15. Jovanovic SV, Hara Y, Steenken S, Simic MG. Antioxidant potential of theaflavins. A pulse radiolysis study. J Am Chem Soc 1997; 119:5337–5343.
16. Balentine DA, Wiseman SA, Bouwens LCM. The chemistry of tea flavonoids. Crit Rev Food Sci Nutr 1997; 37:693–704.
17. Afanas'ev IB, Dorozhko AI, Brodksii AV, Kostyuk VA, Potapovitch AI. Chelating and free radical scavenging mechanisms of inhibitory action of rutin and quercetin in lipid peroxidation. Biochem Pharmacol 1989; 38:1763–1769.
18. Muira YH, Tomita I, Watanabe, Hirayama T, Fukui S. Active oxygen generation by flavonoids. Biol Pharm Bull 1998; 21:93–96.
19. van Acker SABE, van der Berg DJ, Tromp NMJL, Griffioen DH, van Bennekom WP, van der Vijgh WJF, Bast A. Structural aspects of antioxidant activity of flavonoids. Free Radic Biol Med 1996; 20:331–342.
20. Namiki M, Osawa T. Antioxidants/antimutagens in foods. Basic Life Sci 1986; 39:131–142.
21. Vinson JA, Dabbagh YA, Serry MM, Jang J. Plant flavonoids, especially tea flavonols, are powerful antioxidants using an in vitro oxidation model for heart disease. J Agric Food Chem 1995; 43:2800–2802.
22. Wiseman SA, Balentine DA, Frei B. Antioxidants in tea. Crit Rev Food Sci Nutr 1997; 37:705–718.
23. van Acker SABE, Plemper van Balen G, van den Berg DJ, Bast A, van der Vijgh WJF. Influence of iron chelation on the antioxidant activity of flavonoids. Biochem Pharmacol 1998; 56:935–943.
24. Esterbauer H, Jurgens G. Mechanistic and genetic aspects of susceptibility of LDL to oxidation. Curr Opin Lipidol 1993; 4:114–124.
25. Ingold K, Bowry VW, Stocker R, Walling C. Autoxidation of lipids and antioxidation by α-tocopherol and ubiquinol in homogeneous solution and in aqueous dispersions of lipids: unrecognised consequences of lipid particle size as exemplified by oxidation of human low density lipoproteins. Proc Natl Acad Sci USA 1993; 90:45–49.
26. Roginsky VA, Barsukova TK, Remorova AA, Bors W. Moderate antioxidative efficiencies of flavonoids during peroxidation of methyl linoleate in homogeneous and micellar solutions. J Am Oil Chem Soc 1996; 73:777–786.
27. Terao J, Piskula M, Yao Q. Protective effect of epicatechin, epicatechin gallate, and quercetin on lipid peroxidation in phospholipid bilayers. Arch Biochem Biophys 1994; 308:278–284.
28. Buettner GR. The pecking order of free radicals and antioxidants: lipid peroxidation, α-tocopherol and ascorbate. Arch Biochem Biophys 1993; 300:535–543.
29. van het Hof KH, Wiseman SA, Yang CS, Tijburg LBM. Plasma and lipoprotein levels of tea catechins following repeated tea consumption. Proc Soc Exp Biol Med 1999; 220:203–209.
30. Lee M-J, Wang ZY, Li H, Chen L, Sun Y, Gobbo S, Balentine DA, Yang CS. Analysis of plasma and urinary tea polyphenols in human subjects. Cancer Epidemiol Biomed Prev 1995; 4:393–399.

31. Conquer JA, Maiani G, Azzini E, Raguzini A, Holub BJ. Supplementation with quercetin markedly increases plasma quercetin concentration without effect on selected risk factors for heart disease in healthy subjects. J Nutr 1998; 128:593–597.
32. Gugler R, Leschik M, Dengler HJ. Disposition of quercetin in man after single oral and intravenal doses. Eur J Clin Pharmacol 1975; 9:229–234.
33. Walgren RA, Walle UK, Walle T. Transport of quercetin and its glucosides across human intestinal epithelial Caco-2 cells. Biochem Pharmacol 1998; 55:1721–1727.
34. Boulton DW, Walle UK, Walle T. Fate of the flavonoid quercetin in human cell lines: chemical instability and metabolism. J Pharm Pharmacol 1999; 51:353–359.
35. Kivits GAA, van der Sman FJP, Tijburg LBM. Analysis of catechins from green and black tea in humans: a specific and sensitive colorimetric assay of total catechins in biological fluids. Int J Food Sci Nutr 1997; 48:387–392.
36. Kaneko T, Matsuo M, Baba N. Inhibition of linoleic acid hydroperoxide-induced toxicity in cultured human umbilical vein endothelial cells by catechins. Chem Biol Interact 1990; 114:109–119.
37. Matsuo N, Yamada K, Yamashita K, Shoji K, Mori M, Sugano M. Inhibitory effect of tea polyphenols on histamine and leukotriene B-4 release from rat peritoneal exudate cells. In Vitro Cell Dev Biol 1996; 32:340–344.
38. Chen ZP, Schell JB, Ho CT, Chen KY. Green tea epigallocatechin gallate shows a pronounced growth inhibitory effect on cancerous cells but not on their normal counterparts. Cancer Lett 1998; 129:173–179.
39. Lin YL, Lin JK. (−)-Epigallocatechin-3-gallate blocks the induction of nitric oxide synthase by downregulating lipopolysaccharide-induced activity of transcription factor nuclear factor-kappa B. Mol Pharmacol 1997; 52:465–472.
40. Yokozawa T, Oura H, Nakagawa H, Sakanaka S, Kim M. Effects of a component of green tea on the proliferation of vascular smooth muscle cells. Biosci Biotechnol Biochem 1995; 59:2134–2136.
41. Hibasami H, Komiya T, Achiwa Y, Ohnishi K, Kojima T, Nakanishi K, Akashi K, Hara Y. Induction of apoptosis in human stomach cancer cells by green tea catechins. Oncol Rep 1998; 5:527–529.
42. Kennedy DO, Matsumoto M, Kojima A, Matsui–Yuasa I. Cellular thiol status and cell death in the effect of green tea polyphenols in Ehrlich ascites tumor cells. Chem Biol Interact 1999; 122:59–71.
43. Kuroda Y, Hara Y. Antimutagenic and anticarcinogenic activity of tea polyphenols. Rev Mutat Res 1999; 436:69–97.
44. Rodgers EH, Grant MH. The effect of the flavonoids, quercetin, myricetin and epicatechin on the growth and enzyme activities of MCF7 human breast cancer cells. Chem Biol Interact 1998; 116:213–228.
45. Kobuchi H, Roy S, Sen CK, Nguyen HG, Packer L. Quercetin inhibits inducible ICAM-1 expression in human endothelial cells through the JNK pathway. Am J Physiol Cell Physiol 1999; 46:C403–C411.
46. Musonda CA, Chipman JK. Quercetin inhibits hydrogen peroxide (H_2O_2)-induced NF-kappa B DNA binding activity and DNA damage in HepG2 cells. Carcinogenesis 1998; 19:1583–1589.
47. Kim HK, Cheon BS, Kin YH, Kim SY, Kim HP. Effects of naturally occurring flavonoids on nitric oxide production in the macrophage cell line RAW 264.7 and their structure–activity relationships. Biochem Pharmacol 1999; 58:759–765.
48. Miodini P, Fioravanti L, Di Fronzo G, Cappelletti V. The two phyto-oestrogens genistein and quercetin exert different effects on oestrogen receptor function. Br J Cancer 1999; 80:1150–1155.
49. Lean MEJ, Noroozi M, Kelly I, Burns J, Talwar D, Sattar N, Crozier A. Dietary flavonols protect diabetic human lymphocytes against oxidative damage to DNA. Diabetes 1999; 48:176–181.
50. Kawada N, Seki S, Inoue M, Kuroki T. Effects of antioxidants, resveratrol, quercetin and N-acetylcysteine on the functions of cultured rat hepatic stellate cells and Kupffer cells. Hepatology 1998; 27:1265–1274.
51. Shen F, Weber G. Synergistic action of quercetin and genistein in human ovarian carcinoma cells. Oncol Res 1997; 9:597–602.
52. Kuhlmann MK, Burkhardt G, Horsch E, Wagner M, Kohler H. Inhibition of oxidant-induced lipid peroxidation in cultures renal tubular epithelial cells (LLC-PK1) by quercetin. Free Radic Res 1998; 29:451–460.
53. Uchida S, Ozaki M, Suzuki K, Shikita M. Radioprotective effect of (−)-epigallocatechin 3-O-gallate (green-tea tannin) in mice. Life Sci 1992; 50:147–152.

54. Shimoi K, Masuda S, Furugori M, Esaki S, Kinae N. Radioprotective effect of antioxidant flavonoids in γ-ray-irradiated mice. Carcinogenesis 1994; 15:2669–2672.
55. Wang ZY, Huang M-T, Ferraro T, Wong C-Q, Lou Y-R, Reuhl K, Iatropoulos M, Yang CS, Conney AH. Inhibitory effect of green tea in the drinking water on tumorigenesis by ultraviolet light and 12-O-tetradecanoylphorbol-13-acetate in the skin of SKH-1 mice. Cancer Res 1992; 52:1162–1170.
56. Wang ZY, Huang M-T, Lou Y-R, Jian-Guo X, Reuhl KR, Newmark HL, Ho C-T, Yang CS, Conney AH. Inhibitory effects of black tea, green tea, decaffeinated black tea and decaffeinated green tea on ultraviolet B light-induced skin carcinogenesis in 7,12-dimethylbenz[a]anthracene-initiated SKH-1 mice. Cancer Res 1994; 54:3428–3435.
57. Record IR, Dreosti IE. Protection by black tea and green tea against UVB and UVA+B induced skin cancer in hairless mice. Mutat Res 1998; 422:191–199.
58. Yozokawa T, Oura H, Sakanaka S, Kim M. Effect of tannins in green tea on the urinary methyl-guanidine excretion in rats indicating a possible radical scavenging action. Biosci Biotechnol Biochem 1992; 56:896–899.
59. Nanjo F, Honda M, Okushio K, Matsumoto N, Ishigaki F, Ishigami T, Hara Y. Effects of dietary tea catechins on α-tocopherol levels, lipid peroxidation, and erythrocyte deformability in rats fed on high palm oil and perilla oil diets. Biol Pharm Bull 1993; 16:1156–1159.
60. Sano M, Takahashi Y, Yoshino K, Shimoi K, Nakamura Y, Tomita I, Oguni I, Konomoto H. Effect of tea (*Camellia sinensis* L.) on lipid peroxidation in rat liver and kidney: a comparison of green and black tea feeding. Biol Pharm Bull 1995; 18:1006–1008.
61. Yoshino K, Tomita I, Sano M, Oguni I, Hara Y, Nakano M. Effects of long-term dietary supplement of tea polyphenols on lipid peroxide levels in rats. Age 1994; 17:79–85.
62. Kenny MT, Balistreri FJ, Torney HL. Flavonoid modulation of murine neutrophil cytokinesis. Immunopharmacol Immunotoxicol 1990; 12:527–541.
63. Lin YL, Tsai SH, Lin-Shiau SY, Ho CT, Lin JK. Theaflavin-3,3'-digallate from black tea blocks the nitric oxide synthase by down-regulating the activation of NF-kappaB in macrophages. Eur J Pharmacol 1999; 367:379–388.
64. Agarwal R, Katiyar SK, Khan SG, Mukhtar H. Protection against ultraviolet B radiation-induced effects in the skin of SKH-1 hairless mice by a polyphenolic fraction isolated from green tea. Photochem Photobiol 1993; 58:695–700.
65. Yang F, de Villiers WJ, McClain CJ, Varilek GW. Green tea polyphenols block endotoxin-induced tumor necrosis factor-production and lethality in a murine model. J Nutr 1998; 128:2334–2340.
66. Tijburg LBM, Wiseman SA, Meijer GW, Weststrate JA. Effects of green tea, black tea and dietary lipophilic antioxidants on LDL oxidizability and atherosclerosis in hypercholesterolaemic rabbits. Atherosclerosis 1997; 135:37–47.
67. Crawford RS, Kirk EA, Rosenfeld ME, LeBoeuf RC, Chait A. Dietary antioxidants inhibit development of fatty streak lesions in the LDL receptor-deficient mouse. Arterioscler Thromb Vasc Biol 1998; 18:1506–1513.
68. Beretz A, Cazenave J-P, Anton R. Inhibition of aggregation and secretion of human platelets by quercetin and other flavonoids: structure activity relationships. Agents Actions 1982; 12:382–387.
69. Janssen PLTMK, Mensink RP, Cox FJJ, Harryvan JL, Hovenier R, Hollman PCH, Katan MB. Effects of the flavonoids quercetin and apigenin on haemostasis in healthy volunteers: results from an in vitro and a dietary supplement study. Am J Clin Nutr 1998; 67:255–262.
70. Folts JD. Flavonoids in tea but not coffee given by gastric tube inhibit in vivo platelet activity and thrombus formation in stenosed dog coronary arteries [abstr]. FASEB J 1996; 10:A793; 4579.
71. Hasegawa R, Chujo T, Sai-Kato K, Umemura T, Tanimura A, Kurokawa Y. Preventive effects of green tea against liver oxidative DNA damage and hepatotoxicity in rats treated with 2-nitropropane. Food Chem Toxicol 1995; 33:961–970.
72. Xu Y, Ho CT, Amin SG, Han C, Chung FL. Dietary inhibitors of chemical carcinogenesis. XVII. Inhibition of tobacco-specific nitrosamine-induced lung tumorigenesis in A/J mice by green tea and its major polyphenol as antioxidants. Cancer Res 1992; 52:3875–3879.
73. Yang CS, Wang ZY. Tea and cancer. J Natl Cancer Inst 1993; 85:1038–1049.
74. Katiyar SK, Mukhtar H. Tea consumption and cancer. World Rev Nutr Diet 1996; 79:154–184.
75. Swiercz R, Skrzypcak-Jankun E, Merrell MM, Selman SH, Jankun J. Angiostatic activity of synthetic inhibitors of urokinase type plasminogen activator. Oncol Rep 1999; 6:523–526.

76. Paschka AG, Butler R, Young CY. Induction of apoptosis in prostate cancer cell lines by the green tea components, (−)-epigallocatechin-3-gallate. Cancer Lett 1998; 14:1–7.
77. Serafini M, Ghiselli A, Fero–Luzzi A. In vivo antioxidant effect of green and black tea in man. Eur J Clin Nutr 1996; 50:28–32.
78. Benzie IFF, Szeto YT, Strain JJ, Tomlinson B. Consumption of green tea causes rapid increase in plasma antioxidant power in humans. Nutr Cancer 1999; 34:83–87.
79. Leenen R, Roodenburg AJC, Tijburg LBM, Wiseman SA. A single dose of tea with or without milk increases plasma antioxidant activity in humans. Eur J Clin Nutr 2000; (in press).
80. van het Hof KH, Kivits GAA, Weststrate JA, Tijburg IBM. Bioavailability of catechins from tea: the effect of milk. Eur J Clin Nutr 1998; 52:356–359.
81. Maxwell S, Thorpe G. Tea flavonoids have little short-term impact on serum antioxidant activity. Br Med J 1996; 313:229.
82. Diplock AT, Charleux J–L, Crozier–Willi G, Kok FJ, Rice–Evans C, Roberfroid M, Stahl W, Viňa–Ribes J. Functional food science and defence against reactive oxidative species. Br J Nutr 1998; 80(suppl 1):S77–S112.
83. van het Hof KH, de Boer HSM, Wiseman SA, Lien N, Weststrate JA, Tijburg LBM. Consumption of green or black tea does not increase the resistance of LDL to oxidation in humans. Am J Clin Nutr 1997; 66:1125–1132.
84. Princen HMG, van Duyvenvoorde W, Buytenhek R, Blonk C, Tijburg LBM, Languis JAE, Meinders AE, Pijl H. No effect of consumption of green and black tea on plasma lipid and antioxidant levels and on LDL oxidation in smokers. Arterioscler Thromb Vasc Biol 1998; 18:833–841.
85. Cherubini A, Beal MF, Frei B. Black tea increases the resistance of human plasma to lipid peroxidation in vitro but not ex vivo. Free Radic Biol Med 1999; 27:381–387.
86. Ishikawa T, Suzukawa M, Toshimitsu I, Yoshida H, Ayaori M, Nishiwaki M, Yonemura A, Hara Y, Nakamura H. Effect of tea flavonoid supplementation on the susceptibility of low-density lipoprotein to oxidative modification. Am J Clin Nutr 1997; 66:261–266.
87. Freese R, Basu S, Hietanen E, Nair J, Nakachi K, Bartsch H, Mutanen M. Green tea extract decreases plasma malondialdehyde concentration but does not affect other indicators of oxidative stress, nitric oxide production, or hemostatic factors during a high-linoleic acid diet in healthy females. Eur J Nutr 1999; 38:149–157.
88. Klaunig JE, Xu Y, Han C, Kamendulis LM, Chen J, Heiser C, Gordon MS, Mohler ER. The effect of tea consumption on oxidative stress in smokers and nonsmokers. Proc Soc Exp Biol Med 1999; 220:249–254.
89. Nakagawa K, Ninomiya M, Okubo T, Aoi N, Juneja LR, Kim M, Yamanaka K, Miyazawa T. Tea catechin supplementation increases antioxidant capacity and prevents phospholipid hydroperoxidation in plasma of humans. J Agric Food Chem 1999; 47:3967–3973.
90. Shim JS, Kang MH, Kim YH, Roh JK, Roberts C, Lee IP. Chemopreventive effects of green tea (*Camellia sinensis*) among cigarette smokers. Cancer Epidemiol Biomarkers Prev 1995; 4:387–391.
91. Xue K, Wang S, Ma G, Zhou P, Wu P, Xu Z, Chen W, Wang Y. Micronucleus formation in peripheral-blood lymphocytes from smokers and the influence of alcohol- and tea-drinking habits. Int J Cancer 1992; 50:702–705.
92. Bingham SA, Vorster H, Jerling JC, Magee L, Mulligan A, Runswick S, Cummings JH. Effect of tea drinking on blood lipids, blood pressure and aspects of bowel habit. Br J Nutr 1997; 78:41–55.
93. Vorster H, Jerling J, Oosthuizen W, Cummings J, Bingham S, Magee L, Mulligan A, Ranswick S. Tea drinking and haemostasis: a randomized, placebo-controlled, crossover study in free-living subjects. Haemostasis 1996; 26:58–64.
94. Loktionov A, Bingham SA, Vorster H, Jerling JC, Runswick SA, Cummings JH. Apolipoprotein E genotype modulates the effect of black tea drinking on blood lipids and blood coagulation factors: a pilot study. Br J Nutr 1998; 79:133–139.
95. James JE. Understanding Caffeine: A Behavioral Analysis. California: Sage Publications, 1997.
96. Sung BH, Whitset TL, Wilson MF. Prolonged increase in blood pressure by a single oral dose of caffeine in mildly hypertensive men. Am J Hypertens 1994; 7:755–758.
97. Zahn TP, Rapoport JL. Autonomic nervous system effects of acute doses of caffeine in caffeine users and abstainers. Int J Psychophysiol 1987; 5:33–41.
98. Quinlan PT, Lane JL, Aspinall L. The effects of hot tea, coffee and water ingestion on physiological responses and mood: the role of caffeine, water and beverage type. Psychopharmacology 1997; 134:164–173.

99. Bingham SA, Magee L, Mulligan A, Runswick S, Cummings JH. Effect of tea drinking on blood lipids, blood pressure and aspects of bowel habit. Br J Nutr 1997; 78:41–55.
100. Van Dusseldorp M, Smits P, Lenders JWM, Temme T, Thien T, Katan M. Effects of coffee on cardiovascular response to stress: a 14 week controlled trial. Psychosom Med 1992; 54:344–353.
101. Barone JJ, Roberts HR. Caffeine consumption. Food Chem Toxicol 1996; 34:119–129.
102. Lieberman HR, Wurtman RJ, Emde GG, Roberts C, Coviella ILG. The effects of low doses of caffeine on human performance and mood. Psychopharmacology 1987; 92:308–312.
103. Hindmarch L, Quinlan PT, Moore KL, Parkin C. The effects of black tea and other beverages on aspects of cognition and psychomotor performance. Psychopharmacology 1998; 139:230–238.
104. Quinlan PT, Lane J, Moore KL, Aspen J, Rycroft JA, O'Brien DC. The acute physiological and mood effects of tea and coffee: the role of caffeine level. Pharmacol Biochem Behav 2000; (in press).
105. Cook NC, Samman S. Flavonoids—chemistry, metabolism, cardioprotective effects and dietary sources. J Nutr Biochem 1996; 7:66–76.
106. Zhu M, Phillipson D, Greengrass PM, Bowery N, Cai Y. Plant polyphenols—biologically active compounds or non-selective binders to protein? Phytochemistry 1997; 44:441–447.
107. Rycroft JA, Quinlan PT, Burggraaf J, van Haarst AD, Schoemaker HC, Cohen AF. Effect of chronic black tea intake on the physiological responses to isoprenaline infusion and a mental performance task in human volunteers. Bioflavonoids and Health, Dinard, France, Dec 1–4, 1999.
108. Medina JH, Viola H, Wolfman C, Marder M, Wasowski C, Calvo D, Paladini AC. Flavonoids: a new family of benzodiazepine receptor ligands. Neurochem Res 1997; 22:419–425.
109. Chu DC. Green tea. In: Yamamoto T, Juneja LR, Chu DC, Kim M, eds. Chemistry and Applications of Green Tea. New York: CRC Press, 1997:1–12.
110. Yokogashi H, Kato Y, Sagesaka YM, Takihar–Mitsuraa T, Kakuda T, Tkeuchi N. Reduction effect of theanine on blood pressure and brain 5-hydroxyindoles in spontaneously hypertensive rats. Biosci Biotechnol Biochem 1995; 59:615–618.
111. Kimura R, Murata T. Effect of theanine on norepinephrine and serotonin levels in rat brain. Chem Pharm Bull 1986; 34:3053–3057.
112. Launer LJ, Kalmijn S. Anti-oxidants and cognitive function: a review of clinical and epidemiologic studies. J Neural Transmis Suppl 1988; 53:1–8.
113. Jama JW, Launer LJ, Witteman JCM, den Breeijen JH, Breteler MMB, Grobbee DE, Hofman A. Dietary antioxidants and cognitive function in a population-based sample of older persons—the Rotterdam study. Am J Epidemiol 1996; 144:275–280.
114. Le Bars PL, Katz MM, Berman N, Itil MD, Freedman AM, Schatzburg AF. A placebo controlled double-blind randomised trial of an extract of *Ginkgo biloba* for dementia. JAMA 1997; 278:1327–1332.
115. World Health Organization. 1995 World Health Statistics. Geneven, 1996.
116. FAO, Food Balance Sheets 1995. http://apps.fao.org/lim500/nph-wrap.pl?FoodBalanceSheet&Domain
117. Boston Collaborative Surveillance Program. Coffee drinking and acute myocardial infarction. Lancet 1972; 2:1278–1281.
118. Rosenberg L, Palmer JR, Kelly JP, Kaufman DW, Shapiro S. Coffee drinking and nonfatal myocardial infarction in men under 55 years of age. Am J Epidemiol 1988; 128:570–578.
119. Sesso HD, Gaziano JM, Buring JE, Hennekens CH. Coffee and tea intake and the risk of myocardial infarction. Am J Epidemiol 1999; 149:162–167.
120. Klatsky AL, Armstrong MA, Friedman GD. Coffee, tea and mortality. Ann Epidemiol 1993; 3:375–381.
121. Stensvold I, Tverdal A, Solvoll K, Foss OP. Tea consumption. Relationship to cholesterol, blood pressure and coronary and total mortality. Prev Med 1992; 21:546–553.
122. Hertog GLM, Feskens EJM, Hollman PCH, Katan MB, Kromhout D. Dietary antioxidant flavonoids and risk of coronary heart disease: the Zutphen Elderly Study. Lancet 1993; 342:1007–1011.
123. Keli SO, Hertog MGL, Feskens EJM, Kromhout D. Dietary flavonoids, antioxidant vitamins, and incidence of stroke. Arch Intern Med 1996; 154:637–642.
124. Hertog MGL, Sweetnam PM, Fehily AM, Elwood PC, Kromhout D. Antioxidant flavonols and ischaemic heart disease in a Welsh population of men. The Caerphilly Study. Am J Clin Nutr 1997; 65:1489–1494.

125. Marmot MG, Shipley MJ, Rose G. Inequalities in death-specific explanations of a general pattern. Lancet 1984; 1:1003–1006.
126. Woodward M, Tunstall–Pedoe H. Coffee and tea consumption in the Scottish Heart Health Study follow-up: conflicting relations with coronary risk factors, coronary disease and all cause mortality. J Epidemiol Community Health 1999; 53:481–487.
127. Brown CA, Bolton–Smith C, Woodward M, Tunstall–Pedoe H. Coffee and tea consumption and the prevalence of coronary heart disease in men and women: results from the Scottish Heart Healthy Study. J Epidemiol Community Health 1993; 47:171–175.
128. Yochum L, Kushi LH, Meyer K, Folsom AR. Dietary flavonoid intake and risk of cardiovascular disease in postmenopausal women. Am J Epidemiol 1999; 149:943–949.
129. Sato Y, Nakatsuka H, Watanabe T, Hisamichi S, Shimizu H, Fujisaku S, Chinowatari Y, Ida Y, Suda S, Kato K, Ikeda M. Possible contribution of green tea drinking habits to the prevention of stroke. Tohoku J Exp Med 1989; 157:337–343.
130. Huang B, Rodriguez BL, Burchfiel CM, Curb JD, Yano K, Chen R, Sharp DS. Association of green tea consumption with coronary heart disease in the Japanese–American men. Am J Epidemiol 1997; 145:30.
131. Yang CS, Lee MJ, Chen L, Yang GY. Polyphenols as inhibitors of carcinogenesis. Environ Health Perspect 1997; 105:971–976.
132. Zheng W, Doyle TJ, Kushi LH, Sellers TA, Hong C–P, Folsom AR. Tea consumption and cancer incidence in a prospective cohort study of postmenopausal women. Am J Epidemiol 1996; 14:175–182.
133. Gao C–M, Takezaki T, Ding J–H, Li M–S, Tajima K. Protective effect of allium vegetables against both esophageal and stomach cancer: a simultaneous case–referent study of a high-epidemic area in Jiangsu Province, China. Jpn J Cancer Res 1999; 90:614–621.
134. Severson RK, Nomura AMY, Grove JS, Stemmerman GN. A prospective study of demographics, diet, and prostate cancer among men of Japanese ancestry in Hawaii. Cancer Res 1989; 49:1857–1860.
135. Jain MG, Hislop GT, Howe GR, Burch JD, Ghadirian P. Alcohol and other beverage use and prostate cancer risk among Canadian men. Int J Cancer 1998; 78:707–711.
136. Zatonski WA, Boyle P, Przewozniak K, Maisonneuve P, Drosik K, Walker AM. Cigarette smoking, alcohol, tea and coffee consumption and pancreas cancer risk: a case–control study from Opole, Poland. Int J Cancer 1993; 53:601–607.
137. Shibata A, Mack TM, Paganini–Hill A, Ross RK, Henderson BE. A prospective study of pancreatic cancer in the elderly. Int J Cancer 1994; 58:46–49.
138. Chyou P–H, Nomura AMY, Stemmerman GN. A prospective study of diet, smoking, and lower urinary tract cancer. Ann Epidemiol 1993; 3:211–216.
139. Michaud DS, Spiegelman D, Clinton SK, Rimm EB, Curhan GC, Willett WC, Giovanucci EL. Fluid intake and the risk of bladder cancer in men. N Engl J Med 1999; 340:1390–1397.
140. Goldbohm RA, Hertog MGL, Brants HAM, Van Poppel G, Van den Brandt PA. Consumption of black tea and cancer risk: a prospective cohort study. J Natl Cancer Inst 1996; 88:93–100.
141. Hunter DJ, Manson JE, Stampfer MJ, Colditz GA, Rosner B, Hennekens CH, Speizer FE, Willett WC. A prospective study of caffeine, coffee, tea, and breast cancer. Am J Epidemiol 1992; 136:1000–1001.
142. Nakachi K, Imai K, Suga K. Cancer-preventive effects of drinking green tea in a Japanese population. Proc Am Assoc Cancer Res 1997; 38:261.
143. Forster DP, Newens AJ, Kay DWK, Edwardson JA. Risk factors in clinically diagnosed presenile dementia of the Alzheimer type: a case–control study in northern England. J Epidemiol Commun Health 1995; 49:253–258.
144. Rogers MAM, Simon DG. A preliminary study of dietary aluminum intake and risk of Alzheimer's disease. Age Ageing 1999; 28:205–209.
145. Morano A, Jimenez–Jimenez FJ, Molina JA. Risk factors for Parkinson's disease: case–control study in the province of Caceres, Spain. Acta Neurol Scand 1994; 89:164–170.
146. Hellenbrand W, Seidler A, Boeing H, Robra BP, Vieregge P, Nischan P, Joerg J, Oertel WH, Schneider E, Ulm G. Diet and Parkinson's disease I: a possible role for the past intake of specific foods and food groups. Neurology 1996; 47:636–643.
147. Tavani A, Negri E, LaVecchia C. Food and nutrient intake and risk of cataract. Ann Epidemiol 1996; 6:41–46.

148. Robertson J, Donner AP, Trevithick JR. A possible role for vitamins C and E in cataract prevention. Am J Clin Nutr 1991; 53:346S–351S.
149. Cooper C, Atkinson EJ, Wahner HW, O'Fallon WM, Riggs BL, Judd HL, Melton LJ III. Is caffeine consumption a risk factor for osteoporosis? J Bone Min Res 1992; 7:465–471.
150. Hernandez–Avila M, Stampfer MJ, Ravnikar VA, Willett WC, Schiff I, Francis M, Longscope C, McKinlay SM. Caffeine and other predictors of bone density among pre- and perimenopausal women. Epidemiology 1993; 4:128–134.
151. Kreiger N, Gross A, Hunter G. Dietary factors and fracture in postmenopausal women: a case–control study. Int J Epidemiol 1992; 21:953–958.
152. Johnell O, Gullberg B, Kanis JA, Allander E, Elffors L, Dequeker J, Dilsen G, Gennari C, Lopes Vaz A, Liritis G, Mazzuoli G, Miravet L, Passeri M, Perez Cano R, Rapado A, Ribot CJ. Risk factors for hip fracture in European women—the MEDOS study. Bone Min Res 1995; 10:1802–1815.

20
The Phenolic Wine Antioxidants

Andrew L. Waterhouse
University of California, Davis, California

I. INTRODUCTION

Wine contains many phenolic antioxidant substances; most all these originate in the grape berry. If oak is used, additional and different phenolic compounds will also be found in the wine, and a few small phenols of low concentration have microbial origins, such as tyrosol and 4-ethylphenol. Wine also contains other antioxidants, in particular the sulfites, added as a preservative in most wine at levels between 20 and 50 mg/L, and occasionally, ascorbate is added.

Phenolic compounds are found in all foods of plant origin, and rich sources are tea, coffee, nuts, and chocolate, but especially fruit, including preserved fruit, such as wine, juices, and dried fruits. A simple indicator that a food is high in phenolics is bitterness or astringency (when sugar is absent). Foods that exhibit these properties include strong tea or dark red wine, unsweetened chocolate, strong coffee, white citrus peels, and the best example of astringency, an unripe persimmon. The amounts of these substances in the diet are highly variable, depending on personal choice, and reliable data on population intake is limited, but recent reviews have contributed greatly to accessible information (1–8). Estimates of daily intake have varied from 25 mg to 1 g/day, depending on personal dietary preferences. Processing alters the quantity and quality of these substances and can cause drastic chemical changes.

A. Definitions

To understand phenolic nomenclature, it is helpful to understand the basis of the general terms used. Phenols or phenolics includes all the substances. *Simple phenols* include those compounds that have a single aromatic ring containing one or more hydroxyl groups, a common example being caffeic acid. *Polyphenolic* compounds are those that have multiple phenol rings within the structure, and examples include catechin and ellagic acid. *Flavonoids* have a very specific three-ring structure. *Tannin* is a functional term that describes substances that are used to tan hide to leather. Many phenolic compounds have this property; although traditional phenol-containing tannins are natural plant extracts that contain a complex mixture of high molecular weight polyphenolic compounds. Tannin is often used loosely to describe high molecular weight phenolic mixtures. The term *condensed tannin* refers to mixtures of polymers of flavonoids, and *hydrolyzable tannin* refers to gallic or ellagic acid-based mixtures, also called gallotannins or ellagitannins, respectively.

The simple phenols in Table 1 are not found in wine, but their nomenclature is a key to understanding more complex names. These names are used in the nomenclature of many

Table 1 Basic Phenols

Structure	Name	Notes
(phenol)	Phenol (hydroxybenzene)	Rare in natural products but abundant in sore throat sprays
(1,2-dihydroxybenzene)	Pyrocatechol, (1,2 dihydroxybenzene). Note: when a 1,2 dihydroxy functional group is present, it is called a catechol group	Easily oxidized to o-quinone. Also called catechol: this same term has been used for catechin, a complex flavonoid described below.
(methoxybenzene)	Anisole (methoxybenzene)	
(2-methoxyphenol)	Guaiacol (2-methoxyphenol). Note: when a 1-hydroxy-2-methoxy group is present, it is called a guaiacyl group	
(1,3-dihydroxybenzene)	Resorcinol (1,3 dihydroxybenzene)	Not as easily oxidized as the *ortho* or *para* dihydroxybenzenes
(1,4-dihydroxybenzene)	1,4 dihydroquinone (1,4 dihydroxybenzene)	Also easily oxidized to quinone, but this form unusual in natural products.
(1,2,3-trihydroxybenzene)	Pyrogallol 1,2,3-trihydroxy. Note: when a 1,2,3 trihydroxy functional group is present it is called a gallol or galloyl group	

different phenolic substances and are helpful to interpret those other names (i.e., *res*veratrol contains a resorcinol functional group).

B. Basis of Antioxidant Activity

Compounds that are easier to oxidize are often better antioxidants, and that is true here. The catechol group reacts very readily with oxidants in the form of free radical reactive oxygen species to form a very stable radical, the semiquinone radical. The compounds with catechol or 1,4-dihydroquinone functionality are especially easy to oxidize because the resulting phenoxyl radical can be stabilized on another oxygen (Fig. 1). It is stable enough that it does not abstract hydrogens from other substances and will persist long enough to react with another semiquinone radical, resulting in a disproportionation reaction that yields a quinone and a phenol, in total quenching two radicals. Wine is rich in substances with the catechol group, and these compounds impart an antioxidant activity to wine that is its natural preservative. The use of sulfites in winemaking enhances this antioxidant property by reducing and recycling the quinone product back to the phenol. If this quinone is not removed, it will eventually react with other nucleophiles—when this is other phenols, browning results.

C. Wine and Grape Phenolic Levels

The following description is based on the compounds and levels found in grapes and wine from *Vitis vinfera*, the European wine grape, as this grape dominates wine production. There are significant varietal differences within *V. vinifera*, and other *Vitis* species will have some different compounds as well as different levels.

1. Phenolic Levels in Grapes and Distribution

The phenolic compounds in wine come largely from the grape, although their structures are altered during fermentation and further processing. In grapes, the skin and seed are the primary sources of these compounds, whereas free-run juice is relatively low. The distribution of these in typical grapes is listed in Table 2 (9). Although similar otherwise, the higher levels in red grape skins is due to the colored anthocyanins.

Being secondary metabolites, the levels of these substances is subject to a large variability depending on grape variety and climate, and the variation between grapes in a vineyard can be quite high. Thus grape sampling in any experiment to study phenolics must be tested to ensure the validity and significance of the samples analyzed.

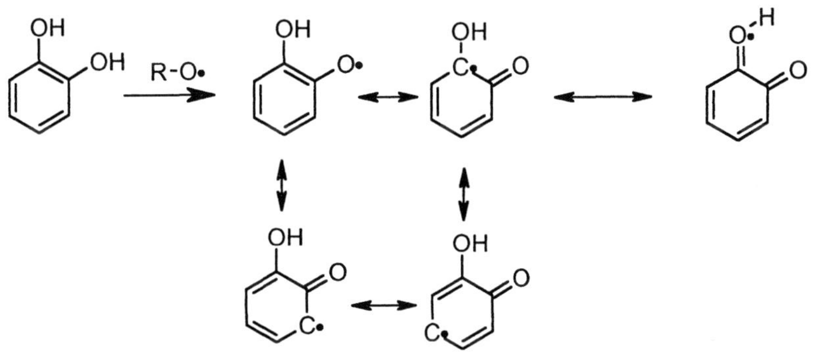

Figure 1 Resonance stabilization of semiquinone radical.

Table 2 Total Phenols (mg/kg FW)

Tissue	% Fresh weight	Red	White
Skins	15	1800	900
Pulp	1	40	35
Juice	78	210	175
Seeds	6	3500	2800
Total		5600	3900

2. Phenolic Levels in Wines

The levels of the phenolics in wines is also highly variable owing to both differences in fruit sources as well as processing. The first and most important factor to understand is that white wines are made by quickly pressing the juice away from the grape solids, whereas reds are made by fermenting the juice in the presence of the grape solids (skin and seeds). Because the skins and seeds contain the vast majority of the phenols, red wine is a whole-berry extract, whereas white wine is a juice product. In addition, because of the significant sensory effects of these substances on bitterness and astringency, they are controlled by winemakers. The methods of control involve the manipulation of extraction as well as fining with protein to precipitate and remove tannin from finished wine; ultrafiltration is now seeing some use. Typical levels for red and white wines are listed in Table 3, based on literature sources noted in the following sections but, in some cases, on unpublished data. Keep in mind there is a wide range of variation.

Table 3 Typical Levels of Phenolics in Red and White Table Wine[a]

	White wine		Red wine	
Phenol class	Young	Aged	Young	Aged
Nonflavonoids				
Hydroxycinnamates	154	130	165	60
Benzoic acids	10	15	60	60
Hydrolyzable tannins (from oak)	0	100	0	250
Stilbenes (resveratrol)	0.5	0.5	7	7
Total mg/L	164.5	245.5	232	377
Flavonoids				
Flavanol monomers	25	15	200	100
Proanthocyanidins and condensed tannins	20	25	750	1000
Flavonols	—	—	100	100
Anthocyanins	—	—	400	90
Others	—	—	50	75
Total mg/L	45	40	1500	1365
Total all phenols	209.5	285.5	1732	1742

[a]Young means new wine < 6-months aged; not having been aged or fermented in oak barrels. Age implies ~1 year for white, ~2 years for red, and some oak barrel aging or other oak contact.

II. NONFLAVONOIDS

Wine phenolics are grouped into two categories, the flavonoids and nonflavonoids, and the major subgroups will be surveyed. In summary, the nonflavonoids are listed with examples and general comments.

Hydroxycinnamic acids (i.e., caffeic acid)
Ubiquitous in fruits and all plants tissues, and found as esters in fruit–tartrate esters in grapes, but quinic esters (i.e., cholorgenic acids) in most other fruits

Benzoic acids (i.e., gallic acid)
Ester forms are found in fruit sources, but few free acids are found in fresh sources. Hydrolysis yields the free acids in wine.

Hydrolyzable tannins (i.e., vescaligin)
Ester-linked oligomers of gallic acid or ellagic acid with glucose or other sugars. These are not present in grapes, only in oak-treated wine.

Stilbenes (i.e., resveratrol)
Hydroxylated stilbenes are found as the glycosides in grapes and very few other dietary sources.

A. Hydroxycinnamates

Hydroxycinnamates are the major phenols in grape juice and the major class of phenolics in white wine. Similar levels are found in red and white wine. These materials are also the first to be oxidized, and subsequently, initiate browning, a problem in white wines. There are three common hydroxycinnamates in grapes and wine: those based on coumaric acid (mono 4-hydroxy), caffeic acid (catechol substitution), and ferulic acid (guaiacyl substitution) (Fig. 2).

In grape berries the simple hydroxycinnamic acids noted in the foregoing are not found. Instead these acids exist as esters of tartaric acid. Enologists have adopted trivial names for these compounds: *p*-coutaric acid, caftaric acid, fertaric acid, respectively. These substances are found in the flesh of the fruit, and thus are found in all grape juices and, consequently, in all wines. The levels of these compounds vary in grapes, but caftaric acid is, by far, the predominant cinnamate in grapes, averaging about 170 mg/kg in *V. vinifera* grapes, whereas the *p*-coutaric and fertaric occur at about 20 and 5 mg/kg, respectively (10,11), and these relative proportions are maintained in wine.

The naturally occurring esters are susceptible to hydrolysis, and this occurs in the aqueous acidic solution of wine, releasing the simple hydroxycinnamic acids, such that they are readily detected in wine of a few weeks old. In addition, the free acids will partially esterify with the ethanol in wine. The rate of these reactions is variable, depending on the pH of the wine, which typically varies between 3.0 and 3.9. Hydrolysis of the caffeic acids esters of tartaric

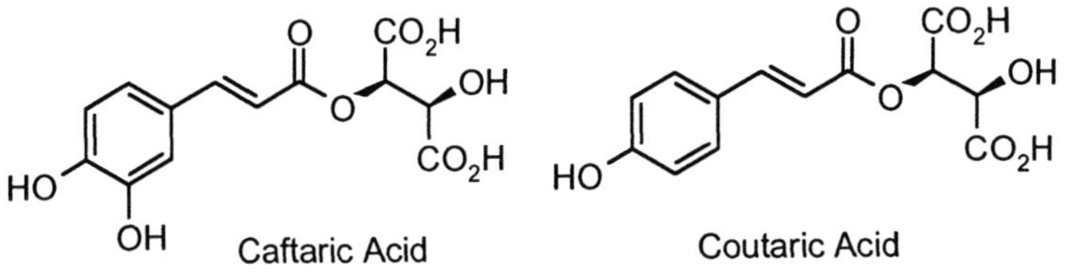

Figure 2 Two of the hydroxycinnamates in wine.

acid can be catalyzed by an enzyme HCEH (12). Levels of total hydroxycinnamates in finished wine are typically 130 mg/L in whites and 60 mg/L in reds.

In terms of wine sensory qualities, the hydroxycinnamates appear to have no perceptible bitterness or astringency at the levels found in wine. The caftaric and coutaric esters have taste thresholds of 50 and 10–25 ppm in water, with bitterness and astringency being the descriptors (13), but work by Noble and others (14) showed that in wine the levels of these compounds were below threshold.

B. Browning

Browning caused by cinnamates is their most important effect in winemaking, in particular the color of white wine. When grapes are crushed, polyphenol oxidase enzymes are released, and these enzymes rapidly oxidize the hydroxycinnamates to quinones. Glutathione (GSH) will quickly react with the quinone forming a colorless product called grape reaction product (GRP), so juices that have high glutathione have lower browning potential in the short run. Thus the browning potential of musts can be characterized by whether or not they have high relative amounts of GSH present (15). In raisins, the GSH adduct is not formed, and thus they brown quite a bit more (16). It is possible that the elimination of sulfide aromas by aeration of wine is due largely to the efficient reaction of these quinones with thiols (17).

Analysis of wines of different ages shows that GRP is slowly hydrolyzed to the GSH–caffeic acid derivative (the tartrate ester is hydrolyzed), but the amides are only partially hydrolyzed (18). This acid will also be partially converted to the ethyl ester. The specific brown products are not well characterized, but it appears that the hydroxycinnamate quinones react further with flavanols to form the actual pigmented products (19).

C. Benzoic Acids

The benzoic acids are a minor component in new wines. Gallic acid appears from the hydrolysis of gallate esters of hydrolyzable tannins and condensed tannin after standing for at least a few months. Gallic acid appears to be stable during aging, as it is one phenolic compound readily visible by chromatographic analysis of older red wines. Its levels in red wine average near 70 mg/L, whereas white wines average near 10 mg/L (20).

D. Hydrolyzable Tannins

In wine hydrolyzable tannins come from oak, and levels are near 100 mg/L for white wines aged for about 6 months in barrels, whereas red wines will have levels in the range of 250 mg/L after aging 2 or more years (21). These phenols are composed of gallic acid and ellagic acid esters with glucose or related sugars (Fig. 3). Because of the ester linkage, they are referred to as "hydrolyzable." There are two categories, the gallotannins and the ellagitannins, which contain gallic acid or ellagic acid. Hydrolyzable tannins are not found in *V. vinfera*, but can be found in other fruits, such as raspberries or muscadine grapes. When hydrolyzed in wine from ellagitannins, the ellagic acid will precipitate if it is at high levels, as in muscadine wine. Gallic acid is quite soluble and is found in all aged red wines, and it comes from both hydrolyzable tannins and the condensed tannins found in grape seeds. The sensory impact of oak-derived tannins is controversial (22).

E. Stilbenes

Stilbenes are another minor class. The principal stilbene in grapes resveratrol, is produced by vines in response to *Botrytis* infection and other fungal attacks. The actual antifungal

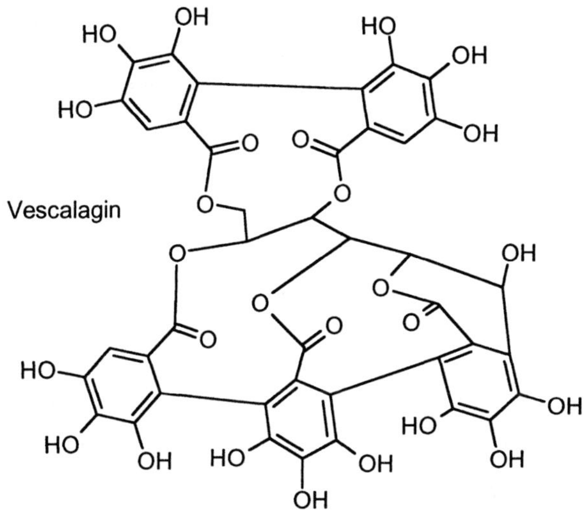

Figure 3 An ellagitannin from oak.

compounds are the oligomers of resveratrol called the viniferins. Several forms of resveratrol exist including the *cis*- and *trans*-isomers, as well as the glucosides of both isomers. All are found in wine (Fig. 4), but in grapes *cis*-resveratrol is absent. Light causes the *cis–trans*-isomerization (23). Resveratrol derivatives are found only in the skin of the grape, thus, much more is found in red wine. The total levels of all forms average about 7 mg/L for reds (24), 2 mg/L for roses, and 0.5 mg/L for white wines (25). Resveratrol has been implicated as a wine component that may reduce heart disease or cancer, but bioavailability data have not been reported, so it is difficult to assess physiological significance. The interest in the health effects of resveratrol has been greatly stimulated by a report in *Science* (26) implicating anticancer activity and in 1999 there were over 60 papers published on resveratrol.

III. FLAVONOIDS

The wine flavonoids are all polyphenolic compounds, having multiple aromatic rings possessing hydroxyl groups. A specific three-ring system defines flavonoids, there being a central oxygen-

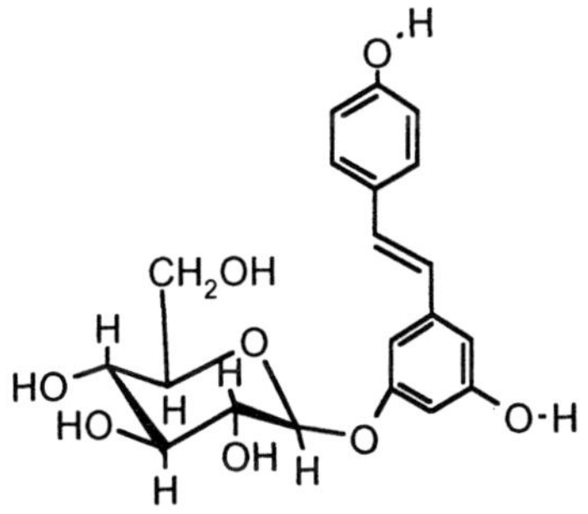

Figure 4 Piceid.

containing pyran ring (C-ring) of different oxidation states. It is fused to an aromatic ring (A-ring) along one bond and attached to another aromatic ring with a single bond (B-ring) as seen in Figure 5. The flavonoids found in grapes and wine all have the same hydroxyl substitution groups on ring-A, at positions 5 and 7. Differences in the oxidation state and substitution on ring-C defines the different *classes* of flavonoids. For instance a saturated C-ring defines the flavans, a keto at position 4 (and unsaturation between 2 and 3) defines the flavones, and the fully aromatic ring, which also has a positive charge, defines the anthocyanidins. The -ol ending further specifies an alcohol substituent on the C-ring, as in flavan-3-ol, where the position is distinguished because it could alternatively exist in the 4-position.

The substitution pattern on ring-B defines the member of the class. Normal substitution patterns are a hydroxyl at the 4′-position, with additional oxygen substitution at 3′ or 5′, or both. Those oxygens can be hydroxyls (phenols) or methoxyls at positions 3′ or 5′. Thus the number of class members is relatively short; however, the "free" flavonoid structure can also be substituted further (usually with sugar conjugation on the oxygens); this gives rise to many additional compounds.

The flavonoid comprise most of the phenols in red wine and are derived from extraction of the skins and seeds of grapes during the fermentation process. Because red wines are produced by fermentation of the juice's sugar into alcohol, a good solvent for polyphenol extraction, in the presence of the skins and seed over a period of 4–10 or more days, there is ample opportunity for extraction of much of the polyphenols into a red wine, and in typical winemaking, about half these substance are extracted during the maceration process. The major classes of wine flavonoids are the flavanols, flavonols, and the anthocyanins.

Flavan-3-ols (i.e., catechin)
Flavanols constitute the most abundant class, and include simple monomeric catechins, but most exist in the oligomeric and polymeric proanthocyanidin forms from the skins and seeds.

Flavonols (i.e., quercetin)
Flavonols are found in the berry skin, appear to function as a sunscreen, and are increased by high sunlight exposure.

Anthocyanins (i.e., malvidin-3-glucoside)
These are the red-colored phenols.

A. Flavanols

Flavonols are the most abundant class of flavonoids in grapes and wine and, in the grape, are found in both the seed and skin. These are often specifically called the flavan-3-ols to identify the location of the alcohol group on the C-ring. The flavan-3-ols are the most reduced form

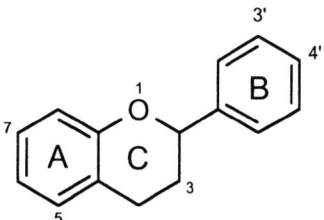

Figure 5 The flavonoid ring system.

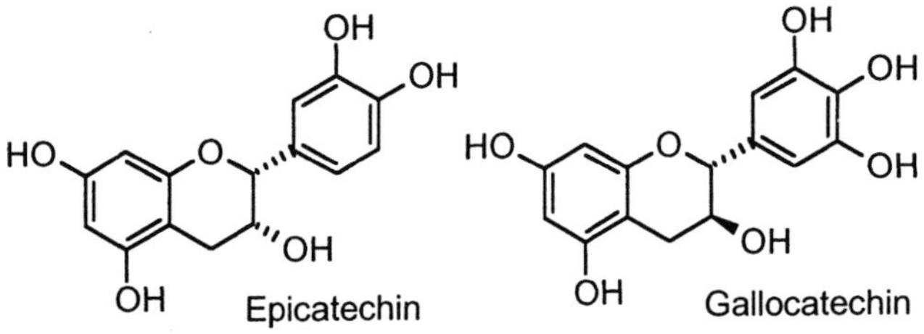

Figure 6 *cis*- and *trans*-forms of flavan-3-ols.

of the flavonoids. Because positions 2 and 3 on the C-ring are saturated, stereoisomers exist, and two are found in grapes (Fig. 6). The *trans*-form is (2R,3S) (+)-catechin and the *cis*-form is (2R,3R) (−)-epicatechin. Both catechin and epicatechin have the $3',4'$-catechol substitution on the B-ring. The only other B-ring substitution pattern found in the wine flavan-3-ols is the $3'4'5'$-trihydroxy form, appropriately called the gallocatechins. Some epigallocatechin is found in grape skin, but gallocatechin is not found in significant amounts. The wine flavan-3-ols are not found as glycosides, typical for the other classes, but instead gallate esters are found, and the gallic acid is esterified at the 3-position of the epi- series only. Epicatechin gallate is a small, but significant proportion of the flavan-3-ol pool in grapes in the seeds. Thus, for the simple series of monomeric flavanols, there are four different ones found in wine. A few others exist in different foods; of particular note, is epigallocatechin gallate in tea. These monomeric flavan-3-ols are sometimes referred to as the "catechins." The levels of total monomeric flavan-3-ols in typical red wine is in the range of 40–120 mg/L, with the majority usually being catechin (27). The other compounds exist only in very small amounts in wine. The levels are strongly affected by seed extraction techniques and are higher when extended maceration techniques are used.

Most phenolic compounds in red wine are from the condensation of flavan-3-ol units to yield the oligomers (proanthocyanidins) and polymers (condensed tannins). The condensation occurs to form covalent bonds between flavan-3-ol units: the most common linkages being 4→8 and 4→6 positions (Fig. 7). On average, epicatechin is the predominant unit in condensed tannins from grapes and wine, catechin is the next most abundant (often found at the end or terminal units—those with no bonds at the 4 position). In typical red wines, the amount of polymer plus oligomer is a sizable fraction of the total phenolic level, being in the range of

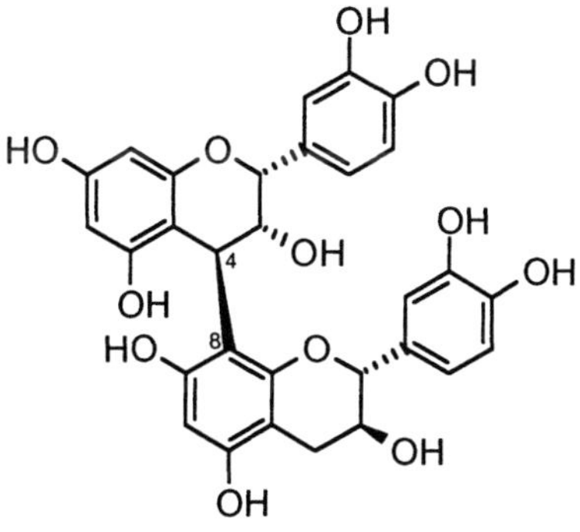

Figure 7 Procyanidin B_1.

25–50% in new wines and a higher proportion in older wines. Levels are between 0.5 and 1.5 g/L or even higher in some red wines, whereas in white wine, levels are in the range of 10–50 mg/L and are highly dependent on pressing techniques.

There are two types of proanthocyanidins, the procyanidins and the prodelphinidins. These names arise from the fact that when these substances are treated with acid, they break down into two specific anthocyanidins with the related substitution on the B-ring (i.e., the $3'4'$-dihydroxycatechin and epicatechin yield cyanidin, whereas the $3'4'5'$-trihydroxy gallocatechins yield delphinidin (see anthocyanins; Sec. III.C). This treatment hydrolyzes the gallate esters. A milder degradation, called thiolysis, yields all subunits with their original stereochemical configurations and substitutions retained (28).

The polymeric-condensed tannin polyphenols arise from two sources. First, these are found in sizable quantities in the seeds and skins of grapes, and they are extracted into the wine during fermentation. Second, processing, in particular those steps that incorporate oxygen into the must or wine, can initiate oxidation reactions of the flavan-3-ols. The oxidation yields o-quinone products from the catechol groups, and these then react with other phenols to create new bonds; these products have not been well characterized, such reactions lead to higher molecular weight phenols in the wine. Another important reaction is that between the proanthocyanidins and the anthocyanins to produce red-pigmented polymer, discussed further later. A recently described reaction shows that acetaldehyde acts to condense the flavan-3-ols (Fig. 8); these reactions can lead to yellow products (29).

The catechins are bitter and astringent. In the polymer, the bitterness is minimal, but the astringency remains (30). Over long aging (many years), a disproportionation reaction can occur, perhaps with some oxidation, so the polymers continue to increase in size until they are no longer soluble in wine and form the precipitate common in older red wines. So, on long aging, the amount of phenols in a wine decreases.

The distribution of the flavanols in grape berries is not the same in all varieties and, in fact, has a wide range of differences between the seed and skin. The proportion of the flavanols

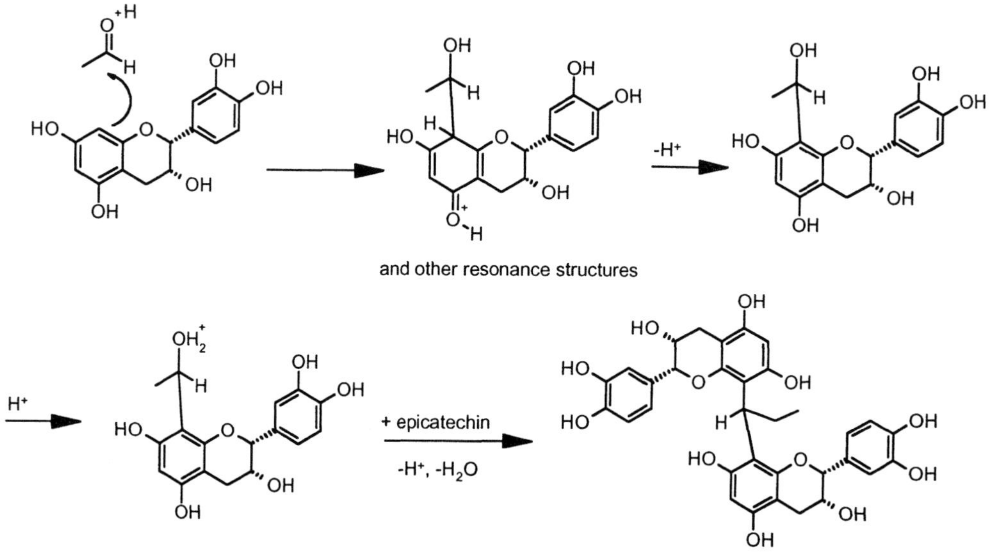

Figure 8 Flavan-3-ol dimerization.

Table 4 Distribution of Flavan-3-ols Within the Grape

Varieties	Monomers (mg/kg)	% in Seeds	Procyanidins (mg/kg)	% in Seeds
Alicante–Bouchet	360	64	287	50
Aramon	213		182	
Syrah	190		176	
Mourvedre	164	58	169	53
Grenache noir	137		125	
Cinsaut	136	37	116	32
Carignan	77	54	73	40
Cabernet sauvignon	344	83	546	68
Pinot noir	1165	94	1609	86

Table 5 Tissue Distribution

Average grape	Catechin proportion in each tissue (%)	Cat/epi ratio in tissues	Procyanidin proportion in each tissue (%)	Procyanidin distribution (%)
Stems	27	C 94, E 6	33	B_1, 71; B_2, 5; B_3, 20; B_4, 4
Seeds	56	C 42, E 58	38	B_1, 14; B_2, 37; B_3, 16; B_4, 33
Skins	17	C 84, E 16	28	B_1, 68; B_2, 8; B_3, 18; B_4, 6
Pulp	0		1	

in the seed goes from a low of less than 40% to a high of over 90%, as shown in Tables 4 and 5 (31).

B. Flavonols

Flavonols occur in a wide range of vegetable food sources. This class of compounds is always found in a glycoside form in plants, including in grape berries, where it is found in grape skin. There are only three forms of the simple flavonoid aglycones in grapes, quercetin (Fig. 9), myricetin ($3'4'5'$-trihydroxy) and kaempferol ($4'$-hydroxy), but because these compounds occur with a diverse combination of glycosidic forms, there are many individual compounds present. The identity of the glycosides has not been established in many different grape varieties, but they have been shown to be mostly the 3-glucosides as well as the 3-glucuronides and small amounts of diglycosides in Cinsault (32).

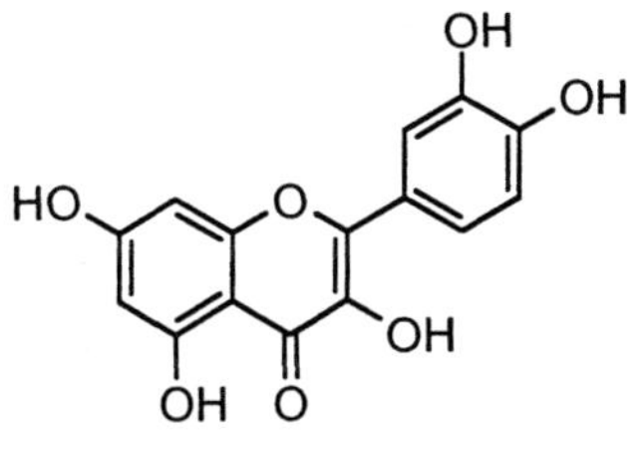

Figure 9 Quercetin.

A study on Pinot noir has shown that sunlight on the berry skin strongly enhances the levels of the flavonols (33). Because flavonols absorb UV light strongly at 360 nm, and they appear mostly in the outermost layer of cells in the berry, it appears that the plant produces these compounds as a natural sunscreen. Although this has not been studied in other grape varieties, a study of the levels of phenolic compounds in wine has shown that expensive Cabernet Sauvignon wines expected to come from lower-yielding vines with better sun exposure of the fruit has threefold or higher levels of flavonols, suggesting that the levels of these compounds in grapes may be a useful indicator of grape sun exposure, and perhaps quality. The levels of total flavonols are near 53 mg/L for widely sold Cabernet wine, but over 200 mg/L in the more expensive wine (27).

C. Anthocyanins

Anthocyanins provide the color in red wine and the red and blue colors found in the skins of red or black grapes, but also in many other plants including other foods in the diet. The color is based on the fully conjugated ten-electron A–C-ring π-system. If that is disrupted, the color is lost, as when anthocyanins are bleached by bisulfite. The anthocyanins react with the tannins to produce a "stabilized" anthocyanin or pigmented tannin, which persist much longer in wine than the initial form, and it is this stabilized color that persists in most red wines past a few years, although in some wines the monomeric forms found in the grape are still found after this time.

The term for the simple flavonoid ring system is *anthocyanidin*. However, anthocyanidins are never found in grapes or wine, except in trace quantities, because they are unstable. There are five basic anthocyanidins in wine: cyanidin, peonidin, delphindin, petunidin, and malvidin, the most abundant in red wines (Fig. 10).

Anthocyanin implies a glycoside. In *V. vinifera*, this is the single 3-glucoside (**1** in Fig. 11). In American species and hybrids, the 3,5-diglucoside is found, and its presence is the basis of identifying the use of these grapes in making a wine. The glucose conjugates are further substituted, however. At the 6-hydroxyl of the glucose, acyl substitution is also found, with ester linkages connecting either an acetyl group **2** or a coumaryl **3** group, and a small amount of caffeoyl substitution is also observed.

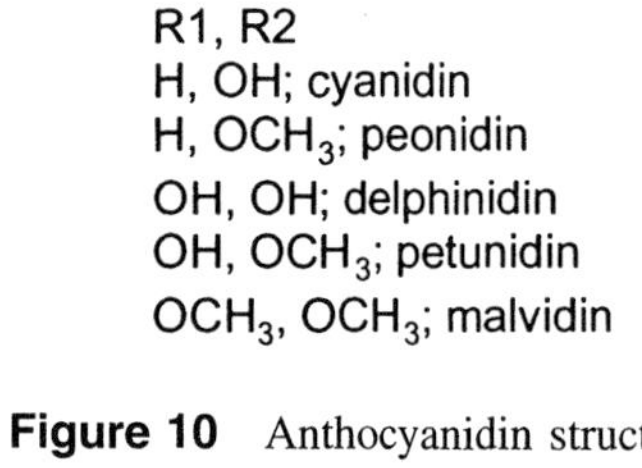

R1, R2
H, OH; cyanidin
H, OCH$_3$; peonidin
OH, OH; delphinidin
OH, OCH$_3$; petunidin
OCH$_3$, OCH$_3$; malvidin

Figure 10 Anthocyanidin structures.

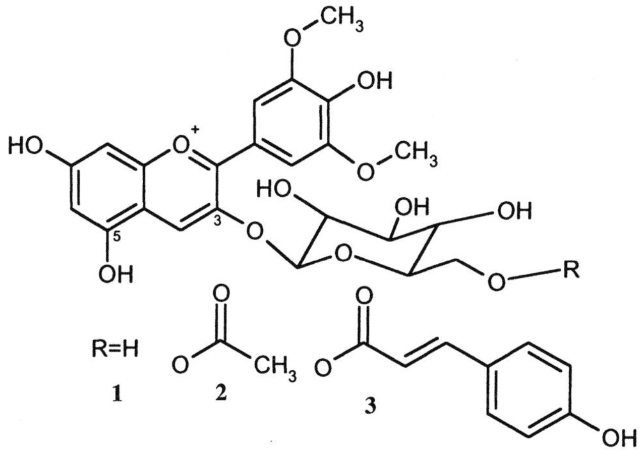

Figure 11 Anthocyanidin conjugate forms (anthocyanins).

In wine and similar solutions there are several forms of anthocyanins and the proportions strongly affect the color of a solution containing these substances (Fig. 12). The charged C-ring is an electrophilic center, and it can react with nucleophiles. Common reactions are with water, a pH-dependent reaction, and with bisulfite. In both cases, the red color is lost as the C-ring conjugation is disrupted. The pK_a of the flavylium pseudobase form is 2.7. At low pH (<1), all forms are converted to the flavylium form, and this treatment is used to assess total anthocyanin content. In addition, there is a quinone form that has a violet hue, and its pK_a is 4.7, so it is present in small amounts at high wine pH values.

Anthocyanins interact with other phenolic compounds in solution to create the effect known as copigmentation. This is a transient interaction; no chemical bonds are formed. It is a result of the chemical phenomenon called charge-transfer complex formation, or $\pi-\pi$ interactions (34). This occurs when there are two aromatic-ring substances in solution that have very different electron densities. The extreme examples are rings with positive charges and those with negative charges. When these differences exist, the rings associate by a weak "bond," and electron density is transferred from the electron-rich ring to the electron-poor ring. Because the flavylium anthocyanin has a positive charge, it is a very good candidate for a charge-transfer complex with electron-rich substrates. In addition, the other phenolic compounds in wine are almost all electron-rich because the phenol group is a strong electron donor; thus, they are likely to act as partners. As an example in Figure 13, pyrocatechol is used as the electron-rich partner for simplicity, but other phenolic compounds cause the copigmentation effect in wine.

The overall effect of copigmentation is based on two effects. First, the formation of the $\pi-\pi$-complex causes changes in the spectral properties of the molecules in the flavylium from, in particular, increasing absorption (hyperchromic shift) and increasing the wavelength of the absorption (bathochromic shift) (35). But also, the stabilization of the flavylium form by the π-complex shifts the equilibrium to better favor the flavylium, thereby boosting the proportion of anthocyanin molecules in the red-colored form (see Fig. 13). So, the magnitude of the copigmentation effect is pH-dependent because at very low pH values, all the anthocyanin molecules are already in the flavylium form, and at high pH, the flavylium form is not accessible. There is some speculation that the formation of the $\pi-\pi$-complex enhances the reactions between anthocyanins and the tannins, which produce the covalent bonds of pigmented tannins (36).

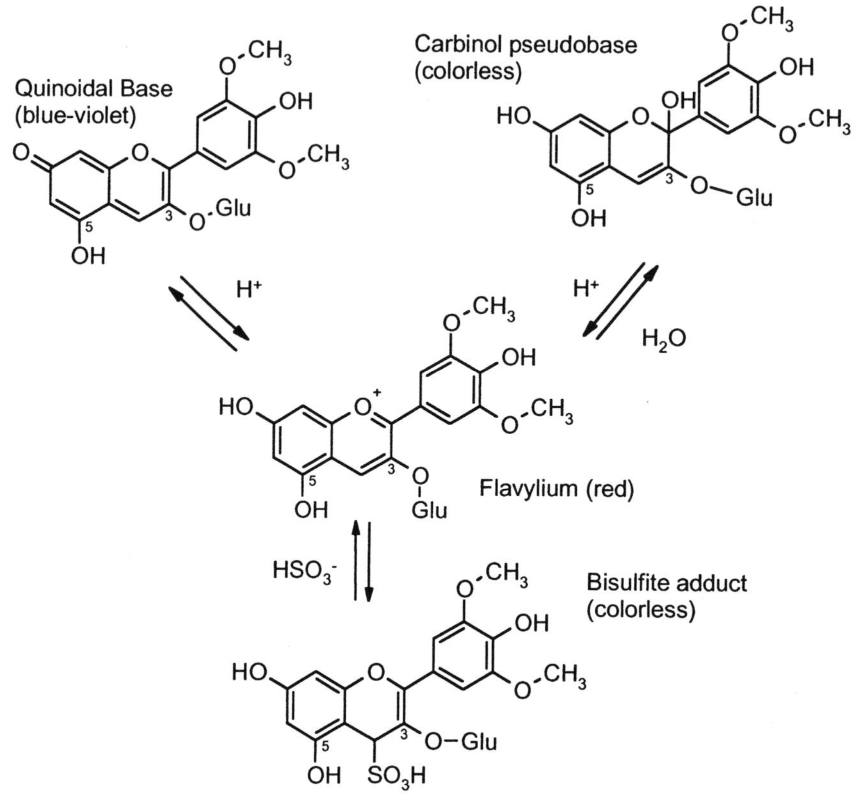

Figure 12 Anthocyanin forms present in wine.

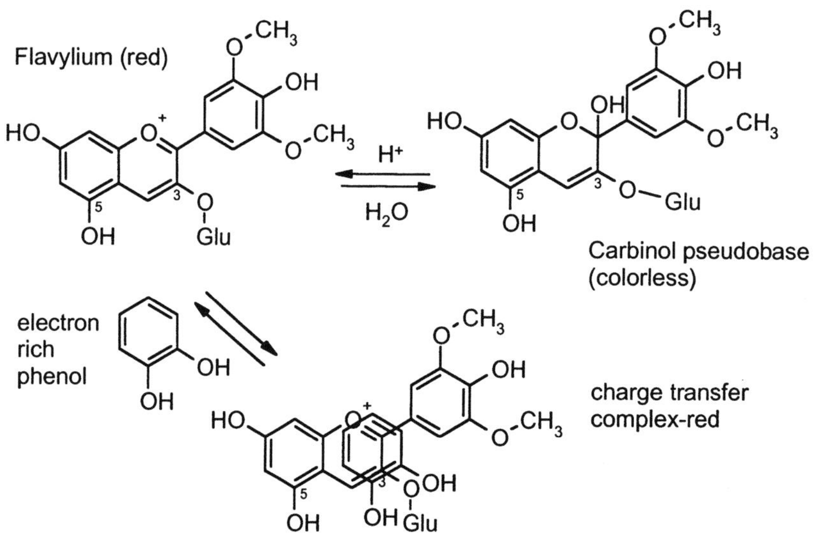

Figure 13 Copigmentation of wine anthocyanins.

Because the effect is bimolecular, it is highly dependent on concentration. It typically occurs in new red wine where the effect can increase apparent color by double. The partners in wine appear to include all other phenols and the anthocyanin itself. Because most of the anthocyanin molecules in a wine solution are in the uncharged, electron-rich pseudobase form, the anthocyanins act as self-copigmentors.

Another important factor in wine color is the formation of *pigmented tannins*. These are products formed by bond-forming reactions between the condensed tannins and anthocyanins. These compounds increase during aging at the expense of the monomeric anthocyanins, although the conversion is not very efficient. Consequently, after a wine has aged for 3–8 years, the monomeric anthocyanins have all but disappeared from most red wines. The remaining color is caused solely by the pigmented tannins. The pigmented tannins are also known by the name *polymeric anthocyanins*.

The chemical linkages between the anthocyanin and tannin molecules are not well known, but some scientists have suggested possibilities. The first proposal was made by Timberlake and Bridle who suggested that reactions between acetaldehyde, tannins, and anthocyanins created a link (37). Similar reactions have been observed between flavan-3-ols more recently (38).

Another type of anthocyanin product has been described recently, involving a reaction with pyruvate. This gives a simple monomeric product, but one that is not susceptible to sulfite bleaching, one of the characteristics of "pigmented tannin" (39); hence, related reactions may be important in the formation of pigmented tannin.

REFERENCES

1. Cassidy A, Hanley B, Lamuela–Raventós RM. Isoflavones, lignans and stilbenes–origins, metabolism and potential importance to human health. J Sci Food Agric 2000; 80:1044–1062.
2. Clifford MN. Anthocyanins—nature, occurrence and dietary burden. J Sci Food Agric 2000; 80:1063–1072.
3. Clifford MN. Chlorogenic acids and other cinnamates—nature, occurrence, dietary burden, absorption and metabolism. J Sci Food Agric 2000; 80:1033–1042.
4. Clifford MN. Miscellaneous phenols in foods and beverages—nature, occurrence and dietary burden. J Sci Food Agric 2000; 80:1126–1137.
5. Clifford MN, Scalbert A. Ellagitannins—nature, occurrence and dietary burden. J Sci Food Agric 2000; 80:1118–1125.
6. Hollman PCH, Arts ICW. Flavonols, flavones, and flavanols—nature, occurrence and dietary burden. J Sci Food Agric 2000; 80:1081–1093.
7. Santos–Buelga C, Scalbert A. Proanthocyanidins and tannin-like compounds—nature, occurrence, dietary intake and effects on nutrition and health. J Sci Food Agric 2000; 80:1094–1117.
8. Tomás–Barberán FA, Clifford MN. Dietary hydroxybenzoic acid derivatives—nature, occurrence and dietary burden. J Sci Food Agric 2000; 80:1073–1080.
9. Singleton VL. Tannins and the qualities of wines. In: Hemingway RW, Laks PE, eds. Plant Polyphenols. New York: Plenum Press, 1992:859–880.
10. Ong BY, Nagel CW. Hydroxycinnamic acid–tartaric acid ester content in mature grapes and during the maturation of white riesling grapes. Am J Enol Vitic 1978; 29:277–281.
11. Singleton VL, Zaya J, Trousdale E. Compositional changes in ripening grapes: caftaric and coutaric acids. Vitis 1986; 25:107–117.
12. Somers TC, Vérette E, Pocock KF. Hydroxycinnamate esters of *V. vinifera*: changes during white vinification and effects of exogenous enzyme hydrolysis. J Sci Food Agric 1987; 40:67–78.
13. Okamura S, Watanabe M. Agric Biol Chem 1981; 45:2063.
14. Verette E, Noble AC, Somers CT. Hydroxycinnamates of *Vitis vinifera*: sensory assessment in relation to bitterness in white wine. J Sci Food Agric 1988; 45:267–272.
15. Cheynier V, Rigaud J, Souquet JM, Duprat F, Moutounet M. Must browning in relation to the behavior of phenolic compounds during oxidation. Am J Enol Vitic 1990; 41:346–349.

16. Singleton VL, Trousdale E, Zaya J. One reason sun-dried raising brown so much. Am J Enol Vitic 1985; 36:111–113.
17. Cillier JJL, Singleton VL. Caffeic acid autoxidation and the effects of thiols. J Agric Food Chem 1990; 38:1789–1796.
18. Cheynier VF, Trousdale EK, Singleton VL, Salgues MJ, Wylde R. Characterization of 2-S-glutathioylcaftaric acid and its hydrolysis in relation to grape wines. J Agric Food Chem 1986; 34:217–221.
19. Rigaud J, Cheynier V, Souquet JM, Moutounet M. Influence of most composition on phenolic oxidation kinetics. J Sci Food Agric 1991; 57:55–63.
20. Waterhouse AL, Teissedre PL. Levels of phenolics in California varietal wine. In: Watkins T, ed. Wine: Nutritional and Therapeutic Benefits. Washington, DC: American Chemical Society, 1997:12–23.
21. Quinn KM, Singleton VL. Isolation and identification of ellagitannins from white oak and an estimation of their roles in wine. Am J Enol Vitic 1985; 36:148–155.
22. Pocock KF, Sefton MA, Williams JP. Taste threshold of phenolic extracts of French and American oakwood: the influence of oak phenols on wine flavor. Am J Enol Vitic 1994; 45:429–434.
23. Trela BC, Waterhouse AL. Resveratrol: isomeric molar absorptivities and stability. J Agric Food Chem 1996; 44:1253–1257.
24. Lamuela–Raventós RM, Romero–Pérez AI, Waterhouse AL, de la Torre–Boronat MC. Direct HPLC analysis of cis- and trans-resveratrol and piceid isomers in Spanish red Vitis vinifera wines. J Agric Food Chem 1995; 42:281–283.
25. Romero–Perez AI, Lamuela–Raventos RM, Waterhouse AL, de la Torre–Boronat MC. Levels of cis- and trans-resveratrol and their glycosides in white and rose Vitis vinifera wines from Spain. J Agric Food Chem 1996; 44:2124–2128.
26. Jang M, Cai L, Udeani GO, Slowing KV, Thomas CF, Beecher CWW, Fong HHS, Farnsworth NR, Kinghorn AD, Mehta RG, Moon RC, Pezzuto JM. Cancer chemopreventive activity of resveratrol, a natural product derived from grapes. Science 1997; 275:218–220.
27. Ritchey JG, Waterhouse AL. A standard red wine: monomeric phenolic analysis of commercial cabernet sauvignon wines. Am J Enol Vitic 1999; 50:91–100.
28. Rigaud J, Escribano–Bailon MT, Prieur C, Souquet JM, Cheynier V. Normal-phase high-performance liquid chromatographic separation of procyanidins from cacao beans and grape seeds. J Chromatogr A 1993; 654:255–260.
29. Es-Safi N, Fulcrand H, Cheynier V, Moutounet M. Competition between (+)-catechin and (−)-epicatechin in acetaldehyde-induced polymerization of flavanols. J Agric Food Chem 1999; 47:2088–2095.
30. Robichaud JL, Noble AC. Astringency and bitterness of selected phenolics in wine. J Sci Food Agric 1990; 53:343–353.
31. Bourzeix M, Weyland D, Heredia N, Desfeux C. A study of catechins and procyanidins of grape clusters, the wine and other by products of the vine. Bull OIV 1986; 59:1171–1254.
32. Cheynier V, Rigaud J. HPLC separation and characterization of flavonols in the skins of Vitis vinfera var. Cinsault. Am J Enol Vitic 1986; 37:248–252.
33. Price SF, Breen PJ, Valladao M, Watson BT. Cluster sun exposure and quercetin in pinot noir grapes and wine. Am J Enol Vitic 1995; 46:187–194.
34. Foster R. Organic Charge–Transfer Complexes. New York: Academic, 1969.
35. Dangles O, Brouillard R. Polyphenols interactions. The copigmentation case: thermodynamic data from temperature and relaxation kinetics. Medium effect. Can J Chem 1992; 70:2174–2189.
36. Mirabel M, Saucier C, Guerra C, Glories Y. Copigmentation in model wine solutions: occurrence and relation to wine aging. Am J Enol Vitic 1999; 50:211–218.
37. Timberlake CF, Bridle P. Interactions between anthocyanins, phenolic compounds, and acetaldehyde and their significance in red wines. Am J Enol Vitic 1976; 27:97–105.
38. Saucier C, Guerra C, Pianet I, Laguerre M, Glories Y. (+)-Catechin–acetaldehyde condensation products in relation to wine aging. Phytochemistry 1997; 46:229–234.
39. Bakker J, Bridle P, Honda T, Kuwano H, Saito N, Terahara N, Timberlake CF. Identification of an anthocyanin occurring in some red wines. Phytochemistry 1997; 44:1375–1382.

21
French Maritime Pine Bark: Pycnogenol

Gerald Rimbach and Fabio Virgili
University of California, Berkeley, California
Lester Packer
University of Southern California School of Pharmacy, Los Angeles, California

I. INTRODUCTION

The term *pycnogenols* was coined to describe an entire class of flavonoids composed of flavan-3-ol derivatives (from the ancient Greek *puknos*, which means condensed, and *genos*, which means class, family). This term was originally intended to serve as a scientific name for this class of polyphenols (1), but now refers to a specific blend of procyanidins extracted from the bark of the French maritime pine (*Pinus maritima*), which is patented under the trade name of Pycnogenol (PYC) (Horphag Research, Geneva, Switzerland). Pycnogenol is now utilized throughout the world as a nutritional supplement and as a phytochemical remedy for various diseases, ranging from chronic inflammation, to circulatory dysfunction. Studies that have been done consistently indicate that this flavonoid mixture has tremendous antioxidant capacity as well as other bioactivities not directly associated with its free radical-scavenging activity, such as inhibition of enzyme activity and modulation of gene expression. For a general review that covers all points in this chapter, see Ref. 2.

Pine bark extract is obtained by water extraction of the raw bark of *P. maritima*, followed by washing with ethanol to eliminate some of non–water-soluble substances, as described in both U. S. patent (4,698,360) and in the early paper by Masquelier and Triaud (3). Although its chemical composition is still not completely elucidated, the main constituents of PYC are phenolic compounds, broadly divided into monomers (catechin, epicatechin, and taxifolin) and condensed flavonoids (classified as procyanidins or proanthocyanidins because they release anthocyanins when heated in acidic conditions). The presence of flavonoids belonging to the family of procyanidins in PYC can be easily detected by means of the Bates–Smith reaction (4). The chromatographic profile (Fig. 1) after size separation by normal-phase high-performance liquid chromatography (HPLC) on a silica gel column (5), kindly provided by Drs. Shirley and Waterhouse of the Department of Viticulture and Enology of the University of California at Davis, shows that PYC is mainly composed of oligomers of five to seven units. These con-

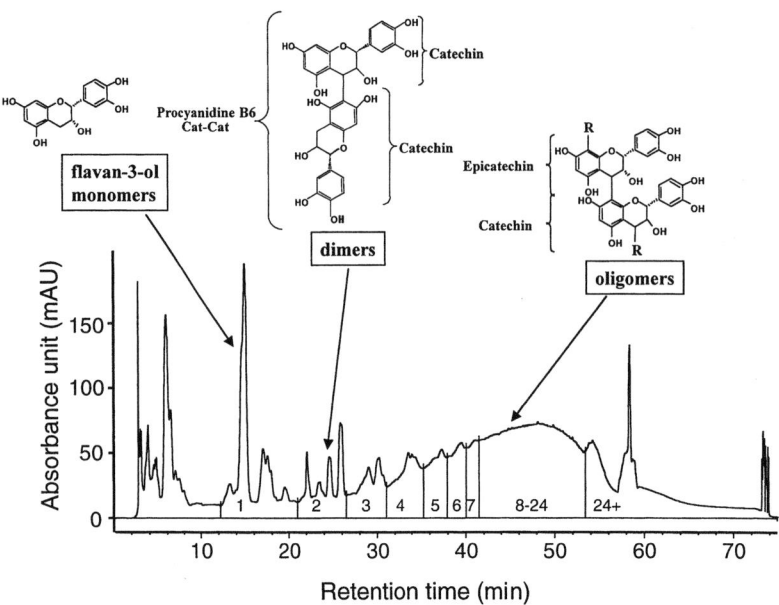

Figure 1 The separation of groups of compounds of PYC by normal-phase silica gel HPLC using an acidic polar solvent system and UV detection as described by Cheynier and co-workers (5). Chemical structures of catechin and procyanidine B_1 and B_6 are shown as examples. (Courtesy of Dr. J. Shirley and A. Waterhouse, Department of Viticulture and Enology, University of California, Davis.)

densed polyphenols, composed of "bricks" of the flavan-3-ols catechin and epicatechin linked together into lengths ranging from dimers to heptamers, are classified as procyanidins B_1, B_3, B_7, and others. Pine bark extract also contains phenolic acids (such as caffeic, ferulic, and *p*-hydroxybenzoic acids) as minor constituents and glycosylation products (i.e., glucopyranosyl derivatives of either flavanols or phenolic acids as minute constituents). Many of these components are also found in commonly ingested fruits and vegetables, in plant-derived substances from grapes and berries, and in beverages such as green and black tea and red wine. From epidemiological evidence, the consumption of such polyphenols has frequently been associated with low incidence of degenerative diseases (6,7), and experimental evidence is accumulating about phenolic compounds acting as natural phytochemical antioxidants important for human health (8).

II. BIOAVAILABILITY OF PYCNOGENOL

Bioavailability can be defined as the result of a sequence of properties and complex metabolic events for a given compound to be available for use in the body; these properties and events include solubility, digestion, absorption, tissue distribution and retention, enzymatic transformation, and, finally, secretion and excretion mechanisms. The actual bioavailability of complex mixtures of flavonoids, and in particular of PYC, has not yet been completely elucidated. Supplementation studies are currently being performed in our laboratory and in others to assess which components, and in what form, are absorbed by humans and are able to exert bioactivity.

The presence of the procyanidin-B_3 in human urine has been demonstrated after PYC administration (9). However, the same study reported that the administration of purified dimeric procyanidins (B_1 and B_3) is not followed by the appearance of the corresponding chromatographic peaks in urine, and that the new chromatographic profile found in urine following ingestion of PYC does not match that of the PYC. These observations indicate that modification of flavonoids occurs during digestion and absorption and that compounds exerting an effect in vivo may be different from those composing the raw extract.

Preliminary data from a controlled study in humans performed in our laboratory, in collaboration with Rice–Evans and colleagues at the United Medical and Dental School of Guy's and St. Thomas' Hospital of London (U.K.), indicate that ferulic acid is bioavailable in humans after PBE supplementation. After a 48-h washout period, during which eight adult subjects abstained from the ingestion of any kind of phenolics, a single dose of 200 mg of PYC was orally administered. Urine was collected for the next 24 h and analyzed for the presence of phenolic compounds by HPLC coupled with the diode-array detection and spectra characterization as described by Bourne and Rice–Evans (10). The urine of all subjects contained ferulic acid, which is a component of PYC, and other hydroxycinnamic esters, with a maximum peak of excretion at about 18 h after ingestion (Fig. 2). The total cumulative excretion of hydroxycinnamic acids ranged between 1 and 4 mg over 24 h (i.e., about 1% of the total dose of PYC administered). These data indicate that PYC can be considered highly bioavailable in humans, at least in terms of its component ferulic acid.

Even though few data are available about the metabolism of PYC, evidence exists that other more complex components of PYC, such as oligomeric procyanidins, undergo some biological modification after ingestion in humans (9). These observations bring up an important general

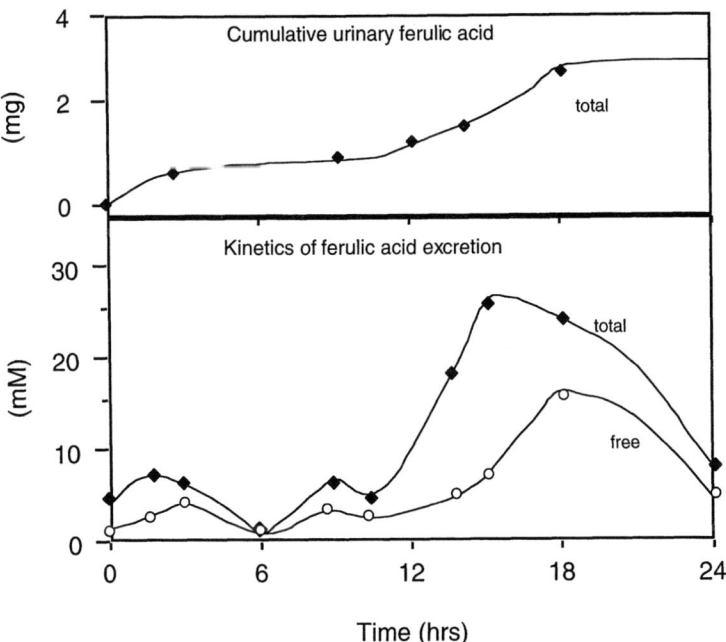

Figure 2 Kinetic study of urinary ferulic acid concentration and cumulative ferulic acid excretion after administration of a single dose of 200 mg PYC in human volunteers: Urine was collected over 24 h after PYC administration. Ferulic acid was determined by HPLC, coupled with diode array detection and spectra characterization as described by Bourne and Rice–Evans (10). ◆, total ferulic acid [free plus glucuronide]; ○, free ferulic acid.

issue in the study of flavonoid activity. In vitro studies have to be interpreted with caution and, eventually, reconsidered in light of supplementation studies in vivo, because the compounds in the supplementation mixture may not be the compounds that eventually exert biological activity. Finally, an indirect indication of flavonoid bioavailability is that flavonoid supplementation, in general, and of PYC, in particular, both in animals and in humans, is associated with biological effects, such as enhancement of antioxidant capacity and anti-inflammatory effects. These observations will be discussed in the appropriate section of this review. Further studies on flavonoid bioavailability are needed to obtain a more accurate estimate of the physiologically achievable concentrations of polyphenols in humans and to fully understand which components of PYC are absorbed, transported through the blood, taken up by various tissues, and perhaps metabolized.

III. MOLECULAR BASIS OF PYCNOGENOL ACTIVITY

A. Free Radical-Scavenging Activity

Owing to the basic chemical structure of its components, the most obvious feature of PYC is its strong antioxidant activity. Phenolic acids, polyphenols, and in particular, flavonoids, are composed of one (or more) aromatic rings bearing one or more hydroxyl groups and, therefore, are potentially able to quench free radicals by forming resonance-stabilized phenoxyl radicals (11). Superoxide radical anion ($O_2^{\cdot-}$), hydroxyl radical ($HO^{\cdot}$), lipid peroxyl radical, and the reactive nitrogen species, such as nitric oxide radical ($^{\cdot}NO$) and peroxynitrite ($ONOO^-$), which are among the most important free radicals in the biological environment and in human health and disease, have been investigated either in vitro or in vivo. Moreover, as suggested by the early reports from the laboratory of Szent-Gyorgyi (12), flavonoids may have a fundamental role in the antioxidant network interplaying together with other antioxidants and, in particular, with ascorbic acid, thus significantly contributing to cellular and extracellular defenses against oxidative stress.

Various studies have addressed the antioxidant capacity of PYC in simplified assay systems in vitro, cultured cell models, perfused organs, and in vivo.

1. Studies In Vitro

One of the earliest studies addressing the antioxidant activity of various procyanidins in vitro reported strong scavenging activity against free radicals, such as the stable radical, 1,1-diphenyl-2-picrylhydrazyl (DPPH), and the oxygen free radicals $O_2^{\cdot-}$ and $HO^{\cdot}$, as assessed by electron-spin resonance (ESR) spectroscopy (13). The 1,1-diphenyl-2-picrylhydrazyl radical has been more recently reported to be efficiently reduced by PYC in vivo, displaying an activity comparable with that of both purified catechin and α-tocopherol (14).

Blazso and co-workers (15) tested the in vivo $O_2^{\cdot-}$-scavenging activity of PYC as well as three different chromatographic fractions separated by molecular sieve filtration through Sephadex LH. These three fractions, which have also been used for other studies described in this review, were characterized by thin-layer chromatography (TLC) and nuclear magnetic resonance spectrometry (NMRS) as containing: fraction 1, monomeric flavonoids (taxifolin, catechin, epicatechin) and phenolic acids (caffeic, ferulic, vanillic); fraction 2, procyanidins dimers (B_1, B_3, B_6, B_7, and others), trimers, and tetramers; and fraction 3, oligomers larger than four subunits. The whole extract and each of its fractions were reported to inhibit superoxide-induced reduction of nitroblue tetrazolium (NBT) to formazan in a dose-dependent fashion. The most active fraction was fraction 3, containing oligomeric procyanidins. Other investigators have reported PYC to be an efficient scavenger of both $O_2^{\cdot-}$ and $HO^{\cdot}$ (16,17). The $O_2^{\cdot-}$ scavenging activity of PYC was studied by utilizing EST techniques and reported as superoxide dismutase (SOD) equivalents, and was on the order of hundreds units of SOD per milligram of PYC (16). In the same investigation, the specific scavenging activity of PYC toward HO$^{\cdot}$ (generated by an iron–ascorbate system) was also studied by means of ESR spectroscopy. Utilizing EPC-K1, a water-soluble synthetic ascorbate tocopherol ester, as a reference, the antioxidant activity of PYC was in the order of moles EPC-K1 per milligram of PYC. Both HO$^{\cdot}$- and O$_2^{\cdot -}$-scavenging activities were maintained after treatment with ascorbate oxidase, indicating that ascorbate, possibly present in the mixture, was not responsible for the observed antioxidant activity. On the other hand, O$_2^{\cdot -}$-scavenging activity was partially affected by ultrafiltration, implying a contribution to the antioxidant activity by high molecular weight compounds present in the mixture. When compared with other phytochemicals and plant extracts the before-reported values render PYC among the highest-ranking oxygen free radical scavenger in vitro (18). A PBE radical generated from the oxidation of PBE by the horseradish peroxidase–hydrogen peroxide system has been recently described for the first time by Guo and co-workers (19). In addition to acting as a free radical scavenger, PBE has been also reported to reduce cytochrome c reversibly, possibly by donation of electrons to the iron of the heme group, and competitively inhibit mitochondrial electron transport chain activity (20).

Macrides and co-workers (21), have also studied the HO$^{\cdot}$-scavenging activity of different compounds and plant extracts, including PYC, using inhibition of the degradation of deoxyribose challenged by iron–ascorbate as an assay. PYC was the most potent procyanidin-containing plant extract tested in this system; its protective effect was of the same order of that displayed by Trolox, but lower than that of scymnol, a 27-carbon alcohol extracted from the bile of sharks and rays, and 5-scymnol-sulfate.

Elstner and co-workers (17) studied the scavenging activity of PYC in various models, using several in vitro models to mimic physiological conditions associated with oxidative stress (namely, xanthine/xanthine oxidase [X/XO], reduced nicotinamide adenine dinucleotide [NADH]/diaphorase, copper/dihydroxyfumarate, and rose bengal activation by light). They reported that pine bark procyanidins preferentially react with both hydroxyl radical and singlet oxygen, and they suggested a possible role of PYC flavonoids in the therapy of pathologies related to the formation of these aggressive oxygen species.

Nelson and co-workers (22) investigated the capacity of PYC to protect the low-density lipoprotein (LDL) fraction of human plasma from copper-induced oxidation and have reported a dose-dependent decrease in lipid peroxide generation, starting with PYC concentrations as low as 2 μg/mL. In this model, to achieve a comparable degree of protection, about 100 μg/mL of tocopherol succinate had to be added. In the same investigation, the ability to protect DNA from iron–ascorbate-induced damage was also studied. Furthermore, in the same study (22), a decrease in single- and double-strand DNA breaks, known as a possible factor in carcinogenesis (23), was reported, suggesting a potentially important role of PYC in protection of genetic material against free radical-induced injury.

2. Studies on Cultured Cells

The capacity of PYC to protect cellular systems has also been investigated, in particular in cultured endothelial cells and macrophages. In a bovine line of cultured normal endothelial cells (pulmonary artery endothelial cells; PAEC), preincubation with 20–80 μg/mL PYC is associated with significant protection from both lipid peroxidation and cell damage induced by tert-butylhydroperoxide (t-BHP). At 60 μg/mL, PYC completely inhibited the release of lactate dehydrogenase after t-BHP treatment, suggesting significant protection from oxidative stress-induced cytotoxicity. The generation of thiobarbituric acid-reactive substances (TBARS) was also significantly decreased, indicating that the protective effect was, at least partly, due to the antioxidant activity of PYC (24).

Studies currently in progress strongly suggest that PYC can affect cell death and survival after various types of proapoptotic stimuli. A high glutamate concentration induces oxidative stress in murine hippocampal HT4 cells (neuronal cells that lack glutamate receptors) by inhibiting cystine transport. This inhibition results in glutathione (GSH) depletion, lipid peroxidation, and finally, cell death, as was described in PC12 cells (25). When HT-4 cells are pretreated with PYC, as well as with other antioxidants, such as α-tocopherol, a significant increase in cell survival is observed without any effect on cellular GSH levels. In this model of glutamate-induced cytotoxicity, protection by PYC appears to be mediated either by a bona fide scavenging activity, which substitutes for decreased GSH, or by modulating calcium concentrations and signal transduction (26).

In the murine macrophage cell line J774, preincubation with PYC significantly decreased the extent of the oxidative burst, induced by zymosan treatment, in a dose-dependent fashion (22). This observation corroborates a possible therapeutic role for PYC and other related substances in chronic inflammatory and cardiovascular disease and agrees with other reports more directly addressed to the effects of PYC on the modulation of macrophage activity and on inflammation (16,27).

A protective activity has also been reported for the eye, which is constantly exposed to photooxidative stress. PYC, in concentrations as low as 2.5 μg/mL, protected both purified rod outer segments and the pigment epithelium of the retina from lipid peroxidation induced in vitro by ferric iron (28). Not surprisingly, ascorbate did not protect against such iron-driven lipid peroxidation, whereas flavonoids related to PYC components, such as the gallic ester of catechin, enhanced the protective effect of α-tocopherol in concentrations on the order of 50 μg/mL. The nature of the inhibitory activity reported in this study was not investigated; therefore, it is not clear if PYC and other tested compounds reduced lipid peroxidation owing their free radical-quenching ability or by chelating ferric ions, or both.

3. Studies In Vivo

Studies in vivo are fundamental in assessing the real efficacy of ingested flavonoids as antioxidants and to determine if they are bioavailable, or at least if their administration results in a detectable outcome. In hearts isolated from rats after dietary supplementation of PYC (50 mg/day for 4 weeks and then 30 mg/day for 3 weeks) subjected to ischemia–reperfusion injury, neither dietary PYC nor addition of PYC to the perfusate significantly decreased tissue damage, assessed both as release of low molecular weight iron and mitochondrial oxidative phosphorylation (14). In the same study, when catechin was added to the perfusate, a significant protection of the heart from ischemia–reperfusion injury was observed.

These data indicate that the antioxidant potential of PYC is at least partially available in vivo, but also suggest that the pattern of absorption and distribution of PYC's flavonoid components is complex. PYC components may exert important activity in selected target organs and tissues. A fuller understanding of in vivo targets of PYC and, in general, of polyphenols deserves further study, utilizing other animal models and as clinical studies with human subjects.

4. Participation to the Antioxidant Network

It is now clear that the various antioxidants, either in a single cell or in a complete tissue or organism, do not work in an isolated manner; rather their activities interact, and complex pathways of reciprocal oxidation–reduction and recycling occur, assisting overall system homeostasis (29). Flavonoids and, in general, polyphenols, may play an important role in such interplay. Because their average redox potential is 700–540 mV (30), they are capable of reducing many of the oxygen free radical species having redox potentials in the range of 2300–1000 mV (31). The resulting radical can be reduced back to the parental nonradical species by ascorbic acid, uric acid, or tocopherol (280, 590, and 500 mV redox potential, respectively).

The effect of various flavonoids and flavonoid blends on the lifetime of the ascorbate radical has been investigated in our laboratory by means of ESR spectroscopy. In the presence of flavonoids both the lifetime and the ESR signal intensity of ascorbyl radical generated by ascorbate oxidase is significantly prolonged (32). Among the natural plant extracts tested, PYC displayed the strongest effect on the ascorbyl radical lifetime (Fig. 3), increasing it from a control value of 20 min to a maximum of 80 with 200 μg/mL PYC. We propose that PYC, and in general polyphenols, may regenerate ascorbic acid from its corresponding radical. The apparent contradiction between these experiments and the redox potentials presented can be explained by taking into consideration that because of the complex structure of flavonoids, the recovery process of free radicals is not necessarily driven by the reduction potential of the couples involved. Given the study of Yamasaki and Grace (33), it is also possible that the prolongation of the ascorbate radical lifetime in the presence of PYC results from a one-electron reduction of dehydroascorbic acid. Future experiments, possibly performed by pulse radiolysis, will provide substantial information on the actual mechanism of electron transfer and on the synergistic interaction of flavonoids with ascorbate in biological systems (34).

PYC has been reported to interact with cellular antioxidants. In our laboratory we have challenged ECV 304 cells with cocultured, activated macrophages and with purified $ONOO^-$. We have demonstrated (Fig. 4) that the preincubation of ECV 304 cells with PYC, in concentrations as low as 10 μg/mL, is associated with an increase of the endogenous steady-state levels of α-tocopherol and with protection of α-tocopherol in conditions of oxidative stress, induced either by $ONOO^-$ or from activated macrophages (35). With this model we have also

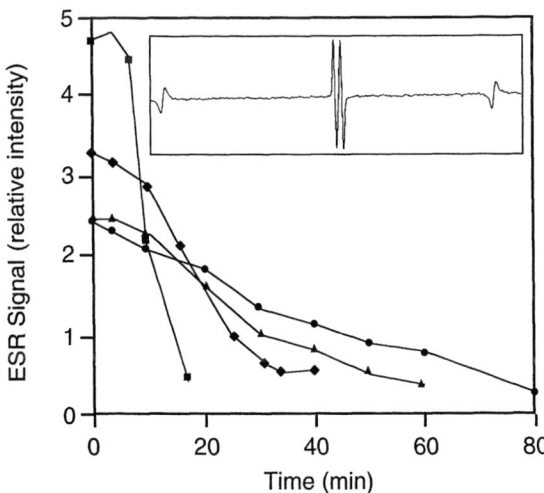

Figure 3 Effect of PYC on ascorbate radical lifetime: Ascorbic acid was incubated in the presence of ascorbate oxidase and, thereby, an ascorbyl radical was generated that has a distinct ESR spectrum as shown in the insert. PYC prolongs in a dose-dependent fashion the lifetime of the ascorbyl radical. ■, control; ●, 50 μg/mL; ◆, 100 μg/mL; ▲, 200 μg/mL.

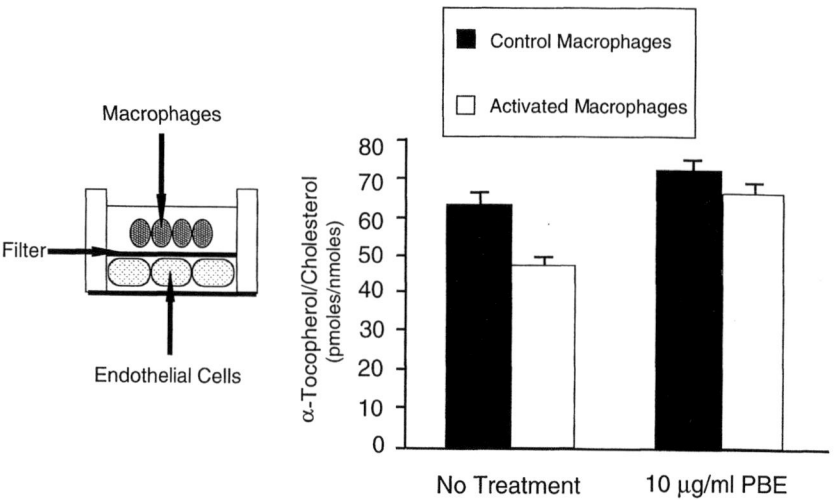

Figure 4 Effect of PYC on vitamin E content in endothelial cells: Pretreatment with PYC increases α-tocopherol content in endothelial cells (line ECV 304) both under basal conditions and after challenge by activated macrophages (line RAW 264.7). Macrophages were cocultured with endothelial cells on a 0.45-m filter and activated by LPS and IFN-γ. Bars represent the mean ± SD.

demonstrated that PYC protected endothelial cells from activated macrophage-induced GSH depletion (36).

In other laboratories, supplementation with PYC in the diet was associated with a significant increase in α-tocopherol levels in rat hearts. No effects, with the exception of a significant decrease of ascorbic acid level in the lungs, were observed in other organs (14).

Taken together, all these data demonstrate that polyphenols, and in particular PYC, may play a central and pivotal role in not only the network of antioxidants inside the cell, but also in the body as a whole.

B. Specific Binding to Proteins and Enzyme Inhibition

The biological effects of polyphenols, and in particular of flavonoids, are thought to result from their most widely studied property, their antioxidant activity. Furthermore, information demonstrating the ability of bioflavonoids to bind to proteins is likely to be another important factor in determining their biological activity. Interaction of small molecules, such as phenolic acids and polyphenols, with macromolecules in biological systems may result in a modification of their physicochemical properties, thereby affecting the characteristics of the entire biological system.

Baxter and collaborators (37) have demonstrated that polyphenols, particularly the procyanidin B_2, form complexes with proline-rich proteins. Other studies have shown that procyanidins present in PYC have multiple sites for association with proteins and that the o-dihydroxyphenol groups in natural tannin molecules are the sites for the formation of protein–polyphenol complexes (38).

In all of these studies, it is evident that the nature of the flavonoid–protein interaction is selective and specific, rather than due to random hydrogen bonds. Studies in progress in our laboratory indicate that PYC significantly inhibits the activity of enzymes that produce free radicals in biological systems; namely, horseradish peroxidase (HRP), lipoxygenase, and

XO. Horseradish peroxidase activity was inhibited in vivo by about 70% by 30 μg/mL PYC, whereas oxygen consumption, owing to lipoxygenase activity, was reduced by about 30% in the presence of PYC. In vitro XO activity was also significantly inhibited by PYC in a dose-dependent fashion, with an IC_{50} of about 50 μg/mL (Moini H, personal communication).

Nardini and co-workers (39) have recently studied the mode of action of PYC and caffeic acid (CA) on the activity of some protein kinases, such as phosphorylase kinase (PhK), protein kinase A (PKA), and protein kinase C (PKC), known to be involved in the regulation of fundamental cellular processes. At 20 μg/mL PBE activity of PKA, PhK, and PKC were inhibited by 90, 59, and 57%, respectively, whereas 100 μM (18 μg/mL) caffeic acid were inhibited by 37, 52, and 54%, respectively. Considerable inhibitions have been observed at still even lower concentrations of CA and PBE. For PhK and PKA, the inhibition followed a noncompetitive mechanism. CA also inhibits PKC activity in a partially purified cellular extract. These data suggest a direct and specific involvement of CA and PBE in the modulation of cellular functions.

The inhibitory effect of procyanidins on enzyme activities has also been reported for other plant extracts, with characteristics similar to those of PYC. Facino and co-workers (86) reported that procyanidins from *V. vinifera* inhibit xanthine oxidase, elastase, collagenase, β-glucuronidase, and hyaluronidase, which are considered key enzymes in the microvascular endothelium and extravascular matrix.

Other enzymes have been studied in our laboratory. We have demonstrated that PYC significantly affects inducible nitric oxide synthase (iNOS) activity both in vivo (40) and in murine macrophages (RAW 264.7 cell line) activated by lipopolysaccharide (LPS) and interferon (IFN)-γ (16). In vitro, we found that PYC had a remarkable modulatory effect on iNOS enzyme activity, producing a slight stimulatory effect at low concentrations (10 μg/mL) while acting as a powerful inhibitor of iNOS activity at higher, although still physiologically achievable, concentrations (50–100 μg/mL). As with many polyphenols, the inhibitory activity of PYC on iNOS is likely to be nonspecific, or partially specific, owing to the high affinity of phenolics to proteins. This is supported by the noncompetitive type of inhibitory activity. Interestingly, purified catechin and epicatechin, which are the basic blocks of procyanidin structure, inhibit iNOS activity to a significantly lesser extent (41).

IV. PYCNOGENOL AND PATHOLOGICAL CONDITIONS

A. Cardiovascular Effects

Pycnogenol is commonly suggested to lower the risk of cardiovascular diseases and also as a therapeutic alternative to established pharmacological therapy for mild pathological conditions of blood vessels. The rationale behind this is the link between cardiovascular disease and free radical-induced stress. However, besides its strong antioxidant capacity, PYC has been reported to have other activities related to cardiovascular function, such as a vasorelaxant activity, inhibition of angiotensin-converting enzyme, and the ability to enhance microcirculation by increasing capillary resistance. In this section, these PYC activities, independent of its antioxidant capacity, will be described and evaluated.

1. Vasorelaxation and Vasoconstriction

The effects of PYC on circulation can be seen as the outcome of two different activities: relaxation of arterial walls and increase of capillary resistance. The combination of these effects results in an increase of peripheral blood flow and a facilitation of the microcirculation.

Early studies suggested a strong vasoactivity of procyanidins extracted from sources such as wine and grape seed, which has recently been confirmed for PYC. Masquelier and collaborators reported, about 40 years ago (42), that the injection of leucocyanidin (leucocyanidol), a proanthocyanidin extracted from red wine, in the marginal ear vein of the rabbit was associated with a dramatic fall of carotid blood pressure, proportional to the injected dose.

A recent study by Fitzpatrick and collaborators (43) has investigated the possibility that PYC might produce vascular effects by inducing vasorelaxation. Isolated intact rat aortic rings were contracted by either epinephrine or norepinephrine. Exposure to PYC resulted in a dose-dependent relaxation. When the endothelial lining was removed, no vasorelaxation was observed after PYC treatment, suggesting that the effect of PYC on vascular tone depends on the endothelial cells. The authors also suggest that PYC's effects should be secondary to the increase of NO levels, because pretreatment of the aorta ring with an inhibitor of nitric oxide synthase totally prevented PYC-induced vasorelaxation. However, because PYC is a powerful scavenger for superoxide anion radicals, it might be that it prevents the formation of peroxynitrite, thereby maintaining higher levels of nitric oxide, known to be involved in vasorelaxation. The results of the study showed that the rate and extent of PYC-induced vasorelaxation is enhanced by adding 50 U/L of superoxide dismutase at every concentration of PYC tested (42). This supports our hypothesis that the antioxidant activity of PYC plays a significant role in its vasorelaxing properties. In this study, as in other studies described previously (15), PYC was fractionated through a gel permeation column, and the most effective fraction was the one containing oligomeric procyanidins. No experiments were addressed to the mechanisms on the basis of PYC activity, but the same authors have reported a similar activity for various plant extracts (42) associated with a significant effect on tissue levels of cGMP, the mediator of vascular smooth-muscle relaxation. Other mechanisms are also probably involved in the vasorelaxant activity, such as inhibition of PKC, inhibition of cyclic nucleotide phosphodiesterases, and a decrease in calcium influx (44). Interestingly, not all the flavonoid families have been reported to be vasorelaxants. For example, the flavonol myricetin has been reported to potentiate the contraction of aortic rings (45).

2. Inhibition of Platelet Aggregation

A new pharmaceutical use of PYC, recently submitted (46) and patented (47), involves the possibility of its use to inhibit platelet aggregation induced by cigarette smoking, without the adverse effect on bleeding time that characterizes aspirin use. Putter and collaborators (46) have observed that, in a group of heavy smokers, platelet aggregation was prevented by either 500 mg of acetyl salicylic acid (aspirin) or 100 mg of PYC. At the highest dose (200 mg), the inhibition of platelet aggregation by PYC remained effective for over 3 days after administration. The authors, according to the studies by Minuz and collaborators (48), suggest that the activity of PYC on platelet aggregation may be mediated by a stimulation of NO production by endothelial cells which, in turn, would inhibit the synthesis of thromboxane A_2. Moreover, unpublished data suggest that, in contrast to aspirin, which prolongs bleeding time by its ability to irreversibly inhibit cyclooxygenase, PYC did not prolong bleeding time (46). Even though more studies are needed to clarify the mechanism of the antiaggregation mechanism of PYC, these observation indicate that it is a valid alternative to aspirin, with an advantageous risk–benefit ratio in controlling platelet aggregation. Other flavonoids and isoflavones have been reported to affect platelet aggregation triggered by different inducers (49–51) in the concentration range reported for PYC. Several mechanisms have been proposed to mediate these effects on aggregation. Inhibition of cyclooxygenase by PYC, with a subsequent decrease of tromboxane A_2 synthesis (51), or the inhibition of calcium ions traffic across the plasma membrane (50) may be an important role, and the values are in agreement with the data reported by Putter and co-workers. Furthermore, in a study with 60 patients who met the diagnostic criteria of coronary heart disease: PYC administration over 4 weeks inhibited the adhesion and aggregation of platelets, enhanced the capillary diameter, and improved the microcirculation (52).

3. Inhibition of Angiotensin-Converting Enzyme

Angiotensin-converting enzyme (ACE) is a key enzyme in the regulation of the homeostasis of blood pressure. It converts the inactive protein angiotensin I into the biologically active angiotensin II, which has vasoconstrictive activity. ACE inhibitors, normally designed on the basis of a component present in the venom of some species of snakes, are widely used to pharmacologically control various types of hypertension.

Many polyphenols and polyphenol-containing plants have been reported to inhibit ACE activity (53) in a fashion more specific than a simple protein–polyphenols interaction. PYC and its different fractions from molecular sieve filtration has been reported to inhibit ACE activity in vivo (54). The IC_{50} value for the whole extract was 35 µg/mL, whereas that for the most active fraction, composed of higher oligomeric procyanidins, was about 3 µg/mL. This value is in the same range as that reported for other plant extracts (53–55), but appears quite high when compared with the IC_{50} of 0.005 for the established antihypertensive drug captopril (54). In the same paper, an in vivo study is described showing a slight but significant decrease of both systolic and diastolic pressure in Sprague Dawley rats. A 40% decrease was achieved after 36 min of timed intravenous (IV) injections of PYC, up to a cumulative dose of 32 mg/kg body weight (b.wt.). The effect of PYC on blood pressure became significant when the cumulative dose exceeded 8 mg/kg b.wt. and lasted for 30 min after the last PYC administration. It must be considered that the dose necessary for a significant effect was exceedingly high (corresponding to about 600 mg in an average adult man) and that the IV route of administration bypasses any restriction of the bioavailability of PYC. Thus, the authors conclude that the hypotensive action of PYC in humans is likely to be moderate. More studies could possibly be addressed to the effects of long-term oral administration in spontaneously hypertensive animals and in mild hypertension in humans, to establish the contribution of PYC to the modulation of blood pressure.

4. Microcirculation

One of the beneficial activities of PYC is its capacity to enhance microcirculation and capillary resistance. Gabor and colleagues (56) observed a decrease in vascular resistance in spontaneous hypertensive rats after treatment with procyanidins from pine bark, supporting the use of PYC in this context. The beneficial effect of procyanidins on capillary resistance was stronger and lasted longer than that observed after treatment with either purified hydroxyethylrutin or hesperidinchalcon (56). In addition, the effects of hydroxyethylrutoside were not linear. The increase of capillary resistance after treatment with the highest concentration (150 mg/kg b.wt.) was lower than that after a dose of 100 mg/kg. This biphasic effect, attributed by the authors to histamine liberation and edema formation caused by high doses of hydroxyethylrutoside, was not observed after PYC treatment.

Vascular diseases of the eye represent an important pathology associated with glucose homeostasis dysfunction in diabetes, and with other degenerative diseases (57). Effects of oligomeric procyanidins on capillary and vascular disorders were reported in the early 1970s (58). Several observations obtained from patients suffering from different venous diseases (e.g., phlebitis, hemorrhoids, ocular lesions, either primary or secondary to diabetes, or others) and receiving therapy based on oral administration of procyanidins extracted either from *P. maritima* bark or from other sources were presented. Significant improvements of capillary resistance and other objective and subjective parameters were reported in all cases treated, and a particular emphasis was given to the results obtained with diabetic retinopathies. This set of data, although lacking appropriate controls, is in agreement with anecdotal evidence for beneficial effects of PYC on peripheral vasculopathies.

In normal rats, intraperitoneal administration of anthocyanins from *P. maritima* was associated with a significant delay in the disappearance of Evans blue dye from the blood (59), indicating an increase in capillary resistance. Even though the dose administered was very high, corresponding to a load of about 15 g in an adult man, and the method chosen to assess the angioprotective activity is imperfect, the data indicate that PYC administration reduces the disappearance of Evans blue from the circulation to about 40%, relative to the controls. The authors also report a significant inhibition of elastase enzyme activity, considered in the following section.

5. Inhibition of Elastase Enzyme Activity

The fragmentation of elastic fibers is a classic histological hallmark of the inflammatory response associated with several pathological conditions and the aging process. The dramatic proteolytic activity results from an imbalance between natural inhibitors, such as α_1-antitrypsin and α_2-macroglobulin, and leads to elastolysis. Elastin, together with collagen, is an important component of blood vessels, contributing to their integrity, elasticity, and permeability (60). Studies have reported an inhibitory effect of procyanidins on elastase activity in vitro (59,61,62) and in vivo (62). In vitro, Tixier and co-workers (62) found that both procyanidins and (+)-catechin bound to insoluble elastine in a quasi-specific fashion, significantly affecting its rate of degradation by either purified porcine pancreatic elastase or human leukocyte elastase. The authors suggest that the mechanism for the inhibition of elastase cleavage was the binding of procyanidins to proline residues which, in turn, increases the nonproductive (i.e., nonenzymatically active) binding of elastase to the substrate. These authors (62) also report that the presence of procyanidins in an intradermal injection of a solution of fuschin and ferric chloride to rabbits significantly reduces the proteolysis subsequent to the injection of porcine pancreatic elastase, thereby confirming in vivo their observations in vitro. Similarly, collagen from calf skin or guinea pig skin treated with (+)-catechin has been reported to be more resistant to the action of mammalian collagenase, but not to the action of bacterial collagenase (63). A direct inhibiting effect on elastase, rather than enzyme binding to the substrate, has been reported in vitro (59), possibly owing to the formation of a complex between elastase and procyanidins. The noncompetitive character of the observed inhibition indicates that the attachment of procyanidins to the enzyme does not occur on the serine residues of the active center. Procyanidins extracted from *V. vinifera* have also been reported to be potent noncompetitive inhibitors of elastase, whereas purified catechin had no effect on amidolytic activity (37).

B. Regulation of Inflammatory Response

Inflammation is a multifactorial cellular response that is of fundamental importance in the maintenance of homeostasis when the organism is challenged by noxious agents (e.g., bacteria, viruses, or irritating agents) or by tissue mechanical injury. Inflammation is associated with a dramatic rise in the number of polymorphonuclear leukocytes and monocytes in the affected tissue and with the release of inflammatory mediators, such as prostaglandins and cytokines. Under ideal conditions, inflammation results in the complete recovery of the integrity of the affected tissue, but if the response to the triggering stimulus is not subjected to tight regulation, cellular and extracellular components of the organism adjacent to the inflammation site can be injured, inducing a condition known as chronic inflammatory disease. Indeed, a chronic inflammatory-like environment characterizes the pathogenesis of various diseases, such as atherosclerosis, arthritis, and Crohn's disease, and it is thought to be among the causative factors of more than 30% of human cancers. Thus, it is tremendously important to localize the inflammatory response which, on one hand, increases the ability of the immune machinery to destroy the noxious agent and, on the other hand, provides an efficient defense from self-induced damage. In this scenario, PYC has been reported to be able to play an important role either as immunomodulator or as anti-inflammatory agent.

Retrovirus, such as human immunodeficiency virus (HIV), and chronic ethanol consumption are two different pathophysiological conditions that share the common feature of inducing abnormalities in the function and structure of cells involved in humoral and cellular immunity, resulting in an increased susceptibility to infectious agents. Cheshier and collaborators (64) used an animal model to mimic these two conditions and to test the ability of PYC to enhance the immune profile. Mice were either infected by LP-BM5 retrovirus (a valid model HIV) or fed ethanol. Eight weeks of diet enriched with 75 mg/kg diet per day of PYC normalized the increase of interleukin (IL)-6 and IL-10 in ethanol-fed mice. In addition, PYC reduced IL-6 production in splenocytes isolated from retrovirus-infected mice and significantly increased the lymphoproliferative response to concanavalin-A.

Pretreatment with PYC restored the impaired natural killer cell activity in retrovirus-infected, but not in ethanol-fed, mice. The same study (64) reported no effect on hepatic α-tocopherol levels after PYC supplementation, in agreement with van Jaarsveld and co-workers (14), indicating that the improvements of immune functions were not mediated by an effect on vitamin E status. This study, although it used a high dose that is probably not achievable in humans, clearly suggests that PYC may delay the development of immune dysfunctions secondary to retrovirus infection by restoring the imbalanced cytokine secretion by Th1 and Th2 cells. It is also interesting to pair these observations with the inhibitory effect of flavan-3-ols on HIV reverse transcriptase activity, already mentioned (65). These data also indirectly support the hypothesis that flavonoids and, in particular, procyanidins, may affect gene expression. This important aspect of PYC bioactivity will be addressed in the conclusion of this chapter.

Aging is a normal physiological process, but it presents some features characteristic of immune diseases, in that immune functions are depressed and often the capacity to respond to infection is significantly impaired. Nutrition and nutritional supplementation may play an important role in the maintenance of the normal immune function in aged people (66). The senescence-accelerated strain of mice (SAMP8), which displays some of the dysfunctions of the immune system characteristic of senescence, has been used by Liu and collaborators (67) to demonstrate that PYC may restore the immune and hemopoietic functions that are altered in the aging process. Supplementation with 5 or 10 mg/kg b.wt. per day of PYC by intragastric perfusion was associated with a significant improvement in the severely depressed B- and T-lymphocyte response to mitogens and with an increased number of antibody-forming cells. Moreover, the colony-forming unit of granulocyte–macrophage, the erythroid colony-forming unit, and the erythroid burst-forming unit, which are parameters associated with the number and the in vivo proliferative capacity of immunocompetent cells typically affected by aging, were significantly improved by PYC supplementation. These impressive results strongly suggest a significant effect of PYC and warrant further clinical studies to assess if these effects also occur in humans.

1. Inhibition of Localized Inflammation

Blazso and co-workers (15) tested the capacity of PYC in inhibiting a localized inflammatory response. Four days of oral administration of up to 160 mg/kg b.wt. of PYC then intraperitoneal injections just before treatment with a proinflammatory agent, significantly inhibited the formation of the edema induced by injection of croton oil in the mouse ear, in a dose-dependent fashion. PYC chromatographic fractions had the same effect. As with the antioxidant activity already discussed, the most active fraction was that containing oligomeric procyanidins, suggesting that the anti-inflammatory and antioxidant activities may be related.

The same authors have recently reported that the oral supplementation of either PYC or its chromatographic fractions at a dose of 100 mg/animal per day for 10 days significantly inhibited the formation of edema induced either by croton oil in the mouse ear or by compound 48/80 (a proinflammatory substance) in the rat paw model (27). They observed that the extent of edema inhibition of both animal models paralleled the content of oligomeric procyanidins in the PYC fraction administered, suggesting that the anti-inflammatory activity is associated with the procyanidin moiety. Topical application of PYC or its fractions, incorporated into hydroxyethylcellulose, significantly protected rat skin from UV-induced irritation. Furthermore, oral administration of PYC was associated with a protective effect against UV-induced erythema (Watson R, Packer L, unpublished).

More recently, Saito and co-workers (68) reported a significant protective effect of both PYC and grape seed extract on acute gastric injury induced by ethanol–HCl administration in rats. In agreement with previous findings (15,27) the protective activity appears to be dependent on the content of procyanidin oligomers. Longer procyanidins, such as pentamers and hexamers, bind bovine serum albumin in vitro, supporting the idea that their protective activity is due to the ability to cover the surface of the stomach, assessed by histology. It has been proposed that ethanol–HCl-induced gastric injury may have a free radical component (69); therefore, the protective effects of procyanidins could result from a combination of the physical protection of the gastric mucosa together with the ability to efficiently scavenge reactive oxygen and nitrogen species.

2. Ultraviolet-Induced Tissue Injury

Pycnogenol has also been studied in relation to its ability to act as a protective factor against UV radiation-induced injury, either by virtue of its antioxidant capacity, or by its ability to modulate the inflammatory response induced by high-energy radiation. Blazso and collaborators (27) have reported that the topical application of PYC incorporated into hydroxyethylcellulose gel as a 0.3–1% solution inhibited, in a dose-dependent fashion, the increase of capillary permeability induced by UV radiation in the shaved back of rats. Oral supplementation of PYC failed to prevent UV-induced skin irritation, whereas the local application of the chromatographic fractions of PYC, described earlier (see Sec. III.A), was associated with a strong protective activity. The fraction corresponding to oligomeric procyanidins displayed the strongest activity, resulting in a 70% inhibition of the capillary damage when applied at a concentration of 1% to rat skin. These investigators (27) concluded that the protective activity of PYC and its fractions results from the combination of an enhancement of capillary resistance (56) and the free radical-scavenging activity of PYC.

Recent, unpublished studies performed in our laboratory offer new insight into the capacity for PYC to protect tissues from UV-induced damage. One of the molecular features of the UV-induced inflammatory response is the activation of the transcription factor nuclear factor-kappa B (NF-κB) which, in turn, regulates the expression of different inflammatory cytokines and triggers the inflammatory response. By use of the technique of electrophoretic mobility band shift and dual gene reporter assays, PYC was shown to significantly inhibit the activation, the binding to DNA, and the NF-κB-dependent gene expression of the NF-κB transcription factors in HaCaT cells, an immortalized human keratinocyte line (Saliou C, personal communication).

3. Modulation of Macrophage Activity

Nitrogen monoxide (NO) has diverse physiological roles and also contributes to the immune defense against viruses, bacteria, and other parasites. However, excess production of NO is associated with various diseases, such as arthritis, diabetes, stroke, septic shock, autoimmune, and chronic inflammatory diseases, and atherosclerosis. Cells respond to activating or depressing stimuli by enhancing or inhibiting the expression of the enzymatic machinery that produces NO. Thus, maintenance of a tight regulation of NO production is important for human health. Phytochemicals have traditionally been used in ways to treat a family of pathologies that have in common the dysregulation of NO production. Macrophages activated with lipopolysaccharide (LPS) and IFN-γ produce large amounts of NO. Preincubation of RAW 264.7 macrophages with increasing concentrations of PYC significantly decreased NO generation (Fig. 5a). This effect was due to the combination of several different biological activities [i.e., its ROS- and NO-scavenging activity, inhibition of iNOS activity (see Fig. 5b), and inhibition of iNOS mRNA expression (see Fig. 5c)] (16). No effects of PYC pretreatment were observed on the activation of either NF-κB or IRF-1, the transcription factors involved in LPS- and IFN-γ-induced expression of iNOS (70); thus, the modulation of iNOS expression by PYC is likely to occur at the posttranscriptional level. The effect on mRNA expression may be due to a specific effect on mRNA stability, or may be mediated by an effect on some still unknown modulatory step in the cellular regulation of gene expression. Finally, because cellular responses may be indirectly regulated by their redox status (71), the antioxidant activity of PYC and its contribution to the antioxidant network may result in a modulation of inducible gene expression.

V. CONCLUSIONS AND FUTURE DIRECTIONS

Pycnogenol is a complex mixture composed mainly of oligomeric procyanidins and other flavonoids and polyphenols. A wide spectrum of biological activities has been described for the mixture. PYC has been reported to significantly affect circulation, inflammation, and the immune response. The molecular bases of PYC activity are manyfold, but appear to depend mainly on its capacity to efficiently scavenge reactive oxygen and reactive nitrogen species. Other major biological effects are probably due to its ability to specifically bind to proteins, thereby affecting both structural and functional characteristics. Finally, PYC participates in the cellular antioxidant network and is able to affect the expression of those genes that are regulated by cell redox status. Also anticancer effects of PYC have recently been described (72,73). The next challenge in flavonoid research will be the identification and understanding of the molecular mechanisms responsible for each different biological activity. An interesting characteristic emerging from some of the studies described herein is that the complete mixture of PYC displays greater biological effects than a similar amount, on a weight basis, of any single purified component. This is clearly suggested by studies on enzyme inhibition (40) and from studies on its antioxidant capacity (18,32). This means that no "magic bullets" are likely to be present in PYC, but rather, the whole extract is most biologically effective, probably

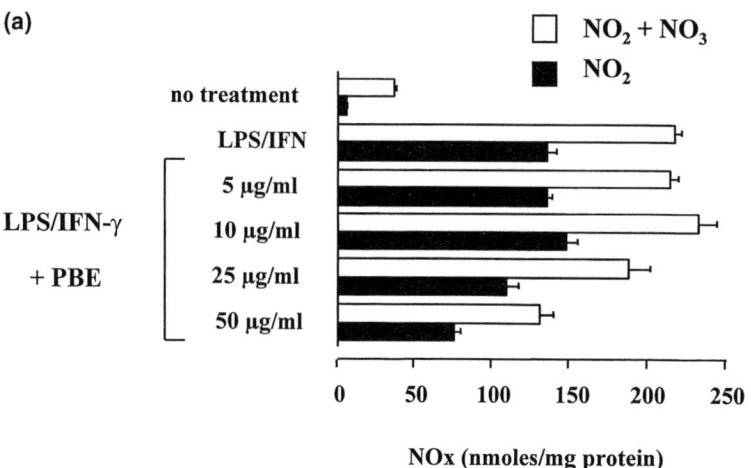

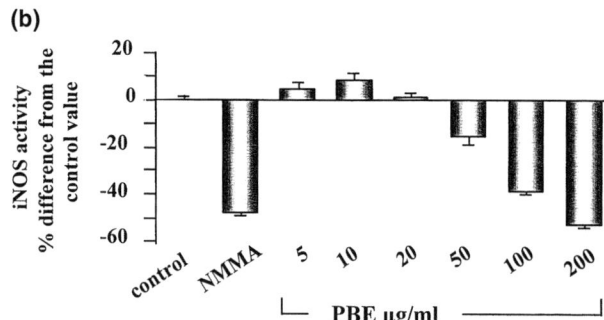

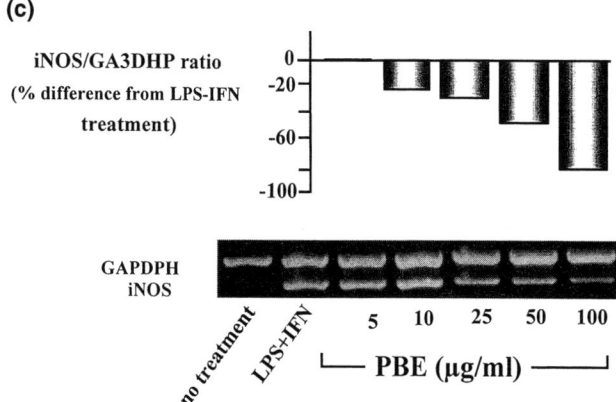

Figure 5 (a) Effect of PYC on NO_2^- and NO_3^- accumulation; (b) iNOS enzyme activity; and (c) iNOS mRNA expression in RAW 264.7 macrophages activated with LPS and IFN-γ.

owing to complex synergistic interactions between its various components. Because most of the studies presented herein on the beneficial effects of PYC have been conducted either in vitro, using cell cultures, or using animal models, additional data on its antioxidant activity and biological properties in humans are warranted.

ACKNOWLEDGMENTS

The authors thank H. Moini, C. A. Rice–Evans, C. Saliou, J. R. Shirley, and A. L. Waterhouse for their generous contributions of unpublished observations. G. R. is supported by the German Research Society (DFG-Forschungsstipendium Ri 884/3-1).

REFERENCES

1. Masquelier J, Michaud J, Laparra J, Dumon MC. Flavonoids and pycnogenols. Int J Vit Nutr Res 1979; 49:307–311.
2. Packer L, Rimbach G, Virgili F. Antioxidant activity and biologic properties of a procyanidin-rich extract from pine (*Pinus maritima*) bark, Pycnogenol. Free Radic Biol 1999; 27:704–724.
3. Masquelier J, Triaud J. Fractionation of wine leucoanthocyanidins. Soc Pharm Bordeaux 1965; 104:81–85.
4. Bates–Smith EC. Phytochemistry of proanthocyanidins. Phytochemistry 1975; 14:1107–1113.
5. Cheynier V, Souquet J–M, Le Roux E, Guyrot S, Rigaud J. Size separation of condensed tannins by normal phase high performance liquid chromatography. Methods Enzymol 1998; 299:178–184.
6. Steinmetz KA, Potter JD. Vegetable, fruit and cancer prevention: a review. J Am Diet Assoc 1996; 96:1027–1039.
7. Hertog MG, Kromhout D, Aravanis C, et al. Flavonoid intake and long-term risk of coronary heart disease and cancer in the seven countries study. [Published erratum appears in Arch Intern Med 1995 Jun 12; 155:1184.] Arch Intern Med 1995; 155:381–386.
8. Halliwell B. Antioxidants in human health and disease. Annu Rev Nutr 1996; 16:33–50.
9. Rohdewald P. Pycnogenol. In: Rice–Evans C, Packer L, eds. Flavonoids in Health and Disease. New York: Marcel Dekker, 1997:405–419.
10. Bourne LC, Rice–Evans CA. Detecting and measuring bioavailability of phenolics and flavonoids in humans: pharmacokinetics of urinary excretion of dietary ferulic acid. Methods Enzymol 1998; 299:91–106.
11. Rice–Evans CA, Miller NJ, Pananga G. Structure–antioxidant activity relationship of flavonoids and phenolic acids. Free Radic Biol Med 1996; 20:933–956.
12. Benthsath A, Rusznyak S, Szent-Gyorgyi A. Vitamin nature of flavones. Nature 1936; 138:798.
13. Uchida S, Edamatsu R, Hiramatsu M, Mori A, Nonaka GI, Nishioka I, Niwa M, Ozaki M. Condensed tannins scavenge active oxygen radicals. Med Sci Res 1987; 15:831–832.
14. van Jaarsveld H, Kuyl JM, Schulemburg DH, Wiid NM. Effect of flavonoids in the outcome of myocardial mitochondrial ischemia/reperfusion injury. Res Commun Mol Pathol Pharmacol 1996; 91:65–75.
15. Blazso G, Gabor M, Sibbel R, Rohdewald P. Antiinflammatory and superoxide radical scavenging activities of procyanidins containing extract from the bark of *Pinus pinaster* Sol. and its fractions. Pharm Pharmacol 1994; 3:217–220.
16. Virgili F, Kobuchi H, Packer L. Procyanidins extracted from *Pinus maritima* (Pycnogenol): scavengers of free radical species and modulators of nitrogen monoxide metabolism in activate murine RAW 264.7 macrophages. Free Radic Biol Med 1998; 24:1120–1129.
17. Elstner EF, Kleber E. Radical scavenger properties of leucocyanidine. In: Das NP, ed. Flavonoids in Biology and Medicine III: Current Issues in Flavonoids Research. Singapore: National University of Singapore Press, 1990:227–235.
18. Noda Y, Anzai K, Mori A, Kohno M, Shinmei M, Packer L. Hydroxyl and superoxide anion radical scavenging activities of natural source of antioxidants using the computerized JES-FR30 ESR spectrometer system. Biochem Mol Biol Int 1997; 42:35–44.

19. Guo Q, Zhao B, Packer L. Electron spin resonance study of free radicals formed from a procyanidin-rich pine (*Pinus maritima*) bark extract. Free Radic Biol Med 1999; 27:(in press).
20. Moini H, Arroyo A, Vaja J, Packer L. Bioflavonoid effects on the mitochondrial respiratory electron transport chin and cytochrome *c* redox state. Redox Rep 1999; 4:37–41.
21. Macrides TA, Shihata A, Kalafatis N, Wright PFA. A comparison of the hydroxyl radical scavenging properties of the shark bile steroid 5-β-scymnol and plant pycnogenols. Biochem Mol Biol Int 1997; 42:1249–1260.
22. Nelson AB, Lau BHS, Ide N, Rong Y. Pycnogenol inhibits macrophage oxidative burst, lipoprotein oxidation and hydroxyl radical induced DNA damage. Drug Dev Ind Med 1998; 24:1–6.
23. Emerit I. Reactive oxygen species, chromosome mutation, and cancer: possible role of clastogenic factors in carcinogenesis. Free Radic Biol Med 1994; 16:99–109.
24. Rong Y, Li L, Lau BH. Pycnogenol protects vascular endothelial cells from *t*-butyl-hydroperoxide induced oxidant injury. Biotechnol Ther 1994–95; 5:117–126.
25. Pereira CM, Oliveira CR. Glutamate toxicity on a PC12 cell line involves glutathione (GSH) depletion and oxidative stress. Free Radic Biol Med 1997; 23:637–647.
26. Kobayashi M, Han D, Packer L. Antioxidants and herbal extracts protect HT-4 neuronal cells against glutamate-induced cytotoxicity. Free Radic Res 1999; (in press).
27. Blazso G, Gabor M, Rohdewald P. Antiinflammatory activities of procyanidin-containing extract from *Pinus pinaster* Ait after oral and cutaneous application. Pharmazie 1997; 52:380–382.
28. Ueda T, Ueda T, Armstrong D. Preventive effect of natural and synthetic antioxidants on lipid peroxidation in the mammalian eye. Ophthalmol Res 1996; 28:184–192.
29. Packer L. Interactions among antioxidants in health and disease: vitamin E and its redox cycle. Proc Soc Exp Biol Med 1991; 200:271–276.
30. Jovanovic SV, Steeken S, Tosic M, Marjanovic B, Simic MG. Flavonoids as antioxidants. J Am Chem Soc 1994; 116:4846–4851.
31. Buettner GR. The pecking order of free radicals and antioxidants lipid peroxidation alpha-tocopherol and ascorbate. Arch Biochem Biophys 1993; 300:535–543.
32. Cossins E, Lee R, Packer L. ESR studies of vitamin C regeneration, order of reactivity of natural source phytochemical preparations. Biochem Mol Biol Int 1998; 45:583–598.
33. Yamasaki H, Grace SC. EPR detection of phytophenoxyl radicals stabilized by zinc ions: evidence for the redox coupling of plant phenolics with ascorbate in the H_2O_2-peroxidase system. FEBS Lett 1998; 422:377–380.
34. Bors WC, Michel C, Schikora S. Interaction of flavonoids with ascorbate and determination of their univalent redox potentials—a pulse radiolysis study. Free Radic Biol Med 1995; 19:45–52.
35. Virgili F, Kim D, Packer L. Procyanidins extracted from pine bark protect a-tocopherol in ECV 304 endothelial cells challenged by activated RAW 264.7 macrophages: role of nitric oxide and peroxynitrite. FEBS Lett 1998; 431:315–318.
36. Rimbach G, Virgili F, Park YC, Packer L. Effect of procyanidins from *Pinus maritima* on glutathione levels in endothelial cells challenged by 3-morpholinosyndonimine or activated macrophages. Redox Rep 1999; (in press).
37. Baxter NJ, Lilley TH, Haslam E, Williamson MP. Multiple interactions between polyphenols and a salivary proline-rich protein repeat result in complexation and precipitation. Biochemistry 1997; 36:5566–5577.
38. Haslam E. Polyphenol–protein interaction. Biochem J 1974; 139:285–288.
39. Nardini M, Scaccini C, Packer L, Virgili F. Inhibitory effect of caffeic acid and a procyanidin rich pine bark (*Pinus maritima*) extract on the activity of phosphorylase kinase, protein kinase C and protein kinase A. Biochim Biophys Acta 1999; (in press).
40. Kobuchi H, Droy–Lefaix MT, Christen Y, Packer L. *Ginkgo biloba* extract (EGb761): inhibitory effect on nitric oxide production in the macrophage cell line RAW 264.7. Biochem Pharmacol 1997; 53:897–903.
41. Kobuchi H, Virgili F, Packer L. Assay of the inducible form of nitric oxide synthase activity: effect of flavonoids and plant extracts. Methods Enzymol 1999; 301:504–513.
42. Fitzpatrick DF, Hirschfield SL, Ricci T, Jantzen P, Coffey RG. Endothelium-dependent vasorelaxation caused by various plant extracts. J Cardiovasc Pharmacol 1995; 26:90–95.
43. Fitzpatrick DF, Bing B, Rohdewald P. Endothelium-dependent vascular effects of Pycnogenol. J Cardiovasc Pharmacol 1998; 32:509–515.

44. Fitzpatrick DF, Bing B, Rohdewald P. Endothelium dependent vascular effects of Pycnogenol. J Cardiovasc Pharmacol 1998; (in press).
45. Herrera MD, Zarzuelo A, Jimenez J, Marhuenda E, Duarte J. Effects of flavonoids on aortic smooth muscle contractility: structure–activity relationship. Gen Pharmacol 1996; 27:273–277.
46. Putter M, Grotemayer KHM, Wurthwein G, Araghi–Nikam M, Watson RR, Hosseini S, Rohdewald P. Inhibition of smoking-induced platelet aggregation by aspirin and Pycnogenol; (in press).
47. Rohdewald P. U.S. Patent 5,720,956, 1998.
48. Minuz P, Lechi C, Gaino S, Bonapace S, Fontana L, Garbin U, Paluani F, Cominacini L, Zatti M, Lechi A. Oxidized LDL and reduction of the antiaggregating activity of nitric oxide derived from endothelial cells. Thromb Haemost 1995; 74:1175–1179.
49. Manach C, Regerat F, Texier O, Agullo G, Demigne C, Remsey C. Bioavailability, metabolism and physiological impact of 4-oxo-flavonoids. Nutr Res 1996; 16:517–544.
50. Ozaki Y, Yatomi Y, Jinnai Y, Kume S. Effects of genistein, a tyrosine kinase inhibitor, on platelet functions. Genistein attenuates thrombin-induced Ca^{2+} mobilization in human platelets by affecting polyphosphoinositide turnover. Biochem Pharmacol 1993; 46:395–403.
51. Tzeng SH, Ko WC, Ko FN, Teng MC. Inhibition of platelet aggregation by some flavonoids. Throm Res 1991; 64:91–100.
52. Wang S, Tan D, Zhao Y, Gao G, Gao X, Hu L. The effect of Pycnogenol on the microcirculation, platelet function and ischemic myocardium in patients with coronary artery disease. Eur Bull Drug Res 1999; 7:19–25.
53. Inokuchi J–I, Okabe H, Yamauchi T, Nagamatzu A. Inhibitors of angiotensin converting enzyme in crude drugs. I. Chem Pharm Bull 1984; 32:3615–3619.
54. Blazso G, Gaspar R, Gabor M, Ruve H–J, Rohdewald P. ACE inhibition and hypotensive effect of a procyanidins containing extract from the bark of *Pinus pinaster* Sol. Pharm Pharmacol Lett 1996; 6:8–11.
55. Inokuchi J–I, Okabe H, Yamauchi T, Nagamatsu A, Nonaka GI, Nishioka I. Antihypertensive substance in seeds of *Areca carecu*. Life Sci 1986; 38:1375–1382.
56. Gabor M, Engi E, Sonkodi S. Die Kapillarwandresistenz und ihre Beeinflussung durch wasserlösliche Flavonderivate bei spontan hypertonischen Ratten. Phlebologie 1993; 22:178–182.
57. Anderson RE, Kretzer FL, Rapp LM. Free radicals and ocular medicine. Adv Exp med Biol 1994; 366:73–86.
58. Magnard G, Franck J–P, Dorne P–A. Interet du tetrahydroxy flavanne diol en ophtalmologie. Lyon Med 1970; 4:1–18.
59. Jonadet M, Meunier MT, Bastide P. Anthocyanosides extraits de vitis vinifera, de vaccinium myrtillus et *Pinus maritimus*. Pharm Belg 1983; 38:41–46.
60. Hay ED. Cell Biology of Extracellular Matrix. New York: Plenum Press, 1993.
61. Maffei Facino R, Carini M, Aldini G, Bombardelli E, Morazzoni P, Morelli R. Free radical scavenging action and anti-enzyme activities of procyanidins from *Vitis vinifera*. Drug Res 1994; 44:592–601.
62. Tixier JM, Godeau G, Robert AM, Hornebeck W. Evidence by in vivo and in vitro studies that binding of pycnogenols to elastin affects its rate of degradation by elastase. Biochem Pharmacol 1984; 33:3933–3939.
63. Kuttan R, Donnelly PV, Di Ferrante N. Collagen treated with (+)-catechin becomes resistant to the action of mammalian collagenase. Experientia 1981; 37:221–223.
64. Cheshier JE, Ardestani–Kaboudanian S, Liang B, Araghiniknam M, Chung S, Lane S, Castro A, Watson RR. Immunomodulation by Pycnogenol in retrovirus infected or ethanol fed mice. Life Sci 1996; 58:87–96.
65. Nakane H, One K. Differential inhibitory effects of some catechin derivatives on the activities of human immunodeficiency virus reverse transcriptase and cellular deoxyribonucleic and ribonucleic acid polymerase. Biochemistry 1992; 29:2841–2945.
66. Lesourd BM, Meaume S. Cell mediated immunity changes in ageing, relative importance of cell subpopulation switches and of nutritional factors. Immunol Lett 1994; 40:235–242.
67. Liu FJ, Zhang YX, Lau BH. Pycnogenol enhances immune and haemopoietic functions in senescence-accelerated mice. Cell Mol Life Sci 1998; 54:1168–1172.
68. Saito M, Hosoyama H, Ariga T, Kataoka S, Yamaji N. Antiulcer activity of grape seed extract and procyanidins. J Agric Food Chem 1998; 46:1460–1464.

69. Pihan G, Regillo C, Szabo S. Free radicals and lipid peroxidation in ethanol- or aspirin-induced gastric mucosal injury. Dig Dis Sci 1987; 32:1395–1401.
70. Nathan C, Xie QW. Regulation of biosynthesis of nitric oxide. J Biol Chem 1994; 269:13725–13728.
71. Suzuki YJ, Forman HJ, Sevanian A. Oxidants as stimulators of signal transduction. Free Radic Biol Med 1997; 22:269–285.
72. Huynh HT, Teel RW. Effects of Pycnogenol on the microsomal metabolism of the tobacco-specific nitrosamine NNK as a function of age. Cancer Lett 1998; 132:135–139.
73. Huynh HT, Teel RW. Effects of intragastrically administered Pycnogenol on NNK metabolism in F344 rats. Anticancer Res 1999; 19:2095–2099.

22
Spices as Potent Antioxidants with Therapeutic Potential

Bharat B. Aggarwal
The University of Texas M.D. Anderson Cancer Center, Houston, Texas
Nihal Ahmad and Hasan Mukhtar
Case Western Reserve University, Cleveland, Ohio

I. INTRODUCTION

Most beneficial or harmful physiological responses are regulated by the balance between pro-oxidants and antioxidants. Many compounds derived from several commonly used spices block production of reactive oxygen species (ROS) in several in vitro and in vivo systems. Owing to their antioxidant properties, various therapeutic effects have been assigned to these spices and spice-derived ingredients. These effects stem from their ability to interfere with signal transduction pathways involving various transcription factors, protein kinases, phosphatases, and other metabolic enzymes. The antioxidant activity of the spices plays a role in suppression of cell growth, viral replication, inflammation, inhibition of allergy and arthritis, prevention of cancer and heart diseases, and in abrogation of several other pathological conditions. Some of the known in vitro and in vivo effects of the ingredients derived from spices are discussed in this chapter.

In the West, they say "beef it up" whereas in the East they say "spice it up." Whether you talk about Texan salsa, Indian curry, Hungarian paprika, or Italian olive oil, the history of spice use goes back thousands of years. While bringing color and taste to the food, some spices have long been considered to possess medicinal value. In every culture, particularly in the Orient, India, and Africa, various plant-derived products have been used for centuries to treat different diseases. In the United States and Europe, the benefits of botanicals for humans are increasingly gaining recognition. In countries with hot climates, spices prevent cooked food from turning rancid. The active principals in spices responsible for these properties are none other than chemical metabolites produced by plants. These phytochemicals include organosulfides, monoterpenes, flavonoids, polyphenols, indoles, and isothiocyanates (Table 1) (1). These common ingredients of herbs and spices exhibit health-promoting properties (2).

Table 1 Chemical Composition of Most Common Spices

Spice	Botanical name	Part of plant	Major constituents
Turmeric	*Curcuma longa*	Rhizome	Essential oils 5%: tumerone (58%), borneol (6.5%), cineole (1%), α-phellandrene (1%), curcumin (0.6%), zingerone, zingiberene (25%)
Pepper (red)	*Capsicum frutescens*	Fruit	Pigments: carotene, zeaxanthin, cryptoxanthin; oleoresin (1.5%); capsaici
Cloves	*Syzgium aromaticum* (*Caryophyllu aromaticus, Eugenia caryophyllata*)	Buds	Essential oils 17%: eugenol (93%), caryophyllin, vanillin, eugenin, methylamylketone
Coriander	*Coriandrum sativum*	Seeds	Essential oils 1%: (+)-linalool (60–70%), α-pinene, β-pinene, α-terpinene, β-terpinene, geraniol, borneol, decylaldehyde, dipentene, cymene
Cumin	*Cuminum cyminum*	Seeds	Essential oil 4.5%: cuminaldehyde (40–65%), thymol, cymol, cymene
Cinnamon	*Cinnamomum zeylanicum*	Bark	Essential oils 1.5–2.5%: cinnamaldehyde (65–75%), (−)-linalool, furfural, methylamylketone, nonylaldehyde, benzaldehyde, hydrocinnamaldehyde, cuminaldehyde, eugenol, caryophyllene, (−)-phellandrene, p-cymene, α-pinene
Allspice	*Pimenta dioica* (*P. officinalis*)	Berry	Volatile oil 4.5%; eugenol (80%), O-methyleugenol, cineole, phellandrene, caryophyllene
Fennel	*Foeniculum vulgare*	Seeds	Essential oils 6%: anethole (50–60%), (+)-fenchone (15–20%), α-pinene, camphene, (+)-α-phellandrene, dipentene, p-hydroxyphenylacetone, estragole, anisaldehyde, anisic acid, 1,3-dimethylbutadiene
Anise	*Pimpinella anisum*	Seeds	Fixed oil 8–20%; essential oil 1.5%; anethole (90–96%), estragole (2%), p-methoxyphenylacetone
Star anise	*Illicium verum*	Seeds	Essential oils 8–9%: anethole (88%), limonine (5%), estragole, safrole, p-methoxyphenylacetone
Ginger	*Zingiber officinale*	Rhizome	Essential oils 1–2.5%: zingerone, shogaol, gingerol, cineole, borneol, geraniol, linalool, farnesene, citral, zingiberene, zingiberol, camphene, phellandrene, methylheptanone

(*continued*)

Table 1 (Continued)

Spice	Botanical name	Part of plant	Major constituents
Cardamon	Elettaria cardomonum	Seeds	Fixed oils 1–2%: fatty acid glycerides; essential oils 2–10%: cineole (25–40%), methylheptanone, terpenene, α-terpinyl acetate (28–34%), β-terpineol, borneol, nerylacetate, geraniol, nerolidol, α-pinene, sabinene, mycrene, limonene, p-cymene
Basil	Ocimum basilicum		Essential oil: (+)-linalool (40%), estragole (25%), eugenol, cineole, geraniol
Capers	Capparis sppinosa	Seeds	Fixed oil 15%: fatty acids; essential oil 7.5%: (+)-carvone (60%), carvol, (+)-limonene, carveol, diacetyl, furfural
Caraway	Carum carvi		
Curry leaves	Murraya koenigii	Leaves	Essential oils 4.0%: carvone (60%), dihydrocarvone, (+)-limonene, α-phellandrene, α-pinene, dipentene
Dill	Anethum graveolens		
Fenugreek	Trigonella foenumgraecum	Seeds	Fixed oils 7%: trigonelline, choline
Garlic	Allium sataivum	Bulb	Essential oils 0.2%: diallyldisulfide (60%), diallyltrisulfide (20%); allylpropyldisulfide (6%), alliin, allicin
Lemon grass	Andropogon nardus (A. citratus); Cymbopogon citratus (C. flexuosus)	Grass	Essential oils 0.3–0.55%: citral (70–85%) geraniol
Licorice	Glycyrrhiza glabra	Rhizome	Water extract: glycyrrhizin 12–20%
Mace	Myristica fragrans	Aril	Essential oils 11–15%: monoterpenes (88%), monoterpenols (55%)
Mint (black)	Mentha vulgaris (M. piperita)		Essential oils 1%: α-pinene, β-pinene, limonene, cineole, ethylamylcarbinol, (−)-menthol, menthone, menthylacetate, piperitone
Mint (white)	M. officinalis		
Mustard (white)	Brassica alba (B. hirta, B. juncea, Sinapsis alba)	Seeds	Fixed oils 30–35%; sinalbin
Mustard (black)	B. Nigra (S. nigra)	Seeds	Sinigrin
Nutmeg	Myristica fragens	Seeds	Fixed oils 24–30%; essential oils 16%; elemicin (2%), eugenol, isoeugenol, o-methyleugenol, safrole (0–6%), myristic acid, α-pinene, sabinene, (+)-camphene (60–80%), dipentene (8%), geranioil, (+)-borneol, (−)-terpeneol, myristicin (4%)
Oregano	Oreganum vulgare		Essential oils: thymol 50%, α-pinene 7–8%, cineole, linalyl acetate, linalool, dipentane, p-cymene, β-cymene, β-cryophyllene

(continued)

Table 1 (*Continued*)

Spice	Botanical name	Part of plant	Major constituents
Pepper (black)	*Piper nigrum*	Unripe fruit	Essential oils 1.5%: monoterpenes (70–80%)
Pepper (white)		Ripe fruit	Sesquiterpenes (20–30%), chavicine; oleoresin: piperine, piperidine
Rosemary	*Rosmarinus officinalis*	Twigs	Essential oils 2%: borneol (16–20%), cineole (27–30%), camphor (10%), borny acetate (2–7%), α-pinene, camphene, terpinol, verbenone
Saffron	*Crocus sativus*	Stigmas	Essential oils 1%: 2,2,6-trimethyl-4,6-cyclohexadienal, crocin, picrocrocin, crocetin
Sesame	*Sesamum indicum*	Seeds	Fixed oils: 45–65%
Spearmint	*Mentha spicata*		Essential oils 0.6%: (−)-carvone (56%), dihydrocuminyl esters, dihydrocarveyl acetate

Source: Ref. 1.

It has been reported that 80% of the world population relies on plant-derived products for their primary health care needs (3).

This long tradition has led scientists to try to identify spices and herbs with therapeutic activity and, ultimately, to identify a role for them in Western medicine. To find a therapeutic phytochemical by random screening is labor-intensive, expensive, and not very effective. For instance the National Cancer Institute failed to find a compound with clinical anticancer activity among 114,000 plant extracts derived from 35,000 species (4). On the other hand, use of folk-belief and traditional healers to identify therapeutic agents has been a short-cut to the discovery and isolation of pharmacologically active compounds. In the United States today, almost 25% of the drug prescriptions are for compounds derived from plants that were discovered through scientific investigation of folklore claims. Several folkloric claims of enormous medicinal value for spices require further investigation. For instance pennyroyal, an aromatic mint plant (*Mentha pulegium*), was considered to be an abortifacient in ancient and mediaeval times. Recent studies have confirmed that the active ingredient, pulegone, in mint can indeed induce abortion in animals and humans (5).

Because they prevent rancidity, antioxidants are of great interest to the food industry. For example, butylated hydroxytoluene (BHT), butylated hydroxyanisole (BHA), and EDTA are frequently used to preserve various foods, such as cheese or fried products. Some of the active antioxidant components in spices include carnosic acid, carnosol, rosmarinic acid, thymol, carvacrol, 6-gingerol, 6-shogaol, zingerone, curcumin, capsaicin, vanillin, eugenol, caffeic acid, and ferulic acid. The nutrient compositions of several commonly consumed spices have been analyzed (6), including those for red chillies (*Capsicum annum*), black pepper (*Piper nigrum*), coriander seeds (*Coriandrum sativum*), cumin seeds (*Cuminum cyminum*), garlic (*Allium sativum*), asafoetida (*Ferula foetida*), dry ginger (*Zingiber officinale*), and ajowan (*Carum copticum*). The nutrients analyzed were proximate principals, minerals, starch, sugars, dietary fiber components, tannins, phytic acid, enzyme inhibitors, and amino acids. Dry ginger, ajowan, and asafoetida have high calcium (1.0–1.5%) and iron (54–62 mg/100 g) levels. The tannin content of spices is also high (0.9–1.3% of dry mass). Dietary fiber ranges from 14–53%. Spices have appreciable amounts of such essential amino acids as lysine and threonine.

Many of the spice-derived ingredients are potent antioxidants and are of great interest to biologists and clinicians because they may help protect the human body against damage by reactive oxygen species. Free radicals generated in vivo damage many targets including lipids, proteins, DNA, and small molecules. The various free radicals generated in vivo may include superoxide radicals, singlet oxygen, hydrogen peroxide, lipid peroxides, hypochlorous acid, alkoxyl radicals, peroxyl radicals, nitric oxide, nitrogen dioxide, peroxynitrite, nitrous oxide, and hydroxyl radicals. Based on their ability to prevent rancidity, various spices have been given an antioxidant index (7). There are studies to show the effect of spice components on scavenging of superoxide anion (8). The superoxide anions, as measured by nitroblue tetrazolium (NBT) reduction in a xanthine–xanthine oxidase system, were inhibited by superoxide dismutase (SOD), the spice principals eugenol (cloves) and cuminaldehyde (cumin), antioxidants, BHT, and BHA in a dose-dependent manner. The $K(i)$ values for the inhibition of NBT reduction by eugenol and cuminaldehyde were 64 and 120 μM, respectively. Zingerone (ginger) and linalool (coriander) inhibited NBT reduction to a maximum of 23 and 28%, respectively.

Similarly various spice-derived ingredients are potent inhibitors of lipid peroxidation (9). Polyunsaturated fatty acids (PUFA) are vulnerable to peroxidative attack. Protecting PUFA from peroxidation is essential to utilize their beneficial effects in health and in preventing disease. Several spice principles, for example, curcumin (5–50 μM) from turmeric, eugenol (25–150 μM) from cloves, and capsaicin (25–150 μM) from red chilies inhibited ascorbate/Fe^{2+}-induced lipid peroxidation in a dose-dependent manner. Zingerone from ginger inhibited lipid peroxidation at high concentrations (greater than 150 μM), whereas linalool (coriander), piperine (black pepper), and cuminaldehyde (cumin) had only marginal inhibitory effects, even at high concentrations (600 μM).

Several effects of spices are mediated through quenching of reactive oxygen intermediates, (ROI). The latter play a major role in activation of various pathways in the cell. The role of ROI has been implicated in inflammation, carcinogenesis, tumorigenesis, chronic heart diseases, allergy, arthritis, and autoimmune diseases. At the cellular level, ROI have been implicated in cell replication and the activation of various transcription factors, protein kinases, protein phosphatases, and various other metabolic enzymes. The role of activation of various redox-sensitive protein kinases (10,11), transcription factor (12,13), and apoptosis (14) in human health and diseases was recently reviewed. For instance, overexpression of antioxidant enzymes can block activation of the nuclear transcription factors NF-κB and AP-1, the stress-activated protein kinases, and apoptosis (15,16), suggesting the critical role of ROI. Furthermore, the activation of certain transcription factors regulate carcinogenesis, inflammation, and other diseases (17,18). Thus, antioxidant ingredients derived from the spices, by blocking transcription factors and kinases, have potential in blocking various diseases, including cancer and cardiovascular diseases, two major causes of death in the United States. Various activities that have been assigned to the antioxidant ingredients derived from spices are the listed in Table 2 (19–215). Descriptions of some of the biological effects of spice ingredients, reported in vitro and in vivo model systems follow.

II. TURMERIC

Turmeric (*Curcuma longa*) is a major component of the commonly called yellow curry powder. Turmeric contains curcumin (also called diferuloyl methane), a peptide called turmerin,

Table 2 Biological Effects of Various Spices

Biological effects	Ref.
1. Turmeric	
Scavenges oxygen radical	19–24
Scavenges hydroxyl radical generation through Fenton reaction	25
Inhibits singlet oxygen-induced DNA damage	26
Inhibits nitrite-induced methemoglobin formation	27
Inhibits NO_2-induced oxidation of hemoglobin	28
Inhibits lipid peroxidation	29
Inhibits lipid peroxide–induced DNA damage	30
Induces glutathione S-transferase in mice	31
Water-soluble peptide with antioxidant activity	32
Inhibits TNF-, PMA-, and LPS-induced NFk-κB activation	33
Inhibits LPS-induced NF-κB activation in macrophages	34
Inhibits PMA-induced c-*Jun*/AP-1 in mouse fibroblasts	35
Inhibits PMA-induced c-*Jun*, c-*fos*, and c-*myc* proto-oncogene mRNA	36
Inhibits TNF-induced IκBa kinase	37
Inhibits TNF-expression of adhesion molecules on endo cells	38
Inhibits LPS-induced TNF and IL-1 production from macrophages	39
Inhibits LPS and IFN-γ-induced nitric oxide synthase mRNA	40
Down-regulates chemokine expression in stromal cells	41
Inhibits TNF-induced JE gene expression	42
Inhibits PMA-induced 5-LPO, 12-LPO, and COX activity	43,44
Inhibits HIV-1-LTR-directed gene expression and viral replication	45
Inhibits HIV-1 integrase	46
Inhibits colonic epithelial cell proliferation	47
Inhibits PMA-induced ornithine decarboxylase	48
Inhibits proliferation of Dalton lymphoma	49
Inhibits proliferation of endothelial cells	50
Inhibits proliferation of smooth-muscle cells	51
Induces apoptosis in human leukemic cells	52
Induces apoptosis in NIH 3T3, S180, HT-29 cells	53
Induces apoptosis in breast cancer cell lines	54
Inhibits EGF-induced activation of EGF receptor tyrosine kinase	55–57
Inhibits PMA-induced PKC	58
Inhibits cAMP-dependent protein kinase	59
Inhibits initiation and promotion of carcinogen-induced carcinogenesis	60–64
Chemoprevention of colon carcinogenesis	65–67
Prevention of oral carcinogenesis	68
Inhibits PMA-induced tumor promotion	69
Inhibits forestomach, duodenal, and colon carcinogenesis	70
Inhibits SOS gene and mutagenesis induced by UV irradiation	71
Protects against fuel smoke condensate-induced DNA damage in lymphocytes	72
Protects against 4-hydroxy-2-*trans*-nonenal-induced cataract	73
Inhibits neutrophil function via Ca^{2+}-dependent mechanism	74
Suppression of fungal infection by turmeric oil	75
Inhibits leukotriene-B_4 formation in PMN	76
Stabilizes lysosomal membranes and uncouples oxidative phosphorylation	77
Inhibits ADP-, epinephrine, and collagen-induced platelet aggregation in monkeys	78

(continued)

SPICES AS ANTIOXIDANTS AND THERAPEUTICS

Table 2 (*Continued*)

Biological effects	Ref.
Exhibits antirheumatic property	79
Exhibits anti-inflammatory property	80–84
Exhibits cholesterol-lowering effects in rats	85–86
Inhibits isoproteranol-induced myocardial infarction in rats	87
Exhibits antithrombotic effects	88
Inhibits glutathione S-transferase activity in rat liver	89
Induces cholersis (i.e., increases the secretion of bile)	90
Increases brain Na/K ATPase	91
Inhibits the kidney microsomal membrane Na/K ATPase	92
2. Red pepper (capsaicin)	
Inhibits superoxide production	93
Inhibits NADH oxidase and growth of transformed cells	94
Inhibits TNF-induced NF-κB activation	95
Regulates expression of substance P in macrophages	96
Used to alleviate symptoms such as pain and itching	97
Acts on pain-linked neurons through vanilloid receptors	98,99
Vanilloid receptors expressed on primary sensory neuron	100
Stimulates the secretion of substance P. tachykinin, calcitonin gene-related protein, and platelet-activating factor	101
Prolonged exposure to capsaicin decreases neurohormone secretion	102
Desensitization/death of the afferent neurons that secrete immunogenic neurohormones leads to suppression of inflammation	103–105
Used for treatment of cluster headache	106
Used for treatment of herpes zoster	107
Used for treatment of vasomotor rhinitis	108
Induces mitochondrial swelling	109,110
Induces adenylate cyclase in different brain regions	111
Causes selective degeneration of afferents in several mammalian species	112
3. Allium (onions, garlic, shallot, chives, Chinese chives, and leeks): organosulfur compounds	
Contain: diallyl sulfide (DAS), glutathione, quercetin, and kaempferol	
DAS increases GST, GSH peroxidase, GSH reductase, in mice	113
Garlic powder potentiates the immune system	114
Allyl compounds selectively kill HIV-1-infected cells	115
Garlic and onion oil are anticarcinogenic	116
Allyl group containing organosulfur are anticarcinogenic	117–119
Implicated in prevention of cancer in humans	120
DAS inhibits neoplasia of forestomach and lung in mice	
DAS inhibits dimethylhydrazine-induced colon cancer	121
Garlic powder is effective in inhibiting DMBA-induced mammary tumors	122
4. Honeybee hive product (propolis)	
Contains CAPE; quercetin, cinnamic acid derivatives, clerodane diterpenoid	
CAPE is a potent antioxidant	123
CAPE inhibits 5-LPO and XO	124
CAPE inhibits TNF-, PMA-, LPS-induced NF-κB activation	125
CAPE induces apoptosis	126
CAPE inhibits proliferation and transformation	127–130

(*continued*)

Table 2 (*Continued*)

Biological effects	Ref.
CAPE inhibits proliferation of human keratinocytes and EGF-induced ODC	131
CAPE inhibits HIV integrase	132–134
CAPE inhibits PMA-induced tumor promotion in mouse skin	135,136
CAPE inhibits colon carcinogenesis	137–139
5. Aloe family (*Aloe barbadensis, Polygonum cuspidatum*): emodin	
Inhibits TNF-induced NF-κB and expression of adhesion molecules	140
Inhibits p56^{lck}	141
Inhibits PI$_3$ kinase	142
Inhibits *Ras*-transformed epithelial cells	143
Inhibits proliferation of leukemic cells	144
Sensitizes HER2 overexpressing NSCLC to chemotherapeutic agents	145
Suppresses transformation and induced differentiation of HER2 overexpressing breast cancer cells	146,147
Antioxidant and radical-scavenging effects of anthraquinones and anthrones	148
6. Cloves: eugenol	
Inhibits hydroxyl radical formation	149
Inhibits lipid peroxidation	150
Inhibits TNF-induced NF-κB activation	151
Modulate GSH metabolism	152
Inhibits arachidonic acid-induced thromboxane B$_2$	153,154
Garam masala (black pepper, cardamom), bay leaves, dry ginger, clove, mace, and nutmeg	
Inhibits DMBA-induced transplacental and translactational carcinogenesis	155
7. Ginger	
Inhibits superoxide radical production	156
Inhibits lipid peroxidation	157
Inhibits thromboxane synthetase and stimulates prostacyclin	158
Inhibits platelet aggregation	159
Inhibits prostaglandin release	160,161
Inhibits pregnancy-induced nausea and vomiting	162
Inhibits chemotherapy-induced nausea and vomiting	163
Inhibits arthritis-induced inflammation and pain	164–166
Inhibits cholesterol biosynthesis	167,168
Exhibits antiulcer effects	169
Exhibits thermogenic effects	170
Exhibits abortive and prophylactic effects on migraine headache	171
Exhibits gastroprotective activity	172
Exhibits antimycotic activity	173
Exhibits antifilarial effects	174
8. Black cumin (*Nigella sativa*)	
Selectively toxic to cancer cells in culture	175
Caffeine (3,7-dihydro-1,3,7-trimethyl-1*H*-purine-6,6-dione)	
Prevents apoptosis and cell cycle effects induced by camptothecin	176
9. Anise (*Pimpinella anisum*): anethole (a chief constituent of anise, camphor, and fennel)	
Inhibits superoxide radical production	177,178
Act as hydroxyl radical scavengers	179

(*continued*)

Table 2 (*Continued*)

Biological effects	Ref.
Inhibit lipid peroxidation	180,181
Increase the intracellular levels of GSH and GST	182–184
Exhibits chemopreventive activity	185–190
10. Saffron (*Crocus sativus*)	
Extracts inhibit growth of tumor cells in vitro and in vivo	191,192
Anticarcinogenic	193
11. Crocetin (*Gardenia fructus*)	
Inhibits tumor promotion in benzo[*a*]pyrene-initiated CD1 mouse skin	194
12. Ellagic acid (grapes, strawberries, raspberries, and certain nuts)	
Antimutagenic	195
Anticarcinogenic	196
Inhibits lipid peroxidation	197
13. Resveratrol	
An agonist for the estrogen receptor	198
Inhibits low-density lipoprotein (LDL) oxidation	199,200
Suppresses pulmonary artery endothelial cell proliferation	201
Blocks human platelet aggregation	202,203
Cell cycle effects and control of gene expression in human breast carcinoma and human prostate cancer cell lines	204,205
Inhibits cyclooxygenase-2 transcription	206
Cancer chemopreventive	207
Inhibits transcription of CYP1A1	208
Decreases the incidence of coronary heart disease	209
14. Parsley leaf oil (myristicin)	
Inhibits benzo[*a*]pyrene-induced tumorigenesis	210
15. Hypericum family: hypericin	
Inhibits PMA-induced superoxide generation	211,212
Anti-HIV activity	213,214
Inhibits PKC	215

and turmeric oil. Curcumin, which gives specific flavor and yellow color to curry, has been studied extensively. The anti-inflammatory and antioxidant properties of curcumin have been well documented (25,82). Most of these activities are mediated through suppression of NF-κB activation, a ubiquitous transcription factor involved intimately in host defense against disease. The inappropriate regulation of NF-κB and its dependent genes has been associated with various pathological conditions, including toxic or septic shock, graft-vs.-host reaction, acute inflammatory conditions, acute-phase response, viral replication, radiation damage, atherosclerosis, and cancer (216,217). With activation of NF-κB, expression of a large number of genes is induced, including various inflammatory cytokines and adhesion molecules, all of which are suppressed by curcumin. Another transcription factor, AP-1, involved in carcinogenesis and cell proliferation, is down-modulated by curcumin (35).

In vitro, curcumin has also been a potent antiproliferative agent against a variety of tumor cell types, including human breast tumor cells (54). Compounds that are pharmacologically safe and can inhibit the proliferation of tumor cells have potential as anticancer agents. Curcumin exhibits anticarcinogenic properties in vivo. The growth inhibitory effects of curcumin are mediated through ornithine deoxycarboxylase (ODC) activity, a rate-determining enzyme needed for cell proliferation. Curcumin also inhibits type 1 human immunodeficiency virus long terminal repeat (HIV-LTR)-directed gene expression and virus replication.

Treatment of endothelial cells with curcumin completely blocks the cell surface expression of ICAM-1, VCAM-1, and ELAM-1 (38), adhesion molecules that mediate tumor metastasis and inflammation. Their importance lies in the role they play in recruitment of leukocytes by endothelial cells and their subsequent migration from the vasculature into the tissue and thus in mediating inflammation. This effect of curcumin on adhesion molecules is mediated through the suppression of the transcription factor NF-κB activation (33,34), which may contribute to the anti-inflammatory properties of curcumin. The anti-inflammatory effects of curcumin are also mediated through its ability to inhibit cyclooxygenase and lipoxygenase (43,44). The compound displays anticarcinogenic properties in animals, as indicated by its ability to inhibit both tumor initiation induced by benzo[a]pyrene and 7,12-dimethylbenz[a]anthracene and tumor promotion induced by phorbol esters (60–64).

Many in vivo studies have shown that curcumin could be useful against many pathological conditions. A dietary administration of turmeric (0.05%) as well as curcumin (0.005%) to rats significantly reduced the number of γ-glutamyl transpeptidase-positive foci induced by aflatoxin B_1, a precursor of hepatocellular neoplasia (218).

Sony and Kuttan (219) studied the effect of curcumin (500 mg/day of curcumin for 7 days) on serum levels of cholesterol and lipid peroxides in healthy human volunteers. Curcumin administration significantly decreased the level of serum lipid peroxides (33%), increased high-density lipoprotein (HDL) cholesterol (29%), and decreased total serum cholesterol (11.63%). In another study, Soudamini et al. (220) assessed the effect of oral administration of curcumin on carbon tetrachloride-, paraquat-, and cyclophosphamide-mediated lipid peroxidation in liver, lung, kidney, and brain of experimental mice. Oral administration of curcumin reduced the peroxidation of lipids in these tissues. The administration of curcumin also lowered the serum and tissue cholesterol levels in these animals, suggesting that curcumin could be used to treat, for example, liver damage and arterial diseases.

Nagabhushan and Bhide (221) studied the effect of curcumins (curcumin I and curcumin III) on different stages of development of cancer. Curcumin I inhibited benzopyrene-induced forestomach tumors in female Swiss mice, whereas curcumin III inhibited dimethylbenzanthracene (DMBA)-induced skin tumors in Swiss bald mice. Curcumin I also inhibited DMBA-initiated, phorbol ester-promoted skin tumors in female Swiss mice (64). This study suggested that curcumin inhibits cancer at the initiation, promotion, and progression stages of development.

In a study by Huang et al. (69), the effects of topically applied curcumin on 12-O-tetradecanoylphorbol-13-acetate (TPA)-induced epidermal ornithine decarboxylase activity, epidermal DNA synthesis, and the promotion of skin tumors were evaluated in female CD-1 mice. Topical application significantly inhibited the induction of epidermal ornithine decarboxylase activity, and stimulated the incorporation of [^{3}H]thymidine into epidermal DNA and 7,12-dimethylbenz[a]anthracene-initiated TPA-promoted skin tumors. In another study (64) the effects of topically applied curcumin on the formation of benzo[a]pyrene (B[a]P)–DNA adducts and the tumorigenic activities of B[a]P and 7,12-dimethylbenz[a]anthracene (DMBA) in epidermis were evaluated in female CD-1 mice. Topical application of curcumin before [^{3}H]B[a]P treatment inhibited the formation of [^{3}H]B[a]P–DNA adducts in epidermis. In a two-stage skin tumorigenesis model (B[a]P-TPA model) a topical application of curcumin 5 min before each application of B[a]P reduced the number of tumors per mouse and the percentage of tumor-bearing mice. Similar results were obtained when curcumin was used with the DMBA–TPA tumor protocol. Lu et al. demonstrated that a topical application of curcumin inhibited TPA-induced epidermal hyperplasia and c-Jun and c-Fos expression in CD-1 mouse skin (223).

Huang et al. also studied the effects of curcumin feeding on carcinogen-induced tumorigenesis in the forestomach, duodenum, and colon of mice (70). The feeding of curcumin in the diet inhibited benzo[a]pyrene-induced forestomach tumorigenesis in A/J mice, N-ethyl-N'-nitro-N-nitrosoguanidine-induced duodenal tumorigenesis in C57BL/6 mice, and azoxymethane (AOM)-induced colon tumorigenesis in CF-1 mice (70).

Kakar et al. investigated the effect of curcumin on the expression of c-*fos*, c-*jun*, and c-*myc* oncogenes in TPA-treated mouse skin in CD-1 mice (224). This study implied that TPA (30 nmol) treatment to the mouse skin increased the mRNA levels of c-*fos*, c-*jun*, and c-*myc* oncogenes and a topical application to the skin 30 min before the TPA treatment inhibited the TPA-induced expression of these proto-oncogenes. These data suggested that curcumin may inhibit skin cancer by modulating expression of these proto-oncogenes.

Turmeric and ethanolic turmeric extract containing curcumin protect against the initiation as well as postinitiation phases of DMBA-induced mammary tumorigenesis in female Sprague–Dawley rats (225). A study by Menon et al. (226) assessed the effects of curcumin on lung metastasis induced by B16F-10 melanoma cells in female C57BL/6 mice. The findings suggested that curcumin inhibited the invasion of B16F-10 melanoma cells by inhibiting metalloprotease activity, thereby inhibiting lung metastasis.

In animal models, curcumin has been reported to impart an ameliorating influence on diabetic nephropathy (227), wound repair in diabetic-impaired healing (228), and advanced glycation end products (AGE)-induced complications of diabetes mellitus (229). Studies have also suggested curcumin is effective for attenuation of acute doxorubicin (Adriamycin) myocardial toxicity (230) and modulation of collagen metabolism in isoproterenol-induced myocardial necrosis in rats (231).

III. RED PEPPER

Capsaicin, a homovanillic acid derivative (8-methyl-N-vanillyl-6-nonenamide; MW 305.42), is an active component of the red pepper of the genus *Capsaicin*. It inhibits superoxide anion generation (93) and alters the redox state of the cell (94), blocks NF-κB activation (95), induces mitochondrial swelling (109), inhibits NADH oxidase, induces apoptosis of transformed cells (94), stimulates adenylate cyclase (111), and activates protein kinase C (PKC) (232). In vitro capsaicin modulates cellular growth, collagenase synthesis, and prostaglandin secretion from rheumatoid arthritis synoviocytes (233). Capsaicin has also been shown to be immunomodulatory as indicated by its ability to modulate lymphocyte proliferation, antibody production, and neutrophil chemotaxis (234–236). These effects play an important role in capsaicin's use for treatment of arthritis (237). Capsicum has been used in humans for topical treatment of cluster headache, herpes zoster, and vasomotor rhinitis (238,106–108). Various effects of capsaicin are mediated through a specific cellular receptor, referred to as vanilloid receptor (239) that is shared by resiniferatoxin (RTX). Similar to capsaicin, RTX is an alkaloid derived from plants of the genus *Euphorbia*, in particular *E. resinifera* (240,241). It is present in the latex of *E. resinifera* and interacts with the vanilloid receptor expressed by primary sensory neurons mediating pain perception as well as neurogenic inflammation. A structural homologue of capsaicin, RTX is also structurally similar to phorbol esters (PMA). It interacts with distinct binding sites and activates PKC (235,242). Unlike RTX, capsaicin has no homology to PMA, but similar to RTX, it too activates PKC (235,243), suggesting that the latter activation is not due to the phorbol ester-like moiety on RTX. RTX mimics many of the actions of capsaicin.

Capsaicin and the compounds related to it, collectively referred to as vanilloids, are increasingly appreciated as a promising therapeutic approach to mitigate neuropathic pain and pathological conditions such as vasomotor rhinitis, in which neuropeptides released from primary sensory neurons play a major role. Many capsaicin-containing preparations are already commercially available. However, the use of capsaicin is severely limited by its irritant nature; therefore, the synthesis of novel vanilloids with an improved efficacy are being pursued in many laboratories around the world. The therapeutic potential of *E. resinifera*, from which RTX is derived, can be traced back to the reign of the Roman Emperor Augustus. Desensitization to RTX is believed to be a promising approach to mitigate neuropathic pain and other pathological conditions in which sensory neuropeptides released from capsaicin-sensitive neurons play a critical role. Clinical trials to investigate the potential of RTX to relieve pain associated with diabetic polyneuropathy and postherpetic neuralgia are in progress.

Topical capsaicin is safe and effective pain management adjunct for rheumatoid arthritis, osteoarthritis, neuralgias, and diabetic neuropathy (244). To determine the effectiveness of capsaicin for painful cutaneous disorders and neural dysfunction, Hautkappe et al. analyzed data from 33 reports from a MEDLINE search of the medical literature for the period 1966–1996 on the efficacy of capsaicin (244). They found that pain relief for postmastectomy syndrome and cluster headache was greater with capsaicin than with placebo; also, psoriasis and pruritus responded better to capsaicin. An evaluation of uncontrolled studies and case reports indicated that pain or dysfunction was less at the end of capsaicin therapy for neck pain, loin pain/hematuria syndrome, rhinopathy, oral mucositis, reflex sympathetic dystrophy syndrome, detrusor hyperreflexia, and cutaneous pain caused by a tumor of the skin. This study (244) concluded that capsaicin is effective for psoriasis, pruritus, and cluster headache; it is often helpful for the itching and pain of postmastectomy pain syndrome, oral mucositis, cutaneous allergy, loin pain/hematuria syndrome, neck pain, amputation stump pain, and skin tumor; and it may be beneficial for neural dysfunction (detrusor hyperreflexia, reflex sympathetic dystrophy, and rhinopathy).

Because alterations in the cutaneous vascular system are prominent in psoriasis and may play an important role in the pathogenesis of this disorder, Bernstein et al. (1986) evaluated the effects of topically applied capsaicin, a known inhibitor of cutaneous vasodilation, on moderate and severe psoriasis (245). Under a double-blind study, 44 patients with symmetrically distributed psoriatic lesions applied topical capsaicin to one side of their body and identical-appearing vehicle to the other side for 6 weeks. This treatment significantly improved the appearance of lesions on sides treated with capsaicin compared with sides treated with vehicle. About 50% of patients reported burning, stinging, itching, and redness of the skin on initial applications of study medication, but these diminished or vanished after continued application. These results suggested that topical application of capsaicin may be a useful new treatment for psoriasis.

Pruritus (itching of the skin without visible eruption) is a significant problem for many patients undergoing long-term hemodialysis. In an open-label, uncontrolled trial and a double-blind vehicle-controlled trial, the efficacy and safety of capsaicin (0.025% cream) was evaluated for the treatment of pruritus in patients undergoing long-term hemodialysis. In this study, capsaicin was very effective against itching. Similarly, many other human studies have shown that capsaicin is effective against pruritus (246–251). Nodular prurigo is a chronic skin disease causing severe itch of unknown origin in restricted skin areas surrounded by healthy skin areas. Studies by Gronroos et al. (1997) demonstrated that capsaicin treatment is effective against this disease (252).

In many studies and trials conducted around the world, capsaicin has been effective for the treatment of cluster headache (253–257). In another study by Watson et al., a topical application of capsaicin (0.025%) was used to treat 33 patients with postherpetic neuralgia. This treatment was useful, particularly in the elderly, who often poorly tolerated oral medications (107). Capsaicin has also been proved useful in patients with vasomotor rhinitis. In a study by Marabini et al. (258) capsaicin markedly reduced the mean symptom score involving nasal obstruction and nasal secretion in patients with vasomotor rhinitis.

Many studies have evaluated mutagenic and carcinogenic activities of capsaicin and chili extracts. For example, De et al. (259) demonstrated that capsaicin significantly inhibits cyclophosphamide-induced chromosomal aberrations and DNA strand breakage. This protective action of capsaicin against cyclophosphamide-induced toxicity may possibly be linked with its "desensitization" effect against chemical irritant-induced damages. Capsaicin appears to interact with xenobiotic-metabolizing enzymes, particularly microsomal cytochrome P450-dependent monooxygenases, involved in activation as well as detoxification of various chemical carcinogens and mutagens. Results from recent studies indicate that capsaicin possesses the chemoprotective activity against some chemical carcinogens and mutagens (260). Surh et al. (261) determined the effect of capsaicin on vinyl carbamate (VC)- and N-nitrosodimethylamine (NDMA)-induced mutagenesis in *Salmonella typhimurium* TA100. Capsaicin treatment significantly attenuated the bacterial mutagenicity of VC and NDMA. This suppression by capsaicin (and diallyl sulfide) correlated with their inhibition of P-450 IIE1-mediated p-nitrophenol hydroxylation and NDMA N-demethylation. In this study, the topical application of capsaicin on the skin of female ICR mice inhibited of VC-induced skin tumors by 62%. In another study, Park and Surh (262) assessed the tumor-initiating and promotional effects of capsaicin in a two-stage mouse skin carcinogenesis model. A single topical application of capsaicin (10 mM) followed by twice-weekly applications of 12-O-tetradecanoylphorbol-13-acetate on the dorsal skin of female ICR mice did not cause any increases in incidence and multiplicity of skin tumors. However, the repeated topical applications of capsaicin inhibited the formation of skin papilloma, when given before each topical application of phorbol ester.

Some studies have also shown carcinogenic effects for capsaicin. In one study rats were fed red chili powder or a colonic carcinogen 1,2-dimethylhydrazine or both, and the histopathological changes occurring in the colonic mucosa were studied (263). All three groups showed polyps and dysplasia, malignant tumors, and malignant tumors with transitional areas of dysplasia. In a population-based case–control study conducted in Mexico City during 1989–1990, the relation between chili pepper consumption and gastric cancer risk was evaluated (264). This study demonstrated that chili pepper consumers were at high risk for gastric cancer compared with nonconsumers. This study suggested that chili pepper consumption might be a strong risk factor for gastric cancer.

In a study by Toth and Gannett, the carcinogenicity of lifelong administration of hot pepper capsaicin in mice was evaluated (265). Capsaicin was administered in a semisynthetic powdered diet at 0.03125% level for the whole lifespan of Swiss mice, starting from 6 weeks of age. This treatment resulted in the development of tumors of the cecum in 22% of females and 14% of males, whereas the corresponding tumor incidences in untreated female and male controls were both 8%. The tumors were histopathologically classified as benign polypoid adenomas. In another study, Agarwal et al. (266) found that chili extract acts as a promoter of chemically induced stomach and liver carcinogenesis in BALB/c mice. The promoter effect of chili extract was also seen in the BHC-induced hepatocarcinogenesis system.

In another study, Jang et al. (267) evaluated the modifying potential of capsaicin on lesion development in a rat multiorgan carcinogenesis model. The rats were treated sequentially with diethylnitrosamine (DEN) (100 mg/kg, i.p., single dose at commencement), N-methylnitrosourea (MNU) (20 mg/kg, i.p., on days 2, 5, 8, and 11), and N,N-dibutylnitrosamine (DBN) (0.05% in drinking water). After this initiating procedure, the animals were administered a diet containing 0.01% capsaicin. All surviving animals were killed 20 weeks after the beginning of the experiment and the target organs examined histopathologically. In this study, capsaicin treatment significantly inhibited the induction of hepatic foci in rats treated with carcinogens. Capsaicin treatment decreased lung adenoma incidence, but increased the incidence of papillary or nodular hyperplasia of the urinary bladder. The tumor incidence in other organs, such as the kidney and thyroid, was not significantly different from the corresponding controls. These results suggested that concurrent treatment with capsaicin can inhibit or enhance carcinogenesis, depending on the organ.

IV. GARLIC

Diallyl sulfide is a flavor component of garlic and onion that has been used as a food additive for generations. Many studies have implicated diallyl sulfide as a chemopreventive agent against a variety of cancer types. Wargovich (121) demonstrated that diallyl sulfide inhibited dimethylhydrazine-induced colon cancer in C57BL/6J mice (117,121). In a study by Sadhana et al. garlic oil topically applied during the initiation phase of B(a)P-induced skin carcinogenesis in female Swiss albino mice depressed the number of tumor-bearing mice and the mean number of tumors per mouse (268). In another study by Perchellet et al., garlic oil and onion oil inhibited tumor-promotion stages in SENCAR mice (270). This study also demonstrated the inhibition of DMBA-induced mouse skin tumorigenesis by garlic oil (269). Athar et al. showed that topical application of diallyl sulfide inhibited benzoyl peroxide-mediated tumor promotion in DMBA-initiated skin of SENCAR mice (271). Dwivedi et al. demonstrated that topical application of diallyl sulfide significantly inhibited DMBA-induced and TPA-promoted skin tumor formation in SENCAR mice (272). Singh and Shukla demonstrated that diallyl sulfide inhibits B(a)P- and DMBA-induced carcinogenesis (273) and DMBA–TPA two-stage skin carcinogenesis in mice (274). Diallyl sulfide completely inhibited N-nitrosomethylbenzylamine-mediated esophageal tumor formation in rats and substantially reduced hepatic microsomal metabolism of the carcinogen (275). Oral or parenteral pretreatment with diallyl sulfide significantly reduced N-methyl-N'-nitro-N-nitrosoguanidine (MN-NG)-induced nuclear aberrations and ODC activity in glandular stomach mucosa of the Wistar rat (276), diallyl sulfide prevented aristolochic acid-induced formation of squamous cell carcinomas in the forestomach of BD-6 rats (277). Liu et al. showed DMBA-induced mammary tumors and DNA adducts were inhibited by garlic powder in rats. Hong et al. demonstrated that diallyl sulfide prevents tobacco-specific carcinogen 4-(methylnitrosamino)-1-(3-pyridyl)-1-butanone (NNK)-induced lung tumorigenesis in A/J mice, probably by inhibiting the metabolic activation of NNK (278). Takahashi et al. evaluated the modifying effects of diallyl sulfide and diallyl disulfide in a liver and multiorgan carcinogenesis rat model (279). In this study, diallyl disulfide inhibited colon and renal carcinogenesis, whereas diallyl sulfide promoted hepatocarcinogenesis (279).

Kim et al. demonstrated an enhanced effectiveness of dimethyl-4,4'-dimethoxy-5,6,5',6'-dimethylene dioxybiphenyl-2,2'-dicarboxylate in combination with garlic oil against experimental hepatic injury in rats and mice (280). Wang et al. showed that fresh garlic homogenate containing diallyl sulfide protects against acetaminophen-induced hepatotoxicity in Swiss–Webster mice (281), possibly mainly owing to its inhibition of P450-mediated acetaminophen bioactivation. In another study, Lin et al. demonstrated that diallyl sulfone, a metabolite of diallyl sulfide, protects against acetaminophen-induced hepatoxicity by blocking acetaminophen bioactivation mainly by the inactivation and inhibition of cytochrome P450 2E1 (282).

Several studies have shown the potential of garlic compounds to prevent cardiovascular disease. Bordia et al. found that garlic oil administration to healthy subjects and patients with coronary artery disease inhibited platelet aggregation ex vivo (283).

V. PROPOLIS

Caffeic acid (3,4-dihydroxy cinnamic acid) phenethyl ester (CAPE), a structural relative of flavonoids, is an active component of propolis from honeybee hives. It is an antioxidant that alters the redox status of the cell and inhibits lipid peroxidation (126,284,285). It has antiviral, anti-inflammatory, and immunomodulatory properties (127) and inhibits the growth of different types of transformed cells (127–130,133,286). It inhibits ODC, protein tyrosine kinase, and lipoxygenase activities (124,131,137,138). CAPE can also inhibit phorbol ester-induced production and tumor promotion (123,135). Although the molecular basis for the multiple activities assigned to CAPE have not been defined, most of the activities inhibited by CAPE may be mediated through the suppression of NF-κB activation.

Caffeic acid was shown to ameliorate glomerular disease. In a study (287), the efficacy of a herbal prescription containing caffeic acid on renal diseases was examined using an experimental model system of glomerular lesions in mice induced by *Agkistrodon acutus* venom (Acl-P). The effect was suggested to be caused by caffeic acid inhibiting the proteolytic enzyme activity of Acl-P.

Studies have shown anticarcinogenic potential of caffeic acid for certain neoplasms. In a study by Tanaka et al. (288), caffeic acid significantly reduced the incidences of tongue neoplasms (squamous cell papilloma and carcinoma) and preneoplastic lesions (hyperplasia and dysplasia) induced by 4-NQO in male F344 rats. In a study by Rao et al. (138), the inhibitory effect of caffeic acid esters—methyl caffeate (MC) and phenylethyl caffeate (PEC)—on AOM-induced biochemical changes and aberrant crypt foci formation in rat colon was investigated in male F344 rats. The caffeic acid derivatives inhibited AOM-induced colonic preneoplastic lesions, ODC, protein tyrosine kinase, and lipoxygenase activities, which are relevant to colon carcinogenesis. Another study demonstrated a potent inhibitory effect of caffeic acid on TPA-induced tumor promotion and the formation of 5-hydroxymethyl-2′-deoxyuridine in DNA of mouse skin (136). Michaluart et al. investigated the mechanisms by which caffeic acid inhibits the stimulation of prostaglandin (PG) synthesis in an animal model of acute inflammation (289). In the rat carrageenan air pouch model of inflammation, caffeic acid caused dose-dependent suppression of PG synthesis. Caffeic acid also markedly suppressed cyclooxygenase-2 in this model. These data could be relevant for understanding the anticancer and anti-inflammatory properties of caffeic acid.

Many studies have also shown that caffeic acid possesses cancer-enhancing potential in the forestomach. One study has shown that caffeic acid induced pronounced hyperplasia throughout the forestomach epithelium in F344 male rats (290). In other studies, the development of chemically induced forestomach tumors was enhanced by caffeic acid in animal models (291–293). Another study showed that caffeic acid exerted carcinogenic activity for the forestomach squamous cell epithelium in both sexes of F344 rats and C57BL/6N × C3H/HeN F$_1$ mice, for the renal tubular cell in male rats and female mice, and for the alveolar type II cell in male mice (294). These responses of caffeic acid were associated with stimulation of cell division (295). In a study by Hepsen et al. (296), the effectiveness of caffeic acid was evaluated for the prevention of posterior capsule opacification (PCO) in rabbits by suppressing the transformation of the lens epithelial cells. The results from this study suggested that caffeic acid is effective in suppressing PCO in pigmented rabbits and may be beneficial in clinical use in humans. A recent study demonstrated that prophylactic administration of caffeic acid in ischemic condition prevents reperfusion injuries in rat intestine by eliminating oxygen radicals and inhibiting polymorphonuclear leukocyte infiltration (397). Another study suggested that caffeic acid may be effective in protecting the spinal cord from ischemia–reperfusion injury (298).

VI. ALOE

Emodin (3-methyl-1,6,8-trihydroxyanthraquinone) is an active component from the roots of *Polygonum cuspidatum* that has been reported to exhibit anti-inflammatory properties. Emodin displays several biological activities, such as antiviral, antimicrobial, immunosuppressive, hepatoprotective, anti-inflammatory, and antiulcerogenic ones (299,300). It also inhibits the activity of PKC and of c-*src*, p56^{lck}, and HER-2 protein tyrosine kinases (141,142,145). Emodin has also been reported to induce the differentiation of HER-2/neu-overexpressing breast cancer cells (147) and inhibit the growth of v-*ras*-transformed human bronchial epithelial cells (143). Treatment of human umbilical vein endothelial cells (EC) with emodin inhibited NF-κB activation, which led to suppression of expression of the adhesion molecules ICAM-1, VCAM-1, and ELAM-1. This may explain the anti-inflammatory effects of emodin.

Goel et al. have shown that emodin imparts anti-inflammatory activity against carrageenin-induced pedal inflammation in rats (301). It demonstrated antiulcer activity against 4-h pylorus-ligated, aspirin, and immobilization stress-induced gastric ulcers in rats. In this study, emodin decreased acid and pepsin output and augmented mucous secretion/protein ratio in the gastric juice of aspirin-treated pylorus-ligated rats, suggesting that the antiulcerogenic effect of emodin may be due to its effect on gastric secretion (301). In still another study emodin exhibited anti-inflammatory effect on carrageenan-induced edema in rats (302). In another recent study, emodin imparted an inhibitory effect on arylamine *N*-acetyltransferase activity in strains of *Helicobacter pylori* from peptic ulcer patients (303).

Emodin also exhibited hepatoprotective effects on CCl_4- and D-galactosamine-induced liver damage in rats (304). In this study, the histopathological examination showed that emodin reduced lymphocyte cells, Kupffer cells, ballooning degeneration, cell necrosis, and hyaline degeneration on CCl_4- and D-galactosamine-induced tests. In another study, emodin inhibited effect the pathogenicity of *Trichomonas vaginalis* in mice (305). Emodin treatment delayed the development of subcutaneous abscesses caused by this parasite and cured the intravaginal infestation of trichomonas (305).

VII. GINGER

The effects of ginger are well known. Ginger sticks or gingerol consumed during travel provide relief from motion sickness (306,307). The efficacy of ginger rhizome for the prevention of nausea, dizziness, and vomiting as symptoms of motion sickness, and for postoperative vomiting and vomiting of pregnancy, has been well documented and proved beyond doubt in numerous high-quality clinical studies (306). In a study by Kobayashi et al., gingerol, isolated from the rhizome of ginger was found to be a cardiotonic agent (308).

The use of this ancient medicine for gastrointestinal problems has also been given scientific approval. The antiulcer effects of ginger constituents have been appreciated (163). In a study by Micklefield et al., the effect of a ginger rhizome extract on fasting and postprandial gastroduodenal motility with stationary manometry in 12 healthy volunteers demonstrated that oral ginger improves gastroduodenal motility in the fasting state and after a standard test meal (309) Al-Yahya et al. demonstrated that oral ginger extract exerted highly significant cytoprotection against chemically induced gastric lesions (172). The extract also prevented the occurrence of gastric ulcers induced by nonsteroidal anti-inflammatory drugs (NSAIDs) and hypothermic restraint stress. These observations suggest that ginger has cytoprotective and antiulcerogenic effects (172).

This antiemetic effects of ginger are also well appreciated. In 60 women who had major gynecological surgery in a double-blind, randomized study (313), significantly fewer incidents of nausea occurred in subjects receiving ginger root or metoclopramide compared with placebo ($p < 0.05$). It also worked well as a prophylactic antiemetic for day case surgery (314). Ginger taken before 8-methoxypsoralen (8-MOP), which is given to patients undergoing photopheresis, may substantially reduce nausea caused by this drug (315). Study by Aikins showed ginger as alternative therapies for nausea and vomiting of pregnancy (316). Ginger also protected against rheumatic and musculoskeletal disorders (310,311). Eugenol and ginger oil were effective in arthritic rats (166).

The antitumor effects of ginger have been widely studied. The ethanol extract of ginger (GE) applied to the skin of SENCAR mice significantly inhibited TPA-caused induction of epidermal ODC, cyclooxygenase, and lipoxygenase activities, and ODC mRNA expression. GE also inhibited TPA-caused epidermal edema and hyperplasia (317). In long-term tumor studies, topical application of GE 30 min before each TPA application to DMBA-initiated SENCAR mice resulted in a highly significant protection against skin tumor incidence and multiplicity. This study suggested that GE possesses antiskin tumor-promoting effects, and that the mechanism of such effects may involve inhibition of tumor promoter-caused cellular, biochemical, and molecular changes in mouse skin.

In another study, Park et al. determined the antitumor promotional activity of [6]-gingerol, the major pungent principle of ginger, using a two-stage mouse skin carcinogenesis model (318). In this study, the topical application of [6]-gingerol onto shaven backs of female ICR mice before each topical dose of TPA significantly inhibited DMBA-induced papilloma formation and TPA-induced epidermal ODC activity and inflammation in mouse skin (318).

VIII. ANISE

Anethole,1-methoxy-4-(1-propenyl) benzene, is the chief constituent of anise oil, fennel oil, and camphor (319). This compound and related ones, such as eugenol and isoeugenol, have striking metabolic effects. These compounds act similar to antioxidants (177,178), inhibit lipid peroxidation (180,181,332) and act as hydroxyl radical scavengers (179). Because eugenol and isoeugenol inhibit arachidonic acid-induced thromboxane B_2, they are extensively used as anti-inflammatory compounds (323,324). For example, anethole and its derivative, anethole dithiolethione (ADT), increase the intracellular levels of glutathione (GSH) and glutathione S-transferase (GST) (182–184). Eugenol and isoeugenol, which are found in clove oil, also modulate GSH metabolism (319,320). As well as their anti-inflammatory properties, anethole and its analogues exhibit chemopreventive activities, as indicated by suppression of the incidence and multiplicity of both invasive and noninvasive adenocarcinomas (185–190). The mechanism underlying these effects has not been established. As anethole exhibits anticarcinogenic and anti-inflammatory properties, the effects may be mediated through suppression of NF-κB and AP-1 activation. Anethol inhibits activation of various SAPK and apoptosis.

Although skin-sensitizing and irritating properties of anise oil are reported (321), studies have shown the cancer chemopreventive potential of anethole. The chemopreventive actions of 40 and 80% maximum tolerated doses (MTD) of anethole trithione administered in AIN-76A diet, on azoxymethane (AOM)-induced neoplasia were investigated in male F344 rats (185). Also, the effects of anethole trithione on the activities of phase II enzymes—namely, GST—NAD(P)H-dependent quinone reductase, and UDP-glucuronosyl transferase, in the liver and colonic mucosa and tumors was assessed. The results indicated that administration of 200 ppm (80% MTD) anethole trithione significantly inhibited the incidence and multiplicity of both invasive and noninvasive adenocarcinomas, whereas feeding of 100 ppm (40% MTD) anethole trithione suppressed only invasive adenocarcinomas of the colon. GST, NAD-(P)H-dependent quinone reductase, and UDP-glucuronosyl transferase activities in colonic mucosa and tumor and liver were significantly elevated in animals fed anethole trithione. This study suggested that the inhibition of AOM-induced colon carcinogenesis by anethole trithione may be partly associated with increased activities of phase II enzymes, such as GST, NAD(P)H-dependent quinone reductase, and UDP-glucuronosyl transferase in the liver and colon.

In another study, dietary supplemented anethole trithione significantly reduced the multiplicity of DMBA-induced mammary tumors in Sprague–Dawley rats. However, a recent study has shown that synthetic *trans*-anethole oxide, prepared from *trans*-anethole and dimethyldioxirane, is not only mutagenic for *Salmonella* tester strains, but is also carcinogenic in the induction of hepatomas in B6C3F1 mice and skin papillomas in CD-1 mice (322).

IX. SAFFRON

Saffron obtained from the dried stigmas of *Crocus sativus* is an important spice, rich in carotenoids, that is commonly consumed in different parts of the world. A growing body of evidence indicates that carotenoids possess anticarcinogenic, antimutagenic, and immunomodulating effects. Salomi et al. showed that the topical application of *C. sativus* extracts inhibited two-stage initiation–promotion (DMBA–croton oil) skin carcinogenesis and 20-methylcholanthrene (MCA)-induced soft tissue sarcomas in mice (193). Nair et al. studied the antitumor activity of saffron extract against intraperitoneally transplanted sarcoma-180 (S-180), Ehrlich ascites carcinoma (EAC), and Dalton's lymphoma ascites (DLA) tumors in mice. Oral administration of the extract significantly increased the life span of S-180-, EAC-, and DLA tumor-bearing mice (191).

That same year, Nair et al. showed that an extract of *C. sativus* prevented the decreases in body weight, hemoglobin levels, and leukocyte counts caused by cisplatin, which is a chemotherapeutic drug against cancer known to have many side effects (192). This treatment also significantly prolonged the life span of cisplatin-treated mice. Other studies demonstrated protection against cisplatin-induced toxicity in rats (325) and against the impairment of learning and memory by ethanol (326).

X. CROCETIN

Crocetin is a major component in the fruit of *Gardenia jaminoides* Ellis, a Chinese herbal medicine. Its protective potential against oxidative damage is well studied. Crocetin has been found to prevent skin cancer. Wang et al. (194) showed that topical application of crocetin on TPA-induced mice prevented skin tumors, hyperplasia, hydrogen peroxide and ODC formation, and inflammation. Topical application of crocetin with TPA to mice previously initiated with B[*a*]P inhibited the number of TPA-induced tumors per mouse. Crocetin also afforded significant protection against TPA-induced hyperplasia in the ear skin and inhibited tumor promoter-caused induction of epidermal ODC activity, hydrogen peroxide, and myeloperoxidase production. Gainer (328) showed crocetin increased the diffusion speed of oxygen through plasma, and provided a net increase in oxygen at the level of the capillary endothelial cell in dogs with spinal cord injury. The treated animals showed a significant improvement in recovery rates. In another study Gainer et al. showed that crocetin protected against hemorrhagic shock in rats by modulating whole-body oxygen consumption. Crocetin treatment increased survival rates in this study (329).

Crocetin and its relatives have other effects. Crocetin (crocetin digentiobiose ester) can prevent the ethanol-induced impairment of hippocampal synaptic plasticity in vivo (330). Gentiobioses attached to the fatty acid chain were important for this activity. The intravenous injection of *Gardeniae fructus* extract significantly lowered the systemic arterial pressure in rats that was related to a decreased cardiac output with decreased stroke volume (331). *Gardeniae fructus* extract also decreased the myocardial contractility of perfused isolated rat heart (331).

XI. ELLAGIC ACID

The compound has important hepatotoxicity effects. Ellagic acid administered orally to Wistar rats circumvented carbon tetrachloride hepatotoxicity (332). It also inhibited liver fibrosis, as seen from pathological analysis elevations in liver hydroxyproline (332). In a study by Tanaka et al., exposure to N-2-fluorenylacetamide (FAA) in male ACI/N rats induced a substantial number of altered foci, producing an incidence of hepatocellular neoplasms of 100%. Treatment with ellagic acid plus FAA resulted in a substantial decrease in the number of altered foci, and the final incidence of hepatocellular neoplasms was reduced to 30% (333).

Ellagic acid inhibits NMBA-induced esophageal tumorigenesis in F344 rats (334–336). It also inhibits cytochrome P450-mediated activation of NMBA in this animal model of esophageal tumorigenesis (334).

Ellagic acid protects the skin. When applied topically to mouse skin, the compound inhibited TPA-induced ODC activity, hydroperoxide population, and DNA synthesis, which are regarded as the markers of skin tumor promotion (337). Moreover, ellagic acid inhibited the incidence and yield of skin tumors promoted by TPA (337). In another study, chronic oral feeding of small amounts of ellagic acid to BALB/c mice in drinking water afforded significant protection against skin tumorigenesis induced by 3-methylcholanthrene (338). In this study, it was suggested that the protection against tumor induction by ellagic acid might be due to inhibition of the metabolic activation of the polycyclic aromatic hydrocarbon because epidermal aryl hydrocarbon hydroxylase activity was significantly inhibited (196). In another study by Mukhtar et al., the topical application of ellagic acid significantly protected BALB/c mice against 3-methylcholanthrene (MCA)-induced skin tumorigenesis (339). In this study ellagic acid significantly inhibited the aryl hydrocarbon hydroxylase activity in skin and liver and the extent of [^{3}H]BP-binding to skin, liver, and lung DNA. These results further suggested that ellagic acid can inhibit the metabolism of polyaromatic hydrocarbons and modulate skin carcinogenesis.

Ellagic acid has been tested against several other compounds for efficiency. In a study by Lesca (340), ellagic acid proved most potent antagonist of B[*a*]P-induced pulmonary adenoma formation in A/J mice and on DMBA-induced skin tumorigenesis in NMRI Swiss mice. Ferulic acid and chlorogenic acid were less active than ellagic acid against the lung carcinogenesis by benzo[*a*]pyrene and totally ineffective against the formation of skin tumors by DBMA. Ellagic

acid also proved to be more potent than quercetin in inhibiting the tumor formation induced by
N-nitrosodiethylamine. Both of these agents suppressed the tumor incidence, mainly by acting
at the initiation phase of carcinogenesis, for continuing the feeding of polyphenols until the
termination of the experiment did not cause any apparent change in tumor incidence or tumor
burden (341). Ellagic acid and quercetin both increased GSH and decreased in NADPH- and
ascorbate-dependent lipid peroxidation (341), but ellagic acid was more effective. This difference was suggested to be one of the reasons for the better anticarcinogenic effects of ellagic
acid as compared with quercetin (341). Finally, ellagic acid provided better protection than vitamin E succinate against 2,3,7,8-tetrachlorodibenzo-*p*-dioxin-induced fetal growth retardation
and increases in lipid peroxidation in embryonic and placental tissues of the C57BL/6J mice
(342).

XII. RAISINS

Resveratrol is a polyphenol (*trans*-3,4′,5-trihydroxystilbene) found in various fruits and vegetables and is abundant in grapes. It is also a potent antioxidant. The root extracts of the weed
Polygonum cuspidatum, an important constituent of Japanese and Chinese folk medicine, is also
an ample source of resveratrol (338). In plants, resveratrol functions as a phytoalexin that protects against fungal infections (345,346). Several studies within the last few years have shown
that resveratrol exhibits cardioprotective and chemopreventive effects (344). This constituent
has been suggested to account for the reduced risk of coronary artery disease that has been
associated with moderate wine consumption in humans (219,347). A constituent of the skin of
grapes, its concentration reaches 10–20 mM in red wine, but is absent in white wines (347).
How exactly resveratrol exerts its cardioprotective effects is not understood, but they have been
ascribed to its ability to block platelet aggregation (202,203), inhibit oxidation of low-density
lipoprotein (LDL) (199,200), and induce nitric oxide production (201). Resveratrol's ability
to inhibit ribonucleotide reductase and DNA polymerase and to suppress cell growth has also
been suggested to play a role in cardioprotection (201,348–350).

In 1997, resveratrol was reported to be one of the most potent chemopreventive agents
able to block all three phases of tumor development: initiation, promotion, and progression,
induced by the aryl hydrocarbon DMBA (207). How reseveratrol exerts its anticarcinogenic
effects is only partially understood. This polyphenol inhibits the growth of a wide variety of
tumor cells, including leukemic, prostate, breast, and endothelial cells (201,204,205,351). The
ability of resveratrol to induce the expression of CD95L (also called FasL), p53, and p21 may
contribute to its growth inhibitory effects (201,204). The suppression of cyclooxygenase 2,
cytochrome P450, and c-*fos* expression by resveratrol may account for its ability to inhibit
tumor promotion (206,208,352). Recently, the drug was reported to be a phytoestrogen that
behaves as superagonist of estrogen receptor and thereby an inducer of tumor cell proliferation (198). Its structural similarity with estrogen may also account for its cardioprotective
effects. It also inhibited SAPK activation and caspase-induced apoptosis through inhibition of
ROI generation. Lipid peroxidation was also suppressed by resveratrol. The suppression of
NF-κB and AP-1 may explain resveratrol's activity against carcinogenesis, inflammation, and
cell growth modulation, all dependent on the production of reactive oxygen species (353–356).

Resveratrol possesses anticarcinogenic potential. It inhibits the development of preneoplastic lesions in carcinogen-treated mouse mammary glands in culture and tumorigenesis in
a mouse skin cancer model, suggesting that this dietary compound merits investigation as
a potential cancer chemopreventive agent in humans (298). A recent study suggested that
resveratrol inhibits tumorigenesis in mouse skin through interference with pathways of reactive

oxidants and possibly by modulating the expression of c-*fos* and TGF-β_1 (358). In another study, resveratrol administration to rats inoculated with Yoshida AH-130 ascites hepatoma significantly decreased the tumor cell content (359). This response was associated with an increase in the number of cells in the G_2/M cell cycle phase and apoptosis of the tumor cell population.

Recent studies provided evidence that *trans*-resveratrol (3,4′,5-trihydroxystilbene), found in high concentrations in some red wines, may decrease the risk of death from coronary artery disease (360–364). A study by Jager et al. (360), performed with large epicardial porcine coronary artery strips, demonstrated a relaxant effect of *trans*-resveratrol on isolated porcine coronary arteries. The data from the study suggested that the relaxation is based on a nongenomic interaction with steroid-like receptors located on the cell membrane. In a recent study, Ray et al. (365) investigated the potential cardioprotective effects of resveratrol in the face of ischemia–reperfusion injury. The results of this study suggested that resveratrol's cardioprotective effects may be attributable to its peroxyl radical-scavenging activity.

XIII. CONCLUSION

From the foregoing descriptions, it is evident that spice ingredients have antioxidant properties. Most of these phytochemicals exhibit a wide variety of therapeutic activities. Whether all the effects of spices are mediated through the antioxidant mechanism, however, is still unclear. It is known that consumption of spices lowers the incidence of certain types of cancers and cardiovascular diseases. For instance, epidemiological studies have revealed that the incidence of large- and small-bowel adenomas and cancers are extremely low in East Indians, and this was attributed to the high intake of natural antioxidants, such as curcumin (343). Thus, it is reasonable to assume that natural antioxidants have chemopreventive effects. Overall an age-old saying that "you are what you eat" is not all that far off.

ACKNOWLEDGMENTS

We wish to thank for Mr. Walter Pagel for editorial suggestions and Ms. Linda Ford for assistance in preparation of this manuscript. This research was supported, in part, by The Clayton Foundation of Research.

REFERENCES

1. Max B. This and that: the essential pharmacology of herbs and spices. Trends Pharmacol Sci 1992; 13:15–20.
2. Craig WJ. Health-promoting properties of common herbs. Am J Clin Nutr 1999; 70(3 suppl):491S–499S.
3. Farnsworth NR, Akerele O, Bingel AS, Soejarto DD, Guo Z. Medicinal plants in therapy. Bull WHO 1985; 63:965–981.
4. Reynolds T. Tropical rain forest conservation tied to drug development [news]. J Natl Cancer Inst 1991; 83:594–596.
5. Thomassen D, Pearson PG, Slattery JT, Nelson SD. Partial characterization of biliary metabolites of pulegone by tandem mass spectrometry. Detection of glucuronide, glutathione, and glutathionyl glucuronide conjugates. Drug Metab Dispos 1991; 19:997–1003.
6. Uma PK, Geervani P, Eggum BO. Common Indian spices: nutrient composition, consumption and contribution to dietary value. Plant Foods Hum Nutr 1993; 44:137–148.
7. Halliwell B, Aeschbach R, Loliger J, Aruoma OI. The characterization of antioxidants [review]. Food Chem Toxicol 1995; 33:601–617.
8. Krishnakantha TP, Lokesh BR. Scavenging of superoxide anions by spice principles. Ind J Biochem Biophys 1993; 30:133–134.

9. Reddy AC, Lokesh BR. Studies on spice principles as antioxidants in the inhibition of lipid peroxidation of rat liver microsomes. Mol Cell Biochem 1992; 111:117–124.
10. Kumar A, Aggarwal BB. Assay for redox sensitive kinases. Methods Enzymol 1999; 300:339–345.
11. Lo YYC, Wong JMS, Cruz TF. Reactive oxygen species mediate cytokine activation of c-Jun NH$_2$-terminal kinases. J Biol Chem 1996; 271:15703–15707.
12. Chaturvedi MM, Mukhopadhyay A, Aggarwal BB. Assay for redox sensitive transcription factors. Methods Enzymol 2000; 319:585–601.
13. Li N, Karin M. Is NF-κB the sensor of oxidative stress? FASEB J 1999; 13:1137–1143.
14. Buttke TM, Sandstrom PA. Oxidative stress as a mediator of apoptosis. Immunol Today 1994; 15:7–10.
15. Manna SK, Zhang HJ, Ya T, Oberley LW, Aggarwal BB. Overexpression of Mn-superoxide dismutase suppresses TNF induced apoptosis and activation of nuclear transcription factor-κB and activated protein-1. J Biol Chem 1998; 273:13245–13254.
16. Manna SK, Kuo MT, Aggarwal BB. Overexpression of γ-glutamylcysteine synthetase abolishes tumor necrosis factor-induced apoptosis and activation of nuclear transcription factor-κB and activator protein-1. Oncogene 1999; 18:4371–4382.
17. Sharma HW, Narayanan R. The NF-κB transcription factor in oncogenesis. Anticancer Res 1996; 16:589–596.
18. Waddick KG, Uckun FM. Innovative treatment programs against cancer: II. Nuclear factor-κB (NF-κB) as a molecular target. Biochem Pharmacol 1999; 57:9–17.
19. Sharma OP. Antioxidant activity of curcumin and related compounds. Biochem Pharmacol 1976; 25:1811–1812.
20. Toda S, Ohnishi M, Kimura M, Nakashima K. Action of curcuminoids on the hemolysis and lipid peroxidation of mouse erythrocytes induced by hydrogen peroxide. J Ethnopharmacol 1988; 23:105–108.
21. Kunchandy E, Rao MNA. Oxygen radical scavenging activity of curcumin. Int J Pharm 1990; 58:237–240.
22. Tonnesen HH, de Vries H, Karlsen J, Beijersberge van Henegouwen G. Studies on curcumin and curcuminoids. IX: Investigation of the photobiological activity of curcumin using bacterial indicator systems. J Pharm Sci 1987; 76:371–373.
23. Reddy AC, Lokesh BR. Studies on anti-inflammatory activity of spice principles and dietary n-3 polyunsaturated fatty acids on carrageenan-induced inflammation in rats. Ann Nutr Metab 1994; 38:349–358.
24. Grinberg LN, Rachmilewitz EA, Kitrossky N, Chevion M. Hydroxyl radical generation in beta-thalassemic red blood cells. Free Radic Biol Med 1995; 18:611–615.
25. Kunchandy E, Rao MNA. Oxygen radical scavenging activity of curcumin. Int J Pharm 1989; 58:237–240.
26. Subramanian M, Sreejayan, Rao MN, Devasagayam TP, Singh BB. Diminution of singlet oxygen-induced DNA damage by curcumin and related antioxidants. Mutat Res 1994; 311:249–255.
27. Unnikrishnan MK, Rao MN. Curcumin inhibits nitrite-induced methemoglobin formation. FEBS Lett 1992; 301:195–196.
28. Unnikrishnan MK, Rao MN. Curcumin inhibits nitrogen dioxide induced oxidation of hemoglobin. Mol Cell Biochem 1995; 146:35–37.
29. Sreejuayan Rao MNA. Curcuminoids as potent inhibitors of lipid peroxidation. J Pharm Pharmacol 1994; 46:1013–1016.
30. Shalini VK, Srinivas L. Lipid peroxide induced DNA damage: protection by turmeric (*Curcuma longa*). Mol Cell Biochem 1987; 77:3–10.
31. Susan M, Rao MN. Induction of glutathione S-transferase activity by curcumin in mice. Arzneimittelforschung 1992; 42:962–964.
32. Srinivas L, Shalini VK, Shylaja M. Turmerin: a water soluble antioxidant peptide from turmeric [Curcuma longa]. Arch Biochem Biophys 1992; 292(2):617–623.
33. Singh S, Aggarwal BB. Activation of transcription factor NF-kappa B is suppressed by curcumin (diferuloylmethane) [corrected]. J Biol Chem 1995; 270:30235.
34. Chan MM. Inhibition of tumor necrosis factor by curcumin, a phytochemical. Biochem Pharmacol 1995; 49:1551–1556.
35. Huang TS, Lee SC, Lin JK. Suppression of c-Jun/AP-1 activation by an inhibitor of tumor promotion in mouse fibroblast cells. Proc Natl Acad Sci USA 1991; 88:5292–5296.

36. Kakar SS, Roy D. Curcumin inhibits TPA induced expression of c-*fos*, c-*jun* and c-*myc* proto-oncogenes messenger RNAs in mouse skin. Cancer Lett 1994; 87:85–89.
37. Jobin C, Bradham CA, Russo MP, Juma B, Narula AS, Brenner DA, Sartor RB. Curcumin blocks cytokine-mediated NF-kappa B activation and proinflammatory gene expression by inhibiting inhibitory factor I-kappa B kinase activity. J Immunol 1999; 163:3474–3483.
38. Kumar A, Dhawan S, Hardegen NJ, Aggarwal BB. Curcumin (diferuloylmethane) inhibition of TNF-mediated adhesion of monocytes to endothelial cells by suppression of cell surface expression of adhesion molecules and of nuclear factor-κB activation. Biochem Pharmacol 1998; 55:775–783.
39. Chan MM, Ho CT, Huang HI. Effects of three dietary phytochemicals from tea, rosemary and turmeric on inflammation-induced nitrite production. Cancer Lett 1995; 96:23–29.
40. Brouet I, Ohshima H. Curcumin, an anti-tumour promoter and anti inflammatory agent, inhibits induction of nitric oxide synthase in activated macrophages. Biochem Biophys Res Commun 1995; 206:533–540.
41. Xu YX, Pindolia KR, Janakiraman N, Chapman RA, Gautam SC. Curcumin inhibits IL-1-alpha and TNF-alpha induction of AP-1 and NF-κB DNA binding activity in bone marrow stromal cells. Hematopathol Mol Hematol 1997–1998; 11:49–62.
42. Hanazawa S, Akeshita A, Amano S, Matumoto T, Kitano S. IL-1 induces expression of monocyte chemoattractant JE in clonal mouse osteoblastic cell line MC3T3-E1. J Immunol 1993; 150:1554–1562.
43. Huang MT, Lysz T, Ferraro T, Abidi TF, Laskin JD, Conney AH. Inhibitory effects of curcumin on in vitro lipoxygenase and cyclooxygenase activities in mouse epidermis. Cancer Res 1991; 51:813–819.
44. Ammon HP, Safayhi H, Mack T, Sabieraj J. Mechanism of antiinflammatory actions of curcumine and boswellic acids. J Ethnopharmacol 1993; 38:113–119.
45. Li CJ, Zhan LJ, Dezube BJ, Crumpacker CS, Pardee AB. Three inhibitors of type 1 human immunodeficiency virus long terminal repeat-directed gene expression and virus replication. Proc Natl Acad Sci USA 1993; 90:1839–1842.
46. Mazumder A, Burke TR Jr, Fesen MR, Wang J, Carothers AM, Grunberger D, Driscoll J, Kohn K, Pommier Y. Hydroxylated aromatic inhibitors of HIV 1 integrase. J Med Chem 1995; 38:4171–4178.
47. Huang MT, Deschner EE, Newmark HL, Wang ZY, Ferraro TA, Conney AH. Effect of dietary curcumin and ascorbyl palmitate on azoxymethanol induced colonic epithelial cell proliferation and focal areas of dysplasia. Cancer Lett 1992; 64:117–121.
48. Lu YP, Chang RL, Huang MT, Conncy AH. Inhibitory effect of curcumin on 12-*O*-tetradecanoyl-phorbol-13-acetate-induced increase in ornithine decarboxylase mRNA in mouse epidermis. Carcinogenesis 1993; 14:293–297.
49. Kuttan R, Bhanumathy P, Nirmala K, George MC. Potential anticancer activity of turmeric (*Curcuma longa*). Cancer Lett 1985; 29:197–202.
50. Singh AK, Sidhu GS, Deepa T, Maheshwari RK. Curcumin inhibits the proliferation and cell cycle progression of human umbilical vein endothelial cell. Cancer Lett 1996; 107:109-115.
51. Huang HC, Jan TR, Yeh SF. Inhibitory effect of curcumin, an anti-inflammatory agent, on vascular smooth muscle cell proliferation. Eur J Pharmacol 1992; 221:381–384.
52. Kuo ML, Huang TS, Lin JK. Curcumin, an antioxidant and anti-tumor promoter, induces apoptosis in human leukemia cells. Biochim Biophys Acta 1996; 1317:95–100.
53. Jiang MC, Yang–Yen HF, Yen JJ, Lin JK. Curcumin induces apoptosis in immortalized NIH 3T3 and malignant cancer cell lines. Nutr Cancer 1996; 26:111–120.
54. Mehta K, McQueen T, Neamati N, Collins S, Andreeff M. Activation of retinoid receptors RAR alpha and RXR alpha induces differentiation and apoptosis, respectively, in HL-60 cells. Cell Growth Differ 1996; 7:179–186.
55. Korutla L, Kumar R. Inhibitory effect of curcumin on epidermal growth factor receptor kinase activity in A431 cells. Biochim Biophys Acta 1994; 1224:597–600.
56. Reddy SAG, Chaturvedi MM, Darnay BG, Chan H, Higuchi M, Aggarwal BB. Reconstitution of NF-κB activation induced by tumor necrosis factor requires membrane-associated components: comparison with pathway activated by ceramide. J Biol Chem 1994; 269:25369.
57. Korutla L, Cheung JY, Mendelsohn J, Kumar R. Inhibition of ligand-induced activation of epidermal growth factor receptor tyrosine phosphorylation by curcumin. Carcinogenesis 1995; 16:1741–1745.

58. Liu JY, Lin SJ, Lin JK. Inhibitory effects of curcumin on protein kinase C activity induced by 12-O-tetradecanoyl-phorbol-13-acetate in NIH 3T3 cells. Carcinogenesis 1993; 14:857–861.
59. Hasmeda M, Polya GM. Inhibition of cyclic AMP-dependent protein kinase by curcumin. Phytochemistry 1996; 42:599–605.
60. Nagabhushan M, Bhide SV. Nonmutagenicity of curcumin and its antimutagenic action versus chili and capsaicin. Nutr Cancer 1987; 8:201–210.
61. Huang MT, Smart RC, Wong CQ, Conney AH. Inhibitory effect of curcumin, chlorogenic acid, caffeic acid, and ferulic acid on tumor promotion in mouse skin by 12-O-tetradecanoylphorbol-13-acetate. Cancer Res 1988; 48:5941–5946.
62. Lundquist F, Quistorff B, Huang MT. Deuterium isotope effects on ethanol oxidation in perfused rat liver and in rats and rabbits in vivo: application to determine the contribution of various pathways. Pharmacol Toxicol 1989; 65:55–62.
63. Nagabhushan M, Bhide SV. Curcumin as an inhibitor of cancer. J Am Coll Nutr 1992; 11:192–198.
64. Huang MT, Wang ZY, Georgiadis CA, Laskin JD, Conney AH. Inhibitory effects of curcumin on tumor initiation by benzo[a]pyrene and 7,12-dimethylbenz[a]anthracene. Carcinogenesis 1992; 13:2183–2186.
65. Rao CV, Desai D, Kaul B, Amin S, Reddy BS. Effect of caffeic acid esters on carcinogen-induced mutagenicity and human colon adenocarcinoma cell growth. Chem Biol Interact 1992; 84:277–290.
66. Rao CV, Rivenson A, Simi B, Reddy BS. Chemoprevention of colon cancer by dietary curcumin. Ann NY Acad Sci 1995; 768:201–204.
67. Azuine MA, Bhide VS. Chemopreventive effect of turmeric against stomach and skin tumors induced by chemical carcinogens in Swiss mice. Nutr Cancer 1992; 17:77–83.
68. Tanaka T, Kojima T, Kawamori T, Wang A, Suzui M, Okamoto K, Mori H. Inhibition of 4-nitroquinoline-1-oxide-induced rat tongue carcinogenesis by the naturally occurring plant phenolics caffeic, ellagic, chlorogenic and ferulic acids. Carcinogenesis 1993; 14:1321–1325.
69. Huang MT, Ma W, Yen P, Xie JG, Han J, Frenkel K, Grunberger D, Conney AH. Inhibitory effects of topical application of low doses of curcumin on 12-O-tetradecanoylphorbol-13-acetate-induced tumor promotion and oxidized DNA bases in mouse epidermis. Carcinogenesis 1997; 18:83–88.
70. Huang MT, Lou YR, Ma W, Newmark HL, Reuhl KR, Conney AH. Inhibitory effects of dietary curcumin on forestomach, duodenal, and colon carcinogenesis in mice. Cancer Res 1994; 54:5841–5847.
71. Oda Y. Inhibitory effect of curcumin on SOS functions induced by UV irradiation. Mutat Res 1995; 348:67–73.
72. Shalini VK, Luthra M, Srinivas L, Rao SH, Basti S, Reddy M, Balasubramanian D. Oxidative damage to the eye lens caused by cigarette smoke and fuel smoke condensates. Indian J Biochem Biophys 1994; 31:261–266.
73. Awasthi S, Srivatava SK, Piper JT, Singhal SS, Chaubey M, Awasthi YC. Curcumin protects against 4-hydroxy-4-trans-nonenal-induced cataract formation in rat lenses. Am J Clin Nutr 1996; 64:761–766.
74. Srivastava R. Inhibition of neutrophil response by curcumin. Agents Actions 1989; 8:298–303.
75. Apisariyakul A, Vanittanakom N, Buddhasukh D. Antifungal activity of turmeric oil extracted from Curcuma longa (Zingiberaceae). J Ethnopharmacol 1995; 49:163–169.
76. Ammon HP, Anazodo MI, Safayhi H, Dhawan BN, Srimal RC. Curcumin: a potent inhibitor of leukotriene B4 formation in rat peritoneal polymorphonuclear neutrophils (PMNL). Planta Med 1992; 58:226.
77. Srivastava R, Dikshit M, Srimal RC, Dhawan BN. Anti-thrombotic effect of curcumin. Thromb Res 1985; 40:413–417.
78. Srivastava R, Puri V, Srimal RC, Dhawan BN. Effect of curcumin on platelet aggregation and vascular prostacyclin synthesis. Arzneimittelforschung 1986; 36:715–717.
79. Deodhar SD, Sethi R, Srimal RC. Preliminary study on antirheumatic activity of curcumin (diferuloyl methane). Indian J Med Res 1980; 71:632–634.
80. Ghatak N, Basu N. Sodium curcuminate as an effective anti-inflammatory agent. Indian J Exp Biol 1972; 10:235–236.
81. Srivastava R. Inhibition of neutrophil response by curcumin. Agents Actions 1989; 28:298–304.
82. Srimal RC, Dhawan BN. Pharmacology of diferuloyl methane (curcumin), a non-steroidal anti-inflammatory agent. J Pharm Pharmacol 1973; 25:447–452.

83. Rao TS, Basu N, Siddiqui HH. Anti-inflammatory activity of curcumin analogues. Indian J Med Res 1982; 75:574–578.
84. Srivastava R, Srimal RC. Modification of certain inflammation-induced biochemical changes by curcumin. Indian J Med Res 1985; 81:215–223.
85. Patil TN, Srinivasan M. Hypocholesteremic effect of curcumin in induced hypercholesteremic rats. Indian J Exp Biol 1971; 9:167–169.
86. Rao DS, Sekhara NC, Satyanarayana MN, Srinivasan M. Effect of curcumin on serum and liver cholesterol levels in the rat. J Nutr 1970; 100:1307–1315.
87. Nirmala C, Puvanakrishnan R. Effect of curcumin on certain lysosomal hydrolases in isoproterenol-induced myocardial infarction in rats. Biochem Pharmacol 1996; 51:47–51.
88. Srivastava R, Srimal RC. Modifications of certain inflammation-induced biochemical changes by curcumin. Indian J Med Res 1985; 81:215–223.
89. Oetari S, Sudibyo M, Commandeur JN, Samhoedi R, Vermeulen NP. Effects of curcumin on cytochrome P450 and glutathione S-transferase activities in rat liver. Biochem Pharmacol 1996; 51:39–45.
90. Ramparsad , Sirsi M. Studies on Indian medicinal plants: *Curcuma longa* Linn.—effect of curcumin and the essential oils of *C. longa* on bile secretion. J Sci Ind Res 1956; 15C:262–265.
91. Kaul S, Krishnakanth TP. Effect of retinol deficiency and curcumin or turmeric feeding on brain Na(+)-K$^+$ adenosine triphosphatase activity. Mol Cell Biochem 1994; 137:101–107.
92. Shantha K, Krishnakanth TP. Microisomal Na$^+$–K$^+$ activated adenosine triphosphatase activity in retinol deficient albino rats. Nutr Rep Int 1987; 36:573–580.
93. Joe B, Lokesh BR. Studies on the inactivation of superoxide dismutase activity by nitric oxide from rat peritoneal macrophages. Mol Cell Biochem 1997; 168:87–93.
94. Morre DJ, Wu LY, Morre DM. The antitumor sulfonylurea N-(4-methylphenylsulfonyl)-N'-(4-chlorophenyl) urea (LY181984) inhibits NADH oxidase activity of HeLa plasma membranes. Biochim Biophys Acta 1995; 1240:11–17.
95. Singh S, Chainy GB, Raju U, Aggarwal BB. Differential activation of the nuclear factor-kappa B by TNF muteins specific for the p60 and p80 TNF receptors. J Immunol 1996; 157:2410–2417.
96. Ho W, Kim E, Han J, Earm YE. Modulation of ATP-sensitive K$^+$ channels in rabbit ventricular myocytes by adenosine A$_1$ receptor activation. Am J Physiol 1997; 272(1 pt 2):H325–333.
97. Szallasi A, Blumberg PM. Vanilloid (capsaicin) receptors and mechanisms [review]. Pharmacol Rev 1999; 51:159–212.
98. Marsh SJ, Stansfeld CE, Parcej DN, Dolly JO, Brown DA. Mast cell degranulating peptide and dendrotoxin selectively inhibit a fast-activating potassium current and bind to common neuronal proteins. Neuroscience 1987; 23:893–902.
99. Liu L, Simon SA. A rapid capsaicin-activated current in rat trigeminal ganglion neurons. Proc Natl Acad Sci USA 1994; 91:738–741.
100. Caterina MJ, Schumacher MA, Tominaga M, Rosen TA, Levine JD, Julius D. The capsaicin receptor: a heat-activated ion channel in the pain pathway [see comments]. Nature 1997; 389:816–824.
101. Jhamandas K, Yaksh TL, Harty G, Szolcsanyi J, Go VL. Action of intrathecal capsaicin and its structural analogues on the content and release of spinal substance P: selectivity of action and relationship to analgesia. Brain Res 1984; 306:215–225.
102. Santicioli P, Del Bianco E, Tramontana M, Maggi CA. Adenosine inhibits cation potential-dependent release of calcitonin gene-related peptide- and substance P-like immunoreactivities from primary afferents in rat spinal cord. Neurosci Lett 1992; 144:211–214.
103. Helme RD, Eglezos A, Andrews PV. The effects of capsaicin denervation on leucocyte and complement components of the inflammatory response. Clin Exp Neurol 1987; 24:207–211.
104. Girolomoni G, Tigelaar RE. Capsaicin-sensitive primary sensory neurons are potent modulators of murine delayed-type hypersensitivity reactions. J Immunol 1990; 145:1105–1112.
105. Nagahisa A, Kanai Y, Suga O, Taniguchi K, Tsuchiya M, Lowe JA, Hess HJ. Antiinflammatory and analgesic activity of a non-peptide substance P receptor antagonist. Eur J Pharmacol 1992; 217:191–195.
106. Sicuteri F. Antiandrogenic medication of cluster headache. Int J Clin Pharmacol 1988; 8:21–24.
107. Watson CP, Evans RJ, Watt VR. Post-herpetic neuralgia and topical capsaicin. Pain 1988; 33:333–340.

108. Marabini S, Ciabatti G, Polli G. Effect of topical nasal treatment with capsaicin in vasomotor rhinitis. Regul Pept 1988; 22:1.
109. Chiba T, Masuko S, Kawano H. Correlation of mitochondrial swelling after capsaicin treatment and substance P and somatostatin immunoreactivity in small neurons of dorsal root ganglion in the rat. Neurosci Lett 1986; 64:311–316.
110. Joo F, Szolcsanyi J, Jancso–Gabor A. Mitochondrial alterations in the spinal ganglion cells of the rat accompanying the long-lasting sensory disturbance induced by capsaicin. Life Sci 1969; 8:621–626.
111. Jancso G, Wollemann M. The effect of capsaicin on the adenylate cyclase activity of rat brain. Brain Res 1977; 123:323–329.
112. Vanner S, MacNaughton WK. Capsaicin-sensitive afferent nerves activate submucosal secretomotor neurons in guinea pig ileum. Am J Physiol 1995; 269:G203–G209.
113. Maurya AK, Singh SV. Differential induction of glutathione transferase isoenzymes of mice stomach by diallyl sulfide, a naturally occurring anticarcinogen. Cancer Lett 1991; 57:121–129.
114. Morioka N, Sze LL, Morton DL, Irie RF. A protein fraction from aged garlic extract enhances cytotoxicity and proliferation of human lymphocytes mediated by interleukin-2 and concanavalin A. Cancer Immunol Immunother 1993; 37:316–322.
115. Shoji S, Furuishi K, Yanase R, Miyazaka T, Kino M. Allyl compounds selectively killed human immunodeficiency virus (type 1)-infected cells. Biochem Biophys Res Commun 1993; 194:610–621.
116. Belman S. Onion and garlic oils inhibit tumor promotion. Carcinogenesis 1983; 4:1063–1065.
117. Sumiyoshi H, Wargovich MJ. Chemoprevention of 1,2-dimethylhydrazine-induced colon cancer in mice by naturally occurring organosulfur compounds. Cancer Res 1990; 50:5084–5087.
118. Sparnins VL, Mott AW, Barany G, Wattenberg LW. Effects of allyl methyl trisulfide on glutathione S-transferase activity and BP-induced neoplasia in the mouse. Nutr Cancer 1986; 8:211–215.
119. Sparnins VL, Barany G, Wattenberg LW. Effects of organosulfur compounds from garlic and onions on benzo[*a*]pyrene-induced neoplasia and glutathione S-transferase activity in the mouse. Carcinogenesis 1988; 9:131–134.
120. Dorant E, van den Brandt PA, Goldbohm RA, Hermus RJ, Sturmans F. Garlic and its significance for the prevention of cancer in humans: a critical view [review]. Br J Cancer 1993; 67:424–429.
121. Wargovich MJ. Diallyl sulfide, a flavor component of garlic (*Allium sativum*), inhibits dimethylhydrazine-induced colon cancer. Carcinogenesis 1987; 8:487–489.
122. Liu J, Lin Ri, Milner JA. Inhibition of 7,12-dimethylbenz[*a*]anthracene-induced mammary tumors and DNA adducts by garlic powder. Carcinogenesis 1992; 13:1847–1851.
123. Bhimani RS, Troll W, Grunberger D, Frenkel K. Inhibition of oxidative stress in HeLa cells by chemopreventive agents. Cancer Res 1993; 53:4528–4533.
124. Sud'ina GF, Mirzoeva OK, Pushkareva MA, Korshunova GA, Sumbatyan NV, Varfolomeev SD. Caffeic acid phenethyl ester as a lipoxygenase inhibitor with antioxidant properties. FEBS Lett 1993; 329:21–24.
125. Natarajan K, Singh S, Burke TR Jr, Grunberger D, Aggarwal BB. Caffeic acid phenethyl ester is a potent and specific inhibitor of activation of nuclear transcription factor NF kappa B. Proc Natl Acad Sci USA 1996; 93:9090–9095.
126. Chiao C, Carothers AM, Grunberger D, Solomon G, Preston GA, Barrett JC. Apoptosis and altered redox state induced by caffeic acid phenethyl ester (CAPE) in transformed rat fibroblast cells. Cancer Res 1995; 55:3576–3583.
127. Grunberger D, Banerjee R, Eisinger K, Oltz K, Efros EM, Caldwell M, Estevez V, Nakanishi K. Experientia 1988; 44:230–232.
128. Su ZZ, Grunberger D, Fisher PB. Suppression of adenovirus type 5 E1A-mediated transformation and expression of the transformed phenotype by caffeic acid phenethyl ester (CAPE). Mol Carcinog 1991; 4:231–242.
129. Guarini L, Su ZZ, Zucker S, Lin J, Grunberger D, Fisher PB. Growth inhibition and modulation of antigenic phenotype in human melanoma and glioblastoma multiforme cells by caffeic acid phenethyl ester (CAPE). Cell Mol Biol 1992; 38:513–527.
130. Su ZZ, Lin J, Grunberger D, Fisher PB. Growth suppression and toxicity induced by caffeic acid phenethyl ester (CAPE) in type 5 adenovirus-transformed rat embryo cells correlate directly with transformation progression Cancer Res 1994; 54:1865–1870.

131. Zheng ZS, Xue GZ, Grunberger D, Prystowsky JH. Caffeic acid phenethyl ester inhibits proliferation of human keratinocytes and interferes with the EGF regulation of ornithine decarboxylase. Oncol Res 1995; 7:445–452.
132. Fesen MR, Kohn KW, Leteurtre F, Pommier Y. Inhibitors of human immunodeficiency virus integrase. Proc Natl Acad Sci USA 1993; 90:2399–2403.
133. Burke TR Jr, Fesen MR, Mazumder A, Wang J, Carothers AM, Grunberger D, Driscoll J, Kohn K, Pommier Y. Hydroxylated aromatic inhibitors of HIV-1 integrase. J Med Chem 1995; 38:4171–4178.
134. Mazumder A, Raghavan K, Weinstein J, Kohn KW, Pommier Y. Inhibition of human immunodeficiency virus type-1 integrase by curcumin. Biochem Pharmacol 1995; 49:1165–1170.
135. Frenkel K, Wei H, Bhimani R, Ye J, Zadunaisky JA, Huang MT, Ferraro T, Conney AH, Grunberger D. Inhibition of tumor promoter-mediated processes in mouse skin and bovine lens by caffeic acid phenethyl ester. Cancer Res 1993; 53:1255–1261.
136. Huang MT, Ma W, Yen P, Xie JG, Han J, Frenkel K, Grunberger D, Conney AH. Inhibitory effects of caffeic acid phenethyl ester (CAPE) on 12-*O*-tetradecanoylphorbol-13-acetate-induced tumor promotion in mouse skin and the synthesis of DNA, RNA and protein in HeLa cells. Carcinogenesis 1996; 17:761–765.
137. Rao CV, Desai D, Kaul B, Amin S, Reddy BS. Effect of caffeic acid esters on carcinogen-induced mutagenicity and human colon adenocarcinoma cell growth. Chem Biol Interact 1992; 84:277–290.
138. Rao CV, Desai D, Simi B, Kulkarni N, Amin S, Reddy BS. Inhibitory effect of caffeic acid esters on azoxymethane-induced biochemical changes and aberrant crypt foci formation in rat colon. Cancer Res 1993; 53:4182–4188.
139. Rao CV, Rivenson A, Simi B, Reddy BS. Chemoprevention of colon carcinogenesis by dietary curcumin, a naturally occurring plant phenolic compound. Cancer Res 1995; 55:259–266.
140. Kumar K, Dhawan S, Aggarwal BB. Emodin (3-methyl-1,6,8-trihydroxyanthraquinone) inhibits the TNF-induced NF-κB activation, IκB degradation and expression cell surface adhesion protein in human vascular endothelial cells. Oncogene 1998; 17:913–918.
141. Jayasuriya H, Koonchanok NM, Geahlen RL, McLaughlin JL, Chang CJ. Emodin, a protein tyrosine kinase inhibitor from *Polygonum cuspidatum*. J Nat Prod 1992; 55:696–698.
142. Frew T, Powis G, Berggren M, Abraham RT, Ashendel CL, Zalkow LH, Hudson C, Qazia S, Gruszecka–Kowalik E, Merriman R. A multiwell assay for inhibitors of phosphatidylinositol-3-kinase and the identification of natural product inhibitors. Anticancer Res 1994; 14:2425–2428.
143. Chan TC, Chang CJ, Koonchanok NM, Geahlen RL. Selective inhibition of the growth of ras-transformed human bronchial epithelial cells by emodin, a protein–tyrosine kinase inhibitor. Biochem Biophys Res Commun 1993; 193:1152–1158.
144. Kupchan SM, Karim A. Tumor inhibitors. 114. Aloe emodin: antileukemic principle isolated from *Rhamnus frangula* L. Lloydia 1976; 39:223–224.
145. Zhang L, Hung MC. Sensitization of HER-2/neu-overexpressing non-small cell lung cancer cells to chemotherapeutic drugs by tyrosine kinase inhibitor emodin. Oncogene 1996; 12:57157–57166.
146. Yeh SF, Chou TC, Liu TS. Effects of anthraquinones of *Polygonum cuspidatum* on HL-60 cells. Planta Med 1988; 54:413–414.
147. Zhang L, Chang CJ, Bacus SS, Hung MC. Suppressed transformation and induced differentiation of HER-2/neu-overexpressing breast cancer cells by emodin. Cancer Res 1995; 55:3890–3896.
148. Malterud KE, Farbrot TL, Huse AE, Sund RB. Antioxidant and radical scavenging effects of anthraquinones and anthrones. Pharmacology 1993; 47(suppl 1):77–85.
149. Reddy AC, Lokesh BR. Studies on the inhibitory effects of curcumin and eugenol on the formation of reactive oxygen species and the oxidation of ferrous iron. Mol Cell Biochem 1994; 137:1–8.
150. Reddy AC, Lokesh BR. Studies on spice principles as antioxidants in the inhibition of lipid peroxidation of rat liver microsomes. Mol Cell Biochem 1992; 111:117–124.
151. Chainy GBN, Manna SK, Chaturvedi MM, Aggarwal BB. Anethole blocks both early and late cellular responses transduced by tumor necrosis factor: effect on NF-κB, AP-1, JNK, MAPKK and apoptosis. Oncogene 2000; 19:2943–2950.
152. Stohs SJ, Lawson TA, Anderson L, Bueding E. Effects of oltipraz, BHA, ADT and cabbage on glutathione metabolism, DNA damage and lipid peroxidation in old mice. Mech Ageing Dev 1986; 37:137–145.
153. Naidum KA. Eugenol—an inhibitor of lipoxygenase-dependent lipid peroxidation. Prostaglandins Leuko Essent Fatty Acids 1995; 53:381–383.

154. Sharma JN, Srivastava KC, Gan EK. Suppressive effects of eugenol and ginger oil on arthritic rats. Pharmacology 1994; 49:314–318.
155. Rao AS, Hashim S. Modulatory effect of food seasoning spices mixture, garam massalla, on DMBA-induced transplacental and translactational carcinogenesis in mice. School of Life Sciences, Jawaharial Nehru University, New Delhi, India, 1995.
156. Krishnakantha TP, Lokesh BR. Scavenging of superoxide anions by spice principals. Indian J Biochem Biophys 1993; 30:133–134.
157. Reddy AC, Lokesh BR. Studies on spice principles as antioxidants in the inhibition of lipid peroxidation of rat liver microsomes. Mol Cell Biochem 1992; 111:117–124.
158. Backon J. Ginger: inhibition of thromboxane synthetase and stimulation of prostacyclin: relevance for medicine and psychiatry [review]. Med Hypotheses 1986; 20:271–278.
159. Verma SK, Singh J, Khamesra R, Bordia A. Effect of ginger on platelet aggregation in man. Indian J Med Res 1993; 98:240–242.
160. Mascolo N, Jain R, Jain SC, Capasso F. Ethnopharmacologic investigation of ginger (*Zingiber officinale*). J Ethnopharmacol 1989; 27:129–140.
161. Kiuchi F, Shibuya M, Sankawa U. Inhibitors of prostaglandin biosynthesis from ginger. Chem Pharm Bull 1982; 30:754–757.
162. Backon J. Ginger in preventing nausea and vomiting of pregnancy; a caveat due to its thromboxane synthetase activity and effect on testosterone binding [letter; comment]. Eur J Obstet Gynecol Reprod Biol 1992; 42:163–164.
163. Yamahara J, Rong HQ, Naitoh Y, Kitani T, Fujimura H. Inhibition of cytotoxic drug-induced vomiting in suncus by a ginger constituent. J Ethnopharmacol 1989; 27:353–355.
164. Srivastava KC. Isolation and effects of some ginger components of platelet aggregation and eicosanoid biosynthesis. Prostaglandins Leukotr Med 1986; 25:187–198.
165. Srivastava KC, Mustafa T. Ginger (*Zingiber officinale*) in rheumatism and musculoskeletal disorders. Med Hypotheses 1992; 39:342–348.
166. Sharma JN, Srivastava KC, Gan EK. Suppressive effects of eugenol and ginger oil on arthritic rats. Pharmacology 1994; 49:314–318.
167. Tanabe M, Chen YD, Saito K, Kano Y. Cholesterol biosynthesis inhibitory component from *Zingiber officinale* Roscoe. Chem Pharm Bull 1993; 41:710–713.
168. Srinivasan K, Sambaiah K. The effect of spices on cholesterol 7 alpha-hydroxylase activity and on serum and hepatic cholesterol levels in the rat. Int J Vit Nutr Res 1991; 61:364–369.
169. Yamahara J, Mochizuki M, Rong HQ, Matsuda H, Fujimura H. The anti-ulcer effect in rats of ginger constituents. J Ethnopharmacol 1988; 23:299–304.
170. Eldershaw TP, Colquhoun EQ, Dora KA, Peng ZC, Clark MG. Pungent principles of ginger (*Zingiber officinale*) are thermogenic in the perfused rat hindlimb. Int J Obes Relat Metab Disord 1992; 16:755–763.
171. Mustafa T, Srivastava KC. Ginger (*Zingiber officinale*) in migraine headache. J Ethnopharmacol 1990; 29:267–273.
172. al-Yahya MA, Rafatullah S, Mossa JS, Ageel AM, Parmar NS, Tariq M. Gastroprotective activity of ginger *Zingiber officinale* Rosc. in albino rats. Am J Chin Med 1989; 17:51–56.
173. Llewellyn GC, Burkett ML, Eadie T. Potential mold growth, aflatoxin production, and antimycotic activity of selected natural spices and herbs. J Assoc Off Anal Chem 1981; 64:955–960.
174. Datta A, Sukul NC. Antifilarial effect of *Zingiber officinale* on *Dirofilaria immitis*. J Helminthol 1987; 61:268–270.
175. Traganos F, Kapuscinski J, Gong J, Ardelt B, Darzynkiewicz RJ, Darzynkiewicz Z. Caffeine prevents apoptosis and cell cycle effects induced by camptothecin or topotecan in HL-60 cells. Cancer Res 1993; 53:4613–4618.
176. Medenica RD, Mukerjee S, Huschart T, Corbitt W. Interferon inhibitor factor predicting success of plasmapheresis in patients with multiple sclerosis. J Clin Apheresis 1994; 9:216–221.
177. Rajakumar DV, Rao MN. Dehydrozingerone and isoeugenol as inhibitors of lipid peroxidation and as free radical scavengers. Biochem Pharmacol 1993; 46:2067–2072.
178. Ko FN, Liao CH, Kuo YH, Lin YL. Antioxidant properties of demethyldiisoeugenol. Biochim Biophys Acta 1995; 1258:145–152.
179. Taira J, Ikemoto T, Yoneya T, Hagi A, Murakami A, Makino K. Essential oil phenyl propanoids. Useful as ·OH scavengers? Free Radic Res Commun 1992; 16:197–204.
180. Nagababu E, Lakshmaiah N. Inhibition of microsomal lipid peroxidation and monooxygenase activities by eugenol. Free Radic Res 1994; 20:253–266.

181. Mansuy D, Sassi A, Dansette PM, Plat M. A new potent inhibitor of lipid peroxidation in vitro and in vivo, the hepatoprotective drug anisyldithiolthione. Biochem Biophys Res Commun 1986; 135:1015–1021.
182. Drukarch B, Schepens E, Stoof JC, Langeveld CH. Anethole dithiolethione prevents oxidative damage in glutathione-depleted astrocytes. Eur J Pharmacol 1997; 329:259–262.
183. Rompelberg CJ, Verhagen H, van Bladeren PJ. Effects of the naturally occurring alkenylbenzenes eugenol and *trans*-anethole on drug-metabolizing enzymes in the rat liver. Food Chem Toxicol 1993; 31:637–645.
184. Bouthillier L, Charbonneau M, Brodeur J. Assessment of the role of glutathione conjugation in the protection afforded by anethol dithiolthione against hexachloro-1,3-butadiene induced nephrotoxicity. Toxicol Appl Pharmacol 1996; 139:177–185.
185. Reddy BS, Rao CV, Rivenson A, Kelloff G. Chemoprevention of colon carcinogenesis by organosulfur compounds. Cancer Res 1993; 53:3493–3498.
186. Reddy BS. Antioxidant properties of demethyldiisoeugenol. Prev Med 1996; 25:48–50.
187. Reddy BS. Antioxidant properties of demethyldiisoeugenol. Adv Exp Med Biol 1997; 400B:931–936.
188. Al-Harbi MM, Qureshi S, Raza M, Ahmed MM, Giangreco AB, Shah AH. Influence of anethole treatment on the tumour induced by Ehrlich ascites carcinoma cells in paw of Swiss albino mice. Eur J Cancer Prev 1995; 4:307–318.
189. Lubet RA, Steele VE, Eto I, Juliana MM, Kelloff GJ, Grubbs CJ. Chemopreventive efficacy of the anethole trithione, *N*-acetyl-L-cysteine, miconazole and phenethylisothiocyanate in the DMBA-induced rat mammary cancer model. Int J Cancer 1997; 72:95–101.
190. Miller EC, Swanson AB, Phillips DH, Fletcher TL, Liem A, Miller JA. Structure–activity studies of the carcinogenicities in the mouse and rat of some naturally occurring and synthetic alkenylbenzene derivatives related to safrole and estragole. Cancer Res 1983; 43:1124–1134.
191. Nair SC, Pannikar B, Panikkar KR. Antitumour activity of saffron (*Crocus sativus*). Cancer Lett 1991; 57:109–114.
192. Nair SC, Salomi MJ, Panikkar B, Panikkar KR. Modulatory effects of *Crocus sativus* and *Nigella sativa* extracts on cisplatin-induced toxicity in mice. J Ethnopharmacol 1991; 31:75–83.
193. Salomi MJ, Nair SC, Panikkar KR. Inhibitory effects of *Nigella sativa* and saffron (*Crocus sativus*) on chemical carcinogenesis in mice. Nutr Cancer 1991; 16:67–72.
194. Wang CJ, Lee MJ, Chang MC, Lin JK. Inhibition of tumor promotion in benzo[*a*]pyrene-initiated CD-1 mouse skin by crocetin. Carcinogenesis 1995; 16:187–191.
195. Wood AW, Huang MT, Chang RL, Newmark HL, Lehr RE, Yagi H, Sayer JM, Jerina DM, Conney AH. Inhibition of the mutagenicity of bay-region diol epoxides of polycyclic aromatic hydrocarbons by naturally occurring plant phenols: exceptional activity of ellagic acid. Proc Natl Acad Sci USA 1982; 79:5513–5517.
196. Mukhtar H, Del Tito B Jr, Marcelo CL, Das M, Bickers DR. Ellagic acid: a potent naturally occurring inhibitor of benzo[*a*]pyrene metabolism and its subsequent glucuronidation, sulfation and covalent binding to DNA in cultured BALB/c mouse keratinocytes. Carcinogenesis 1984; 5:1565–1571.
197. Majid S, Khanduja KL, Gandhi RK, Kapur S, Sharma RR. Influence of ellagic acid on antioxidant defense system and lipid peroxidation in mice. Biochem Pharmacol 1991; 42:1441–1445.
198. Gehm BD, McAndrews JM, Chien PY, Jameson JL, Resveratrol, a polyphenolic compound found in grapes and wine, is an agonist for the estrogen receptor. Proc Natl Acad Sci USA 1997; 94:14138.
199. Frankel EN, Waterhouse AL, Kinsella JE. Inhibition of human LDL oxidation by resveratrol. Lancet 1993; 341:1103–1104.
200. Kerry NL, Abbey M. Red wine and fractionated phenolic compounds prepared from red wine inhibit low density lipoprotein oxidation in vitro. Atherosclerosis 1997; 135:93.
201. Hsieh TC, Juan G, Darzynkiewicz Z, Wu JM. Resveratrol increases nitric oxide synthase, induces accumulation of p53 and p21 (WAF1/CIP1), and suppresses cultured bovine pulmonary artery endothelial cell proliferation by perturbing progression through S and G_2. Cancer Res 1999; 59:2596–2601.
202. Pace–Asciak CR, Hahn S, Diamandis EP, Soleas G, Goldberg DM. The red wine phenolics *trans*-resveratrol and quercetin block human platelet aggregation and eicosanoid synthesis: implications for protection against coronary heart disease. Clin Chim Acta 1995; 235:207.
203. Bertelli A, Giovannini AL, Giannessi D, Migliori M, Bernini W, Fregoni M, Bertelli A. Antiplatelet activity of synthetic and natural resveratrol in red wine. Int J Tissue React 1995; 17:1.

204. Hsieh TC, Burfeind P, Laud K, Backer JM, Traganos F, Darzynkiewicz Z, Wu M. Cell cycle effects and control of gene expression by resveratrol in human breast carcinoma cell lines with different metastatic potentials. Int J Oncol 1999; 15:245.
205. Hsieh TC, Wu JM. Differential effects on growth, cell cycle arrest, and induction of apoptosis by resveratrol in human prostate cancer lines. Exp Cell Res 1999; 249:109.
206. Subbaramaiah K, Chung WJ, Michaluart P, Telang N, Tanabe T, Inoue H, Jang M, Pezzuto JM, Dannenberg AJ. Resveratrol inhibits cyclooxygenase-2 transcription and activity in phorbol ester-treated human mammary epithelial cells. J Biol Chem 1998; 273:21875.
207. Jang M, Cai L, Udeani GO, Slowing KV, Thomas CF, Beecher CW, Fong HH, Farnsworth NR, Kinghorn AD, Mehta RG, Moon RC, Pezzuto JM. Cancer chemopreventive activity of resveratrol, a natural product derived from grapes. Science 1997; 275:218.
208. Ciolino HP, Daschner PJ, Yeh GC. Resveratrol inhibits transcription of CYP1A1 in vitro by preventing activation of the aryl hydrocarbon receptor. Cancer Res 1998; 58:5707.
209. Rimm EB. Alcohol consumption and coronary heart disease: good habits may be more important than just good wine. Am J Epidemiol 1996; 143:1094.
210. Zhang W, Lawa RE, Hintona DR, Su Y, Couldwell WT. Growth inhibition and apoptosis in human neuroblastoma SK-N-SH cells induced by hypericin, a potent inhibitor of protein kinase C. Cancer Lett 1995; 96:31–35.
211. Utsumi T, Okuma M, Kanno T, Takehara Y, Yoshioka T, Fujita Y, Horton AA, Utsumi K. Effect of the antiretroviral agent hypericin on rat liver mitochondria. Biochem Pharmacol 1995; 50:655–662.
212. Nishiuchi T, Utsumi T, Kanno T, Takehara Y, Kobuchi H, Yoshioka T, Horton AA, Yasuda T, Utsumi K. Inhibition of neutrophil superoxide generation by hypericin, an antiretroviral agent. Arch Biochem Biophys 1995; 323:335–342.
213. Tang J, Colacino JM, Larsen SH, Spitzer W. Virucidal activity of hypericin against enveloped and non-enveloped DNA and RNA viruses. Antiviral Res 1990; 13:313–325.
214. Schinazi RF, Chu CK, Babu JR, Oswald BJ, Saalmann V, Cannon DL, Eriksson BF, Nasr M. Anthraquinones as a new class of antiviral agents against human immunodeficiency virus. Antiviral Res 1990; 13:265–272.
215. Lavie G, Valentine F, Levin B, Mazur Y, Gallo G, Lavie D, Weiner D, Meruelo D. Studies of the mechanisms of action of the antiretroviral agents hypericin and pseudohypericin. Proc Natl Acad Sci USA 1989; 86:5963–5967.
216. Siebenlist U, Franzo G, Brown K. Structure, regulation and function of NF-kappa B. Annu Rev Cell Biol 1994; 10:405–455.
217. Baeuerle PA, Henkel T. Function and activation of NF-κB in the immune system. Annu Rev Immunol 1994; 12:141.
218. Soni KB, Lahiri M, Chackradeo P, Bhide SV, Kuttan R. Protective effect of food additives on aflatoxin-induced mutagenicity and hepatocarcinogenicity. Cancer Lett 1997; 19:115,129–133.
219. Soni KB, Kuttan R. Effect of oral curcumin administration on serum peroxides and cholesterol levels in human volunteers. Indian J Physiol Pharmacol 1992; 36:273–275.
220. Soudamini KK, Unnikrishnan MC, Soni KB, Kuttan R. Inhibition of lipid peroxidation and cholesterol levels in mice by curcumin. Indian J Physiol Pharmacol 1992; 36:239–243.
221. Nagabhushan M, Bhide SV. Curcumin as an inhibitor of cancer. J Am Coll Nutr 1992; 11:192–198.
222. Huang MT, Smart RC, Wong CQ, Conney AH. Inhibitory effect of curcumin, chlorogenic acid, caffeic acid, and ferulic acid on tumor promotion in mouse skin by 12-O-tetradecanoylphorbol-13-acetate. Cancer Res 1988; 48:5941–5946.
223. Lu YP, Chang RL, Lou YR, Huang MT, Newmark HL, Reuhl KR, Conney AH. Effect of curcumin on 12-O-tetradecanoylphorbol-13-acetate- and ultraviolet B light-induced expression of c-Jun and c-Fos in JB6 cells and in mouse epidermis. Carcinogenesis 1994; 15:2363–2370.
224. Kakar SS, Roy D. Curcumin inhibits TPA induced expression of c-*fos*, c-*jun* and c-*myc* proto-oncogenes messenger RNAs in mouse skin. Cancer Lett 1994; 87:85–89.
225. Deshpande SS, Ingle AD, Maru GB. Chemopreventive efficacy of curcumin-free aqueous turmeric extract in 7,12-dimethylbenz[*a*]anthracene-induced rat mammary tumorigenesis. Cancer Lett 1998; 123:35–40.
226. Menon LG, Kuttan R, Kuttan G. Anti-metastatic activity of curcumin and catechin. Cancer Lett 1999; 141:159–165.
227. Suresh BP, Srinivasan K. Amelioration of renal lesions associated with diabetes by dietary curcumin in streptozotocin diabetic rats. Mol Cell Biochem 1998; 181:87–96.

228. Sidhu GS, Mani H, Gaddipati JP, Singh AK, Seth P, Banaudha KK, Patnaik GK, Maheshwari RK. Curcumin enhances wound healing in streptozotocin induced diabetic rats and genetically diabetic mice. Wound Repair Regen 1999; 7:362–374.
229. Sajithlal GB, Chithra P, Chandrakasan G. Effect of curcumin on the advanced glycation and crosslinking of collagen in diabetic rats. Biochem Pharmacol 1998; 56:1607–1614.
230. Venkatesan N. Curcumin attenuation of acute Adriamycin myocardial toxicity in rats. Br J Pharmacol 1998;124:425–427.
231. Nirmala C, Anand S, Puvanakrishnan R. Curcumin treatment modulates collagen metabolism in isoproterenol induced myocardial necrosis in rats. Mol Cell Biochem 1999; 197:31–37.
232. Harvey JS, Davis S, James IF, Burgess GM. Activation of protein kinase C by the capsaicin analogue resiniferatoxin in sensory nerves. J Neurochem 1995; 65:1309.
233. Matucci–Cerinic M, Marabini S, Jantsch S, Cagnini M, Partsch G. Effects of capsaicin on the metabolism of rheumatoid arthritis synoviocytes in vitro. Ann Rheum Dis 1990; 49:598.
234. Nilsson G, Ahlstedt S. Altered lymphocyte proliferation of immunized rats after neurological manipulation with capsaicin. J Immunopharmacol 1988; 10:747.
235. Nilsson G, Alving K, Ahlstedt S. Effects of immune responses in rats after neuromanipulation with capsaicin. J Immunopharmacol 1991; 13:21.
236. Eglezos A, Andrews PV, Boyd RL, Helme RD. Effects of capsaicin treatment on immunoglobulin secretion in the rat: further evidence for involvement of tachykinin-containing afferent nerves. J Neuroimmunol 1990; 26:131.
237. Matucci–Cerinic M, McCarthy G, Lombardi A, Pignone A, Partsch G. Neurogenic influences in arthritis: potential modification by capsaicin. J Rheum 1995; 22:1447.
238. Holzer P. Capsaicin: cellular targets, mechanisms of action, and selectivity for thin sensory neurons. Pharmacol Rev 1994; 43:143.
239. Szallasi A. The vanilloid (capsaicin) receptor: receptor types and species differences. Gen Pharmacol 1994; 25:223.
240. Szallasi A, Sharkey NA, Blumberg PM. Structure/activity analysis of resiniferatoxin analogs. Phytother Res 1989; 3:253.
241. Szallasi A, Blumberg PM. Specific binding of resiniferatoxin, an ultrapotent capsaicin analog, by dorsal root ganglion membranes. Brain Res 1990; 524:106.
242. Szallasi A, Blumberg PM. Resiniferatoxin, a phorbol-related diterpene, acts as an ultrapotent analog of capsaicin, the irritant constituent in red pepper. Neuroscience 1989; 30:515.
243. Acs G, Lee J, Marquez VE, Wang S, Milne GWA, Du L, Lewin NE, Blumberg PM. Resiniferatoxin-amide and analogues as ligands for protein kinase C and vanilloid receptors and determination of their biological activities as vanilloids. J Neurochem 1995; 65:301.
244. Hautkappe M, Roizen MF, Toledano A, Roth S, Jeffries JA, Ostermeier AM. Review of the effectiveness of capsaicin for painful cutaneous disorders and neural dysfunction. Clin J Pain 1998; 14:97–106.
245. Bernstein JE, Parish LC, Rapaport M, Rosenbaum MM, Roenigk HH Jr. Effects of topically applied capsaicin on moderate and severe psoriasis vulgaris. J Am Acad Dermatol 1986; 15:504–507.
246. Tarng DC, Cho YL, Liu HN, Huang TP. Hemodialysis-related pruritus: a double-blind, placebo-controlled, crossover study of capsaicin on 0.025% cream. Nephron 1996; 72:617–622.
247. Szeimies RM, Stolz W, Wlotzke U, Korting HC, Landthaler M. Successful treatment of hydroxyethyl starch-induced pruritus with topical capsaicin. Br J Dermatol 1994; 131:380–382.
248. Knight TE, Hayashi T. Solar (brachioradial) pruritus—response to capsaicin cream [see comments]. Int J Dermatol 1994; 33:206–209.
249. Lotti T, Teofoli P, Tsampau D. Treatment of aquagenic pruritus with topical capsaicin cream. J Am Acad Dermatol 1994; 30:232–235.
250. Goodless DR, Eaglstein WH. Brachioradial pruritus: treatment with topical capsaicin. J Am Acad Dermatol 1993; 29:783–784.
251. Ellis CN, Berberian B, Sulica VI, Dodd WA, Jarratt MT, Kazt HI, Prawer S, Krueger G, Rex IH Jr, Wolf JE. A double-blind evaluation of topical capsaicin in pruritic psoriasis [see comments]. J Am Acad Dermatol 1993; 29:438–442.
252. Gronroos MA, Reunala T, Kartamaa M, Pertovaara A. Altered skin sensitivity in chronic itch: role of peripheral and central mechanisms. Neurosci Lett 1997; 228:199–202.
253. Stovner LJ, Sjaastad O. Treatment of cluster headache and its variants. Curr Opin Neurol 1995; 8:243–247.

254. Liano H, Lopez–Zuazo I. [Prophylactic treatment of episodic forms of cluster headache]. Rev Neurol 1995; 23(suppl 4):S525–S529.
255. Titus F. [Symptomatic treatment of cluster headache]. Rev Neurol 1995; 23(suppl 4):S519-S524.
256. Kumar KL. Recent advances in the acute management of migraine and cluster headaches. J Gen Intern Med 1994; 9:339–348.
257. Stammberger H, Wolf G. Headaches and sinus disease: the endoscopic approach. Ann Otol Rhinol Laryngol Suppl 1988; 134:3–23.
258. Marabini S, Ciabatti PG, Polli G, Fusco BM, Geppetti P. Beneficial effects of intranasal applications of capsaicin in patients with vasomotor rhinitis. Eur Arch Otorhinolaryngol 1991; 248:191–194.
259. De AK, Agarwal K, Mukherjee A, Sengupta D. Inhibition by capsaicin against cyclophosphamide-induced clastogenicity and DNA damage in mice. Mutat Res 1995; 335:253–258.
260. Surh YJ, Lee SS. Capsaicin, a double-edged sword: toxicity, metabolism, and chemopreventive potential. Life Sci 1995; 56:1845–1855.
261. Surh YJ, Lee RC, Park KK, Mayne ST, Liem A, Miller JA. Chemoprotective effects of capsaicin and diallyl sulfide against mutagenesis or tumorigenesis by vinyl carbamate and N-nitrosodimethylamine. Carcinogenesis 1995;16:2467–2471.
262. Park KK, Surh YJ. Effects of capsaicin on chemically-induced two-stage mouse skin carcinogenesis. Cancer Lett 1997; 19:114,183–184.
263. Chitra S, Viswanathan P, Nalini N, Sabitha K, Menon VP. Role of redchilli (*Capsaicin*) in the formation of colonic carcinoma. Indian J Pathol Microbiol 1997; 40:21–25.
264. Lopez–Carrillo L, Hernandez AM, Dubrow R. Chili pepper consumption and gastric cancer in Mexico: a case–control study. Am J Epidemiol 1994; 139:263–271.
265. Toth B, Gannett P. Carcinogenicity of lifelong administration of capsaicin of hot pepper in mice. In Vivo 1992; 6:59–63.
266. Agrawal RC, Wiessler M, Hecker E, Bhide SV. Tumour-promoting effect of chilli extract in BALB/c mice. Int J Cancer 1986; 38:689–695.
267. Jang JJ, Cho KJ, Lee YS, Bae JH. Different modifying responses of capsaicin in a wide-spectrum initiation model of F344 rat. J Korean Med Sci 1991; 6:31–36.
268. Sadhana AS, Rao AR, Kucheria K, Bijani V. Inhibitory action of garlic oil on the initiation of benzo[*a*]pyrene-induced skin carcinogenesis in mice. Cancer Lett 1988; 40:193–197.
269. Perchellet JP, Perchellet EM, Belman S. Inhibition of DMBA-induced mouse skin tumorigenesis by garlic oil and inhibition. Nutrition Cancer 1990; 14:183–193.
270. Perchellet JP, Gali HU, Perchellet EM, Klish DS, Armbrust AD. Antitumor-promoting activities of tannic acid, ellagic acid, and several gallic acid derivatives in mouse skin. Basic Life Sci 1992; 59:783–801.
271. Athar M, Raza H, Bickers DR, Mukhtar H. Inhibition of benzoyl peroxide-mediated tumor promotion in 7,12-dimethylbenz(*a*)anthracene-initiated skin of Sencar mice by antioxidants nordihydroguaiaretic acid and diallyl sulfide. J Invest Dermatol 1990; 94:162–165.
272. Dwivedi C, Rohlfs S, Jarvis D, Engineer FN. Chemoprevention of chemically induced skin tumor development by diallyl sulfide and diallyl disulfide. Pharm Res 1992; 9:1668–1670.
273. Singh A, Shukla Y. Antitumour activity of diallyl sulfide on polycyclic aromatic hydrocarbon-induced mouse skin carcinogenesis. Cancer Lett 1998; 131:209–214.
274. Singh A, Shukla Y. Antitumor activity of diallyl sulfide in two-stage mouse skin model of carcinogenesis. Biomed Environ Sci 1998; 11:258–263.
275. Wargovich MJ, Woods C, Eng VW, Stephens LC, Gray K. Chemoprevention of N-nitrosomethylbenzylamine-induced esophageal cancer in rats by the naturally occurring thioether, diallyl sulfide. Cancer Res 1988; 48:6872–6875.
276. Hu PJ, Wargovich MJ. Effect of diallyl sulfide on MNNG-induced nuclear aberrations and ornithine decarboxylase activity in the glandular stomach mucosa of the Wistar rat. Cancer Lett 1989; 47:153–158.
277. Hadjiolov D, Fernando RC, Schmeiser HH, Wiessler M, Hadjiolov N, Pirajnov G. Effect of diallyl sulfide on aristolochic acid-induced forestomach carcinogenesis in rats. Carcinogenesis 1993; 14:407–410.
278. Hong JY, Wang ZY, Smith TJ, Zhou S, Shi S, Pan J, Yang CS. Inhibitory effects of diallyl sulfide on the metabolism and tumorigenicity of the tobacco-specific carcinogen 4-(methylnitrosamino)-1-(3-pyridyl)-1-butanone (NNK) in A/J mouse lung. Carcinogenesis 1992; 13:901–904.

279. Takahashi S, Hakoi K, Yada H, Hirose M, Ito N, Fukushima S. Enhancing effects of diallyl sulfide on hepatocarcinogenesis and inhibitory actions of the related diallyl disulfide on colon and renal carcinogenesis in rats. Carcinogenesis 1992; 13:1513–1518.
280. Kim SG, Nam SY, Chung HC, Hong SY, Jung KH. Enhanced effectiveness of dimethyl-4,4′-dimethoxy-5,6,5′,6′-dimethylene dioxybiphenyl-2,2′-dicarboxylate in combination with garlic oil against experimental hepatic injury in rats and mice. J Pharm Pharmacol 1995; 47:678–682.
281. Wang EJ, Li Y, Lin M, Chen L, Stein AP, Reuhl KR, Yang CS. Protective effects of garlic and related organosulfur compounds on acetaminophen-induced hepatotoxicity in mice. Toxicol Appl Pharmacol 1996; 136:146–154.
282. Lin MC, Wang EJ, Patten C, Lee MJ, Xiao F, Reuhl KR, Yang CS. Protective effect of diallyl sulfone against acetaminophen-induced hepatotoxicity in mice. J Biochem Toxicol 1996; 11:11–20.
283. Bordia A, Verma SK, Srivastava KC. Effect of garlic on platelet aggregation in humans: a study in healthy subjects and patients with coronary artery disease. Prostaglandins Leukotr Essent Fatty Acids 1996; 55:201–205.
284. Laranjinha J, Vieira O, Madeira V, Almeida L. Two related phenolic antioxidants with opposite effects on vitamin E content in low density lipoproteins oxidized by ferrylmyoglobin: consumption vs. regeneration. Arch Biochem Biophys 1995; 323:373–381.
285. Kimura Y, Okuda H, Okuda T, Hatano T, Agata I, Arichi S. Studies on the activities of tannins and related compounds from medicinal plants and drugs. VII. Effects of extracts of leaves of *Artemisia* species, and caffeic acid and chlorogenic acid on lipid metabolic injury in rats fed peroxidized oil. Chem Pharm Bull 1985; 33:2028–2034.
286. Hlandon B, Bylka W, Ellnain–Wojtaszek M, Skrzypczak L, Szafarek P, Chodera A, Kowalevski Z. In vitro studies on the cytostatic activity of propolis extracts. Arzneimmittelforschung Drug Res 1980; 30:1847–1848.
287. Sugimoto K, Sakurai N, Fujise Y, Shirasawa H, Shibata K, Matsuo M, Takahashi T, Komori Y, Nikai T, Sugihara H. Identification of effective component from a traditional herbal medicine and the inhibitory effects on experimental glomerular lesion in mice. J Vet Med Sci 1992; 54:111–118.
288. Tanaka T, Kojima T, Kawamori T, Wang A, Suzui M, Okamoto K, Mori H. Inhibition of 4-nitroquinoline-1-oxide-induced rat tongue carcinogenesis by the naturally occurring plant phenolics caffeic, ellagic, chlorogenic and ferulic acids. Carcinogenesis 1993; 14:1321–1325.
289. Michaluart P, Masferrer JL, Carothers AM, Subbaramaiah K, Zweifel BS, Koboldt C, Mestre JR, Grunberger D, Sacks PG, Tanabe T, Dannenberg AJ. Inhibitory effects of caffeic acid phenethyl ester on the activity and expression of cyclooxygenase-2 in human oral epithelial cells and in a rat model of inflammation. Cancer Res 1999; 59:2347–2352.
290. Hirose M, Masuda A, Imaida K, Kagawa M, Tsuda H, Ito N. Induction of forestomach lesions in rats by oral administrations of naturally occurring antioxidants for 4 weeks. Jpn J Cancer Res 1987; 78:317–321.
291. Hirose M, Masuda A, Fukushima S, Ito N. Effects of subsequent antioxidant treatment on 7,12-dimethylbenz[*a*]anthracene-initiated carcinogenesis of the mammary gland, ear duct and forestomach in Sprague–Dawley rats. Carcinogenesis 1988; 9:101–104.
292. Hirose M, Mutai M, Takahashi S, Yamada M, Fukushima S, Ito N. Effects of phenolic antioxidants in low dose combination on forestomach carcinogenesis in rats pretreated with *N*-methyl-*N*′-nitro-*N*-nitrosoguanidine. Cancer Res 1991; 51:824–827.
293. Hirose M, Kawabe M, Shibata M, Takahashi S, Okazaki S, Ito N. Influence of caffeic acid and other *o*-dihydroxybenzene derivatives on *N*-methyl-*N*′-nitro-*N*-nitrosoguanidine-initiated rat forestomach carcinogenesis. Carcinogenesis 1992; 13:1825–1828.
294. Hagiwara A, Hirose M, Takahashi S, Ogawa K, Shirai T, Ito N. Forestomach and kidney carcinogenicity of caffeic acid in F344 rats and C57BL/6N × C3H/HeN F_1 mice. Cancer Res 1991; 51:5655–5660.
295. Lutz U, Lugli S, Bitsch A, Schlatter J, Lutz WK. Dose response for the stimulation of cell division by caffeic acid in forestomach and kidney of the male F344 rat. Fundam Appl Toxicol 1997; 39:131–137.
296. Hepsen IF, Bayramlar H, Gultek A, Ozen S, Tilgen F, Evereklioglu C. Caffeic acid phenethyl ester to inhibit posterior capsule opacification in rabbits. J Cataract Refract Surg 1997; 23:1572–1576.
297. Koltuksuz U, Ozen S, Uz E, Aydinc M, Karaman A, Gultek A, Akyol O, Gursoy MH, Aydin E. Caffeic acid phenethyl ester prevents intestinal reperfusion injury in rats. J Pediatr Surg 1999; 34:1458–1462.

298. Ilhan A, Koltuksuz U, Ozen S, Uz E, Ciralik H, Akyol O. The effects of caffeic acid phenethyl ester (CAPE) on spinal cord ischemia/reperfusion injury in rabbits. Eur J Cardiothorac Surg 1999; 16:458–463.
299. Huang HC, Chang JH, Tung SF, Wu RT, Foegh ML, Chu SH. Immunosuppressive effect of emodin, a free radical generator. Eur J Pharmacol 1992; 211:359–364.
300. Lin CC, Chang CH, Yang JJ, Namba T, Hattori M. Anti-inflammatory effects of emodin from *Ventilago leiocarpa*. Am J Chin Med 1996; 24:139–142.
301. Goel RK, Das GG, Ram SN, Pandey VB. Antiulcerogenic and anti-inflammatory effects of emodin, isolated from *Rhamnus triquerta* Wall. Indian J Exp Biol 1991; 29:230–232.
302. Chang CH, Lin CC, Yang JJ, Namba T, Hattori M. Anti-inflammatory effects of emodin from *Ventilago leiocarpa*. Am J Chin Med 1996; 24:139–142.
303. Chung JG, Wang HH, Wu LT, Chang SS, Chang WC. Inhibitory actions of emodin on arylamine N-acetyltransferase activity in strains of *Helicobacter pylori* from peptic ulcer patients. Food Chem Toxicol 1997; 35:1001–1007.
304. Lin CC, Chang CH, Yang JJ, Namba T, Hattori M. Hepatoprotective effects of emodin from *Ventilago leiocarpa*. J Ethnopharmacol 1996; 52:107–111.
305. Wang HH. Antitrichomonal action of emodin in mice. J Ethnopharmacol 1993; 40:111–116.
306. Langner E, Greifenberg S, Gruenwald J. Ginger: history and use. Adv Ther 1998; 15:25–44.
307. Grontved A, Brask T, Kambskard J, Hentzer E. Ginger root against seasickness. A controlled trial on the open sea. Acta Otolaryngol 1988; 105:45–49.
308. Kobayashi M, Shoji N, Ohizumi Y. Gingerol, a novel cardiotonic agent, activates the Ca^{2+}-pumping ATPase in skeletal and cardiac sarcoplasmic reticulum. Biochim Biophys Acta 1987; 903:96–102.
309. Micklefield GH, Redeker Y, Meister V, Jung O, Greving I, May B. Effects of ginger on gastroduodenal motility. Int J Clin Pharmacol Ther 1999; 37:341–346.
310. Srivastava KC, Mustafa T. Ginger (*Zingiber officinale*) and rheumatic disorders. Med Hypotheses 1989; 29:25–28.
311. Srivastava KC, Mustafa T. Ginger (*Zingiber officinale*) in rheumatism and musculoskeletal disorders. Med Hypotheses 1992; 39:342–348.
312. Sharma JN, Srivastava KC, Gan EK. Suppressive effects of eugenol and ginger oil on arthritic rats. Pharmacology 1994; 49:314–318.
313. Bone ME, Wilkinson DJ, Young JR, McNeil J, Charlton S. Ginger root—a new antiemetic. The effect of ginger root on postoperative nausea and vomiting after major gynaecological surgery [see comments]. Anaesthesia 1990; 45:669–671.
314. Phillips S, Ruggier R, Hutchinson SE. *Zingiber officinale* (ginger)—an antiemetic for day case surgery. Anaesthesia 1993; 48:715–717.
315. Meyer K, Schwartz J, Crater D, Keyes B. *Zingiber officinale* (ginger) used to prevent 8-MOP associated nausea. Dermatol Nurs 1995; 7:242–244.
316. Aikins MP. Alternative therapies for nausea and vomiting of pregnancy. Obstet Gynecol 1998; 91:149–155.
317. Katiyar SK, Agarwal R, Mukhtar H. Inhibition of tumor promotion in SENCAR mouse skin by ethanol extract of *Zingiber officinale* rhizome. Cancer Res 1996; 56:1023–1030.
318. Park KK, Chun KS, Lee JM, Lee SS, Surh YJ. Inhibitory effects of [6]-gingerol, a major pungent principle of ginger, on phorbol ester-induced inflammation, epidermal ornithine decarboxylase activity and skin tumor promotion in ICR mice [published erratum appears in Cancer Lett 1998 Sep 25;131(2):231]. Cancer Lett 1998; 129:139–144.
319. Budavari S, ed. The Merck Index. Rahway NJ: Merck & Co, 1996; 108–109.
320. Stohs SJ, Lawson TA, Anderson L, Bueding E. Effects of oltipraz, BHA, ADT and cabbage on glutathione metabolism, DNA damage and lipid peroxidation in old mice. Mech Ageing Dev 1986; 37:137–145.
321. Rudzki E, Grzywa Z. Sensitizing and irritating properties of star anise oil. Contact Dermatitis 1976; 2:305–308.
322. Kim SG, Liem A, Stewart BC, Miller JA. New studies on *trans*-anethole oxide and *trans*-asarone oxide. Carcinogenesis 1999; 20:1303–1307.
323. Naidum KA. Prostaglandin Leukotr Essen Fatty Acids 1995; 53:381–383.
324. Sharma JN, Srivastava KC, Gan EK. Suppressive effects of eugenol and ginger oil on arthritic rats. Pharmacology 1994; 49:314–318.

325. el Daly ES. Protective effect of cysteine and vitamin E, *Crocus sativus* and *Nigella sativa* extracts on cisplatin-induced toxicity in rats. J Pharm Belg 1998; 53:87–93.
326. Zhang Y, Shoyama Y, Sugiura M, Saito H. Effects of *Crocus sativus* L. on the ethanol-induced impairment of passive avoidance performances in mice. Biol Pharm Bull 1994; 17:217–221.
327. Gainer JL, Wallis DA, Jones JR. The effect of crocetin on skin papillomas and Rous sarcoma. Oncology 1976; 33:222–224.
328. Gainer JV Jr. Use of crocetin in experimental spinal cord injury. J Neurosurg 1977; 46:358–360.
329. Gainer JL, Rudolph DB, Caraway DL. The effect of crocetin on hemorrhagic shock in rats. Circ Shock 1993; 41:1–7.
330. Sugiura M, Shoyama Y, Saito H, Abe K. Crocin (crocetin di-gentiobiose ester) prevents the inhibitory effect of ethanol on long-term potentiation in the dentate gyrus in vivo. J Pharmacol Exp Ther 1994; 271:703–707.
331. Chow HY, Wang JC, Cheng KK. Cardiovascular effects of *Gardenia florida* L. (*Gardeniae fructus*) extract. Am J Chin Med 1976; 4:47–51.
332. Thresiamma KC, Kuttan R. Inhibition of liver fibrosis by ellagic acid. Indian J Physiol Pharmacol 1996; 40:363–366.
333. Tanaka T, Iwata H, Niwa K, Mori Y, Mori H. Inhibitory effect of ellagic acid on N-2-fluorenylacetamide-induced liver carcinogenesis in male ACI/N rats. Jpn J Cancer Res 1988; 79:1297–1303.
334. Stoner GD, Morse MA. Isothiocyanates and plant polyphenols as inhibitors of lung and esophageal cancer. Cancer Lett 1997; 19:114,113–119.
335. Siglin JC, Barch DH, Stoner GD. Effects of dietary phenethyl isothiocyanate, ellagic acid, sulindac and calcium on the induction and progression of N-nitrosomethylbenzylamine-induced esophageal carcinogenesis in rats. Carcinogenesis 1995; 16:1101–1106.
336. Mandal S, Stoner GD. Inhibition of N-nitrosobenzylmethylamine-induced esophageal tumorigenesis in rats by ellagic acid. Carcinogenesis 1990; 11:55–61.
337. Perchellet JP, Gali HU, Perchellet EM, Klish DS, Armbrust AD. Antitumor-promoting activities of tannic acid, ellagic acid, and several gallic acid derivatives in mouse skin. Basic Life Sci 1992; 59:783–801.
338. Mukhtar H, Das M, Bickers DR. Inhibition of 3-methylcholanthrene-induced skin tumorigenicity in BALB/c mice by chronic oral feeding of trace amounts of ellagic acid in drinking water. Cancer Res 1986; 46:2262–2265.
339. Mukhtar H, Das M, Del TB Jr, Bickers DR. Protection against 3-methylcholanthrene-induced skin tumorigenesis in Balb/C mice by ellagic acid. Biochem Biophys Res Commun 1984; 119:751–757.
340. Lesca P. Protective effects of ellagic acid and other plant phenols on benzo[*a*]pyrene-induced neoplasia in mice. Carcinogenesis 1983; 4:1651–1653.
341. Khanduja KL, Gandhi RK, Pathania V, Syal N. Prevention of N-nitrosodiethylamine-induced lung tumorigenesis by ellagic acid and quercetin in mice. Food Chem Toxicol 1999; 37:313–318.
342. Hassoun EA, Walter AC, Alsharif NZ, Stohs SJ. Modulation of TCDD-induced fetotoxicity and oxidative stress in embryonic and placental tissues of C57BL/6J mice by vitamin E succinate and ellagic acid. Toxicology 1997; 19:124,27–37.
343. Mohandas KM, Gopalakrishnan G. Mucocutaneous exposure to body fluids during digestive endoscopy: the need for universal precautions. Indian J Gastroenterol 1999; 18:109–111.
344. Soleas GJ, Diamandis EP, Goldberg DM. Resveratrol: a molecule whose time has come? And gone? Clin Biochem 1997; 30:91.
345. Hain R, Bieseler B, Kindl H, Schroder G, Stocker R. Expression of a stilbene synthase gene in *Nicotiana tabacum* results in synthesis of the phytoalexin resveratrol. Plant Mol Biol 1990; 15:325.
346. Langcake P, Pryce RJ. A new class of phytoalexins from grapevines. Experientia 1977; 33:151.
347. Goldberg DM, Hahn SE, Parkes JG. Beyond alcohol: beverage consumption and cardiovascular mortality. Clin Chim Acta 1995 237:155.
348. Fontecave M, Lepoivre M, Elleingand E, Gerez C, Guittet O. Resveratrol, a remarkable inhibitor of ribonucleotide reductase. FEBS Lett 1998; 421:277.
349. Sun NJ, Woo SH, Cassady JM, Snapka RM. DNA polymerase and topoisomerase II inhibitors from *Psoralea corylifolia*. J Natl Prod 1998; 61:362.
350. Mgbonyebi OP, Russo J, Russo IH. Antiproliferative effect of synthetic resveratrol on human breast epithelial cells. Int J Oncol 1998; 12:865.

351. Clement MV, Hirpara JL, Chawdhury SH, Pervaiz S. Chemopreventive agent resveratrol, a natural product derived from grapes, triggers CD95 signaling-dependent apoptosis in human tumor cells. Blood 1998; 92:996–1002.
352. Jang M, Pezzuto JM. Effects of resveratrol on 12-O-tetradecanoylphorbol-13-acetate-induced oxidative events and gene expression in mouse skin. Cancer Lett 1998; 134:81–89.
353. Manna SK, Zhang HJ, Yan T, Oberley LW, Aggarwal BB. Overexpression of Mn-superoxide dismutase suppresses TNF induced apoptosis and activation of nuclear transcription factor-κB and activated protein-1. J Biol Chem 1998; 273:13245–13254.
354. Manna SK, Mukhopadhyay A, Aggarwal BB. Resveratrol suppresses TNF-induced activation of nuclear transcription factors NF-kB, activator protein-1, and apoptosis: potential role of reactive oxygen intermediates and lipid peroxidation. J Immunol 2000; 164:6509–6519.
355. Li N, Karin M. Is NF-κB the sensor of oxidative stress? FASEB J 1999; 13:1137–1143.
356. Kumar A, Aggarwal BB. Assay for redox sensitive kinases. Methods Enzymol 1999; 300:339–345.
357. Jang M, Cai L, Udeani GO, Slowing KV, Thomas CF, Beecher CW, Fong HH, Farnsworth NR, Kinghorn AD, Mehta RG, Moon RC, Pezzuto JM. Cancer chemopreventive activity of resveratrol, a natural product derived from grapes. Science 1997; 275:218–220.
358. Jang M, Pezzuto JM. Effects of resveratrol on 12-O-tetradecanoylphorbol-13-acetate-induced oxidative events and gene expression in mouse skin. Cancer Lett 1998; 134:81–89.
359. Carbo N, Costelli P, Baccino FM, Lopez–Soriano FJ, Argiles JM. Resveratrol, a natural product present in wine, decreases tumour growth in a rat tumour model. Biochem Biophys Res Commun 1999; 254:739–743.
360. Jager U, Nguyen–Duong H. Relaxant effect of *trans*-resveratrol on isolated porcine coronary arteries. Arzneimittelforschung 1999; 49:207–211.
361. Weisburger JH. Mechanisms of action of antioxidants as exemplified in vegetables, tomatoes and tea. Food Chem Toxicol 1999; 37:943–948.
362. Das DK, Sato M, Ray PS, Maulik G, Engelman RM, Bertelli AA, Bertelli A. Cardioprotection of red wine: role of polyphenolic antioxidants. Drugs Exp Clin Res 1999; 25:115–120.
363. Soleas GJ, Diamandis EP, Goldberg DM. Wine as a biological fluid: history, production, and role in disease prevention. J Clin Lab Anal 1997; 11:287–313.
364. Goldberg DM, Hahn SE, Parkes JG. Beyond alcohol: beverage consumption and cardiovascular mortality. Clin Chim Acta 1995; 237:155–187.
365. Ray PS, Maulik G, Cordis GA, Bertelli AA, Bertelli A, Das DK. The red wine antioxidant resveratrol protects isolated rat hearts from ischemia reperfusion injury. Free Radic Biol Med 1999; 27:160–169.

23

Lipoic Acid: Cellular Metabolism, Antioxidant Activity, and Clinical Relevance

Oren Tirosh and Sashwati Roy
University of California, Berkeley, California

Lester Packer
University of Southern California School of Pharmacy, Los Angeles, California

I. INTRODUCTION

R-α-Lipoic acid (R-LA) is a naturally occurring compound present as a cofactor in several mitochondrial enzymes that are involved in metabolism and energy production. α-Lipoic acid (LA) was first isolated in 1951 by Reed and colleagues (1). It is an eight-carbon compound containing two sulfur atoms in a dithiolane ring structure. The two enantiomers of LA are the S form and the R form (Fig. 1). In its free form, LA is a powerful antioxidant, functioning as a reactive oxygen species scavenger.

When taken orally as a supplement or administered in vitro, LA is rapidly adsorbed and taken up into cells where it is reduced to the more active form, dihydrolipoic acid (DHLA). The uptake of LA has been studied in the perfused rat liver and isolated hepatocytes (2). Two different transport mechanisms were reported: carrier-mediated uptake, which is prominent below 75 μM, and passive diffusion, which is prominent at higher concentrations (2). Recently, the pharmacokinetic properties of LA were elucidated and reported in healthy human adults (3). These investigators reported a nonsaturable clearance kinetics of LA up to 600 mg of oral dose. Therefore, area under the curve (AUC) recovered following 200- or 600-mg oral dose of LA was the same. The absolute bioavailability after the 200-mg dose was 29.1 $\pm$ 10.3% and the plasma $t_{1/2}$ was approximately 30 min for intravenous or oral administration (3).

II. LIPOIC ACID IN BIOENERGETICS: ENZYMES CONTAINING R-LIPOIC ACID AND THEIR BIOLOGICAL ROLE

Energy production by mitochondria is primarily dependent on several enzymatic dehydrogenase complexes possessing the ability to utilize different substrates that are imported to the mitochon-

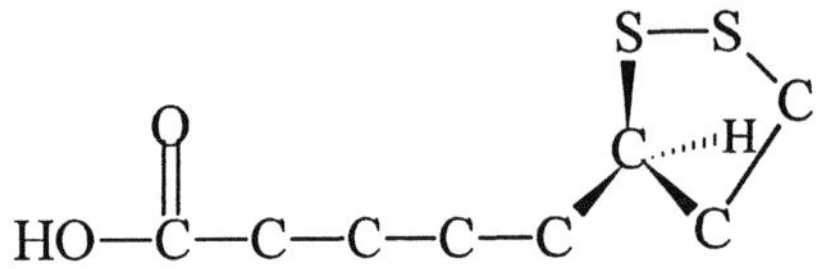

Figure 1 Molecular structures of R- and S-α-lipoic acid.

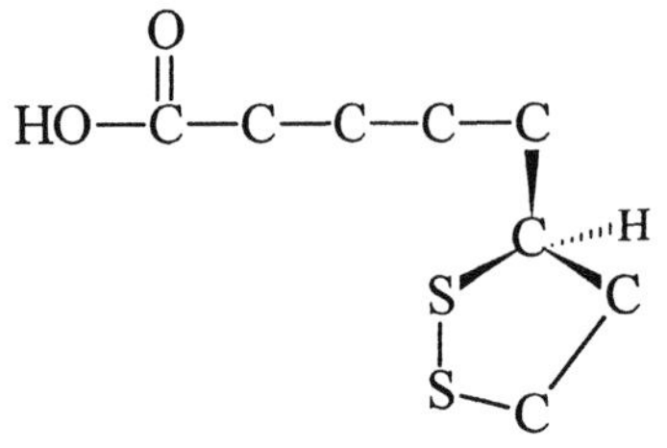

dria for NAD$^+$ and FAD reduction to NADH and FADH$_2$, respectively. These molecules are capable of donating electrons to the mitochondrial electron transport chain system embedded along the mitochondria inner membrane.

In human cells, R-LA is present in a bound lipoyllysine form in mitochondrial proteins that play a central role in oxidative metabolism (4). R-LA is the naturally occurring cofactor in five mitochondrial proteins: acyltransferase component of the pyruvate complex; α-ketoglutarate; branched-chain α-ketoacid dehydrogenase complexes (E2P, E2O, and E2B, respectively); protein X of the pyruvate dehydrogenase complex; and the H-protein of the glycine cleavage system. Reed et al. (5) found that lipoyl-AMP is the intermediate for the activation of R-LA-containing proteins. Lipoyltransferases I and II both catalyzed the lipoylation of the apoH-protein in a reaction that is absolutely dependent on lipoyl-AMP. K_m values obtained with lipoyltransferases I and II for lipoyl-AMP were 13 and 16 μM and for apoH protein were 0.29 and 0.17 μM, respectively. Recently, it has been shown that lipoyltransferases I and II lipoylate not only H-protein of the glycine cleavage system, but also lipoyl domains of E2P, E2O, and E2B (6). Incorporation of R-LA into these proteins is always in the ε-amino group of a specific lysine residue of the protein by an amide linkage. This lipoyllysine residue functions as a carrier for intermediates and products of the protein-specific reaction, and also as a redox agent interacting with other reducing equivalents in the active sites of the complexes.

The family of the 2-oxo acid dehydrogenase multienzyme complexes is located in the mitochondria of living eukaryotic cells and catalyzes the oxidative decarboxylation of various 2-oxo acid substrates in glycolysis, the citric acid cycle, and branched-chain amino acid metabolism (7,8). The pyruvate dehydrogenase (PDH) complex comprises three enzymes that make up the assembly. These enzymes are: pyruvate decarboxylase (E1P), dihydrolipoyl acetyltransferase (E2P), and dihydrolipoyl dehydrogenase (E3). For the 2-oxoglutarate dehydrogenase (2OGDH) complex, the corresponding enzymes are 2-oxoglutarate decarboxylase (E1O), dihydrolipoyl succiniltransferase (E2O), and dihydrolipoamide dehydrogenase (E3). The three, short, branched-chain 2-oxo acids produced by transamination of the amino acid leucine, isoleucine, and valine are oxidatively decarboxylated by a single multienzyme complex of comparable structure.

Lipoic acid is a cofactor of pyruvate dehydrogenase complex (PDC) that catalyzes the overall reaction

$$\text{Pyruvate} + \text{CoA} + \text{NAD}^+ \leftrightarrow \text{acetyl-CoA} + \text{NADH} + \text{H}^+$$

The PDH (E1) is the first catalytic component of the PDC. E1 catalyzes the following two partial reactions: thiamin pyrophosphate (TPP)-dependent decarboxylation of pyruvic acid to 2-hydroxyethylidene-TPP (HETPP) and reductive acetylation of lipoic acid residues covalently linked to the second catalytic component of the dihydrolipoamide acetyltransferase (E2).

PDC in many higher eukaryotes is regulated by the phosphorylation–dephosphorylation cycle carried out by specific regulatory enzymes: E1-kinase (E2-X-kinase) and phospho-E1-phosphatase (8). Three serine residues [site 1 (ser-204), site 2 (ser-271), and site 3 (ser-203)] belonging to the E1α subunit of mammalian PDC are phosphorylated (9). Phosphorylation of site 1 correlated with major inactivation of the enzyme. However, the role of sites 2 and 3 phosphorylation in the inactivation of the enzyme in the presence of active site 1 is unclear (10).

The E2 enzyme of the mammalian PDC contains a lipoyllysine residue and an organized acetyltransferase activity in its COOH-terminal inner domain. The E2 subunit of mammalian PDC has four domains connected by a relatively large (2–3 kDa) and highly mobile linker region. In an E2 assembly, 60 inner domains, $E2_I$, associate to form a dodecahedral inner core structure. Three globular domains outside the core are connected by the linker or hinge regions. The globular domains consist of two 10-kDa lipoyl domains designated $E2_{L1}$ and $E2_{L2}$ (L1 or L2) and an E1-binding domain, designated $E2_B$ (11).

The high rate of the kinase and phosphatase function is regulated by whether they or their appropriate E1 substrates are bound to the E2 core. The enhanced activity of the kinase is due to its ability to move between L2 domains by a reversible Ca^{2+}-requiring association. Feedback shutdown of PDC reaction is mediated by marked stimulation of the kinase activity owing to an NADH-dependent reduction and acetyl-CoA-dependent acetylation of the lipoyl group of L2 (11).

The third part of the PDH complex is dihydrolipoamide dehydrogenase (12). Dihydrolipoamide dehydrogenase belongs to the family of the homodimeric FAD-dependent disulfide oxidoreductases, and its main function is to reoxidize DHLA at the prosthetic group of the E2P enzyme back to lipoate utilizing NAD^+ and producing NADH. The enzyme is insensitive to inhibition by NADH (13). Enzyme 3 or E3 is usually a common name for the enzyme that can reduce LA to DHLA, although the acid form of LA compared with the amide-bearing form of LA is a very poor substrate for the enzyme (12,14). Other lipoamide dehydrogenases that are not part of the PDH complex have been reported; for example, two lipoamide dehydrogenases from Archaebacteria have been purified and characterized (15–17). These enzymes were not associated with any of the ketoacid dehydrogenase complexes, but could be associated with the glycine cleavage complex.

The *R*-enantiomer is the natural substrate of the complex. The biphasic kinetic profile of the reduction of racemic-LA was explained by a rapid reaction with the *R*-enantiomer, while the slow phase could be due to much slower reduction of the *S*-enantiomer. However, the *S*-enantiomer has previously been shown to be a better substrate for mammalian glutathione reductase (18). In humans, a single gene codes for lipoamide dehydrogenase (19). Therefore, E3 deficiency causes reduction in the activities of all three α-ketoacid dehydrogenase complexes involved as well as in the glycine cleavage system (12).

An important question is whether a direct supplementation of LA can induce higher incorporation into the relevant proteins in the different tissues. Free LA (racemic mixture) sup-

Table 1 Lipoyllysine Content in Rat Liver[a]

	Control rest	LA rest	Control ex	LA ex
Untrained	0.543 ± 0.105	0.409 ± 0.062	0.675 ± 0.202	0.209 ± 0.066
Trained	1.107 ± 0.731	0.479 ± 0.148	1.123 ± 0.285	1.408 ± 0.406

[a]The lipollysine (μM/g dry wt) was measured in resting rats and following exercise (Ex). Two groups of animal were tested for the effect of lipoate (LA): untrained and trained rats were subjected to endurance treadmill exercise training.
Source: Ref. 20.

plementation to rats did not induce an increase in the incorporation of LA into proteins in different tissues. However, physical exercise dramatically increased lipoyllysine content in rat liver (Table 1), but not that in rat muscles. These data, as suggested by the authors of the study, imply that proteins containing LA are up-regulated following physical exercise (20).

III. ANTIOXIDANT ACTIVITY OF LIPOIC ACID

Lipoic acid in its free form and its reduced form DHLA can function together as a strong redox couple. It has been suggested that the antioxidant properties of LA are due to its reduced form (21). Antioxidant effects of DHLA and LA were investigated in vitro based on their interactions with (1) peroxyl radicals, which are essential for the initiation of lipid peroxidation; (2) chromanoxyl radicals of vitamin E; and (3) ascorbyl radicals of vitamin C. It was demonstrated that (1) DHLA (but not LA) was an efficient, direct scavenger of peroxyl radicals generated in the aqueous phase by the water-soluble azoinitiator 2,2'-azobis(2-amidinopropane)dihydrochloride (AAPH), and in liposomes or in microsomal membranes by the lipid-soluble azoinitiator 2,2'-azobis(2,4-dimethylvaleronitrile) (AMVN); (2) neither DHLA or LA interacts directly with chromanoxyl radicals of vitamin E (or its synthetic homologues) generated in liposomes or in the membranes either by UV-irradiation, peroxyl radicals of 2,2'-azobis(2,4-dimethylvaleronitrile), or peroxyl radicals of linolenic acid formed by the lipoxygenase-catalyzed oxidation; and (3) DHLA (but not LA) recycled ascorbyl radicals and reduced dehydroascorbate generated in the course of ascorbate oxidation by chromanoxyl radicals. This interaction resulted in ascorbate-mediated DHLA-dependent reduction of the vitamin E chromanoxyl radicals (i.e., vitamin E recycling). Therefore, dihydrolipoic acid may act as a strong chain-breaking antioxidant and may enhance the antioxidant potency of other antioxidants (ascorbate and vitamin E) in both the aqueous as well as in the hydrophobic membrane phase (21). The ability of LA to function as an antioxidant and its ability to protect has also been demonstrated in vivo. Using an animal model for vitamin E deficiency in adult animals (hairless mice), LA supplementation was reduced to DHLA in tissues, protecting the animals against vitamin E-deficiency symptoms (22).

One of the important properties of LA as an antioxidant in living cells is that its activation and reduction to an antioxidant is regulated by metabolic pathways of the cell. Reduction of LA in cells to its antioxidant from DHLA can modulate the rest of the cellular-reducing equivalent homeostasis. Direct evidence describing the influence of LA on the levels of cellular-reducing equivalents and homeostasis of the NAD(P)H/NAD(P)$^+$ ratio has been reported (23). Twenty-four–hour treatment of the human T-cell line with LA (0.5 mM) resulted in a decrease in cellular NADH, NADPH levels, NADH/NAD$^+$, lactate/pyruvate, and an increase in glucose uptake. A decrease in the NADH/NAD$^+$ ratio following treatment with LA may have direct implications in diabetes, ischemia–reperfusion injury, and other pathologies where reductive (high NADH/NAD$^+$ ratio) and oxidant (excess reactive oxygen species) imbalances are considered as major factor contributing to metabolic disorders. Under conditions of reductive stress, LA decreases high NADH levels in the cell by utilizing it as a cofactor for its own reduction process, whereas in oxidative stress, both α-lipoate and its reduced form, dihydrolipoate, may protect by direct scavenging of free radicals and the recycling of other antioxidants from their oxidized forms (21). The metabolic antioxidant properties of LA were demonstrated by its ability to up-regulate the overall free thiol status in T cells treated with LA (24) and to specifically increase the synthesis of the ubiquitous thiol-bearing tripeptide glutathione in cultured human Jurkat T cells, human erythrocytes, C6 glial cells, NB41A3 neuroblastoma cells, and peripheral blood lymphocytes (25). The metabolic antioxidant effect of LA was dependent on reduction of LA to DHLA following its release into the culture medium where it reduces cystine to cysteine (Fig. 2). Cysteine thus formed is readily taken up by the neutral amino acid transport system and used for glutathione (GSH) synthesis. The antioxidant protective effects of LA were also demonstrated in the brain damage model in which C6 glial (26) and HT4 neuronal cells (14,27) exposed to high levels of glutamate were protected by micromolar concentrations of LA. LA was also effective as a neuron protector in vivo. The effect of thiol antioxidants (such as LA and the isopropyl ester of GSH) was examined on the morbidity and mortality of rats subjected to reperfusion following cerebral ischemia induced by occlusion of the bilateral carotid artery and hypotension. The GSH isopropyl ester had no significant protective effect, but after pretreatment of rats, LA was detected in the rat brain and dramatically reduced the mortality rate (28). LA also was reported to improve the memory of old mice, probably by a partial compensation of NMDA receptor deficits. A possible mode of action of LA was assumed to be based on its free radical scavenger and antioxidant properties (29) (reviewed in Ref. 30).

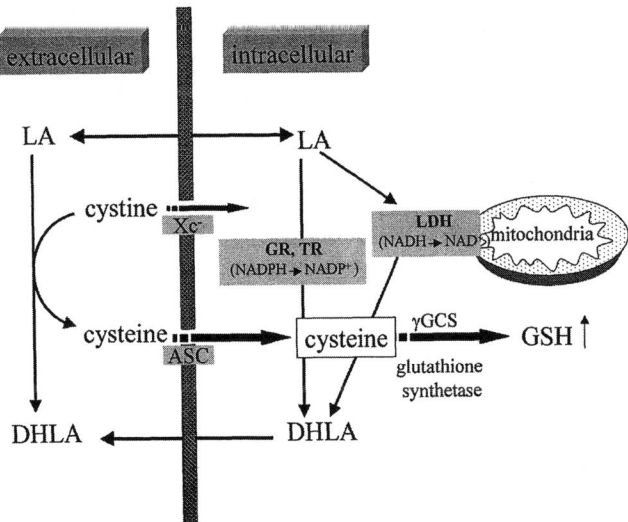

Figure 2 Cellular pathways for the bioreduction of α-lipoic acid (LA) to dihydrolipoic acid (DHLA) and lipoate-mediated up-regulation of cellular glutathione (GSH) biosynthesis by increase in cysteine bioavailability. TR, thioredoxin reductase; GR, glutathione reductase; γGCS, γ-glutamyl cysteine synthetase; LDH, lipoamide dehydrogenase.

In living cells, reduction of LA to DHLA, the potent antioxidant form, take place by enzymatic processes; therefore, the stereochemistry of LA obviously plays an important role. Several enzymes have been reported to reduce LA to DHLA. These enzymes are lipoamide dehydrogenase, an enzyme highly specific to the R-enantiomer of LA; glutathione reductase, which has higher specificity for the S-enantiomer (18,31); and thioredoxin reductase (32). In various tissues the reduction of LA to DHLA is a crucial process for its antioxidant activity. Haramaki et al. (33) investigated mechanisms of LA reduction. In the mitochondria, NADH-dependent dihydrolipoamide dehydrogenase exhibited a marked preference for $R(+)$-lipoate, whereas NADPH-dependent glutathione reductase showed slightly greater activity toward the $S(-)$-lipoate stereoisomer. In the rat liver cytosol, NADPH-dependent reduction was greater than NADH. In rat heart, kidney, and brain—whole cell-soluble fractions—NADH-dependent reduction was more pronounced (70–90%) than NADPH, whereas in liver extracts, NADH and NADPH contributed equally to the reduction. An intact organ study showed that in isolated perfused rat heart, the reduction of R-LA was six to eight times higher than that of S-LA. These data correlate with high mitochondrial dihydrolipoamide dehydrogenase activity in isolated cardiac mitochondria. On the other hand, erythrocytes, which lack mitochondria, reduced S- more actively than R-LA. These results demonstrate stereospecific differences in the rate of reduction by various cells and tissues. Mechanisms of reduction of α-lipoate are highly tissue-specific, and effects of exogenously supplied α-lipoate are determined by tissue glutathione reductase and dihydrolipoamide dehydrogenase activity (33).

IV. CELLULAR GLUCOSE METABOLISM

Non–insulin-dependent diabetes mellitus (NIDDM), also referred to as type II diabetes, is the most common of all metabolic disorders. NIDDM affects about 6–7% of the U.S. population, with a cumulative risk of 17% by age 80. The metabolic derangement created by chronic hyperglycemia, in addition to a strong association between NIDDM, obesity, hypertension, and hyperlipidemia, lead to an extensive list of long-term complications. This complication includes a high rate of cardiovascular death and amputation owing to accelerated atherosclerosis, as well as the typical complications of diabetes, such as retinopathy, nephropathy, and neuropathy (34).

Normal glucose homeostasis depends on several factors: the ability of tissues to take up glucose in response to insulin (insulin sensitivity; S_i); the ability of cells to take up glucose in the absence of insulin (insulin-independent glucose uptake, sometimes referred to as glucose sensitivity; S_g); and the ability of the pancreatic β-cells to control this process by both rapid and sustained insulin secretion (i.e., first- and second-phase insulin secretion). Pathophysiologically, patients with NIDDM exhibit two defects: the first is a decrease in response of peripheral tissues to insulin (i.e., insulin resistance); the second is a failure of the β-cell to compensate for the insulin resistance by appropriately increasing insulin secretion (34).

The effects of LA on glucose metabolism and utilization has been the subject of several investigations. In general LA can be designated as a natural (the R-enantiomer) low molecular weight compound that can alleviate the side effects of diabetes (e.g., diabetic polyneuropathy) (35–39). However, LA has been considered also as a glucose-lowering agent in diabetic conditions (40–43). The hypoglycemic effect of LA may be independent of its antioxidant properties.

A. Lipoic Acid as a Hypoglycemic Agent

Lipoic acid improves insulin action of skeletal muscle glucose transport and metabolism in both human and animal models of diabetes. One of the cases in which LA is beneficial is in patients who develop insulin resistance. Insulin resistance of skeletal muscle glucose uptake is a prominent feature of type II diabetes (NIDDM). In one of the first clinical studies to show that LA increases insulin-stimulated glucose disposal in NIDDM, Jacob et al. (41) demonstrated that LA enhances glucose utilization. *R*-LA supplementation (1000 mg/day) to 13 patients resulted in a significant increase of insulin-stimulated glucose disposal. The metabolic clearance rate (MCR) for glucose rose by about 50%. This suggested that *R*-LA has a potential use as a hypoglycemic agent.

In obese Zucker (*fa/fa*) rats, an animal model of muscle insulin resistance, treatments with a racemic mixture of LA improved glucose metabolism in insulin-resistant skeletal muscle. Glucose transport activity, net glycogen synthesis, and glucose oxidation were significantly improved. Prolonged LA treatment increased both insulin-stimulated glucose oxidation (33%) and glycogen synthesis (38%) and was associated with a significantly greater (21%) in vivo muscle glycogen concentration. These adaptive responses after long-term LA administration were also associated with significantly lower (15–17%) plasma levels of insulin and free fatty acids. No significant effects on glucose transporter (GLUT4) protein level or on the activities of hexokinase and citrate synthase were observed (40). These findings indicate that LA significantly enhances the capacity of the insulin-stimulatable glucose transport system and of both oxidative and nonoxidative pathways of glucose metabolism in insulin-resistant rat skeletal muscle.

In a study conducted in L6 myotubes, the *R*-enantiomer of LA was able to stimulate glucose uptake in cytokine-treated cells that are insulin-resistant. This study shows that cytokine-induced glucose uptake in skeletal muscle cells is redox sensitive and that, under the conditions of acute infection that often accompanies insulin resistance, LA may have therapeutic implications in restoring glucose availability in tissues such as the skeletal muscle (44).

Facilitation of glucose uptake by the different enantiomers of LA was studied in L6 muscle cells and 3T3-L1 adipocytes in culture (45). Glucose uptake was rapidly increased by *R*-LA, which was superior to the effect elicited by the *S*-isomer or the racemic mixture and was comparable with that caused by insulin. In parallel to insulin action, the stimulation of glucose uptake by LA dependent on phosphatidylinositol-3-kinase (PI-3k) and the stimulatory effect of *R*-LA on glucose uptake was associated with an intracellular redistribution of GLUT1 and GLUT4 glucose transporters. LA stimulates basal glucose transport and has a positive effect on insulin-stimulated glucose uptake (45). A similar effect of LA in streptozocin (STZ)-induced diabetic rats was observed in vivo. Blood glucose concentration in STZ-diabetic rats following 10 days of intraperitoneal injection of LA (30 mg/kg) was reduced and crude membrane GLUT4 protein was elevated both in control and in diabetic rats treated with LA by 1.5- and 2.8-fold, respectively, without significant changes in GLUT4 mRNA levels. LA treatment prevented the impairment in insulin stimulation of 2-deoxyglucose (2-DG) uptake in soleus muscle isolated from diabetic rats compared with nondiabetic control animals. The insulin-response of glucose uptake after LA treatment was, in fact, comparable with that of nondiabetic animals (42).

B. Lipoic Acid as an Antidiabetic Neuropathy Agent

Peripheral neuropathy affects at least 15% of all patients with diabetes and 37% of 18 years or older patients with insulin-dependent diabetes mellitus (46). The hallmark of diabetic neuropathy is distal sensorimotor polyneuropathy. Clinical neuropathy is the culmination of progressive damage and loss of nerve fibers and is detectable by nerve conduction and autonomic nervous system tested (47,48).

A growing body of evidences suggests that oxidative stress resulting from enhanced free radical formation or defects in antioxidant defense is implicated in the development of diabetic complication (49–51). Treatment with LA results in prevention of some neurovascular abnormalities associated with experimental diabetic neuropathy (52). One mechanism of reduced nerve blood flow is the inhibitory effect of superoxide anions on NO concentrations, and LA might prevent this inhibition by reducing oxidative stress (52).

The effects of LA on diabetic neuropathy were studied in two multicenter, randomized, double-blind placebo-controlled trials. In one study, 328 patients with NIDDM and symptomatic peripheral neuropathy were orally supplemented by 1200 mg/day for 19 days. This regimen reduced the total symptom score (pain, burning, paresthesia, and numbness) in the feet. In patients with NIDDM and cardiac autonomic neuropathy diagnosed by reduced heart rate variability, 800 mg/day of LA for 4 months improved heart rate variability at rest (37–39).

V. REGULATION OF THE AGING PROCESS

Micronutrients, such as lipoic acid, folic acid, vitamins B_{12}, B_6, niacin, C, E, and iron or zinc, are required in the human diet. Remedying the micronutrient deficiencies is likely to lead to a major improvement in health and an increase in longevity. Aging appears to be due, in good part, to the oxidants produced by mitochondria as by-products of normal metabolism (53). In old rats mitochondrial membrane potential, cardiolipin levels, respiratory control ratio, and overall cellular O_2 consumption are lower than these in the young rats, and the level of oxidants (per unit O_2) is higher. The level of mutagenic aldehydes from lipid peroxidation is also increased. Ambulatory activity declines markedly in old rats (53). A diet supplemented with R-LA or S-LA was fed to old rats to determine their efficacy in reversing the decline in metabolism seen with age. Young and old rats supplemented with R-LA (0.5% w/w) were also studied for age-related biochemical and behavioral parameters (54). Hepatocytes from untreated old rats versus young controls had significantly lower oxygen consumption and mitochondrial membrane potential. R-LA, but not S-LA, supplementation reversed the age-related decline in O_2 consumption and increased mitochondrial membrane potential. Ambulatory activity, a measure of general metabolic activity, was almost threefold lower in untreated old rats versus controls, but this decline was reversed in old rats that were fed R-LA. The increase of oxidants with age, as measured by the fluorescence produced on oxidizing $2',7'$-dichlorofluorescin, was significantly lower in R-LA-supplemented old rats. Lipid peroxidation was increased fivefold with age in cells from unsupplemented rats. R-LA diet reduced lipid peroxidation levels markedly. Both glutathione and ascorbic acid levels declined in hepatocytes with age, but their loss was completely reversed with R-LA supplementation. Thus, R-LA supplementation was shown to improve indices of metabolic activity and lower the oxidative stress and damage, as evidenced in aging (54).

VI. REDOX REGULATION OF GENE EXPRESSION AND CELL FUNCTION

A. Effect of LA on Transcription Factor NF-κB

The redox-sensitive transcription factor NF-κB is a pleiotropic regulator of many genes involved in immune and inflammatory responses, including cell adhesion molecules, such as intracellular adhesion molecule 1 (ICAM-1). Treatment of cells with thiol antioxidants inhibit agonist-induced activation of NF-κB (55–57). LA treatment in combination with α-tocopherol inhibited ultraviolet radiation-induced activation of NF-κB better than the use of the antioxidants separately (58). Oxidatively modified human low-density lipoproteins (LDL) can also serve as a signal for activation of inflammatory responses in endothelial and other cells by activating the nuclear transcription factor NF-κB. Lipoate was observed to substantially decrease Cu^{2+}-induced oxidative modification of LDL (59).

Oxidative stress-dependent NF-κB activation in patients with diabetic nephropathy in ex vivo, isolated peripheral blood mononuclear cells was demonstrated to occur (60). Patients with diabetic nephropathy showed higher NF-κB–binding activity in electrophoretic mobility shift assays and stronger immunohistological staining for activated NF-κB p65 than in patients without renal complications (Fig. 3). Following a 3-day intervention study in which 600 mg of LA per day was given to nine patients with diabetic nephropathy, oxidative stress in plasma was decreased by 48% and NF-κB–binding activity in ex vivo, isolated peripheral blood mononuclear cells was inhibited by 38% (see Fig. 3) (60).

B. Regulation of Cell Adhesion Processes by LA

Cell adhesion molecule expression and adhesive properties of cells are greatly modified in several conditions such as cancer, atherosclerosis, diabetes, chronic inflammation, and ischemia–reperfusion injury. LA, at clinically relevant doses (50–100 μM) down-regulated phorbol-12-myristate-13-acetate–induced adhesion molecule (e.g., intracellular adhesion molecule-1; ICAM-1) expression and adhesion of leukocytes to endothelial cells. Inhibition of agonist-induced ICAM-1 expression and cell–cell adhesion was more pronounced when a combination of LA and tocopherol was used compared with the use of either of these antioxidants alone (61). These results are consistent with the findings showing that LA inhibits agonist-induced NF-κB activation, as NF-κB is known to positively regulate agonist-induced ICAM expression.

C. LA and Programmed Cell Death

Somatic cells possess the potential for self-destruction by activation of an intrinsic death pathway, which is usually turned on when cells are no longer needed or have become seriously

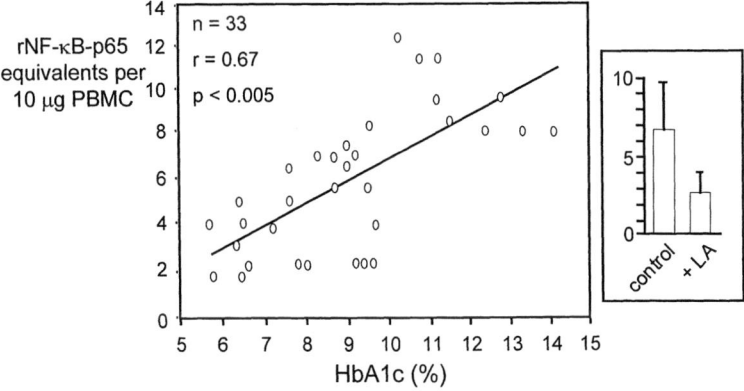

Figure 3 (Right) 10 μg nuclear extract of PBMC from 33 IDDM patients with normoalbuminuria and without any diabetic late complications were assayed for NF-κB–binding activity using EMSA. The signal was expressed as microgram (μg)rNF-κBp65 equivalents by using the internal standard curves of rNF-κBp65. Correlation of NF-κB–binding activity with HbA1c values was 0.67, $p < 0.005$. (Left) Effect of 600-mg lipoic acid treatment of IDDM patients for 2 weeks on NF-κB activation in PBMC. (From Ref. 60.)

damaged. This death-execution biological cascade, which was designated as apoptosis, is often associated with morphological and biochemical changes (62,63). During apoptosis the nucleus and cytoplasm are condensed, and the dying cells are disintegrated into membrane-bound apoptotic bodies. Nucleases are activated, and cause the degradation of chromosomal DNA, at first into large chromosomal DNA (50–300 kb), and finally into very small oligonucleosomal fragments (62,63).

Recent reports have implicated the involvement of intracellular excess of reactive oxygen species in the initiation of apoptotic cell death in acquired immune deficiency syndrome (AIDS). In AIDS patients, chronic inflammation and elevated levels of cytokines seem to be associated with reduced levels of glutathione (GSH). Antioxidant and especially thiol antioxidant treatment may thus prevent, or at least slow down, such apoptotic death of T cells. Indeed GSH and N-acetylcysteine inhibit the reverse transcriptase (RT) process of HIV-1 (24,64–66). LA is a potent inhibitor of the human immunodeficiency virus-1 (HIV-1) replication in immune system cells. This effect of LA was attributed to its potent antioxidant activity (67–69). Because the death of T cells in AIDS can be seen as an apoptotic cell death process, it is of significance to elucidate the effect of LA in apoptotic cell death.

Rat thymocytes that were pretreated with low and clinically relevant concentrations of LA for 2 h, after which apoptosis was induced by treating the cells with etoposide (25 μM). Lipoate at concentrations (50–100 μM) was able to protect against typical nuclear alterations that occur in etoposide-treated cells, suggesting protective effects of lipoate in etoposide-induced apoptosis (unpublished data). The antiapoptotic effect of LA was extensively augmented by a chemical modification of LA. A novel positively charged amide–amine analogue of R-LA (R-LA-plus) was effective in preventing thymocytes' apoptosis at concentration of 5 μM (70).

Fas receptor-mediated killing of tumor cells is a novel strategy that is being explored for cancer therapy. Activation of cysteine death proteases, caspases, is required in all apoptosis. Maintenance of a reducing environment inside the cell has been suggested to be necessary for caspase activity during apoptosis. Exploring the possibility to potentiate Fas-mediated killing of tumor cells by LA revealed that treatment of cells with 100 μM lipoate for 72 h markedly potentiated Fas-mediated apoptosis of leukemic Jurkat cells, but not that of peripheral blood lymphocytes from healthy humans. This work provides evidence that a commonly used nutritional antioxidant potentiates Fas-mediated apoptosis of leukemic cells. With recombinant caspase-3, it was observed that DHLA can markedly enhance this enzyme's activity (71).

The data from the different cell death models suggest that LA is a unique compound that, in some cases, can exacerbate cell death; however, it can also rescue cells and protect against apoptotic insults. The redox-signaling and cell function regulation were studied mainly using the racemic lipoate. Further studies are currently in progress to elucidate whether the R- and S-enantiomers have the same biological activity and potency.

VII. CATARACT AND LIPOIC ACID

Over 95% of the dry mass of the eye lens consists of specialized proteins called crystallins. Lenses are subject to cataract formation (especially during aging and in diabetes), in which damage, cross-linking, and precipitation of crystallins contribute to loss of lens clarity. Cataract is one of the major causes of blindness, and it is estimated that over 50 million people suffer from this disability. In young lens, the combination of antioxidants and proteases serves to prevent crystallin damage and precipitation involved in cataract formation (72).

There are ample amounts of experimental evidence that free radicals are involved in the development of cataractogenesis. Supporting experimental evidence are (1) H_2O_2 is significantly increased two- to threefold in ocular humors in several experimental cataract models and in human senile (age-related) cataract. Various cataractogenic agents also increase H_2O_2 in ocular humors in vivo before cataract formation. (2) Enzymatic defenses against $O_2^{-\cdot}$ and H_2O_2 provided by superoxide dismutase, catalase, and glutathione peroxidase were impaired in lenses with cataracts. (3) Malondialdehyde (MDA), a breakdown product of lipid peroxides significantly increased (two- to fourfold) in human senile cataract, in cataract induced in rabbit and rat, and in hereditary cataract in mice. (4) Biological antioxidants, such as vitamin E, afforded prevention of lipid peroxidation in lens and in arresting experimental cataract induced in rabbits by 3-aminotriazole (5). A connection has been made between improved uptake of antioxidant and mitigation of the cataract prognosis (73–77).

Oxygen free radicals appear to impair not only lens crystallins, which will aggregate and precipitate forming lens opacities, but also proteolytic enzyme activity, the function of which is to eliminate the damaged proteins (78). Crystallins that experience mild oxidative damage are rapidly degraded by a system of lenticular proteases. However, extensive oxidation and cross-linking severely decrease proteolytic susceptibility of lens crystallins (72).

Several studies have demonstrated beneficial effects of LA in prevention and treatment of cataract. Cysteine-elevating precursor drugs (prodrugs) were tested on lens damage occurring after in vitro exposure to low levels of ^{60}Co-gamma-irradiation, R-α-lipoic acid (1 mM), protected against radiation-associated protein leakage, indicating that antioxidants and prodrugs of cysteine appear to offer protection against lens damage caused by low level radiation (79).

The effect of R, S, and racemic forms of LA was tested on the formation of opacity in normal rat lenses incubated with 55.6 mM of glucose, as a model for ex vivo diabetic cataractogenesis. Opacity formation and LDH leakage, resulting from incubation in medium containing 55.6 mM of glucose, were both suppressed by the addition of 1 mM R-lipoic acid. Compared with R-LA, addition of 1 mM racemic lipoic acid reduced these damaging effects to the lens by one-half, whereas S-LA potentiated LDH leakage. These data are consistent with the hypothesis that R-LA is the active form. Stereospecific protection against hyperglycemia-induced opacity is consistent with specific reduction of R-LA in mitochondria of the vulnerable cells at the lens equator where the first globular degeneration is seen in glucose cataract (80). Two hypotheses were investigated for the mechanism of prevention of opacity by R-LA: (1) increased glucose uptake by the lens, leading to increased glycolysis and release of lactate into the incubation medium, or (2) maintenance of glutathione levels by the R-LA. The data did not support the former hypothesis, but was consistent with the later one. The concentrations of glutathione in normal lenses or lenses incubated with R- or racemic-LA were not significantly different from each other, but the concentration of glutathione in lenses incubated with S-LA was significantly lower than that of the R-LA-incubated lenses (81). In newborn rats, R- and racemic LA decreased cataract formation induced by buthionine sulfoximine (BSO) by 55 and 40%, respectively. S-LA had no effect on cataract formation induced by BSO. BSO lowers cellular glutathione by inhibiting the glutathione synthesis. The lens antioxidants glutathione, ascorbate, and vitamin E were depleted to 45, 62, and 23% of control levels, respectively, by BSO treatment, but were maintained at 84–97% of control levels when R-LA or racemic-LA were coadministered with BSO. S-LA administration had no protective effect on lens antioxidants. When enantiomers of LA were administered to animals, R-LA was taken up by lens and reached concentrations two- to sevenfold higher than those of S-LA, with racemic-LA reaching levels midway between the R-isomer and racemic form. DHLA, reached the highest levels in lens of the racemic-LA-treated animals and the lowest levels in S-LA-treated animals. The stereospecificity in the protective effect of R-LA was probably due to selective uptake and reduction of R-LA by the lens cells (82).

VIII. CONCLUDING REMARKS

This chapter summarized in part half a century of LA research. Some of the beneficial properties of this micronutrient were not addressed. Since, the popularity and the interest in LA as an antioxidant are rising, there is, therefore, a need for better understanding of the pharmacology of this compound. Frequently, the two enantiomers of LA the *R*- and the *S*-forms do not have the same potency and biological efficacy. Occasionally, the biological effects exerted by one enantiomer were contradicted by the other form. However, so far *R*-LA, which is the natural form of LA, was superior and with more potent pharmacological activity than *S*-LA in all of in vitro models and clinical experiments. The two enantiomers of LA should be looked on as two different pharmacological agents, antioxidants, or drugs.

REFERENCES

1. Reed JL, et al. (1951) Crystalline α-lipoic acid: a catalitic agent associated with pyruvate dehydrogenase. Science 114:93–94.
2. Peinado J, H Sies, TP Akerboom. (1989) Hepatic lipoate uptake. Arch Biochem Biophys 273:389–395.
3. Teichert J, J Kern, HJ Tritschler, H Ulrich, R Preiss. (1998) Investigations on the pharmacokinetics of alpha-lipoic acid in healthy volunteers. Int J Clin Pharmacol Ther 36:625–628.
4. Reed LJ. (1998) From lipoic acid to multi-enzyme complexes. Protein Sci 7:220–224.
5. Reed LJ, FR Leach, M Koike. (1958) Studies on a lipoic acid-activating system. J Biol Chem 232:123–142.
6. Fujiwara K, K Okamura–Ikeda, Y Motokawa. (1996) Lipoylation of acyltransferase components of alpha-ketoacid dehydrogenase complexes. J Biol Chem 271:12932–12936.
7. Perham RN. (1991) Domains, motifs, and linkers in 2-oxo acid dehydrogenase multienzyme complexes: a paradigm in the design of a multifunctional protein. Biochemistry 30:8501–8512.
8. Patel MS, TE Roche. (1990) Molecular biology and biochemistry of pyruvate dehydrogenase complexes. FASEB J 4:3224–3233.
9. Yeaman SJ, ET Hutcheson, TE Roche, FH Pettit, JR Brown, LJ Reed, DC Watson, GH Dixon. (1978) Sites of phosphorylation on pyruvate dehydrogenase from bovine kidney and heart. Biochemistry 17:2364–2370.
10. Sugden PH, AL Kerbey, PJ Randle, CA Waller, KB Reid. (1979) Amino acid sequences around the sites of phosphorylation in the pig heart pyruvate dehydrogenase complex. Biochem J 181:419–426.
11. Roche TE, S Liu, S Ravindran, JC Baker, L Wang. (1996) Role of the E2 core in the dominant mechanisms of regulatory control of mammalian pyruvate dehydrogenase complex. In: M Patel, TE Roche, RA Harris, eds. alpha-Keto Acid. Dehydrogenase Complexes. Basel: Birkhauser, 33–52.
12. de Kok A, WJH van Berkel. (1996) Lipoamide dehydrogenase. In: M Patel, TE Roche, RA Harris, eds. alpha-Keto Acid Dehydrogenase Complexes. Basel: Birkhauser, 53–67.
13. Snoep JL, M van Bommel, F Lubbers, MJ Teixeira de Mattos, OM Neijssel. (1993) The role of lipoic acid in product formation by *Enterococcus faecalis* NCTC 775 and reconstitution in vivo and in vitro of the pyruvate dehydrogenase complex. J Gen Microbiol 139:1325–1329.
14. Tirosh O, CK Sen, S Roy, MS Kobayashi, L Packer. (1999) Neuroprotective effects of alpha-lipoic acid and its positively charged amide analogue. Free Radic Biol Med. 26:1418–1426.
15. Vettakkorumakankav N, MJ Danson, DW Hough, KJ Stevenson, M Davison, J Young. (1992) Dihydrolipoamide dehydrogenase from the halophilic archaebacterium *Haloferax volcanii*: characterization and *N*-terminal sequence. Biochem Cell Biol 70:70–75.
16. Vettakkorumakankav NN, KJ Stevenson. (1992) Dihydrolipoamide dehydrogenase from *Haloferax volcanii*: gene cloning, complete primary structure, and comparison to other dihydrolipoamide dehydrogenases. Biochem Cell Biol 70:656–663.
17. Danson MJ, R Eisenthal, S Hall, SR Kessell, DL Williams. (1984) Dihydrolipoamide dehydrogenase from halophilic Archaebacteria. Biochem J 218:811–818.
18. Pick U, N Haramaki, A Constantinescu, GJ Handelman, HJ Tritschler, L Packer. (1995) Glutathione reductase and lipoamide dehydrogenase have opposite stereospecificities for alpha-lipoic acid enantiomers. Biochem Biophys Res Commun 206:724–730.

19. Otulakowski G, BH Robinson, HF Willard. (1988) Gene for lipoamide dehydrogenase maps to human chromosome 7. Somat Cell Mol Genet 14:411–414.
20. Khanna S, M Atalay, JK Lodge, DE Laaksonen, S Roy, O Hanninen, L Packer, CK Sen. (1998) Skeletal muscle and liver lipoyllysine content in response to exercise, training and dietary alpha-lipoic acid supplementation. Biochem Mol Biol Int 46:297–306.
21. Kagan VE, A Shvedova, E Serbinova, S Khan, C Swanson, R Powell, L Packer. (1992) Dihydrolipoic acid—a universal antioxidant both in the membrane and in the aqueous phase. Reduction of peroxyl, ascorbyl and chromanoxyl radicals. Biochem Pharmacol 44:1637–1649.
22. Podda M, HJ Tritschler, H Ulrich, L Packer. (1994) alpha-Lipoic acid supplementation prevents symptoms of vitamin E deficiency. Biochem Biophys Res Commun 204:98–104.
23. Roy S, CK Sen, HJ Tritschler, L Packer. (1997) Modulation of cellular reducing equivalent homeostasis by alpha-lipoic acid. Mechanisms and implications for diabetes and ischemic injury. Biochem Pharmacol 53:393–399.
24. Sen CK, S Roy, D Han, L Packer. (1997) Regulation of cellular thiols in human lymphocytes by alpha-lipoic acid: a flow cytometric analysis. Free Radic Biol Med 22:1241–1257.
25. Han D, G Handelman, L Marcocci, CK Sen, S Roy, H Kobuchi, HJ Tritschler, L Flohe, L Packer. (1997) Lipoic acid increases de novo synthesis of cellular glutathione by improving cystine utilization. Biofactors 6:321–338.
26. Han D, CK Sen, S Roy, MS Kobayashi, HJ Tritschler, L Packer. (1997) Protection against glutamate-induced cytotoxicity in C6 glial cells by thiol antioxidants. Am J Physiol 273:R1771–R1778.
27. Kobayashi MS, D Han, L Packer. (1999) Antioxidants and herbal extracts protect HT-4 neuronal cells against glutamate-induced cytotoxicity. Free Radic Res (in press).
28. Panigrahi M, Y Sadguna, BR Shivakumar, SV Kolluri, S Roy, L Packer, V Ravindranath. (1996) alpha-Lipoic acid protects against reperfusion injury following cerebral ischemia in rats. Brain Res 717:184–188.
29. Stoll S, H Hartmann, SA Cohen, WE Muller. (1993) The potent free radical scavenger alpha-lipoic acid improves memory in aged mice: putative relationship to NMDA receptor deficits. Pharmacol Biochem Behav 46:799–805.
30. Packer L, HJ Tritschler, K Wessel. (1997) Neuroprotection by the metabolic antioxidant alpha-lipoic acid. Free Radic Biol Med 22:359–378.
31. Constantinescu A, U Pick, GJ Handelman, N Haramaki, D Han, M Podda, HJ Tritschler, L Packer. (1995) Reduction and transport of lipoic acid by human erythrocytes. Biochem Pharmacol 50:253–261.
32. Arner ES, J Nordberg, A Holmgren. (1996) Efficient reduction of lipoamide and lipoic acid by mammalian thioredoxin reductase. Biochem Biophys Res Commun 225:268–274.
33. Haramaki N, D Han, GJ Handelman, HJ Tritschler, L Packer. (1997) Cytosolic and mitochondrial systems for NADH- and NADPH-dependent reduction of alpha-lipoic acid. Free Radic Biol Med 22:535–542.
34. Kahn CR, D Vincent, A Doria. (1996) Genetics of non–insulin-dependent (type-II) diabetes mellitus. Annu Rev Med 47:509–531.
35. Biewenga G, GR Haenen, A Bast. (1997) The role of lipoic acid in the treatment of diabetic polyneuropathy. Drug Metab Rev 29:1025–1054.
36. Wiznitzer A, N Ayalon, R Hershkovitz, M Khamaisi, EA Reece, H Trischler, N Bashan. (1999) Lipoic acid prevention of neural tube defects in offspring of rats with streptozocin-induced diabetes. Am J Obstet Gynecol 180:188–193.
37. Ziegler D, FA Gries. (1997) alpha-Lipoic acid in the treatment of diabetic peripheral and cardiac autonomic neuropathy. Diabetes 46(suppl 2):S62–S66.
38. Ziegler D, H Schatz, F Conrad, FA Gries, H Ulrich, G Reichel. (1997) Effects of treatment with the antioxidant alpha-lipoic acid on cardiac autonomic neuropathy in NIDDM patients. A 4-month randomized controlled multicenter trial (DEKAN study). Deutsche Kardiale Autonome Neuropathie [see comments]. Diabetes Care 20:369–373.
39. Ziegler D, M Hanefeld, KJ Ruhnau, HP Meissner, M Lobisch, K Schutte, FA Gries. (1995) Treatment of symptomatic diabetic peripheral neuropathy with the anti-oxidant alpha-lipoic acid. A 3-week multicentre randomized controlled trial (ALADIN study). Diabetologia. 38:1425–1433.
40. Jacob S, RS Streeper, DL Fogt, JY Hokama, HJ Tritschler, GJ Dietze, EJ Henriksen. (1996) The antioxidant alpha-lipoic acid enhances insulin-stimulated glucose metabolism in insulin-resistant rat skeletal muscle. Diabetes. 45:1024–1029.

41. Jacob S, EJ Henriksen, AL Schiemann, I Simon, DE Clancy, HJ Tritschler, WI Jung, HJ Augustin, GJ Dietze. (1995) Enhancement of glucose disposal in patients with type 2 diabetes by alpha-lipoic acid. Arzneimittelforschung 45:872–874.
42. Khamaisi M, R Potashnik, A Tirosh, E Demshchak, A Rudich, H Tritschler, K Wessel, N Bashan. (1997) Lipoic acid reduces glycemia and increases muscle GLUT4 content in streptozotocin-diabetic rats. Metabolism 46:763–768.
43. Khamaisi M, A Rudich, R Potashnik, HJ Tritschler, A Gutman, N Bashan. (1999) Lipoic acid acutely induces hypoglycemia in fasting nondiabetic and diabetic rats. Metabolism 48:504–510.
44. Khanna S, S Roy, L Packer, CK Sen. (1999) Cytokine-induced glucose uptake in skeletal muscle: redox regulation and the role of alpha-lipoic acid. Am J Physiol 276:R1327–1333.
45. Estrada DE, HS Ewart, T Tsakiridis, A Volchuk, T Ramlal, H Tritschler, A Klip. (1996) Stimulation of glucose uptake by the natural coenzyme alpha-lipoic acid/thioctic acid: participation of elements of the insulin signaling pathway. Diabetes 45:1798–1804.
46. Dyck PJ, PC O'Brien. (1989) Meaningful degrees of prevention or improvement of nerve conduction in controlled clinical trials of diabetic neuropathy. Diabetes Care 12:649–652.
47. Greene DA, AF Sima, MA Pfeifer, JW Albers. (1990) Diabetic neuropathy. Annu Rev Med 41:303–317.
48. American Diabetes Association, American Academy of Neurology. (1988) Consensus statement: report and recommendations of the San Antonio conference on diabetic neuropathy. Diabetes Care. 11:592–607.
49. Baynes JW. (1991) Role of oxidative stress in development of complications in diabetes. Diabetes 40:405–412.
50. Cameron NE, MA Cotter. (1994) The relationship of vascular changes to metabolic factors in diabetes mellitus and their role in the development of peripheral nerve complications. Diabetes Metab Rev 10:189–224.
51. Cameron NE, MA Cotter, V Archibald, KC Dines, and EK Maxfield. (1994) Anti-oxidant and pro-oxidant effects on nerve conduction velocity, endoneurial blood flow and oxygen tension in non-diabetic and streptozotocin-diabetic rats. Diabetologia 37:449–459.
52. Nagamatsu M, KK Nickander, JD Schmelzer, A Raya, DA Wittrock, H Tritschler, PA Low. (1995) Lipoic acid improves nerve blood flow, reduces oxidative stress, and improves distal nerve conduction in experimental diabetic neuropathy. Diabetes Care 18:1160–1167.
53. Ames BN. (1998) Micronutrients prevent cancer and delay aging. Toxicol Lett 102–103:5–18.
54. Hagen TM, RT Ingersoll, J Lykkesfeldt, J Liu, CM Wehr, V Vinarsky, JC Bartholomew, AB Ames. (1999) (R)-alpha-Lipoic acid-supplemented old rats have improved mitochondrial function, decreased oxidative damage, and increased metabolic rate. FASEB J 13:411–418.
55. Sen CK, L Packer. (1996) Antioxidant and redox regulation of gene transcription [see comments]. FASEB J 10:709–720.
56. Packer L, S Roy, CK Sen. (1997) alpha-Lipoic acid: a metabolic antioxidant and potential redox modulator of transcription. Adv Pharmacol 38:79–101.
57. Packer L. (1998) alpha-Lipoic acid: a metabolic antioxidant which regulates NK-kappa B signal transduction and protects against oxidative injury. Drug Metab Rev 30:245–275.
58. Saliou C, M Kitazawa, L McLaughlin, JP Yang, JK Lodge, T Tetsuka, K Iwasaki, J Cillard, T Okamoto, L Packer. (1999) Antioxidants modulate acute solar ultraviolet radiation-induced NF-kappa-B activation in a human keratinocyte cell line. Free Radic Biol Med. 26:174–183.
59. Lodge JK, MG Traber, L Packer. (1998) Thiol chelation of Cu^{2+} by dihydrolipoic acid prevents human low density lipoprotein peroxidation. Free Radic Biol Med. 25:287–297.
60. Hofmann MA, S Schiekofer, B Isermann, M Kanitz, M Henkels, M Joswig, A Treusch, M Morcos, T Weiss, V Borcea, AK Abdel Khalek, J Amiral, H Tritschler, E Ritz, P Wahl, R Ziegler, A Bierhaus, PP Nawroth. (1999) Peripheral blood mononuclear cells isolated from patients with diabetic nephropathy show increased activation of the oxidative-stress sensitive transcription factor NF-kappaB. Diabetologia 42:222–232.
61. Roy S, CK Sen, H Kobuchi, L Packer. (1998) Antioxidant regulation of phorbol ester-induced adhesion of human Jurkat T-cells to endothelial cells. Free Radic Biol Med 25:229–241.
62. Steller H. (1995) Mechanisms and genes of cellular suicide. Science 267:1445–1449.
63. Nagata S. (1997) Apoptosis by death factor. Cell 88:355–365.
64. Kameoka M, Y Okada, M Tobiume, T Kimura, K Ikuta. (1996) Intracellular glutathione as a possible direct blocker of HIV type 1 reverse transcription. AIDS Res Hum Retroviruses 12:1635–1638.

65. Opalenik SR, Q Ding, SR Mallery, JA Thompson. (1998) Glutathione depletion associated with the HIV-1 TAT protein mediates the extracellular appearance of acidic fibroblast growth factor. Arch Biochem Biophys 351:17–26.
66. Repetto M, C Reides, ML Gomez Carretero, M Costa, G Griemberg, S Llesuy. (1996) Oxidative stress in blood of HIV infected patients. Clin Chim Acta 255:107–117.
67. Merin JP, M Matsuyama, T Kira, M Baba, T Okamoto. (1996) alpha-Lipoic acid blocks HIV-1 LTR-dependent expression of hygromycin resistance in THP-1 stable transformants. FEBS Lett 394:9–13.
68. Grieb G. (1992) [alpha-Lipoic acid inhibits HIV replication]. Med Monatsschr Pharm 15:243–244.
69. Baur A, T Harrer, M Peukert, G Jahn, JR Kalden, B Fleckenstein. (1991) alpha-Lipoic acid is an effective inhibitor of human immuno-deficiency virus (HIV-1) replication. Klin Wochenschr 69:722–724.
70. Sen CK, O Tirosh, S Roy, MS Kobayashi, L Packer. (1998) A positively charged alpha-lipoic acid analogue with increased cellular uptake and more potent immunomodulatory activity. Biochem Biophys Res Commun 247:223–228.
71. Sen CK, R Sashwati, L Packer. (1999) Fas mediated apoptosis of human jurkat T-cells: Intracellular events and potentiation by redox-active alpha-lipoic acid. Cell Death Differ 6:481–491.
72. Taylor A, K Davies. (1987) Protein oxidation and loss of protease activity may lead to cataract formation in the aged lens. Free Radic Biol Med 3:371–377.
73. Bhuyan KC, DK Bhuyan. (1984) Molecular mechanism of cataractogenesis: III. Toxic metabolites of oxygen as initiators of lipid peroxidation and cataract. Curr Eye Res 3:67–81.
74. Taylor A, T Nowell. (1997) Oxidative stress and antioxidant function in relation to risk for cataract. Adv Pharmacol 38:515–536.
75. Taylor A. (1992) Effect of photooxidation on the eye lens and role of nutrients in delaying cataract. Exs. 62:266–279.
76. Taylor A. (1993) Cataract: relationship between nutrition and oxidation. J Am Coll Nutr 12:138–146.
77. Taylor A, PF Jacques, EM Epstein. (1995) Relations among aging, antioxidant status, and cataract. Am J Clin Nutr 62:1439S–1447S.
78. Gerster H. (1989) Antioxidant vitamins in cataract prevention. Z Ernahrungswiss 28:56–75.
79. Bantseev V, R Bhardwaj, W Rathbun, H Nagasawa, JR Trevithick. (1997) Antioxidants and cataract: (cataract induction in space environment and application to terrestrial aging cataract). Biochem Mol Biol Int 42:1189–1197.
80. Kilic F, GJ Handelman, E Serbinova, L Packer, JR Trevithick. (1995) Modelling cortical cataractogenesis 17: in vitro effect of a lipoic acid on glucose-induced lens membrane damage, a model of diabetic cataractogenesis. Biochem Mol Biol Int 37:361–370.
81. Kilic F, GJ Handelman, K Traber, K Tsang, L Packer, JR Trevithick. (1998) Modelling cortical cataractogenesis XX. In vitro effect of alpha-lipoic acid on glutathione concentrations in lens in model diabetic cataractogenesis. Biochem Mol Biol Int 46:585–595.
82. Maitra I, E Serbinova, HJ Tritschler, L Packer. (1996) Stereospecific effects of R-lipoic acid on buthionine sulfoximine-induced cataract formation in newborn rats. Biochem Biophys Res Commun 221:422–429.

24

Cellular Effects of Lipoic Acid and Its Role in Aging

Régis Moreau, Wei-Jian Zhang, and Tory M. Hagen
Linus Pauling Institute, Oregon State University, Corvallis, Oregon

I. INTRODUCTION

There is increasing and compelling evidence that reactive oxygen species (ROS), produced as by-products of mitochondrial respiration and by reaction with metal ions, are a significant contributor to aging and to pathological conditions associated with aging. Various therapeutic strategies have been proposed to lower the deleterious consequences that age-related oxidative damage has on cell and organ function. These strategies include dietary supplementation of antioxidants, such as vitamins C and E, or chelation therapies to remove redox-active metal ions that would convert rather innocuous ROS (superoxide or hydrogen peroxide) to more reactive and deleterious free radicals (hydroxyl radicals).

Herein, we review the evidence showing the role of ROS in the aging process and how dietary supplementation with lipoic acid (LA), a naturally occurring dithiol compound, may be an effective means to maintain or improve health. The reduced form of lipoic acid, dihydrolipoic acid (DHLA), is a powerful antioxidant, transition metal chelator, and can reverse the age-associated decline in endogenous antioxidants, including vitamin C and glutathione. These properties make lipoic acid a potentially useful compound, not only to combat the effects of aging per se, but also for conditions associated with age. In the last part of this chapter, we discuss the current evidence for the use of lipoic acid to ameliorate certain age-related disorders, which include unwarranted apoptosis, cardiovascular disease, and cataract formation.

II. THE FREE RADICAL THEORY OF AGING

Aging can be defined as the progressive accumulation of structural and functional deleterious changes that commonly begins at maturity and culminates in death (1). Aging is marked by a progressive decline in the capacity of the body to cope with the damaging effects of environmental stressors, and the associated rise in the predisposition to disease and the risk of death. In due time all tissues in the body age, postmitotic tissues in particular, such as the heart, smooth muscle, and brain. The onset of aging and the rate of aging are two important variables in the genesis of the aging process. These variables are influenced by genetic (metabolic capacity, stress response efficiency, and resistance to dysregulation) and environmental factors (such as lifestyle, exposure to chemicals, and radiation). Altogether these attributes confer to organisms a functional potential that correlates with life expectancy (statistically represented by the maximum life span). By acting against reaching maximum life span, deleterious developmental and environmental factors and genetic instability promote imbalances that ultimately lead to functional decline.

The fundamentals of the free radical theory of aging were first described by Harman in 1956 (2). Harman proposed that the continuous generation of reactive oxygen species (ROS), which arise as by-products of cellular respiration and the extensive propagation of free radicals within the cell, is one of the principal underlying factors involved in the process of aging. The theory predicts a negative correlation between the rate of ROS production and longevity [for more information on the free radical theory of aging see Ref. 3]. Free radicals, namely superoxide ($O_2^{·-}$), hydroxyl ($·OH$), and hydroperoxyl ($·OOH$) radicals, have an unpaired electron which reacts with major organic molecules (such as lipids, peptides, nucleic acids, and carbohydrates) and metals (such as iron and copper). In so doing, ROS modify the structure and function of organic cellular constituents, and augment the reactivity of metal ions. Newly formed organic radicals can propagate free radical chain-reactions with neighboring organic molecules, a process that may ultimately impair cellular function and lead to cell death.

It is now known that oxidants are produced in vivo, and they can cause significant harm (4–9). Sources of ROS have been identified, which include peroxisomal β-oxidation of fatty acids in the liver (10–13), microsomal cytochrome P450 enzymes (14,15), and activated phagocytic cells (16–18). In 1972, Harman (19) further proposed that mitochondria were the major intracellular source of ROS generation and damage causing aging. About 1% of oxygen (O_2) consumed by mitochondria is converted to primarily $O_2^{·-}$ in the mitochondrial matrix (20,21). Most $O_2^{·-}$ radicals rapidly dismutate to produce hydrogen peroxide (H_2O_2) and O_2, either spontaneously or enzymatically by mitochondrial Mn-superoxide dismutase. Although H_2O_2 is a weak oxidant, its half-life is relatively long. Thus, H_2O_2 can leak from the mitochondrion, diffuse throughout the cell, including the nucleus. Upon reaction with reduced metal ions (by the Fenton chemistry), H_2O_2 is converted to highly reactive and deleterious $·OH$, which can damage a wide array of biomolecules. In addition, $O_2^{·-}$ can reduce free metal ions to a more reactive state, produce peroxynitrite ($ONOO^-$) by reaction with nitric oxide (NO), and also release metal ions from metal-bound proteins, such as ferritin (22). With age, the extent of metal–ROS interaction is believed to intensify as total iron and copper contents increase in most tissues studied (23–32). This would increase the likelihood of converting less potent ROS into highly reactive free radicals and thereby cause a proportionately greater level of oxidative damage. DNA may be particularly susceptible to metal-catalyzed oxidative damage owing to the propensity for free metal ions to transiently bind to nucleobases.

Mitochondria not only may be the chief intracellular source for ROS generation, but also may be a principal target for oxidative damage and consequent functional decline with age. Because of its proximity to the source of ROS and lack of protecting histones, mitochondrial DNA is also prone to oxidant-induced base modification (33–36). Mitochondrial DNA damage, if not repaired, may be converted into deleterious mutations. These mutations would affect electron transport efficiency, thereby reducing the capacity to synthesize ATP, and further increasing ROS generation. With age, the proportion of O_2 partially reduced to ROS by the mitochondrion increases to 2–4% (37–39), which would contribute to heightened ROS damage to biomolecules (proteins, lipids, and DNA). Thus, aging results in a vicious cycle of ever-increasing levels of ROS leaking from mitochondria that lead to elevated cell damage followed by ever-decreasing electron transport efficiency, which may cause further reduction of O_2 to ROS.

The modern concept of the free radical theory of aging recognizes a shift in the antioxidant–pro-oxidant balance that leads to increased oxidative stress and dysregulation of cellular function with age. A significant perturbation in the antioxidant defense systems is observed in aging organs. Antioxidant enzymes (glutathione peroxidase, superoxide dismutases, and catalase) and low molecular weight ROS scavengers (ascorbate and thiol compounds) show a general decline in the blood, liver, brain, and heart with age (40–45). In the elderly, low levels of circulating antioxidants are associated with greater numbers of illnesses and higher illness risk factors. Age-associated degenerative and chronic diseases, such as cancer, cardiovascular diseases, cataracts, and brain dysfunction, are increasingly found to have an oxidative origin (46). Considerable evidence is available to support the notion that dietary antioxidants, such as vitamin C, vitamin E, carotenoids, bioflavonoids, and more recently, lipoic acid, can lessen or prevent oxidative damage.

Lipoic acid is a natural coenzyme involved in cellular energy production and antioxidant defense mechanisms. The view that lipoic acid may protect against oxidative damage with age is based on its properties to regenerate water- and lipid-soluble endogenous antioxidants (vitamin C, E, and thiol compounds), to scavenge ROS, and prevent lipid peroxidation. Moreover, lipoic acid is a metal ion chelator that may be effective against the age-associated increase of iron and copper content in biological systems.

III. CHEMICAL NATURE OF LIPOIC ACID RELATIVE TO THE FREE RADICAL THEORY OF AGING

A. Biochemistry of Lipoic Acid

α-Lipoic acid (1,2-dithiolane-3-pentanoic acid) is a thiol-containing compound, which is naturally occurring in pro- and eukaryotes, and is biosynthesized from octanoic acid (47). Lipoic acid contains a chiral center at the 3-position on the 1,2-dithiolane moiety (a disulfide in a five-membered ring system), making possible the artificial synthesis of two stereoisomers: R- and S-lipoic acid (Fig. 1). In tissues, lipoate is a coenzyme bound covalently to lysine residues in α-ketoacid dehydrogenases (pyruvate dehydrogenase complex, α-ketoglutarate dehydrogenase complex, and the branched-chain α-ketoacid dehydrogenase). R-Lipoate is the "natural" stereoisomer and is preferentially used by α-ketoacid dehydrogenases (48,49). Kidney, heart, and skeletal muscle tissues contain the highest concentrations of protein-bound lipoate. Accordingly, concentrations of free lipoate are very low in vivo (50–52). However, following dietary supplementation, there is a transient increase in unbound lipoate inside all cells of the body, especially the heart, brain, and liver. Orally administered lipoic acid is absorbed and transported to tissues, taken up by the cells (53,54) as lipoate (LA; 1,2-dithiolane in oxidized state), and reduced to dihydrolipoate (DHLA) enzymatically (49,55–57). Because of its high hydrophobicity lipoate can penetrate biological membranes and enter the mitochondrial matrix (58). [For a more complete review on lipoic acid metabolism see Ref. 59.]

B. Roles of Lipoic Acid Relevant to the Aging Process

Several experimental and clinical studies have documented the potential of lipoic acid as a therapeutic antioxidant in such conditions as diabetes, ischemia–reperfusion injury, heavy

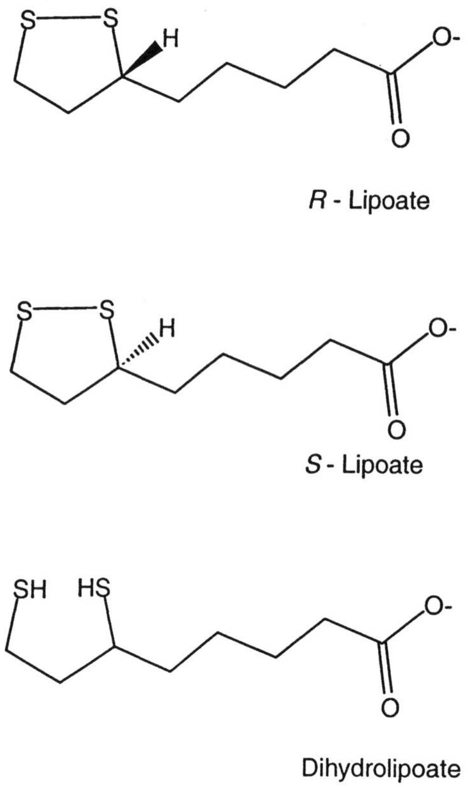

Figure 1 Chemical structures of *R*- and *S*-lipoate, and the reduced form, dihydrolipoate.

metal poisoning, radiation damage, neurodegenerative diseases, and HIV infection. Because of the oxidative nature of many age-related disorders, lipoic acid supplementation has been increasingly considered for the elderly. The restorative properties of lipoic acid are attributable to the ability of its thiol groups to reduce cellular compounds and to scavenge ROS. Unlike vitamins C, E, and carotenoids, lipoic acid also chelates transition metals that are found to accumulate with age. Furthermore, lipoate has both lipid and water solubility. For that reason it can access the source of antioxidant perturbation in any compartment of the tissue. The chemical nature of lipoic acid with relevance to age-associated pathophysiologies will now be discussed.

1. Reducing Agent

DHLA/LA acts as a redox couple with a standard reduction potential of −0.325 V (60,61). Packer et al. (62) have reviewed the antioxidant properties of DHLA. In vitro, DHLA is a more potent antioxidant than L-ascorbic acid, and other biologically relevant thiol compounds (glutathione and cysteine).

The low redox potential of DHLA/LA suggests that DHLA can easily reduce a wide array of oxidized metabolites, thereby contributing to the reducing power of the cell. The potency of DHLA to the maintenance of cellular redox homeostasis becomes even more critical in aging organs when antioxidant defense mechanisms collapse. Thus, lipoic acid supplementation emerges as a means to compensate for this decline. The reduction potential of DHLA/LA also suggests that DHLA can reduce, in vivo, low molecular weight antioxidants, such as reduced glutathione (GSH), cysteine, coenzyme Q10, vitamin C, and vitamin E (62–67), thereby preserving ever-decreasing concentrations of endogenous antioxidants with age.

Lipoic acid was reported to increase GSH content in cell culture (68) and in rat tissues (52), which may protect aged cells against enhanced oxidative damage. Such increase in GSH could not, however, be explained by the reduction of intracellular GSSG because of its low concentration (69,70). A lipoic acid-induced expression of γ-glutamylcysteine synthetase, the first enzyme in GSH synthesis, was also excluded (70). Rather, Han et al. (71) proposed that, in cell culture, lipoic acid stimulates GSH synthesis by supplying γ-glutamylcysteine synthetase with cysteine, the rate-limiting substrate in GSH biosynthesis. On incubation with LA, LA is rapidly reduced enzymatically in the cell and released into the culture medium as DHLA where it reduces cystine to cysteine. Intravenous administration of LA in rats resulted in enhanced circulating levels of cysteine and GSH, and decreased level of cystine (72). Protection by lipoic acid against oxidative damage exacerbated by the age-associated decline of GSH synthesis (44) has been demonstrated in rats (73).

2. ROS Scavenger

Lipoic acid or DHLA scavenge various ROS in reconstituted systems (62,64). LA preferentially quenches hydroxyl radical, hypochlorous acid, and singlet oxygen, whereas DHLA readily reacts with peroxyl and hydroxyl radicals, and hypochlorous acid. Whether LA or DHLA can scavenge superoxide is still debated. Also, there is no direct evidence that LA or DHLA can react with peroxynitrite and hydrogen peroxide in vivo (74). Clues come from studies that showed that LA or DHLA prevented peroxynitrite-driven α_1-antiprotease inactivation and tyrosine nitration (75), and that cysteine can reduce peroxynitrite and hydrogen peroxide (76,77). Because DHLA has higher reductive properties than cysteine, it was suggested that DHLA might also react with superoxide and hydrogen peroxide.

Hydroxyl radicals, superoxide, and hydrogen peroxide, have long been recognized as potentially highly damaging ROS for eukaryotic cells. Any increase in the steady-state levels of these ROS will elevate the oxidative threat to a cell. Such an imbalance is believed to occur in aging tissues as a result of an enhanced generation of ROS from the mitochondrial electron transport chain, or a decrease in the antioxidant capacity of cells. This age-associated oxidative stress could be alleviated through the increase of cellular levels of a ROS scavenger such as lipoic acid. Lipoic acid has been used as a therapeutic agent in liver and neurological disorders where enhanced free radical peroxidation of membrane phospholipids was reported. In biomembranes, the ROS-scavenging capacity of lipoic acid paralleled that of vitamin E. Because the rate of de novo synthesis of lipoic acid in the body is limited, dietary or supplemental intake is required to enhance ROS-eliminating capacity of cells.

3. Metal Chelator

Our body contains transition metals—iron and copper—that promote the generation of one of the most reactive ROS, hydroxyl radical ($^{\cdot}OH$). In vivo metal–protein complexation is designed to prevent metal-induced oxidative damage to circulating lipoproteins, polyunsaturated fatty acids, polypeptides, and nucleobases. Little free metal is normally present in the body. Once unbound, metals are readily oxidized by H_2O_2, a reaction that generates $^{\cdot}OH$ (Fenton chemistry). It is believed that iron is the main metal ion responsible for the formation of $^{\cdot}OH$ in vivo. The increase of redox active iron in tissues represents a significant risk factor for enhanced oxidative stress, and is currently believed to play a central role in conditions such as coronary heart disease, neurodegenerative diseases, and in aging.

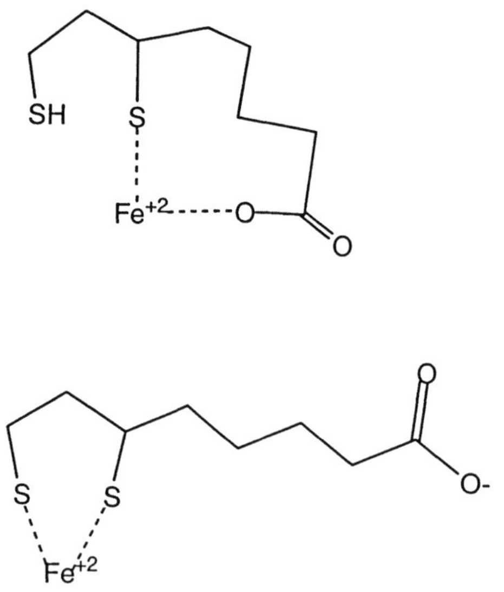

Figure 2 Tentative schematization of iron (II) complexation by dihydrolipoate.

Lipoic acid or DHLA can chelate metals through their carboxylate moiety or their sulfur atoms (Fig. 2). In vitro LA binds Cu^{+2} and Fe^{+2} (64). LA-bound iron was unable to oxidize ascorbate (Suh JH, Hagen TH, personal communication, 2000) which suggests that chelated iron would no longer be a pro-oxidant. Furthermore, DHLA inhibited Cu^{+2}-dependent liposomal (78) and low density lipoprotein (LDL) (79) peroxidation by chelating copper. In contrast, LA had no copper-chelating effect under certain experimental conditions (79). DHLA preferentially chelates copper, mercury, aluminum, and iron. DHLA and dihydrolipoamide (the amide form of DHLA) could remove iron from ferritin in vitro (80,81). DHLA may also prevent cadmium-catalyzed lipid peroxidation (82), partly by affecting cadmium cellular uptake (72).

Over the past 5 years, research on lipoic acid has increased and diversified dramatically. Lipoic acid is now viewed as being both an antioxidant and a metal chelator, the quite unique versatility of which makes it a potentially outstanding dietary supplement. Already lipoic acid supplementation has proved beneficial in the treatment of the complications of diabetes (see Chap. 5). Given its demonstrated antioxidant function, lipoic acid would be expected to be an effective agent against age-associated conditions in which oxidative stress might play a role, such as cancer, cardiovascular diseases, and cataracts. Although little knowledge is yet available on the specific mechanisms of action, we have reviewed the contribution played by lipoic acid in conditions affecting the elderly: unwarranted apoptosis, cardiovascular diseases (heart dysfunction and atherosclerosis), and cataracts.

IV. ROLES OF LIPOIC ACID IN AGING

A. ROS-Induced Apoptosis

Apoptosis is a natural process essential to the development, survival, and turnover of cells and tissues. It is characterized by a sudden decrease in cell volume (owing to loss of water and electrolytes), a blebbing of the cell surface, a reorganization of phospholipids in the plasma membrane, and a collapse of chromatin structure (83,84). Apoptosis can be initiated by a variety of endogenous and exogenous signals, including oxidants, viral infection, extracellular survival factors, cell interactions, and hormones (85). Although beneficial to the organism, the unwanted activation of apoptosis may cause or contribute to normal aging and a variety of degenerative diseases. Currently, mitochondria are considered one of the principal gatekeepers that govern whether a cell irreversibly undergoes apoptosis (86). Because the mitochondrion is the major site of ROS generation, age-related mitochondrial dysfunction may become a major determinant of tissue atrophy through unwarranted apoptosis, particularly in postmitotic tissues. In mammals, cell death is regulated by proteins of the Bcl-2 family. Although Bcl-2 and Bcl-xL are antiapoptotic members of the family, Bax and Bad are proapoptotic. Bcl-2 and Bcl-xL are predominantly localized to the outer mitochondrial membrane, whereas Bax and Bad translocate from the cytosol to the mitochondria on activation by oxidative stress, proteolytic cleavage, or dephosphorylation. In cultured neonatal rat myocytes exposed to H_2O_2, translocation of Bad to the mitochondria was followed by the release of cytochrome c into the cytosol, and the collapse of the inner mitochondrial membrane potential ($\Delta\Psi$) (87,88). Collapse of $\Delta\Psi$ involves the opening of a mitochondrial pore, which markedly affects the permeability of mitochondria (89,90). This so-called mitochondrial permeability transition (MPT) appears to be a hallmark of cells entering into irreversible apoptosis (91). MPT appears to activate caspase-3, an aspartyl protease that has been called the "death protease," because its activation is believed to be one of the first committed steps leading to cell death (90).

Reactive oxygen species induce normal and unscheduled apoptosis (92–95), whereas antioxidants, metal chelators, and catalase have been identified as active antiapoptotic factors (96–99). As powerful antioxidants, lipoic acid and its derivatives have been considered effective inhibitors of oxidative stress-induced apoptosis. Bustamante et al. (100) reported that DHLA, and to some extent lipoamide, but not LA, inhibited cell shrinkage, chromatin condensation, and subsequent DNA fragmentation in apoptosis-induced rat thymocytes. Because other unrelated antioxidants demonstrated the same property, it was suggested that DHLA inhibits thymocyte apoptosis by a redox mechanism yet to be identified (101).

Furthermore, as a coenzyme in mitochondrial energy-producing pathways, lipoic acid may boost mitochondrial function. Cysteine's thiol group is the most reactive of any amino acid side chain, and disulfide bond formation is involved in protein conformational change. ATP synthesis by mitochondria requires membrane fluidity as well as polypeptide chain mobility. ATPase efficiency was lessened on disulfide bond formation in ATP-synthase β-subunit, and the impairment was reversed with lipoic acid (102). Owing to its ability to reduce disulfide bonds established between peptide subunits, and to scavenge free radicals that otherwise would induce membrane component cross-linkings, it has been speculated that DHLA could prevent uncoupling of oxidation from phosphorylation, a phenomenon observed after oxidative damage to mitochondria (103).

B. Heart Dysfunction

1. ROS-Induced Changes to the Aging Myocardium

Aging is associated with an increased incidence of cardiac arrythmias, as well as diastolic and systolic dysfunction, which may ultimately lead to heart failure. Heart failure alone is the leading cause of hospitalization, permanent disability, and death in individuals older than 65 in the United States (104).

General age-related changes to the myocardium, such as a loss of distensibility, a decline in myocyte number, and a decreased basal metabolic rate (Fig. 3A), all have been implicated as underlying events that account for increased cardiac dysfunction (105–108). To maintain

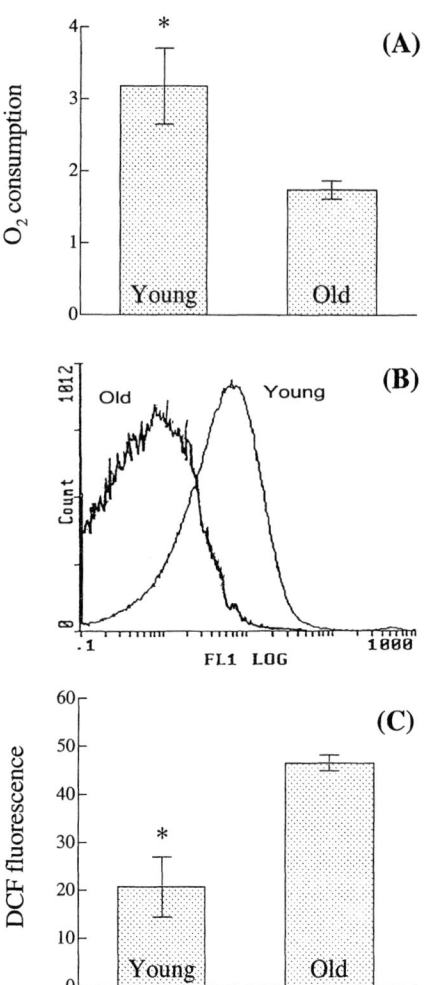

Figure 3 Parameters of mitochondrial function in cardiac myocytes isolated from young (2–5 mo) and old (24–28 mo) male rats: The hearts were dispersed into single cells by collagenase perfusion. Only cell preparations with initial viability (determined by trypan blue exclusion) higher than 70% were used. (A) Oxygen consumption (expressed as nmol O_2/min per 10^6 cells) is shown as mean ± SEM for five young and old rats. (B) Mitochondrial membrane potential ($\Delta\Psi$) evaluated using rhodamine 123, a fluorescent dye that accumulates specifically in the mitochondria based on the inner $\Delta\Psi$. Fluorescence distribution of stained myocytes is presented. A shift of fluorogram to lower fluorescence intensities indicates a decline in mitochondrial $\Delta\Psi$. (C) Oxidant production of cardiac myocytes is expressed as fluorescence units/min per 10^6 cells per nmol O_2 consumed. Data are shown as mean ± SEM for four young and three old rats. Cellular oxidant production was measured by monitoring spectrofluorometrically the oxidation of dichlorofluorescin diacetate (DCFH). *$p < 0.05$ compared with old rats following Mann–Whitney U test. (Source: Ref. 104a.)

myocardial integrity and function, a constant supply of ATP is required, and little reserves are maintained. The major driving force of ATP synthesis is the mitochondrial membrane potential ($\Delta\Psi$). Yet, myocytes from old rats have a significantly lower mitochondrial $\Delta\Psi$ when compared with young animals (see Fig. 3B). Any decrement in $\Delta\Psi$ can significantly impair myocyte energy production (109) which, in turn, appreciably affects myocardial stiffness and relaxation (105,110–115).

Part of the age-associated changes to the heart is due to an antioxidant–pro-oxidant imbalance, which might either cause or result from exacerbated ROS generation. There is growing evidence that oxidative damage to the electron transport chain plays a critical role in the age-related decline of mitochondrial $\Delta\Psi$ (116–118). Recently, we showed that cardiac myocytes isolated from old rats produce abnormally high quantities of ROS (see Fig. 3C). Concomitantly, heart concentrations of antioxidant enzymes decrease with age, including glutathione peroxidase, Mn-superoxide dismutase, and catalase (119,120). A decline in low molecular weight antioxidants, ascorbate, and GSH, is also apparent in the heart of aging rats (104a,121). Thus, recent data suggest that the aging heart is under oxidative stress.

2. Role of Lipoic Acid in Improving Heart Dysfunction

It has been proposed that dietary supplementation with antioxidants could improve cardiac function in old animals. Once taken up by the cells, supplemental antioxidants may quench oxidants on formation before they damage important biomolecules in the heart.

Because lipoic acid is a potent antioxidant and a coenzyme in energy-producing pathways located in the mitochondrion, the effects of lipoic acid supplementation on the antioxidant capacity of the aging myocardium was studied. As a means to rectify the age-associated oxidative stress in the heart, *R*-LA (0.2%, w/w) was added to the diet of aged male rats for 2 weeks, and compared with control groups of young and old rats (104a). *R*-LA reversed the age-related decrease in cardiac ascorbate levels, as well as the rise of mutagenic base modifications (8-oxo-2′-deoxyguanosine) in nuclear DNA (Table 1). This implies that *R*-LA acted in part through regeneration or sparing of endogenous antioxidants. A direct scavenging of ROS, ˙OH in particular, by lipoate inside the myocytes is also possible. Further studies are required to elucidate the mechanisms of action of lipoic acid in preventing oxidative stress in the aging rat heart, and to evaluate the effects of lipoic acid supplementation on heart

Table 1 Effects of Age and *R*-Lipoic Acid (LA) Supplementation on Redox Status in the Rat Heart[a]

	Young		Old	
	Control	LA	Control	LA
Ascorbate[b]	2.9 ± 0.7 (3)	2.8 ± 0.02 (2)	1.4 ± 0.3 (10)	2.9 ± 0.4 (12)
8-Oxo-2′-deoxyguanosine[c]	2.1 ± 0.2 (8)	2.5 ± 0.3 (3)	4.0 ± 0.4 (10)	2.8 ± 0.4 (9)

[a] Data are shown as mean ± SE. The number of animal analyzed is indicated in parentheses. Fischer 344 male rats, young (2 mo) and old (28 mo), were fed AIN-93M diet unsupplemented (Control) or supplemented (LA) with 0.2% (w/w) *R*-LA for 2 weeks before sacrifice.
[b] pmol/mg protein.
[c] 8-Oxo-2′-deoxyguanosine/10^5 2′-deoxyguanosines.
Source: Ref. 104a.

performance. Supplementation with lipoic acid may also ameliorate mitochondrial function by increasing pyruvate and α-ketoacid dehydrogenases and, as such, stimulate overall cardiac myocyte metabolism.

C. Vascular Disease: Atherosclerosis

1. Pathophysiology of Atherosclerosis

The vascular system is also markedly affected by aging. Similar to the changes observed in the heart, the aging vascular system (122–127) exhibits lowered arterial distensibility and increased vessel stiffness (127,128). These age-associated changes may eventually lead to pathologies, such as hypertension, coronary artery disease, and atherosclerosis.

Atherosclerosis is the vascular disorder most frequently associated with morbidity and mortality in Western societies (129). Atherosclerotic lesions narrow the arterial lumen and predispose affected individuals to complications such as thrombosis, hemorrhage, and embolism. Smoking, diabetes mellitus, hypercholesterolemia, hypertension, and hyperhomocysteinemia are well-recognized risk factors for atherogenesis (130). Clinical and epidemiological studies have also shown that elevated low-density lipoprotein/high-density lipoprotein ratio (LDL/HDL) is an important risk factor for cardiovascular disease as well.

Oxidative damage to LDL is a significant contributor to atherosclerosis, especially in the early stages of atherogenesis (131,132). Beyond minor alterations that occur in lipoprotein processing during normal aging, severe impaired intracellular processing of completely oxidized LDL in macrophages, with accumulation of lipid-laden foam cells is one of the pathological hallmarks of atherosclerosis. Although the underlying mechanisms by which oxidation initiates atherogenesis remain unclear, various pathways for LDL oxidation have been proposed largely based on the results of in vitro studies. Metal ions, superoxide, peroxynitrite, lipoxygenases, ceruloplasmin, and myeloperoxidase have been studied as potential triggers of these oxidative pathways (133).

Heinecke et al. (134) showed that the oxidative modification of lipid moieties in LDL by cultured cells requires redox-active metal ions, such as iron or copper. Metal chelators and lipid-soluble antioxidants could block the oxidative damage to lipoprotein (135–138). However, such a mechanism seems an unlikely contributing factor in the early stages of atherogenesis, because iron and copper are normally found in blood plasma bound to transport proteins, rendering them unable to catalyze lipid peroxidation (139). Also, albumin, the major blood plasma protein, inhibits copper-stimulated LDL oxidation (140). Conversely, the interior of advanced atherosclerotic lesions contains iron and copper ions that are available to initiate free radical reactions (141).

One pathway by which oxidative stress might promote the dysfunction of vascular endothelial cells leading to the development of atherosclerotic lesions is through the activation of nuclear factor (NF)-κB. Endothelial cells, cells of the immune system, epithelial cells, and keratinocytes, rely on NF-κB activity to modulate responses to pathogenic conditions. Following its translocation to the nucleus, NF-κB stimulates the transcription of genes involved in immune, inflammatory, and acute-phase responses. Age-related alterations of endothelial oxidant defense capacity may be responsible for the activation of NF-κB, a central event in the pathogenesis of atherosclerosis (142). Agents, such as oxidized lipids, can induce endothelial oxidative stress by lowering endothelial glutathione levels leading to enhanced lipid peroxidation.

It is possible that the dietary intake of micronutrient antioxidants (vitamin E, vitamin C, β-carotene) may modulate the rate of development of coronary heart disease (141,143–145); although some of the latest clinical trials dispute earlier ones relevant to vitamin E. Placebo-controlled clinical trials looking into the roles of antioxidant vitamin supplementation in the prevention of cardiovascular disease have been mostly inconclusive (146–150), showing no benefit with β-carotene and a possible benefit with vitamins E and C (151).

Because of its role as an antioxidant and a metal ion chelator, lipoic acid may contribute to the maintenance of interstitial and cellular redox status, thereby hindering oxidant-induced atherogenesis.

2. Role of Lipoic Acid in Preventing Atherosclerosis

Early studies have documented that lipoic acid implanted subcutaneously could prevent atherogenesis in the Japanese quail (152). The findings that lipoic acid inhibited metal-dependent LDL peroxidation in vitro (64,79) provide a rationale for the beneficial effect of lipoic acid.

Although lipoic acid supplementation has yet to be experimentally examined for reversing age-related loss of endothelial cell function, recent work (153) reported that lipoic acid directly inhibited NF-κB activation in human T cells, a pathway believed to be stimulated by a pro-oxidant environment (154–156). Lipoic acid increases cellular redox status and maintains mitochondrial function in isolated endothelial cells. A recent study showed that addition of lipoic acid to endothelial cells in culture decreased the levels of advanced glycation end products (AGE), prevented the depletion of GSH and ascorbate, and lowered AGE-dependent activation of NF-κB (157). Although the redox-sensitive component has not been identified, it was proposed that lipoic acid prevents the oxidant-dependent dissociation of NF-κB p50 and p65 subunits from their cytoplasmic inhibitor IκB.

The initial step in the formation of the atherosclerotic lesion involves the adherence of circulating monocytes to the endothelium and their migration into the arterial intima (129). Because monocyte adherence would take place subsequently to radical-dependent activation of NF κB (158), the inhibition of NF-κB activation pathway by lipoic acid is relevant to early atherogenesis. Vascular and endothelial cells produce adhesion molecules as well as chemotactic agents for monocytes, lymphocytes, and neutrophils. When exposed to oxidized LDL, monocytes produce factors that stimulate endothelial cells to express leukocyte adhesion molecules and chemotactic agents. Cybulski and Gimbrone (159) reported that the expression of endothelial adhesion molecules was increased in endothelium adjacent to atherosclerosis lesions in the rabbit aorta. The expression of vascular cell adhesion molecule-1 (VCAM-1), stimulated on AGE-induced NF-κB activation, was significantly decreased in human umbilical vein endothelial cells pretreated with lipoic acid, and coincided with lower monocyte attachment to endothelium (158). Moreover, lipoic acid also inhibited, dose dependently, the tumor necrosis factor-alpha (TNF-α)-induced expression of VCAM-1, E-selectin, and intercellular adhesion molecule-1 (ICAM-1) in human aorta endothelial cells (Fig. 4) (160). Thus, lipoic acid may decrease overall monocyte adhesion and recruitment to the vascular wall and inhibit the progression of atherogenesis.

Endothelin-1 is a vasoconstrictive peptide with chemotactic properties that is elevated in patients with atherosclerosis and hyperlipidemia (161). In cell culture, lipoic acid inhibits the chemotactic activity of endothelin-1 (162), thereby lessening monocyte migration.

Furthermore, lipoic acid may indirectly inactivate NF-κB by regenerating vitamin E. Boscoboinik et al. (163) demonstrated that α-tocopherol inhibits protein kinase C, and protein

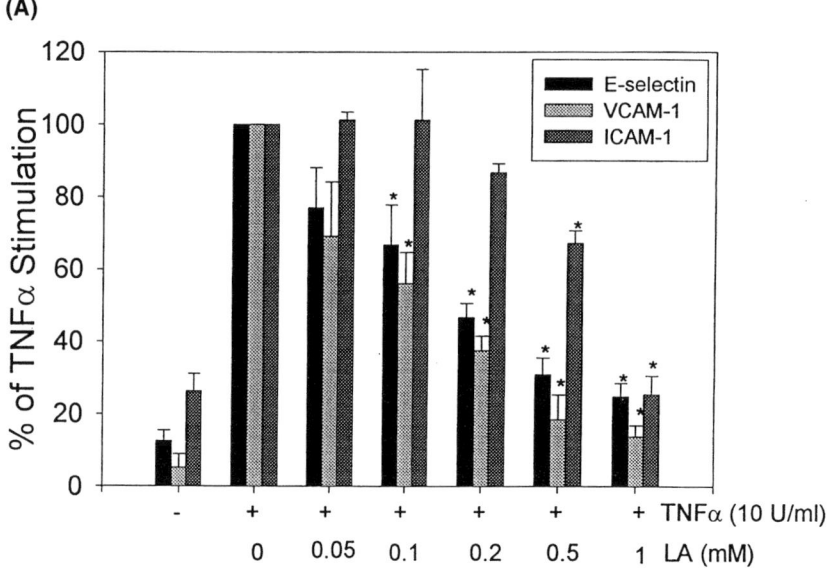

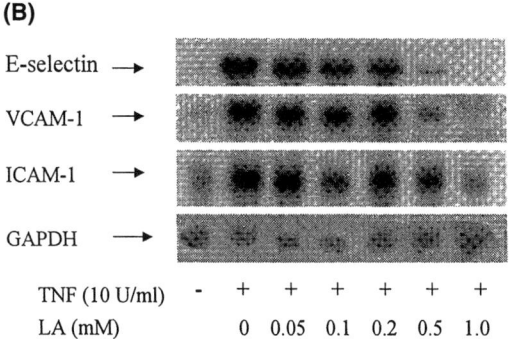

Figure 4 (A) Lipoic acid inhibited dose dependently tumor necrosis factor-alpha (TNF-α)-induced cell surface protein expression of E-selectin, vascular cell adhesion molecule-1 (VCAM-1), and intercellular adhesion molecule-1 (ICAM-1) in cultured human aorta endothelial cells (HAEC). Cells were preincubated for 48 h with 0, 0.05, 0.1, 0.2, 0.5, or 1 mM lipoic acid in medium 199 containing 20% fetal calf serum. The cells were then washed twice with medium 199 and coincubated with lipoic acid (same concentrations as those used in preincubation) and TNF-α (10 U/mL) for 4.5 h. The extent of adhesion molecules displayed at the endothelium surface was measured by enzyme-linked immunosorbent assay (ELISA). Data are shown as means $\pm$ SD. *p < 0.05 compared with TNF-α alone. (B) Lipoic acid inhibited TNF-α-induced up-regulation of E-selectin, VCAM-1, and ICAM-1 mRNA levels in HAEC. Cells were preincubated and washed as above and coincubated with lipoic acid and TNF-α (10 U/mL) for 2 h. Northern blot analysis of total RNA extracts was performed using ^{32}P-labeled cDNA probes for E-selectin, VCAM-1, ICAM-1, and glyceraldehyde-3-phosphate dehydrogenase (GAPDH) mRNAs. (From Ref. 160.)

kinase C is known to phosphorylate IκB in vitro (164), which is a necessary step in NF-κB activation.

D. Cataracts

1. Pathophysiology of Cataracts

Cataracts are conditions characterized by an increasing opacity and light scattering of the eye's lens that interferes with vision. Senile cataract is the leading cause of blindness in the world, according to the World Health Organization, and the third cause of legal blindness in the United States (165). A variety of factors, either physical (radiation), chemical (toxicants, oxidants), or physiological (metabolic impairments resulting from diabetes or aging) may cause cataracts. Cataractogenesis affects the central or outer lens differently. Opacity of the lens nucleus results from the cellular aggregation of lens proteins termed crystallins (166). Cellular changes causing light-scattering in the cortical lens, however, involve the formation of cell surface globules or intracellular vacuoles filled with fluid of different refractive index (167). Various biochemical modifications have been observed during cataractogenesis, including Na^+/K^+ ATPase inhibition (168), ion-transport impairment (169,170), actin inhibition (171), defective protein synthesis (172), and oxidative stress (173–175). Water- and fat-soluble antioxidants, glutathione, vitamin C, vitamin E, and melatonin, were effective in preventing cataracts in tissue and trial studies (175–179).

Oxidative stress, causing damage to the lens membranes and proteins, has been associated with opacities (180). In vitro incubation of α-crystallins with H_2O_2 or $FeCl_3$ provoked the extensive oxidation of methionine residues to methionine sulfoxide, resulting in a loss of chaperone activity that correlates with the development of cataract (181). The finding that cataract can be induced in the newborn rat by inhibiting glutathione synthesis with buthionine sulfoximine (BSO) pointed at the key role of a cellular antioxidant in preventing cataract (182). In diabetic cataract, the origin of the oxidative stress was linked to a compensatory decrease of intracellular antioxidants, GSH and ascorbate (183), orchestrated by the cell to cope with sorbitol-driven osmotic stress. In both BSO and diabetic cataracts, antioxidants were effective in restoring antioxidant status and preventing cataractogenesis.

Because DHLA is a powerful antioxidant, able to regenerate several cellular reducing agents (ascorbate, GSH, α-tocopherol) normally found in the eye, lipoic acid has been studied as a potential factor of cataract prevention.

2. Role of Lipoic Acid in Preventing Cataractogenesis

The treatment of BSO-induced cataract with lipoic acid led to a significant decrease in cataract incidence, and restored ascorbate and α-tocopherol contents as well as antioxidant enzyme system activities (182). R-LA, but not S-LA, was effective in protecting lens clarity. On the contrary, S-LA potentiated lactate dehydrogenase leakage and lens damage in diabetic cataract (184). Lens glutathione level was maintained after R-LA incubation, but not with S-LA (185). Kilic et al. (184) suggested that the enantiomer unequivalency was due to the preferred reduction of R-LA to DHLA by mitochondrial lipoamide dehydrogenase (49). Because DHLA is viewed as a more potent reductant than LA in vivo (64), and can convert GSSG to GSH directly in vitro (186), these studies indicated that lipoic acid protects the eye lens against cataract formation partly through the antioxidant properties of its reduced form, DHLA (187). The metal-chelating properties of lipoic acid were invoked in the protection against diabetic cataract. Ou et al. (188) reported that lipoic acid prevented the rise in sorbitol by inhibiting aldose reductase activity in glucose-incubated rat lenses, in a manner resembling that of copper-chelating aldolase reductase inhibitors.

Although both *R*- and *S*-LA are taken up by the cell, only the *R*-form is incorporated in the mammalian pyruvate dehydrogenase complex or the α-ketoacid dehydrogenase complexes from *Escherichia coli* (48). Thus, *R*-LA treatment would favor mitochondrial ATP synthesis, which is required for GSH synthesis. Because the loss of GSH was invoked as a possible cause of cataracts (182,189), another aspect of lipoic acid participation in cataract prevention would come from its role as a coenzyme in ATP production.

V. CONCLUSION

As reviewed, the aging process and many age-related diseases are characterized by a marked increase in oxidative stress. This may be due to mitochondrial decay, which causes increased release of ROS. Enhanced ROS production may be further exacerbated by a decline in cytosolic low molecular weight antioxidant status and decreased antioxidant enzyme function, which would be expected to increase damage to important cellular biological constituents. Also, iron accumulates in several organs with age, thereby causing an increased probability for superoxide or hydrogen peroxide to be converted to more deleterious hydroxyl radicals. Thus, agents that can restore antioxidant status or chelate redox-active metals may be an effective means of lowering oxidative insult and maintaining or improving cell and organ function. Lipoic acid may be an ideal dietary supplement here, because it is a powerful antioxidant in its reduced form, it increases the levels of other important antioxidants, such as glutathione and ascorbate, and it chelates redox active transition metals. Thus, lipoic acid may be considered a "complete" antioxidant in that it not only terminates ROS, but also prevents free radical formation by effectively removing redox-active transition metals.

Although there have been no long-term studies examining whether lipoic acid supplementation actually improves the mean life span or more importantly the "health span" of an animal, short-term studies point to a marked improvement in cellular antioxidant capacity and an overall decline in oxidative stress. These results are particularly evident in age-associated pathophysiologies, such as cardiovascular diseases and cataracts, which have been reviewed herein. Other disease states where lipoic acid supplementation may also have direct therapeutic implications, include brain disorders, such as Parkinson's syndrome and Alzheimer's disease. Subjects with these diagnoses evidence increased oxidative stress and iron accumulation in subregions of the brain controlling motor or cognitive function. Long-term feeding studies using experimental animals will be necessary to determine whether dietary supplementation with lipoic acid markedly improves or maintains organ function in the aging animal.

ACKNOWLEDGMENTS

We thank Drs. Baltz Frei and Rosemary Wander for critically reading the manuscript, and Jung Suh for graphic design.

REFERENCES

1. Arking R. (1991) Biology of Aging: Observations and Principles. Englewood Cliffs, NJ: Prentice-Hall.
2. Harman D. (1956) Aging: a theory based on free radical and radiation chemistry. J Gerontol 11:298–300.

3. Beckman KB, Ames BN. (1998) The free radical theory of aging matures. Physiol Rev 78:547–581.
4. Chance B, Sies H, Boveris A. (1979) Hydroperoxide metabolism in mammalian organs. Physiol Rev 59:527–605.
5. Halliwell B. (1989). Free radicals, reactive oxygen species, and human disease: a critical evaluation with special reference to atherosclerosis. Br J Exp Pathol 70:737–757.
6. Beyer W, Imlay J, Fridovich I. (1991) Superoxide dismutases. Prog Nucl Acids Res 40:221–253.
7. Yu BP. (1994) Cellular defenses against damage from reactive oxygen species. Physiol Rev 74:139–162.
8. Davies KJ. (1995) Oxidative stress: the paradox of aerobic life. Biochem Soc Symp 61:1–31.
9. Fridovich I. (1995) Superoxide radical and superoxide dismutases. Annu Rev Biochem 64:97–112.
10. Kasai H, Okada Y, Nishimura S, Rao MS, Reddy JK. (1989) Formation of 8-hydroxydeoxyguanosine in liver DNA of rats following long-term exposure to a peroxisome proliferator. Cancer Res 49:2603–2605.
11. Ockner RK, Kaikaus RM, Bass NM. (1993) Fatty-acid metabolism and the pathogenesis of hepatocellular carcinoma: review and hypothesis. Hepatology 18:669–676.
12. Arnaiz SL, Travacio M, Llesuy S, Boveris A. (1995) Hydrogen peroxide metabolism during peroxisome proliferation by fenofibrate. Biochim Biophys Acta 1272:175–180.
13. Lake BG. (1995) Mechanisms of hepatocarcinogenicity of peroxisome-proliferating drugs and chemicals. Annu Rev Pharmacol Toxicol 35:483–507.
14. Koop DR. (1992) Oxidative and reductive metabolism by cytochrome P450 2E1. FASEB J 6:724–730.
15. Goeptar AR, Scheerens H, Vermeulen NP. (1995) Oxygen and xenobiotic reductase activities of cytochrome P450. Crit Rev Toxicol 25:25–65.
16. Chanock SJ, el Benna J, Smith RM, Babior BM. (1994) The respiratory burst oxidase. J Biol Chem 269:24519–24522.
17. Molsen MT. (1994) Reactive oxygen species in normal physiology, cell injury and phagocytosis. Adv Exp Med Biol 366:17–27.
18. Robinson JM, Badwey JA. (1994) Production of active oxygen species by phagocytic leukocytes. Immunol Ser 60:159–178.
19. Harman D. (1972) The biologic clock: the mitochondria? J Am Geriat Soc 20:145–147.
20. Boveris A, Cadenas E. (1975) Mitochondrial production of superoxide anions and its relationship to the antimycin insensitive respiration. FEBS Lett 54:311–314.
21. Dionisi O, Galeotti T, Terranova T, Azzi A. (1975) Superoxide radicals and hydrogen peroxide formation in mitochondria from normal and neoplastic tissues. Biochim Biophys Acta 403:292–300.
22. Paz MA, Baynes JW, Frei B, Schweiger M, Sohal RS, Stadtman ER, Stahl U, Swartz HM, Thorpe SR, Yu BP. (1995) Group report: do research findings from diverse model systems support oxidative damage theories of aging? In: Esser K, Martin GM, eds. Molecular Aspects of Aging. Chichester: John Wiley & Sons, pp 145–161.
23. Massie HR, Aiello VR, Banziger V. (1983) Iron accumulation and lipid peroxidation in aging C57BL/6J mice. Exp Gerontol 18:277–285.
24. Massie HR, Aiello VR, Shumway ME, Armstrong T. (1990) Calcium, iron, copper, boron, collagen, and density changes in bone with aging in C57BL/6J male mice. Exp Gerontol 25:469–481.
25. Madaric A, Ginter E, Kadrabova J. (1994) Serum copper, zinc and copper/zinc ratio in males: influence of aging. Physiol Res 43:107–111.
26. Joshi JG, Fleming JT, Dhar M, Chauthaiwale V. (1995) A novel ferritin heavy chain messenger ribonucleic acid in the human brain. J Neurol Sci 134:S52–S56.
27. Ghio AJ, Pritchard RJ, Dittrich KL, Samet JM. (1997) Non-heme (Fe^{3+}) in the lung increases with age in both humans and rats. J Lab Clin Med 129:53–61.
28. Sanchez DJ, Gomez M, Llobet JM, Corbella J, Domingo JL. (1997) Effects of aluminium on the mineral metabolism of rats in relation to age. Pharmacol Toxicol 80:11–17.
29. Schipper HM, Vininsky R, Brull R, Small L, Brawer JR. (1998) Astrocyte mitochondria: a substrate for iron deposition in the aging rat substantia nigra. Exp Neurol 152:188–196.
30. Cook CI, Yu BP. (1998) Iron accumulation in aging: modulation by dietary restriction. Mech Ageing Dev 102:1–13.
31. Mezzetti A, Pierdomenico SD, Costantini F, Romano F, De Cesare D, Cuccurullo F, Imbastaro T, Riario-Sforza G, Di Giacomo F, Zuliani G, Fellin R. (1998) Copper/zinc ratio and systemic oxidant load: effect of aging and aging-related degenerative diseases. Free Radic Biol Med 25:676–681.

32. Sohal RS, Wennberg–Kirch E, Jaiswal K, Kwong LK, Forster MJ. (1999) Effect of age and caloric restriction on bleomycin-chelatable and nonheme iron in different tissues of C57BL/6 mice. Free Radic Biol Med 27:287–293.
33. Hofer H, Haltmann H. (1971) gamma Irradiation of a DNA-Cu^{2+} complex. Int J Radiat Biol Relat Stud Phys Chem Med 19:459–465.
34. Shearman CW, Kalf GF. (1977) DNA replication by a membrane DNA complex from rat liver mitochondria. Arch Biochem Biophys 182:573–586.
35. Shigenaga MK, Hagen TM, Ames BN. (1994) Oxidative damage and mitochondrial decay in aging. Proc Natl Acad Sci USA 91:10771–10778.
36. Giulivi C, Boveris A, Cadenas E. (1995) Hydroxyl radical generation during mitochondrial electron transfer and the formation of 8-hydroxydesoxyguanosine in mitochondrial DNA. Arch Biochem Biophys 316:909–916.
37. Nohl H, Hegner D. (1978) Do mitochondria produce oxygen radicals in vivo? Eur J Biochem 82:563–567.
38. Sawada M, Carlson JC. (1987) Changes in superoxide radical and lipid peroxide formation in the brain, heart, and liver during the lifetime of the rat. Mech Aging Dev 41:125–137.
39. Sohal RS, Ku HH, Agarwal S, Forster MJ, Lal H. (1994) Oxidative damage, mitochondrial oxidant generation and antioxidant defenses during aging and in response to food restriction in the mouse. Mech Ageing Dev 74:121–133.
40. Hazelton GA, Lang CA. (1980) Glutathione contents of tissue in the aging mouse. Biochem J 188:25–30.
41. Hazelton GA, Lang CA. (1985) Glutathione peroxidase and reductase activities in the aging mouse. Mech Ageing Dev 29:71–81.
42. Ji LL. (1993) Antioxidant enzyme response to exercise and aging. Med Sci Sports Exerc 25:225–231.
43. Julius M, Lang CA, Gleiberman L, Harburg E, DiFranceisco W, Schork A. (1994) Glutathione and morbidity in a community-based sample of elderly. J Clin Epidemiol 47:1021–1026.
44. Ohkuwa T, Sato Y, Naoi M. (1997) Glutathione status and reactive oxygen generation in tissues of young and old exercised rats. Acta Physiol Scand 159:237–244.
45. Calabrese V, Spadaro F, Dinotta F, Ravagna A, Randazzo F, Randazzo G, Ragusa N, Rizza V. (1998) Long-term ethanol administration enhances urinary ultraweak luminescence and age-dependent modulation of redox in central and peripheral organs of the rat. Int J Tissue React 20:57–62.
46. Ames B, Shigenaga MK, Hagen TM. (1993) Oxidants, antioxidants, and the degenerative diseases of aging. Proc Natl Acad Sci USA 90:7915–7922.
47. Carreau JP. (1979) Biosynthesis of lipoic acid via unsaturated fatty acids. Methods Enzymol 62:152–158.
48. Oehring R, Bisswanger H. (1992) Incorporation of the enantiomers of lipoic acid into the pyruvate dehydrogenase complex from *Escherichia coli* in vivo. Biol Chem Hoppe–Seyler 373:333–335.
49. Pick U, Haramaki N, Constantinescu A, Handelman G, Tritschler H, Packer L. (1995) Glutathione reductase and lipoamide dehydrogenase have opposite stereospecificities for alpha-lipoic acid enantiomers. Biochem Biophys Res Commun 206:724–730.
50. Kamata K, Akiyama K. (1990) High-performance liquid chromatography with electrochemical detection for the determination of thioctic acid and thioctic acid amine. J Pharm Biomed Anal 8:453–456.
51. Podda M, Tritschler HJ, Ulrich H, Packer L. (1994) alpha-Lipoic acid supplementation prevents symptoms of vitamin E deficiency. Biochem Biophys Res Commun 204:98–104.
52. Khanna S, Atalay M, Laaksonen DE, Gul M, Roy S, Sen CK. (1999) α-Lipoic acid supplementation: tissue glutathione homeostasis at rest and after exercise. J Appl Physiol 86:1191–1196.
53. Sanders DC, Leach FR. (1964) Studies on lipoic acid uptake by bacteria. I. Characterization of the reaction. Biochim Biophys Acta 82:41–49.
54. Peinado J, Sies H, Akerboom TPM. (1989) Hepatic lipoate uptake. Arch Biochem Biophys 273:389–395.
55. Constantinescu A, Pick U, Handelman GJ, Haramaki N, Han D, Podda M, Tritschler HJ, Packer L. (1995) Reduction and transport of lipoic acid by human erythrocytes. Biochem Pharmacol 50:253–261.
56. Biewenga GP, Dorstijn MA, Verhagen JV, Haenen GR, Bast A. (1996) Reduction of lipoic acid by lipoamide dehydrogenase. Biochem Pharmacol 51:233–238.

57. Haramaki N, Han D, Handelman GJ, Tritschler HJ, Packer L. (1997) Cytosolic and mitochondrial systems for NADH- and NADPH-dependent reduction of alpha-lipoic acid. Free Radic Biol Med 22:535–542.
58. Harrison EH, McCormic DB. (1974) The metabolism of dl-[1,6-^{14}C]lipoic acid in the rat. Arch Biochem Biophys 160:514–522.
59. Bustamante J, Lodge JK, Marcocci L, Tritschler HJ, Packer L, Rihn BH. (1998) α-Lipoic acid in liver metabolism and disease. Free Radic Biol Med 24:1023–1039.
60. Ke B. (1957) The polarographic behavior of α-lipoic acid. Biochem Biophys Acta 25:650–651.
61. Reed LJ. (1966) Chemistry and function of lipoic acid. In: Florkin M, Stoltz EH, eds. Comprehensive Biochemistry: Biological Oxidants. Amsterdam: Elsevier, pp 99–127.
62. Packer L, Witt EH, Tritschler HJ. (1995) alpha-Lipoic acid as a biological antioxidant. Free Radic Biol Med 19:227–250.
63. Haenen GR, Bast A. (1991) Scavenging of hypochlorous acid by lipoic acid. Biochem Pharmacol 42:2244–2246.
64. Scott BC, Aruoma OI, Evans PJ, O'Neill C, Van Der Vliet A, Cross CE, Tritschler H, Halliwell B. (1994) Lipoic and dihydropiloic acids as antioxidants: a critical evaluation. Free Radic Res 20:119–133.
65. Biewenga GP, Bast A. (1995) Reaction of lipoic acid with ebselen and hypochlorous acid. Methods Enzymol 251:303–314.
66. Schoneich C. (1995) Kinetics of thiol reaction. Methods Enzymol 251:45–55.
67. Kozlov AV, Gille L, Staniek K, Nohl H. (1999) Dihydrolipoic acid maintains ubiquinone in the antioxidant active form by two-electron reduction of ubiquinone and one-electron reduction of ubisemiquinone. Arch Biochem Biophys 363:148–154.
68. Busse E, Zimmer G, Schopohl B, Kornhuber B. (1992) Influence of α-lipoic acid on intracellular glutathione in vitro and in vivo. Arzneimittelforschung 42:829–831.
69. Halliwell B, Gutteridge JMC. (1989) Free Radicals in Biology and Medicine. Oxford: Clarendon.
70. Han D, Tritschler HJ, Packer L. (1995) α-Lipoic acid increases intracellular glutathione in a human T-lymphocyte Jurkat cell line. Biochem Biophys Res Commun 207:258–264.
71. Han D, Handelman G, Marcocci L, Sen CK, Roy S, Kobuchi H, Tritschler HJ, Flohe L, Packer L. (1997) Lipoic acid increases de novo synthesis of cellular glutathione by improving cystine utilization. Biofactors 6:321–328.
72. Gregus Z, Stein AF, Varga F, Klaassen C. (1992) Effect of lipoic acid on biliary excretion of glutathione and metals. Toxicol Appl Pharmacol 114:88–96.
73. Hagen TM, Vinarsky V, Wehr CM, Ames BN. (2000) (R) α Lipoic acid reverses the age associated increase in oxidant vulnerability of hepatocytes isolated from old rats, both in vitro and in vivo, when added to the diet. Antioxid Redox Signal 2:473–483.
74. Dikalov S, Khramtsov VV, Zimmer G. (1997) Reaction of lipoate and its derivatives with reactive oxygen species. In: Fuchs J, Packer L, Zimmer G, eds. Lipoic Acid in Health and Disease. New York: Marcel Dekker, pp 47–66.
75. Whiteman M, Tritschler H, Halliwell B. (1996) Protection against peroxynitrite-dependent tyrosine nitration and $α_1$-antiproteinase inactivation by oxidized and reduced lipoic acid. FEBS Lett 379:74–76.
76. Augusto O, Gatti RM, Radi R. (1994) Spin trapping studies of peroxynitrite decomposition and of 3-morpholinosydnonomine N-ethylcarbamide autooxidation: direct evidence for metal-independent formation of free radical intermediates. Arch Biochem Biophys 310:118–125.
77. Radi R, Beckman JS, Bush KM, Freeman BA. (1991) Peroxynitrite oxidation of sulfhydryls: the cytotoxic potential of superoxide and nitric oxide. J Biol Chem 266:4244–4250.
78. Ou PM, Tritschler HJ, Wolff SP. (1995) Thiotic (lipoic) acid: a therapeutic metal-chelating antioxidant? Biochem Pharmacol 50:123–126.
79. Lodge JK, Traber MG, Packer L. (1998) Thiol chelation of Cu^{+2} by dihydrolipoic acid prevents human low density lipoprotein peroxidation. Free Radic Biol Med 25:287–297.
80. Bonomi F, Pagani S. (1986) Removal of ferritin-bound iron by dl-dihydrolipoate and dl-dihydrolipoamide. Eur J Biochem 155:295–300.
81. Bonomi F, Cerioli A, Pagani S. (1989) Molecular aspects of the removal of ferritin-bound iron by DL-dihydrolipoate. Biochim Biophys Acta 994:180–186.
82. Müller L, Menzel H. (1990) Studies on the efficacy of lipoate and dihydrolipoate in the alteration of $cadmium^{2+}$ toxicity in isolated hepatocytes. Biochim Biophys Acta 1052:386–391.

83. Kerr JFR, Wyllie AH, Currie AR. (1972) Apoptosis: a basic biological phenomenon with wide-ranging implication in tissue kinetics. Br J Cancer 26:239–257.
84. Williams JR, Little JB, Shipley WU. (1974) Association of mammalian cell death with a specific endonucleolytic degradation of DNA. Nature 252:754–756.
85. Steller H. (1995) Mechanisms and genes of cellular suicide. Science 267:1445–1449.
86. Murphy AN, Fiskum G, Beal MF. (1999) Mitochondria in neurodegeneration: bioenergetic function in cell life and death. J Cereb Blood Flow Metab 19:231–245.
87. Zamzami N, Marchetti P, Castedo M, Zanin C, Vayssiere J–L, Petit PX, Kroemer G. (1995) Reduction in mitochondrial potential constitutes an early irreversible step of programmed lymphocyte death in vivo. J Exp Med 181:1661–1672.
88. Cook SA, Sugden PH, Clerk A. (1999) Regulation of Bcl-2 family proteins during development and in response to oxidative stress in cardiac myocytes: association with changes in mitochondrial membrane potential. Circ Res 85:940–949.
89. Zoratti M, Szabo I. (1995) The mitochondrial permeability transition. Biochim Biophys Acta 1241:139–176.
90. Cai J, Jones DP. (1998) Superoxide in apoptosis. Mitochondrial generation triggered by cytochrome c loss. J Biol Chem 273:11401–11404.
91. Petit PX, Zamzami N, Vayssiere J–L, Mignotte B, Kroemer G, Castedo M. (1997) Implication of mitochondria in apoptosis. Mol Cell Heart Biochem 174:185–188.
92. Halliwell B, Gutteridge JMC. (1990) Role of free radicals and catalytic metal ions in human disease: an overview. Methods Enzymol pp 1–85.
93. Pierce GB, Parchment RE, Lewellyn AL. (1991) Hydrogen peroxide as a mediator of programmed cell death in the blastocyst. Differentiation 46:181–186.
94. Forrest VJ, Kang YH, McClain DE, Robinson DH, Ramakrishnan N. (1994) Oxidative stress-induced apoptosis prevented by Trolox. Free Radic Biol Med 16:675–684.
95. Terawi M, Dixit VM. (1995) Fas- and tumor necrosis factor-induced apoptosis is inhibited by the poxvirus crmA gene product. J Biol Chem 270:3255–3260.
96. Morel Y, Cillard J, Lescoat G, Sergent O, Pasdeloup N, Ocaktan AZ, Abdallah MA, Brissot P, Cillard P. (1992) Antioxidant and free radical scavenging activities of the iron chelators pyoverdin and hydroxypyrid-4-ones in iron-loaded hepatocyte cultures: comparison of their mechanism of protection with that of desferrioxamine. Free Radic Biol Med 13:499–508.
97. Sandstrom PA, Butke TM. (1993) Autocrine production of extracellular catalase prevents apoptosis of human CEM T-cell line in serum-free medium. Proc Natl Acad Sci USA 90:4708–4712.
98. Sandstrom PA, Roberts B, Folks TM. (1993) HIV gene expression enhances T cell susceptibility to hydrogen peroxide-induced apoptosis. AIDS Res Hum Retroviruses 911:107–113.
99. Slater AF, Nobel SI, Maellaro E, Bustamante J, Kimland M, Orrenius S. (1995) Nitrone spin traps and a nitroxide antioxidant inhibit a common pathway of thymocyte apoptosis. Biochem J 306:771–778.
100. Bustamante J, Slater AFG, Orrenius S. (1995) Antioxidant inhibition of thymocyte apoptosis by dihydrolipoic acid. Free Radic Biol Med 19:339–347.
101. Bustamante J, Slater AFG, Orrenius S. (1997) Lipoic acid and the redox regulation of apoptosis. In Fuchs J, Packer L, Zimmer G, eds. Lipoic Acid in Health and Disease. New York: Marcel Dekker, pp 99–111.
102. Sheer B, Zimmer G. (1993) Dihydrolipoic acid prevents hypoxic/reoxygenation and peroxidative damage in rat heart mitochondria. Arch Biochem Biophys 302:385–390.
103. Zimmer G, Beikler T–K, Schneider M, Ibel J, Tritschler H, Ulrich H. (1995) Dose/response curves of lipoic acid R- and S-forms in the working heart during reoxygenation: superiority of the R-enantiomer in enhancement of aortic flow. J Mol Cell Cardiol 27:1895–1903.
104. Cohn JN, Bristow MR, Chien KR, Colucci WS. Frazier OH, Leinuond LA, Lorell BH, Moss AJ, Sonnenblick EH, Walsh RA, Mockrin SC, Reinlib L. (1997) Report of the National Heart, Lung, and Blood Institute special emphasis panel on heart failure research. Circulation 95:766–770.
104a. Suh JH, Shigeno ET, Morrow JD, Cox B, Rocha AE, Frei B, Hagen TM. (2001) Oxidative stress in the aging rat heart is reversed by dietary supplementation with (R)-α-lipoic acid. FASEB J 15:700–706.
105. Katz AM. (1988) Cellular mechanisms of heart failure. Am J Cardiol 62:3A–8A.
106. Carré F, Rannou F, Sainte Beuve C, Chevalier B, Moalic JM, Swynghedauw B, Charlemagne D. (1993) Arrhythmogenicity of the hypertrophied and senescent heart and relationship to membrane proteins involved in the altered calcium handling. Cardiovasc Res 27:1784–1789.

107. Tresch DD, McGough MF. (1995) Heart failure with normal systolic function: a common disorder in older people. J Am Geriatr Soc 43:1035–1042.
108. Colucci WS. (1997) Molecular and cellular mechanisms of myocardial failure. Am J Cardiol 80:15L–25L.
109. Davey GP, Clark JB. (1996) Threshold effects and control of oxidative phosphorylation in nonsynaptic rat brain mitochondria. J Neurochem 66:1617–1624.
110. Neeley JR, Morgan HE. (1974) Relationship between carbohydrate and lipid metabolism and energy balance of heart muscle. Annu Rev Physiol 36:413–459.
111. Frolkis VV, Frolkis RA, Mkhitarian LS, Shevchuk VG, Fraifeld VE, Vakulenko LG, Syrovy I. (1988) Contractile function in Ca^{+2} transport system of myocardium in ageing. Gerontology 34:64–74.
112. Morgan JP, Erny RE, Allen PD, Grossman W, Gwathmey JK. (1990) Abnormal intracellular calcium handling, a major cause of systolic and diastolic dysfunction in ventricular myocardium from patients with heart failure. Circulation 81(suppl 3):21–23.
113. Siri FM, Krueger J, Nordin C, Ming Z, Aronson RS. (1991) Depressed intracellular calcium transients and contraction in myocytes from hypertrophied and failing guinea pig hearts. Am J Physiol 261:H514–H530.
114. Negretti N, O'Neill SC, Eisner DA. (1993) The relative contributions of different intracellular and sarcolemmal systems to relaxation in rat ventricular myocytes. Cardiovasc Res 27:1826–1830.
115. Grynberg A, Demaison L. (1996) Fatty acid oxidation in the heart. J Cardiovasc Pharmacol 28(suppl):S11–S17.
116. Sohal RS, Dubey A. (1994) Mitochondrial oxidative damage, hydrogen peroxide release, and aging. Free Radic Biol Med 16:621–626.
117. Dykens JA. (1997) Mitochondrial free radical production and oxidative pathophysiology: implications for neurodegenerative disease. In: Beal MF, Howell N, eds. Mitochondria and Free Radicals in Neurodegenerative Diseases. New York: Wiley-Liss.
118. Hagen TM, Yowe DL, Bartholomew JC, Wehr CM, Do KLM, Park J-Y, Ames BA. (1997) Mitochondrial decay in hepatocytes from old rats: membrane potential declines, heterogeneity and oxidants increase. Proc Natl Acad Sci USA 94:3064–3069.
119. Boucher F, Tanguy S, Besse S, Tresallet N, Favier A, de Leiris J. (1998) Age-dependent changes in myocardial susceptibility to zero flow ischemia and reperfusion in isolated perfused rat hearts: relation to antioxidant status. Mech Ageing Dev 103:301–316.
120. Abete P, Napoli C, Santoro G, Ferrara N, Tritto I, Chiariello M, Rengo F, Ambrosio G. (1999) Age-related decrease in cardiac tolerance to oxidative stress. J Mol Cell Cardiol 31:227–236.
121. Vega JA, Cavallotti C, Collier WL, De Vincentis G, Rossodivita I, Amenta F. (1992) Changes in glutathione content and localization in rat heart as a function of age. Mech Ageing Dev 64:37–48.
122. Cox RH. (1977) Effects of age on the mechanical properties of rat carotid artery. Am J Physiol 233:H256–H263.
123. Wadsworth RM. (1990) Calcium and vascular reactivity in ageing and hypertension. J Hypertens 8:975–983.
124. Yin FCP. (1980) The aging vasculature and its effect on the heart. In: Weisfeldt ML, ed. The Aging Heart. New York: Raven Press, pp 137–214.
125. Goldberg ID, Shapiro H, Stemerman MB, Wei J, Hardin D, Christenson L. (1984) Frequency of tetraploid nuclei in the rat aortae increases with age. Ann NY Acad Sci 435:422–424.
126. Epstein FH. (1992) Age and cardiovascular system. N Engl J Med 327:1735–1739.
127. Benetos A, Huget F, Albalagejo P, Brisac A–M, Pappo M, Safar ME, Levy BI. (1993) Role of adrenergic tone in mechanical and functional properties of carotid artery during aging. Am J Physiol 26:H1132–H1138.
128. Abrams WB. (1988) Pathophysiology of hypertension in older patients. Am J Med 85(suppl 3B):7–13.
129. Munro JM, Cotran RS. (1988) The pathogenesis of atherosclerosis: atherosclerosis and inflammation. Lab Invest 58:249–261.
130. Ross R. (1986) The pathology of atherosclerosis—an update. N Engl J Med 314:488–500.
131. Henning B, Chow CK. (1988) Lipid peroxidation and endothelial cell injury: implications in atherosclerosis. Free Radic Biol Med 4:99–105.
132. Steinberg D, Parthasarathy S, Carew TE, Khoo JC, Witztum JL. (1989) Beyond cholesterol: modifications of low-density lipoproteins that increase its atherogenicity. N Engl J Med 320:915–924.

133. Heinecke JW, Stocker R. (1995) Lipoprotein oxidation and atherosclerosis. In: Esser K, Martin GM, eds. Molecular Aspects of Aging. Chichester: John Wiley & Sons, pp 254–263.
134. Heinecke JW, Rosen H, Chait A. (1984) Iron and copper promote modification of low-density lipoprotein by human arterial smooth muscle cells in culture. J Clin Invest 74:1890–1894.
135. Morel DW, DiCorleto PE, Chisolm GM. (1984) Endothelial and smooth muscle cells alter low-density lipoprotein in vitro by free radical oxidation. Arteriosclerosis 4:357–364.
136. Steinbrecker UP, Parthasarathy S, Leake DS, Witztum JL, Steinberg D. (1984) Modification of low-density lipoprotein by endothelial cells involves lipid peroxidation and degradation of low density lipoprotein phospholipids. Proc Natl Acad Sci USA 81:3883–3887.
137. Reaven PD, Khouw A, Beltz WF, Parthasarathy S, Witztum JL. (1993) Effect of dietary anitoxidant combinations in humans: protection of LDL by vitamin E but not beta-carotene. Arterioscler Thromb 13:590–600.
138. Reaven PD, Parthasarathy S, Beltz WF, Witztum JL. (1992) Effect of probucol dosage on plasma lipid and lipoprotein levels and on protection of low density lipoprotein against in vitro oxidation in humans. Arterioscler Thromb 12:318–324.
139. Dabbagh AJ, Frei B. (1995) Human suction blister interstitial fluid prevents metal ion-dependent oxidation of low density lipoprotein by macrophages and in cell-free systems. J Clin Invest 96:1958–1966.
140. Thomas CE. (1992) The influence of medium components on co-dependent oxidation of low-density lipoproteins and its sensitivity to superoxide dismutase. Biochim Biophys Acta 1128: 50–57.
141. Offermann MK, Medford RM. (1994) Antioxidants and atherosclerosis: a molecular perspective. Heart Dis Stroke 3:52–57.
142. Collins T. (1993) Biology of disease: endothelial nuclear factor-κB and the initiation of atherosclerotic lesion. Lab Invest 68:499–507.
143. Hennekens CH, Gaziano MJ. (1993) Antioxidants and heart disease: epidemiology and clinical evidence. Clin Cardiol 16:10–15.
144. Rimm EB, Stampfer MJ, Ascherio A, Giovannuci E, Willett GA, Colditz WC. (1993) Vitamin E consumption and the risk of coronary heart disease in men. N Engl J Med 328:1450–1456.
145. Stampfer MJ, Hennekens CH, Manson JE, Colditz GA, Rosner B, Willett WC. (1993) Vitamin E consumption and the risk of coronary heart disease in women. N Engl J Med 328:1444–1449.
146. Brown KM, Morrice PC, Duthie GG. (1994) Vitamin E supplementation suppresses indexes of lipid peroxidation and platelet counts in blood of smokers and nonsmokers but plasma lipoprotein concentrations remain unchanged. Am J Clin Nutr 60:383–387.
147. ATBC—The alpha-tocopherol, beta Carotene Cancer Prevention Study Group (1994) The effect of vitamin E and beta carotene on the incidence of lung cancer and other cancers in male smokers. N Engl J Med 330:1029–1035.
148. Hennekens CH, Buring JE, Manson JE, Stampfer M, Rosner B, Cook NR, Belanger C, LaMotte F, Gaziano JM, Ridker PM, Willett W, Peto R. (1996) Lack of effect of long-term supplementation with beta carotene on the incidence of malignant neoplasms and cardiovascular disease. N Engl J Med 334:1145–1149.
149. Stephens NG, Parsons A, Schofield PM, Kelly F, Cheeseman K, Mitchinson MJ. (1996) Randomised controlled trial of vitamin E in patients with coronary disease: Cambridge Heart Antioxidant Study (CHAOS). Lancet 347:781–786.
150. Virtamo J, Rapola JM, Ripatti S, Heinonen OP, Taylor PR, Albanes D, Huttunen JK. (1998) Effect of vitamin E and beta carotene on the incidence of primary nonfatal myocardial infarction and fatal coronary heart disease. Arch Intern Med 158:668–675.
151. Diaz MN, Frei B, Vita JA, Keaney JF Jr. (1997) Antioxidants and atherosclerotic heart desease. N Engl J Med 337:408–416.
152. Shih JCH. (1983) Atherosclerosis in Japanese quail and the effect of lipoic acid. Fed Proc 42:2492–2497.
153. Suzuki YJ, Aggarwal BB, Packer L. (1992) α-Lipoic acid is a potent inhibitor of NF-kB activation in human T cells. Biochem Biophys Res Commun 189:1709–1715.
154. Schreck R, Rieber P, Baeuerle PA. (1991) Reactive oxygen intermediates as apparently widely used second messengers in the activation of the NFkB transcription factor and HIV-1. Eur Mol Biol Organ J 10:2247–2258.
155. Los M, Dröge W, Stricker K, et al. (1995) Hydrogen peroxide as a potent activator of T lymphocyte functions. Eur J Immunol 25:159–165.

156. Sen CK, Packer L. (1996) Antioxidant and redox regulation of gene transcription. FASEB J 10:709–720.
157. Bierhaus A, Chevion S, Chevion M, Hofmann M, Quehenberger P, Illmer T, Luther T, Berentshtein E, Tritschler H, Muller M, Wahl P, Ziegler R, Nawroth PP. (1997) Advanced glycation end product-induced activation of NF-κB is suppressed by α-lipoic acid in cultured endothelial cells. Diabetes 46:1482–1490.
158. Kunt T, Forst T, Wilhelm A, Tritschler H, Pfuetzner A, Harzer O, Engelbach M, Zschaebitz A, Stofft E, Beyer J. (1999) α-Lipoic acid reduces expression of vascular cell adhesion molecule-1 and endothelial adhesion of human monocytes after stimulation with advanced glycation end products. Clin Sci 96:75–82.
159. Cybulski MI, Gimbrone MA Jr. (1991) Endothelial expression of a mononuclear leukocyte adhesion molecule during atherogenesis. Science 251:788–791.
160. Zhang W, Frei B. (1999) Effect of antioxidants on TNFa-induced adhesion molecule expression in human endothelial cells. Free Radic Biol Med 27(suppl 1):S46.
161. Lerman A, Hallet JW, Henblein DM, Burnett JC Jr. (1991) Circulating and tissue endothelin immunoreactivity in advanced atherosclerosis. N Engl J Med 325:997–1001.
162. Achmad TH, Rao GS. (1992) Chemotaxis of human blood monocytes toward endothelium-1 and the influence of calcium channel blockers. Biochem Biophys Res Commun 189:994–1000.
163. Boscoboinik D, Szewczyk A, Hensey C, Azzi A. (1991) Inhibition of cell proliferation by alpha-tocopherol: role of protein kinase C. J Biol Chem 266:6188–6194.
164. Ghosh S, Baltimore D. (1990) Activation in vitro of NF-kappa B by phosphorylation of its inhibitor I kappa B. Nature 344:678–682.
165. National Society to Prevent Blindness. (1980) Vision Problems in the USA. New York.
166. Benedek GB. (1971) Theory of transparency of the eye. Appl Opt 10:459–473.
167. Creighton MO, Trevithick JR, Mousa GY, Percy DH, McKinna AJ, Dyson C, Maisel H, Bradley R. (1978) Globular bodies: a primary cause of the opacity in senile and diabetic posterior subcapsular cataracts? Can J Ophthalmol 13:166–181.
168. Iwata S, Kinoshita JH. (1971) Mechanism of development of hereditary cataract in mice. Invest Ophthalmol 10:504–512.
169. David LL, Shearer TR, Shih M. (1993) Sequence analysis of lens β-crystallins suggests involvement of caplain in cataract formation. J Biol Chem 268:1937–1940.
170. Duncan G, Williams MR, Riach RA. (1994) Calcium, cell signaling and cataract. Prog Ret Eye Res 13:623–652.
171. Mousa GY, Creighton MO, Trevithick JR. (1979) Eye lens capacity in cortical cataracts associated with actin-related globular degeneration. Exp Eye Res 29:379–391.
172. Shinohara T, Piatigorsky J. (1980) Persistence of crystallin messenger RNA's with reduced translation in hereditary cataracts in mice. Science 210:914–916.
173. Ross WM, Creighton MO, Inch WR, Trevithick JR. (1983) Radiation cataract in vitro reduced by vitamin E. Exp Eye Res 36:645–653.
174. Creighton MO, Ross WM, Stewart–DeHaan PJ, Sanwal M, Trevithick JR. (1985) Modeling cortical cataractogenesis: VII. Effects of vitamin E treatment on galactose-induced cataracts. Exp Eye Res 40:213–222.
175. Linklater HA, Dzialoszynski T, McLeod HL, Sanford SE, Trevithick JR. (1986) Modeling cortical cataractogenesis: VIII. Effects of butylated hydroxytoluene (BHT) in reducing protein leakage from lenses in diabetic rats. Exp Eye Res 43:305–313.
176. Creighton MO, Trevithick JR. (1979) Cortical cataract formation prevented by vitamin E and glutathione. Exp Eye Res 29:680–693.
177. Trevithick JR, Creighton MO, Ross WM, Stewart–DeHaan PJ, Sanwal M. (1981) Modeling cortical cataractogenesis: 2. In vitro effects on the lens of agents preventing glucose- and sorbitol-induced cataract. Can J Ophthalmol 16:32–38.
178. Abe M, Reiter RJ, Orhii PB, Hara M, Poeggeler B. (1994) Inhibitory effect of melatonin on cataract formation in newborn rats: evidence for an antioxidative role for melatonin. J Pineal Res 17:94–100.
179. Leske MC, Wu S-Y, Hyman L, Sperduto R, Underwood B, Chylack LT, Mitton RC, Srivastava S, Ansari N. (1995) Biochemical factors in the lens opacities case–control study. Arch Ophthalmol 113:1113–1119.
180. Babizhayev MA, Costa EB. (1994) Lipid peroxide and reactive oxygen species generating systems of the crystalline lens. Biochim Biophys Acta 1225:326–337.

181. Smith JB, Jiang X, Abraham EC. (1997) Identification of hydrogen peroxide oxidation sites of α-A- and α-B-crystallins. Free Radic Res 26:103–111.
182. Maitra I, Serbinova E, Tritschler H, Packer L. (1995) α-Lipoic acid prevent buthionine–sulfoximine-induced cataract formation in newborn rats. Free Radic Biol Med 18:823–829.
183. Mitton KP. (1994) Antioxidant and ATP loss in the diabetic rat lens. PhD dissertation, University of Western Ontario.
184. Kilic F, Handelman GJ, Serbinova E, et al. (1995) Modeling cortical cataractogenesis: XVII. In vitro effect of α-lipoic acid on glucose-induced lens membrane damage, a model of diabetic cataractogenesis. Biochem Mol Biol 37:361–370.
185. Trevithick JR. (1997) α-Lipoic acid and cataract risk reduction. In: Fuchs J, Packer L, Zimmer G, eds. Lipoic Acid in Health and Disease. New York: Marcel Dekker, pp 227–242.
186. Jocelyn PC. (1967) The standard redox potential of cysteine–cystine from the thiol–disulfide exchange reaction with glutathione and lipoic acid. Eur J Biochem 2:327–331.
187. Packer L. (1993) The role of anti-oxidative treatment of diabetes mellitus. Diabetologia 36:1212–1213.
188. Ou P, Nourooz–Zadeh J, Tritschler HJ, Wolff S. (1996) Activation of aldolase reductase in rat lens and metal-ion chelation by aldolase reductase inhibitors and lipoic acid. Free Radic Res 25:337–346.
189. Mitton KP, Dean PAW, Dzialoszynski T, Xiong H, Sanford SE, Trevithick JR. (1993) Modeling cortical cataractogenesis: 13. Early effects on lens ATP/ADP and glutathione in streptozotocin rat model of diabetic cataract. Exp Eye Res 56:187–198.

25
Vascular Complications in Diabetes: Mechanisms and the Influence of Antioxidants

Peter Rösen
Diabetes Research Institute, Düsseldorf, Germany

Hans-Jürgen Tritschler
Asta Medica AG, Frankfurt Am Main, Germany

Lester Packer
University of Southern California School of Pharmacy, Los Angeles, California

I. INTRODUCTION

Diabetes and its complications is one of the major disorders worldwide, and the number of patients with this disease is increasing worldwide (1). According to an estimation of the World Health Organization (WHO) the number of diabetic patients will double between 1990 and the beginning of the next millennium. The large majority of these patients consists of type 2 or non–insulin-dependent (NIDDM) patients. The life expectancy and quality of life of these patients is no longer determined by the acute complications of diabetes, but the development of vascular complications. Thus, diabetes is the main cause for blindness in adults; most of the patients who undergo dialysis or kidney transplantation are diabetic, the cardiovascular risk is two- to fourfold increased when compared with the nondiabetic population (2,3).

There is emerging evidence that diabetes leads to depletion of the cellular antioxidant defense system and increased levels of reactive oxygen species (ROS). This new concept of oxidation stress as an important trigger in the onset and progression of diabetes may offer a unique therapeutic option to treat the disease and its complications by using antioxidants or nutrients with high antioxidant capacity.

II. OXIDATIVE STRESS AND OXIDATION DAMAGE IN DIABETES AND ITS COMPLICATIONS

There is emerging evidence that free ROS make a significant contribution to the progression of diabetes and its complications (4–9). The term *oxidative stress*, widely used in the literature, refers to a serious imbalance between the production of free radicals and antioxidant defense, leading to potential tissue damage (10). Free radical reactions are essential for host defense mechanisms, as with neutrophils, macrophages, and other cells of the immune system, but if free radicals are overproduced, they cause tissue injury and cell death (11–13). To avoid the free radical overproduction, antioxidants are present in tissues to neutralize them (12–15) and to protect biological tissues from free radical damage. The most prominent members of antioxidants are vitamin E (*RRR*-α-tocopherol), vitamin C (ascorbate), α-lipoic acid (thioctic acid), and glutathione (16–19). Recent research has shown that these four substances compose an antioxidant network, which enables them to be recycled and regenerated in a coordinated way (20–22). Importantly, oxidative stress can be derived either from an increased formation of ROS or by a diminished ability to inactivate the ROS.

A. Evidence for an Increased Stress in Diabetes

There is now convincing evidence hat the oxidative stress is increased in diabetic patients. In the recommendations for the nutritional management of patients with diabetes mellitus, the Diabetes and Nutrition Study Group (DNSG) of the European Association for the Study of Diabetes (EASD) declares that the equilibrium between pro- and antioxidants is disturbed in patients with diabetes mellitus and that this increased oxidative stress increases the cardiovascular risk (23).

A manifold of clinical studies shows increases in levels of oxidative stress markers (Fig. 1), such as of lipid peroxidation, oxidatively damaged DNA (8-hydroxydeoxyguanosine, 8-hydroxyadenine, 7-methyl-8-hydroxyguanine), and reduced levels of antioxidants (glutathione, vitamin E, and vitamin C).

Increased levels of lipid peroxides and lipid hydroperoxides, oxidized low-density lipoproteins (LDL), and thiobarbituric acid-reactive compounds (TBARS) have been observed in the plasma of both types of diabetic patients (24–29). Very recently, the formation of isoprostanes

Evidence for the Generation of ROI in Diabetes

- increased formation of isoprostanes
- increased generation of lipidhydroperoxides
- elevated oxidized and glycoxidized LDL
- formation of MDA
- changes in the antioxidative enzymes
- alterations in the redox systems (NADPH, glutathione, antioxidative vitamines, etc.)
- increased oxidative breakdown of DNA

Figure 1 Markers of oxidative stress that are described to be increased in patients with diabetes mellitus.

has been suggested as a more specific parameter of oxidative stress (30). Isoprostanes such as the 8-epi-isoprostaglandin F_{2a} are synthesized nonenzymatically from arachidonic acid by autoxidative processes. In recent studies evidence has been presented that the formation of these specific markers of oxidative stress is increased in diabetic patients (31–33). Furthermore, the levels of isoprostanes measured in the urine became reduced if the metabolic control was improved or if the patients were treated with antioxidative vitamins (33). Thus, these and other data suggest a clear dependency of the oxidative stress on the metabolic control as originally postulated from experimental observations (34).

Several studies have demonstrated increased LDL oxidation in diabetic patients when compared with their corresponding controls (24,25,35–44), an observation that is of much importance, for oxidized lipoproteins (oxLDL) contribute to the development of cardiovascular complications.

In addition, the glycation of proteins increases their susceptibility for oxidative modifications. Thus, glycated LDLs are much more easily oxidized than nonglycated LDL. Both fractions of LDL—oxidized and glycoxidized LDL—are increased in diabetic patients. This high susceptibility can be reduced by treatment of diabetic patients with tocopherol (37,39,45).

Reactive oxygen species (ROS) cause strand breaks in DNA and base modifications, including the oxidation of guanine residues as to 8-oxo-2′deoxyguanosine (8-oxodG) (46). 8-OxodG was increased in the kidney of diabetic rats, and insulin treatment reduced the urinary albumin excretion as well as the generation of 8-oxodG. Very recently, an increase in the 8-oxodG content in mononuclear cells of type 1 and type 2 diabetic patients was observed when compared with control subjects (47). The urinary excretion of 8-oxodG was higher in type 2 diabetic patients than in control subjects and correlated with glycated hemoglobin (48). Furthermore, Hinokio et al. (49) could show that the excretion and the content of 8-oxodG was higher in mononuclear cells of diabetic patients with vascular complications than in those from patients without complications.

In addition to these alterations in specific markers of oxidative stress, a decrease in antioxidant capacity has been observed in the plasma of diabetic patients by several research groups. The total radical-trapping antioxidant parameter (TRAP) reflecting the antioxidative activity of the network of antioxidants was clearly diminished in diabetes of both types (50,51). That the concentration of specific antioxidants in the plasma of diabetic patients is reduced has been shown by various clinical studies (25,51–64). Thornally et al. reported (65) a decrease of the endogenous antioxidant glutathione in the erythrocytes of diabetic patients. The decline in the plasma levels of the antioxidants *RRR*-α-tocopherol or glutathione may be explained as a result of the increased production of free radicals in diabetic patients. However, also other explanations need to be taken into considerations. Rösen et al. presented data of two nutritional studies (Fig. 2; Table 1) showing a dietary-induced *RRR*-α-tocopherol deficiency in older subjects and especially in diabetic patients (66,67). Dietary recommendations are for diabetic patients aiming to reduce their fat intake to decrease weight. The lipophilic antioxidant *RRR*-α-tocopherol is present in the fat-soluble phase of food ingredients and, therefore, may be underrepresented in a fat-reduced diabetic diet. In addition, the *RRR*-α-tocopherol content of dietary recommendations of diabetic patients was analyzed in food records of 100 such patients, those values were compared with the recommended dietary allowance (RDA) of *RRR*-α-tocopherol. In 50% of the eating plans and dietary recommendations, the *RRR*-α-tocopherol intake was lower than what the RDA would achieve. Furthermore, there was a negative relation in the energy content of the diabetic diet and the dietary *RRR*-α-tocopherol intake, resulting in a potentially severe α-tocopherol deficiency in those diabetic patients who were obese and received a slimming diet. Long-term dietary restriction of *RRR*-α-tocopherol leads to reduced *RRR*-α-tocopherol

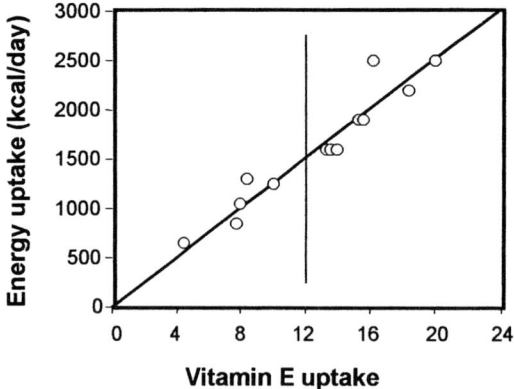

Figure 2 Intake of vitamin E by type 2 diabetic patients: Intake of vitamin E is dependent on the energy uptake. The intake of vitamin E was calculated as described in the reference. A significant number of patients (43%) consumed less vitamin E than the recommended allowance of 12 mg/day. (From Ref. 66.)

plasma levels in men (66,67). A reduced uptake of vitamin C has also been described in diabetic patients (61–63). Most studies have found that persons with diabetes mellitus have at least 30% lower circulating ascorbic acid concentrations than those without diabetes (6). Nevertheless, the reported data do not allow the conclusion that there is a general vitamin C deficit in diabetic patients. This is very clearly shown by a very recent report about the data from the third National Health and Nutrition Examination Survey (NHANES III) (64). The data rather suggest that the oxidative stress and the supply with antioxidative vitamins varies with the disease state and especially with the age. Therefore, we would assume that a deficit in antioxidative vitamins is detected only in subgroups of patients and, specifically, in elderly ones, those on diets for weight reduction, and with progression of the disease (65). Independently from the observed plasma levels, the demand for antioxidative vitamins might be increased in diabetic patients.

The effects of antioxidant supplementation on oxidative stress measures is an indirect way to further prove the pathogenic concept of elevated free radicals and antioxidant depletion leading to diabetic complications. Despite the arguments that can be raised about the validity of

Table 1 Intakes of Vitamins E and C by a Sample of the German Population Older than 40 Years (Nationale Verzehrstudie)

Vitamin	Nondiabetics (N, $n = 4958$)	Diabetics (D, $n = 383$)	Intake equal or more than RDA
Provitamin A/β-carotin (mg/day)	1.55 (1–2.6)	1.58 (0.9–2.6)	N 37%; D 38%
Vitamin E/total tocopherol (mg/day)	12.5 (10–16)	12.7 (9–17)	N 54%; D 55%
Vitamin C/total ascorbic acid (mg/day)	78 (52–114)	80 (55–109)	N 53%; D 55%
Intake of vitamin supplements (n%)	14%	17%	

The intake of the vitamins was assessed from standardized nutritional protocols in an age and diabetes duration stratified sample of individuals with type 1 diabetes. A significant number of individuals consumed less vitamins than the recommended daily allowance.
Source: Ref. 67.

some individual biomarkers, the sum of evidence from biomarkers reporting oxidative damage to DNA and lipids proteins supports the concept of increased oxidative stress in diabetes.

III. VASCULAR COMPLICATIONS

Microvascular complications are one of the most serious burdens of diabetes that determine the life quality and expectancy of diabetic patients. Diabetic retinopathy and nephropathy are typical complications, but it became clear in the last years that microvascular complications can also affect the heart and contribute to the development of diabetic neuropathy by limiting the endoneuronal blood flow. Our knowledge about the mechanisms leading to microvascular complications in diabetes are still limited, but it is very well known that reactive oxygen intermediates (ROI) contribute to vascular disease by promoting

- Vascular tone alterations
- Vascular permeability
- Monocyte–macrophage infiltration
- Smooth-muscle cell proliferation
- Activation of metalloproteases

Thus, it is to be expected that oxidative stress has a large effect on the function and structure of the vessel wall and the stability of already existing plaques in diabetic patients. We will at first discuss mechanisms that may lead to oxidative stress in diabetes; secondly, mechanisms that alter cellular-signaling pathways and may contribute to changes in gene expression; and lastly, more specifically, the consequences for the function of the vessel wall and the vascular risk of diabetic patients.

A. Generation of Reactive Oxygen Species (ROS) and Activation of PKC

There is a lot of evidence from experimental studies that the formation of reactive oxygen species (ROS) is a direct consequence of hyperglycemia. Incubation of endothelial and smooth-muscle cells with increasing concentrations of glucose initiates the formation of ROS (68–74). A significant increase was already observed at glucose concentrations as high as 10 mM (68). In addition, advanced glycolation end products (AGE) stimulate the formation of ROS by a receptor-mediated process (75–78). Recently, Giardino et al. (71) have shown that the intracellular formation of AGEs and lipid peroxidation are closely dependent processes. Inhibition of lipid peroxidation also prevented the formation AGE products. That the autoxidation of glucose leads to the formation of ROS has already been shown (79,80). Furthermore, the regeneration of glutathione is delayed in the presence of high glucose levels, causing an impairment of the antioxidant defense (81). Thus, there are various pathways known by which ROS may be generated in diabetes, and a lot of experimental evidence has been accumulated that various types of vascular cells are able to produce ROS under hyperglycemic conditions.

However, the exact mechanisms and sources by which ROS are generated in the vasculature are not yet known in detail. In hypercholesterolemic as well as hypertonic animal models, several groups have shown that the endothelium is one of the major sources for the generation of ROS. In parallel with the vascular dysfunction the formation of superoxide anions became augmented, and removal of endothelium completely abolished the production of ROS (82–85). Furthermore, the generation of ROS is largely dependent on the activation of a NADH-oxidase that is present not only in mononuclear cells, but also in endothelial cells. A similar scenario seems to exist in diabetes (Fig. 3). High glucose levels stimulate the generation of superoxide anions in various types of endothelial cells (68,86), and this process is initiated by the release of calcium from intracellular stores (86). Because the production of superoxide anions is not inhibited by inhibitors of P450-dependent oxygenases, and lipo- and cyclooxygenases, but by inhibition of NADH-oxidase, we have concluded that in addition to autoxidation (78,79), NADH-oxidases become activated as a consequence of hyperglycemia and presumably also of incubation of endothelial cells with AGE-products. Activation of NADH-oxidase would be supported by the accelerated conversion of glucose to fructose through the sorbitol-pathway. Because in vascular cells the uptake of glucose is not limited by the glucose transporter (87), a significant amount of glucose is metabolized by this pathway. This metabolic pathway has a large influence on the redox state of a cell, because conversion of glucose by this pathway consumes NADPH, but leads to an increase in NADH (88). Thus, a cofactor of NADH-oxidase is available, whereas NADPH as an important cofactor for glutathione peroxidase is diminished, which may impair the regeneration of glutathione and limit the antioxidative capacity of the cells (76,81).

Alternatively, the endothelial nitric oxide synthase (eNOS) might be considered an important source for the generation of ROS. A reduced availability of L-arginine or reduced regeneration of biopterin, which is an essential cofactor of NOS, causes a partial uncoupling of the electron flux in the NOS complex and leads to an enhanced production of superoxide anions instead of nitric oxide (89). In line with this hypothesis, we observed that the hyperglycemia-induced formation of ROS could be inhibited by L-NAME, an inhibitor of NOS (68). Furthermore, the impaired endothelium-dependent vasodilatation was at least partially prevented by supplementation of diabetic rats with high doses of L-arginine (90).

Irrespective of the mechanism of ROS production, the increased formation of ROS in diabetes has severe consequences:

1. Quenching of Nitric Oxide

There is considerable evidence that nitric oxide reacts in a diffusion-controlled way with superoxide anions to peroxynitrite (91). Thus, a simultaneous formation of ROS would reduce the amount of biologically active nitric oxide and lead to an impairment of endothelium-dependent vasodilation. That such a mechanism may be operative has been demonstrated in hypertension

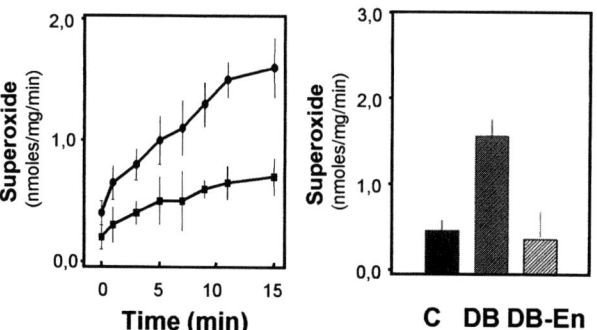

Figure 3 The generation of superoxide anions by isolated aortas from control and diabetic rats: The aortas were isolated and incubated in a glucose-containing phosphate buffer. Superoxide anions were determined by the cytochrome c assay. Diabetes was induced by streptozocin (94), the diabetes duration was 12 weeks. C, controls; DB, diabetes; DB-end, aortas from diabetic rats from which the endothelium has been removed.

and hypercholesterolemia (92,93). We have suggested that a similar mechanism is acting in the heart, as the impaired endothelium-dependent relaxation was restored by the addition of superoxide dismutase, an enzyme that inactivates superoxide anions very effectively (Fig. 4), and by pretreatment of diabetic animals with tocopherol (94). Furthermore, in endothelial cells exposed to high glucose concentrations, the formation of peroxynitrite has been shown directly by immunoblotting (95). Experimental studies using various types of vessels are in line with this hypothesis (5–9,94). In addition to superoxide anions, AGE have been shown (96) to quench nitric oxide and may thereby be important modulators of endothelium-dependent relaxation. Recent clinical studies show consistently that antioxidants are able to reverse or to improve the disturbed endothelium-dependent vasodilation in diabetic patients, in patients with coronary artery disease, hypercholesterolemia, hypertension, or high, remnant lipoproteins levels using various types of antioxidants (97–107).

Quenching of nitric oxide, however, affects not only the vasotone, but additionally the antithrombotic properties of endothelium, because nitric oxide inhibits the expression of adhesion molecules (VCAM-1 and ICAM-1) and the proliferation of smooth-muscle cells (108). Thus, the antithrombotic and antiatherosclerotic defense becomes defective if the bioavailability of nitric oxide is diminished by oxidative stress.

2. *Activation of Redox-Sensitive Transcription Factors by AGE and Hyperglycemia*

The generation of ROS in the presence of hyperglycemia and AGE results in depletion of cellular antioxidant defense mechanisms (e.g., glutathione, ascorbate) and the activation of redox-sensitive transcription factors, such as NF-κB (68,109–113).

Nawroth et al. reported increased activation of NF-κB in monocytes of type 1 diabetic patients when compared with healthy controls (114,115). Additionally, a positive correlation

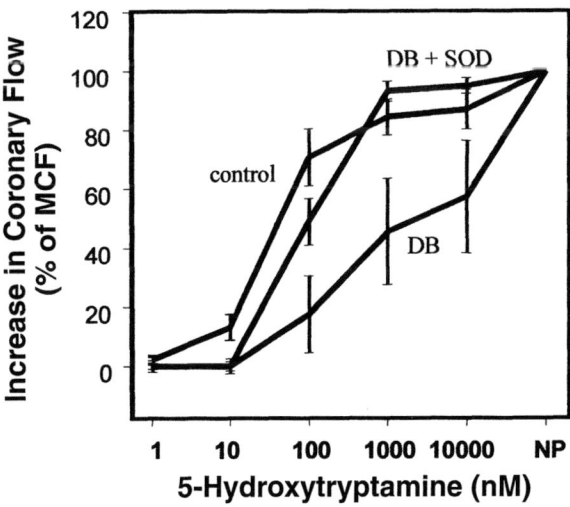

Figure 4 Endothelium-dependent vasodilation in response to 5-hydroxytryptamine: impairment by diabetes and normalization by perfusion with superoxide dismutase: Hearts were isolated from control and diabetic (streptozocin; 16 weeks) rats and perfused retrogradely. The increase in coronary flow was determined by dependence on 5-hydroxytryptamine. Diabetes caused a shift of the dose–response curve, indicating an impairment in the endothelium-dependent relaxation of coronary vessels. Addition of superoxide dismutase nearly normalized this defect. (From Ref. 94.)

between metabolic control and NF-κB was seen (114). A positive correlation between the endothelial dysfunction marker thrombomodulin and NF-κB activation has been observed. A similar correlation was found between urinary albuminuria and NF-κB activation (115). The correlation of thrombomodulin plasma levels, urinary albumin, and NF-κB–binding activity suggests a link between NF-κB activation, endothelial dysfunction as well as diabetic nephropathy.

Activation of NF-κB even by short-term high concentrations of glucose might indicate a link between elevated postprandial glucose levels ("glucose spikes") and the development of vascular complications (69). Ceriello et al. (116) demonstrated recently that free radicals are produced in diabetic patients in the absorptive state. These observations suggest that the postprandial state is associated with an increase in the generation of ROS that may be linked to the activation of NF-κB. Activation of NF-κB, on the other hand, can contribute to the increased cardiac risk, changing the dynamic endothelial balance from an anti- to a procoagulant state, and favoring vasoconstriction instead of vasodilation (Fig. 5).

In line with the concept that ROS play an important role for NF-κB activation, its activation could be inhibited by antioxidants, such as *RRR-α*-tocopherol, acetylcysteine, and α-lipoic acid (Fig. 6) (68,111,114–116). In a clinical trial a decrease in NF-κB binding activity in mononuclear blood cells was observed in diabetic patients receiving 600 mg of α-lipoic acid per day (114,115). This effect was independent of the level of glycemic control, the degree of endothelial dysfunction, as well as different stages of diabetic nephropathy. In an 18-month pilot study, the effect of 600 mg α-lipoic acid supplementation on the progression of diabetic nephropathy was studied (117). Plasma thrombomodulin levels (as a marker for endothelial dysfunction) and urinary albuminuria (as a marker for nephropathy) were compared between a group treated with α-lipoic acid and a control group who received no treatment. α-Lipoic acid significantly reduced the time-dependent decrease of plasma thrombomodulin and urinary albuminuria seen in control patients. Treatment with α-lipoic acid was the only significant factor predicting the decrease of plasma thrombomodulin and urinary albuminuria in multiple regression analysis.

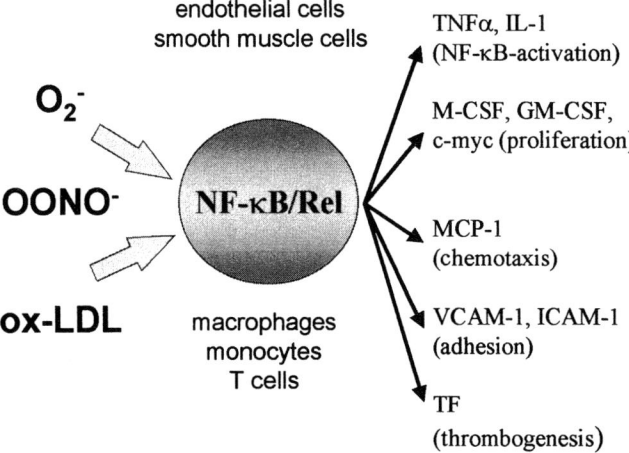

Figure 5 Activation of the transcription factor NF-κB by various oxygen radicals and the consequences for the vasculature: increased adhesivity and thrombogenicity, increased proliferation and induction of an inflammatory response were observed.

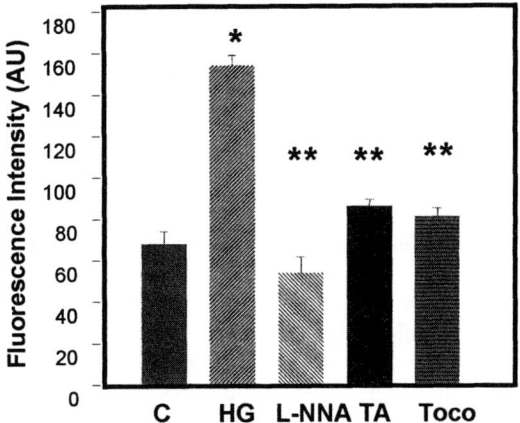

Figure 6 Activation of NF-κB by high glucose concentration and its inhibition by antioxidants: Human endothelial cells were incubated in the presence of a high glucose level (30 mM) for 4 h. Thereafter, the activation of NF-κB was determined by the electrophoretic mobility shift assay. C, control; HG, high-glucose; L-NNA, L-nitroarginine; TA, α-lipoic acid; Toco, α-tocopherol. (From Ref. 68.)

In summary, experimental and clinical results provide increasing evidence that redox-sensitive transcription factors are activated by AGE or hyperglycemia, which may play a central role in the development of hyperglycemia-induced "late" complications.

3. Activation of Protein Kinase C Isoforms

Various experimental observations and the use of the selective protein kinase (PKC) inhibitors, such as LY 333531 and *RRR*-α-tocopherol, suggest that in diabetes various isoform of PKC, such as PKC-β and PKC-α are activated in vascular tissue and may be responsible for many vascular dysfunctions occurring in diabetes (118–124). In increase in diacylglycerol (DAG), a strong activator of PKC (125,126) has been suggested to underlie this activation of PKC in diabetes, because an increase in DAG has been observed in hyperglycemia and diabetes by several investigators, especially in those tissues and cells that take up glucose independently from insulin (125,126). The observation that α-tocopherol specifically inhibits the hyperglycemia-mediated activation of PKC suggests that redox-sensitive mechanisms may be important. For example, the regulation of diacylglycerol kinase (118,127)—activation would lead to reduced levels of DAG—or activation of specific proteinphosphatases that cause PKC-α dephosphorylation and inhibition (128), may prevent activation of PKC isoforms in diabetes. These observations suggest that activation of PKC might be a common downstream mechanism to which multiple cellular and functional abnormalities in the diabetic vascular tissue can be attributed, including changes in vascular blood flow, vascular permeability, extracellular matrix components, and cell growth. However, much more work has to be done to understand the complex interactions between redox-sensitive and PKC–dependent-signaling pathways.

B. Vascular Blood Flow

Abnormalities in the vascular blood flow and contractility have been found in many organs of diabetic animals and patients, including kidney, retina, heart, peripheral arteries, and microvessels of peripheral nerves.

In the retina of diabetic patients and animals with short duration of diabetes, but also in peripheral nerves of diabetic rats, a decrease in blood flow has been described that was normalized by α-tocopherol or inhibition of PKC (122,129–136), although there are also reports claiming an increased retinal and neuronal blood flow (137). In line with the assumption of a disturbed retinal blood flow, the effect of 1800 mg *RRR*-α-tocopherol on retinal blood flow and renal function has been evaluated in IDDM patients in a placebo-controlled double-shielded trial (138). After 6 months there was an increase in retinal blood flow and improvement of renal function in the *RRR*-α-tocopherol-treated group, which was statistically significant when compared with placebo.

Another mechanism by which a ROS-mediated activation of PKC may contribute to vasoconstriction is an increase in the expression of endothelin-1 (ET-1) (139). The expression of ET-1 is dependent on the binding of nuclear proteins to the GATA motif and on activation of the redox-sensitive transcription factor AP-1 (140). Furthermore, hypoxia, which is associated with the increased formation of ROS, induces the expression of ET-1 and of the vascular endothelial growth factor (VEGF) (141). That the expression of ET-1 is increased in the retina of diabetic rats, and that the decrease in retinal blood flow is prevented by an endothelin receptor antagonist (141), supports this hypothesis. ROS may, therefore, directly and indirectly contribute to reduction in retinal blood flow, to local hypoxia, and induce VEGF, causing increases in vascular permeability and microaneurysms (142,143).

In the kidney, various abnormalities in hemodynamics have been clearly documented to precede diabetic nephropathy (144,145). Elevated renal glomerular filtration rate (GFR) and increases in renal flow are typically found in IDDM patients and animals with experimental diabetes (144–146). It is assumed that a decrease in arteriolar resistance, especially at the level of arterioles (147,148) results in an elevation of glomerular filtration pressure. Various mechanisms have been suggested to explain the increases in the generation of vasodilatory prostanoids (PGE_2, PGI_2) and the increases in the generation of NO (149–154) that are assumed to be responsible for the reduced arteriolar resistance. We know that oxidative stress induces the expression of transforming growth factor-β (TGF-β), which is consistently increased in the kidney in diabetes (155). Because TGF-β has already been shown to be not only able to increase the PGE_2 and NO generation by α-tocopherol-sensitive mechanisms (156), but also to have a profound effect on the mesangial expansion (157)—another characteristic of diabetic nephropathy—we assume that the expression of TGF-β caused by an increased oxidative stress plays a significant role for the development of abnormalities in hemodynamics and the structural adaptation processes in the diabetic kidney.

In resistance and larger vessels, the endothelium-dependent vasodilation has been reported to be impaired (4–9,72,74,94). This defect seems of special importance in type 2 diabetic patients because it seems to be related to the incidence of type 2 diabetes (158) and to precede the presence of microalbuminuria as a very early indicator for the development of vascular complications in diabetes (159). An impairment of endothelium-dependent vasodilation (4–9,94) has been observed in school children between 9 and 11 years of age (160), and there is considerable evidence that this defect precedes the onset of type 2 diabetes (159). In diabetic patients and animals with experimental diabetes, it has consistently been shown that application of antioxidants (α-tocopherol, probucol, vitamin C, and others) at least partially normalized the impaired endothelium vasodilation similar (see Fig. 4) to that of patients with other types of vascular diseases (hypertension, hypercholesterolemia, cigarette smoking, and others) (94,97–107,161). As those defects have been described, even under conditions with an enhanced NOS activity, it seems that this is less of a defect in the NOS system itself, but rather, an accelerated degradation of NO under hyperglycemic conditions is of importance.

Taken together, there is a lot of experimental and clinical evidence that the formation of ROS has a large influence on the blood flow and structure of the vessel wall in diabetes. These observations, however, do not exclude that other mechanisms may be operative in addition, such as the activation of specific isoforms of PKC, the enhanced formation of the endothelium-constricting factor, or vasoconstricting prostaglandin peroxides. For a complete understanding we have to know the network of mediators determining the fine-tuning of blood flow and the influence of diabetes on this network.

C. Vascular Permeability and Proliferation of Vascular Cells

Increased vascular permeability and vascular cell proliferation are early manifestations of endothelial dysfunction leading to microvascular and macrovascular complications (162–167). The mechanism accounting for increased endothelial permeability in diabetes is unclear. Ultrastructural studies presented little evidence of endothelial denudation, implying endothelial dysfunction rather than injury (168). Because strict glycemic control is able to prevent or to delay the increase in vascular permeability (169), it has been postulated that elevated glucose concentrations play an important role in the alteration of permeability typically seen in diabetes. Abnormalities in endothelial proliferation, leading to neovascularization, represent another important characteristic of endothelial dysfunction in diabetes (170). The development of diabetic microangiopathy can be delayed by strict glycemic control, suggesting that hyperglycemia may be an important stimulus for the development of neovascularization and microangiopathy (171–173). VEGF is an attractive candidate as a mediator for the increases in endothelial permeability and other endothelial dysfunctions observed in diabetes (6,170). In addition to its potent capacity to increase endothelial permeability and promote angiogenesis, VEGF also stimulates the release of von Willebrand's factor, another characteristic feature of diabetic microangiopathy, and induces a procoagulant state of the endothelial surface (174). In line with this hypothesis, the release of VEGF is increased by high glucose levels and advanced glycation end products (AGEs) (176). Additionally, topical application of a superoxide-generating system increased albumin permeation and blood flow in diabetic rats, changes that were strongly attenuated by VEGF antibodies (6). The AGE-induced increases in VEGF were dose- and time-dependent and were inhibited by antioxidants, suggesting a prominent role of ROS. That ROS stimulate the expression of VEGF has been clearly demonstrated by others (176). There is also some evidence that activation of PKC-β contributes to the alterations in vascular permeability and neovascularization, for application of PKC-β-specific inhibitors decreased endothelial proliferation, angiogenesis, and permeability induced by VEGF (177). Williams et al. (143) have additionally shown that, in smooth-muscle cells, a high glucose level increases the release and expression of VEGF by a PKC-dependent mechanism indicating again a complex interrelation between oxidative stress and activation of specific isoforms of PKC.

However, it cannot be excluded that other mechanisms may also contribute to the observed changes in endothelial permeability. Thus, there is a lot of evidence that ROS directly induce a contraction of endothelial cells that is associated with an opening of endothelial junctions (178). In addition, Haller et al. (179) presented evidence that high glucose levels reduce the endothelial barrier function by a PKC-α- and calcium-dependent process.

D. Extracellular Matrix Components

Thickening of capillary basement membrane is one of the early structural abnormalities observed in tissues including the vascular system in diabetes (180). Histologically increases in type IV and VI collagen, fibronectin, and laminin, as well as decreases of proteoglycans are observed not only in mesangium (181–187), but also in the heart (94) and other vascular beds of diabetic patients (189). Experimental studies show that these alterations in the vascular bed can be prevented by high doses of antioxidants, such as tocopherol and inhibition of PKC (94,118,119). Several lines of evidence suggest that the expression of transforming growth factor-β (TGF-β) is of major importance for the observations typically seen in the kidney and the vessel wall of diabetic patients and animals. In the kidney and in the vessel wall the expression of TGF-β is increased in diabetes (155). There is also some evidence that the expression of TGF-β is elevated in mesangial cells exposed to high glucose levels (155) and that ROS play an important role for the induction of this growth factor (156). Furthermore, Ziyadeh et al. (189) and Sharma et al. (190) reported that neutralizing TGF-β antibodies significantly reduced collagen synthesis and gene expression of type IV collagen and fibronectin in the renal cortex of diabetic rats and in cultured mesangial cells exposed to high glucose levels.

IV. MACROVASCULAR COMPLICATIONS: THE ROLE OF MODIFIED LIPOPROTEINS, OXIDATIVE STRESS MEASURES, AND ANTIOXIDANT DEPLETION IN THE ONSET AND PROGRESSION OF CARDIOVASCULAR DISEASE

The imbalance between oxidative stress measures and antioxidant levels in diabetes is present because of the generation of ROS during glycation and glucose and lipid oxidation. These elevated levels of free radicals may be at least partly responsible for the observed depletion of antioxidants, such as glutathione, *RRR*-α-tocopherol, and ascorbate, in the plasma of diabetic patients (25,45,52,65). In addition, there is sufficient evidence of an *RRR*-α-tocopherol and ascorbic acid deficiency in the diet of diabetic patients (63–67), which may account for the decrease in plasma levels of both antioxidants in diabetic patients when compared with controls. *RRR*-α-Tocopherol is the major antioxidant in the LDL particle accounting for over 90% of LDL protection against lipid peroxidation (191). Therefore, it is reasonable to suggest that enhanced LDL oxidation in diabetic patients derives not only from glucose-induced free radical production, but also from insufficient antioxidant protection. Hyperglycemia not only leads to increased susceptibility of LDL oxidation, but also to increased nonenzymatic glycation of LDL (36,192). These modified LDL particles are increased in the plasma of diabetic patients compared with healthy controls (36–45,191,192). Elevated levels of autoantibodies against these modified LDL particles have also been detected in diabetic patients (36,37). Modified LDL exhibits biological properties that promote atherogenesis. Unlike other lipoproteins, oxidized or glycated LDL is also able to transform macrophages and perhaps also smooth-muscle cells into foam cells as well as modulate the growth factor and cytokine expression, thereby leading to the formation of atherogenic plaques (191). Salonen et al. (193) could demonstrate that the titer of autoantibodies to MDA-LDL (as an epitope of oxLDL) in asymptomatic middle-aged men predicted the rate of carotid arteriosclerosis. Since this initial report, there have been several studies demonstrating a relation between such autoantibody titers and clinical manifestations of atherosclerosis (36,194,195).

That *RRR*-α-tocopherol reduces the proatherogenic risk factors such as oxidized LDL, which are thought to be responsible for the onset and progression of coronary heart disease in diabetic patients, is demonstrated by several observations. Clinical studies have shown an inhibitory effect of *RRR*-α-tocopherol supplementation on the hyperglycemia-induced LDL modifications in IDDM and NIDDM patients (39,196,197). Reaven evaluated the effect 1600 IU of *RRR*-α-tocopherol supplementation daily for 10 weeks on the hyperglycemia-induced LDL modifications in a placebo-controlled randomized trial (39). There was a reduction of plasma

LDL oxidation of approximately 60% in diabetic patients, which was statistically significant when compared with healthy controls. These results could be confirmed by other groups. Jialal et al. (197) found that doses equal or higher than 450 IU are sufficient to significantly ameliorate the susceptibility of LDL to oxidation, indicating that relatively high doses of *RRR*-α-tocopherol for supplementation are needed. Furthermore, the effects of *RRR*-α-tocopherol supplementation on LDL oxidation is accompanied by a concomitant reduction in autoantibody levels against hyperglycemia-induced LDL modifications (36,37). Hyperglycemia-induced LDL modifications are antigens and induce autoantibodies against these epitopes. Several studies also point to the importance of ascorbate for LDL-protection (198,199). The best protection might be achieved by a combination of both antioxidants, as ascorbic acid is necessary for the regeneration of reduced tocopherol at the surface of the LDL particle and to finally detoxify the oxygen radicals.

There is epidemiological and clinical evidence in nondiabetic individuals that *RRR*-α-tocopherol supplementation is associated with a reduction of coronary heart disease. The evidence for other antioxidants is less convincing. The WHO-sponsored Monica Study found an inverse correlation between plasma *RRR*-α-tocopherol levels and coronary heart disease (CHD) mortality in different European populations (200). The Physician Health Study, investigating the beneficial effects of *RRR*-α-tocopherol supplementation in 80,000 women and 40,000 men, found an approximate 40% reduction in death from coronary heart disease in those ingested 200–400 IU of α-tocopherol daily when compared with those who received less than 10 IU/day (201,202). The hypothesis of cardioprotective effects of *RRR*-α-tocopherol is further supported by the results of the CHAOS study, showing a 77% reduction of nonfatal myocardial infarction rate in those receiving α-tocopherol, compared with the placebo group (203). The subgroup analysis of the approximate 170 diabetic patients also enrolled in this study showed a marked 50% reduction of the nonfatal heart infarction rate, which was not statistically significant ($p = 0.14$) owing to the small sample size of the diabetic patient group (204). The cardioprotective effects of *RRR*-α-tocopherol seen in epidemiological and clinical studies may relate to its inhibitory effects on LDL oxidation (205). Whereas there is no evidence for a cardioprotective effect of ascorbic acid alone, the results of Established Populations for Epidemiological Studies of the Elderly clearly demonstrate that the simultaneous use of both antioxidants is associated with a lower risk of total and coronary mortality (Table 2) (206).

In summary, there is increasing evidence that hyperglycemia-induced LDL modifications are one major factor in the pathogenesis of artherosclerosis. Elevated levels of reactive oxygen species and insufficient antioxidant protection of the LDL particle lead to the enhanced LDL oxidation in diabetes. Supplementation with the antioxidants reduces LDL oxidation in diabetic patients. The idea of cardioprotective effects of antioxidant supplementation in diabetic patients is further supported by epidemiological and clinical studies showing a decrease in

Table 2 Effect of Vitamins E and C on Coronary Heart Mortality: Age- and Sex-Adjusted Relative Risk of Death

Supplement	All-cause mortality	Coronary disease mortality
Vitamin E	0.80	0.64
Vitamin C	1.04	1.0
Vitamin E + C	0.58	0.47
Multivitamins/minerals	1.04	1.14

Source: Ref. 206.

the myocardial infarction rate in the nondiabetic patient population. However, more placebo-controlled clinical trials are needed to assess the cardioprotective effects of in nondiabetic as well as diabetic patients to establish the value of antioxidant supplementation for primary prevention.

V. CONCLUSIONS

There is emerging evidence that the generation of reactive oxidative species (ROS) is one major factor in the onset and the development of diabetes and its complications. Research over the last 10 years suggests that oxidative stress plays a role in this pathway as a link between hyperglycemia and the typical observed pathophysiological features of diabetes, associated with the onset and progression of late diabetic complications.

Antioxidants might therefore be helpful for treating diabetic patients and their complications. Among the variety of antioxidants α-lipoic acid, ascorbic acid, and *RRR*-α-tocopherol have been shown in several experimental and clinical studies to have beneficial effects on diabetes and its complications. *RRR*-α-Tocopherol and ascorbic acid reduce LDL oxidation and the autoantibody titers against LDL modification proteins that are prominent and established risk factors for the manifestation of artherosclerosis. Clinical and epidemiological studies have shown an inverse relation between the *RRR*-α-tocopherol and myocardial infarction rate. *RRR*-α-tocopherol and ascorbic acid have been further shown to exert beneficial effects on blood flow in diabetic patients. α-Lipoic acid reduces the imbalance between oxidative stress measures and antioxidant capacity in diabetic patients. In addition to inhibiting LDL oxidation, the vascular-protective effects of antioxidants can be explained by an inhibition of activation of transcription factors, such as NF-κB, in smooth-muscle, endothelial, and plasma mononuclear cells, and the consequent reduction of the proadhesive, prothrombogenic, and proliferative environment in the vessel of diabetic patients. The available experimental and clinical results suggest the importance of studies to further evaluate the potential value of antioxidants for the treatment of diabetes and its complications. Large clinical trials, such as the DCCT Study or the UKPDS Study (171–173) are needed to evaluate the long-term effects of these antioxidants in diabetic patients. The medical and socioeconomic burden of diabetes and its complications in the near future demands further innovation in diabetes therapy. However, it should be taken into consideration that it is important to strengthen the antioxidative network in the cell as a whole, not just a single component.

REFERENCES

1. Zimmet P. (1991) Diabetes care and prevention—around the world in 80 days. In: Rifkin H, Colwell JA, Taylor SI, eds. Diabetes. Amsterdam: Elsevier, pp. 721–729.
2. Schernthaner G. (1996) Cardiovascular mortality and morbidity in type-2 diabetes mellitus. Diabetes Res Clin Pract 31(suppl):S3–S14.
3. Laakso M, Lehtoo S, Penttilä I, Pyörälä K. (1993) Lipids and lipoproteins predicting coronary heart disease mortality and morbidity in patients with non–insulin-dependent diabetes. Circulation 88:1421–1430.
3a. Kannel WB, McGee DL. (1979) Diabetes and cardiovascular risk factors. The Framingham Study. Circulation 1:8–13.
4. Tesfamariam B. (1994) Free radicals in diabetic endothelial cell dysfunction. Free Radic Biol Med 16:383–391.
5. Jones AF, Winkles JW, Jennings PE. (1988) Serum antioxidant activity in diabetes mellitus. Diabetes Res 7:89–92.

6. Tilton RG, Kawamura T, Chang KC, Ido Y, Bjercke RJ, Stephan CC, Brock TA, Williamson JR. (1997) Vascular dysfunction induced by elevated glucose levels in rats is mediated by vascular endothelial growth factor. J Clin Invest 99:2192–2202.
7. Cohen RA. (1993) Dysfunction of vascular endothelium in diabetes mellitus. Circulation 87(suppl 5):V67–V76.
8. Pieper GM, Gross GJ. (1998) Oxygen free radicals abolish endothelium dependent relaxation in diabetic rat aorta. Am J Physiol 255:H825–H833.
9. Lyons T. (1991) Oxidised low density lipoproteins: a role in the pathogenesis of atherosclerosis in diabetes? Diabetes Med 8:411–419.
10. Halliwell B. (1995) Antioxidant characterization; methodology and mechanism. Biochem Pharmacol 49:1341–1348.
11. Southorn PA. (1988) Free radicals in medicine. II: Involvement in human disease. Mayo Clin Proc 63:390–408.
12. Halliwell B, Cross CE, Gutteridge JMC. (1992) Free radicals, antioxidants and human disease: where are we now? J Lab Clin Med 119:598–620.
13. Halliwell B. (1996) Antioxidants in human health and disease. Annu Rev Nutr 16:33–50.
14. Sies H. (1997) Antioxidants in Disease Mechanisms and Therapy. San Diego, CA: Academic.
15. Bendich A. (1990) Antioxidant nutrients and immune functions: introduction. Adv Exp Med Biol 262:1–12.
16. Scott BC, Aruoma OI, Evans PJ, O'Neill C, van der Vliet A, Cross CE, Tritschler HJ, Halliwell B. (1994) Lipoic and dihydrolipoic acid as antioxidants. A critical evaluation. Free Radic Res Commun 20:119–133.
17. Stahl W, Sies H. (1997) Antioxidant defense: vitamins E and C and carotenoids. Diabetes 46(suppl 2):14–18.
18. Bendich A, Machlin LJ, Scandurra O, Burton GW, Wayner DDM. (1986) The antioxidant role of vitamin C. Free Radic Biol Med 2:419–444.
19. Traber MG, Sies H. (1996) Vitamin E in humans: demand and delivery. Annu Rev Nutr 16:321–347.
20. Nicki E. (1987) Antioxidants in relation to lipid peroxidation. Chem Phys Lipids 44:227–253.
21. Packer L. (1992) New horizons in vitamin E research—the vitamin E cycle, biochemistry and clinical applications. In: Ong ASH, Packer L, eds. Lipid Soluble Antioxidants: Biochemistry and Clinical Applications. Boston: Birkhauser, pp. 1–16.
22. Packer L, Witt EH, Tritschler HJ. (1995) alpha-Lipoic acid as a biological antioxidant. Free Radic Biol Med 19:227–250.
23. Diabetes and Nutrition Study Group of the EASD. (1995) Recommendations for the nutritional management of patients with diabetes mellitus. Diabetes Nutr Metab 8:1–4.
24. Nourooz-Zadeh J, Tajaddini-Sarmadi J, McCarthy S, Betteridge DJ, Wolff SP. (1995) Elevated levels of authentic plasma hydroperoxides in NIDDM. Diabetes 44:1054–1058.
25. Nourooz-Zadeh J, Rahimi A, Tajaddini-Sarmadi J, Tritschler HJ, Rösen P, Halliwell B, Betteridge DJ. (1997) Relationships between plasma measures of oxidative stress and metabolic control in NIDDM. Diabetologia 40:647–653.
26. Nishigaka I, Hagihara M, Tsunekawa H, Maseki M, Yagi K. (1981) Lipid peroxide levels of serum lipoprotein fractions of diabetic patients. Biochem Med 25:373–378.
27. Bellomo G, Maggi E, Polli M, Agosta FG, Bollati P, Finardi G. (1991) Autoantibodies against oxidatively modified low density lipoproteins in NIDDM. Diabetes 44:60–66.
28. Roesen P, Tchoepe D. (1991) Vitamin E and diabetes. Fat Sci Technol 11:425–431.
29. Hunt JV, Smith CT, Wolff SP. (1990) Autoxidative glycosylation and possible involvement of peroxides and free radicals in LDL modification by glucose. Diabetes 39:1420–1424.
30. Pratico D, Lawson JA, Fitzgerald GA. (1995) Cyclooxygenase-dependent formation of the isoprostane, 8-epiprostaglandin $F_{2\alpha}$. J Biol Chem 270:9800–9808.
31. Gopaul NK, Nourooz-Zadeh J, Mallet AI, Anggard EE. (1994) Formation of F_2-isoprostanes during aortic endothelial cell-mediated oxidation of low density lipoprotein. FEBS Lett 348:297–300.
32. Davi G, Ciaboattoni G, Consoli A, Mezetti A, Falco A, Santarone S, Pennese E, Vitacolonna E, Bucciarelli T, Costantini F, Capani F, Patrono C. (1999) In vivo formation of 8-iso-prostaglandin $F_{2\alpha}$ and platelet activation in diabetes mellitus: effects of improved metabolic control and vitamin E supplementation. Circulation 99:224–229.

33. Gopaul NK, Anggard EE, Mallet AI, Betteridge DJ, Wolff SP, Nourooz–Zadeh J. (1995) Plasma 8-epi PGF$_{2\alpha}$ levels are elevated in individuals with non–insulin dependent diabetes mellitus. FEBS Lett 368:225–229.
34. Jain SK, MeVie R, Duett J, Herbst JJ. (1989) Erythrocyte membrane lipid peroxidation and glycosylated hemoglobin in diabetes. Diabetes 38:1539–1543.
35. Haffner SM, Agil A, Mykkanen L, Stern M, Jialal I. (1995) Plasma oxidisability in subjects with normal glucose tolerance, impaired glucose tolerance and NIDDM. Diabetes Care 18:646–653.
36. Bellomo G, Maggi E, Poli M, Agosta FG, Bollati P, Finardi G. (1995) Autoantibodies against oxidatively modified low-density lipoproteins in NIDDM. Diabetes 44:60–66.
37. Bellomo G, Maggi E, Palladini G, Perugini C, Seccia M. (1997) Oxidation of low density lipoproteins and vitamin E status in non insulin dependent diabetes mellitus (NIDDM). Diabetes Stoffwechsel 6 (suppl 2):29–33.
38. Cominacini L, Garbin U, Pastorino AM, Fratta–Pasini A, Campagnola M, De-Sanits A, Davoli A. (1994) Increased susceptibility of LDL to in vitro oxidation in patients with insulin dependent diabetes mellitus. Diabetes Res 26:173–184.
39. Reaven PD, Herold DA, Barnett J, Edelman S. (1995) Effects of vitamin E on susceptibility of low-density lipoprotein subfractions to oxidation and protein glycation in NIDDM. Diabetes Care 18:807–816.
40. Babiy AV, Gebicki JM, Sullivan DR, Willey K. (1992) Increased oxidizability of plasma lipoproteins in diabetic patients can be decreased by probucol therapy and is not due to glycation: Biochem Pharmacol 43:995–1000.
41. Bowie A, Owens D, Collins P, Johnson A, Tomkin GH. (1993) Glycosylated low-density protein is more sensitive to oxidation: implications for the diabetic patients. Arteriosclerosis 102:63–67.
42. Dimitriadis E, Griffin M, Owens D, Johnson A, Collin P, Tomkin GH. (1995) Oxidation of low-density lipoprotein in NIDDM: its relationship to fatty acid composition. Diabetologia 38:1300–1306.
43. Beaudeux JL, Guillausseau PJ, Peynet J, Flourie F, Assayag M, Tielmans D, Warnet A, Rousselet F. (1995) Enhanced susceptibility of low-density lipoprotein to in vitro oxidation in type 1 and type 2 diabetic patients. Clin Chim Acta 239:131–141.
44. Rabini RA, Fumelli P, Galassi R, Dousset N, Taus M, Ferretti G, Mazzanti L, Curatola G, Solera ML, Valdiguie P. (1994) Increased susceptibility to lipid oxidation of low-density lipoproteins and erythrocyte membranes from diabetic patients. Metab Clin Exp 43:1470–1474.
45. Leonhardt W, Hahnefeld M, Lattke P, Jaross W. (1997) Vitamin E Mangel und Oxidierbarkeit der Low-Density-Lipoproteine bei Typ-I- und Typ-II-Diabetes: Einfluss der Qualiät der Stoffwechselkontrolle. Diabetes Stoffwechsel 6 (suppl 2): 24–29.
46. Loft S, Fischer–Nielsen A, Jeding IB, Vistisen K, Poulsen HE. (1993) 8-Hydroxydeoxyguanosine as a urinary biomarker of oxidative DNA damage. J Toxicol Environ Health 40:391–404.
47. Dandona P, Thusu K, Cook S, Snyder B, Makowski J, Armstrong D, Nicotera T. (1996) Oxidative damage to DNA in diabetes mellitus. Lancet 347:444–445.
48. Leinonen J, Lehtimaki T, Toyokuni S, et al. (1997) New biomarker evidence of oxidative DNA damage in patients with non–insulin-dependent diabetes mellitus. FEBS Lett 417:150–152.
49. Hinokio Y, Suzuki S, Hirai M, Chiba M, Toyota T. (1999) Oxidative DNA damage in diabetes mellitus: its association with diabetic complications. Diabetologia 42:995–998.
50. Ceriello A. (1997) Acute hyperglycemia and oxidative stress generation 3. Diabetic Med 14:S45–S49.
51. Tsai EC, Hirsch IB, Brunzell JD, Chait A. (1994) Lower plasma peroxyl radical trapping capacity and higher sensitivity of LDL to oxidation in poorly controlled IDDM. Diabetes 43:1010–1014.
52. Leonhardt W, Hahnefeld M, Müller G, Hora C, Meissner D, Lattke P, Paetzold A, Jaross W, Schröder HE. (1996) Impact of concentrations of glycated hemoglobin, alpha-tocopherol, copper, and manganese on oxidation of low-density lipoproteins in patients with type I diabetes, type II diabetes and control subjects. Clin Chim Acta 254:173–186.
53. Tsai EC, Hirsch IB, Brunzell JD, Chait A. (1994) Reduced plasma peroxyl radical trapping capacity and increased susceptibility of LDL to oxidation in poorly controlled IDDM. Diabetes 43:1010–1014.
54. Chari SN, Nath N, Rathi AB. (1984) Glutathione and its redox system in diabetic polymorphonuclear leukocytes. Am J Med Sci 287:14–15.

55. Jennings PE, Chirico S, Jones AF, Lunec J, Barnett AH. (1987) Vitamin C metabolites and microangiopathy in diabetes mellitus. Diabetes Res 6:151–154.
56. Karpen CW, Cataland S, O'Dorisio TM, Panganamala RV. (1985) Production of 12 HETES and vitamin E status in platelets from type 1 human diabetic subjects. Diabetes 34:526–531.
57. Paolisso G, D'Amore A, Balbi V, Volpe C, Galzerano D, Guigliano D, Sgambato S, Varricchio M, D'Onofino F. (1994) Plasma vitamin C affects glucose homeostasis in healthy subjects and in non–insulin-dependent diabetics. Am J Physiol 266:E261–E268.
58. Olmedilla B, Granado F, Gilmartinez E, Blanco I, Rojashidalgo E. (1997) Reference values for retinol, tocopherol and main carotenoids in serum of control and insulin dependent diabetic Spanish subjects. Clin Chem 43:1066–1071.
59. Maxwell SRJ, Thomason H, Sandler D, Leguen C, Baxter MA, Thrope GHG, Jones AF, Barnett AH. (1997) Antioxidant status in patients with uncomplicated insulin-dependent and non insulin-dependent diabetes mellitus. Eur J Clin Invest 27:484–490.
60. Dyer RG, Stewart MW, Mitcheson J, George K, Alberti MM, Laker MF. (1997) 7-Ketocholesterol, a specific indicator of lipoprotein oxidation, and malondialdehyde in non–insulin dependent diabetes and peripheral vascular disease. Clin Chim Acta 260:1–13.
61. Sinclair AJ, Girling AJ, Gray L, LeGuen C, Lunec J, Barnett AH. (1997) Disturbed handling of ascorbic acid in diabetic patients with and without microangiopathy during high dose ascorbate supplementation. Diabetologia 34:171–175.
62. Srinivasan KN, Pugalendi KV, Sambandam G, Rao MR, Menon PV. (1997) Diabetes mellitus, lipid peroxidation and antioxidant status in rural patients. Clin Chim Acta 259:183–186.
63. Will JC, Byers T. (1996) Does diabetes mellitus increase the requirement for vitamin C? Nutr Rev 54:193–202.
64. Will JC, Ford ES, Bowmann BA. (1999) Serum vitamin C concentrations and diabetes: findings from the third National Health and Nutrition Examination Survey, 1988–1994. Am J Nutr 70:49–52.
65. Thornalley P, McLean AC, Lo TW, Benn J, Sonksen PH. (1996) Negative association between erythrocytes, reduced glutathione concentration and diabetic complications. Clin Sci 91:572–582.
66. Simon–Schnass I, Rosak CH, Tritschler HJ, Rösen P. (1997) alpha-Tocopherolaufnahme und -zufuhr bei Typ-ii-Diabetikern. Diabetes Stoffwechsel 6(suppl 2):16–20.
67. Rösen P, Toeller M. (1999) Vitamin E in diabetes: increased oxidative stress and its prevention as a strategy to prevent vascular complications? Int Vit Nutr Res 69:206–213.
68. Du XL, Stockklauser–Färber K, Rösen P. (1999) Generation of reactive oxygen intermediates, activation of NF-κB, and induction of apoptosis in human endothelial cells by glucose: role of nitric oxide synthase? Free Radic Med Biol 27:752–763.
69. Graier WF, Simecek S, Kukovetz WR, Kostner GM. (1996) High glucose-induced changes in endothelial Ca^{2+}/EDRF signaling are due to generation of superoxide anions. Diabetes 45:1386–1395.
70. Wascher TC, Toplak H, Krejs GJ, Simecek S, Kukovetz WR, Graier WF. (1994) Intracellular mechanisms involved in D-glucose-mediated amplification of agonist-induced Ca^{2+} response and EDRF formation in vascular endothelial cells. Diabetes 43:984–991.
71. Giardino I, Fard AK, Hatchell DL, Brownlee M. (1998) Aminoguanidine inhibits reactive oxygen species formation, lipid peroxidation, and oxidant-induced apoptosis. Diabetes 47:1114–1120.
72. Rösen P, Du XL, Tschöpe D. (1998) Role of oxygen derived radicals for vascular dysfunction in the diabetic heart: prevention by α-tocopherol? Mol Cell Biochem 188:103–111.
73. Diedrich D, Skopec J, Diedrich A, Dai FX. (1994) Endothelial dysfunction in mesenteric resistance arteries of diabetic rats: role of free radicals. Am J Physiol 266:H1153–H1161.
74. Tesfamariam B, Brown ML, Deykin D, Cohen RA. (1990) Elevated glucose promotes generation of endothelium-dependent vasoconstrictive prostanoids in rabbit aorta. J Clin Invest 85:929–932.
75. Mullarkey C, Edelstein D, Brownlee M. (1990) Free radical generation by early glycation products: a mechanism for accelerated arteriogenesis in diabetes. Biochem Biophys Res Commun 173:932–939.
76. Sakurai T, Tsuchiya S. (1988) Superoxide production from nonenzymatically glycated protein. FEBS Lett 236:406–410.
77. Schmidt AM, Zhang JH, Crandall J, Cao R, Yan SD, Brett J, Stern D. (1994) Interaction of advanced glycation end products with their endothelial cell receptor leads to enhanced expression of VCAM-1: a mechanism for augmented monocyte–vessel wall interactions in diabetes. FASEB J 8:3841.

78. Schmidt AM, Hori O, Brett J, Yan SD, Wautier JL, Stern D. (1994) Cellular receptors for advanced glycation end products. Implications for induction of oxidant stress and cellular dysfunction in the pathogenesis of vascular lesions. Arterioscler Throm 14:1521–1528.
79. Wolff SP. (1993) Diabetes mellitus and free radicals. Br Med Bull 49:642–652.
80. Wolff SP, Jiang ZY, Hunt JV. (1991) Protein glycation and oxidative stress in diabetes mellitus and ageing. Free Radic Biol Med 10:339–352.
81. Kashiwagi A, Asahina T, Ikebuchi M, Tanaka Y, Takagi Y Nishio Y, Kikkawa R, Shigeta Y. (1994) Abnormal glutathion metabolism and increased cytotoxicity caused by H_2O_2 in human umbilical vein endothelial cells cultured in high glucose medium. Diabetologia 37:264–269.
82. Nakazono K, Watanabe N, Matsuno K, Sasak J, Sato T. (1991) Does superoxide underlie the pathogenesis of hypertension? Proc Natl Acad Sci USA 88:1045–1048.
83. Minor RL, Myers PR, Guerra R, Bates JN, Harrison DG. (1990) Diet-induced atherosclerosis increases the release of vascular relaxing factor. J Clin Invest 86:2109–2116.
84. Keaney JF, Gaziano JM, Xu A, Frei B, Curran–Celentano J, Shwaery GT, Loscalzo J, Vita JA. (1994) Low dose α-tocopherol improves and high tocopherol worsens endothelial vasodilator function in cholesterol-fed rabbits. J Clin Invest 93:844–851.
85. Ohara Y, Peterson TE, Harrison DG. (1993) Hypercholesterolemia increases endothelial superoxide anion production. J Clin Invest 91:2546–2551.
86. Graier W, Simececk S, Kukovetz WR, Kostner GM. (1996) High D-glucose induced changes in endothelial Ca^{2+} EDRF signalling are due to generation of superoxide anions. Diabetes 45:1386–1395.
87. Vinals F, Gross A, Testar X, Palacin M, Rösen P, Zorzano A. (1999) High glucose concentrations inhibit glucose phosphorylation but not glucose transport in human endothelial cells. Biochim Biophys Acta 1450:112–129.
88. Tilton RG, Kwamura T, Chang KC, Ido Y, Bjercke RJ, Stephan CC, Brock TA, Williamson JR. (1999) Vascular dysfunction induced by elevated glucose levels in rats is mediated by vascular endothelial growth factor. J Clin Invest 99:2192–2202.
89. Ignarro LJ. (1990) Physiology and pathophysiology of nitric oxide. Kidney Int 55:S2–S5.
90. Pieper GM. (1998) A review of alterations in endothelial nitric oxide production in diabetes: protective role of arginine on endothelial dysfunction. Hypertension 31:1047–1060.
91. Beckmann J, Koppenol WH. (1996) Nitric oxide, superoxide, and peroxynitrite: the good, the bad, and the ugly. Am J Physiol 271:C1424–C1437.
92. Ohara Y, Petersen TE, Harrison DG. (1993) Hypercholesterolemia increases endothelial superoxide anion production. J Clin Invest 91:844–851.
93. Bouloumie A, Bauersachs J, Linz W, Schölkens BA, Wiemer G, Fleming I, Busse R. (1997) Endothelial dysfunction coincides with an enhanced nitric oxide synthase expression and superoxide anion production. Hypertension 30:934–941.
94. Rösen P, Ballhausen T, Bloch W, Addicks K. (1995) Endothelial relaxation is disturbed by oxidative stress in the diabetic heart: the influence of tocopherol as antioxidant. Diabetologia 38:1157–1168.
95. Sui GZ, Du XL, Rösen P. (1998) High glucose increases the formation of nitrotyrosine as marker of oxidative stress in human endothelial cells. Diabeteologia 41:A317.
96. Bucala R, Tracey KJ, Ceramin A. (1991) Advanced glycation products quench nitric oxide and mediate defective endothelium-dependent vasodilatation in experimental diabetes. J Clin Invest 87:432–438.
97. Ting HH, Timimi FK, Boles KS, Creager SJ, Ganz P, Creager MA. (1997) Vitamin C improves endothelium-dependent vasodilatation in patients with non–insulin-dependent diabetes mellitus. J Clin Invest 97:22–28.
98. Ting HH, Timimi FK, Haley EA, Roddy MA, Ganz P, Creager MA. (1997) Vitamin C improves endothelium-dependent vasodilatation in forearm resistance vessels of humans with hypercholesterolemia. Circulation 95:2617–2622.
99. Vita JA, Frei B, Holbrook M, Gokse N, Leaf C, Keaney JF. (1998) L-2-Oxothizolidine-4-carboxylic acid reverses endothelial dysfunction in patients with coronary artery disease. J Clin Invest 101:1408–1414.
100. Kugiyama K, Motoyama T, Doi H, Kawano H, Hirai N, Soejima H, Miyao Y, Takazoe K, Moriyama Y, Mizuno Y, Tsunoda R, Ogawa H, Sakamoto T, Sugiyama S, Yasue H. (1999) Improvement of endothelial vasomotor dysfunction by treatment with α-tocopherol in patients with high remnant lipoprotein levels. J Am Coll Cardiol 33:1512–1518.

101. Anderson TJ, Meredith IT, Yeung AC, Frei B, Selwyn AP, Ganz P. (1995) The effect of cholesterol-lowering and antioxidant therapy on endothelium-dependent coronary vasomotion. N Engl J Med 332:488–493.
102. Gokce N, Keaney JF, Frei B, Holbrook M, Olesiak M, Zachariah BJ, Leeuwenburg C, Heinecke JW, Vita JA. (1999) Long-term ascorbic acid administration reverses endothelial vasomotor dysfunction in patients with coronary artery disease. Circulation 99:3234–3240.
103. Ting HH, Timimi FK, Haley EA, Roddy MA, Ganz P, Creager MA. (1997) Vitamin C improves endothelium-dependent vasodilation in forearm resistance vessels of human with hypercholesterolemia. Circulation 95:2617–2622.
104. Taddei S, Virdis A, Ghiadoni L, Magagna A, Salvetti A. (1998) Vitamin C improves endothelium-dependent vasodilation by restoring nitric oxide activity in essential hypertension. Circulation 97:2222–2229.
105. Ting HH, Timimi FK, Boiles KS, Creager SJ, Ganz P, Creager MA. (1996) Vitamin C improves endothelium-dependent vasodilation in patients with non–insulin-dependent diabetes mellitus. J Clin Invest 97:22–28.
106. Solzbach U, Hornig B, Jeserich M, Just H. (1997) Vitamin C improves endothelial dysfunction of epicardial coronary arteries in hypertensive patients. Circulation 96:1513–1519.
107. Motoyama M, Kawano H, Kugiyama K, Hirashima O, Ohgushi M, Yoshimura M, Ogawa H, Yasue H. (1997) Endothelium-dependent vasodilation in the brachial artery is impaired in smokers: effect of vitamin C. Am J Physiol 273:H1644–H1650.
108. Lefer AM, Lefer DJ. (1996) The role of nitric oxide and cell adhesion molecules on the microcirculation in ischemia–reperfusion. Cardiovasc Res 32:743–751.
109. Schmidt AM, Yan SD, Stern DM. (1995) The dark side of glucose. Nature Med 1:1002–1004.
110. Bierhaus A, Illmer T, Kasper M, Luther T, Quehenberger P, Tritschler HJ, Wahl P, Ziegler R, Müller M, Nawroth PP. (1996) Advanced glycation endproducts (AGEs) mediated induction of tissue factor in cultured endothelial cells is dependent on RAGE. Circulation 96:2262–2271.
111. Bierhaus A, Chevion S, Chevion M, Quehenberger P, Hofmann M, Illmer T, Luther T, Berentsthein E, Tritschler HJ, Müller M, Wahl P, Ziegler R, Nawroth PP. (1997) Advanced glycation end products (AGEs) induced activation of NF-κB is suppressed by alpha-lipoic acid in cultured endothelial cells. Diabetes 46:1481–1490.
112. Morigi M, Angioletti S, Imberti B, Donadeli R, Micheletti G, Figliuzzi M, Remuzzi A, Zoja C, Remuzzi G. (1998) Leukocyte-endothelial interaction is augmented by high glucose concentrations and hyperglycaemia in an NF-κB-dependent fashion. J Clin Invest 101:1905–1915.
113. Pieper GM. (1997) Activation of nuclear factor-kappaB in cultured endothelial cells by increased glucose concentration: prevention by calphostin C. J Cardiovasc Pharmacol 30:528–532.
114. Hofmann MA, Schiekofer S, Kanitz M, Klevesatz MS, Joswig M, Lee V, Morcos M, Tritschler HJ, Ziegler R, Wahl P, Bierhaus A, Nawroth PP. (1998) Insufficient glycemic control increases NF-κB binding activity in peripheral blood mononuclear cells isolated from patients with type-1 diabetes. Diabetes Care 21:1–7.
115. Hofmann MA, Schiekofer S, Isermann B, Kanitz M, Henkels M, Joswig M, Treusch A, Morcos M, Weiss T, Borcea V, Khalek A, Amiral J, Tritschler HJ, Ritz E, Wahl P, Ziegler P, Bierhaus A, Nawroth PP. (1999) Peripheral blood mononuclear cells isolated from patients with diabetic nephropathy demonstrate increased activation of the oxidative stress sensitive transcription factor NF-κB. Diabetologia 42:222–232.
116. Ceriello A, Bortolotti N, Motz E, Crescentini A, Lizzio S, Russo A, Tonutti L, Taboga C. (1998) Meal-generated oxidative stress in type 2 diabetic patients. Diabetes Care 21:1529–1533.
117. Morcos M, Borcea V, Isermann B, Gehre S, Henkels M, Schiekofer S, Hoffmann M, Amiral J, Tritschler HJ, Ziegler R, Wahl P, Nawroth PP. (2001) Effect of the antioxidant lipoic acid on the progression of endothelial cell damage and albuminuria in patients with diabetes mellitus. Diabetes Res Clin Pract 52:175–183.
118. Koya D, King GL. (1998) Protein kinase C activation and the development of diabetic complications. Diabetes 47:859–866.
119. King GL, Ishii H, Koya D. (1997) Diabetic vascular dysfunctions: a model of excessive activation of protein kinase C. Kidney Int 52:S77–S85.
120. Inoguchi T, Battan R, Handler E, Sportsman JR, Heath W, King GLI. (1992) Preferential elevation of protein kinase C isoform β II and diacylglycerol levels in aorta and heart of diabetic rats:

differential reversibility to glycemic control by islet cell transplantation. Proc Natl Acad Sci USA 89:11059–11063.
121. Kunisaki M, Bursell SE, Umeda F, Nawata H, King GL. (1994) Normalization of diacylglycerol–protein kinase C activation by vitamin E in aorta of diabetic rats and cultured rat smooth muscle cells exposed to elevated glucose levels. Diabetes 43:1372–1377.
122. Ishii H, Jirousek MR, Koya D, Takagi C, Xia P, Clermont A, Bursell SE, Kern TS, Ballas LM, Heath WF, Stramm LE, Feener EP, King GL. (1996) Amelioration of vascular dysfunctions in diabetic rats by an oral PKCβ inhibitor. Science 272:728–731.
123. Kunisaki M, Bursell SE, Clermont AC, Ishii H, Ballas LM, Jirousek MR, Umeda F, Nawata H, King GL. (1995) Vitamin E prevents diabetes-induced abnormal retinal blood flow via the diacyglycerol–protein kinase C pathway. Am J Physiol 269:E239–E246.
124. Boscoboinik D, Szewczyk A, Hensey C, Azzi A. (1991) Inhibition of cell proliferation by alpha-tocopherol. Role of protein kinase C. J Biol Chem 266:6188–6194.
125. Nishizuka Y. (1992) Intracellular signaling by hydrolysis of phospholipids and activation of protein kinase C. Science 258:607–614.
126. Nishizuka Y. (1995) Protein kinase C and lipid signaling for sustained cellular responses. FASEB J 9:484–496.
127. Bursell SE, Takagi C, Clermont AC, Takagi H, Mori F, Ishii H, King GL. (1997) Specific retinal diacylglycerol and protein kinase C beta isoform modulation mimics abnormal retinal hemodynamics in diabetic rats. Invest Ophthalmol Vis Sci 38:2711–2720.
128. Azzi A, Boscoboinik D, Chatelain E, Ozer NK, Stauble B. (1993) D-Tocopherol control of cell proliferation. Mol Aspects Med 14:265–271.
129. Feke GT, Buzney SM, Ogasawara H, Fujio N, Goger DG, Spack NP, Gabbay KH. (1994) Retinal circulatory abnormalities in type 1 diabetes. Invest Ophthalmol Vis Sci 35:2968–2975.
130. Bursell S-E, Takagi C, Clermont AC. (1997) Specific retinal DAG and PKC-β isoform modulation mimics abnormal retinal hemodynamics in diabetic rats. Invest Ophthalmol Vis Sci 38:2711–2720.
131. Small KW, Stefansson E, Hatchell D. (1987) Retinal blood flow in normal and diabetic dogs. Invest Ophthalmol Vis Sci 28:672–675.
132. Clermont AC, Brittis M, Shiba T, McGovern T, King GL, Bursell SE. (1994) Normalization of retinal blood flow in diabetic rats with primary intervention using insulin pumps. Invest Ophthalmol Vis Sci 35:981–990.
133. Miyamoto K, Ogura Y, Nishiwaki H, Matsuda N, Honda Y, Kato S, Ishida H, Seino Y. (1996) Evaluation of retinal microcirculatory alterations in the Goto–Kakizaki rat. Invest Ophthalmol Vis Sci 37:898–905.
134. Shiba T, Inoguchi T, Sportsman JR, Heath W, Bursell S, King GL. (1993) Correlation of diacylglycerol and protein kinase C activity in rat retina to retinal circulation. Am J Physiol 265:E783–E793.
135. Tesfaye S, Malik R, Ward JD. (1994) Vascular factors in diabetic neuropathy. Diabetologia 37:847–851.
136. Cameron NE, Cotter MA, Lai K, Hohman TC. (1997) Effect of protein kinase C inhibition on nerve function, blood flow and Na^+,K^+ ATPase defects in diabetic rats. Diabetes 46(suppl 1):31A.
137. Kohner EM. (1995) Role of blood flow and impaired autoregulation in the pathogenesis of diabetic retinopathy. Diabetes 44:603–607.
138. Bursell SE, Clermont AC, Aiello LP, Aiello LM, Schlossmann DK, Feener EP, Laffel L, King GL. (1999) High-dose vitamin E supplementation normalizes retinal blood flow and creatinine clearance in patients with type 1 diabetes. Diabetes Care 22:1245–1251.
139. Lee TS, Saltsman LA, Onishi H, King GL. (1989) Activation of protein kinase C by elevation of glucose concentration: proposal for a mechanism in the development of diabetic vascular complications. Proc Natl Acad Sci USA 86:5141–5145.
140. Kawana M, Lee ME, Quertemous EE, Quertermous T. (1995) Cooperative interaction of GATA-2 and AP1 regulates transcription of endothelin-1 gene. Mol Cell Biol 15:4225–4231.
141. Takagi C, Bursell SE, Lin YW, Takagi H, Duh E, Jiang Z, Clermont AC, King GL. (1996) Regulation of retinal hemodynamics in diabetic rats by increased expression and action of endothelin-1. Invest Ophthalmol Vis Sci 37:2504–2518.
142. Aiello LP, Avery RL, Arrigg PG, Keyt BA, Jampel HD, Shah ST, Pasquale LR, Thieme H, Iwamoto MA, Park JE, Ngyuen HV, Aiello LM, Ferrara N, King GL. (1994) Vascular endothelial growth factor in ocular fluids of patients with diabetic retinopathy and other retinal disorders. N Engl J Med 331:1480–1487.

143. Williams B, Gallachen B, Patel H, Orme C. (1997) Glucose-induced protein kinase C activation regulates vascular permeability factor mRNA expression and peptide production by vascular smooth muscle cells in vitro. Diabetes 46:1497–1503.
144. Ditzel J, Schwartz M. (1967) Abnormally increased glomerular filtration rates in short-term insulin treated diabetic subjects. Diabetes 16:264–267.
145. Christiansen JS, Gammelgaard J, Fraandsen M, Parving HH. (1991) Increased kidney size, glomerular filtration rate and renal plasma flow in short-term insulin dependent diabetes. Diabetologia 20:451–456.
146. Hostetter TH, Troy JL, Brenner BM. (1981) Glomerular hemodynamics in experimental diabetes mellitus. Kidney Int 19:410–415.
147. Viberti GC. (1979) Early functional and morphological changes in diabetic nephropathy. Clin Nephrol 12:47–53.
148. O'Donnell MP, Kasiske BL, Keane WF. (1988) Glomerular hemodynamic structural alterations in experimental diabetes mellitus. FASEB J 2:2339–2347.
149. Ruan X, Arendshorst WJ. (1996) Role of protein kinase C in angiotensin II-induced vasoconstriction in genetically hypertensive rats. Am J Physiol 265:F477–F486.
150. Craven PA, Caines MA, DeRubertis FR. (1987) Sequential alterations in glomerular prostaglandin and thromboxane synthesis in diabetic rats: relationship to the hyperfiltration of early diabetes. Metabolism 36:95–103.
151. Perico N, Benigni A, Gabanelli M, Piccinelli A, Rog M, Riva CD, Remuzzi G. (1992) Atrial natriuretic peptide and prostacyclin synthesis synergistically mediate hyperfiltration and hyperfusion of diabetic rats. Diabetes 41:533–538.
152. Bank N, Aynedjan HS. (1993) Role of EDRF (nitric oxide) in diabetic renal hyperfiltration. Kidney Int 43:1306–1312.
153. Tolins JP, Shultz PJ, Raij L, Brown DM, Mauer SM. (1993) Abnormal renal hemodynamic response to reduced renal perfusion pressure in diabetic rats: role of NO. Am J Physiol 265:F886–F895.
154. Komers R, Allen TJ, Cooper ME. (1994) Role of endothelium derived nitric oxide in the pathogenesis of the renal hemodynamic changes of experimental diabetes. Diabetes 43:1190–1197.
155. Sharma K, Ziyadeh FN. (1995) Hyperglycemia and diabetic kidney disease. The case for transforming growth factor-β as a key modulator. Diabetes 44:1139–1146.
156. Kuemmerle NB, Brandt RB, Chan W, Krieg RJ, Chan JC. (1997) Inhibition of transforming growth factor beta 1 induction by dietary vitamin E in unilateral ureteral obstruction in rats. Biochem Mol Med 61:82–86.
157. Luft FC, Mervaala E, Muller DN, Gross V, Schmidt F, Park JK, Schmitz C, Lippoldt A, Breu V, Dechend R, Dragun D, Schneider W, Ganten D, Haller H. (1999) Hypertension-induced end-organ damage: a new transgenic approach to an old problem. Hypertension 33:212–218.
158. Tooke JE. (1998) Endotheliopathy precedes type 2 diabetes. Diabetes Care 21:2047–2049.
159. Meeking DR, Cummings MH, Thornet S, Donald A, Clarlson P, Crook JR, Watts GF, Shaw KM. (1999) Endothelial dysfunction in type 1 diabetic subjects with and without microalbuminuria. Diabetic Med 16:841–847.
160. Leson CPM, Whincup PH, Cook DG, Donald AE, Papacosta O, Lucas A, Deanfield JE. (1997) Flow-mediated dilation in 9–11 year old children. Circulation 96:2233–2238.
161. Bursell SE, Clermont AC, Aiello LP, Aiello LM, Schlossmann DK, Feener EP, Laffel L, King GL. (1999) High-dose vitamin E supplementation normalizes retinal blood flow and creatinine clearance in patients with type 1 diabetes. Diabetes Care 22:1245–1251.
162. Gilbert RE, Cox A, Wu LL. (1998) Expression of transforming growth factor beta 1 and type IV collagen in the renal tubulointerstitium in experimental diabetes: effects of ACE inhibition. Diabetes 47:414–422.
163. Park IS, Kiyomoto H, Abboud SL, Abboud HE. (1997) Expression of transforming growth factor-beta and type IV collagen in early streptozotocin-induced diabetes. Diabetes 46:473–480.
164. Sumida Y, Ura H, Yano Y, Misaki M, Shima T. (1997) Abnormal metabolism of type IV collagen in normotensive non–insulin-dependent diabetes mellitus patients. Horm Res 48:23–28.
165. Williamson JR, Chang K, Tilton RG, Prater C, Jeffrey JR, Weigel C, Sherman WR, Eades DM, Kilo C. (1987) Increased vascular permeability in spontaneously diabetic BB/W rats with mild versus severe streptozotocin-induced diabetes. Diabetes 36:813–821.
166. Oliver JA. (1990) Adenylate cyclase and protein kinase C mediate opposite actions on endothelial junctions. J Cell Physiol 145:536–542.

167. Lynch JJ, Ferro TJ, Blumenstock FA, Brockenauer AM, Malik AM. (1990) Increased endothelial albumin permeability mediated by protein kinase C activation. J Clin Invest 85:1991–1998.
168. Dolgov VV, Zaikina OE, Bomdaranko MF, Repin VS. (1982) Aortic endothelium of alloxan diabetic rabbits: a quantitative study using scanning electron microscopy. Diabetologia 22:338–343.
169. Tucker BJ. (1990) Early onset of increased transcapillary albumin escape in awake diabetic rats. Diabetes 39:919–923.
170. Aiello LP, Cavallerano J, Bursell SE. (1996) Diabetic eye disease. Endocrinol Metab Clin North Am 25:271–291.
171. Diabetes Control and Complications Trial Research Group. (1993) The effect of intensive treatment of diabetes on the development and progression of long-term complications in insulin-dependent diabetes mellitus. N Engl J Med 329:977–986.
172. DCCT Research Group. (1995) The effect of intensive diabetes therapy on the development and progression of neuropathy. Ann Intern Med 122:561–568.
173. The UK Prospective Diabetes Study (UKPDS) Group. (1998) Intensive blood-glucose control with sulphonylureas or insulin compared with conventional treatment and risk of complications in patients with type 2 diabetes (UKPDS 33). Lancet 352:837–853.
174. Brock TA, Dvorak HF, Senger DR. (1991) Tumor-secreted vascular permeability factor increases cytosolic calcium and Von Willebrand factor release in human endothelial cells. Am J Pathol 138:213–221.
175. Lu M, Kuroki M, Amano S, Tolentino M, Keough K, Kim I, Bucala R, Adamis AP. (1998) Advanced glycation end products increase retinal vascular endothelial growth factor expression. J Clin Invest 101:1219–1224.
176. Kuroki M, Voest EE, Amano S, Beerepoot LV, Takashima S, Tolentino M, Kim I, Rohan RM, Colby KA, Yeo KT, Adamis AP. (1998) Reactive oxygen intermediates increase vascular endothelial growth factor expression in vitro and in vivo. J Clin Invest 98:1667–1675.
177. Xia P, Aiello LP, Ishii H, Jiang Z, Park DJ, Robinson GS, Takagi H, Newsome WP, Jirousek MR, King GL. (1996) Characterization of vascular endothelial growth factor's effect on activation of protein kinase C, its isoforms, and endothelial cell growth. J Clin Invest 98:2018–2026.
178. Roberts WG, Palade GE. (1995) Increased permeability and endothelial fenestration induced by vascular endothelial growth factor. Mol Cell Biol 108:2369–2379.
179. Haller H. (1997) High glucose concentrations increase endothelial permeability via activation of protein kinase C alpha. Circ Res 81:363–371.
180. Williamson JR, Kilo C. (1984) Extracellular matrix changes in diabetes mellitus. In: Scapelli DG, Migahi G, eds. Comparative Pathobiology of Major Age-Related Diseases. New York: Liss, pp. 269–288.
181. Scheinman JL, Fish AJ, Matas AJ, Michael AF. (1978) The immunohistopathology of glomerular antigens. II. The glomerular basement membrane, actomyosin, and fibroblast surface antigens in normal, diseased and transplanted human kidneys. Am J Pathol 90:71–88.
182. Bruneval P, Foidart JM, Nochy D, Camiller JP, Bariety J. (1985) Glomerular matrix proteins in nodular glomerulosclerosis in association with light chain deposition disease and diabetes mellitus. Hum Pathol 16:477–484.
183. Studer RK, Craven PA, DeRubertis FR. (1993) Role for protein kinase C in the mediation of increased fibronectin accumulation by mesangial cells grown in high glucose medium. Diabetes 42:118–126.
184. Ayo SH, Radnik RA, Garoni J, Glass WF, Kreisberg JI. (1990) High glucose causes an increase in extracellular matrix proteins in cultured mesangial cells. Am J Pathol 136:1339–1348.
185. Ayo SH, Radnik RA, Glass WF, Garoni JA, Rampt ER, Appling DR, Kreisberg JI. (1991) Increased extracellular matrix synthesis and mRNA in mesangial cells grown in high-glucose medium. Am J Physiol 260:F185–F191.
186. Pugliese G, Pricc IF, Pugliese F, Mene P, Lenti L, Andreani D, Galli G, Casini A, Bianchi S, Rotella CM, Mario UD. (1994) Mechanisms of glucose-enhanced extracellular matrix accumulation in rat glomerular mesangial cells. Diabetes 43:478–490.
187. Haneda M, Kikkawa R, Horide N, Togawa M, Koya D, Kajiwara N, Ooshima A, Shigeta Y. (1991) Glucose enhances type IV collagen production in cultured rat glomerular mesangial cells. Diabetologia 34:198–200.

188. Walker JD, Viberti GC. (1994) Pathophysiology of microvascular disease: an overview. In Pickup JC, Williams G, eds. Chronic Complications of Diabetes. Oxford: Blackwell Scientific, pp. 11–19.
189. Zidayeh N, Sharma K, Ericksen M, Wolf G. Stimulation of collagen gene expression and protein synthesis in murine mesangial cells by high glucose is mediated by autocrine activation of transforming growth factor-β. J Clin Invest 93:536–542.
190. Sharma K, Jin Y, Guo J, Zidayeh FN. (1996) Neutralization of TGF-β by anti-TGF-β antibody attenuates kidney hypertrophy and the enhanced extracellular matrix gene expression in STZ-induced diabetic mice. Diabetes 45:522–530.
191. Packer L. (1997) Protection of human low density lipoprotein from oxidation by vitamin E and the antioxidant network: interaction with vitamin C and lipoic (thioctic) acid. Diabetes Stoffwechsel 6(suppl 2):4–10.
192. Bowie A, Owens D, Collins P, Johnson A, Tomkin GH. (1993) Glycosylated low density lipoprotein is more sensitive to oxidation: implications for the diabetic patient. Arteriosclerosis 102:63–67.
193. Salonen JT, Yla-Herttuala S, Yamamoto R, Butler S, Korpela H, Salonen R, Nysonen K, Palinski W, Witztum JL. (1992) Autoantibody against oxidized LDL and progression of carotid arteriosclerosis. Lancet 339:883–887.
194. Puurunen M, Manttari M, Manninen V, Tenkanen L, Alfthan G, Ehnholm C, Vaarala O, Aho K, Palosuo T. (1994) Antibody against oxidized low-density lipoprotein predicting myocardial infarction. Arch Intern Med 154:2605–2609.
195. Parums DV, Brown DL, Mitchinson MJ. (1990) Serum antibodies to oxidized lipoprotein and ceroid in chronic periaortitis. Arch Pathol Lab Med 114:383–387.
196. Fuller CJ, Chandalia M, Garg A, Grundy SM, Jialal I. (1996) *RRR*-alpha-Tocopheryl acetate supplementation at pharmacologic doses decreases low-density-lipoprotein oxidative susceptibility but not protein glycation in patients with diabetes mellitus. Am J Clin Nutr 63:753–759.
197. Jialal I, Fuller CJ, Huet BA. (1995) The effect of α-tocopherol supplementation on LDL oxidation: a dose dependent study. Arterioscler Throm Vasc Biol 15:190–198.
198. Jialal I, Vega GL, Grundy SM. (1990) Physiologic levels of ascorbate inhibit the oxidative modification of low density lipoprotein. Atherosclerosis 82:185–191.
199. Fuller CJ, Grundy SM, Norkus EP, Jialal I. (1996) Effect of ascorbate supplementation on low density lipoprotein oxidation in smokers. Atherosclerosis 119:139–150.
200. Gey KF, Puska P, Jordan P, Maser UK. (1991) Inverse correlation between plasma vitamin E and mortality from ischemic heart disease in cross-cultural epidemiology. Am J Clin Nutr 53:326S–334S.
201. Stampfer MJ, Hennekens CH, Manson JE, Colditz GA, Rosner B, Willett WC. (1993) Vitamin E consumption and the risk of coronary disease in women. N Engl J Med 328:1444–1449.
202. Rimm EB, Stampfer MJ, Ascherio A, Giovannucci E, Colditz GA, Willett WC. (1993) Vitamin E consumption and the risk of coronary heart disease in men. N Engl J Med 328:1450–1456.
203. Stephens NG, Kelley FJ. (1997) Vitamin E and coronary artery disease. Diabetes Stoffwechsel 6(suppl 2):41–44.
204. Stephens NG, Parsons A, Schofield PM, Kelly FJ, Cheeseman K, Mitchinson MT, Brown MJ. (1996) A randomized controlled trial of vitamin E in patients with coronary diseases: the Cambridge Heart Antioxidant Study (CHAOS). Lancet 347:781–786.
205. Buring JE. (1997) Epidemiologic evidence on vitamin E in the prevention and treatment of cardiovascular disease. Diabetes Stoffwechsel 6(suppl 2):38–40.
206. Losonczy KG, Harris TB, Havlik RJ. (1996) Vitamin E and vitamin C supplement use and risk of all-cause and coronary heart disease mortality in older persons: the Established Populations for Epidemiologic Studies of the Elderly. Am J Clin Nutr 64:190–196.

26

Therapeutic Effects of Lipoic Acid on Hyperglycemia and Insulin Resistance

Erik J. Henriksen
University of Arizona College of Medicine, Tucson, Arizona

I. INTRODUCTION

A. Regulation of Glucose Homeostasis

The maintenance of whole-body glucose homeostasis involves the interplay between the disposal of blood glucose in the periphery, primarily in skeletal muscle, and the delivery of glucose to the blood, either endogenously from the liver (hepatic glucose production) or exogenously from dietary sources (Fig. 1A). Disruptions in the normal regulation of either process—hepatic glucose production or skeletal muscle glucose disposal—will lead to chronic elevations of blood glucose and the development of diabetes mellitus (see Fig. 1B).

Skeletal muscle, which makes up about 40% of the body mass of humans and other mammalian species, is the major tissue responsible for the peripheral disposal of glucose in response to a glucose or insulin challenge, or during an exercise bout (1,2). Skeletal muscle glucose transport activity is acutely regulated by insulin through the activation of a series of intracellular proteins (Fig. 2A), including insulin receptor autophosphorylation and tyrosine kinase activation, tyrosine phosphorylation of insulin receptor substrate-1 (IRS-1), activation of phosphotidylinositol-3-kinase (PI3-kinase), and, finally, activation of Akt/protein kinase B (Akt/PKB). The activation of these steps ultimately results in the translocation of a glucose transporter protein isoform, GLUT-4, to the sarcolemmal membrane, where glucose transport takes place by a facilitative diffusion process (3–5). Defects in these signaling steps and in the translocation of GLUT-4 protein are thought to underlie most conditions of insulin resistance in humans (see Fig. 2B) (6,7).

In addition, glucose transport into skeletal muscle is stimulated by an insulin-independent mechanism that is activated by contractions (8–10) or hypoxia (11,12). The translocation mechanism for increasing plasma membrane GLUT-4 glucose transporters appears to function in response to contractions (13,14) and hypoxia (12) as well. In most conditions of insulin resistance, glucose transport stimulated by contractions or hypoxia is normal (15,16) or near-normal (17).

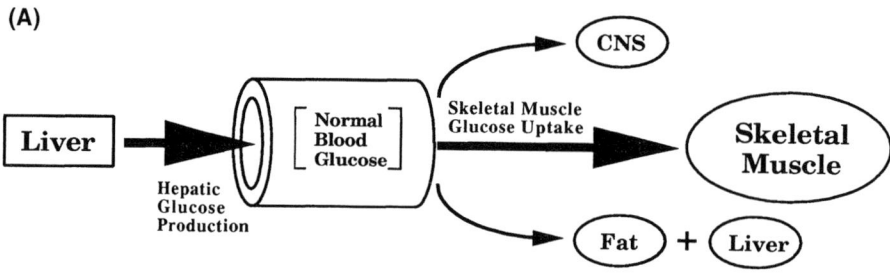

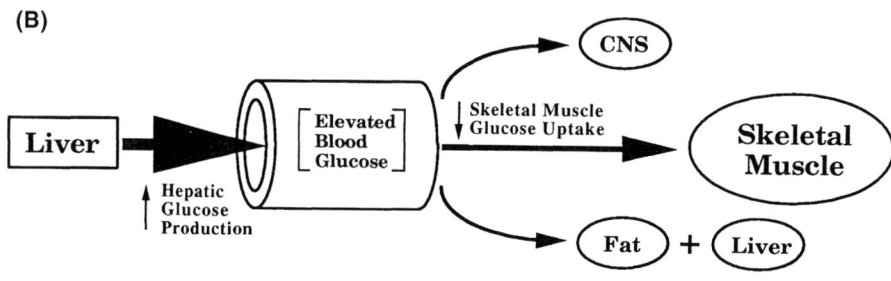

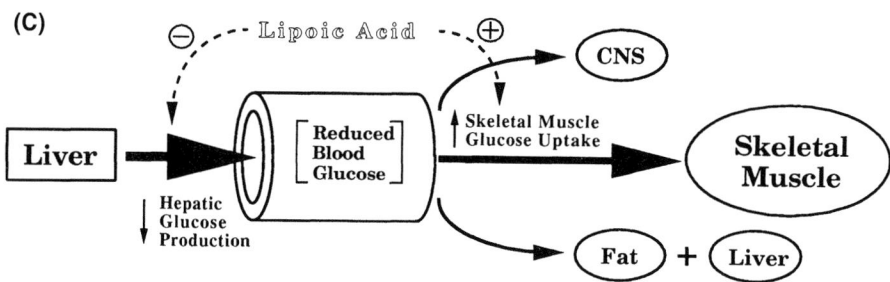

Figure 1 (A) Regulation of blood glucose levels in normal individuals; (B) in insulin-resistant diabetic individuals; and (C) in insulin-resistant diabetic individuals treated with lipoic acid.

B. Insulin Resistance and Hyperglycemia

The total diagnosed cases of diabetes mellitus in the United States numbered over 16 million in 1998 (18). There are two major forms of diabetes mellitus: type 1 and type 2. Type 1 diabetes mellitus, which represents about 5–10% of all cases of diabetes, is an autoimmune disorder in which the insulin-producing cells (β-cells) of the pancreas are destroyed, rendering the individual completely dependent on insulin injections for regulation of blood glucose levels. The primary intervention in type 1 diabetes is frequent blood glucose monitoring and appropriate insulin replacement for normalization of glucose control. Ideally, this should be accomplished by intensive insulin therapy, with frequent assessment of blood glucose concentration and appropriate insulin treatments (19).

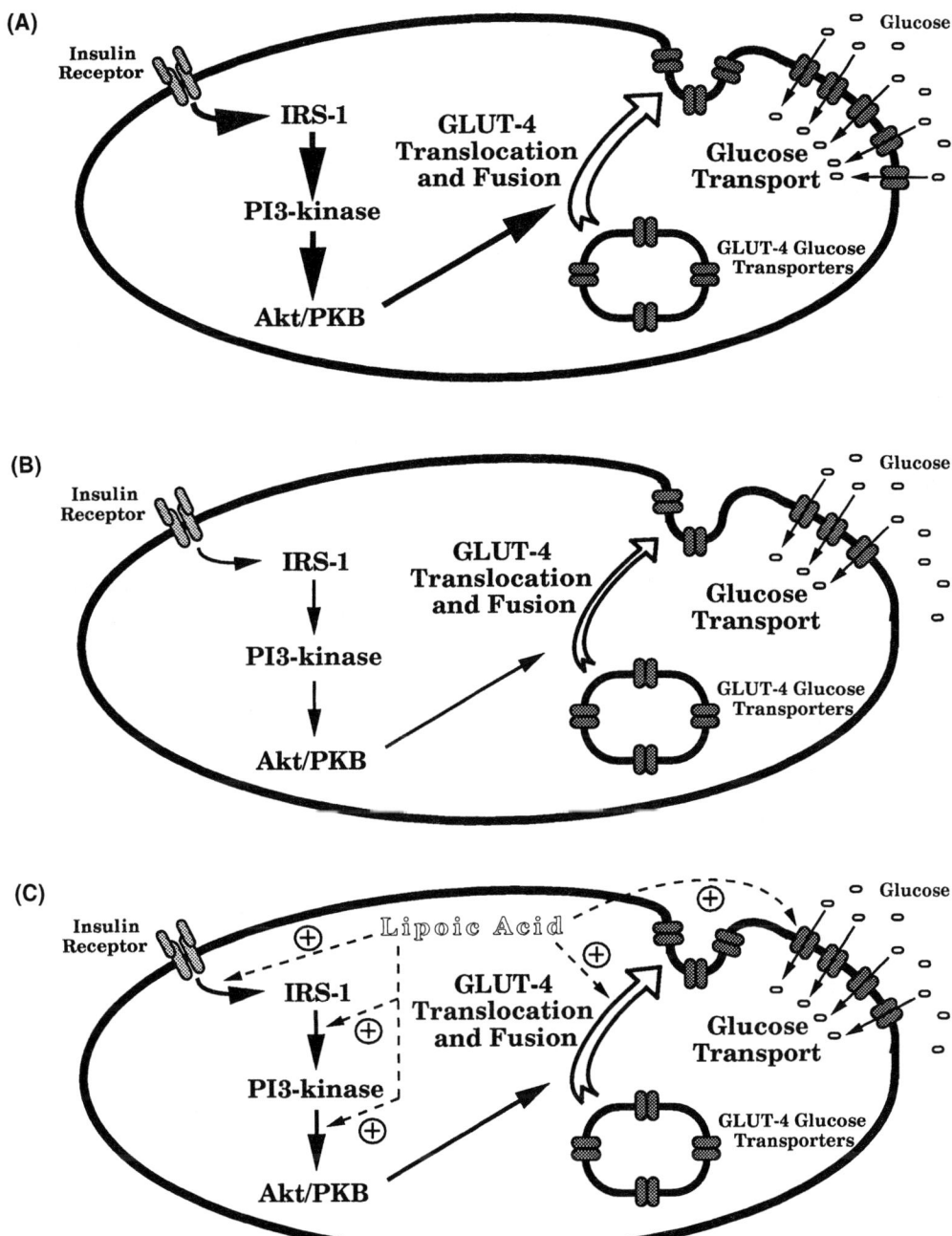

Figure 2 (A) Regulation by insulin of glucose transport in skeletal muscle of normal subjects; (B) in skeletal muscle of insulin-resistant diabetic subjects; and (C) in skeletal muscle of insulin-resistant diabetic subjects treated with lipoic acid.

Type 2 diabetes mellitus, which represents over 90% of all cases, is a multifactorial condition hallmarked by a reduced ability of insulin to stimulate glucose transport into skeletal muscle. This insulin resistance of skeletal muscle glucose transport represents a major defect in the normal maintenance of euglycemia (20,21) and is often accompanied by a variety of metabolic abnormalities, including hypertension, hyperinsulinemia, dyslipidemia, atherosclerosis, and central obesity, a condition referred to variously as "syndrome X" (22,23) or the "insulin-resistance syndrome" (24). The link among these disorders has been attributed to hyperinsulinemia, a consequence of the insulin resistance (24). Indeed, the increased cardiovascular mortality associated with this condition has been directly attributed by some leading investigators to the hyperinsulinemia itself (25–27). The ability to improve insulin action on skeletal muscle glucose metabolism in insulin-resistant individuals is, therefore, expected to decrease conversion rates to overt diabetes, as well as to reduce cardiovascular mortality in this population.

There are essentially three general approaches for enhancing insulin action in mammalian skeletal muscle. Although exercise training (28,29) and caloric restriction and fat mass loss (30,31) are certainly effective in eliciting cardiovascular and metabolic improvements in insulin-resistant individuals, a large percentage of these subjects are resistant to these dramatic changes in their lifestyles. A third approach, therefore, would involve treatment of the insulin resistance and the accompanying pathophysiological conditions with pharmaceutical interventions. Among the many pharmaceutical compounds that are known to beneficially modify glucose metabolism in type 2 diabetics are ones that decrease hepatic glucose production (metformin), increase insulin secretion (sulfonylureas), and increase insulin-stimulated skeletal muscle glucose transport (thiazolidenediones). The usefulness of other types of pharmaceutical interventions, such as antioxidants, is now increasingly recognized, and will be discussed in the following.

C. Antioxidants as a Modulator of Glucose Metabolism

It is well recognized that diabetic states are characterized by an imbalance in the oxidant–antioxidant status. Increased reactive oxygen species (ROS) production, reduced antioxidant defenses, and increased levels of biomarkers of oxidative stress damage have been described in several experimental animal models of diabetes (32-38) and also in type 2 diabetic subjects (39–42). Particularly compelling are the data of Nourooz–Zadeh et al. (42), who demonstrated in a population of type 2 diabetic subjects a significant relation between hyperglycemia and elevated indices of oxidative stress, including plasma hydroperoxides. In addition, Salonen et al. (43) showed that vitamin E, a lipid-soluble antioxidant vitamin, is significantly reduced in a Finnish population of type 2 diabetics. Even in individuals with impaired glucose tolerance, but no frank hyperglycemia (a condition immediately preceding type 2 diabetes), antioxidant status is impaired, as evidenced by reduced erythrocyte levels of the antioxidant enzymes, superoxide dismutase and catalase, and by reduced levels of glutathione and ascorbic acid (41).

Recent evidence concerning the role of oxidative stress in the pathogenesis of insulin resistance has led to suggestions that antioxidants may be effective treatments for reducing insulin resistance (34,40,44–46). Indeed, several studies have shown that treatment with antioxidants can beneficially modulate insulin-stimulated glucose disposal in type 2 diabetic subjects. For example, treatment with high doses of vitamin E (900 mg/day for 3–4 months) causes significant improvements in several of the deleterious conditions associated with type 2 diabetes, including glucose intolerance during an oral glucose tolerance test, insulin resistance of whole-body glucose disposal during a euglycemic clamp, and dyslipidemia (47–49).

D. Focus of This Chapter

The remainder of this chapter will review the available evidence from the peer-reviewed scientific literature on the effect of the water-soluble antioxidant lipoic acid (also called thioctic acid) on glucose metabolism in skeletal muscle, the myocardium, and the liver. The potential cellular mechanisms underlying the action of lipoic acid in modulating glucose metabolism in insulin-resistant states will also be incorporated into this discussion. Finally, some speculation on the future potential of lipoic acid as an intervention in conditions of type 1 and type 2 diabetes and in prediabetic conditions of insulin resistance will be presented.

II. MODULATION OF GLUCOSE METABOLISM BY THE ANTIOXIDANT LIPOIC ACID

A. Studies Using Muscle and Adipocyte Cell Lines

Rudich et al. (50,51) have recently demonstrated in 3T3-L_1 adipocytes and L_6 myocytes that prolonged exposure to low-grade oxidative stress (induced using hydrogen peroxide) markedly decreased insulin-stimulated glucose metabolism. This decreased insulin responsiveness was associated with increased GLUT-1 protein and mRNA and decreased GLUT-4 protein and mRNA (50,52), and with a decrease in insulin-stimulated Akt/PKB (53). Thus, these findings are consistent with the hypothesis that oxidative stress can directly and negatively affect the insulin-signaling cascade and the glucose transport system in insulin-responsive cells.

The effect of the antioxidant lipoic acid on insulin signaling and glucose transport in these cell lines has been addressed by several investigators. A direct stimulatory effect of lipoic acid on glucose transport activity has been shown in L_6 myocytes (54,55). This stimulatory effect of lipoic acid was much more pronounced in the R-(+)-enantiomer, the biologically active form of the compound, compared with the S-(−)-enantiomer, which is present at low levels in tissues (55). Importantly, the full stimulatory effect of lipoic acid on glucose transport activity is dependent on activation of PI3-kinase (56) and Akt/PKB (53), as well as increased translocation of GLUT-4 protein to the plasma membrane (53,55). These findings indicate that lipoic acid interacts with the insulin-signaling cascade in these insulin-responsive cell lines.

B. Normal Animal Model Studies

As early as 1970, it was known that lipoic acid could stimulate in vitro glucose transport activity in diaphragms (57) and hearts (58) isolated from normal rats. In 1997, it was first demonstrated that lipoic acid enhances glucose transport activity in skeletal muscle from insulin-sensitive lean Zucker rats in a dose-dependent fashion, with a maximally effective dose of approximately 2 mM (59), similar to observations in L_6 myocytes (55). In addition, the effect of lipoic acid on activation of glucose transport in skeletal muscle was partially inhibitable by wortmannin, which inhibits PI3-kinase (59), suggesting that lipoic acid does indeed interact with the insulin-signaling pathway in mammalian skeletal muscle, again in agreement with muscle cell line studies (55,56).

Lipoic acid also has dramatic effects on liver function. In isolated hepatocytes from fasted rats, lipoic acid causes a concentration-dependent reduction in gluconeogenesis from precursors such as lactate, pyruvate, alanine, and glycerol (60). This effect of lipoic acid in reducing hepatic glucose output was attributed to sequestration of coenzyme A in the mitochondrion, thereby inhibiting carbon flux through the gluconeogenic pathway in these cells (60).

C. Insulinopenic Animal Models

The primary animal model of type 1 diabetes is one in which the insulin-secreting cells of the pancreas (β-cells) have been destroyed. This is done most commonly by treating normal rats with agents such as streptozotocin or alloxan. Numerous investigations on the metabolic actions of lipoic acid have been conducted in this model of insulinopenia and hyperglycemia. This diabetic animal model is characterized by oxidative stress, as evidenced by markedly reduced tissue levels of reduced glutathione (61). This defect is completely reversed by prolonged treatment with a high dose of lipoic acid (100 mg/kg body weight) (61). In addition, either brief intravenous administration (60–100 mg/kg body weight) (62) or long-term intraperitoneal (30 mg/kg body weight for 10 days) treatment (63) with lipoic acid significantly lowers the otherwise elevated blood glucose level in these animals.

The level of GLUT-4 protein in skeletal muscle of the streptozotocin-diabetic rat is significantly reduced (63–65), and this alteration in GLUT-4 expression is associated with insulin resistance of skeletal muscle glucose transport (63,65). Extended treatment of streptozotocin-diabetic rats with lipoic acid (30 mg/kg body weight for 10 days) leads not only to an increase in the muscle level of GLUT-4 protein, but also to a normalization of insulin-stimulated glucose transport activity (63). Supplementation of lipoic acid in these diabetic animals also improves whole-body glucose disposal (66) and glucose oxidation (66,67).

The streptozotocin-diabetic rat is characterized by acute cardiomyopathies, including a markedly decreased glucose transport capacity, decrease oxygen uptake, altered energy status, and reduced cardiac output (68,69). The brief administration of lipoic acid (0.5 mg/mL in the perfusate) to isolated working heart preparations from these animals causes a significant enhancement of glucose transport activity and normalization of myocardial oxygen uptake, ATP levels, and cardiac output (69).

In streptozotocin-diabetic animals, endogenous levels of lipoic acid in hepatocytes are diminished (66), which may impair pyruvate dehydrogenase activity. Moreover, the enhanced hepatic conversion of alanine to glucose by the liver in these animals is completely inhibited by short-term intravenous administration of lipoic acid (62), and this intervention is associated with reductions in both liver coenzyme A and acetyl-CoA levels (62). These alterations in gluconeogenic flux may underlie the inhibition of hepatic glucose production elicited by lipoic acid treatment in this animal model of type 1 diabetes.

D. Insulin-Resistant Animal Models

The obese Zucker (*fa/fa*) rat is an animal model of severe skeletal muscle insulin resistance that is also characterized by marked hyperinsulinemia, glucose intolerance, dyslipidemia, hypertension, and central adiposity (17,70–72). Insulin-stimulated GLUT-4 protein translocation (73,74) and glucose transport activity (17,74,75) are substantially impaired in isolated skeletal muscle from these obese animals. Anai et al. (76) have recently shown that in skeletal muscle from the obese Zucker rat there are significant defects in crucial aspects of the insulin-signaling cascade (see Fig. 2B). This animal model of obesity-associated insulin resistance can be considered a precursor to overt type 2 diabetes and, therefore, is appropriate for the study of interventions designed to improve insulin action, including antioxidants.

The direct treatment of muscle preparations from the obese Zucker rat with lipoic acid significantly enhances glucose transport activity. For example, lipoic acid increases glucose transport in a dose-dependent manner in isolated epitrochlearis muscle of these insulin-resistant animals, an effect that is partially dependent on activation of PI3-kinase (59). Furthermore, a similar activation of glucose transport can be elicited by direct perfusion of lipoic acid in isolated heart preparations from the obese Zucker rat (77). These latter effects were associated with enhanced translocation of GLUT-4 protein to the plasma membrane (77) and were elicited with the racemic mixture and the pure R-(+)-enantiomer of lipoic acid, but not the S-(−)-enantiomer (77).

Studies designed to assess the metabolic effects of short- and long-term treatment of obese Zucker rats with lipoic acid have demonstrated the effectiveness of these interventions as a treatment against insulin resistance. The rapid intraperitoneal administration of a high dose of lipoic acid (100 mg/kg body weight) to the obese Zucker rat causes a significant enhancement of skeletal muscle glucose transport activity (78). It is noteworthy that this acute effect of lipoic acid on insulin action can be attributed entirely to the R-(+)-enantiomer, as treatment with the S-(−)-isoform elicits no significant effect (79).

Prolonged intraperitoneal administration of lipoic acid to this animal model of insulin resistance elicits improvements in whole-body and skeletal muscle glucose metabolism. Ten to 42 days of treatment with lipoic acid (30–50 mg/kg body weight) significantly improves glucose tolerance during an oral glucose tolerance test (80,81), likely due to an increase in skeletal muscle glucose transport activity (78–81). Extended treatment with lipoic acid also brings about small, but significant, reductions in fasting plasma levels of insulin and free fatty acids (78–80). These lipoic acid-induced improvements of whole-body and skeletal muscle glucose disposal are dose-dependent, with an apparent 50% effective dose (ED_{50}) of about 15 mg/kg body weight and a maximally effective dose of 30 mg/kg body weight (78–80). Furthermore, continued treatment of obese Zucker rats with lipoic acid improves both nonoxidative (glycogen synthesis) and oxidative metabolism of the glucose taken up into the muscle cells (78,79). Interestingly, this lipoic acid treatment does not appear to modify the effect of insulin to enhance protein synthesis and inhibit protein degradation in skeletal muscle of normal or insulin-resistant Zucker rats (82).

The aforementioned metabolic improvements following prolonged treatment with lipoic acid are stereospecific and are restricted to the R-(+)-enantiomer (79,81). In fact, such treatment with the S-(−)-enantiomer can have deleterious metabolic consequences, including further worsening of the existing hyperinsulinemia and a reduction in skeletal muscle GLUT-4 protein levels (79).

Recent studies have demonstrated that lipoic acid can be effective in combination with other beneficial interventions against the insulin resistance that characterizes the obese Zucker rat. For example, a unique conjugate consisting of equimolar parts of lipoic acid and the n-6 essential fatty acid γ-linolenic acid has been developed and administered over a long period to obese Zucker rats (80). This conjugate of lipoic acid and γ-linolenic acid elicits significant dose-dependent improvements in whole-body and skeletal muscle insulin action, and these actions of the conjugate appear to be due to the additive effects of its individual components (80). This same additivity of effects on whole-body and skeletal muscle glucose metabolism is seen when long-term lipoic acid [R-(+)-enantiomer] treatment is combined with 6 weeks of endurance exercise training of the obese Zucker rat (81). These findings provide strong experimental evidence that lipoic acid can be used as an adjunct therapy in combination with other interventions to optimize treatment of insulin resistance and its associated pathophysiological conditions.

E. Clinical Investigations with Type 2 Diabetics

Several clinical investigations have confirmed that treatment with lipoic acid can improve insulin-stimulated glucose metabolism in insulin-resistant type 2 diabetic human subjects. In an initial placebo-controlled study, Jacob and colleagues (83) demonstrated in type 2 diabetic subjects that a single intravenous administration of lipoic acid (1000 mg) significantly enhances whole-body insulin-stimulated glucose disposal, as assessed using the isoglycemic, hyperinsulinemic clamp. This finding that lipoic acid can rapidly enhance insulin action in human type 2 diabetics was confirmed by others using a lower dose (500 mg) of the antioxidant (84). Moreover, the beneficial actions of intravenous lipoic acid administration on insulin-mediated whole-body glucose disposal were shown in an open study in which type 2 diabetics received daily infusions of the compound (500 mg/day) over a 10-day period (85). The improvements in the metabolic clearance rate for glucose in these intravenous studies were all close to 30% (83–85).

More recently, the results of two studies in Germany involving the oral administration of lipoic acid to type 2 diabetic patients have been published. In a multicenter, placebo-controlled study, Jacob et al. (86) report that 4 weeks of oral administration of lipoic acid (600, 1200, or 1800 mg/day) to older (about 60 years of age) insulin-resistant type 2 diabetic subjects resulted in an approximately 30% net improvement in insulin-mediated glucose disposal, as assessed using the metabolic clearance rate during an isoglycemic, hyperinsulinemic glucose clamp. In addition, Konrad et al. (87) conducted an oral treatment study involving lean and obese type 2 diabetic subjects. In this investigation, the diabetic subjects received 600-mg doses of lipoic acid twice daily for 4 weeks. Following the treatment period, significant improvements in insulin sensitivity during an intravenous glucose tolerance test were observed in the lean type 2 diabetic subjects, and significant improvements in glucose effectiveness during an intravenous glucose tolerance test and significant reductions in serum lactate and pyruvate levels during an oral glucose tolerance test were noted in both lean and obese type 2 diabetic subjects. Taken together, these oral studies provide promising evidence for continued investigation on the usefulness of lipoic acid as an intervention against the insulin resistance associated with type 2 diabetes.

III. CONCLUSIONS

It is clear that lipoic acid elicits a variety of effects that modulate carbohydrate metabolism in skeletal muscle. These effects are summarized in Table 1. In the markedly hyperglycemic and insulinopenic streptozotocin-diabetic rat, lipoic acid can reduce blood glucose levels as a result of both an increase in skeletal muscle glucose transport activity and a reduction in glucose production by the liver (see Fig. 1C). These adaptations likely underlie the increased glucose tolerance following lipoic acid treatment of these animals. Improved glucose metabolism and bioenergetics in the myocardium of the streptozotocin-diabetic rat also results from lipoic acid treatment.

In the insulin-resistant, hyperinsulinemic, glucose-intolerant, and dyslipidemic obese Zucker rat, lipoic acid treatment improves insulin action on skeletal muscle and myocardial glucose uptake, and this is associated with improved glucose tolerance in these animals (see Table 1). Moreover, decreases in blood insulin and lipids are also realized with lipoic acid treatment. Importantly, both intravenous and oral administration of lipoic acid in insulin-resistant human type 2 diabetic subjects improve insulin action on whole-body glucose disposal.

From the data available from a variety of insulin-responsive cell lines and tissues and from whole-body investigations, one can speculate on the potential mechanisms of action of lipoic acid on insulin-resistant skeletal muscle (see Fig. 2C). Results to date are consistent with the concept that lipoic acid interacts with various defective steps in insulin-signaling factors in the cell, ultimately leading to enhanced GLUT-4 protein translocation and glucose transport activity. There may also be a role of lipoic acid directly enhancing glucose transport, possibly

Table 1 Beneficial Metabolic Actions of Lipoic Acid in Animal and Human Diabetes

Condition	Effect of lipoic acid treatment	Ref.
Insulinopenic rat	Lowering of elevated blood glucose levels	62,63
	Increased skeletal muscle GLUT-4 protein	63
	Increased skeletal muscle glucose transport	63
	Increased cardiac muscle glucose transport	69
	Enhanced glucose tolerance	66
	Reduced hepatic glucose output	62
Obese Zucker rat	Increased skeletal muscle glucose transport	59,78–81
	Increased cardiac muscle glucose transport	77
	Enhanced glucose tolerance	80,81
	Lowering of elevated plasma insulin levels	59,78–81
	Lowering of elevated plasma lipid levels	59,78–81
Human type 2 diabetes	Increased skeletal muscle glucose disposal	83–87
	Decreased glucose-derived plasma lactate and pyruvate levels	87

by its actions to reduce circulating free fatty acids and thereby lessen the inhibitory effect of these free fatty acids on the glucose transport process (88). It should be emphasized, however, that direct evidence in mammalian skeletal muscle for most of these potential actions of lipoic acid is still forthcoming.

The prospect of lipoic acid as an adjunct therapy in conditions of hyperglycemia and insulin resistance is intriguing. Future research on the metabolic actions of lipoic acid in diabetes should be focused on the cellular and molecular mechanisms associated with the improvements in insulin-mediated skeletal muscle glucose transport activity. Direct evidence in skeletal muscle on the interactions of lipoic acid with proteins of the insulin-signaling pathway is needed. Moreover, the actions of lipoic acid on hepatic glucose production in models of insulin resistance need to be more thoroughly investigated. Finally, more comprehensive clinical trials in human type 1 and type 2 diabetic subjects are needed to document the efficacy of lipoic acid administration in bringing about metabolic improvements.

ACKNOWLEDGMENTS

I wish to thank the current and former members of my laboratory (Donovan Fogt, Dr. Jason Hokama, Tyson Kinnick, Tony Peth, Vitoon Saengsirisuwan, Melanie Schmit, Dr. Ryan Streeper, and Erik Youngblood) and my German collaborators (Dr. Stephan Jacob, Dr. Hans J. Tritschler, and Dr. Günther J. Dietze) who have contributed to many of the studies mentioned in this chapter.

REFERENCES

1. DeFronzo RA, Ferrannini E, Hendler R, Felig P, Wahren J. (1983) Regulation of splanchnic and peripheral glucose uptake by insulin and hyperglycemia in man. Diabetes 32:32–45.
2. Baron AD, Brechtel G, Wallace P, Edelman SV. (1988) Rates and tissue sites of non–insulin- and insulin-mediated glucose uptake in humans. Am J Physiol 255:E769–E774.
3. Cheatham B, Kahn CR. (1995) Insulin action and the insulin signaling network. Endocr Rev 16:117–142.

4. Ueki K, Yamamoto–Honda R, Kaburagi Y, Yamauchi T, Tobe K, Burgering BMT, Coffer PJ, Komuro I, Akanuma Y, Yazaki Y, Kadowaki T. (1998) Potential role of protein kinase B in insulin-induced glucose transport, glycogen synthesis, and protein synthesis. J Biol Chem 273:5315–5322.
5. Hajduch E, Alessi DR, Hemmings BA, Hundal HS. (1998) Constitutive activation of protein kinase B_α by membrane targeting promotes glucose and system A amino acid transport, protein synthesis, and inactivation of glycogen synthase kinase-3 in L_6 muscle cells. Diabetes 47:1006–1013.
6. Zierath JR, Krook A, Wallberg–Henriksson H. (1998) Insulin action in skeletal muscle from patients with NIDDM. Mol Cell Biochem 182:153–160.
7. Krook A, Roth RA, Jiang XJ, Zierath JR, Wallberg–Henriksson H. (1998) Insulin-stimulated Akt kinase activity is reduced in skeletal muscle from NIDDM subjects. Diabetes 47:1281–1286.
8. Holloszy JO, Narahara HT. (1965) Studies of tissue permeability. X. Changes in permeability to 3-methylglucose associated with contraction of frog muscle. J Biol Chem 240:3493–3500.
9. Garetto LP, Richter EA, Goodman MN, Ruderman NB. (1984) Enhanced muscle glucose metabolism after exercise in the rat: the two phases. Am J Physiol 246:E471–E475.
10. Nesher R, Karl IE, Kipnis DM. (1985) Dissociation of effects of insulin and contraction on glucose transport in rat epitrochlearis muscle. Am J Physiol 249:C226–C232.
11. Chaudry IH, Gould MK. (1970) Effect of externally added ATP on glucose uptake by isolated rat soleus muscle. Biochim Biophys Acta 196:327–335.
12. Cartee GD, Douen AG, Ramlal T, Klip A, Holloszy JO. (1991) Stimulation of glucose transport in skeletal muscle by hypoxia. J Appl Physiol 70:1593–1600.
13. Goodyear LJ, Hirshman MF, Horton ES. (1991) Exercise-induced translocation of skeletal muscle glucose transporters. Am J Physiol 261:E795–E799.
14. Gao J, Ren J, Gulve EA, Holloszy JO. (1994) Additive effect of contractions and insulin on GLUT-4 translocation into the sarcolemma. J Appl Physiol 77:1587–1601.
15. Brozinick JT Jr, Etgen GJ, Yaspelkis BB, Ivy JL. (1992) Contraction-activated glucose uptake in normal in insulin-resistant muscle of the obese Zucker rat. J Appl Physiol 73:382–387.
16. Azevedo JL Jr, Carey JO, Pories WJ, Morris PG, Dohm GL. (1995) Hypoxia stimulates glucose transport in insulin-resistant human skeletal muscle. Diabetes 44:695–698.
17. Henriksen EJ, Jacob S. (1995) Effects of captopril on glucose transport activity in skeletal muscle of obese Zucker rats. Metabolism 44:267–272.
18. National Institute of Diabetes and Digestive and Kidney Diseases Website. (1999) http://www.niddk.nih.gov.
19. Diabetes Control and Complications Trial Research Group. (1993) The effect of intensive treatment of diabetes on the development and progression of long-term complications of insulin-dependent diabetes mellitus. N Engl J Med 329:977–986.
20. Dohm GL, Tapscott EB, Pories WJ, Dabbs DJ, Flickinger EG, Meelheim D, Fushiki T, Atkinson SM, Elton CW, Carol JF. (1988) An in vitro human muscle preparation suitable for metabolic studies: decreased insulin stimulation of glucose transport in muscle from morbidly obese and diabetic subjects. J Clin Invest 82:486–494.
21. Mueckler M. (1990) Family of glucose-transport genes. Implications for glucose homeostasis and diabetes. Diabetes 39:6–13.
22. Reaven GM. (1988) Role of insulin resistance in human disease. Diabetes 37:1595–1607.
23. Reaven GM. (1993) Role of insulin resistance in human disease (syndrome X): an expanded definition. Annu Rev Med 44:121–131.
24. DeFronzo RA, Ferrannini E. (1991) Insulin resistance: a multifaceted syndrome responsible for NIDDM, obesity, hypertension, dyslipidemia, and atherosclerotic cardiovascular disease. Diabetes Care 14:173–194.
25. Ferrannini E, Haffner SM, Mitchell BD, Stern MP. (1991) Hyperinsulinaemia: the key feature of a cardiovascular and metabolic syndrome. Diabetologia 34:416–422.
26. Reaven GM. (1995) The fourth Musketeer—from Alexandre Dumas to Claude Bernard. Diabetologia 38:3–13.
27. King GL. (1996) The role of hyperglycaemia and hyperinsulinaemia in causing vascular dysfunction in diabetes. Ann Med 28:427–432.
28. Holloszy JO, Schultz J, Kuznierkiewicz J, Hagberg JM, Ehsani AA. (1986) Effects of exercise on glucose tolerance and insulin resistance. Acta Med Scand Suppl 711:55–65.
29. Rogers MA, Yamamoto C, King DS, Hagberg JM, Ehsani AA, Holloszy JO. (1988) Improvements in glucose tolerance after 1 week of exercise in patients with mild NIDDM. Diabetes Care 11:613–618.

30. Hughes TA, Gwynne JT, Switzer BR, Herbst C, White G. (1984) Effects of caloric restriction and weight loss on glycemic control, insulin resistance, and atherosclerotic risk in obese patients with type II diabetes mellitus. Am J Med 77:7–17.
31. Laakso M, Uusitupa M, Takala J, Majander H, Reijonen T, Penttilä I. (1988) Effects of hypocaloric diet and insulin therapy on metabolic control and mechanisms in obese non–insulin-dependent diabetic subjects. Metabolism 37:1092–1100.
32. Woollard A, Bascal ZA, Armstrong GR, Wolff SP. (1990) Abnormal redox status without increased lipid peroxidation in sugar cataract. Diabetes 39:1347–1352.
33. Wolff SP, Jiang ZY, Hunt JV. (1991) Protein glycation and oxidative stress in diabetes mellitus and aging. Free Radic Biol Med 10:339–352.
34. Baynes JW. (1991) Role of oxidative stress in development of complications in diabetes. Diabetes 40:405–412.
35. Armstrong D, Awadi F. (1991) Lipid peroxidation and retinopathy in streptozotocin induced diabetes. Free Radic Biol Med 11:433–436.
36. Schmidt AM, Hori O, Brett J, Yan SD, Wautier JL, Stern D. (1994) Cellular receptors for advanced glycation end products. Implications for induction of oxidant stress and cellular dysfunction in the pathogenesis of vascular lesions. Arterioscler Thromb 14:1521–1528.
37. Yan SD, Schmidt AM, Anderson GM, Zhang J, Brett J, Zou YS, Pinsky D, Stern D. (1994) Enhanced cellular oxidant stress by the interaction of advanced glycation end products with their receptors/binding proteins. J Biol Chem 269:9889–9897.
38. Nourooz-Zadeh J. (1998) Antioxidant and prooxidant profile in diabetes mellitus and its relevance to the onset of the syndrome. Oxygen Club of California World Congress, Santa Barbara, CA, February 6–8.
39. Jones AW, Winkles JW, Jennings PE, Florkowski CM, Lunec J, Barnett AH. (1988) Serum antioxidant activity in diabetes mellitus. Diabetes Res 7:89–92.
40. Paolisso G, D'Amore A, Volpe C, Balbi V, Saccomanno F, Galzerano D, Giugliano D, Varricchio M, D'Onofrio F. (1994) Evidence for a relationship between oxidative stress and insulin action in NIDDM patients. Metabolism 43:1426–1429.
41. Vijayalingam S, Parthiban A, Shanmugasundaram KR, Mohan V. (1996) Abnormal antioxidant status in impaired glucose tolerance and non–insulin-dependent diabetes mellitus. Diabetes Med 13:715–719.
42. Nourooz-Zadeh J, Rahimi A, Tajaddini-Sarmadi J, Tritschler H, Rosen P, Halliwell B, Betteridge DJ. (1997) Relationships between plasma measures of oxidative stress and metabolic control in NIDDM. Diabetologia 40:647–653.
43. Salonen JT, Nyyssonen K, Tuomainen TP, Maenpaa PH, Korpela H, Kaplan G, Lynch J, Helmrich SP, Salonen R. (1995) Increased risk of non–insulin-dependent diabetes mellitus at low plasma vitamin E concentrations: a four year follow-up study in men. Br Med J 311:1124–1127.
44. Johnson MB, Heineke EW, Rhinehart BL, Sheetz MJ, Barnhart RL, Robinson KM. (1993) Antioxidant with marked lipid- and glucose-lowering activity in diabetic rats and mice. Diabetes 42:1179–1186.
45. Cominacini L, Garbin U, Cascio L. (1996) The need for a free radical initiative. Diabetologia 39:364–366.
46. Paolisso G, Giugliano D. (1996) Oxidative stress and insulin action: is there a relationship? Diabetologia 39:357–364.
47. Paolisso G, D'Amore A, Giugliano D, Ceriello A, Varricchio M, D'Onofrio F. (1993) Pharmacologic doses of vitamin E improve insulin action in healthy subjects and non–insulin-dependent diabetic patients. Am J Clin Nutr 57:650–656.
48. Paolisso G, D'Amore A, Galzerno D, Balbi V, Giugliano D, Varricchio M, D'Onofrio F. (1993) Daily vitamin E supplements improve metabolic control but not insulin secretion in elderly type II diabetic patients. Diabetes Care 16:1433–1437.
49. Caballero B. (1993) Vitamin E improves the action of insulin. Nutr Rev 51:339–340.
50. Rudich A, Kazlovsky N, Potashnik R, Bashan N. (1997) Oxidant stress reduces insulin responsiveness in 3T3-L_1 adipocytes. Am J Physiol 272:E935–E940.
51. Rudich A, Tirosh A, Potashnik R, Hemi R, Kanety H, Bashan N. (1998) Prolonged oxidative stress impairs insulin-induced GLUT4 translocation in 3T3-L_1 adipocytes. Diabetes 47:1562–1569.
52. Kozlovsky N, Rudich A, Potashnik R, Ebina Y, Murakami T, Bashan N. (1997) Transcriptional activation of the GLUT1 gene in response to oxidative stress in L_6 myotubes. J Biol Chem 272:33367–33372.

53. Bashan N, Rudich A, Tirosh A, Potashnik R, Khamaisi M. (1999) Lipoic acid protects against oxidation-induced insulin resistance in 3T3-L$_1$ adipocytes. Diabetes 48(suppl 1):A261.
54. Bashan N, Burdett E, Guma A, Klip A. (1993) Effect of thioctic acid on glucose transport. In: Gries FA, Wessel K, eds. The Role of Antioxidants in Diabetes Mellitus. PMI-Verl.-Gruppe, pp. 2291–2299.
55. Estrada DE, Ewart HS, Tsakiridis T, Volchuk A, Ramlal T, Tritschler H, Klip A. (1996) Stimulation of glucose uptake by the natural coenzyme α-lipoic acid/thioctic acid: participation of elements of the insulin signaling pathway. Diabetes 45:1798–1804.
56. Tsakiridis T, Estrada DE, Tritschler H, Klip A. (1995) Thioctic (lipoic) acid induces protein tyrosine phosphorylation and phosphotidylinositol 3-kinase activation in muscle cells. Diabetologia 38:A132.
57. Haugaard N, Haugaard ES. (1970) Stimulation of glucose utilization by thioctic acid in rat diaphragm incubated in vitro. Biochim Biophys Acta 222:583–586.
58. Singh HP, Bowman RH. (1970) Effect of DL-alpha-lipoic acid on the citrate concentration and phosphofructokinase activity of perfused hearts from normal and diabetic rats. Biochem Biophys Res Commun 41:555–561.
59. Henriksen EJ, Jacob S, Streeper RS, Fogt DL, Hokama JY, Tritschler HJ. (1997) Stimulation by α-lipoic acid of glucose transport activity in skeletal muscle of lean and obese Zucker rats. Life Sci 61:805–812.
60. Blumenthal SA. (1984) Inhibition of gluconeogenesis in rat liver by lipoic acid. Evidence for more than one site of action. Biochem J 219:773–780.
61. Nagamatsu M, Nickander KK, Schmelzer JD, Raya A, Wittrock DA, Tritschler H, Low PA. (1995) Lipoic acid improves nerve blood flow, reduces oxidative stress, and improves distal nerve conduction in experimental diabetic neuropathy. Diabetes Care 18:1160–1167.
62. Khamaisi M, Rudich A, Potashnik R, Tritschler HJ, Gutman A, Bashan N. (1999) Lipoic acid acutely induces hypoglycemia in fasting nondiabetic and diabetic rats. Metabolism 48:504–510.
63. Khamaisi M, Potashnik R, Tirosh A, Demshchak E, Rudich A, Tritschler H, Wessel K, Bashan N. (1997) Lipoic acid reduces glycemia and increases muscle GLUT4 content in streptozotocin-diabetic rats. Metabolism 46:763–768.
64. Shepherd PR, Kahn BB. (1994) Expression of the GLUT4 glucose transporter in diabetes. In: Draznin B, LeRoith D, eds. Molecular Biology of Diabetes. Insulin Action, Effects on Gene Expression and Regulation, and Glucose Transport. vol 2. Totowa, NJ: Humana Press, pp. 529–546.
65. Klip A, Tsakiridis T, Marette A, Ortiz PA. (1994) Regulation of expression of glucose transporters by glucose: a review of studies in vivo and in cell cultures. FASEB J 8:43–53.
66. Natraj CV, Gandhi VM, Menon KKG. (1984) Lipoic acid and diabetes. Effects of dihydrolipoic acid administration in diabetic rats and rabbits. J Biosci 6:37–46.
67. Wagh SS, Natraj CV, Menon KKG. (1987) Mode of action of lipoic acid in diabetes. J Biosci 11:59–74.
68. Strödter D, Willmann P, Willmann J, Federlin K, Schaper W. (1991) Results of a balance of energy in the diabetic heart. In: Nagano M, Dhalla NS, eds. The Diabetic Heart. New York: Raven Press, pp 383–399.
69. Strödter D, Lehmann E, Lehmann U, Tritschler HJ, Bretzel RG, Federlin K. (1995) The influence of thioctic acid on metabolism and function of the diabetic heart. Diabetes Res Clin Pract 29:19–26.
70. Mathe D. (1995) Dyslipidemia and diabetes: animal models. Diabetes Metab 21:106–111.
71. Turner NC, Gudgeon C, Toseland N. (1995) Effects of genetic hyperinsulinemia on vascular reactivity, blood pressure, and renal structure in the Zucker rat. J Cardiovasc Pharmacol 26:714–720.
72. Van Zwieten PA, Kam KL, Pijl AJ, Hendriks MG, Beenen OH, Pfaffendorf M. (1996) Hypertensive diabetic rats in pharmacological studies. Pharmacol Res 33:95–105.
73. King PA, Horton ED, Hirshman MF, Horton ES. (1993) Insulin resistance in obese Zucker rat (*fa/fa*) is associated with a failure of glucose transporter translocation. J Clin Invest 90:1568–1575.
74. Etgen GJ, Wilson CM, Jensen J, Cushman SW, Ivy JL. (1996) Glucose transport and cell surface GLUT-4 protein in skeletal muscle of the obese Zucker rat. Am J Physiol 271:E294–E301.
75. Crettaz M, Prentki M, Zaninetti D, Jeanrenaud B. (1980) Insulin resistance in soleus muscle from obese Zucker rats: involvement of several defective sites. Biochem J 186:525–534.
76. Anai M, Funaki M, Ogihara T, Terasaki J, Inukai K, Katagiri H, Fukushima Y, Yazaki Y, Kikuchi M, Oka Y, Asano T. (1998) Altered expression levels and impaired steps in pathways to phosphotidylinositol-3-kinase activation via insulin receptor substrates 1 and 2 in Zucker fatty rats. Diabetes 47:13–23.

77. Loeblein K, Rett K, Maerker E, Tritschler HJ, Wessel K, Wicklmayr M, Häring HU. (1995) Thioctic acid stimulates translocation of glucose transports in hearts of insulin resistant Zucker rats. Diabetologia 38:A132.
78. Jacob S, Streeper RS, Fogt DL, Hokama JY, Tritschler HJ, Dietze GJ, Henriksen EJ. (1996) The antioxidant α-lipoic acid enhances insulin-stimulated glucose metabolism in insulin-resistant skeletal muscle. Diabetes 45:1024–1029.
79. Streeper RS, Henriksen EJ, Jacob S, Hokama JY, Fogt DL, Tritschler HJ, Dietze GJ. (1997) Differential effects of stereoisomers of alpha-lipoic acid on glucose metabolism in insulin-resistant rat skeletal muscle. Am J Physiol 273:E185–E191.
80. Peth JA, Kinnick TR. Youngblood EB, Tritschler HJ, Henriksen EJ. (2000) Effects of a unique conjugate of alpha-lipoic acid and gamma-linolenic acid on insulin action in the obese Zucker rat. Am J Physiol 279:R453–R459.
81. Saengsirisuwan V, Kinnick TR, Schmit MB, Henriksen EJ. (2000) Interactions of exercise training and lipoic acid on insulin action in obese Zucker rats. FASEB J 14:A435.
82. Weinstein RB, Tritschler HJ, Henriksen EJ. (2001) Antioxidant alpha-lipoic acid and protein turnover in insulin-resistant rat muscle. Free Radic Biol Med 30:383–388.
83. Jacob S, Henriksen EJ, Schiemann AL, Simon I, Clancy DE, Tritschler HJ, Jung WI, Augustin HJ, Dietze GJ. (1995) Enhancement of glucose disposal in patients with type 2 diabetes by alpha-lipoic acid. Drug Res 45:872–874.
84. Rett K, Wicklmayr M, Maerker E, Ruus P, Nehrdich D, Herrmann R, Standl E. (1995) Effect of acute infusion of thioctic acid on oxidative and non-oxidative metabolism in obese subjects with NIDDM. Diabetologia 38:A41.
85. Jacob S, Henriksen EJ, Tritschler HJ, Augustin HJ, Dietze GJ. (1996) Improvement of insulin-stimulated glucose disposal in type 2 diabetes after repeated parenteral administration of thioctic acid. Exp Clin Endocrinol Diabetes 104:284–288.
86. Jacob S, Ruus P, Hermann R, Tritschler HJ, Maerker E, Renn W, Augustin HJ, Dietze GJ, Rett K. (1999) Oral administration of rac-α-lipoic acid modulates insulin sensitivity in patients with type 2 diabetes mellitus—a placebo controlled pilot trial. Free Radic Biol Med 27:309–314.
87. Konrad T, Vicini P, Kusterer K, Hoflich A, Assadkhani A, Bohles HJ, Sewell A, Tritschler HJ, Cobelli C, Usadel KH. (1999) alpha-Lipoic acid treatment decreases serum lactate and pyruvate concentrations and improves glucose effectiveness in lean and obese patients with type 2 diabetes. Diabetes Care 22:280–287.
88. Boden G. (1997) Role of fatty acids in the pathogenesis of insulin resistance and NIDDM. Diabetes 46:3–10.

27
Bioavailability of Glutathione

Dean P. Jones
Emory University, Atlanta, Georgia

I. INTRODUCTION

Glutathione (GSH) is among the most important antioxidants in biological systems, and several strategies have been used to increase GSH and thereby protect against oxidants and reactive electrophiles (1). The simplest approach is to supply glutathione directly as an oral preparation (2). The present chapter is an update of previous reviews, which discuss in detail glutathione content in foods (3,4), cell transport of glutathione (5–7), and absorption and utilization of orally supplied glutathione (2).

Glutathione is present at up to 150 mg/day in the human diet (8) and can be absorbed intact in the small intestine (9,10). Quantitative evaluation indicates that in healthy individuals with ample sulfur amino acids (1–2 g/day) in their diets, the amount of GSH is probably insufficient to have an important effect systemically. In individuals with limiting sulfur amino acid intake, however, dietary and supplemental GSH may enhance systemic GSH supply by improving sulfur amino acid balance. Accumulating data indicates that dietary and supplemental glutathione can be absorbed by epithelial cells in the oral cavity and gastrointestinal tract and provide specific health benefits in these tissues (11,12). In addition, a variety of preparations are now available to enhance synthesis of glutathione by supply of precursors (1) or by supplying chemicals that induce the enzymatic machinery responsible for synthesizing glutathione in cells (13).

II. METABOLISM AND FUNCTIONS

A. Distinct Pathway from Protein Metabolism

Glutathione is a tripeptide composed of the amino acids, glutamate, cysteine, and glycine (Fig. 1). The linkage of the glutamate to the cysteine is through the γ-carboxylate, rather than the usual α-carboxylate found in proteins, and this linkage renders the GSH (γ-glutamyl-cysteinyl-glycine) resistant to proteases and peptidases that function in protein degradation. Synthesis occurs independently of ribosomal protein synthesis by a pathway consisting of two

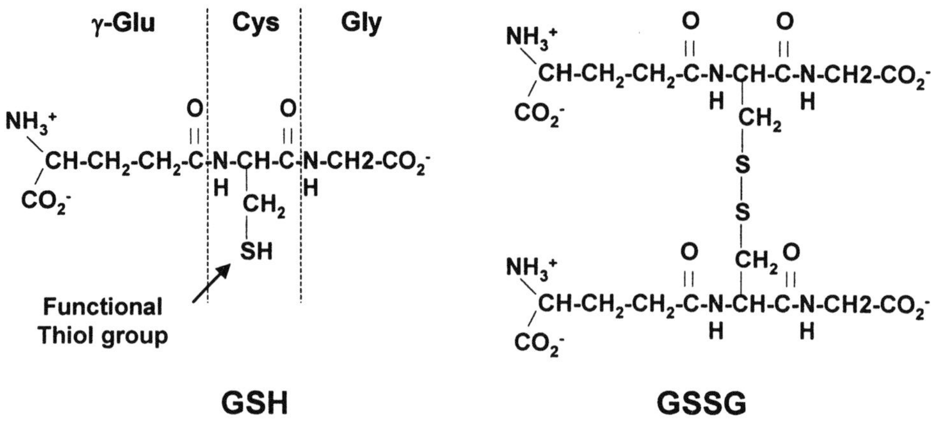

Figure 1 Structures of GSH and GSSG: Glutathione is a tripeptide composed of the amino acids glutamate, cysteine, and glycine. The linkage of glutamate and cysteine is an isopeptide bond between the γ-carboxyl group of glutamate and the α-amino group of cysteine. This unique bond makes glutathione resistant to degradation by proteases and peptidases that function in protein turnover. The thiol group of the cysteine is the functional portion of the molecule, undergoing oxidation to form the disulfide in GSSG and reacting with electrophiles in conjugation reactions.

enzymes, γ-glutamylcysteine synthetase and glutathione synthetase. Both are ATP-dependent and are present in the cytoplasm of all mammalian cells. The intermediate, γ-glutamylcysteine, is present in all cells, typically at a low micromolar concentration.

Degradation of GSH occurs by a unique enzyme, γ-glutamyltransferase (GGT), also known as γ-glutamyltranspeptidase, which removes glutamate and yields cysteinylglycine. This enzyme is present mostly as an ectoenzyme associated with the plasma membrane of epithelial cells, with very high activity in the renal proximal tubules. Cysteinylglycine is present at micromolar concentrations in the plasma and is degraded by at least three different enzymes with dipeptidase activity. Thus, most of the degradation of GSH occurs extracellularly, and the combined pathways of enzymes allow GSH turnover to be independent of protein synthesis and degradation.

B. The Thiol Group Provides the Functional Portion of the Molecule

The sulfur of the cysteine provides the functional portion of GSH. Cysteine is an amino acid that provides a great flexibility in chemical reactivity owing to the sulfur atom present as a thiol (–SH). This thiol is critical for the biological functions of perhaps half of all enzymes. The sulfur of cysteine, whether it is in free cysteine, in a protein, or in glutathione, is present as a thiol (–SH) that can be oxidized to a disulfide. In GSH, cysteine is oxidized to form a disulfide (GSSG) when GSH serves as a reductant. The thiol is also used for detoxification of reactive electrophilic chemicals, often catalyzed by glutathione S-transferases.

C. Distinction from Cysteine

In principle, cysteine itself can function as a reductant and as a nucleophile so that it could have been used in place of glutathione for detoxification in biological systems. However, the thiol in cysteine is about ten times more reactive than GSH and rapidly oxidizes to produce reactive oxygen species (ROS). This reactivity of the thiol in cysteine is due to the free amino group on the α-carbon, which withdraws electron density from the thiol group on the β-carbon. This reactivity is decreased in GSH because of the glutamate attached to the amino group (see Fig. 1). Thus, a function of the glutamate in GSH is to decrease the reactivity of the thiol so that high concentrations can be maintained in cells without generation of ROS.

D. Function as a Short-Term Store of Cysteine

Although GSH has a very critical role in detoxification, the decreased reactivity compared with cysteine suggests that the primordial function of GSH may have been to serve as a short-term reservoir for cysteine. Cysteine is required for synthesis of most proteins, and as cysteine becomes limiting for protein synthesis, GSH degradation provides additional cysteine (14). The liver is especially important in this short-term supply, and diurnal variation in hepatic GSH in mice has been observed in association with dietary intake of sulfur amino acids (15). In humans, the total body content of GSH, about 10 g, is about five times the daily intake of sulfur amino acids. Thus, at most, this is only a short-term reservoir. Although cysteine that is released from protein degradation can be reutilized, cysteine is also used for production of taurine and sulfate. Taurine and sulfate are needed for a variety of biological functions, including detoxification. Thus, a continual supply of cysteine is required to replace this loss.

Maintenance of GSH as a reservoir for cysteine is energy-requiring because GSH synthesis requires two molecules of ATP per molecule of GSH synthesized. However, an issue that is more fundamental than the energetic cost of maintaining this reservoir is that the provision of GSH for detoxification appears to be secondary to the use for maintenance of the cysteine pools. When cysteine becomes limiting for protein synthesis, GSH pools decrease and detoxification functions that are dependent on GSH become impaired. Thus, after only a few days of fasting or protein malnutrition, GSH-dependent detoxification mechanisms may become compromised. This period of time can be important, for instance, following illness, surgery, or antitumor therapy that results in prolonged nutritional insufficiency. These may represent conditions for which supplemental GSH or sulfur amino acid precursors are particularly needed.

III. ORAL GSH SUPPLY

A. Glutathione in Foods

Glutathione is present in the plant and animal products that form the basis of the human diet (8,16). Because the concentration of glutathione is in the millimolar range in most cells, this means that many foods contain 15 mg or more per 100 g. Among the foods that are high in glutathione are fresh or freshly prepared vegetables, such as asparagus, potatoes, spinach, tomato, and avocado; fruits such as oranges, grapefruit, and peaches; and freshly prepared meat, poultry, and fish (Table 1). Freshly frozen foods often contain glutathione in amounts similar to fresh foods. However, cereals and other grain products have little glutathione, and many canned foods have lost most of their glutathione during processing (8). Thus, for individuals consuming fresh fruits and vegetables and freshly prepared meats, glutathione consumption is in a relatively high range of 100–150 mg/day. On the other hand, individuals who consume mostly prepared foods may consume as little as 5 mg/day.

B. Utilization of Dietary Glutathione

Several studies have shown that glutathione can be transported across the brush border membrane of the small intestine and absorbed into the bloodstream (17–19). The transport across the

Table 1 GSH Contents of Selected Foods

Food group	GSH mg/100 g	GSH mg/serving
Fruit, fresh		
Apples	3.3	4.6
Bananas	4.1	4.8
Grapefruit	7.9	14.6
Oranges	7.3	10.6
Watermelon	6.6	28.3
Vegetables, fresh		
Asparagus, cooked	28.3	26.3
Avocado, raw	27.7	31.3
Broccoli spears, cooked	9.1	7.8
Carrots, raw	7.9	5.9
Tomatoes, raw	9.0	10.9
Meats		
Hamburger, pan fried	17.5	14.9
Boiled ham	23.3	13.0
Chicken, fried	13.1	13.4
Cereal grains		
Cornflakes	0.0	0.0
Bread, whole wheat	1.2	0.6
Bread, white	0.0	0.0
Rice, white, enriched, cooked	1.6	2.1
Dairy products		
Milk, whole	0.0	0.0
Cheese, American	0.0	0.0
Yogurt, plain, lowfat	0.0	0.0
Ice cream, 10% fat	0.0	0.0

Source: Ref. 16.

brush border and into the epithelium occurs by both sodium-dependent and sodium-independent mechanisms. Appearance of intact glutathione in the mesenteric circulation has been detected in isolated perfused intestine (9), and increased glutathione has been measured in vivo following oral glutathione administration (5,20,21).

With administration of 1 g or more of glutathione, only a small percentage of the GSH is absorbed intact into general circulation. Lauterburg and co-workers (22) found no significant increase in plasma GSH in humans following oral administration of 3 g. Hagen et al. (5,20) found a 2.5-fold increase in GSH following an oral load of 15 mg/kg, but this increase was transient and represented only a small fraction of the total GSH administered.

In studies in rats, absorption was stimulated by stress hormones (19). α-Adrenergic agonists, including epinephrine, caused a substantial increase in circulating GSH concentrations. When GSH was administered alone in small-intestinal preparations, the rate of GSH absorption exceeded the rate of cysteine absorption when GSH concentration was greater than 200 μM (9). Thus, under conditions of stress, supplemental GSH appears to be more effectively utilized.

C. Measurement of Increase in Plasma and Tissue GSH

Oral administration of GSH (100 mg/kg) to mice yielded plasma GSH concentrations of 75 μM, compared with control values of 30 μM (21). A significant increase in tissue GSH was found only in the lung. However, in mice pretreated for 5 days with buthionine sulfoximine to inhibit GSH synthesis and deplete tissue GSH, oral administration of GSH gave statistically significant increases in GSH in kidney, heart, lung, brain, small intestine, and skin, but not in liver (21). Administration of the equivalent amount of the constituent amino acids, glutamate, cysteine, and glycine, resulted in little increase in tissue GSH. Thus, the results indicated that orally supplied GSH could increase tissue GSH concentrations under conditions of GSH depletion by impaired synthesis.

The amount of glutathione present in the diet is normally small relative to the amount of glutathione present in tissues in vivo. For instance, an adult individual contains 30–40 L of tissue water containing about 1 mM GSH. At 307 mg/mM, that is about 10 g of glutathione. Thus, 100 mg of glutathione per day in the diet is only about 1% of the glutathione in the body. Consequently, even if all of the dietary glutathione were absorbed intact, a supplemental amount of glutathione would be needed to significantly boost the total amount of glutathione in the body. However, most cells cannot directly utilize GSH. Thus, cell types with active GSH uptake systems, such as type 2 cells of the lung, may be able to effectively utilize the small fraction of GSH that is absorbed intact.

Under nonstressed conditions, only a small amount of the ingested GSH is absorbed as the intact tripeptide. The rest is degraded by γ-glutamyltransferase in the small intestine and the cysteine is absorbed. Because cysteine is converted to glutathione in tissues, dietary GSH can boost tissue GSH by providing a source of cysteine. Early research showed that GSH can completely replace other nutritional sources of cysteine to maintain sulfur amino acid balance (23). Taken in context with the usual human intake of 0.5–1 g each of methionine and cysteine derived from dietary protein, however, dietary GSH can contribute only a small fraction of the total sulfur amino acid (i.e., 150 mg of GSH is only about 10% of the usual cysteine consumption). This means that GSH needs to be supplemented above the 150 mg/day range i.e., 1–4 g/day) to substantially enhance systemic GSH by improving cysteine supply. However, in individuals consuming low-protein diets, sulfur amino acid intake may be in the 200-mg range so that even 150 mg of GSH would represent an important contribution to the sulfur balance.

D. Glutathione Utilization in the Gastrointestinal Tract

In contrast to evidence indicating that dietary or supplemental GSH may be systemically useful only at doses of 1 g or more, available evidence indicates that glutathione at levels found in normal diets can be very important in the alimentary canal. Glutathione is secreted from liver into bile at millimolar concentrations (Fig. 2). Part of the glutathione is degraded in transit to the small intestine, but the remaining biliary glutathione is sufficient to maintain about 200 μM of GSH in the lumen (9). As indicated before, a small fraction is absorbed and transported intact into circulation. Of perhaps greater importance, recent evidence indicates that luminal GSH functions directly in detoxification in the small intestine.

Earlier research showed that glutathione is transported intact from the lumen into the small-intestinal epithelium at a rate that exceeds GSH synthetic capacity in the small intestine. This transported glutathione enhances the detoxification capacity over that provided by glutathione synthesis (Fig. 3). The capacity to detoxify luminal-peroxidized lipids is greatly stimulated by

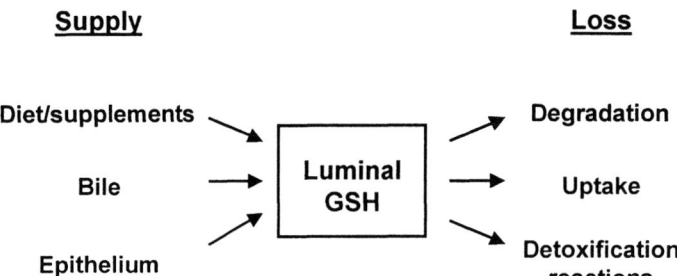

Figure 2 Glutathione supply and removal from the intestinal lumen: GSH is supplied to the lumen of the intestine by oral consumption, by the bile, and by secretion from the intestinal epithelium. The amount supplied by the bile is sufficient to maintain about 200 μM in the rat, but is probably lower in humans owing to degradation in the bile duct. The amount consumed in the diet is variable and normally would provide less than 200 μM. The amount supplied by the epithelium is only about 10% or less than the amount provided by bile. Removal occurs by degradation by γ-glutamyltranspeptidase and dipeptidases on the surface of the epithelial cells, transport into cells by sodium-dependent and sodium-independent mechanisms, and conjugation with reactive electrophiles, catalyzed by glutathione S-transferases associated with the mucus.

exogenously supplied glutathione (24), available from either the bile or the diet (25,26). If the normal glutathione concentration is 200 μM in the lumen, consumption of about 50 mg of glutathione can be expected to double that amount. Consequently, dietary glutathione can be expected to have a protective function by enhancing lipid peroxide detoxification in the small intestine even if it provides no systemic benefit.

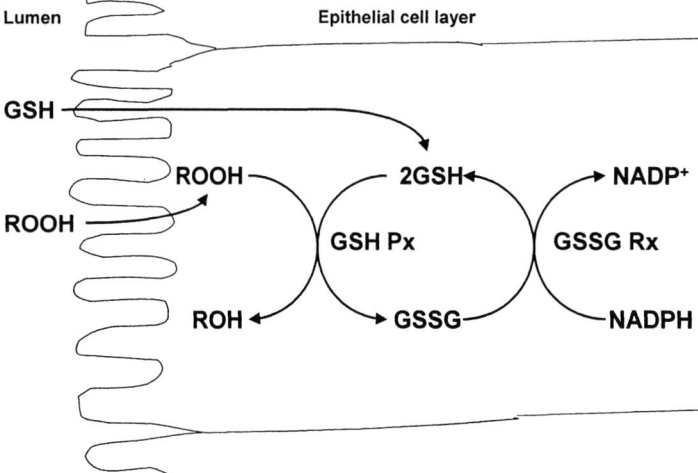

Figure 3 Detoxification of lipid hydroperoxides in the small intestine: GSH supplied to the lumen of the small intestine is used for detoxification of dietary peroxides by intracellular glutathione peroxidase (GSH Px). This requires that both the peroxide and the glutathione be taken up by the epithelial cells for the detoxification to occur. The GSSG produced is reduced back to GSH by GSSG reductase (GSSG Rx), using NADPH as the reductant.

IV. TARGETS FOR USE OF SUPPLEMENTAL GLUTATHIONE

A. Detoxification by Glutathione S-transferase in Mucus of the Small Intestine

Glutathione S-transferases are a family of enzymes that detoxify reactive electrophiles by conjugating them with glutathione (27). The intestinal epithelium contains members of this family that function in protection against dietary electrophiles. The amount of dietary electrophiles can be substantial (4), and high concentrations of electrophiles can deplete cells of glutathione and cause cell death.

In a study to determine whether conjugation of electrophiles in the intestinal epithelium is increased by luminal glutathione, Samiec et al. (28) used a model electrophile, 1-chloro-2,4-dinitrobenzene, added to isolated rat intestinal enterocytes with and without added GSH. The results showed that added glutathione stimulated conjugation about threefold over that without glutathione. Addition of the precursor amino acids provided very little stimulation of conjugation. The results, therefore, indicated that the glutathione was transported into the cells, rather than being degraded to amino acids, which would be taken up to support glutathione synthesis. However, experiments with transport inhibitors did not prevent the glutathione-stimulated activity. Furthermore, studies with sodium-free medium indicated that the glutathione-stimulated activity was not sodium-dependent. Because previous studies showed that the inhibitors and sodium-free medium substantially decreased glutathione uptake, the results were inconsistent with uptake of glutathione being the primary mechanism to enhance conjugation.

Experiments were, therefore, performed to determine whether glutathione S-transferase was associated with the plasma membrane. Plasma membranes were isolated and analyzed for glutathione S-transferase activity. Results showed no detectable activity above that which could be accounted for by contamination by other subcellular fractions. Experiments in which cells were suspended in medium and then removed by centrifugation showed that a substantial glutathione S-transferase activity was released from the cells into the medium without cell death. Mucus isolated from the rat small intestine and contained glutathione S-transferase activity even though no cells were present. The association of glutathione S-transferase with the mucus was further confirmed by immunohistochemistry (28).

These results show that the intestine contains an extracellular detoxification system (Fig. 4) in which glutathione S-transferase associated with the mucus utilizes glutathione from bile and from the diet to allow detoxification of electrophiles before they have a chance to reach the epithelial cell layer. Taken together with the studies showing that dietary glutathione can be used to detoxify dietary peroxides, these results indicate that dietary glutathione can play an important detoxification function in the small intestine. Because mucus lines the nasopharyngeal cavity, glutathione may be an important component of saliva and fluids that line the epithelium surfaces, especially if the mucous layers contain detoxification enzymes such as glutathione S-transferase.

B. Dietary Glutathione Intake Is Associated with Decreased Risk of Oral and Pharyngeal Cancer

To study the association between risk of oral and pharyngeal cancer and dietary intake of glutathione, food consumption data from a large case–control study were combined with the database for glutathione in commonly consumed foods (16). Glutathione intakes and food sources of glutathione among the study participants were estimated, and the risk of oral and pharyngeal cancer was assessed at different levels of glutathione intake (11). Data on oral and pharyngeal cancer risk factors, including food and nutrient intakes, were used to evaluate

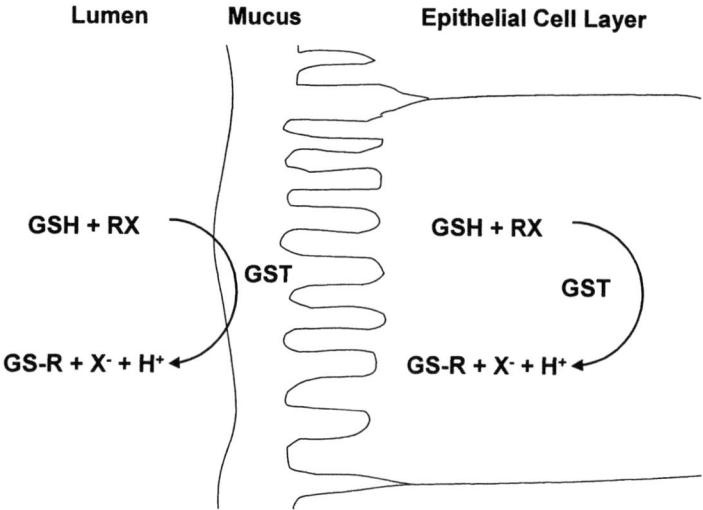

Figure 4 Detoxification of reactive electrophiles in the diet: The mucus of the small intestine contains glutathione S-transferase, an enzyme that functions to eliminate reactive electrophiles. Utilizing GSH provided by the bile, diet, or epithelial cells, this mucus-associated enzyme can detoxify reactive compounds before their uptake into cells. Cells also contain glutathione S-transferase activity and GSH so that intracellular detoxification also occurs.

whether risk associated with dietary glutathione was affected by other factors. The estimated relative risk of cancer among persons with the highest quartile of glutathione intake from all sources was 0.5 (95% confidence interval 0.3–0.7). When analyzed by dietary source, however, glutathione intakes derived from all vegetables and from meat were not related to cancer risk. Only glutathione derived from fruit and from vegetables commonly consumed raw was associated with reduced oral cancer risk. Relative to the lowest level of combined intake of fruit and fruit-derived glutathione, the risk of cancer decreased slightly with increasing intake of glutathione. This analysis was limited by the small number of subjects with extreme combinations of intakes. Further studies are needed to distinguish between the potential effect of glutathione from that of fruit and raw vegetables per se or from the influence of other constituents in these foods.

This case–control study raises the possibility that glutathione intake from fruit and from vegetables could protect the lining of the mouth against oral cancer risk. Because of the findings described earlier that glutathione S-transferase is present in mucus, the results could indicate that GSH in foods or supplied as a supplement, can be directly used to detoxify reactive electrophilic compounds that come into contact with these epithelial surfaces and protect against cancer-causing mutations. Thus, additional studies are needed to determine whether supplemental glutathione, fortification of food or beverages with GSH, or other preparations could protect against risk of oral and pharyngeal cancer.

C. Anti-Influenza Activity of Glutathione

Influenza viral infection in mice was shown to result in an oxidation of the lung GSH pool (29–30). Although the basis for this oxidation is unclear, this oxidation may be important in the infectious process (31) and may specifically function in influenza virus activation (12). In some strains of influenza, viral particles are released from cells in an inactive form that must undergo limited proteolysis for activation (29). Such activation occurs by enzymes that are inhibited by host protease inhibitors (Fig. 5). These inhibitors contain a methionine residue that can be oxidized to a sulfoxide, with an associated loss of inhibitory activity. Thus, oxidizing conditions are likely to enhance the proteolytic activity and increase virus activation. Consequently, the antioxidant GSH, which can protect against the oxidation of the protease inhibitor, can function to block virus activation.

To determine whether added glutathione affected production of the active influenza virus particles, cultured MDCK cells and normal human small airway epithelial cells were inoculated with influenza A/WSN strain at multiplicity of infection of 0.1 plaque-forming units per cell (12). Viral production was determined 3 days after inoculation by both plaque-forming assay and hemagglutinin antigen assay. When included in the culture medium, GSH showed a dose-dependent antiviral effect at concentrations higher than 5 mM. Incubation of virus with 30 mM glutathione either before or during the inoculation period did not affect the viral production, indicating that GSH does not directly inactivate the virus. Neither viral protein synthesis nor viral-induced apoptosis was inhibited by GSH. Protection against viral particle production was not seen at high multiplicity of infection. These results indicate that the viral particle production following low multiplicity infection was due to decreased production of active viral particles.

To determine whether GSH could protect against virus production in vivo, BALB/c mice were infected with influenza A/X-31 strain by intranasal inoculation (12). Virus titers were measured as the tissue culture infection dose in both lung and trachea homogenates 4 days after infection. Results showed that 50 mM of glutathione in the drinking water resulted in significantly lower virus levels in the lungs, although there was no difference in lung glutathione levels between groups. These results combined with those of the cell culture experiments

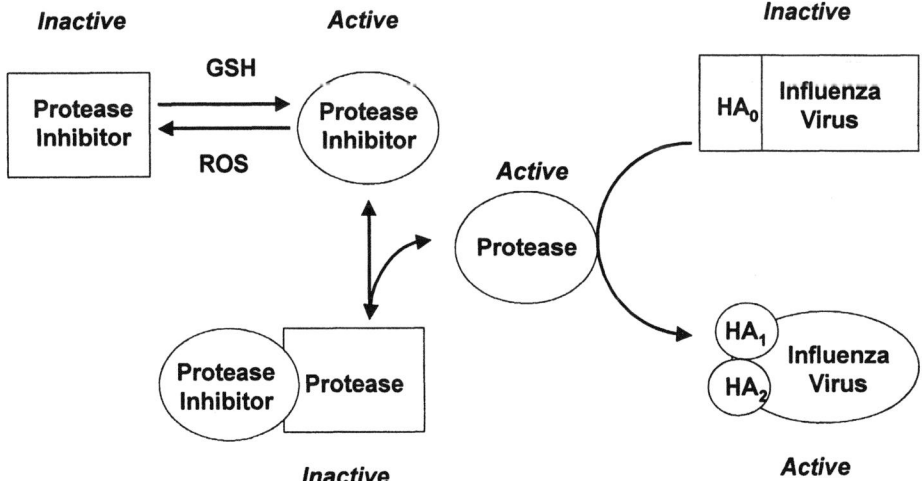

Figure 5 Exogenously supplied GSH can protect against influenza virus activation: Influenza virus contains a protein, hemagglutinin (HA_0) that must undergo limited proteolysis to proteins (HA_1 and HA_2) for activation. If this does not occur in the secretory pathway during intracellular processing, it can occur extracellularly by proteases in the fluid lining the epithelium. However, protease inhibitors are also present in the lining fluid, and these must be oxidized to allow activation of the proteases. Because GSH blocks or reverses this oxidation of the protease inhibitor, GSH can prevent protease activation and thereby prevent activation of the inactive virus particles.

indicate that exogenously supplied GSH can protect against influenza, at least at low multiplicity of infection. Because a viral infection spreads from initially infected cells by release of viral particles into the epithelial lining fluids, activation by proteolysis, and subsequent infection of other cells, the results indicate that provision of glutathione in an oral or lozenge form could protect against influenza infection.

D. Glutathione Redox State

1. Plasma Redox

Glutathione is oxidized to glutathione disulfide in its function as an antioxidant, and the glutathione disulfide is recycled to glutathione by an NADPH-dependent GSSG reductase. In the presence of oxidants, the balance between glutathione and glutathione disulfide provides a measure of the degree of oxidative stress (Fig. 6). In human plasma, the redox state of the glutathione–glutathione disulfide pool is about -137 ± 9 mV (32). This value is substantially more oxidized than the glutathione pool in tissues, which is about to -250 to -200 mV (33). Thus, the glutathione is rapidly oxidized on being released from tissue into the plasma (Fig. 7).

The major oxidant for the glutathione pool in plasma is probably the large cystine pool. The redox state of the cysteine/cystine pool is about 57 mV more oxidized than the GSH/GSSG pool (32). Consequently, the circulating glutathione pool is intermediate between tissue GSH/GSSG values and plasma cysteine/cystine values. This means that glutathione pool should be responsive to factors affecting tissue glutathione and also extracellular oxidants.

To determine whether the glutathione pool is oxidized in vivo in response to an oxidant challenge, we examined the glutathione redox state in bone marrow transplant patients before and after chemotherapy (34). The results showed a significant oxidation of the plasma glutathione pool by about 15 mV over 2 weeks following the chemotherapy treatment. Thus, plasma glutathione redox appears to provide a measure of oxidation as induced by chemotherapy for bone marrow transplantation. A study of oxidation of the plasma GSH in rats following acute hepatic oxidative stress induced by carbon tetrachloride showed changes occur at early time points under relatively mild conditions but that extensive liver injury results in release of hepatic antioxidants and masks this effect (35).

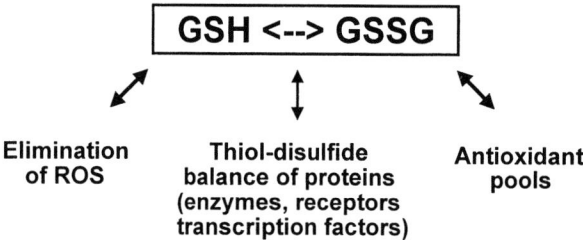

Figure 6 GSH redox provides a central indicator of the balance of oxidative stress and antioxidant systems: Because the GSH/GSSG pool undergoes reversible oxidation–reduction in association with detoxification of reactive oxygen species (ROS), functions in maintenance of other antioxidant pools, and maintains protein thiols in their reduced state, this pool provides a dynamic measure of the oxidant–antioxidant balance in cells and in vivo. Although the ratio GSH/GSSG is most frequently used to express this redox balance, the stoichiometry is 2GSH per GSSG, and therefore expressions incorporating this stoichiometry, such as the redox potential (E_h), are preferred.

BIOAVAILABILITY OF GLUTATHIONE

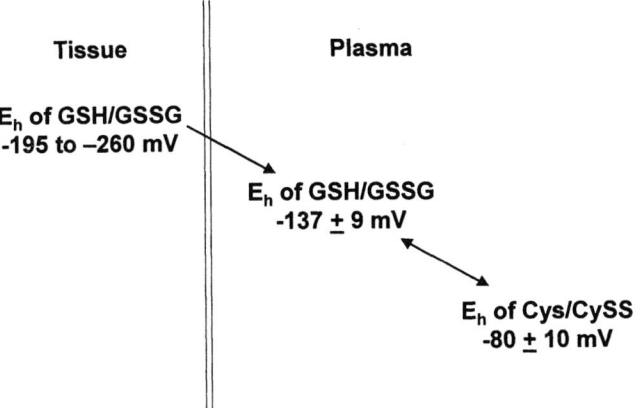

Figure 7 Redox states of plasma thiol–disulfide pools are more oxidized than the cellular GSH–GSSG pool: The redox potential of cellular GSH is about −195 to −260 mV, but that of the GSH–GSSG pool in plasma is considerably more oxidized (−137 mV). Although the oxidant is not known, it may well be cystine, because the cysteine/cystine redox is even more oxidized (−80 mV), and GSH rapidly reacts with cystine. However, if cystine is the oxidant, then that means that a kinetically important oxidation of cysteine occurs in the extracellular compartment. The mechanism responsible for this oxidation is unknown, but thiol oxidases have been identified associated with the plasma membrane of kidney and intestinal cells.

In a study of plasma redox association with disease, the GSH/GSSG pool was oxidized at about 40 mV in individuals older than 60 years compared with individuals younger than 43 years (36). Individuals with type 2 diabetes were about 20 mV more oxidized than age-matched controls (36). Together with the foregoing data, these results indicate that plasma GSH/GSSG redox provides an indicator of the balance between oxidative stress and antioxidant systems in vivo. Moreover, the results suggest that aging individuals, and those with type 2 diabetes, may benefit from supplementation with agents that help maintain the GSH redox state. A supply of 3 g of cysteine orally increased the plasma thiol disulfide ratio (37), but effects of oral supply of GSH are not available.

2. Extracellular Redox Control

The mechanism to control the extracellular redox state in blood plasma appears to involve the release of glutathione from tissue, principally the liver (38). However, in the small intestine, a different mechanism controls the redox state in the lumen. Hagen et al. (9) showed that GSSG in the diet was partially reduced to GSH in the upper jejunum. The mechanism for this reduction was studied in an isolated, vascularly perfused jejunum free from biliary thiols (39). After addition of GSSG to the lumen, GSH was formed with approximately stoichiometric formation of the mixed disulfide of glutathione and cysteine. In the absence of GSSG in lumen, substantial cysteine was released from the epithelium. Thus, the results indicate that cysteine release from the epithelium to the lumen is used to reduce GSSG to GSH. Because cystine is rapidly taken up by the intestinal epithelium, the release of cysteine and uptake of cystine provides a cysteine–cystine shuttle mechanism to reduce disulfides in the lumen (Fig. 8). Thus, in addition to control of redox state within tissues, the tissues are also capable of controlling extracellular redox.

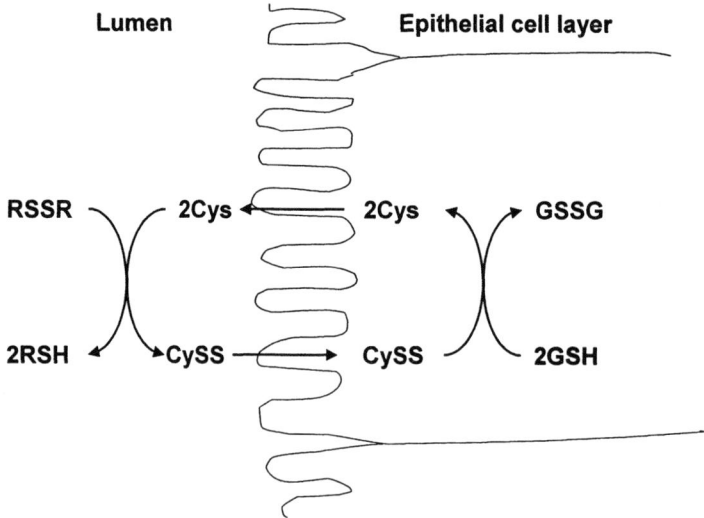

Figure 8 Cysteine–cystine shuttle for reduction of luminal disulfides: Although the plasma redox state appears to be maintained by efflux of GSH from the liver and other organ systems, the redox of the intestinal lumen appears to be maintained by a cysteine–cystine shuttle. Disulfides in the lumen stimulate release of cysteine from the epithelial cells. The cysteine undergoes thiol–disulfide exchange with the luminal disulfide, with generation of cystine. The cystine is rapidly absorbed back into the epithelium and reduced to cysteine, probably by reaction with GSH.

3. Cellular Glutathione Redox

Calculations of glutathione redox in rat liver, small intestine, and colon indicate tissues have a GSH/GSSG redox of −200 to −250 mV (34,40,41). Red blood cells, which are nondividing, have a value of −193 mV (36). Caloric restriction in the rat results in an oxidation in the glutathione pools in the small intestine and colonic epithelium (41). This oxidation is associated with a decrease in indices of intestinal mucosal growth such as mucosal height and crypt depth. Glutathione redox recovers with ad libitum feeding or with keratinocyte growth factor and 25% of ab libitum feeding. These results indicate that thiol redox changes are associated with nutrition and growth.

In dividing HT29 cells, redox changes from −258 to −201 on differentiation induced by 5 mM of sodium butyrate (33). This oxidation and differentiation is associated with a substantial decline in the cell proliferation rate. A similar shift in redox associated with a decline in cell proliferation was found in fibroblasts, which became more oxidized on reaching confluence (42). Thus, the results suggest that proliferating cells have a more reduced thiol–disulfide state than do differentiated and nondividing cells (Fig. 9).

Measurement of redox change in cells undergoing apoptosis show that an extensive oxidation occurs after cytochrome c is released from mitochondria (41). The glutathione redox in murine hybridoma (Do11-10) cells with activation-induced apoptosis is oxidized to −170 mV (43); that of myeloid leukemia (HL60) cells is oxidized to −165 mV during an apoptosis (40). HT29 cells undergoing terminal differentiation and apoptosis are oxidized to −170 mV. Thus, apoptotic cells appear to be more oxidized than nondividing and differentiated cells, and the latter cells are more oxidized then rapidly dividing cells. This indicates that there is a natural progression in redox state from a highly reducing condition during cell proliferation through

BIOAVAILABILITY OF GLUTATHIONE

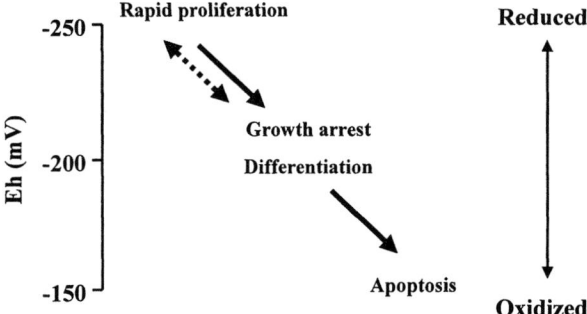

Figure 9 Redox state (E_h) of GSH–GSSG pool becomes oxidized in association with differentiation and apoptosis: Accumulating data on the redox state of GSH–GSSG in cells show that proliferating cells typically are in the range of −230 to −260 mV, whereas growth-arrested and differentiated cells are 30–60 mV more oxidized. Induction of apoptosis results in a further oxidation of 30–50 mV. Thus, there appears to be a progressive cellular oxidation associated with the progression of cells through the life cycle. It is presently unknown whether dietary or supplemental GSH, cysteine, or related precursors can affect these cellular values.

an intermediate oxidized state in differentiated cells to a highly oxidized state in apoptosis (Fig. 9). Such a progression suggests that nutritional or therapeutic manipulations affecting the redox state may affect the balance of cell division and cell death in processes that control the normal tissue homeostasis.

V. SUMMARY AND PERSPECTIVES

Glutathione is present in amounts up to about 150 mg/day in diets consisting largely of fresh fruits and freshly prepared vegetables and meats. In individuals in good health with balanced nutrition, this glutathione probably contributes little to the systemic glutathione available in the body, but is used by glutathione S-transferase, a detoxification enzyme associated with mucus, to detoxify reactive electrophilic compounds found in the diet. Consumption of 25–50 mg of glutathione with a meal is sufficient to support this function. Orally consumed glutathione also functions along with biliary glutathione to support detoxification of peroxidized fats in epithelial cells lining the alimentary canal. Again, consumption of 25–50 mg should be sufficient to protect against toxic compounds in food. However, for protection against reactive compounds, such as those found in tobacco products, more frequent GSH supply would be needed. Although specific disease processes associated with low oral glutathione consumption have not been clearly documented, epidemiological evidence suggests that individuals consuming foods high in glutathione have about a 50% reduction in risk of oral and pharyngeal cancer. Additional studies are needed to confirm this.

Studies of the redox state of glutathione show that cellular glutathione is controlled over a rather narrow range. In proliferating cells, the glutathione redox is about −230 to −260 mV. In nondividing and differentiated cells the redox potential is about −190 to −220 mV. Apoptotic cells have a redox of about −150 to −180 mV. These redox potentials appear to represent a continuum from a reduced state to an oxidized state as cells progress from cell division to cell death. At present it is unclear to what extent these redox potentials can be externally controlled or whether they are important in cell control.

Redox of the extracellular glutathione pool is considerably more oxidized than that of the cellular pool. The value for the plasma glutathione pool in young healthy adults is -137 ± 9 mV, indicating that glutathione is very rapidly oxidized once released from tissues. This oxidation probably occurs by cystine because the redox potential of the cysteine/cystine pool is 57 mV more oxidized than that of glutathione. The glutathione pool becomes oxidized following high-dose chemotherapy and also in association with type 2 diabetes and aging. It is not known whether antioxidant supplementation alters the plasma redox state or can be used to prevent the oxidation with age.

The plasma redox appears to be controlled, at least partly; by glutathione release from tissue, principally the liver. Thus mechanisms to increase glutathione in the liver and other tissues may provide a mechanism to better maintain the redox state in the plasma. Alternatively, nonnutritive compounds in food that increase tissue glutathione by stimulating its synthesis may also be useful to protect against disease-, toxicity-, and age-related oxidation of the circulating glutathione pool.

Control of the redox state in fluids lining the alimentary canal can occur by release of glutathione and also by a cysteine–cystine shuttle mechanism. Both of the systems appear to depend on adequate sulfur amino acid in the diet. Provision of glutathione, which is more stable than the amino acid cysteine, may be useful for maintaining redox state in the oral, nasal, and upper respiratory epithelia. Maintenance of redox can protect against infections that depend on oxidative conditions for activation (e.g., influenza) or entry into cells (e.g., rhinovirus).

Additional research is needed to evaluate the utilization of orally supplied glutathione by the epithelia of the alimentary canal and upper airways in protection against relevant toxicities and disease processes.

REFERENCES

1. Meister A. (1988) Glutathione metabolism and its selective modification. J Biol Chem 263:17205–17208.
2. Jones DP. (1995) Glutathione distribution in natural products: absorption and tissue distribution. Methods Enzymol 252:3–13.
3. Dahm LJ, Samiec PS, Eley JW, Flagg EW, Coates RJ, Jones DP. (1993) Utilization of oral glutathione. In: Poli G, Albano E, Dianzani MU, eds. Free Radicals: From Basic Science to Medicine. Basel: Birkäuser, pp. 506–523.
4. Samiec PS, Dahm LJ, Flagg EW, Coates RJ, Eley JW, Jones DP. (1993) Bioavailability of dietary glutathione. In: Corongiu F, Rice–Evans C, eds. Free Radicals and Antioxidants in Nutrition. London: Richelieu, 7:269–285.
5. Hagen TM, Jones DP. (1989) Role of glutathione in extrahepatic detoxification. In: Sakamoto Y, Higashi T, Taniguchi N, Meister A, eds. Glutathione Centennial: Molecular and Clinical Implications. San Diego: Academic, pp. 423–433.
6. Ookhtens M, Kaplowitz N. (1998) Role of the liver in interorgan homeostasis of glutathione and cyst(e)ine. Semin Liver Dis 18:313–329.
7. Ballatori N, Rebbeor JF. (1998) Roles of MRP2 and oatp1 in hepatocellular export of reduced glutathione. Semin Liver Dis 18:377–387.
8. Wierzbicka GT, Hagen TM, Jones DP. (1990) Glutathione in food. J Food Comp Anal 2:327–337.
9. Hagen TM, Jones DP. (1987) Transepithelial transport of glutathione in vascularly perfused small intestine of rat. Am J Physiol 252:G607–G613.
10. Hagen TM, Wierzbicka GT, Sillau AH, Bowman BB, Jones DP. (1990) Bioavailability of dietary glutathione. Effect on plasma concentration. Am J Physiol 259:G524–G529.
11. Flagg EW, Coates RJ, Jones DP, Byers TE, Greenberg RS, Gridley G, McLaughlin JK, Blot WJ, Haber M, Preston–Martin S, Schoenberg JB, Austin DF, Fraumeni JF Jr. (1994) Dietary glutathione intake and the risk of oral and pharyngeal cancer. Am J Epidemiol 139:453–465.
12. Cai J, Furukawa S, Jones DP. (2000) Anti-influenza activity of glutathione. FASEB J 14:A493.

13. Dinkova–Kostova AT, Abeygunawardana C, Talalay P. (1998) Chemoprotective properties of phenylpropenoids, bis(benzylidene)cycloalkanones, and related Michael reaction acceptors: correlation of potencies as phase 2 enzyme inducers and radical scavengers. J Med Chem 41:5287–5296.
14. Tateishi N, Sakamoto Y. (1983) Nutritional significance of glutathione in rat liver. In: Sakamoto Y, ed. Glutathione: Storage, Transport and Turnover in Mammals. Tokyo: Japan Scientific Societies, pp. 13–38.
15. Jaeschke H, Wendel A. (1985) Diurnal fluctuation and pharmacological alteration of mouse organ glutathione content. Biochem Pharmacol 34:1029–1033.
16. Jones DP, Coates RJ, Flagg EW, Eley JW, Block G, Greenberg RS, Gunter EW, Jackson B. (1992) Glutathione in foods listed in the National Cancer Institute's Health Habits and History Food Frequency Questionnaire. Nutr Cancer 17:57–75.
17. Hunjan MK, Evered DF. (1985) Absorption of glutathione from the gastrointestinal tract. Biochim Biophys Acta 815:184–188.
18. Vincenzini MT, Favilli F, Iantomasi T. (1987) Glutathione-mediated transport across intestinal brush border membranes. Biochim Biophys Acta 942:107–114.
19. Hagen TM, Bai C, Jones DP. (1991) Hormonal regulation of glutathione absorption. Stimulation by α-adrenergic agonists in small intestine. FASEB J 5:2721–2727.
20. Jones DP, Hagen TM, Weber R, Wierzbicka GT, Bonkovsky HL. (1989) Oral administration of glutathione (GSH) increases plasma GSH concentrations in humans. FASEB J 3:A1250.
21. Aw TY, Wierzbicka G, Jones DP. (1991) Oral glutathione increases tissue glutathione in vivo. Chem Biol Interact 80:89–97.
22. Witschi A, Reddy S, Stofer B, Lauterburg BH. (1992) The systemic availability of oral glutathione. Eur J Clin Pharmacol 43:667–669.
23. Dyer HM, du Vigneaud V. (1936) The utilization of glutathione in connection with a cystine-deficient diet. J Biol Chem 115:543–549.
24. Kowalski DP, Feeley RM, Jones DP. (1990) Use of exogenous glutathione for metabolism of peroxidized methyl linoleate in the small intestine. J Nutr 120:1115–1121.
25. Aw TY, Williams MW, Gray L. (1992) Absorption and lymphatic transport of peroxidized lipids by rat small intestine in vivo: role of mucosal GSH. Am J Physiol 262:G99–G106.
26. Aw TY, Williams MW. (1992) Intestinal absorption and lymphatic transport of peroxidized lipids in rats: effect of exogenous GSH. Am J Physiol 263:G665–G672.
27. Eaton DL, Bammler TK. (1999) Concise review of the glutathione S-transferases and their significance to toxicology. Toxicol Sci 49:156–164.
28. Samiec PL, Dahm LJ, Jones DP. (2000) Glutathione S-transferase in mucus of rat small intestine. Toxicol Sci 54:52–59.
29. Buffinton GD, Christen S, Peterhans E, Stocker R. (1992) Oxidative stress in lungs of mice infected with influenza A virus. Free Radic Res Commun 16:99–110.
30. Hennet T, Peterhans E, Stocker R. (1992) Alterations in antioxidant defenses in lung and liver of mice infected with influenza A virus. J Gen Virol 73:39–46.
31. Peterhans E. (1997) Oxidants and antioxidants in viral diseases: disease mechanisms and metabolic regulation. J Nutr 127:962S–965S.
32. Jones DP, Carlson JL, Mody VC Jr, Cai J, Lynn MJ, Sternberg P Jr. (2000) Redox state of glutathione in plasma. Free Radic Biol Med 28:625–635.
33. Kirlin WG, Cai J, Thompson SA, Diaz D, Kavanagh TJ, Jones DP. (1999) Glutathione redox potential during differentiation and enzyme inducers. Free Radic Biol Res 27:1208–1218.
34. Jonas CR, Puckett AB, Jones DP, Griffith DP, Szeszycki EE, Bergman GF, Carlson JL, Galloway JR, Blumberg JB, Ziegler TR. (2000) Plasma antioxidant status after high-dose chemotherapy: a randomized trial of parenteral nutrition in bone marrow transplantation patients. Am J Clin Nutr 72:181–189.
35. Kadiiska MB, Gladen BC, Baird DD, Dikalova AE, Sohal RS, Hatch GE, Jones DP, Mason RP, Barrett CJ. (2000) Biomarkers of oxidative stress study: are plasma antioxidants markers of CCl_4 poisoning? Free Radic Biol Med 28:838–845.
36. Samiec PS, Drews–Botsch C, Flagg EW, Kurtz JC, Sternberg P, Reed RL, Jones DP. (1998) Glutathione in human plasma. Decline in association with aging, age-related macular degeneration and diabetes. Free Radic Biol Med 24:699–704.
37. Tribble DL, Jones DP, Ardehali A, Feeley RM, Rudman D. (1989) Hypercysteinemia and delayed sulfur excretion in cirrhotics following oral cysteine loads. Am J Clin Nutr 50:1401–1406.

38. Adams JD Jr, Lauterburg BH, Mitchell JR. (1984) Plasma glutathione disulfide as an index of oxidant stress in vivo: effects of carbon tetrachloride, dimethylnitrosamine, nitrofurantoin, metronidazole, doxorubicin and diquat. Res Commun Chem Pathol Pharmacol 46:401–410.
39. Dahm LJ, Jones DP. (1993) Control of cysteine and glutathione (GSH) levels in rat intestine. Toxicologist 14:178.
40. Cai J, Jones DP. (1998) Superoxide in apoptosis. Mitochondrial generation triggered by cytochrome c loss. J Biol Chem 273:11401–11404.
41. Jonas CR, Estivariz CF, Jones DP, Gu LH, Wallace TM, Diaz EE, Pascal RR, Cotsonis GA, Ziegler TR. (1999) Keratinocyte growth factor enhances glutathione redox state in rat intestinal mucosa during nutritional repletion. J Nutr 127:1278–1284.
42. Nakamura H, Nakamura K, Yodoi J. (1997) Redox regulation of cellular activation. Annu Rev Immunol 15:351–369.
43. Jones DP, Maellaro E, Jiang S, Slater AFG, Orrenius S. (1995) Effects of *N*-acetyl-L-cysteine on T-cell apoptosis are not mediated by increased cellular glutathione. Immunol Lett 4:205–209.
44. Jonas CR, Estivariz CF, Jones DP, Gu LH, Wallace TM, Diaz EE, Pascal RR, Cotsonis GA, Ziegler TR. (1999) Keratinocyte growth factor enhances glutathione redox state in rat intestinal mucosa during nutritional repletion. J Nutr 127:1278–1284.

28
Antioxidative Capacity of Melatonin

Russel J. Reiter and Dun-xian Tan
The University of Texas Health Science Center, San Antonio, Texas

Lucien C. Manchester
St. Mary's University, San Antonio, Texas

Juan R. Calvo
University of Seville School of Medicine, Seville, Spain

I. INTRODUCTION

N-Acetyl-5-methoxytryptamine, commonly known as melatonin because of its effects on the epidermal pigment melanin in amphibians and reptiles and its derivation from serotonin, was discovered in bovine tissue slightly over 40 years ago (1,2). Once thought to be exclusively of pineal origin, melatonin is now known to be produced in a variety of other tissues as well, including the retina (3,4), some orbital glands (5,6), gastrointestinal tract (7,8), and possibly in some blood cells (9). Although it is commonplace to make judgments related to melatonin's actions based on its levels in the serum (which normally range from 5 to 250 pg/mL), relatively little is known concerning the intracellular concentrations of melatonin, although some studies suggest that nuclear levels of melatonin, for example, in brain cells, are considerably higher than concurrent concentrations in the blood (10,11). Additionally, in tissues where melatonin is produced (e.g., in the retina), it is also anticipated that melatonin levels may be much higher than circulating values. It has been proposed that higher intracellular concentrations of melatonin may be possible because of binding proteins that maintain elevated levels against a gradient (12,13).

In addition to these observations, some cells and body fluids have extraordinary high levels of melatonin. It was recently shown using radioimmunoassay, immunocytochemical, high-performance liquid chromatographic (HPLC), and mass spectral (MS) techniques that cells present in the bone marrow contain melatonin concentrations orders of magnitude greater than those in the blood of several mammals, including humans (14,15). Similarly, ventricular cerebrospinal fluid (CSF) (16–18) and bile (19) contain quantities of melatonin that are also several orders of magnitude higher that those measured in the blood. Considering these findings, the assumption that intracellular concentrations of melatonin are always in the picomolar to nanomolar range may be erroneous. What is obviously required are more extensive investigations into the levels of melatonin in subcellular compartments, particularly in those organelles in which free radical generation is usually considered to be high (e.g., the mitochondria). Besides its uptake by all cells in the organism (19,20), melatonin also crosses all known morphophysiological barriers, including the blood–brain barrier (5,6) and the placenta (21,22).

Even though all vertebrates, from fish to mammals, produce melatonin, it is possibly not their only source of the indole. Melatonin is also found in many plants (23–27), and the consumption of these materials increases circulating (23), and, presumably, tissue concentrations of the indole. As with other antioxidants, the amount of melatonin varies widely among individual plants and also in different parts of the same plant (27,28). At this point, few plants have been investigated relative to their melatonin concentrations, and it is likely that this area of research will develop rapidly in the near future.

Functionally, since its discovery, melatonin has been linked to several physiological processes. Most notably, it mediates seasonal reproductive events in photoperiodically dependent species that exhibit obvious changes in annual reproductive capability (29,30). It alters the function of other endocrine organs (31); strengthens circadian rhythms (32,33); is involved in sleep regulation in at least diurnally active species (34,35); stimulates the immune system (36,37); and controls tumor growth (38,39). Except for the latter two functions, the importance of melatonin in modulating these physiological events probably varies with the species being tested. In general, these regulatory actions of melatonin are believed to rely on specific membrane receptors (40–42) and nuclear-binding sites and their receptors (43–45) for the indole.

The ability of melatonin to neutralize free radicals and prevent tissue damage associated with oxidative stress was almost a serendipitous finding. Ten years ago reports appeared that suggested melatonin had subtle actions on a variety of organs and tissues (46,47), which were not always explainable in terms of its previously described actions. This led us to test the ability of this indole to scavenge the highly toxic hydroxyl radical ($^{\cdot}$OH). The resulting report (48), which used a variety of techniques, including spin-trapping with electron spin resonance spectroscopy (ESR), revealed that melatonin, in fact, did scavenge this toxic agent. This observation has been repeatedly confirmed under a variety of in vitro and in vivo experimental conditions (49–63) and, subsequently, evidence has shown that melatonin may or does neutralize a number of toxic oxygen- and nitrogen-based species, including hypochlorous acid (64,65), singlet oxygen (59,66,67), hydrogen peroxide (28,59), nitric oxide (68), and the peroxynitrite anion or its metabolites (68,73). Besides these actions, which would reduce tissue damage resulting from free radical generation, melatonin possesses indirect means to lower the toxic actions of reactive species. Thus, melatonin has been shown to stimulate either mRNA levels or activities of the superoxide dismutases (SOD) (74), catalase (75), glutathione peroxidase (GPx) (76–78), glutathione reductase (GRd) (78), glucose-6-phosphate dehydrogenase (79), and the rate-limiting enzyme in glutathione synthesis, γ-glutamylcysteine synthase (80). These antioxidative enzymes are important elements in the antioxidative armamentarium of vertebrates. Additionally, melatonin has been reported to reduce the activity of the pro-oxidative enzyme, nitric oxide synthase (81,82). Whereas the direct free radical-scavenging actions of melatonin are obviously receptor-independent, it is possible that its enzymatic effects are mediated by either membrane or nuclear receptors for the indole (78). Finally, there is some evidence that melatonin may serve as a metal chelator, a function that would also have implications in terms of the ability of the indole to reduce oxidative damage (83).

II. EXPERIMENTAL MODELS OF OXIDATIVE STRESS: PROTECTION BY MELATONIN

Melatonin has been widely tested for its ability to reduce oxidative damage to tissue in experimental models in which free radicals are believed to be involved in the molecular destruction (85–87). The following paragraphs summarize the results of some of these investigations that highlight melatonin's protective actions against oxygen- and nitrogen-based radicals and reactive species. Although in the bulk of the studies, summarized herein, pharmacological levels of melatonin were presumably administered to reduce oxidative damage; studies are also included during which animals were deprived, in part, of their ability to endogenously produce physiological quantities of melatonin, and an increased level of oxidative damage was reported.

A. Ischemia–Reperfusion Injury

Temporary ischemia (anoxia, hypoxia), followed by reperfusion and reoxygenation, creates a metabolic state in cells that leads to the generation of free radicals and reactive species, the quantity and type of which may differ somewhat among tissues. The transient interruption of blood flow and the resulting oxygen deprivation forces cells into an anaerobic state, which causes uncoupling of the electron transport chain, the release of catecholamines and the activation of xanthine oxidase, a pro-oxidative enzyme (Fig. 1). When cells are resupplied with oxygen during reperfusion, the superoxide anion radical ($O_2^{\cdot-}$) is abundantly produced during the catalytic breakdown of purines and uric acid. In addition to $O_2^{\cdot-}$, other oxidants, including hydrogen peroxide (H_2O_2), are concomitantly generated owing to uncoupled electron transport, auto-oxidation of catecholamines, and the recruitment and activation of phagocytes. Whereas a variety of cells probably contribute free radicals that lead to cellular dysfunction and death, endothelial cells and the recruited leukocytes may be major contributors (88). The involved endothelial cells supply $O_2^{\cdot-}$ and H_2O_2 from cell membrane-associated enzymes, such as xanthine oxidase, and from dysfunctional mitochondria; whereas activated leukocytes utilize NADPH oxidase to produce large quantities of $O_2^{\cdot-}$.

Other important consequences of ischemia–reperfusion injury include the exaggerated production of inflammatory mediators such as leukotriene-B_4 (LT-B_4) and platelet-activating factor (PAF), as well as the activation of nuclear factor-κB (NFκB), an oxidant-sensitive transcription factor (see Fig. 1). These mediators activate receptors on leukocytes that induce the mobilization of the adhesion molecules that cause leukocytes to adhere to endothelial cells (89); this plugs the capillaries, which leads to endothelial cell destruction and edema. The adherent leukocytes as well as those that are extravasated, release proteases, oxidant mediators, and permeability factors that cause further tissue damage (90,91). This combined onslaught of free radicals and destructive mediators overwhelms the intrinsic antioxidative defense system of cells, causing massive molecular destruction, cellular dysfunction, and in severe cases, cell and tissue death.

1. Central Nervous System

The first report illustrating the protective actions of melatonin on experimentally induced stroke is that of Manev and co-workers (92). When both common carotid and both middle cerebral arteries were occluded for 1 h, followed by restoration of blood flow to the brain of adult rats, large neural infarcts were observed 4–6 h later. The lesions, however, were significantly larger in the brains of melatonin-deficient animals (from an earlier pinealectomy). Because in this study endogenous melatonin levels were reduced as a consequence of pineal removal, the authors concluded that even normal physiological levels of melatonin limit ischemia–reperfusion-induced damage in the brain (92). This finding is of particular interest because of

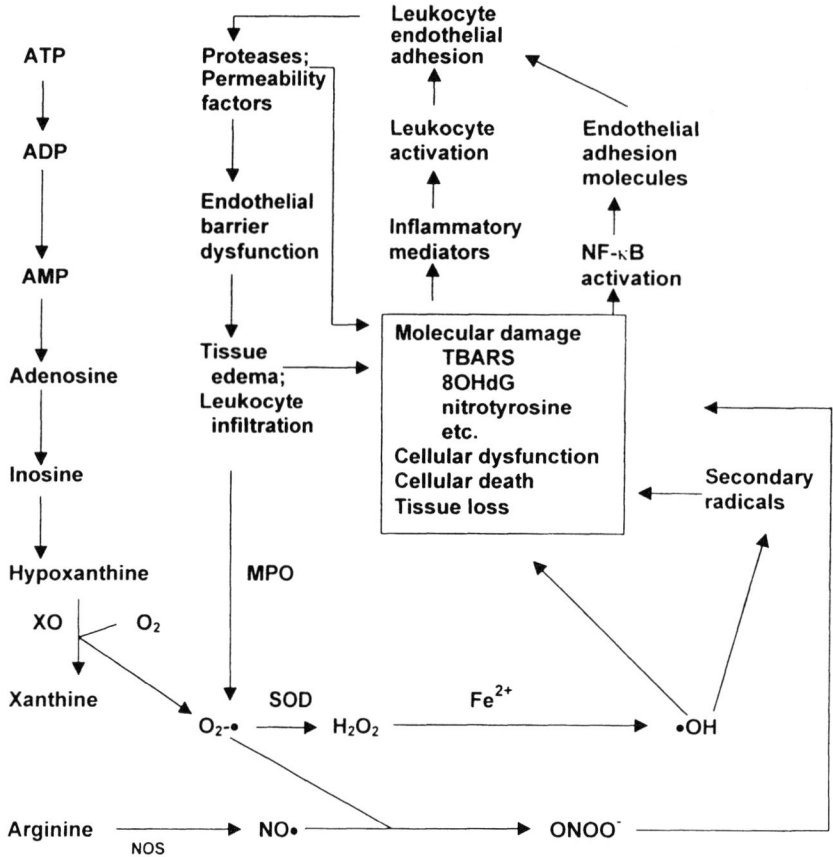

Figure 1 Some of the processes involved in ischemia–reperfusion injury that lead to physiological dysfunction and tissue death. The processes clearly include free radical generation and ancillary events that are activated and that eventually cause damage to key macromolecules. Antioxidants, and melatonin, in particular, act at several sites to abate free radical damage from ischemia–reperfusion and inhibit events that contribute to tissue destruction.

a report showing that infarct size after stroke is increased in the brain of elderly rats relative to those in young animals (93). Aging is associated with a generalized reduction in endogenous melatonin production (94), suggesting that the loss of this antioxidant may be relevant to the amount of damage that the brain of older animals (and possibly humans) sustains after a stroke.

The findings of Manev and co-workers (92) were recently confirmed by Kilic et al. (95). In this study as well, earlier pinealectomy, which leads to diminished levels of circulating melatonin, exaggerated infarct volume in rats after induced focal ischemia–reperfusion in the brain. In this study the hypoxia persisted for 2 h followed by 22 h of reperfusion. Besides the pineal removal that increased lesion size, injecting the rats with 4 mg/kg melatonin reduced the size of the neural infarct by 40%. Given the outcome of these studies the authors believe the most plausible explanation for the beneficial effects of melatonin against stroke is a result of the antioxidative capacity of the indole. Besides melatonin's direct free radical-scavenging activity, they considered that its ability to stimulate antioxidative enzymes may also have been important in reducing infarct volume. The results of Kilic and colleagues (95) are essentially identical with those of Joo et al. (96), who found that pinealectomy aggravated markers of brain injury after induced stroke and that exogenously administered melatonin attenuated the responses. The endpoints used to estimate damage in this study were quantitative measures of DNA damage and determination of infarct volume in Nissl-stained brain sections.

By using what is referred to as four-vessel occlusion ischemia in the rat, Cho and colleagues (97) tested the ability of melatonin administration to reduce loss of CA1 pyramidal neurons in the hippocampus of male Wistar rats. The duration of ischemia was 10, 20, or 30 min; at the onset of reperfusion the initial melatonin injection (10 mg/kg) was given followed 2 and 6 h later by a similar injection. One week thereafter, the neuronal density in the CA1 hippocampal area was estimated using sections stained with cresyl violet. Regardless of the duration of cerebral ischemia, the rats that received melatonin during the early reperfusion period exhibited a significant preservation of CA1 neurons compared with the saline-injected controls. Although the authors claimed that giving only one injection of melatonin 30 min before ischemia onset did not statistically significantly protect the CA1 neurons, these animals had neuronal densities twice those of the control animals.

From the published literature relative to the antioxidant potential of melatonin, Cho et al. (97) surmised that the protective effects of the indole was related to its ability to quickly cross the blood–brain barrier where it functioned as a direct free radical scavenger and indirect antioxidant. They did not, however, provide evidence of reduced oxidatively damaged products in the ischemic brains of the melatonin-treated rats.

Li and co-workers (98) have shown that the number of hydroxyl radicals ($^\cdot$OH) produced in the brain during ischemia–reperfusion is reduced by melatonin. In their study, focal ischemia–reperfusion injury was induced by occluding the left middle cerebral artery of rats that had had a microdialysis probe previously implanted into the ipsilateral striatum of the brain. When the $^\cdot$OH spin trap, salicylate, was injected before interruption of blood flow, the resulting product (dihydrobenzoic acid [DHBA], which represents the number of $^\cdot$OH scavenged) recovered from the microdialysate increased during ischemia–reperfusion (99). This rise in DHBA was attenuated by concurrent administration of melatonin (4 mg/kg). These findings are consistent with the $^\cdot$OH-scavenging activity of melatonin (49–64) and is the first evidence that melatonin functions in this capacity in vivo. This group further investigated the protective role of melatonin during hypoxia–reoxygenation using rat cortical slices and measuring lactate dehydrogenase (LDH), a sensitive indicator in brain cell damage, in the supernatant (100). Again, when melatonin was present during the period of hypoxia and reoxygenation, LDH in the supernatant fluid was reduced, as was the concentration of DHBA.

In their most recent study, this same group showed that middle cerebral artery occlusion (for 60 min) in rats was followed by an increased expression of *bcl*-2 in neurons in the infarct area when melatonin was administered; in the same sections *bax* expression was not altered (101). Up-regulation of *bcl*-2 is generally considered to counteract cell death by apoptosis (102); thus, the authors felt that the stimulatory action of melatonin on *bcl*-2 expression was partly responsible for the protective effects of melatonin against neuronal death normally induced by ischemia–reperfusion.

In addition to the rat, because of the incomplete circle of Willis on the base of the brain of the Mongolian gerbil (*Meriones unguiculatus*), this species is commonly used to investigate the ability of presumed neuroprotective agents to reduce ischemia–reperfusion damage. After transient bilateral carotid artery ligation followed by reperfusion in the brain of gerbils, the nitrite/nitrate ratio was increased, as were the levels of cyclic GMP (103); both these indices are indicative of elevated NO$^\cdot$ synthesis. These changes, as well as the associated morphological alterations (104), were prevented when melatonin (10 mg/kg) was administered intraperitoneally

30 min before the ischemic insult. Excessive NO· is believed to be partially responsible for neural injury during stroke, and the ability of melatonin to reduce the nitrite/nitrate ratio and cGMP levels presumably relates to melatonin's ability to inhibit the pro-oxidative enzyme, NOS (82,83), and to scavenge NO· (105).

With use of several additional endpoints, Cuzzocrea and colleagues (105) followed up on the studies of Guerrero et al. (103) and showed that melatonin's neuroprotective actions in the ischemic gerbil brain probably extended beyond melatonin's ability to inhibit and scavenge NO·. In this study, a 10-mg/kg dose of melatonin, given before ischemia–reperfusion in the Mongolian gerbil, reduced brain edema, attenuated the rise in neural malondialdehyde formation, prevented the increase in neural myloperoxidase activity, reduced the formation of nitrotyrosine, and lowered the activation of poly(ADP-ribose) synthetase (PARS). Finally, neural loss in the CA1 region of the hippocampus was reduced by melatonin treatment of hypoxic–reoxygenated gerbil brains. Cuzzocrea and co-workers (105) invoked a number of known antioxidative actions of melatonin to explain its protective effects; these included melatonin's stimulatory action on antioxidative enzymes (76–81), inhibition of NOS (82,83), and its direct scavenging of NO· (69) and $ONOO^-$ (70–74). The relative significance of each of these actions of melatonin in protecting against stroke-induced damage, however, could not be ascertained.

Even the brain of fetal rats is protected from ischemia–reperfusion-induced oxidative damage when melatonin is given to the mother. For this study, the fetuses of rats were rendered hypoxic on the 19th day of gestation by bilateral occlusion of the utero-ovarian artery for 30 min (106); after this interval the arterial clamp was removed and the fetuses were reperfused for 30 min. The brains of fetal rats had highly elevated levels of thiobarbituric-reactive substances (TBARS) and of the damaged DNA product 8-hydroxydeoxyguanosine (8-OHdG). An injection of melatonin (10 mg/kg to the mother), 1 h before initiation of ischemia, reduced both indices of oxidative stress in a highly significant manner; indicating that melatonin had crossed the placenta and entered the brain of the fetuses in sufficient amounts to abate the induced oxidative stress. These data are consistent with the ready transfer of melatonin through the placenta as demonstrated by this group (22) and by others (23).

In vitro studies have also documented melatonin's ability to reduce oxidative stress-induced molecular injury in the neuroectodermally derived structures. Cazevieille and colleagues (107) rendered fetal rat cortical cultures hypoxic (5 h), followed by reoxygenation (3 h), and measured the release of lactate dehydrogenase (LDH) from the cells. Adding either 100 or 300 μM melatonin to the culture medium significantly reduced LDH release from the cells suggesting reduced oxidative damage. When a melatonin receptor antagonist, luzindole, was also added to the cultures it did not impair the ability of melatonin to afford protection against the ischemia–reperfusion insult, suggesting that the protective actions of melatonin were membrane receptor-independent. The authors felt that the most likely means by which melatonin protected the cortical cells from oxidative destruction was the ability of the indole to neutralize free radicals (107).

Similar studies have been performed using another neurally derived cell, the retinal pigment epithelial (RPE) cells (108). Human RPE cells subjected to ischemic conditions showed signs of apoptosis, including DNA fragmentation. These changes were significantly reduced when the medium contained melatonin, but not when ascorbate was present. Melatonin's inhibitory actions on apoptosis and related events was not reduced in the presence of luzindole, a melatonin receptor blocker. Thus, the ability of melatonin to counteract ischemia-mediated apoptosis in RPE cells was most likely the consequence of a reduced number of reactive species, which can cause programmed cell death.

Physiologically, melatonin has also preserved the integrity of cultured brain cells after a period of hypoxia–reoxygenation. When rat hippocampal slices were rendered hypoxic (with lowered D-glucose concentrations) followed by reoxygenation, synaptic transmission failure occurred in 80–100% of the CA1 neurons when the Schaffer collaterals were stimulated (109,110). When melatonin, in a dose range of 30–100 μM, was present in the medium, synaptic transmission was significantly preserved. The aminosteroid U-74389G and the pyridoindole stobadine also protected the cells from functional degeneration caused by hypoxia–reoxygenation. Because each of the molecules (i.e., melatonin, stobadine, and the aminosteroid) are antioxidants, the authors postulated that this action was relevant to the preserved synaptic transmission, although other beneficial actions of the agents cannot be ruled out. On the other hand, Trolox had little protective action in this system.

2. Gastrointestinal Tract and Adnexa

All organs suffer from oxidative damage when they are transiently deprived of an oxygen supply and after reoxygenation occurs. Similar to the brain, the gastrointestinal system is highly susceptible to ischemia–reperfusion injury. Also, as in the brain, melatonin reduces the molecular destruction associated with alterations in the oxygen supply.

The clamping of the celiac artery for 30 min followed by a 60-min period of reperfusion caused extensive mucosal damage to the stomach of rats (111). The indices measured included lesion size, TBARS, myloperoxidase activity (as an indication of neutrophil infiltration), and the activity of GPx. Except for GPx, these parameters, which were significantly increased after transient interruption of the blood supply, were reduced in a dose–response manner when melatonin was given in advance of the treatment. The drop in GPx activity that was induced during gastric injury was partially restored in the melatonin-treated rats. Because oxygen free radicals have been implicated in gastric injury from ischemia–reperfusion, it is surmised that melatonin protected against the damage owing to its diverse antioxidant capabilities.

In the series of three papers, Konturek and colleagues (112–114) reported a detailed series of experiments in which they showed that melatonin dose-dependently protects the mucosa of the stomach from the damaging effects of free radicals generated during ischemia–reperfusion. In these studies the blood flow to the stomach was transiently interrupted by clamping the celiac artery. Besides several determinants of oxidative damage, this group also used a fluorescent assay to estimate the number of free radicals in the blood draining the stomach. Melatonin, given by gastric lavage, reduced not only the cellular and molecular damage in the stomach, it also lowered the number of free radicals in the effluent. This being the case, the authors assumed it was the antioxidative capacity of melatonin that afforded protection against the insult imposed. Gastric hyperemia, which was also apparent after ischemia–reperfusion, may have contributed to the protective effects of melatonin, for prostaglandin synthesis was elevated in the stomachs of melatonin-treated rats.

As in the stomach, the ileum was also protected from the ravages of ischemia–reperfusion injury when melatonin was given in advance of reoxygenation. In a thorough study of the associated events (115), clamping both the superior mesenteric artery and the celiac trunk for 45 min and reperfusing the tissue for 60 min caused massive damage to the ileal mucosa, as illustrated by both morphological and biochemical measures. Thus, there was marked tissue damage on histological examination (Fig. 2), a rise in immunoreactive nitrotyrosine (an index of tyrosine nitration by ONOO$^-$), substantial positive staining for P-selectin (especially in the vascular endothelial cells), and for the intercellular adhesion molecule (ICAM) along with rises in myloperoxidase activity and malondialdehyde (MOA) levels, and an increase in the dihydrorhodamine 123 oxidation product rhodamine (a marker of ONOO$^-$-induced oxidative

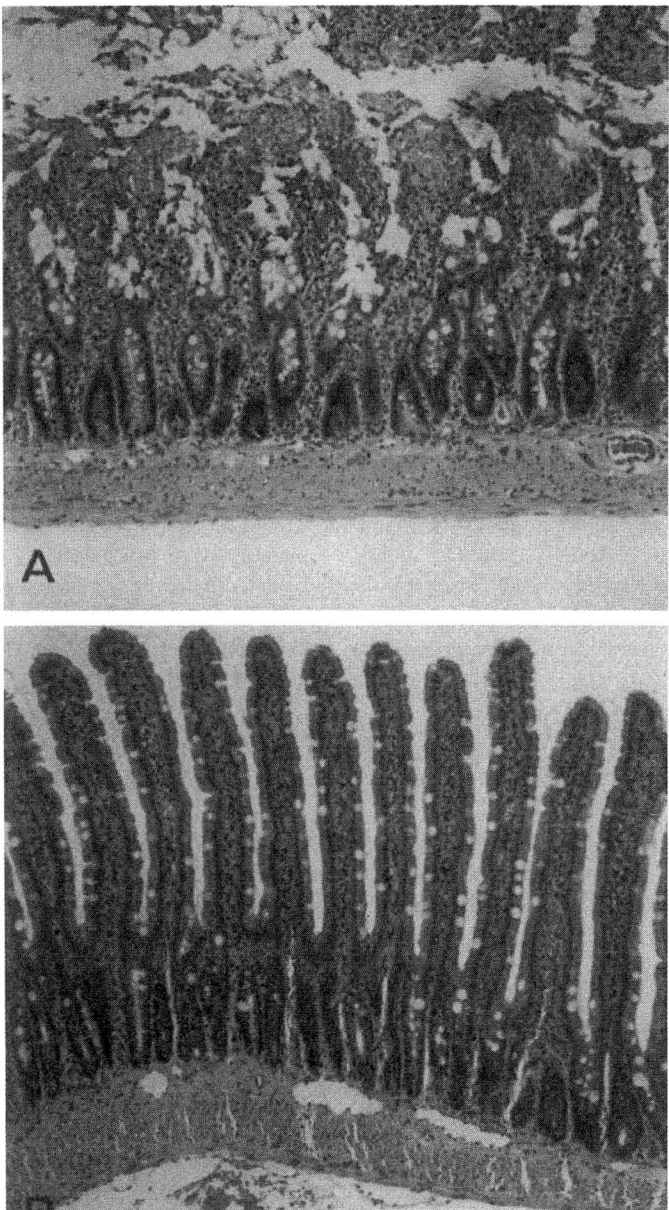

Figure 2 Morphological damage to the ileal mucosa of rats that experience ischemia–reperfusion caused by temporarily interrupting the blood flow in the superior mesenteric artery and celiac trunk: (A) the marked sloughing of the mucosa that occurs in these animals; (B) the protective effects of melatonin in reducing the damage. (From Ref. 115.)

processes) in the plasma. The administration of melatonin (3 mg/kg) just before reperfusion, and an additional 3-mg infusion during the 1-h reperfusion period, substantially reduced oxidative damage and evidence of $ONOO^-$ activity. Furthermore, no up-regulation of either P-selectin or ICAM was noted in the melatonin-treated rats. Excessive P-selectin and ICAM contribute to tissue damage during ischemia–reperfusion injury by assisting leukocytes to adhere to the endothelial cells and contribute to neutrophil recruitment (see Fig. 1). The extra neutrophils then generate free radicals that further tissue destruction. The results of this study show clearly that melatonin possesses marked protective effects against hypoxia–reoxygenation injury and that it does so by several mechanisms that result in the reduction of oxygen- and nitrogen-based oxidants.

Sewerynek et al. (116) tested melatonin's ability to curtail oxidative damage to the liver of rats after its blood supply was interrupted for 40 min followed by a 1-h reperfusion period. Elevated levels of MDA plus 4-hydroxyalkenals were measured at the end of the reperfusion period along with a reduction in reduced glutathione (GSH) and a rise in the glutathione disulfide (GSSG). Also, the activities of the antioxidative enzymes GPx and GRd were diminished as a result of the ischemia–reperfusion insult. In each case melatonin administration restored the endpoints to levels of the controls (i.e., it reduced lipid peroxidation, increased the ratio of GSH to GSSG, and stimulated the activities of the antioxidative enzymes). When the livers were studied morphologically, it was also obvious that melatonin preserved the structure of the hepatocytes and reduced polymorphonuclear leukocyte infiltration. Thus, melatonin's protective action against hepatic ischemia–reperfusion injury seems to be a consequence of a number of antioxidative actions of the indole.

3. Cardiovascular System

Inadequate coronary blood flow leads to the state of myocardial ischemia, the consequences of which are well catalogued (117,118). Reperfusion of the involved tissue reoxygenates the heart muscle, which can extend the damage and destroy cardiomyocytes. The consequences of ischemia–reperfusion injury in the heart are manifested by arrhythmias, fibrillation, and tissue infarction, and there is general agreement that free radicals contribute to these signs (119).

The isolated, perfused rat heart has been used to investigate the effects of melatonin on cardiac ischemia–reperfusion injury. Tan and co-workers (120) ligated the anterior descending coronary artery for 10 min and followed this with a 10-min period of reperfusion. In half of the hearts, melatonin was either continually infused throughout the experimental period or only during reperfusion. During reperfusion in the control hearts ventricular tachycardia (VT) and ventricular fibrillation (VF) were observed in 80 and 90% of the hearts, respectively. These parameters of myocardial dysfunction were markedly reduced in the hearts that were either perfused with melatonin throughout the experimental period or only during reperfusion (Fig. 3). When compared with vitamin C, melatonin proved roughly 30 times more effective in reducing the arrhythmias. The implication of this study is that free radicals are involved in the cardiac dysfunction that occurs with ischemia–reperfusion and that melatonin, owing to its antioxidant activity, can reduce the severity of the changes.

Studies related to the efficacy of melatonin in protecting against cardiac hypoxia–reoxygenation were also performed by Lagneux et al. (121). Rats were injected with 10 mg/kg of melatonin 30 min before the hearts were excised and perfused. In paradigm 1 in which regional ischemia was performed for 5 min with a 30-min reperfusion period, melatonin markedly reduced VT and VF in confirmation of the findings of Tan et al. (120). In a second paradigm (30 min ischemia and 120 min reperfusion) both arrhythmias and infarct size were studied. On this occasion, the authors (121) describe a "spectacular protection" by melatonin against both the irregular contractions and the size of the lesion. Although these studies do not prove

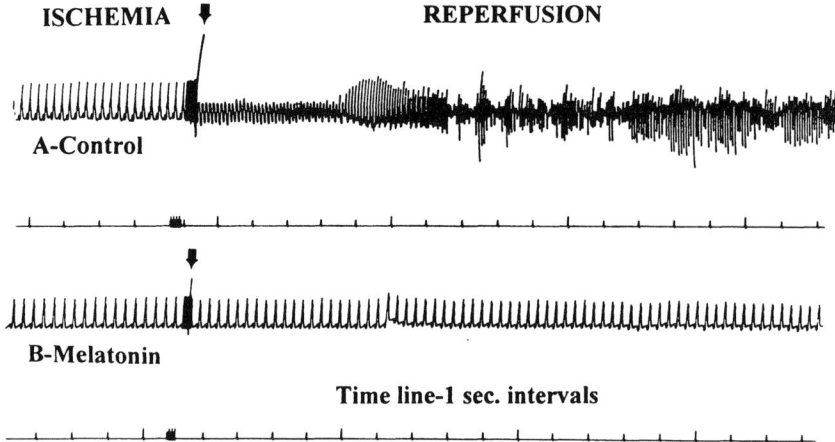

Figure 3 Electrocardiographic recording of the contraction rate of an isolated rat heart during ischemia–reperfusion caused by interruption of blood flow in the left descending branch of the coronary artery: Reperfusion, as illustrated here, is often followed by ventricular tachycardia and fibrillation, processes that are believed to involve, among other factors, free radicals. The lower trace illustrates the absence of these contraction anomalies when the heart is infused with melatonin at the time of cardiac reperfusion.

that melatonin's protective action against the ischemia–reperfusion insult is due exclusively to its detoxification of free radicals, it is likely that the antioxidative capacity of melatonin was involved.

Bertuglia et al. (122) studied the microcirculation in the hamster cheek pouch in response to ischemia–reperfusion (30 min each), with and without the systemic administration or topical application of melatonin. In some cases the cheek pouch was superfused with hypoxanthine plus xanthine. By using computerized in vivo microscopy, capillary permeability, perfused capillary length, leukocyte adhesion, and edema were quantified. In all cases, melatonin inhibited microvascular edema, reduced leukocyte adhesion, prevented the reduction in perfused capillary lengths and generally preserved microvascular perfusion. In a report cited previously (115) melatonin reduced the production of adhesion molecules during ischemia–reperfusion. This probably accounts for the reduced leukocyte sticking and the reduction in edema. The beneficial effects of melatonin in the hamster check pouch model were presumed to be related to the antioxidant properties of the indole.

Of interest to the general issue of ischemia–reperfusion is a process that occurs normally in nature (i.e., hibernation). During the hypothermia associated with hibernation, a 90% reduction in blood flow to all organs occurs. Conversely, during the periodic arousals from torpor during which respiration is markedly increased, heat is generated, energy production is high, and tissues are rapidly reperfused with oxygenated blood, the likelihood of tissue damage from free radicals would be expected to be high. That free radicals are produced during these intervals of arousal is supported by the observations that ascorbate and GSH levels diminish during these times (123). Also, during every arousal period, regardless of the time of day it occurs, pineal melatonin production increases markedly (124). This rise in melatonin, because of the antioxidant properties of the molecule, could be important in protecting against the onslaught of free radicals that occurs. Interestingly, in humans, the phrase "hibernating myocardium" has been used to describe localized impaired myocardial dysfunction that can be restored to normal when the oxygen supply to the area is reestablished (125).

B. Models of Neurodegenerative Diseases

The brain contains large amounts of substrates (e.g., unsaturated lipids and catecholamines) that are readily oxidatively abused by free radicals, and the related molecular damage is generally associated with neurodegenerative diseases (126). Of the oxidative processes that occur in the brain, lipid peroxidative events seem especially hazardous because the lipoperoxyl radical generated during the process can initiate and propagate the oxidative chain reaction. Beyond this, however, neural DNA and proteins are also readily damaged by reactive oxygen- and nitrogen-based toxicants.

Protection against free radical–mediated neural damage is somewhat hampered by the inability of some antioxidants (e.g., vitamin E) to easily cross the blood–brain barrier (127). Also, another antioxidant (i.e., ascorbate), although in high concentrations in certain regions of the brain, can act as a potent pro-oxidative agent in areas enriched with iron. Finally, catalase, an important H_2O_2-metabolizing enzyme in many cells, is virtually absent from the brain (128).

1. Alzheimer's Disease

Alzheimer's disease (AD) is a neurodegenerative condition that is occurring with increasing frequency in the human population, presumably partly because people are living longer, thereby allowing the condition to be expressed. Although the degenerative processes of AD are undoubtedly highly complex, interest in the possible role of free radical destruction has increased in the last decade, and the experimental data generally support a relation between oxidative processes and AD-type neural degeneration and dementia (129,130). Thus, there are a variety of free radical scavengers and antioxidants that are being experimentally tested in an attempt to defer the signs of AD.

Pappolla and colleagues (131,132) were the first to investigate the role of melatonin in reducing oxidative damage to neurons exposed to amyloid-β (Aβ) peptide, a 40- to 42-amino acid peptide that is often prominent in the brain of AD patients (Fig. 4). Amyloid deposits in the brain of AD patients are major components of senile plaques; additionally, they are often found in the walls of cerebral and meningeal blood vessels. When murine N2a neuroblastoma cells were incubated with Aβ(25–35), the segment of the longer peptide that generates free radicals, or with a peptide in which the sequence of the amino acids was scrambled (which does not generate radicals), the former caused increased lipid peroxidation, rises in intracellular Ca^{2+}, and induced cellular death. Coincubation of the Aβ(25-35)-treated neuroblastoma cells with melatonin greatly reduced the degree of lipid breakdown, limited the rise in intracellular Ca^{2+}, and returned cell viability to that of the controls. When the studies were repeated using the entire Aβ molecule, which similar to Aβ(25–35) is highly neurotoxic, melatonin was equally effective in reducing the pro-oxidative effects of the peptide (132). In this study both murine neuroblastoma cells and primary neuronal cultures were used. Although the measurements made in these studies do not definitively prove that the mechanism of inhibition of Aβ toxicity by melatonin involved antioxidative processes, of the actions of the indole that have been described, its ability to scavenge free radicals (133–134) and stabilize membranes (135) seem most likely to explain its protective effects. More recently, Bozner et al. (136) and Pappolla and colleagues (137) also have shown that melatonin reduced mitochondrial DNA damage induced by the entire Aβ peptide or by Aβ(25–35) in culture neurons, a finding consistent with the free radical-scavenging activity of the indole.

Similar to melatonin, an endogenous melatonin-related indole, indole-3-propionic acid, is also at least as effective as melatonin itself in reducing Aβ toxicity from free radical-scavenging

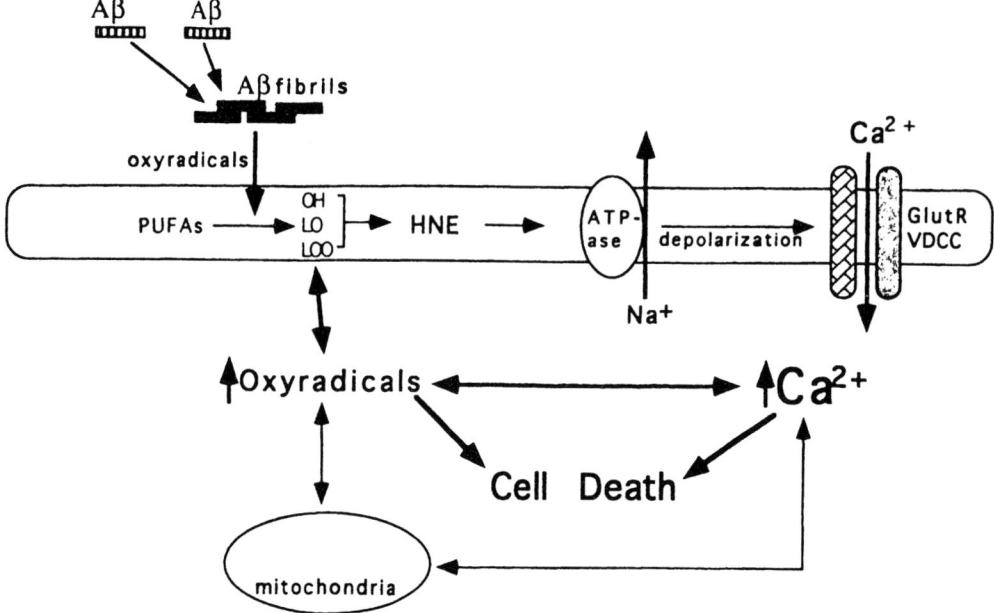

Figure 4 Diagrammatic representation of some of the processes involved in the toxicity of amyloid-β (Aβ) peptide, which is believed to be a contributory factor to neuronal loss in humans with Alzheimer's disease. Melatonin reduces the damage and increases the survival of neurons exposed to Aβ-peptide by several means as summarized in the text.

activity (138). Finally, Daniels et al. (139) showed that melatonin reduced the lipid peroxidative changes in platelet membranes incubated with Aβ.

Beyond melatonin's ability to reduce the direct neurotoxicity of Aβ, it seems to have additional actions, related to Aβ, that may not be free radical-mediated, but may aid this indole in reducing the formation or damaging effects of the peptide. Pappolla et al. (139) have shown that melatonin interacts with Aβ(1–40) and Aβ(1–42) and inhibits the formation of β-sheets and myloid fibrils; this would reduce the toxicity of Aβ in terms of its ability to generate free radicals. Song and Lahiri (140) and Lahiri (141) have reported that the formation of Aβ is also reduced by melatonin.

Heavy metals have also been implicated as potential contributing factors to AD. When SHSY5Y neuroblastoma cells were exposed to 180 nM $HgCl_2$ it caused a 30% reduction of GSH in the cells; this change was reduced by melatonin. In other situations, when neuroblastoma cells were challenged with mercury, melatonin also reduced the toxicity of the heavy metal (143). Furthermore, preincubation of cells with melatonin attenuated Aβ(1–40) and Aβ(1–42) release and also reduced tau phosphorylation. Besides implicating mercury in the pathophysiological mechanisms of AD, the findings showed that melatonin counteracts many of the effects of mercury. To explain the beneficial effects of melatonin in these studies, Olivieri et al. (143) considered several actions of melatonin, including its reported ability to chelate mercury (84). Heavy metal chelators can function as important antioxidants.

Two recent comprehensive reviews have considered these new findings related to AD and melatonin and have proposed the potential usefulness of treating these patients with this nontoxic indole (144,145). The limited clinical data available suggests that melatonin may benefit such patients (146,147).

2. Parkinson's Disease

Parkinson's disease (PD) is the second most common degenerative condition of the central nervous system in the aging population. Although the signs of the disease typically become apparent close to 60 years of age, the initial degenerative processes probably begin decades earlier. Pathologically, the disease is only poorly understood, but there are strong indications that free radicals are involved, although whether they are a cause or a consequence of the condition has not been established (148). Products of dopamine metabolism seem linked to PD; these products include the pro-oxidant agents hydrogen peroxide, aldehydes, and quinones (149).

The most common model used to induce Parkinson-like signs in experimental animals is to inject them with 1-methyl-4-phenyl-1,2,3,6-tetrahydropyridine (MPTP). In the brain, monoamine oxidase type B (MAO-B) converts MPTP to the 1-mthyl-4-phenyl-pyridinium ion (MPP$^+$); this product generates other potential pro-oxidative toxins, including isoquinolines and β-carbolines (150). Among the features of MPP$^+$ toxicity is the loss of the dopaminergic parikarya in the substantia nigra of the brain stem, a finding consistent with PD in humans.

There have been several successful attempts to attenuate MPTP neural toxicity by administering melatonin. In the first of these, products of lipid peroxidation and the level of tyrosine hydroxylase (TH) activity were measured in various brain areas after MPTP administration alone or in combination with melatonin (151). In mice given MPTP alone, products of the breakdown of lipids were increased in several brain areas, whereas striatal TH activity was reduced, as determined immunocytochemically. Both these changes were prevented by co-administering melatonin with MPTP, presumably because the indole neutralized the reactive toxicants generated by MPTP.

Melatonin's protective actions against MPTP toxicity were essentially confirmed by Jin et al. (152). In this case, MPTP was unilaterally sterotoxically injected into the substantia nigra of rats. As in the previous study (151), lipid peroxidation was increased while TH activity dropped in the substantia nigra on the side of MPTP injection; both responses were again prevented by melatonin administration. These observations were made 4 h after the onset of the study. When the experiment was continued for 1 week the protective effects of melatonin were less apparent, perhaps because melatonin was not continually available during this interval, although it was given twice daily. In vitro, melatonin possesses a remarkable ability to rescue DA neurons from cell death in several paradigms, including MPTP exposure, in which oxidative stress is involved (153).

Methamphetamine (METH) is a drug of abuse that causes pronounced release of dopamine (DA). High doses of METH induce long-lasting neurotoxicity by reducing TH activity, DA, and the dopamine transporter (DAT)-binding sites in the striatum. METH administration (5 mg/kg $\times$ 3) to mice depleted striatal DA, its metabolites, and DAT. An injection of melatonin (10 mg/kg before each METH injection and for an additional 2 days) provided full protection against the toxicity of METH (154). Additionally, melatonin diminished METH-induced hypothermia.

In contrast, however, these workers found no protection of melatonin against MPTP neurotoxicity relative to the neural concentrations of DA or its metabolites. Likewise, melatonin did not alter the behavioral sensitization response nor the development of conditioned locomotion caused by METH. This differential effect of melatonin in two models where free radicals are involved was unexpected and may relate to the severity of the damaging actions of the doses of the respective neural toxins used (154).

In a study similar to that of Itzhak et al. (154), Hirata and colleagues (155) studied the deleterious effects of METH on brain monoaminergic systems using autoradiographic techniques. Of interest in this report was the neurotoxic effects of METH on DA and serotoninergic terminals in the striatum and nucleus accumbens of the mouse brain. When mice were injected with 5 mg/kg × 4 METH the number of catecholaminergic terminals was decreased. Although the lowest dose of melatonin used (5 mg/kg) did not prevent the changes, higher doses (40 or 80 mg/kg) did. The authors conclude that METH neurotoxicity, particularly in terms of monoamines, involves free radicals; a corollary of this is that melatonin likely acted as a antioxidant to reduce the toxicity of the drug.

An aspect of MPTP toxicity is a marked reduction in cellular energy depletion by the binding of MPP^+ to complex I in the mitochondrial respiratory chain (156). When hepatic mitochondria were incubated with MPP^+, respiration was inhibited (157). The inclusion of melatonin in the incubation mixture prevented the reduction in respiration induced by MPP^+; however, this effect was seemingly not a consequence of melatonin's free radical-scavenging or antioxidant properties, but rather, was related to the indole's ability to prevent the interaction of MPP^+ with complex I. By preventing this interaction, free radical generation would be reduced. Although the final result of melatonin's action in this case would be a reduction in radical toxicant generation, melatonin here would not function as a direct free radical scavenger.

Another drug commonly used to induce Parkinson-like signs in animals is 6-hydroxydopamine (6-OHDA) (158). The neurotoxicity of 6-OHDA is manifested by the selective destruction of catecholaminergic neurons, with the most marked change being the depletion of DA and its metabolites in the substantia nigra. The loss of DA under these conditions is believed to involve oxygen-based free radicals (159). Mayo and colleagues (160–162) investigated the ability of melatonin to modify the response of neurons to 6-OHDA. In these studies this group found melatonin to sharply reduce apoptosis of both naive (undifferentiated) and neuronal (differentiated) PC12 cells in culture. The endpoints studied included cell viability, counts of apoptotic cells, ultrastructural definition of apoptotic features, and DNA fragmentation studies. The mechanisms by which melatonin reduced apoptosis were believed to be a consequence of the induction of antioxidative enzymes (as deduced from the increases in their mRNA levels) and on inhibition of cell proliferation. In vivo as well, Kim et al. (163) claimed melatonin preserved the integrity of dopaminergic neurons in the substantial nigra and TH activity in the striatum of rats treated with 6-OHDA. The protective action of melatonin in the nigrostriatal dopaminergic system in this study was presumed to relate to the antioxidant actions of melatonin, although the authors provided no direct evidence of this.

Dopamine, similar to other catecholamines, is subject to auto-oxidation, a process known to produce cytotoxic reactive species. The effect of melatonin on the auto-oxidation of DA in the presence of $CuSO_4$ has been investigated using an oxygen radical absorbance capacity (ORAC) assay; in this system the rate of oxidation of the fluorescent protein *Porphyridium cruentum* β-phycoerythrin (β-PE) is estimated. Melatonin significantly impeded the oxidation of β-PE in the presence of DA (164). In a similar study in which metal-catalyzed oxidation of DA was examined, melatonin again was effective in reducing the auto-oxidation of the catecholamine (165). Melatonin was more efficient in reducing DA oxidation than was either deprenyl or vitamin E, whereas vitamin C was totally ineffective. Both groups feel that melatonin's ability to reduce catecholamine auto-oxidation relates to its ability to neutralize the generated free radicals.

3. Huntington's Disease

The tryptophan metabolite quinolinic acid (QA) has been used experimentally in a model of Huntington's disease (HD). It increases in the brain during aging, and it is toxic, having a variety of actions, the best known of which is its function as a selective agonist of the N-methyl-D-aspartate (NMDA) receptor (166). These excitotoxic actions and the resulting neurodegeneration have been examined by several groups to determine whether melatonin would be effective in reducing QA toxicity.

Southgate et al. (167) injected QA directly into the hippocampus of rats; 5 days later the brain was removed for morphological examination of the hippocampal pyramidal neurons and glutamate receptor binding. QA caused a noticeable swelling and minor degenerative changes of the CA1 and CA3 pyramidal neurons; these alterations were not apparent in the neurons of rats that had been given QA in combination with intraperitoneally injected melatonin. A reduction in glutamate receptor numbers in the hippocampus was also partially prevented by melatonin.

A more complete in vivo study was conducted by Behan et al. (168). Intrahippocampal injections of QA, with or without the coadministration of melatonin, was performed in rats and the pyramidal neurons of the hippocampus were histologically examined. The cells were clearly damaged by QA, a response prevented by melatonin. When the melatonin receptor blocker luzindole was given it did not impede the ability of melatonin to protect the neurons from QA; this suggests that melatonin had not preserved the morphology of the pyramidal neurons by acting on a membrane receptor. Besides the morphological changes, melatonin also curtailed the breakdown of lipids by QA. This latter observation is in line with the results of Cabrera and colleagues (169) who have found, both in vitro and in vivo, that melatonin prevents QA-induced lipid peroxidation. The implications of these studies, as both groups agree, is that QA toxicity in the central nervous system involves free radicals, and that melatonin's protective actions are membrane–receptor-independent and likely related to its antioxidant capacity (164,165).

C. Excitotoxicity

Cell death results when neurons are exposed to excitatory neurotransmitters for prolonged periods. The mechanisms underlying the vulnerability of neurons to excitotoxic agents, such as glutamate, are only partially understood. Glutamate receptors of the NMDA subtype, when activated, allow the massive influx of Ca^{+2}, which causes an imbalance in cellular homeostasis and eventually leads to cellular death (170). There is agreement, however, that oxygen is a requirement for excitotoxicity and that free radicals are involved in mediating the subsequent molecular destruction and cell death (Fig. 5) (171,172). This being true, attempts to reduce the damage inflicted by prolonged activation of the glutamate receptor have often investigated the usefulness of antioxidants in this regard. Melatonin has been examined for this action as well.

Kainic acid (KA) is a nondegradable agonist for a subtype of glutamate ionotropic receptor that induces excitotoxicity in in vitro preparations (173) and generalized limbic seizures accompanied by neuronal damage and death in animals (174). When homogenates of brain areas (cerebellum, hippocampus, striatum, and hypothalamus) were incubated with KA, high levels of lipid peroxidation products were induced; these increases were readily inhibited in a dose–response manner by the addition of melatonin to the medium (175). The degree of inhibition of lipid breakdown was particularly dramatic, varying from 10 to 100% and correlating directly with the melatonin concentration. Subsequent studies using homogenates of the brain were equally effective in demonstrating the ability of melatonin to reduce KA-mediated oxidative damage to lipids (176).

When neuronal cell cultures were used in lieu of cell homogenates, the protective actions against kainate-induced molecular damage were equally apparent. Cerebellar granule cells, collected from the brain of newborn rats, were used by Giusti and colleagues (177) to test the antiexcitotoxic effects of melatonin. They showed that melatonin reduced KA toxicity

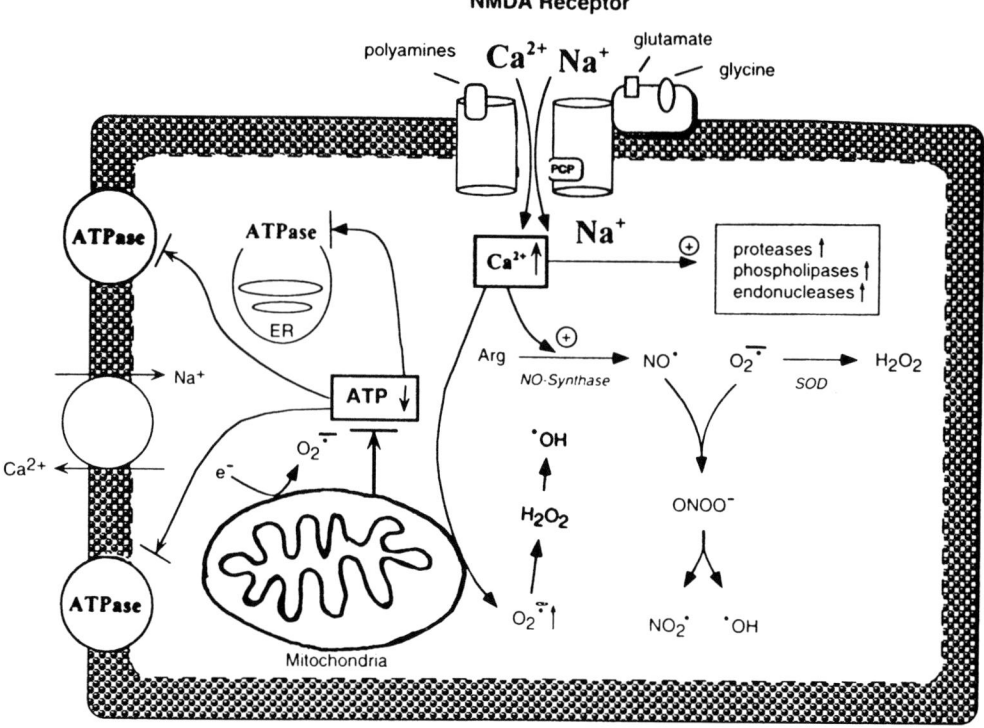

Figure 5 Presumed events in neurons associated with neuronal loss caused by excitotoxicity. The generation of free radicals is believed to account, in part, for the loss of neurons that contain receptors for the excitatory amino acid neurotransmitter, glutamate. A nondegradable analogue of the glutamate receptor, kainic acid, is frequently used to induce excitotoxicity and neuronal death. Melatonin reduces the severity of excitotoxicity by minimizing free radical damage.

and that this action was not a consequence of melatonin's ability to compete with the agonist for the glutamate receptor on the granule neurons. Rather, the authors felt that melatonin worked intracellularly to scavenge radicals that were generated as a result of the influx of massive amounts of Ca^{2+}. Consistent with these observations as well as in the interpretation of the findings, Lezoualc'h et al. (178,179) found that oxidatively mediated apoptosis in cultured hippocampal neurons and in hippocampal slices caused by glutamate treatment was inhibited by melatonin. DNA fragmentation, which accompanies programmed cell death, was also reduced in the presence of melatonin. This group compared the efficacy of melatonin with its metabolic precursor, N-acetylserotonin, in reducing glutamate-induced neuronal damage and found that whereas N-acetylserotonin was more effective than melatonin in reducing cell death, melatonin had greater efficiency in limiting lipid peroxidation in the hippocampus (179,180).

Cazevieille and co-workers (107,181) used both retinal neurons and rat cortical neurons in culture to test the ability of melatonin to protect against excitotoxicity. When cortical neurons were used, glutamate caused a large increase in LDH in the medium, indicative of oxidative damage and leakage of the enzyme from the neurons. Melatonin reduced these aspects of glutamate toxicity, and these workers further showed that this action was membrane receptor-independent, as adding luzindole, a melatonin receptor antagonist, did not diminish melatonin's protective effect. In retinal neurons as well, the presence of melatonin during KA treatment prevented the detrimental actions of the latter molecule.

Primary cell cultures of hippocampal pyramidal neurons underwent degeneration when incubated in a Mg^{2+}-free, glycine-supplemented medium. This treatment enhances excitatory neurotransmission. When melatonin was added after (but not during) exposure to the Mg^{2+}-free medium, it concentration-dependently ($EC_{50} = 19.2 \pm 2.8$ μM) reduced neuronal cell death by 75% 24 h later (182). Because N-tert-butyl-α-phenylnitrone (PBN), a radical spin trap, also reduced hippocampal neuron death under these circumstances, the authors surmised that the protective actions of these agents related to their free radical-scavenging ability. These workers noted that adding melatonin any time up to 4 h after the treatment of the neurons with a Mg^{2+}-free medium conferred protection, although by 6 h the beneficial effects of the indole were lost.

An equally large number of studies have been conducted in vivo to document the antiexcitotoxic effects of melatonin. The initial reports were published by the group of Manev et al. (183–186); however, others have also confirmed and extended their findings. A variety of different endpoints were used to illustrate melatonin's ability to protect against KA in rats. With use of the quantitative dUTP–biotin nick end labeling (TUNEL) technique and Nissl-stained brain sections, Manev and co-workers found that the number of cells containing damaged DNA after KA treatment was reduced by melatonin. Likewise, morphological examination of the affective neurons revealed extensive damage that was abated by melatonin. Melatonin administration also prevented the epileptic seizures normally associated with giving KA. This series of papers convincingly demonstrates that pharmacologically melatonin protects against a variety of negative effects induced by the excitotoxin KA.

The approach used by Floreani et al. (187) also showed that melatonin protects the rat brain from kainate, but their endpoints were different from those in the previously discussed studies. Melatonin negated the inhibitory effect of KA on the GSH content of the hippocampus and amygdala and restored the reduction in GRd caused by KA. Also, in cultured cerebellar granule cells, melatonin reduced the drop in cellular GSH caused by KA treatment. In this study the authors felt that melatonin's protective action was partly due to its ability to preserve levels of the important intracellular antioxidant GSH, in addition to functioning as a direct free radical scavenger.

In confirmation of the work of Manev et al. (92,183), Tang et al. (188) also showed that melatonin protected DNA from oxidative damage induced by KA. In this case, the damaged DNA product 8-hydroxydeoxyguanosine (8-OHdD) was measured. In both the rat brain and liver, melatonin reduced 8-OHdD levels that were elevated after giving the excitotoxin. Likewise, lipid peroxidation in the rat brain is reduced when melatonin is given in conjunction with KA (189).

One of the most convincing illustrations of the beneficial effects of coadministering melatonin with KA comes from observations in mice (190). When CD-F1 mice were given KA subcutaneously, 7 days later there was a profound degeneration of the CA3 pyramidal neurons of the hippocampus. In mice treated with both KA and melatonin the CA3 neurons were, at the light microscopic level, morphologically totally preserved. Additionally, melatonin reduced the severity of the behavioral manifestations (seizures, and such) typical of KA-treated mice.

In birds as in mammals, glutamate provokes excitotoxic neuronal degeneration. When glutamate was injected into the vitelin sac of chick eggs, it interfered with synaptogenesis of the cerebellar Purkinje cells and the development of the glomerular synaptic complexes (19). Additionally, 44% of the embryos died as a result of this treatment. Melatonin prevented the effects of glutamate on the development of synaptic contacts in the cerebellum, and it reduced embryo death to 22%.

Uniformly, studies that have used neuronal excitotoxicity models to examine the protective actions of melatonin have shown that the indole is capable of reducing damage to the brain caused by glutamate and its agonist KA. Although the mechanisms by which excitotoxins damage neurons are not completely clarified, there is widespread agreement that free radicals are partly responsible (192). Given the variety of antioxidative actions of melatonin, its protective effects are generally explainable in terms of free radical suppression.

D. Ionizing Radiation

An estimated 60–70% of the damage inflicted on DNA during exposure to ionizing radiation is a consequence of the ·OH (193). This damage is similar to that produced during normal oxidative metabolism in cells, although the product yields may be somewhat different (194). Given that ionizing radiation induces molecular damage by free radical mechanisms, this model is often used to check the efficacy of antioxidants; those molecules that reduce radiation-induced damage are identified as radioprotectors.

The first evidence that melatonin may have radioprotective actions was provided in 1997, although this report cites unpublished work in which it was claimed that melatonin, given in advance of a lethal dose of ionizing radiation, led to survival of 75% of the mice (195). In their paper, Blinkenstaff et al. tested a number of melatonin homologues for their radioprotective capacity and reported that the survival rate of mice given 950-cGy radiation was best when they were treated with the hexanoic amide **5** and the octanoic amide **6** (see Ref. 195). Later studies also showed that mice were protected, judging from their 30-day–survival rate, by melatonin (196).

Cytogenetic evaluation of isolated human peripheral white blood cells have been used on several occasions to examine the radioprotective potential of melatonin. The cells were typically evaluated for the following abnormalities: exchange aberrations, acentric fragments, and micronuclei. In these in vitro studies, melatonin, in a concentration-dependent manner, always reduced the incidence of the abnormalities, indicating less damage to nuclear DNA (197–201). The workers also compared melatonin's efficacy with that of another known radioprotector, dimethyl sulfoxide (DMSO); invariably, melatonin proved to be a significantly better radioprotector in these studies than did DMSO.

One study involved humans ingesting melatonin followed by isolation of the peripheral lymphocytes and then subjecting them to gamma radiation; the resulting damage was then correlated with circulating levels of melatonin (202). Elevated circulating melatonin levels inversely correlated with the degree of cytogenetic damage. The authors propose that melatonin's radioprotective actions related to direct free radical–scavenging and indirect antioxidant actions (203).

Studies similar to those described in the foregoing were conducted by Badr et al. (204). Again, mice were exposed to gamma irradiation, with and without prior melatonin treatment; melatonin reduced the number of micronuclei in polychromatic erythrocytes from bone marrow. Also, melatonin reduced chromosomal aberration frequency in spermatogonial chromosomes; however, the indole was not effective in protecting either bone marrow or testicular cells from radiation-induced damage when it was given after the radiation exposure had occurred. The authors concluded that melatonin likely confers protection to nuclear DNA by scavenging the radicals that are generated during gamma radiation exposure.

When rats were exposed to 32-cGy gamma radiation continually for 12 h, significant rises in ovarian and blood MDA levels and a reduction in the activities of two antioxidative enzymes,

SOD and GPx, in the erythrocytes were recorded. Rats that received an intraperitoneal injection of melatonin before exposure showed none of these changes (205).

Because the damage done by ionizing radiation is widely considered to be mediated primarily by the resulting free radicals, the evidence that melatonin is pharmacologically effective in reducing the associated molecular destruction is consistent with the indole's antioxidant capacity. In general, melatonin's radioprotective potential seems at least on a par with several other agents used for this purpose.

E. Traumatic Brain Injury

Traumatic brain injury (TBI), also referred to as closed head injury, causes neuronal degradation by mechanisms that are believed to involve free radicals (206). Mésenge and co-workers (207) used a TBI model to compare the efficacies of the antioxidant melatonin and the spin trap PBN to inhibit the behavioral sequelae of blunt head injury. Before and after subjecting mice to a standardized head trauma, melatonin or PBN were given. Twenty-four hours later the mice were examined using a behavioral parameter referred to as the grip test (i.e., the ability of a mouse to remain on a taut string suspended 30 cm above a surface). Mice treated with either melatonin or PBN performed better (remained on the string longer) than did mice treated with diluent. Clearly, both agents had a protective effect, at least from the behavioral standpoint, against head trauma. Because both molecules neutralize free radicals, this mechanism was proposed as a means by which they protected the brain from damage (207). In this study the dose of PBN used exceeded that of melatonin by roughly 40-fold.

F. Lipopolysaccharide

Lipopolysaccharide (LPS; endotoxin), produced by gram-negative bacteria, damages numerous organs in animals by the production of reactive oxygen and nitrogen intermediates and other toxic species (208,209). In severe cases the animal (or human) exhibits multiple organ failure owing to the massive destruction of tissue; this often causes death of the organism. Because of the involvement of free radicals in this condition, Sewerynek et al. (210–213) conducted a series of studies to examine the possible usefulness of melatonin in resisting this type of septic shock.

In the initial study, melatonin did protect against LPS toxicity, as indicated by its effects on glutathione metabolism and the activity of the antioxidative enzyme, GPx (210) in liver and brain. No indices of oxidative damage, however, were actually measured. In another study in which the products of hepatic lipid peroxidation were estimated, melatonin totally blocked the rise in these constituents induced by LPS. Also, melatonin stimulated the levels of total glutathione (tGSH), reduced GSSG, and prevented the degenerative morphological changes seen in the liver after LPS injection (211). In homogenates of lung, liver, and brain, melatonin, in a concentration-dependent manner also prevented peroxidative damage to membrane lipids induced by incubating them with the endotoxin (212).

Besides its obvious ability to damage polyunsaturated fatty acid, LPS also attacks DNA, the destruction of which can be estimated cytogenetically by counting the number of micronuclei in polychromatic erythrocytes collected from bone marrow and peripheral blood. When rats were treated with LPS, micronuclei increased significantly in red blood cells, whereas cotreatment of these animals with melatonin reduced their number (213). This series of studies, similar to a number of others, illustrates that melatonin protects molecules in either a lipid or aqueous environment from oxidative damage.

Maestroni (214) extended these findings by showing that melatonin reduces the death of mice inoculated with what would normally have been a lethal dose of LPS. The reduction in mortality may relate to melatonin's inhibitory action on nitric oxide synthase (NOS), as mice lacking cytokine-inducible NOS are resistant to death caused by endotoxemia.

Melatonin is known to inhibit NOS (82,83,219) and thereby reduce the toxicity of downstream reactive nitrogen species that would have been generated. Similar to Sewerynek et al. (210–213), Maestroni (214) feels melatonin may be a beneficial treatment for individuals with endotoxemic shock. Other aspects of LPS toxicity (i.e., thirst and fever) are also reduced by melatonin (216,217). The authors felt that in reference to these endpoints melatonin's protective effects related to both its free radical-scavenging activities and possibly to some actions mediated by receptors. One of the likely beneficial actions of melatonin, as mentioned by both groups of workers (216,217), is the inhibition of the pro-oxidative enzyme, NOS.

The most complete study documenting the protection of melatonin against LPS-induced multiple organ failure is that of Crespo and colleagues (218). As evidence of liver and renal dysfunction, they found elevated levels of aspartate and alanine aminotransferases, γ-glutamyl transferase, alkaline phosphatase, creatinine, urea, and uric acid in the blood of rats treated with the endotoxin. Also increased were serum levels of cholesterol and triglycerides and reduced concentrations of glucose. These changes were significantly attenuated when melatonin was given in conjunction with LPS. Likewise, dismantling of lipids and the stimulation of iNOS activity induced by LPS in the lungs was inhibited by melatonin. The authors interpreted their findings to mean that a significant portion of melatonin's beneficial actions during endotoxic shock relates to its ability to reduce nitrogen-based radical generation by inhibition of iNOS.

Carrageenan is a shock- and inflammation-inducing agent often used in the experimental setting. The mechanisms by which carrageenan cause the inflammatory response are generally well characterized. In the early phase, edema is associated with the production of histamine, leukotrienes, platelet-activating factor, and cyclooxygenase products, whereas in the late phase, neutrophil infiltration occurs, causing the production of free radicals (219,220). Furthermore, the L-arginine–NO pathway is believed to play a role in the carrageenan-induced inflammatory response (221).

This model has been used extensively by Cuzzocrea et al. (222–224) to define the role of melatonin in inflammation. In their first study, two models of acute inflammation (i.e., carrageenan-induced paw edema and pleurisy) were used. The chief findings in this study were that melatonin reduced the degree of paw edema and attenuated the morphological damage and polymorphoneutrophil (PMN) infiltration. In the pleurisy model, melatonin lowered iNOS expression and NO production and reduced nitrotyrosine staining, indicating the either $ONOO^-$ production was diminished or that it was scavenged before interacting with tyrosine (222).

Follow-up studies produced similar results and added additional information on how melatonin reduces the inflammatory response. When the pleurisy model was again studied, melatonin reduced prostaglandin production and prevented cyclooxygenase-2 (COX-2) expression induced by carrageenan (223). The inhibition of these proinflammatory mediators would reduce free radical production and the resulting tissue damage.

That endogenous melatonin levels are sufficient to reduce carrageenan-induced inflammation is supported by a recent study in which rats were exposed to continuous light for 1 week to reduce pineal melatonin synthesis (9). When these animals were challenged with carrageenan, the resulting inflammatory response was exaggerated compared with that in animals for which endogenous melatonin production had not been suppressed (224). Furthermore, inhibiting melatonin synthesis significantly increased $ONOO^-$ formation as indicated by oxidation of the fluorescent dye dihydrorhodamine 123. Also, the melatonin-depleted rats exhibited elevated DNA damage and reduced mitochondrial respiration. When melatonin was exogenously supplied to these rats, all of the effects of endogenous melatonin depletion were reversed.

Zymosan, a component of the wall of the yeast *Saccharomyces cerevisiae*, produces an intense inflammatory reaction and is a widely used nonseptic model of circulatory shock and multiple organ failure (225). Pathophysiologically, zymosan induces the production of proinflammatory lipid mediators and cytokines as well as free radicals and associated processes (226). When zymosan-activated plasma was given as an intraplantar injection in rats, an inflammatory response followed that included edema, PMN infiltration, increased levels of nitrite and nitrate and myloperoxidase activity, and elevated nitrotyrosine levels (227). The injection of melatonin into the paw suppressed the appearance of all the signs of inflammation and reduced nitrotyrosine formation indicating reduced reactive species generation. When given intraperitoneally, zymosan caused peritoneal exudate formation and increased levels of MDA and 4-hydroxyalkenals in the liver, small intestine, kidney, and lungs. Additionally, the liver exhibited structural damage upon light microscopic examination and immunoreactive nitrotyrosine was observed in several organs, most notably the ileum (228). All of these changes were either significantly reduced or eliminated in zymosan-treated rats that were also given melatonin.

DNA strand breaks and activation of the nuclear enzyme poly(ADP-ribose)synthase (PARS) initiates an energy-consuming, inefficient repair cycle that causes peroxynitrite-mediated molecular injury and can lead to cell death. Zymosan is capable of inflicting cellular injury and killing cells by this means. In macrophages collected from zymosan-shocked rats, melatonin dose-dependently reduced $ONCOO^-$ formation and DNA damage as well as prevented the drop in mitochondrial respiration and loss of cellular NAD^+ (229). Clearly, the antioxidant and anti-inflammatory actions of melatonin are sufficient to provide significant protection against agents, such as zymosan, that are strongly proinflammatory (230).

Ingestion of dextran sodium sulfate (DSS) induces severe colitis associated with mucosal lesions, quantitative changes in intestinal flora, and bloody diarrhea (231). Pentney and Bubenik (232) induced this set of signs by feeding DSS to mice and found that the daily injection of 150 μg/kg melatonin for 7 weeks prevented weight loss, increased food consumption, dramatically reduced the severity and frequency of gastrointestinal mucosal lesions, and virtually eliminated blood in the feces. Melatonin's capability as an anti-inflammatory and antioxidant agent were used to explain the ability of the indole to reduce DSS-induced colitis.

G. Heavy Metals

Chromium (Cr) is a genotoxin that causes tumors in experimental animals and humans (233). Chromium exists in a number of oxidation states with hexavalent Cr [Cr(VI)] being the most genotoxic and carcinogenic (234). Cr(VI) is readily taken up by cells where it is reduced to several intermediate oxidation states; during this reduction process, reactive oxygen species are generated that are believed to be a major culprit in chromium toxicity (235).

The incubation of rat primary hepatocytes with $K_2Cr_2O_7$ markedly increased DNA single-strand breaks, caused the leakage of LDH from the cells, and increased levels of MDA. All of these cytotoxic effects were dose-dependently reduced by the addition of melatonin to the cultures (55). Melatonin did not, however, restore the levels of GSH-metabolizing enzymes, SOD, or alkaline phosphatase that accompanied Cr treatment. In these studies melatonin did not influence the uptake or subcellular distribution of Cr. Susa et al. (55) concluded that melatonin potently protected cultured hepatocytes from Cr toxicity by a combination of preserving endogenous cellular antioxidant levels and by directly scavenging $^{\cdot}OH$, the latter of which was documented in this study using a spin trap and ESR spectroscopy.

Two subsequent reports used purified calf thymus DNA to test melatonin's ability to protect against Cr(III) (236,237) chromium. In these studies the damaged DNA product measured was 8-OHdG. When DNA was incubated with Cr(III) plus H_2O_2, the resulting damage was both time- and concentration-dependent. In comparison with several indoles, melatonin and 6-methoxy-1,2,3,4-tetrhydro-β-carboline (pinoline) were most effective in reducing 8-OHdG levels in DNA treated with Cr(III) (236). This group also compared melatonin with ascorbate and Trolox (vitamin E) in terms of their ability to protect purified DNA from oxidative stress induced by Cr(III) and H_2O_2 (Fig. 6). The concentrations of each required to reduce 8-OHdG levels in DNA by 50% (i.e., the EC_{50} valves, were 0.51, 30.4, and 36.2 μM for melatonin, vitamin C, and vitamin E, respectively (237). Thus, in this system, melatonin was roughly 60 times more effective than vitamin C and 70 times better than vitamin E.

Cadmium (Cd) is another environmental pollutant with considerable hepatotoxicity, inducing lipid peroxidation, a drop in hepatic GSH levels, and hepatocyte necrosis (238). When melatonin was tested for its ability to curtail the negative consequences of Cd, it prevented the drop in hepatic and erythrocyte GSH levels and ameliorated the depression in GRd activity caused by the metal (239). Furthermore, the histopathological areas of focal necrosis observed in the liver of Cd-treated rats were overcome by melatonin. The authors assumed that the antioxidant capacity of melatonin accounted for its protective effects against Cd toxicity, but other possible modes of action of the indole cannot be excluded.

H. Ethanol

Consumption of ethanol predisposes the gastrointestinal tract to acute injury. In the gut ethanol is quickly taken up and induces membrane damage, exfoliation of cells, and erosion of the epithelial covering, leading to ulcers (240). The mechanisms by which ethanol causes this damage are believed to involve free radicals (241), with molecules possessing free radical-scavenging properties generally being protective against the gastric lesions (242). One model used to investigate the ability of ethanol to damage the gastroduodenal mucosa is the instillation of ethanol into the stomach of duodenum-ligated rats. Melchiorri et al. (243) placed 1 mL of absolute ethanol, by gavage, into the stomach of rats with a duodenal ligature, and 1 h later examined the ethanol-bathed tissues. The ethanol caused hemorrhagic streaks that damaged roughly 36 and 25% of the gastric and duodenal mucosa, respectively. Likewise, in both organs PMN infiltration increased several hundredfold and total GSH levels and GRd activity were reduced. For each of these parameters, melatonin injected intraperitoneally 30 min before ethanol instillation reduced the severity of each of the parameters investigated. In a later study, melatonin was less effective in reducing gastric mucosal damage when it was given directly into the stomach (114).

Subsequent studies on melatonin's protective effects against ethanol toxicity, support the beneficial effects of the indole in this situation. Thus, when rats were chronically treated with ethanol and coadministered melatonin, the indole prevented the rises in products of lipid peroxidation seen in the testes, heart, brain, and lungs (244) (Fig. 7). Likewise, simulating a single alcoholic binge in mice (5 g/kg ethanol given intragastrically) led to pronounced hepatic mtDNA degradation that was almost totally overcome by melatonin treatment (245). These studies are consistent with melatonin's antioxidant ability, as alcohol-induced molecular destruction is a result of free radicals.

I. δ-Aminolevulinic Acid

Porphyrias are a group of metabolic disorders wherein there is excessive accumulation and excretion of porphyrins and their precursors. These disorders occur owing to specific acquired enzyme defects in the heme synthetic pathway. In all subtypes of this condition, plasma porphyrins

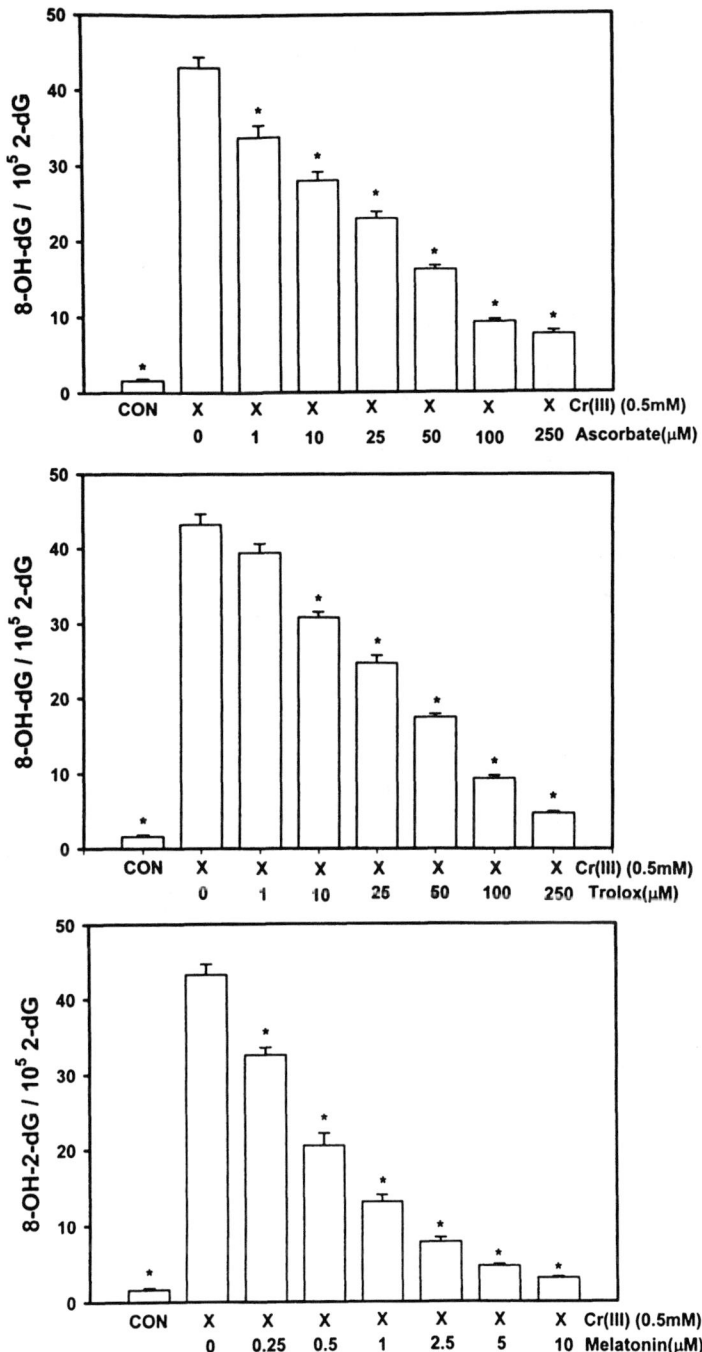

Figure 6 Levels of the damaged DNA product 8-hydroxydeoxyguanosine (8-OHdG) in purified calf thymus DNA after incubating it with a combination of chromium (III) and H_2O_2, which generates the hydroxyl radical. As shown here, increasing concentrations of ascorbate (top panel), Trolox (vitamin E) (middle panel), and melatonin (bottom panel) dose-dependently inhibit the accumulation of the oxidatively damaged product. In this system melatonin was far superior to either vitamins C or E in reducing the damage (note the concentrations of each that were used). (From Ref. 236.)

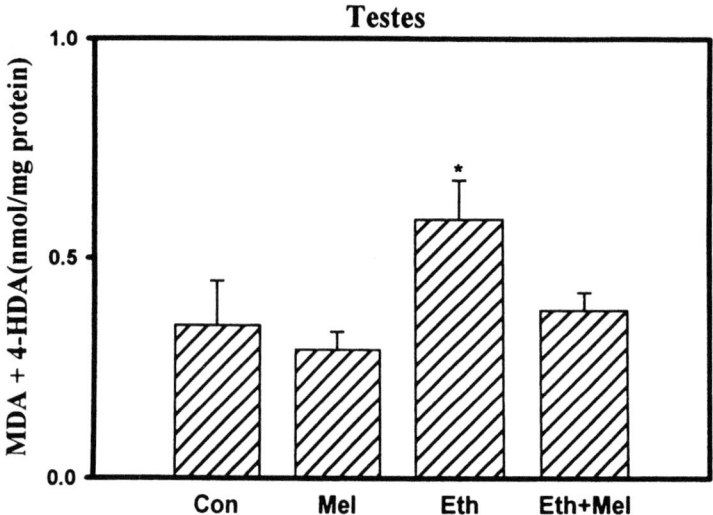

Figure 7 Lipid peroxidation, represented by levels of malondialdehyde (MDA) and 4-hydroxyalkenals (4-HDA), in the testes of rats given a daily subcutaneous injection of ethanol (ETH) for 30 days. In all organs investigated (testes are shown here but also in lung, heart, and brain), melatonin coadministration reduced lipid breakdown products. (From Ref. 244.)

are increased. The primary manifestations of these conditions are cutaneous photosensitivity and neural dysfunction. One of the major heme precursors that accumulates is δ-aminolevulinic acid (ALA) (246). Much of the pathology associated with porphyria has been attributed to ALA (247), and this damage is believed to be related to reactive oxygen- or nitrogen-based species (247). Hepatic carcinoma sometimes occurs in these patients (246).

Because reactive species are presumed to be responsible for the damage and dysfunction associated with ALA, antioxidants would be expected to reduce the molecular destruction and prevent the functional impairment. Princ et al. (248) incubated rat cerebellar tissue with ALA and observed large increases in MDA levels. On the other hand, coincubation of the tissues with ALA plus varying concentrations of melatonin prevented lipid damage; the response to melatonin was concentration-dependent. In a similar study, Carneiro and Reiter (249) revealed essentially the same protection by melatonin against ALA. In this study, PUFA oxidation in rat cerebral cortical, cerebellar, or striatal homogenates treated with ALA was reduced by melatonin. Although both groups hypothesized that the protective actions of melatonin against ALA toxicity related to the indole's ability to directly detoxify radicals and reactive species, Princ and co-workers (250) have also provided evidence that melatonin's stimulatory effect on antioxidative enzymes, particularly GPx, may be important in reducing ALA-mediated tissue damage.

Inasmuch as acute hepatic porphyria is associated with cancer of the liver (246), Carneiro and Reiter (251) extended their studies to include the viscera as well. In both liver and kidney homogenates, melatonin again prevented the accumulation of MDA and related lipid products induced by ALA when melatonin was not present.

The findings presented by these two groups suggest the usefulness of melatonin to treat various porphyric conditions. It is of interest that individuals with acute intermittent porphyria have reduced levels of circulating melatonin relative to individuals without the condition (252,253). This could represent a reduced synthesis or an increased utilization owing to melatonin's scavenging of elevated production of reactive species. The findings that melatonin reduces ALA-related oxidative damage may have applicability to lead poisoning in which ALA also accumulates.

J. Exercise

Prolonged or excessive exercise induces the generation of reactive species, which can result in tissue damage (254,255). When rats were forced to swim with no recourse to rest for 30 min, elevated levels of oxidized lipids were measured in the muscles of their hind legs (256,257). Furthermore, this severe exercise caused increased levels of both reduced and oxidized glutathione levels and a reduction in the ratio of reduced/oxidized isoforms in the liver, indicative of oxidative stress. These changes were prevented if rats were given melatonin before the swimming bout. In another study, running rats to exhaustion on a treadmill caused a significant hypoglycemia and increased levels of lactate and β-hydroxybutyrate, together with a marked reduction of glycogen in muscle and liver. Melatonin administration in advance of the forced run significantly elevated tissue glycogen levels and reduced plasma levels of lactate and β-hydroxybutyrate (258). These changes may also relate to melatonin's antioxidant properties.

K. Hyperoxia

Significant increases in inhaled oxygen not surprisingly leads to increased oxidative damage widely accepted to relate to elevated reactive species generation. Pablos et al. (259) placed rats in an environment of 100% oxygen at 4 atm for 90 min and tested whether melatonin, given before their exposure, would modify their response to hyperbaric hyperoxia. The lungs of untreated rats exhibited increased levels of oxidized lipids at the conclusion of exposure. Likewise, GPx and GRd activities were reduced in the lung and a variety of brain areas, and total glutathione (reduced plus oxidized) and glutathione disulfide levels were increased in the same tissues. Pretreatment with melatonin overcame the changes associated with the hyperbaric, hyperoxic responses, likely related to melatonin's antioxidant capacity.

When bovine cerebral endothelial cells were grown in culture and exposed to a high (95–100%) oxygen atmosphere they exhibited increased levels of DNA fragmentation, DNA laddering, and evidence of apoptotic changes (260). In a dose-dependent manner, melatonin reduced the DNA fragmentation and the apoptotic signs, indicating that exposure of the cells to reactive species was reduced when melatonin was present.

L. Reactive Oxygen- and Nitrogen-Based Species

A single study was uncovered that indicates that melatonin protects against singlet oxygen ($^1O_2$) toxicity. Primary cerebellar granule cell cultures were used to investigate this interaction, and the photosensitizer, rose bengal, followed by bright light exposure was used to generate $^1O_2$. As a consequence of this treatment, the granule cells experienced impaired mitochondrial function (estimated by the rate of reduction of 3-[4,5-dimethylthiazol-2-yl]-2,5-diphenyl tetrazolium bromide into formazan), degradation of the enzyme creatinine kinase, and apoptosis (67). Melatonin counteracted these cytotoxic changes, suggesting that the indole quenches $^1O_2$.

Hydrogen peroxide (H_2O_2) is readily converted to the ·OH and is often used to induce oxidative damage. The incubation of neural homogenates with H_2O_2 causes marked rises in lipid peroxidation that is prevented in a concentration-dependent manner by melatonin (261,262).

An analogue of melatonin (i.e., pinoline) was also protective against H_2O_2 toxicity (262). In cultured cerebellar granule cells, melatonin was also protective against H_2O_2, although the metabolic precursor of melatonin, N-acetylserotonin, proved more effective (179). The reduction of H_2O_2 toxicity was associated with a suppressed NF-κB, a transcription factor previously shown to be inhibited by melatonin (263,264).

Retinal homogenates rapidly undergo peroxidation when incubated with $FeSO_4$ which converts H_2O_2 to ˙OH. The rise in TBARS in these homogenates is reduced in a concentration-dependent manner by melatonin (265,266). When the efficacy of melatonin was compared with vitamin E (266), the EC_{50} of the former compound was lower. Melatonin also reduced MDA levels in rat cell membranes derived from a variety of organs when they were incubated with ferric ammonium citrate (267). This group proposed the potential usefulness of melatonin in iron-overload diseases.

Melatonin reportedly decreased H_2O_2-induced chromosomal aberrations in cultured CHO cells (268); however, it was less efficient in protecting against sister chromatid exchanges. Also using the cytokinesis-block micronucleus technique, Romero et al. (269) found that melatonin effectively reduced H_2O_2-induced micronucleus formation. Furthermore, merely incubating U-937 cells with melatonin reduced the spontaneous formation of micronuclei. In pharmacological concentrations melatonin reduced MCF-7 cell death caused by the addition of H_2O_2 to the medium (270). In this report, the authors claim that melatonin is not a likely physiological antioxidant because only pharmacological concentrations protected the cells against death. However, pharmacological levels of H_2O_2 were also used so it would not be expected that normal intracellular concentrations of any antioxidant could prevent the death of the cells.

Okatani and colleagues (271,272) have investigated whether H_2O_2 potentiates vascular tonic concentrations in the human umbilical arteries. They also evaluated the effects of modulating endogenous production of NO˙- and ˙OH-scavenging activity of melatonin on H_2O_2-induced vasoconstriction in the same preparations. In fact, treating umbilical arteries with H_2O_2 enhanced vascular tension. Melatonin restored relaxation, likely by reducing endothelial NOS activity and by scavenging the ˙OH radical. Melatonin inhibits NOS activity in other tissues (82,83,215) and scavenges ˙OH (29,49,52,273). Melatonin also may have mediated relaxation by directly scavenging NO˙ (69). The results imply that melatonin may have use as a treatment in preeclampsia.

Enzymes that detoxify reactive species and free radicals serve to reduce oxidative stress. Several of these have been stimulated by melatonin. In the fruit fly, inhibition of catalase resulted in a high incidence of death and the formation of protein carbonyls and lipid peroxidation products. Not only was the molecular damage prevented by feeding the flies food containing melatonin, but also death was almost totally averted (274). The findings here are consistent with melatonin functioning as an antioxidant.

GSH is an important intracellular antioxidant that, when depleted, leads to extensive free radical-mediated molecular destruction. One model of GSH depletion has frequently been used to illustrate the role of free radicals in cataractogenesis. When newborn rodents are treated with a GSH synthesis inhibitor, buthionine sulfoxamine (BSO), they develop grossly visible cataracts by the time they reach 2 weeks age (275). Both Abe et al. (276) and Li and co-workers (277) used this model to test whether rats that develop cataracts from GSH deficiency would benefit from melatonin treatment. These studies showed that, in fact, melatonin prevented observable cataracts in rats essentially devoid of GSH, indicating that the depressed antioxidative status was restored by melatonin supplementation. These workers also measured lenticular GSH levels and found that they were not restored by melatonin, suggesting that the antioxidant properties of melatonin per se were responsible in inhibiting cataractogenesis.

M. Stress

One well-known consequence of stress in rats is gastric ulcer formation. Over a decade ago it was shown that pinealectomy exacerbates stress-induced ulcers (278), and melatonin administration reduces gastric ulceration (279) as a consequence of immobilization. These observations actually preceded the knowledge that ˙OH contributes to gastric mucosal damage (280), and that melatonin neutralizes the ˙OH (49) as well as other reactive species. Without this information, Khan et al. (278,279) assumed that the protective actions of melatonin related to its general tranquilizing action.

Subsequent studies (64,114,281) have also shown that melatonin reduces the incidence and size of ulcers in the gastric mucosa of rats subjected to stress associated with restraint and cold exposure. Melatonin was better than GSH and equipotent to α-tocopherol in reducing the stress-induced lesions and, in this case, melatonin's protective actions were related to its ability to scavenge specifically the ˙OH radical (64). Another group of workers, however, claim that melatonin's protective actions against gastric ulcers may also require an interaction with cell bodies in the hypothalamus (280). In these same studies, melatonin reduced the negative effect of both aspirin (114) and indomethacin (64,282), in terms of ulcer formation in the stomach.

N. Drugs

Doxorubicin (Adriamycin), an anthracycline antibiotic, is a well-known and widely used chemotherapeutic agent that is used as a treatment for several blood dyscrasias. Its clinical use is, however, limited because of its collateral toxicity. Although damaging a number of organs, the cardiotoxic effects are especially serious and can lead to congestive heart failure (283). The toxicity of doxorubicin likely relates to its ability to generate free radicals by complex pathways that have been partly identified (284).

When doxorubicin was injected into rats, it increased levels of lipoperoxides in the plasma, cerebral cortex, and hypothalamus, and decreased hypothalamic catalase activity (76). These changes reverted to normal in doxorubicin-treated rats that were also given melatonin. Similarly, the nephropathy associated with doxorubicin administration was prevented by melatonin (285). In reference to the kidney, melatonin's beneficial actions were particularly notable in terms of its ability to reduce doxorubicin-induced lipid peroxidation and loss of proteins in the urine. Additionally, melatonin treatment maintained GSH concentrations that were otherwise depressed by the chemotherapeutic agent (286).

In addition to preserving renal function, melatonin also reduces the toxic reactions of doxorubicin in other organs. Importantly, Morishima et al. (287,288) found that melatonin ameliorated the cardiomyopathy associated with the therapeutic agent. Cardiac changes induced by doxorubicin included decreased heart weight and arterial pressure, left ventricular fractional shortening, accumulation of ascites, accumulation of TBARS, and ultrastructural changes. The morphological, biochemical, and functional changes that accompanied doxorubicin administration were prevented by melatonin. Finally, the toxicity of the drug in the bone marrow (288) and less dramatically in the liver (289,200) was reduced.

Because doxorubicin does not depend on its free radical-generating ability to inhibit cancerous cells, melatonin could possibly be used in conjunction with this therapeutic agent to reduce those side effects that are free radical-based. Also, because melatonin has oncostatic actions (39), it could theoretically synergize with doxorubicin to increase its efficacy as an anticancer drug (Fig. 8).

Another widely used, albeit toxic, chemotherapeutic agent is cisplatin (291). One of its major side effects is damage of the outer hair cells of the organ of Corti resulting in hearing

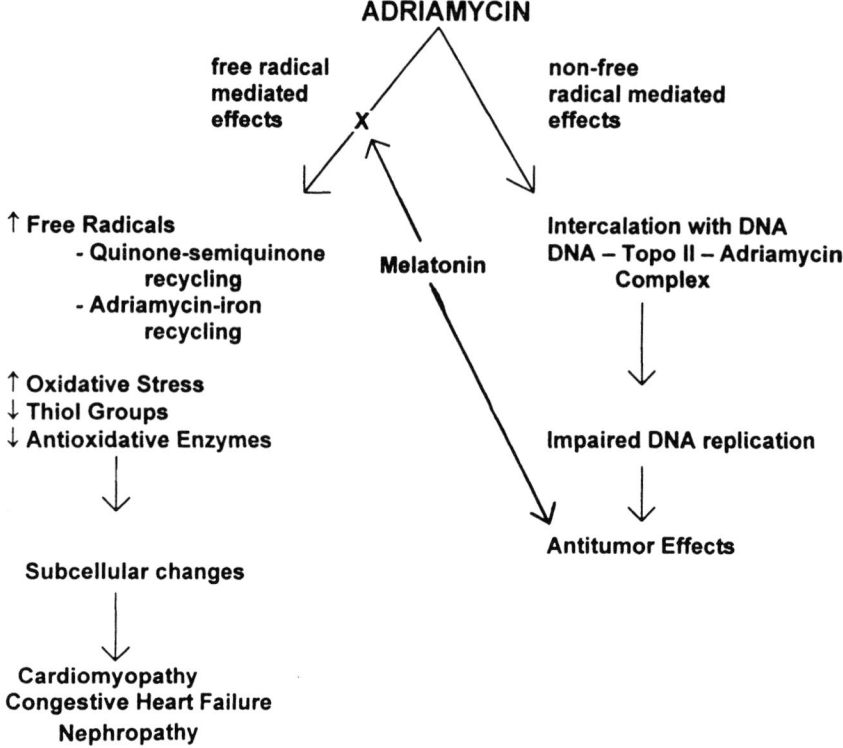

Figure 8 The chemotherapeutic agent doxorubicin (Adriamycin) has side effects, being particularly toxic to the heart and kidneys. The collateral toxicity, which has in part a free radical basis, is inhibited by melatonin in vivo. This action of melatonin does not interfere with the chemotherapeutic efficacy of doxorubicin and may in fact also reduce tumor growth because melatonin has oncostatic actions.

loss. Mechanistically it is known that the ototoxicity caused by cisplatin relates to its generation of free radicals (292). Rats given cisplatin develop functional damage to the auditory apparatus as manifested as distortion product otoacoustic emissions (DPOAEs). After withdrawal of the drug, DPOAEs returned to normal within about 30 days. When melatonin was injected, this time was reduced to 10–12 days (293). This is consistent with the effect of other antioxidants given under similar conditions.

Immunosuppression is another consequence of cisplatin toxicity. When human peripheral mononuclear cells were treated with the chemotherapeutic agent they exhibited an impaired proliferative response to phytohemagglutinin (PHA), and they exhibited GSH depletion and increased DNA fragmentation; in contrast, in cells treated with melatonin the toxicity of cisplatin was significantly diminished (294). In a separate study, the toxicity of the myelosuppressive drug, cytarabine (cytosine arabinoside), was also reversed when melatonin was present (295).

Cyclosporine is a widely used immunosuppressive drug that is helpful in preventing allograft rejection after heart, liver, or kidney transplantation; however, the drug has nephrotoxicity characterized as tubulointerstitial fibrosis (297). In rats treated with cyclosporine, blood urea, serum creatinine, and plasma MDA levels were elevated, and a decrease in renal creatinine and lithium clearance occurred. These changes were significantly antagonized by cotreatment of the animals with melatonin (297). Inasmuch as free radicals are believed to be consequential in cyclosporine toxicity, melatonin's protective actions against the drug were presumed to relate to its antioxidant properties.

The aminoglycosides, gentamicin and tobramycin, are toxic because they generate free radicals in the outer hair cells of the organ of Corti, and antioxidants can be protective when the drugs are used (298). This being so, Lopez–Gonzalez et al. (299) gave melatonin in conjunction with either gentamicin or tobramycin, and in both cases, the damaging effects of the drugs to the inner ear were abated. The reduction in ototoxicity by melatonin may have involved its direct-scavenging activity as well as its indirect antioxidant effects. Importantly, although protective against the side effects of the drug, melatonin did not interfere with their antibiotic capacity.

Haloperidol is used to treat acute as well as chronic psychoses. This neuroleptic drug exhibits cytotoxicity by mechanisms that involve free radicals (300). Incubating HT22 hippocampal cells with haloperidol was followed by a rise in intracellular peroxides and a drop in GSH levels, signs indicative of enhanced oxidative stress. Both melatonin and its precursor N-acetylserotonin in addition to α-tocopherol retarded these changes, with the latter molecule exhibiting the greatest efficacy (301).

A commonly used anticonvulsant drug is carbamazepine. During long-term use it possesses some genotoxic effects, but the evidence that it actually damages DNA by means of free radical mechanisms remains incomplete. Analysis of human lymphocytes treated with carbamazepine showed a significant dose-dependent rise in chromosomal aberrations and sister chromotid exchanges; these increases were prevented when melatonin was added to the culture medium (302).

O. Chemical Toxins

The earliest studies that documented melatonin's ability to protect against free radical-generating toxins utilized safrole. The resulting reports revealed that both pharmacological and physiological levels of melatonin were sufficient to reduce DNA damage caused by the carcinogen safrole (303,304). Other carcinogens against which melatonin has been protective include N-nitroso-N-methylurea (305) and 7,12-dimethylbenz[a]anthracene (306).

Carbon tetrachloride (CCl_4) is a well-known environmental hazard that is a potent agent in damaging the liver. Its toxicity is widely believed to be related to its free radical-generating potential. When rats were treated with CCl_4 in the absence of melatonin, increased levels of TBARS and decreased GSH content were recorded. Despite the high hepatic toxicity of CCl_4, melatonin is able to reduce the resulting lipid peroxidation, although not all aspects of hepatic dysfunction are reversed by giving the indole (307,308). Another hepatotoxicant, 2-nitropropane, when given to rats, induced phospholipid breakdown not only in the liver, but also in the lung and kidney; these changes were both dose- and time-dependent. Additionally, serum sorbital dehydrogenase (SDH) activity is elevated in the serum as a consequence of the liver damage (309). These changes were reduced by melatonin in a dose-dependent manner. Another liver toxicant, α-naphthylisothiocyanate (ANIT) causes free radical damage similar to that seen with a variety of other agents. ANIT toxicity is attenuated by melatonin treatment as well (310).

Tying a ligature around the extrahepatic biliary duct causes hepatic cholestasis, resulting in massive damage to the liver from the backflow of bile. This causes pronounced oxidative damage in the hepatic tissue, with morphological, biochemical, and physiological deterioration of the organ. In a detailed study of the consequences of interruption of bile flow in the bile duct (311), melatonin reduced the degree of hepatic oxidative damage from cholestasis. The treatment with melatonin was so effective that the authors suggested it as a possible therapeutic agent in biliary cholestasis.

Nitrilotriacetic acid (NTA) is a renal toxin that induces acute and subacute renal proximal tubular necrosis and an increased incidence of renal adenocarcinoma. When rats were treated with NTA, the kidneys exhibited oxidative damage in the form of increased renal hydroperoxides and 8-OHdG levels. Treating the animals with melatonin immediately before NTA administration reduced the severity of both parameters of oxidative stress (312). A kidney-specific carcinogen potassium bromate ($KBrO_3$) induces oxidative damage in rats in the form of augmented levels of 8-OHdG. Melatonin partially prevented the free radical damage caused by the administration of $KBrO_3$, similar to the other antioxidants that were tested (313); melatonin was, however, not as effective as resveratrol in ameliorating the oxidative damage.

Colitis is induced in rats by the administration of dinitrobenzene sulfonic acid (DNBS). Prolonged colitis normally is associated with an increased cancer risk at a later date; the tumors are a result of the free radical damage that occurs in DNA during the bout of colitis. DNBS toxicity, as evidenced by the severity of inflammation in the bowel, was reduced by melatonin (314).

A common method for inducing pancreatitis in experimental animals is to give them cerulein, a molecule that induces free radicals. Qi et al. (315) reported that cerulein does indeed cause acute pancreatitis in rats, but its administration also causes gastric oxidative damage. Melatonin reduced the edema as well as lipid peroxidation induced by intraperitoneal injection of cerulein. It was ineffective in reducing the rise in serum amylase activity that was caused by cerulein.

Paraquat is a herbicide that is especially toxic to the lungs because after its uptake by this tissue it undergoes redox recycling. The mortality associated with paraquat as well as the increased levels of lipid peroxidation were greatly reduced by melatonin (316). Likewise, melatonin ameliorated paraquat toxicity in peripheral blood cells, as indicated by reduced evidence of cytological genotoxicity (317).

Collectively, the findings showing that melatonin reduces oxidative stress induced by such a wide variety of chemical toxins strongly suggest that the indole functions as a highly effective free radical scavenger and antioxidant. The results, however, show that not all aspects of oxidative damage are reversed by melatonin administration. This is common when testing the efficacy of other antioxidants as well. In general, melatonin seems to be roughly as effective as other well-known antioxidants in protecting against chemical toxins.

P. Experimental Models of Diabetes

From several perspectives, diabetes mellitus is a free radical-related disease. The destruction of the β-cells of the pancreas by a variety of chemical agents involves free radicals (318,319), and the hyperglycemia associated with the functional and morphological deterioration and loss of the β-cells leads to damage to a number of tissues because of the generation of reactive species (320). The development of autoimmune diabetes (type I) is accelerated in neonatal pinealectomized, nonobese diabetic (NOD) mice and slowed in those animals supplemented with melatonin (321). Although here the actions of melatonin could have been by stimulation of the immune system that led to a preservation of β-cell integrity, melatonin could also have scavenged the free radicals normally released by lymphocytes that invade the islets during autoimmune diabetes (322).

Ebelt and colleagues (323) tested whether melatonin would modify the response of isolated β-cells to two different free radical-generating systems (i.e., alloxan treatment and their exposure to xanthine oxidase–hypoxanthine [XO/HX]). Incubating β-cells with either alloxan and XO/HX causes a transient rise in released insulin. Alloxan also killed some cells by what was presumed to be necrotic processes, whereas XO/HX caused apoptosis of some of the cells. Melatonin prevented the changes induced by alloxan but, unexpectedly, not those caused by XO/HX treatment. With use of a spin trap and ESR, melatonin was shown to readily scavenge ·OH. The failure of melatonin to reduce XO/HX damage to the cells was, in the authors opinion, related to their particular perfusion system that only allowed the generation of $O_2^{·-}$ in or near the β-cells. Melatonin is generally believed to have minimal scavenging effect on $O_2^{·-}$.

Melatonin has also been given in conjunction with another β-cell–specific toxin, streptozocin (STZ). When given to rats STZ causes a variety of predictable changes that are typical of β-cells loss and the resulting hyperglycemia. Melatonin coadministration reduced the severity of diabetes, as indicated by its ability to decrease hyperglycemia, reduce lipoperoxide concentrations in erythrocytes, replenish the erythrocyte GSH, and lower protein glycosylation (324). The authors content that melatonin is a promising antioxidant that may have use in the treatment of complications of diabetes.

In diabetic patients, nephropathy is a common finding. This pathology, which begins as microvascular complications, is initiated by hyperglycemia and is believed to involve free radicals (325). When rats with STZ-induced diabetes were treated with melatonin or another antioxidant, taurine, both agents prevented the increases in glomerular transforming growth factor (TGF)-β_1 and fibronectin mRNAs and proteinuria associated with the diabetic condition, without influencing blood glucose levels (326). Similarly, both antioxidants reduced urinary and blood lipid peroxidation products. These results reemphasize the widely held view that free radical generation contributes to the complications of diabetes and treatment with either melatonin or taurine may ameliorate some of the destructive processes associated with this disease.

This opinion, at least in reference to melatonin, is also shared by Sailaja Devi et al. (327). In rats suffering from diabetes caused by alloxan treatment, these workers observed increased TBARS in plasma and liver, whereas SOD and GPx activities in red blood cells and liver were depressed. Melatonin reversed these changes and did so, as reported also by Ha et al. (326), without depressing hyperglycemia. The authors surmised that melatonin's antioxidant properties accounted for the changes induced.

Q. Ultraviolet Radiation Damage

A major issue in dermatology is damage to the skin by ultraviolet (UV) light. Prolonged and repeated exposure to UV radiation causes accelerated skin aging (photoaging), elastosis, and tumor development (328,329). The most common adverse skin reaction from UV radiation is sunburn (erythema). It is commonly agreed that the damage the skin sustains when exposed to UV rays has its basis in free radical generation (330). This being so, Bangha et al. (331) predicted that melatonin may protect the skin from such damage. A small patch of the skin of human volunteers was exposed to 0.099 J/cm^2 UVB radiation, with and without treatment with topically applied melatonin in a nanocolloidal gel carrier. The degree of erythema was evaluated 5 h later using a visual-scoring method and a more objective method, chromametry. Melatonin significantly reduced the erythema, in a manner consistent with the amount applied. The inhibition of sunburn was observed at a dose of melatonin as low as 0.5% of the applied cream. Although melatonin's protective action could mean it acted as a sun screen, the authors feel that more likely it was the free radical-scavenging properties of the indole that accounted for its beneficial effect.

Melatonin has also been compared with vitamins C and E in terms of their ability to protect the skin from UV radiation damage (332); again humans were the test subjects. In this case the severity of erythema was evaluated visually, using chromametry, by measuring dermal blood flow, by determining transepidermal water loss, and by measuring the electrical capacitance of the skin. When melatonin was topically applied, it caused a dose-dependent inhibition of erythema. A combination of melatonin plus vitamin E was more effective. Maximal protection was achieved using a coformulation of 1% melatonin, 2% vitamin E, and 5% vitamin C. These workers also tested the ability of melatonin to function as a sunscreen and observed that it did in fact show significant UVB/UVC absorption. Thus, the authors concluded that melatonin probably acts by at least two methods; namely, as a scavenger and as a filter, in reducing skin damage by UV radiation.

The observations just summarized were essentially confirmed by Fischer et al. (333). Also using human volunteers this group noted that the topical application of melatonin before UV exposure reduced erythema, as assessed visually and by chromametry. They also observed that melatonin absorbs UV light only in the 225- to 275-nm range (clearly below the wavelength of UVA and UVB, which ranges from 290 to 390 nm). Because of this, they conclude that melatonin resists damage from UV exposure because of its direct radical-detoxifying ability, especially in relation to ·OH (334).

R. Mitochondrial Dysfunction

That melatonin acts to modulate mitochondrial physiology is suggested by several studies. Gilad et al. (335) reported that melatonin protected against $ONOO^-$-induced suppression of mitochondrial respiration. Also, Yamamoto and Tang (336,337) noted that melatonin inhibited seizure activity, brain lipid peroxidation, and the lethality of mice treated with cyanide. Although actions of cyanide are complex, it does function as a mitochondrial toxin (338).

More detailed studies related to melatonin's activity at the level of the mitochondria have been performed as well (339,340). When injected into rats in pharmacological doses, melatonin stimulated the activity of mitochondrial complexes I and IV; these changes were time-dependent and correlated with the levels of melatonin in the blood. Ruthenium red, a mitochondrial toxin, suppressed the activity of complexes I and IV, with these effects being prevented by coadministration of melatonin. Similarly, the rise in lipid peroxidation products induced by ruthenium red was also counteracted by melatonin. Ruthenium red, at the levels used, behaves as a pro-oxidant by acting as a Fenton-type reagent (341). Thus, melatonin's stimulatory and protective effects of mitochondrial complexes I and IV presumably relate to its free radical-scavenging activity, although further studies are required to clarify this point (339).

Because they lack the antioxidative enzyme catalase, mitochondria depend heavily on GPx to detoxify reactive oxygen species. In isolated mitochondria, melatonin was found to promote recycling of GSH, as it increased the activities of both GPx and GRd and, furthermore, the indole elevated total GSH levels (340). Perhaps more importantly, the indole prevented the changes induced by *tert*-butylhydroperoxide (*t*-BPH). In isolated mitochondria incubated with *t*-BHP the level of hydroperoxides increased, 90% of the GSH was reduced to GSSG, and the activities of both GPx and GRd were almost totally suppressed. At a concentration of 100 nM, melatonin counteracted these changes and mediated rises in complexes I and IV in submitochondrial particles isolated from liver and brain. When vitamin C was substituted for melatonin, it had no protective effect at the level of the mitochondria, while vitamin E, only at 1 mM, stimulated total GSH levels and reduced hydroperoxide formation. Thus, melatonin was much better than either vitamin in promoting optimal mitochondrial function and reducing the damage associated with *t*-BHP. In fetal rat brain as well, giving melatonin to the pregnant mother was recently found to protect the mitochondria from oxidative damage (342). Considering

S. Low-Density Lipoprotein Oxidation

A major area of interest for free radical biologists is atherosclerosis and related cardiovascular conditions. Although the etiology of atherosclerosis is multifactorial, free radical damage is believed to be a contributory factor. In particular the oxidation of low-density lipoprotein (LDL) increases its athrogenicity (343).

Several reports show that LDL oxidation can be retarded by melatonin. Three of these reports are based on in vitro studies and show that oxidative modification of LDL is reduced in the presence of high concentrations of melatonin (344–346). In the latter study, melatonin was less effective than vitamin E in reducing LDL oxidation (347). This group did find, however, that the metabolic product of melatonin (i.e., 6-hydroxymelatonin) had a potency equivalent to that of vitamin E in lowering the oxidation of LDL, and N-acetylserotonin was more effective than vitamin E.

Treatment of normolipidemic, postmenopausal women with melatonin (6 mg daily for 2 weeks) provided evidence that it is capable of lowering the susceptibility of LDL to oxidative modification in vivo (348). This treatment paradigm lowered plasma triglycerides, but did not significantly alter total cholesterol, high-density lipoprotein (HDL), or LDL levels in plasma. In an in vivo study that used rats. melatonin attenuate the rises in plasma total cholesterol and in LDL associated with eating a cholesterol-enriched diet and, furthermore, the indole prevented the reduction in HDL normally seen in such cases (349). In the same report, the liver, brain, spleen, and heart contained depressed levels of lipid peroxides at the end of the experiment. These findings are consistent with an early report that claimed that melatonin treatment depressed plasma cholesterol and reduced fatty liver changes in genetically hypercholesterolemic rats (350).

Other data also suggest a beneficial effect of melatonin against the damage inflicted by cholesterol. According to Müller–Wieland et al. (351) melatonin reduces the synthesis of cholesterol from lanosteral and decreases the number of LDL receptor sites. When human umbilical arteries were incubated with oxidized LDL, vascular tension was increased significantly. Melatonin reduced the vasospastic effect of oxidized LDL, presumably related to its ability to scavenge ˙OH that is generated in tissues exposed to oxidized LDL (352). The vasoconstrictor effect of a component of LDL (i.e., lysophosphatidylcholine) is also inhibited by melatonin (353).

III. CONCLUDING REMARKS AND PERSPECTIVE

Since the discovery of melatonin as a free radical scavenger (49), there has been a veritable deluge of papers investigating the antioxidant properties of this indole. Indeed, merely examining reviews on this subject that only recently appeared (354–356), readily emphasizes the rapidity with which this field is developing. Despite the advances, the present reviewers feel we have only uncovered the tip of this "proverbial iceberg." Melatonin's efficacy in reducing free radical damage is not explainable by merely the direct-scavenging activity of the molecule. Rather, it is likely that it has multiple means to reduce oxidative stress. Furthermore, we predict that both receptor-independent and receptor-mediated processes are involved in melatonin's antioxidative actions. The receptors involved may be the well-defined membrane receptors that have been described but, additionally, actions at the level of nuclear receptors should be considered.

A remarkable diversity of studies have been carried out to define melatonin's antioxidative capacity. Rarely, has it failed to perform in protecting molecules from oxidative damage. The pro-oxidant effects of the molecule, based on the data yet published, are negligible, although more effort should be directed at defining any potential in this. Besides its minimal pro-oxidant effects, the molecule has little intrinsic toxicity. Virtually no acute or chronic toxicity has been described in any species, and an LD_{50} (a dose that is lethal to 50% of the animals) has not been established, despite attempts to do so.

One of the major perplexing questions is the role of melatonin as a physiological antioxidant. It is usually argued that the levels (based on measurements of melatonin in blood) are too low to be physiologically relevant in terms of free radical-scavenging. Estimates of blood levels, however, may provide no information on melatonin concentrations within cells and specifically within subcellular compartments. Also, it is already known that some body fluids have melatonin levels orders of magnitude higher than in blood. This indicates that melatonin concentrations throughout the organism are not in equilibrium. Despite what is finally uncovered relative to melatonin's physiological relevance as an antioxidant, there is no doubt pharmacologically it is highly protective during oxidative challenges. Additional research will help further clarify the value of melatonin in the reduction of oxidative stress.

ACKNOWLEDGMENTS

Work by the authors was supported in part by grants from NIH and from Amoun Pharmaceutical Company.

REFERENCES

1. Lerner AB, Case JD, Takahashi Y. (1958) Isolation of melatonin, a pineal factor that lightens melanocytes. J Am Chem Soc 80:2587.
2. Rollag MD. (1988) Response of amphibian melanophores to melatonin. Pineal Res Rev 6:67–95.
3. Pang SF, Allen AE. (1986) Extra-pineal melatonin in the retina: its regulation and physiological function. Pineal Res Rev 4:55–96.
4. Cahill GM, Grace MS, Besharse JC. (1991) Rhythmic regulation of retinal melatonin: metabolic pathways, neurochemical regulation and the ocular circadian clock. Cell Mol Neurobiol 11:529–535.
5. Menendez–Pelaez A, Reiter RJ, Guerrero JM, Puig–Domingo M, Howes KA. (1988) Sexual dimorphism in N-acetyltransferase activity, hydroxyindole-O-methyltransferase activity and melatonin content in the harderian gland of Syrian hamsters: changes following gonadectomy. Proc Soc Exp Biol Med 187:287–291.
6. Mhatre MC, van Jaarsveld AS, Reiter RJ. (1988) Melatonin in the lacrimal gland: first demonstration and experimental manipulation. Biochem Biophys Res Commun 153:1186–1192.
7. Bubenik GA, Ball RO, Pang SF. (1992) The effect of food deprivation on brain and gastrointestinal tissue levels of trypophan, serotonin, 5-hydroxyindoleacetic acid, and melatonin. J Pineal Res 12:7–12.
8. Huether G. (1994) Melatonin synthesis in the gastrointestinal tract and the impact of nutritional factors on circulating melatonin. Ann NY Acad Sci 719:146–151.
9. Reiter RJ. (1991) Pineal melatonin: cell biology of its synthesis and of its physiological interactions. Endocrin Rev 12:151–180.
10. Menendez–Pelaez A, Poeggeler B, Reiter RJ, Barlow–Walden L, Pablos MI, Tan DX. (1993) Nuclear localization of melatonin in different mammalian tissues: immunocytochemical and radioimmunoassay evidence. J Cell Biochem 53:373–382.
11. Menendez–Pelaez A, Reiter RJ. (1993) Distribution of melatonin in mammalian tissues: relative importance of nuclear verses cytosolic localization. J Pineal Res 15:59–69.

12. Laudon M, Zisapel N. (1991) Melatonin binding proteins identified in rat brain by affinity labeling. FEBS Lett 288:105–108.
13. Lahiri DK, Davis D, Nurenberger JI, Jr. (1994) Melatonin-like immunoreactivity in the presence of different chemicals as determined by radioimmunoassay. Biochem Med Metab Biol 51:51–54.
14. Tan DX, Manchester LC, Reiter RJ, Qi W, Zhang M, Weintraub ST, Cabrera J, Sainz RM, Mayo JC. (1999) Identification of highly elevated levels of melatonin in bone marrow: its origin and significance. Biochim Biophys Acta 1472:206–214.
15. Conti A, Conconi S, Hertens E, Skwarlo–Sonta K, Markowska M, Maestroni GJM. (2000) Melatonin synthesis in mouse and human bone marrow. J Pineal Res 28:193–202.
16. Hedlund L, Lischko MM, Rollag MD, Niswender GD. (1977) Melatonin: daily cycle in plasma and cerebrospinal fluid of calves. Science 195:686–687.
17. Kanematsu N, Mori Y, Hayashi S, Hoshino K. (1989) Presence of a distinct 24-hour melatonin rhythm in the ventricular cerebrospinal fluid of the goat. J Pineal Res 7:143–152.
18. Skinner DC, Malpaux B. (1999) High melatonin concentrations in third ventricular cerebrospinal fluid are not due to Galen vein blood recirculating through the choroid plexus. Endocrinology 140:4399–4405.
19. Tan DX, Manchester LC, Reiter RJ, Qi W, Hanes MA, Farley NJ. (1999) High physiological levels of melatonin in the bile of mammals. Life Sci 65:2523–2529.
20. Poeggeler B, Reiter RJ, Tan DX, Chen LD, Manchester LC. (1993) Melatonin, hydroxyl radical-mediated oxidative damage and aging: a hypothesis. J Pineal Res 14:151–168.
21. Reiter RJ. (1996) Functional aspects of the pineal hormone melatonin in combatting cell and tissue damage induced by free radicals: a review. Eur J Endocrinol 134:412–420.
22. Okatani Y, Okamoto K, Hayashi K, Wakatsuki A, Tumura S, Sagara Y. (1998) Maternal–fetal transfer of melatonin in pregnant women near term. J Pineal Res 25:129–134.
23. Schenker S, Yang Y, Perez A, Acuff RV, Papas AM, Henderson G, Lee MP. (1998) Antioxidant transport by the human placenta. Clin Nutr 17:159–167.
24. Hattori A, Migitaka H, Masayaki I, Itoh M, Yamamoto K, Oktani–Kaneko R, Hara M, Suzuki T, Reiter RJ. (1995) Identification of melatonin in plants and its effects on plasma melatonin levels and binding to melatonin receptors. Mol Biol Int 35:627–634.
25. Dubbels R, Reiter RJ, Klenke E, Goebel A, Schnakenberg E, Ehlers C, Schiwara HW, Schloat W. (1995) Melatonin in edible plants identified by radioimmunoassay and high performance liquid chromatography–mass spectrometry. J Pineal Res 18:28–31.
26. Hardeland R, Balzer I, Poeggeler B, Uria H, Behrmann G, Wolf R, Meyer TJ, Reiter RJ. (1995) On the primary functions of melatonin in evolution: mediation of photoperiodic signals in a unicell, photooxidation, and scavenging of free radicals. J Pineal Res 18:104–111.
27. Balzer I, Hardeland R. (1996) Melatonin in algae and higher plants—possible new roles as a phytohormone and antioxidant. Bot Acuta 109:180–183.
28. Murch SJ, Simmons CB, Saxena PX. (1997) Melatonin in feverfew and other medicinal plants. Lancet 350:1598–1599.
29. Tan DX, Manchester LC, Reiter RJ, Qi W, Karbownik M, Calvo JR. (2000) Significance of melatonin in the antioxidant defense system: reactions and products. Biol Signals Recept 9:160–171.
30. Reiter RJ. (1973) Pineal control of a seasonal reproductive rhythm in male golden hamsters exposed to natural daylight and temperature. Endocrinology 92:425–430.
31. Reiter RJ. (1980) The pineal and its hormones in the control of reproduction in mammals. Endocr Rev 1:109–131.
32. Vaughan MK, Vaughan GM. (1993) Metabolic and thyroidal consequences of melatonin administration in mammals. In: Yu HS, Reiter RJ, eds. Melatonin. Boca Raton, FL: CRC Press, pp. 311–348.
33. Reiter RJ. (1993) The melatonin rhythm: both a clock and a calendar. Experientia 49:654–664.
34. Armstrong SM, Redman JR. (1993) Melatonin and circadian rhythmicity. In: Yu HS, Reiter RJ, eds. Melatonin. Boca Raton, FL: CRC Press, pp. 187–224.
35. Wirz–Jurtice A, Armstrong SM. (1996) Melatonin: nature's soporific. J Sleep Res 5:137–141.
36. Dijk DJ, Cajochen C. (1997) Melatonin and circadian regulation of sleep initiation, consolidation, structure, and the sleep EEG. J Biol Rhythms 12:627–635.
37. Guerrero JM, Reiter RJ. (1992) A brief survey of pineal gland–immune system interactions. Endocrin Res 18:91–113.

38. Maestroni GJM, Hertens E, Galli P. (1997) New T-helper cell opioid cytokines as mediators of the immunological and hematopoietic action of melatonin. In: Maestroni GJM, Conti A, Reiter RJ, eds. Therapeutic Potential of Melatonin. Basel: Karger, pp. 62–71.
39. Blask DE, Sauer LA, Dauchy RT, Holowachuk EW, Ruhoff MS, Kopff HS. (1999) Melatonin inhibition of cancer growth in vivo involves suppression of tumor fatty acid metabolism via melatonin receptor-mediated signal transduction events. Cancer Res 59:4693–4701.
40. Lissoni P, Borni S, Mandala M, Ardizyoia A, Paolorossi F, Vaghi M, Longarine R, Malugani F, Tancini G. (1999) Decreased toxicity and increased efficacy of cancer chemotherapy with the pineal hormone melatonin in metastatic solid tumor patients with poor clinical status. Eur J Cancer 12:1672–1688.
41. Stankov B, Reiter RJ. (1990) Melatonin receptors: current status, facts and hypothesis. Life Sci 46:971–982.
42. Morgan RJ, Barrett P, Howell HE, Halliwell R. (1994) Melatonin receptors: localization, molecular pharmacology and physiological significance. Neurochem Int 24:101–146.
43. Reppert SM, Godson C, Mahle CD, Weaver DR, Slaugenhaupt SA, Gusella JF. (1995) Molecular characterization of a second melatonin receptor expressed in human retina and brain: the Mel1b melatonin receptor. Neuron 15:1013–1015.
44. Carlberg C, Wiesenberg I. (1995) The orphan receptor family RZR/ROR, melatonin and 5-lipoxygenase: an unexpected relationship. J Pineal Res 18:171–178.
45. Carlberg C, Wiesenberg I. (1997) Nuclear signaling of melatonin. In: Maestroni GJM, Conti A, Reiter RJ, eds. Therapeutic Potential of Melatonin. Basel: Karger, pp. 25–33.
46. Guerrero JM, Rafii-el-Idrissi M, Garcia–Pergañneda A, Garcia–Maurino S, Gil–Haba M, Pozo D, Calvo JR. (1997) Mechanisms of action of melatonin on human immune system, membrane and nuclear receptors. In: Maestroni GJM, Conti A, Reiter RJ, eds. Therapeutic Potential of Melatonin. Basel: Karger, pp. 43–51.
47. Reiter RJ. (1991) Melatonin: that ubiquitously acting pineal hormone. News Physiol Sci 6:223–227.
48. Ebadi M, Samejima M, Pfeiffer RF. (1993) Pineal gland in synchronizing and refining physiological events. News Physiol Sci 8:30–33.
49. Tan DX, Chen LD, Poeggeler B, Manchester LC, Reiter RJ. (1993) Melatonin: a potent, endogenous hydroxyl radical scavenger. Endocr J 1:57–60.
50. Poeggeler B, Saarela S, Reiter RJ, Tan DX, Chen LD, Manchester LC, Barlow–Walden LR. (1994) Melatonin—a highly potent endogenous radical scavenger and electron donor: new aspects of the oxidation chemistry of this indole assessed in vitro. Ann NY Acad Sci 738:419–420.
51. Poeggeler B, Reiter RJ, Hardeland R, Tan DX, Barlow–Walden LR. (1996) Melatonin and structurally related endogenous indoles act as potent electron donors and radical scavengers in vitro. Redox Rep 2:179–184.
52. Matuszek Z, Reszka K, Chignell CF. (1997) Reaction of melatonin and related indoles with hydroxyl radicals: ESR and spin trapping investigations. Free Radic Biol Med 23:367–372.
53. Roberts JE, Hu DN, Wishart JF. (1997) Pulse radiolysis studies of melatonin and choromelatonin. J Photochem Photobiol 42:125–132.
54. Li XJ, Zhang LM, Gu J, Zhang AZ, Sun FY. (1997) Melatonin decreases production of hydroxyl radical during ischemia–reperfusion. Acta Pharmacol Sinica 18:394–396.
55. Susa N, Ueno S, Furukawa Y, Ueda J, Sugiyama M. (1997) Potent protective effect of melatonin on chromium (VI)-induced DNA single-strand breaks, cytotoxicity and lipid peroxidation in primary cultures of rat hepatocytes. Toxicol Appl Pharmacol 144:377–384.
56. Stasica P, Ulanski P, Rosiak JM. (1998) Melatonin as a hydroxyl radical scavenger. J Pineal Res 25:65–66.
57. Stasica P, Ulanski P, Rosiak JM. (1998) Reactions of melatonin with radicals in deoxygenated aqueous solutions. J Radioanal Nucl Chem 232:107–113.
58. Tan DX, Manchester LC, Reiter RJ, Plummer BF, Hardies LJ, Weintraub ST, Vijayalaxmi, Shepherd AAM. (1998) A novel melatonin metabolite, cyclic 3-hydroxymelatonin: a biomarker of in vivo hydroxyl radical generation. Biochem Biophys Res Commun 253:614–620.
59. Pähkla R, Zilmer M, Kullisar T, Rägo L. (1998) Comparison of the antioxidant activity of melatonin and pinoline in vitro. J Pineal Res 24:96–101.
60. Zang LY, Cosma G, Gardner H, Vallynathan V. (1998) Scavenging of reactive oxygen species by melatonin. Biochim Biophys Acta 1425:467–477.

61. Mahal HS, Sharma HS, Mukherjee T. (1999) Antioxidant properties of melatonin: a pulse radiolysis study. Free Radic Biol Med 26:557–565.
62. Stasica P, Paneth P, Rosiak JM. (2000) Hydroxyl radical reaction with melatonin molecule: a computational study. J Pineal Res 29:125–127.
63. Brömme HJ, Mörke W, Peschkel E, Ebelt H, Peschke D. (2000) Scavenging effect of melatonin on hydroxyl radicals generated by alloxan. J Pineal Res 29:201–209.
64. Bandyopadhyay D, Biswas K, Bandyopadhyay V, Reiter RJ, Banerjee RK. (2000) Melatonin protects against stress-induced gastric lesions by scavenging the hydroxyl radical. J Pineal Res 29:143–151.
65. Marshall KA, Reiter RJ, Poeggeler B, Aruoma OI, Halliwell B. (1996) Evaluation of the antioxidant activity of melatonin in vitro. Free Radic Biol Med 2:307–315.
66. Dellegar SM, Murphy SA, Bourne AE, DiCesare JC, Purser GH. (1999) Identification of the factors affecting the rate of deactivation of hypochlorous acid by melatonin. Biochem Biophys Res Commun 254:431–439.
67. Cagnoli CM, Atabay C, Kharlamova E, Manev H. (1995) Melatonin protects neurons from singlet oxygen-induced apoptosis. J Pineal Res 18:222–226.
68. King M, Scaiano JC. (1997) The excited states of melatonin. Photochem Photobiol 65:538–542.
69. Noda Y, Mori A, Liburty R, Packer L. (1999) Melatonin and its precursors scavenge nitric oxide. J Pineal Res 27:159–163.
70. Gilad E, Cuzzocrea S, Zingarelli B, Salzman AL, Szabo C. (1997) Melatonin is a scavenger of peroxynitrite. Life Sci 60:PL169–PL174.
71. Salzman AL, Szabo C. (1997) Protective effect of melatonin in carrageenan-induced models of local inflammation: relationship to its inhibitory effect on nitric oxide production and its peroxynitrite scavenging activity. J Pineal Res 23:106–116.
72. El-Sokkary GH, Reiter RJ, Cuzzocrea S, Caputi AP, Hassanein AF, Tan DX. (1999) Role of melatonin in reduction of lipid peroxidation and peroxynitrite formation in non-septic shock induced by zymosan. Shock 12:402–208.
73. Zhang H, Squadrito GL, Pryor WA. (1998) The reaction of melatonin with peroxynitrite: formation of melatonin radical cation and absence of stable nitrated products. Biochem Biophys Res Commun 251:83–87.
74. Zhang H, Squadrito GL, Uppu R, Pryor WA. (1999) Reaction of peroxynitrite with melatonin: a mechanistic study. Chem Res Toxicol 12:526–534.
75. Antolin I, Rodriquez C, Sainz RM, Mayo JC, Aria H, Kotler M, Rodriquez–Colunga MJ, Tolivia D, Menendez–Pelaez A. (1996) Neurohormone melatonin prevents cell damage: effect on gene expression for antioxidative enzymes. FASEB J 10:882–890.
76. Montilla P, Tunez I, Munoz MC, Soria JV, Lopez A. (1997) Antioxidative effect of melatonin in rat brain oxidative stress induced by Adriamycin. J Physiol Biochem 53:301–306.
77. Barlow–Walden LR, Reiter RJ, Abe M, Pablos MI, Chen LD, Poeggeler B. (1995) Melatonin stimulates brain glutathione peroxidase activity. Neurochem Int 26:497–502.
78. Pablos MI, Agapito MT, Gutierrez R, Recio JM, Menendez–Pelaez A. (1995) Melatonin stimulates the activity of the detoxifying enzyme glutathione peroxidase in several tissues of chicks. J Pineal Res 19:111–115.
79. Pablos MI, Guerrero JM, Ortiz GG, Agapito MT, Reiter RJ. (1997) Both melatonin and a putative nuclear melatonin receptor agonist CGP 52608 stimulate glutathione peroxidase and glutathione reductase activities in mouse brain in vivo. Neuroendocrinol Lett 18:49–58.
80. Pierrefiche G, Laborit H. (1995) Oxygen radicals, melatonin and aging. Exp Gerontol 30:213–227.
81. Urata Y, Honma S, Goto S, Todoroki S, Iida T, Cho S, Honma K, Kondo T. (1999) Melatonin induces γ-glutamylcysteine synthetase mediated by activator protein-1 in human vascular endothelial cells. Free Radic Biol Med 27:838–847.
82. Pozo D, Reiter RJ, Calvo JM, Guerrero JM. (1994) Physiological concentrations of melatonin inhibit nitric oxide synthase in the cerebellum. Life Sci 55:PL455–PL460.
83. Pozo D, Reiter RJ, Calvo JM, Guerrero JM. (1997) Inhibition of cerebellar nitric oxide synthase and cyclic GMP production by melatonin via complex formation with calmodulin. J Cell Biochem 65:430–442.
84. Limson J, Nyokong T, Daya S. (1998) The interaction of melatonin and its precursors with aluminum, cadmium, copper, iron, lead, and zinc: an adsorptive voltametric study. J Pineal Res 24:15–21.

85. Reiter RJ. (1997) Antioxidant actions of melatonin. Adv Pharmacol 38:103–117.
86. Reiter RJ, Guerrero JM, Escames G, Pappolla MA, Acuña–Castroviejo D. (1997) Prophylactic actions of melatonin in oxidative neurotoxicity. Ann NY Acad Sci 825:70–78.
87. Hardeland R. (1997) New actions of melatonin and their relevance to biometeorology. Int J Biometeorol 41:47–57.
88. Granger DN, Korthius RJ. (1995) Physiologic mechanisms of postischemic tissue injury. Annu Rev Physiol 57:311–332.
89. Horie Y, Wolf R, Anderson DC, Grange DN. (1997) Hepatic leukostasis and hypoxic stress in adhesion molecule deficient mice after gut ischemia/reperfusion. J Clin Invest 99:781–788.
90. Lefer AM, Lefer DJ. (1996) The role of nitric oxide and cell adhesion molecules in the microcirculation in ischemia–reperfusion. Cardiovasc Res 32:743–751.
91. Hurn PD, Kirsch JR, Helfaer MA, Traystman RJ. (1996) Brain damage and free radicals. In: Kamada T, Shirga T, McCuskey RS, eds. Tissue Perfusion and Organ Function: Ischemia/Reperfusion Injury. Amsterdam: Elsevier, pp. 71–84.
92. Manev H, Uz T, Kharlamov A, Joo JY. (1996) Increased brain damage after stroke or excitotoxic seizures in melatonin-deficient rats. FASEB J 10:1546–1551.
93. Davis M, Mendelow AD, Perry RH, Chambers IR, James OF. (1995) Experimental stroke and neuroprotection in the aging rat brain. Stroke 26:1072–1078.
94. Reiter RJ. (1992) The aging pineal gland and its physiological consequences. Bioessays 14:169–175.
95. Kilic E, Özdemir YG, Bolay H, Kelestimur H, Dalkara T. (1999) Pinealectomy aggravates and melatonin administration attenuates brain damage in focal ischemia. J Cerebr Blood Flow Metab 19:511–516.
96. Joo JY, Uz T, Manev H. (1998) Effects of pinealectomy and melatonin administration on brain damage following cerebral focal ischemia in rat. Restor Neurol Neurosci 13:185–191.
97. Cho S, Joh TH, Bails HH, Dibinis C, Volpe BT. (1997) Melatonin administration protects CA1 hippocampal neurons after transient forebrain ischemia in rats. Brain Res 755:335–338.
98. Li XJ, Zhang LM, Gu J, Zhang AZ, Sun FY. (1997) Melatonin decreases production of hydroxyl radical during cerebral ischemia–reperfusion. Acta Pharmacol Sinica 18:394–396.
99. Wei J, Huang NC, Quast MJ. (1997) Hydroxyl radical formation in hyperglycemic rats during middle cerebral artery occlusion/reperfusion. Free Radic Biol Med 23:986–995.
100. Li XJ, Gu J, Pan BS, Sun FY. (1999) Effect of melatonin on production of hydroxyl radical and lactate dehydrogenase during hypoxia in rat cortical slices. Acta Pharmacol Sinica 20:201–205.
101. Ling X, Zhang LM, Lu SD, Li XJ, Sun FY. (1999) Protective effect of melatonin on injured cerebral neurons in associated with *bcl*-2 protein over-expression. Acta Pharmacol Sinica 20:409–414.
102. Zhong LT, Sarafian T, Kane DJ, Charles AC, Mah SP, Edwards RH, Bredeskn DE. (1993) *bcl*-2 Inhibits death of central neural cells induced by multiple agents. Proc Natl Acad Sci USA 90:4533–4537.
103. Guerrero JM, Reiter RJ, Ortiz GG, Pablos MI, Sewerynek E, Chuang JI. (1997) Melatonin prevents increases in nitric oxide and cyclic GMP production after transient ischemia and reperfusion in the Mongolian gerbil (*Meriones unguiculatus*). J Pineal Res 23:24–31.
104. Ortiz GG, Guerrero JM, Sewerynek E, Chuang J, Melchiorri D, Oh CS, Acuña–Castroviejo D, Feria–Velasco A, Reiter RJ. (1997) Melatonin is cytoprotective during neural ischemia–reperfusion injury in the Mongolian gerbil (*Meriones unguiculatus*). In: Webb SM, Puig–Domingo M, Moller M, Pevert P, eds. Pineal Update. Westbury: PJD Publications. pp. 397–401.
105. Cuzzocrea S, Costantino G, Gitto L, Mazzon E, Fulia F, Serraino I, Cordaro S, Berberi I, De Sarro A, Caputi AP. (2000). Protective effects of melatonin in ischemic brain injury. J Pineal Res 29:217–227.
106. Wakatsuki A, Okatani Y, Izumiya C, Ikenoe N. (1999) Melatonin protects against ischemia and reperfusion induced oxidative lipid and DNA damage in fetal rat brain. J Pineal Res 26:147–152.
107. Cazevieille C, Sofa R, Osbourne NN. (1997) Melatonin protects primary cultures or rat cortical neurons from NMDA excitotoxicity and hypoxia/reoxygenation. Brain Res 768:120–124.
108. Osbourne NN, Nash MS, Wood JPM. (1998) Melatonin counteracts ischemia-induced apoptosis in human retinal pigment epithelial cells. Invest Ophthalmol Vis Sci 39:2374–2383.
109. Vlkolinsky R, Stolc S. (1999) Effects of stobadine, melatonin, and other antioxidants on hypoxia/reoxygenation-induced synaptic transmission failure in rat hippocampal slices. Brain Res 850:118–126.

110. Vlkolinsky R, Stolc S, Ross A. (1999) Effects of stobadine, U-74389G, Trolox and melatonin on rat hippocampal slices to oxidative stress. Life Sci 65:1969–1971.
111. Alcaron de la Lastra C, Cabeza J, Motilva V, Martin MJ. (1997) Melatonin protects against gastric ischemia–reperfusion injury in rats. J Pineal Res 23:47–52.
112. Konturek PC, Konturek SJ, Majka J, Zembala M, Hahn EG. (1997) Melatonin affords protection against gastric lesions induced by ischemia–reperfusion possibly due to its antioxidant and mucosal microcirculatory effects. Eur J Pharmacol 322:73–77.
113. Konturek PC, Konturek SJ, Brzozowski T, Deminski A, Zembala M, Mytar B, Hahn EG. (1997) Gastroprotective effect of melatonin and its precursor, L-tryptophan, against stress-induced and ischemia-induced lesions is mediated by scavenging of oxygen free radicals. Scand J Gastroenterol 32:433–438.
114. Brzozowski T, Konturek PC, Konturek SJ, Pajdo R, Bielanski W, Brzozowski I, Stachura J, Hahn EG. (1997) The role of melatonin and L-tryptophan in prevention of acute gastric lesions induced by stress, ethanol, ischemia, and aspirin. J Pineal Res 23:79–89.
115. Cuzzocrea S, Costantino G, Mazzon E, Micali A, De Sarro A, Caputi AP. (2000) Beneficial effects of melatonin in a rat model of splanchnic artery occlusion and reperfusion. J Pineal Res 28:52–63.
116. Sewerynek E, Reiter RJ, Melchiorri D, Ortiz GG, Lewinski AJ. (1996) Oxidative damage to the liver induced by ischemia–reperfusion: protection by melatonin. Hepatogastroenterology 43:898–905.
117. Fishbein MC. (1990) Reperfusion injury. Clin Cardiol 13:213–217.
118. Entman ML, Michael L, Rossen RD, Dreyer WJ, Anderson DS, Taylor AA, Smith CW. (1991) Inflammation in the course of early myocardial ischemia. FASEB J 5:2529–2537.
119. Larner AJ, Conway MA. (1989) Free radicals in acute coronary infarction. Q J Med 263:205–212.
120. Tan DX, Manchester LC, Reiter RJ, Qi W, Kim SJ, El-Sokkary G. (1998) Ischemia/reperfusion-induced arrhythmias in the isolated rat heart: prevention by melatonin. J Pineal Res 25:184–191.
121. Lagneux C, Joyeux M, Demenge P, Ribuot J, Godin-Ribuot D. (2000) Protective effects of melatonin against ischemia-reperfusion injury in the isolated rat heart. Life Sci 66:503–509.
122. Bertuglia S, Marchiafava PL, Colantuoni A. (1996) Melatonin prevents ischemia reperfusion injury in the hamster check pouch. Cardiovasc Res 31:947–952.
123. Drew KL, Osbourne PG, Frericks KU, Hu Y, Koren RE, Hallenbeck JM, Rice ME. (1999) Ascorbate and glutathione regulation in hibernating ground squirrels. Brain Res 851:1–8.
124. Vanecek J, Jansky L, Illnerova H, Hoffmann K. (1984) Pineal melatonin in hibernating and aroused golden hamsters (*Mesocricetus auratus*). Comp Biochem Physiol 77A:759–764.
125. Rahimtoola SH. (1987) The hibernating myocardium. Am Heart J 117:211–221.
126. Sokal RJ, Papas AM. (1999) Antioxidants in neurological diseases. In: Papas AM, ed. Antioxidant Status, Diet, Nutrition and Health. Boca Raton, FL: CRC Press, pp. 567–590.
127. Vatassery GT, Angerhofer CK, Knox CA, Deshmukh DS. (1984) Concentrations of vitamin E in various neuroanatomical regions and subcellular functions, and the uptake of vitamin E by specific areas of rat brain. Biochim Biophys Acta 792:118–122.
128. Marklund SL, Westman NG, Lundgren E, Ross G. (1982) Copper- and zinc-containing superoxide dismutase, maganese-containing superoxide dismutase, catalase, and glutathione peroxidase in normal and neoplastic human cell lines and normal human tissues. Cancer Res 42:1955–1961.
129. Pappolla MA, Omar RA, Kim KS, Robakis NK. (1992) Immunohistochemical evidence of oxidative stress in Alzheimer's disease. Am J Pathol 140:621–628.
130. Smith MA, Kutty RK, Richey PL, Yan SC, Stern D, Chader GJ, Wiggert B, Petersen RB, Perry G. (1994) Heme oxygenase-1 is associated with the neurofibrillary pathology of Alzheimer's disease. Am J Pathol 145:42–47.
131. Pappolla MA, Sos M, Bick RJ, Omar RA, Hickson–Bick DLM, Reiter RJ, Efthimiopoulos S, Sambamurti K, Robakis NK. (1997) Oxidative damage and cell death induced by an amyloid peptide fragment is completely prevented by melatonin. In: Iqbal K, Winblad B, Nishimura T, Takeda M, Wisniewski HM, eds. Alzheimer's Disease: Biology, Diagnosis and Therapeutics. New York: John Wiley & Sons, pp. 741–749.
132. Pappolla MA, Sos M, Omar RA, Bick RJ, Hickson–Bick DLM, Reiter RJ, Efthimiopoulos S, Robakis NK. (1997) Melatonin prevents death of neuroblastoma cells exposed to the Alzheimer amyloid peptide. J Neurosci 17:1683–1690.
133. Reiter RJ, Garcia JJ, Pie J. (1998) Oxidative toxicity in models of neurodegeneration: responses to melatonin. Restr Neurol Neurosci 12:135–142.

134. Reiter RJ. (1998) Oxidative damage in the central nervous system: protection by melatonin. Prog Neurobiol 56:359–384.
135. Garcia JJ, Reiter RJ, Guerrero JM, Escames G, Y BP, Oh CS, Muñoz–Hoyos A. (1997) Melatonin prevents changes in microsomal membrane fluidity during induced lipid peroxidation. FEBS Lett 408:297–300.
136. Bozner P, Grishko V, Le Doux SP, Wilson GL, Chyan YC, Pappolla MA. (1997) The amyloid β protein induces oxidative damage of mitochondrial DNA. J Neuropathol Exp Neurol 56:1356–1362.
137. Pappolla MA, Chyan YJ, Poeggeler B, Bozner P, Ghiso J, Le Doux SP, Wilson GL. (1999) Alzheimer β protein mediated oxidative damage to mitochondrial DNA: prevention by melatonin. J Pineal Res 27:226–229.
138. Chyan YJ, Poeggeler B, Omar RA, Chain DG, Frangione B, Ghiso J, Pappolla MA. (1999) Potent neuroprotective properties against the Alzheimer's β-amyloid by an endogenous melatonin-related indole structure, indole-3-propionic acid. J Biol Chem 274:21937–21942.
139. Daniels WMU, van Rensburg SJ, van Zyl JM, Taljaard JJF. (1998) Melatonin prevents β-amyloid-induced lipid peroxidation. J Pineal Res 24:78–82.
140. Pappolla M, Bozner P, Soto C, Shao H, Robakis NK, Zagorski M, Frangione B, Ghiso J. (1998) Inhibition of Alzheimer β-fibrillogenesis by melatonin. J Biol Chem 273:7185–7188.
141. Song W, Lahiri DK. (1997) Melatonin alters the metabolism of the β-amyloid precursor protein in the neuroendocrine cell line PL12. J Mol Neurosci 9:75–92.
142. Lahiri DK. (1999) Melatonin affects the metabolism of the β-amyloid precursor protein in different cell types. J Pineal Res 26:137–146.
143. Olivieri G, Brack C, Müller–Spahn F, Stahelin HB, Hermann M, Renard P, Brockhaus M, Hock C. (2000) Mercury induces cell cytotoxicity and oxidative stress and increases β-amyloid secretion and tau phosphorylation in SHSY5Y neuroblastoma cells. J Neurosci 74:231–236.
144. Pappolla MA, Chyan YJ, Bozner P, Soto C, Shao H, Reiter RJ, Brewer G, Robakis NK, Zagorski MG, Frangione B, Ghiso J. (1999) Dual anti-amyloidogenic and antioxidant properties of melatonin: a new therapy for Alzheimer's diseases. In: Iqbal K, Swaab DF, Winblad B, Wisniewski HM, ed. Alzheimer's Disease and Related Disorders. New York: John Wiley & Sons, pp. 661–669.
145. Pappolla MA, Chyan YJ, Poeggeler B, Frangione B, Wilson G, Ghiso J, Reiter RJ. (2000) An assessment of the antioxidant and antiamyloidogenic properties of melatonin: implications for Alzheimer's disease. J Neural Transm 107:203–231.
146. Brusco LI, Marquez M, Cardinali DP. (1998) Monozygotic twins with Alzheimer's disease treated with melatonin: case report. J Pineal Res 25:260–263.
147. Brusco LI, Fainstein I, Marquez M, Cardinali DP. (1997) Effect of melatonin in selected populations of sleep-disturbed patients. Biol Signals Recept 8:126–131.
148. Ebadi M, Srinivasan SK, Baxi MD. (1996) Oxidative stress and antioxidant therapy in Parkinson's disease. Prog Neurobiol 48:1–19.
149. Lai CT, Ya PH. (1997) $R(-)$-Deprenyl potentiates dopamine-induced cytotoxicity toward catecholaminergic neuroblastoma SH-SY5Y cells. Toxicol Appl Pharmacol 142:186–191.
150. Jenner P, Olanow CW. (1996) Oxidative stress in Parkinson's disease and other neurodegenerative disorders. Pathol Biol (Paris) 44:57–64.
151. Acuña–Castroviejo D, Coto–Montes A, Monti G, Ortiz GG, Reiter RJ. (1997) Melatonin is protective against MPTP-induced striatal and hippocampal lesions. Life Sci 60:23–29.
152. Jin BK, Shin DY, Jeong MY, Gwag MR, Baik HW, Yoon KS, Cho YH, Joo WS, Kim YS, Baik HH. (1998) Melatonin protects nigral dopaminergic neurons from 1-methyl-4-phenylpyridinium (MPP^+) neurotoxicity in rats. Neurosci Lett 245:61–64.
153. Iacovitti L, Stull ND, Johnston K. (1997) Melatonin rescues dopamine neurons from cell death in tissue models of oxidative stress. Brain Res 768:317–326.
154. Itzhak Y, Martin JL, Block MD, Ali SF. (1998) Effect of melatonin on methamphetamine- and 1-methyl-4-phenyl-1,2,3,6-tetrahydropyridine-induced dopaminergic neurotoxicity and methamphetamine-induced behavior sensitization. Neuropharmacology 37:781–791.
155. Hirata H, Asanuma M, Cadet JL. (1998) Melatonin attenuates methamphetamine-induced toxic effects of dopamine and serotonin terminals in mouse brain. Synapse 30:150–155.
156. Bates TE, Heales SJR, Davies SEC, Boakye P, Clark JB. (1994) Effects of 1-methyl-4-phenylpyridinum on isolated rat brain mitochondria: evidence for a primary involvement of energy depletion. J Neurochem 63:640–648.

157. Absi E, Ayala A, Machado A, Parrado J. (2000) Protective effect of melatonin against the 1-methyl-1-phenyl-pyridinium-induced inhibition of complex I of the mitochondrial respiratory chain. J Pineal Res 29:40–47.
158. Cadet JL, Brannock C. (1998) Free radicals and the pathobiology of brain dopamine systems. Neurochem Int 32:117–131.
159. Perumal AS, Tordzro WK, Katz M, Jackson–Lewis V, Cooper TB, Fahn S, Cadet JL. (1989) Regional effects of 6-hydroxydopamine (6-OHDA) on free radical scavengers in rat brain. Brain Res 504:139–141.
160. Mayo JC, Sainz RM, Uria H, Antolin I, Esteban MM, Rodriquez C. (1998) Melatonin prevents apoptosis induced by 6-hydroxydopamine in neuronal cells: implications for Parkinson's disease. J Pineal Res 24:179–192.
161. Mayo JC, Sainz RM, Antolin I, Rodriquez C. (1999) Ultrastructural confirmation of neuronal protection by melatonin against the neurotoxin 6-hydroxydopamine cell damage. Brain Res 818:221–223.
162. Mayo JC, Sainz RM, Uria M, Antolin I, Esteban MM, Rodriquez C. (1998) Inhibition of cell proliferation: a mechanism likely to mediate the prevention of neuronal cell death by melatonin. J Pineal Res 25:12–18.
163. Kim YS, Joo S, Jin BK, Cho YH, Baik HH, Park CW. (1998) Melatonin protects 6-OHDA-induced neuronal death of nigrostriatal dopaminergic system. Neuroreport 9:2387–2390.
164. Miller JW, Selhub J, Joseph JA. (1996) Oxidative damage caused by free radicals produced during catecholamine auto-oxidation: protective effects of O-methylation and melatonin. Free Radic Biol Med 21:241–249.
165. Khaldy H, Escames G, Leon J, Vivas F, Luna JD, Acuña–Castroviejo D. (2000) Comparative effects of melatonin. L-Deprenyl, Trolox and ascorbate in the suppression of hydroxyl radical formation dring dopamine auto-oxidation in vitro. J Pineal Res 29:100–107.
166. Stone TW. (1993) The neuropharmacology of quinolinic acid and kynurenic acids. Pharmacol Rev 45:309–379.
167. Southgate GS, Daya S, Potgieter B. (1998) Melatonin plays a protective role in quinolinic acid-induced neurotoxicity in the rat hippocampus. J Chem Neuroanat 14:151–156.
168. Behan WMH, McDonald M, Darlington LG, Stone TW. (1999) Oxidative stress as a mechanism for quinolinic acid-induced hippocampal damage: protection by melatonin and deprenyl. Br J Pharmacol 128:1754–1760.
169. Cabrera J, Reiter RJ, Tan DX, Qi W, Sainz RM, Mayo JC, Garcia JJ, Kim SJ, El-Sokkary G. (2000) Melatonin reduces oxidative neurotoxicity due to quinolinic acid: in vitro and in vivo studies. Neuropharmacology 39:507–514.
170. Novelli A, Reilly JA, Lysko PG, Henneberry RC. (1988) Glutamate becomes neurotoxic via the N-methyl-D-aspartate receptor when intracellular energy levels are reduced. Brain Res 451:205–212.
171. Nicholls DG, Bud SL. (1998) Mitochondria and neuronal glutamate cytotoxicity. Biochim Biophys Acta 1366:97–112.
172. Schulz JB, Henshaw DR, Siwek D, Jenkins BG, Ferrante RJ, Cippaloni PB, Kowall NW, Rosen BR, Beal MF. (1995) Involvement of free radicals in excitotoxicity in vivo. J Neurochem 64:2239–2247.
173. Dykens JA, Stern A, Trenker E. (1997) Mechanism of kainate toxicity to cerebellar neurons in vitro is analogous to reperfusion tissue injury. J Neurochem 49:1222–1228.
174. Speck G. (1994) Kainic acid seizures in the rat. Prog Neurobiol 42:1–32.
175. Melchiorri D, Reiter RJ, Sewerynek E, Chen LD, Nistico G. (1995) Melatonin reduces kainate induced lipid peroxidation in homogenates of different brain regions. FASEB J 9:1205–1210.
176. Melchiorri D, Reiter RJ, Chen LD, Sewerynek E, Nistico G. (1996) Melatonin affords protection against kainate-induced in vitro lipid peroxidation. Eur J Pharmacol 305:239–242.
177. Guisti P, Gusella M, Lipartiti M, Milani D, Zhu W, Vincini S, Manev H. (1995) Melatonin protects primary cultures of cerebellar granule neurons from kainate but not from N-methyl-D-aspartate excitotoxicity. Exp Neurol 131:39–46.
178. Lezoualc'h F, Skutella T, Widmann M, Behl C. (1996) Melatonin prevents oxidative stress-induced cell death in hippocampal cells. Neuroreport 7:2071–2077.
179. Lezouchc'h F, Sparapani M, Behl C. (1998) N-Acetylserotonin (normelatonin) and melatonin protect neurons against oxidative challenges and suppress the activity of transcription factor NF-κB. J Pineal Res 24:168–178.

180. Moosman B, Uhr M, Behl C. (1997) Neuroprotective potential of aromatic alcohols against oxidative cell death. FEBS Lett 413:467–462.
181. Cazevieille C, Osbourne NN. (1997) Retinal neurons containing kainate receptors are influenced by exogenous kainate and ischemia while neurons lacking these receptors are not—melatonin counteracts the effect of ischemia and kainate. Brain Res 755:91–100.
182. Skaper SD, Ancona B, Facci L, Franceschini D, Giusti P. (1998) Melatonin prevents the delayed death of hippocampal neurons induced by enhanced excitatory neurotransmission and the nitridergic pathway. FASEB J 12:725–731.
183. Manev H, Uz T, Kharlamov A, Cagnoli CM, Franceschini D, Giusti P. (1996) In vivo protection against kainate-induced apoptosis by the pineal hormone melatonin: effect of exogenous melatonin. Restr Neurol Neurosci 9:251–256.
184. Uz T, Giusti P, Franchschini D, Kharlamov A, Manev H. (1996) Protective effective of melatonin against hippocampal DNA damage induced by intraperitoneal administration of kainate to rats. Neuroscience 73:631–636.
185. Giusti P, Lipartiti M, Franceschini D, Shiavo N, Floreani M, Manev H. (1996) Neuroprotection by melatonin from kainate-induced excitotoxicity in rats. FASEB J 10:891–896.
186. Giusti P, Lipartiti M, Gusella M, Floreani M, Manev H. (1997) In vitro and in vivo protective effects of melatonin against oxidative stress and neurotoxicity. Ann NY Acad Sci 825:79–84.
187. Floreani M, Skaper SD, Facci L, Lipartiti M, Giusti P. (1997) Melatonin maintains glutathione homeostasis in kainic acid-exposed rat brain tissues. FASEB J 11:1309–1315.
188. Tang K, Reiter RJ, Li ZR, Ortiz GG, Yu BP, Garcia JJ. (1998) Melatonin reduces the increase in 8-hydroxydeoxyguanosine levels in the brain and liver of kainic acid-treated rats. Mol Cell Biochem 178:299–303.
189. Kim HJ, Kwon JS. (1999) Effects of placing micro-implants of melatonin in striatum on oxidative stress and neuronal damage mediated by N-methyl-D-aspartate (NMDA) and non-NMDA receptors. Arch Pharmacol Res 22:35–43.
190. Tan DX, Manchester LC, Reiter RJ, Qi W, Kim SJ, El-Sokkary GH. (1998) Melatonin protects hippocampal neurons in vivo against kainic acid-induced damage in mice. J Neurosci Res 54:382–389.
191. Espinar A, Garcia–Oliva A, Isorna M, Quesada A, Prada FA, Guerrero JM. (2000) Neuroprotection by melatonin from glutamate-induced excitotoxicity during development of the cerebellum in the chick embryo. J Pineal Res 28:81–88.
192. Coyle JT, Puttfarcken P. (1993) Oxidative stress, glutamate and neurodegenerative disorders. Science 262:689–695.
193. Ward JF. (1988) DNA damage produced by ionizing radiation in mammalian cells: identities, mechanisms of formation and reparability. Prog Nucleic Acid Res Mol Biol 35:95–125.
194. Dizdaroglu M. (1992) Oxidative damage to DNA in mammalian chromatin. Mutat Res 275:331–342.
195. Blinkenstaff RT, Bradstrader SM, Reddy S, Witt R. (1994) Potential radioprotective agents. 1. Homologs of melatonin. J Pharm Sci 83:216–218.
196. Vijayalaxmi, Meltz ML, Reiter RJ, Herman TS, Kumar KS. (1999) Melatonin and protection from whole body radiation. Mutat Res 425:21–27.
197. Vijayalaxmi, Reiter RJ, Meltz ML. (1995) Melatonin protects human blood lymphocytes from radiation-induced chromosome damage. Mutat Res 346:23–31.
198. Vijayalaxmi, Reiter RJ, Sewerynek E, Poeggeler B, Leal BZ, Meltz ML. (1995) Marked reduction of radiation-induced micronuclei in human blood lymphocytes pretreated with melatonin. Radiat Res 143:102–106.
199. Vijayalaxmi, Reiter RJ, Leal BZ, Meltz ML. (1996) Effect of melatonin on mitotic and proliferation indices, and sister chromatid exchanges in human blood lymphocytes. Mutat Res 351:187–192.
200. Vijayalaxmi, Reiter RJ, Herman TS, Meltz ML. Melatonin reduces gamma-radiation-induced primary DNA damage in human blood lymphocytes. Mutat Res 397:203–208.
201. Vijayalaxmi, Meltz ML, Reiter RJ, Herman TS. (1999) Melatonin and protection from genetic damage in blood and bone marrow: whole body irradiation studies in mice. J Pineal Res 27:221–225.
202. Vijayalaxmi, Reiter RJ, Herman TS, Meltz ML. (1996) Melatonin and radioprotection from genetic damage: in vivo/in vitro studies with human volunteers. Mutat Res 371:221–228.

203. Vijayalaxmi, Reiter RJ, Meltz ML, Herman TS. (1998) Melatonin: possible mechanisms involved in its "radioprotective" effect. Mutat Res 404:187–189.
204. Badr FM, El Habit OHM, Harraz MM. (1999) Radioprotective effect of melatonin assessed by measuring chromosomal damage in mitotic and meiotic cells. Mutat Res 444:367–372.
205. Kaya H, Delibas W, Serteser M, Ulgukaya E, Özkaya O. (1999) The effect of melatonin on lipid peroxidation during radiotherapy in female rats. Strahlenther Onkol 175:285–288.
206. Smith SL, Andrus PK, Zhang JR, Hall ED. (1994) Direct measurement of hydroxyl radicals, lipid peroxidation, and blood–brain barrier disruption following unilateral cortical impact injury. J Neurotrauma 11:393–404.
207. Mésenge C, Margaill I, Verrecchia C, Allix M, Boulu RG, Plotkine M. (1998) Protective effect of melatonin in a model of traumatic brain injury in mice. J Pineal Res 25:41–46.
208. Ghezzi P, Saccardo B, Bianchi M. (1986) Role of reactive oxygen intermediates in the hepatoxicity of endotoxin. Immunopharmacology 12:241–244.
209. Barron RL. (1993) Pathophysiology of septic shock and implications for therapy. Clin Pharmacol 12:829–845.
210. Sewerynek E, Abe M, Reiter RJ, Barlow–Walden LR, Chen LD, McCabe TJ, Roman LJ, Diaz–Lopez B. (1995) Melatonin administration prevents lipopolysaccharide-induced oxidative damage in phenobarbital-treated animals. J Cell Biochem 58:436–444.
211. Sewerynek E, Melchiorri D, Reiter RJ, Ortiz GG, Lewinski A. (1995) Lipopolysaccharide-induced hepatotoxicity is inhibited by the antioxidant melatonin. Eur J Pharmacol 293:327–334.
212. Sewerynek E, Melchiorri D, Chen LD, Reiter RJ. (1995) Melatonin reduces both basal and bacterial lipopolysaccharide-induced lipid peroxidation in vivo. Free Radic Biol Med 19:903–909.
213. Sewerynek E, Ortiz GG, Reiter RJ, Pablos MI, Melchiorri D, Daniels WMU. (1996) Lipopolysaccharide-induced DNA damage is greatly reduced in rats treated with the pineal hormone melatonin. Mol Cell Endocrinol 117:183–188.
214. Maestroni GJM (1996) Melatonin as a therapeutic agent in experimental endotoxic shock. J Pineal Res 20:84–89.
215. Bettahi I, Pozo D, Osuna C, Reiter RJ, Acuña–Castroviejo D, Guerrero JM. (1996) Melatonin reduces nitric oxide synthase activity in rat hypothalamus. J Pineal Res 20:205–210.
216. Nava F, Calapai G, Facciola G, Cuzzocrea S, Giuliani G, De Sarro A, Caputi AP. (1997) Melatonin effects on inhibition of thirst and fever induced by lipopolysaccharide in rat. Eur J Pharmacol 31:267–274.
217. Raghavenda V, Agrewala JN, Kulkarni SK. (1999) Role of centrally administered melatonin and inhibitors of COX and NOS in LPS-induced hyperthermia and adipsia. Prostaglandins Leukotr Essent Fatty Acids 60:249–258.
218. Crespo E, Micias M, Pozo D, Escames G, Martin M, Vives F, Guerrero JM, Acuña–Castroviejo D. (1999) Melatonin inhibits expression of the inducible NO synthase in liver and lung and prevents endotoxema in lipopolysaccharide-induced multiple organ dysfunction syndrome in rats. FASEB J 13:1537–1546.
219. Dawson J, Sedgwick AD, Edwards JC, Lees P. (1991) A comparative study of the cellular, exudative and histological responses to carrageenan, dextran and zymosan in the mouse. Int J Tissue React 13:171–185.
220. Salvemini D, Wang ZQ, Bourdon DM, Stern MK, Currie MG, Manning PT. (1996) Evidence of peroxynitrite involvement in the carrageenan-induced rat paw edema. Eur J Pharmacol 303:217–220.
221. Wei XQ, Charles IG, Smith A, Ure J, Feng GJ, Huang FP, Xu D, Muller W, Moncada S, Liew FT. (1995) Altered immune responses in mice lacking inducible nitric oxide synthase. Nature 375:408–411.
222. Cuzzocrea S, Zingarelli B, Gilad E, Hake P, Salzman AL, Szabo C. (1997) Protective effect of melatonin in carrageenan-induced models of local inflammation: relationship to its inhibitory effect on nitric oxide production and its peroxynitrite scavenging activity. J Pineal Res 23:106–116.
223. Cuzzocrea S, Costantino G, Mazzon E, Caputi AP. (1999) Regulation of prostaglandin production in carrageenan-induced pleurisy by melatonin. J Pineal Res 27:9–14.
224. Cuzzocrea S, Tan DX, Costantino G, Mazzon E, Caputi AP, Reiter RJ. (1999) The protective role of endogenous melatonin in carrageenan-induced pleurisy in the rat. FASEB J 13:1930–1938.
225. Goris RJA, Van Bebber IPT, Mollen RMH, Koopman JP. (1991) Does decontamination of the gastrointestinal tract prevent multiple organ failure? Arch Surg 126:561–565.

226. Rao TS, Currie H, Shaffer AF, Isakson PC. (1993) In vivo characterization of zymosan-induced mouse peritoneal inflammation. J Pharmacol Exp Ther 269:917–925.
227. Costantino G, Cuzzocrea S, Mazzon E, Caputi AP. (1998) Protective effects of melatonin in zymosan-activated plasma-induced paw inflammation. Eur J Pharmacol 363:57–63.
228. El-Sokkary GH, Reiter RJ, Cuzzocrea S, Caputi AP, Hassanein AMM, Tan DX. (1999) Role of oxidation in reduction of lipid peroxidation and peroxynitrite formation in non-septic shock induced by zymosan. Shock 12:402–408.
229. Cuzzocrea S, Costantino G, Caputi AP. (1998) Protective effect of melatonin on cellular energy depletion mediated by peroxynitrite and poly(ADP-ribose)synthase activation in a non-septic shock model induced by zymosan in the rat. J Pineal Res 25:78–85.
230. Cuzzocrea S, Caputi AP. (1999) Protective effect of melatonin on zymosan-induced cellular damage. Biol Signals Recept 8:136–142.
231. Wells CL, Rhame FS. (1990) Effect of oral dextran sulfate on the mouse intestinal tract. J Acquir Immune Def Syndr 3:361–365.
232. Pentney PT, Bubenik GA. (1995) Melatonin reduces the severity of dextran-induced colitis in mice. J Pineal Res 19:31–39.
233. De Flora S, Wetterhahn KE. (1989) Mechanism of chromium (VI) metabolism and genotoxicity. Life Chem Rep 7:169–244.
234. Sugiyama M. (1992) Role of physiological antioxidants in chromium (VI)-induced cellular injury. Free Radic Biol Med 12:397–407.
235. Sugiyama M. (1994) Role of cellular antioxidants in metal-induced damage. Cell Biol Toxicol 10:1–22.
236. Qi W, Reiter RJ, Tan DX, Manchester LC, Sui AW, Garcia JJ. (2000). Increased levels of oxidatively damage DNA induced by chromium (III) and H_2O_2: protection by melatonin and related molecules. J Pineal Res 29:54–61.
237. Qi W, Reiter RJ, Tan DX, Garcia JJ, Manchester LC, Karbownik M, Calvo JR. (2000) Chromium (III)-induced 8-hydroxydeoxyguanosine in DNA and its reduction by antioxidants: comparative effects of melatonin, ascorbate and vitamin E. Environ Health Perspect 108:399–402.
238. Anderson HR, Anderson O. (1988) Effect of cadmium on hepatic lipid peroxidation in mice. Pharmacol Toxicol 63:173–177.
239. Kim CY, Lee MJ, Lee SM, Lee WC, Kim JS. (1998) Effect of melatonin on cadmium-induced hepatotoxicity in male Sprague–Dawley rats. Tohoku J Exp Med 186:205–213.
240. Szabo S. (1987) Mechanisms of mucosal injury in the stomach and duodenum: time-sequence analysis of morphologic, functional, biochemical and histochemical studies. Scand J Gastroenterol Suppl 127:21–28.
241. Pihan G, Regillo C, and Szabo S. (1987) Free radicals and lipid peroxidation in ethanol- or aspirin-induced gastric mucosal injury. Dig Dis Sci 32:1395–1401.
242. Szelenyi K, Brune K. (1988) Possible role of oxygen free radicals in ethanol-induced gastric mucosal damage in rats. Dig Dis Sci 33:865–871.
243. Melchiorri D, Sewerynek E, Reiter RJ, Ortiz GG, Poeggeler B, Nistico G. (1997) Suppressive effect of melatonin administration on ethanol-induced gastrointestinal injury in rats in vivo. Br J Pharmacol 121:264–270.
244. El-Sokkary GH, Reiter RJ, Tan DX, Kim SJ, Cabrera J. (1999) Inhibitory effect of melatonin on products of lipid peroxidation resulting from chronic ethanol administration. Alcohol Alcohol 34:842–850.
245. Mansouri A, Gaou I, de Kerguenec C, Amsellem S, Hauzi D, Berson A, Moreau A, Feldman G, Letteron P, Pessayre D, Fromenty B. (1999) An alcoholic binge causes massive degradation of hepatic mitochondria DNA in mice. Gastroenterology 117:181–190.
246. Battle AMC. (1993) Porphyrins, porphyrias, cancer and photodynamic therapy—a model of carcinogenesis. J Photochem Photobiol B Biol 20:5–22.
247. Monteiro HP, Bechara EJH, Abdalla DSP. (1991) Free radical involvement in neurological porphyrias and lead poisoning. Mol Cell Endocrinol 103:73–83.
248. Princ FG, Juknat AA, Maxit AG, Cardalda C, Battle A. (1997) Melatonin's antioxidant protection against δ-aminolevulinic acid-induced oxidative damage in rat cerebellum. J Pineal Res 23:40–48.
249. Carneiro RCG, Reiter RJ. (1997) Melatonin protects against lipid peroxidation induced by delta-aminolevulinic acid in rat cerebellum, cortex and hippocampus. Neuroscience 82:293–299.

250. Princ FG, Maxit AG, Cardalda C, Battle A, Juknat AA. (1998) In vivo protection by melatonin against δ-aminolevulinic acid–induced oxidative damage and its antioxidant effect on the activity of haem enzymes. J Pineal Res 24:1–8.
251. Carneiro RCG, Reiter RJ. (1998) δ-Aminolevulinic acid-induced lipid peroxidation in rat kidney and liver is attenuated by melatonin: an in vitro and in vivo study. J Pineal Res 24:131–136.
252. Puy H, Deyback JC, Boudry P, Callebert J, Touitou Y, Nordmann Y. (1993) Decreased nocturnal plasma melatonin levels in patients with recurrent acute intermittent porphria attacks. Life Sci 53:621–627.
253. Puy H, Reyback JC, Bogdan A, Callebert J, Baumgarter M, Voisin P, Nordmann Y, Touitou Y. (1996) Increased δ-aminolevulinic acid and decreased pineal melatonin production. J Clin Invest 97:104–110.
254. Zerba E, Komorovsky TE, Faulkner JA. (1990) Free radical injury to skeletal muscle of young, adult and old mice. Am J Pathol 258:C429–C435.
255. Salminen A, Vikko V. (1983) Lipid peroxidation in exercise myopathy. Exp Mol Pathol 38:380–388.
256. Hara M, Abe M, Suzuki T, Reiter RJ. (1996) Tissue changes in glutathione metabolism and lipid peroxidation induced by swimming are partially prevented by melatonin. Pharmacol Toxicol 78:308–312.
257. Hara M, Iigo M, Ohtani–Kaneko R, Nakamura N, Suzuki TK, Reiter RJ, Hirata K. (1997) Administration of melatonin and related indoles prevents exercise-induced cellular oxidative changes in rats. Biol Signals 6:90–100.
258. Mazepa RC, Cuevas MJ, Callado PS, Gonzalez–Gallego J. (2000) Melatonin increases muscle and liver glycogen content in nonexercised and exercised rats. Life Sci 66:153–160.
259. Pablos MI, Reiter RJ, Chuang JI, Ortiz GG, Guerrero JM, Sewerynek E, Agapito MT, Melchiorri D, Lawrence R, Deneke SM. (1997) Acutely administered melatonin reduces oxidative damage in lung and brain induced by hyperbaric oxygen. J Appl Physiol 83:354–358.
260. Shaikh AJ, Xu J, Wu Y, He L, Hsu CY. (1997) Melatonin protects bovine cerebral endothelial cells from hyperoxia-induced DNA damage and death. Neurosci Lett 229:193–197.
261. Sewerynek E, Melchiorri D, Ortiz GG, Poeggeler B, Reiter RJ. Melatonin reduces H_2O_2-induced lipid peroxidation in homogenates of different rat brain regions. J Pineal Res 19:51–56.
262. Pless G, Frederiksen TJP, Garcia JJ, Reiter RJ. (1999) Pharmacological aspects of N-acetyl-5-methoxytryptamine (melatonin) and 6-methoxy-1,2,3,4-tetrahydro-β-carboline (pinoline) as antioxidants: reduction of oxidative damage in brain region homogenates. J Pineal Res 26:236–246.
263. Mohan N, Sadeghi K, Reiter RJ, Meltz ML. (1995) The neurohormone melatonin inhibits cytokine, mitogen and ionizing radiation induced NF-κB. Biochem Mol Biol Int 37:1063–1069.
264. Chuang JI, Mohan N, Meltz ML, Reiter RJ. (1996) Effect of melatonin on NF-κB DNA-binding activity in the rat spleen. Cell Biol Int 20:687–692.
265. Chen LD, Melchiorri D, Sewerynek E, Reiter RJ. (1995) Retinal lipid peroxidation in vitro is inhibited by melatonin. Neurosci Res Commun 17:151–158.
266. Siu AW, Reiter RJ, To CH. (1998) The efficacy of vitamin E and melatonin as antioxidants against lipid peroxidation in rat retinal homogenates. J Pineal Res 24:239–244.
267. Tang PL, Xu MF, Qian ZM. (1997) Differential behavior of cell membranes towards iron-enhanced oxidative damage and the effects of melatonin. Biol Signals 6:291–300.
268. De Salvia R, Fiore M, Aglitti T, Festa F, Recordy R, Cozzi R. (1999) Inhibitory action of melatonin on H_2O_2- and cyclophosphamide-induced DNA damage. Mutagenesis 14:107–112.
269. Romero M, Osuna C, Garcia–Pergañada, Carrillo-Vico AK, Guerrero JM. (1999) The pineal secretory product melatonin reduces hydrogen peroxide-induced DNA damage in U-937 cells. J Pineal Res 26:227–235.
270. Baldwin WS, Barrett JC. (1998) Melatonin attenuates hydrogen peroxide toxicity in MCF-7 cells only at pharmacological concentrations. Biochem Biophys Res Commun 250:602–605.
271. Okatani Y, Watanabe K, Hayashi K, Wakatsuki A, Sagara Y. (1997) Melatonin inhibits vasospastic action of hydrogen peroxide in human umbilical artery. J Pineal Res 22:163–168.
272. Okatani Y, Watanabe K, Hayashi K, Wakatsuki A, Sagara Y. (1997) Melatonin suppresses vasospastic effect of hydrogen peroxide in human umbilical artery: relation to calcium influx. J Pineal Res 22:252–247.
273. Reiter RJ, Tan DX, Kim SJ, and Qi W. (1998) Melatonin as a pharmacological agent against oxidative damage to lipids and DNA. Proc West Pharmacol Soc 41:229–236.

274. Coto–Montes A, Hardeland R. (1999) Antioxidative effects of melatonin in *Drosophila melanogaster* antagonization of damage induced by the inhibition of catalase. J Pineal Res 27:154–158.
275. Laver NM, Robinson WG Jr, Calvin HI, Fu SCJ. (1993) Early epithelial lesions in cataracts of GSH-depleted mouse pups. Exp Eye Res 57:493–498.
276. Abe M, Reiter RJ, Orhii PB, Hara M, Poeggeler B. (1994) Inhibitory effect of melatonin on cataract formation in newborn rats: evidence for an antioxidative role for melatonin. J Pineal Res 17:94–100.
277. Li ZR, Reiter RJ, Fujimori O, Oh CS, Duan YP. (1997) Cataractogenesis and lipid peroxidation in newborn rats treated with buthionine sulfoxamine: preventive actions of melatonin. J Pineal Res 22:117–123.
278. Khan R, Daya S, Potgieter B. (1990) Evidence for a modulation of the stress response by the pineal gland. Experientia 46:860–862.
279. Khan R, Burton S, Morley S, Daya S, Potgieter B. (1990) The effect of melatonin on formation of gastric stress lesions in rats. Experientia 46:88–89.
280. Das D, Bandyopadhyay D, Bhattacharjee M, Banerjee RK. (1997) Hydroxyl radical is the major causative factor in stress-induced gastric ulceration. Free Radic Biol Med 23:8–18.
281. Kato K, Murai I, Asai S, Matsuno Y, Komuro S, Kameda N, Iwaski A, Ishikawa K, Nakagawa S, Arakawa Y, Kuwayama H. (1998) Protective role of melatonin and the pineal gland in modulating water immersion restraint stress ulcer in rats. J Clin Endocrinol Metab 27(suppl 1):S110–S115.
282. Alarcon de la Lastra C, Motilva V, Martin MJ, Nieto A, Barranco MD, Cabeza J, Herrerias JM. (1999) Protective effect of melatonin on indomethacin-induced gastric injury in rats. J Pineal Res 26:101–107.
283. Grotzinger K, Young RC. (1977) Adriamycin: the role of lipid peroxidation in cardiac toxicity and tumor response. Science 197:165–167.
284. Nowak D, Drzewaski J. (1996) Anthracycline-induced oxidative stress—its role in the development of cardiac damage. Cancer J 21:296–303.
285. Montilla P, Tunez I, Munoz MC, Lopez A, Soria JV. (1997) Hyperlipidemic nephropathy induced by Adriamycin: effect of melatonin administration. Nephron 76:345–350.
286. Gascon F, Lopez–Soria JV. (1998) Protective role of melatonin and retinol palmitate in oxidative stress and hyperlipidemic nephropathy induced by Adriamycin in rats. J Pineal Res 25:86–93.
287. Morishima I, Matsui H, Mukawa H, Hayashi K, Toki Y, Okumura K, Ito T, Hayakawa T. (1998) Melatonin, a pineal hormone with antioxidant property, protects against Adriamycin cardiomyopathy in rats. Life Sci 63:511–521.
288. Morishima I, Okumura K, Matsui H, Kaneko S, Numaguchi Y, Kawakami K, Mokuno S, Hayakawa M, Toki Y, Ito T, Hayakawa T. (1999) Zinc accumulation in Adriamycin-induced cardiomyopathy in rats: effects of melatonin, a cardioprotective agent. J Pineal Res 26:204–210.
289. Rapozzi V, Zorget S, Comelli M, Mavelli I, Perissin LK, Giraldi T. (1998) Melatonin decreases bone marrow and lymphatic toxicity of Adriamycin in mice bearing TLX5 lymphoma. Life Sci 63:1701–1713.
290. Rapozzi V, Comelli M, Manelli I, Sentjurc M, Schara M, Perissin L, Giraldi T. (1999) Melatonin and oxidative damage in mice liver induced by the prooxidant antitumor drug, Adriamycin. In Vivo 13:45–50.
291. Zwelling LA, Kahn KW. (1979) Mechanism of action of *cis*-dichlorodiammineplatinum (II). Cancer Treat Res 63:1439–1444.
292. Rybak LP, Husain K, Evenson L, Morris C, Whitworth L, Somani SM. (1997) Protection by 4-methylthiobenzoic acid against cisplatin-induced ototoxicity: the antioxidant system. Pharmacol Toxicol 81:173–179.
293. Lopez–Gonzalez MA, Guerrero JM, Rojas F, Delgado F. (2000) Ototoxicity caused by cisplatin is ameliorated by melatonin and other antioxidants. J Pineal Res 28:73–80.
294. Hassan MI, Ahmed MI, Kassin SK, Rashad A, Khalifa A. (1999) *cis*-Platinum-induced immunosuppression: relationship to melatonin in human peripheral blood mononuclear cells. Clin Biochem 32:621–626.
295. Anwar MM, Mahfouz HA, Sayed AS. (1998) Potential protective effects of melatonin on bone marrow of rats exposed to cytotoxic drugs. Comp Biochem Physiol 119A:493–501.
296. Mihatsh MJ, Ryffel B, Gudat F. (1995) The differential diagnosis between rejection and cyclosporine toxicity. Kidney Int 48:563–571.

297. Vijay Kumar K, Naidu MVR, Shifow AA, Prayag A, Ratnakar KS. (1999) Melatonin: an antioxidant protects against cyclosporine-induced nephrotoxicity. Transplantation 67:1065–1068.
298. Garetz SL, Rhee DJ, Schacht J. (1994) Sulfhydryl compounds and antioxidants inhibit cytotoxicity to outer hair cells of gentamicin metabolite in vitro. Hearing Res 77:75–80.
299. Lopez–Gonzalez MA, Guerrero JM, Torronteras R, Osuna C, Delgado F. (2000) Ototoxicity caused by aminoglycosides is ameliorated by melatonin without interfering with the antibiotic capacity of the drugs. J Pineal Res 28:26–33.
300. Behl C, Lezoualc'h F, Widmann M, Rupprecht F, Holsbaer F. (1996) Oxidative stress-resistant cells are protected against haloperidol toxicity. Brain Res 717:193–195.
301. Post A, Holsbaer F, Behl C. (1998) Induction of NF-κB activity during haloperidol-induced oxidative toxicity in clonal hippocampal cells: suppression of NF-κB and neuroprotection by antioxidants. J Neurosci 18:1–10.
302. Awara WM, El-Gohary M, El-Nabi SH, Fadel WA. (1998) In vivo and in vitro evaluation of the mutagenic potential of carbamezepine: does melatonin have anti-mutagenic activity. Toxicology 125:45–52.
303. Tan DX, Poeggeler B, Reiter RJ, Chen LD, Chen S, Manchester LC, Barlow–Walden LR. (1993) The pineal hormone melatonin inhibits DNA-adduct formation induced by the chemical carcinogen safrole in vivo. Cancer Lett 70:65–71.
304. Tan DX, Reiter RJ, Chen LD, Poeggeler B, Manchester LC, Barlow–Walden LR. (1994) Both physiological and pharmacological levels of melatonin reduce DNA adduct formation induced by the carcinogen safrole. Carcinogenesis 15:215–218.
305. Musatov SA, Anisimov VN, Andre V, Vigreux C, Godard T, Sichel F. (1999) Effects of melatonin on N-nitroso-N-methylurea-induced carcinogenesis in rats and mutagenesis in vivo. Cancer Lett 138:37–44.
306. Musatov SA, Anisimov VN, Andre V, Vigreux C, Godard T, Gauduchon P, Sichel F. (1998) Modulatory effects of melatonin on genotoxic response of reference mutagens in the Ames test and the comet assay. Mutat Res 417:75–84.
307. Daniels WMV, Reiter RJ, Melchiorri D, Sewerynek E, Pablos MI, Ortiz GG. (1995) Melatonin counteracts lipid peroxidation induced by carbon tetrachloride but does not restore glucose-6-phosphatase activity. J Pineal Res 19:1–6.
308. Ohta Y, Kongo M, Sasaki E, Nishida K, Ishiguro I. (2000) Therapeutic effect of melatonin on carbon tetrachloride-induced acute liver injury in rats. J Pineal Res 28:119–126.
309. Kim SJ, Reiter RJ, Rourier–Garay MV, Qi W, El-Sokkary GH, Tan DX. (1998) 2-Nitropropane-induced lipid peroxidation: antitoxic effects of melatonin. Toxicology 130:183–190.
310. Ohta Y, Mutsumi S, Sasaki E, Ishiguro I, Harada N. (2000) Protective effect of melatonin against α-naphthylisocyanate-induced liver injury in rats. J Pineal Res 29:15–23.
311. Montilla P, Tunez I, de Agueda CM, Cabrera ES, Montilla–Munoz MC, Alvarez JP, de la Torro Lozano E. (2000) Protective effective of melatonin against oxidative stress induced by ligature of extra-hepatic biliary duct in rats: comparison with the effect of S-adenosyl-L-methionine. J Pineal Res 28:143–149.
312. Qi W, Reiter RJ, Tan DX, Manchester LC, Kim SJ, Garcia JJ. (1999) Inhibitory effects of melatonin on ferric nitrilotriacetate-induced lipid peroxidation and oxidative DNA damage in the rat kidney. Toxicology 139:81–91.
313. Cadenas S, Barja G. (1999) Resveratol, melatonin, vitamin E and PBN protect against renal oxidative DNA damage induced by the kidney carcinogen $KBrO_3$. Free Radic Biol Med 26:1531–1537.
314. Cuzzocrea S, Mazzon E, Serraino I, Lepore V, Terranova ML, Ciccolo A, Caputi AP. (2001) Melatonin reduces dinitrobenzene sulfonic acid-induced colitis. J Pineal Res 30:1–12.
315. Qi W, Tan DX, Reiter RJ, Kim SJ, Manchester LC, Cabrera J, Sainz RM, Mayo JC. (1999) Melatonin reduces lipid peroxidation and tissue edema in cerulein-induced acute pancreatitis in rats. Dig Dis Sci 44:2257–2262.
316. Melchiorri D, Reiter RJ, Sewerynek E, Hara M, Chen LD, Nistico G. (1996) Paraquat toxicity and oxidative damage: reduction by melatonin. Biochem Pharmacol 51:1095–1099.
317. Melchiorri D, Ortiz GG, Reiter RJ, Sewerynek E, Daniels WMU, Pablos MI, Nistiro G. (1998) Melatonin reduces paraquat-induced genotoxicity in mice. Toxicology 95:103–108.
318. Malaisse WJ. (1982) Alloxan toxicity to the pancreatic B-cell. Biochem Pharmacol 22:3527–3534.

319. Yoon JI, Jun HS, Santamaria P. (1998) Cellular and molecular mechanisms for the initiation and progression of β cell destruction resulting from the collaboration between macrophages and T cells. Autoimmunity 27:109–122.
320. Giugliano D, Ceriello A, Paolisso G. (1996) Oxidative stress and diabetic vascular complications. Diabetes Care 19:257–267.
321. Conti A, Maestroni GJM. (1996) Role of the pineal gland and melatonin in the development of autoimmune diabetes in non-obese diabetic mice. J Pineal Res 20:164–172.
322. Oberley LW. (1988) Free radicals and diabetes. Free Radic Biol Med 5:113–124.
323. Ebelt H, Peschke D, Brömme HJ, Mörke W, Blume R, Peschke E. (2000) Influence of melatonin on free radical induced changes in rat pancreatic beta-cells in vitro. J Pineal Res 28:65–72.
324. Montilla PL, Vargas JF, Tunez TF, de Aguedo MC, Valdelvira ME, Cabrera ES. (1998) Oxidative stress in diabetic rats induced by streptozotocin: protective effects of melatonin. J Pineal Res 25:94–100.
325. Larkins RG, Dunlap ME. (1992) The link between hyperglycemia and diabetic nephropathy. Diabetologia 35:499–504.
326. Ha H, Yu MR, Kim KH. (1999) Melatonin and taurine reduce early glomerulopathy in diabetic rats. Free Radic Biol Med 26:944–950.
327. Sailaja Devi MM, Suresh Y, Das UN. (2000) Preservation of the antioxidant status of chemically-induced diabetes mellitus by melatonin. J Pineal Res 29:108–115.
328. Tyrrell RM. (1991) UVA (320–380 nm) radiation as a oxidative stress. In: Sies H, ed. Oxidative Stress, Oxidants and Antioxidants. San Diego: Academic Press, pp. 57–83.
329. Scharffeter–Kochanek K. (1997) Photoaging of the connective tissue of skin: its prevention and therapy. Adv Pharmacol 38:639–655.
330. Darr D, Fridovich I. (1994) Free radicals in cutaneous biology. J Invest Dermatol 102:671–675.
331. Bangha E, Elsner P, Kistler GS. (1996) Suppression of UV-induced erythema by topical treatment with melatonin (N-acetyl-5-methoxytryptamine): a dose–response study. Arch Dermatol Res 288:522–526.
332. Dreher F, Gabard B, Schwindt DA, Mailback HI. (1998) Topical melatonin in combination with vitamins E and C protects skin from ultraviolet-induced erythema: a human study in vivo. Br J Dermatol 139:332–339.
333. Fischer T, Bangha E, Elsner P, Kistler GS. (1999) Suppression of UV-induced erythema by topical treatment with melatonin. Biol Signals Recep 8:132–135.
334. Taira J, Mimura K, Yoneya T, Higi A, Murikami A, Makino K. (1992) Hydroxyl radical formation by UV-irradiated epidermal cells. J Biochem 111:693–695.
335. Gilad E, Cuzzocrea S, Zingarelli B, Salzman AL, Szabo S. (1997) Melatonin is a scavenger of peroxynitrite. Life Sci 60:PL169–PL14.
336. Yamamoto HA, Tang HW. (1996) Antagonistic effect of melatonin against cyanide-induced seizures and acute lethality in mice. Toxicol Lett 87:19–24.
337. Yamamoto HA, Tang HW. (1997) Preventive effect of melatonin against cyanide-induced seizures and lipid peroxidation in mice. Neurosci Lett 207:89–92.
338. Ballantyne B. (1987) Toxicology of cyanides. In: Ballantyne B, Marrs TC, eds. Clinical and Experimental Toxicology of Cyanides. Bristol: Wright, pp. 41–108.
339. Martin M, Macias M, Escames G, Reiter RJ, Agapito MT, Oritz GG, Acuña–Castroviejo D. (2000) Melatonin-induced increased activity of the respiratory chain complexes I and IV can prevent mitochondrial damage induced by ruthenium red in vivo. J Pineal Res 28:242–248.
340. Martin M, Macias M, Escames G, Leon J, Acuña–Castroviejo D. (2000) Melatonin but not vitamins C and E maintains glutathione homeostasis in t-butylhydroperoxide-induced mitochondrial oxidative stress. FASEB J.
341. Meinicke AA, Bechara EJH, Vercesi AE. (1998) Ruthenium red catalyzed degradation of peroxides can prevent mitochondrial oxidative damage induced by either tert-butyl hydroperoxide or by inorganic phosphate. Arch Biochem Biophys 349:275–280.
342. Wakatsuki A, Okatani Y, Shinohara K, Ikenoue N, Kaneda C, Fukaya T. (2001) Melatonin protects fetal rat brain against oxidative mitochondrial damage. J Pineal Res 30:22–28.
343. Steinberg D. (1997) Low density lipoprotein and its photobiological significance. J Biol Chem 272:20963–20966.
344. Pieri C, Marra M, Gaspar R, Damjanovich S. (1996) Melatonin protects LDL from oxidation but does not prevent the apolipoprotein derivatization. Biochem Biophys Res Commun 222:256–260.

345. Kelly MR, Loo G. (1997) Melatonin inhibits oxidative modification of human low density lipoprotein. J Pineal Res 22:203–209.
346. Walters–Laporte E, Furman C, Fouquet S, Martin–Nizard F, Lestavel S, Gozzo A, Lesieur D, Fruchart JC, Duriez P, Teissier E. A high concentration of melatonin inhibits in vitro LDL peroxidation but not oxidized LDL toxicity toward cultured endothelial cells. J Cardiovasc Pharmacol 32:582–592.
347. Seeger H, Mueck AO, Lippert TH. (1997) Effect of melatonin and metabolites on copper-mediated oxidation of low density lipoprotein. Br J Clin Pharmacol 44:283–284.
348. Wakatsuki A, Okatani Y, Ikenoue N, Izumiya C, Kaneda C. (2000) Melatonin inhibits oxidative modification of low-density lipoprotein particles in normolipidemic post-menopausal women. J Pineal Res (in press).
349. Hoyos M, Guerero JM, Perez–Cano R, Oliva J, Fabiani F, Garcia–Pergañneda A, Osuna C. (2000) Serum cholesterol and lipid peroxidation are decreased by melatonin in diet-induced hypercholesterolemic rats. J Pineal Res 28:150–155.
350. Aoyama H, Mori N, Mori W. (1988) Effects of melatonin on genetic hypercholesterolemia in rats. Atherosclerosis 69:269–272.
351. Müller–Wieland D, Behnke B, Koopmann K, Krone W. (1994) Melatonin inhibits LDL receptor activity and cholesterol synthesis is freshly isolated human mononuclear leukocytes. Biochem Biophys Res Commun 203:416–421.
352. Okatani Y, Wakatsuki A, Watanabe K, Ikenoue N, Fukaya T. (2000) Melatonin inhibits vasospastic action of oxidized low-density lipoprotein in human umbilical arteries. J Pineal Res 29:74–80.
353. Okatani Y, Wakatsuki A, Watanabe K, Fukaya T. (2000) Attenuation by melatonin of human umbilical arterial vasoconstriction induced by lysophosphatidylcholine. J Pineal Res 29:159–165.
354. Reiter J, Carneiro RC, Oh CS. (1997) Melatonin in relation to cellular antioxidative defense mechanisms. Horm Metab Res 29:363–372.
355. Reiter RJ. (1998) Cytoprotective properties of melatonin: association with oxidative damage. Nutrition 14:691–696.
356. Reiter RJ. (1999) Oxidative damage to nuclear DNA: amelioration by melatonin. Neuroendocrinol Lett 20:145–149, 1999.

29
Radical and Reactive Intermediate-Scavenging Properties of Melatonin in Pure Chemical Systems

Maria A. Livrea and Luisa Tesoriere
University of Palermo, Palermo, Italy

Dun-xian Tan and Russel J. Reiter
The University of Texas Health Science Center, San Antonio, Texas

I. INTRODUCTION

Although redox properties of indoles and derivatives have long been known (1–6), studies on the chemical reactivity and redox properties of melatonin are relatively recent. These studies, which developed on finding that melatonin has the ability to neutralize hydroxyl radicals (7), demonstrate that the indoleamine is capable of scavenging a number of free radicals, and led to a postulate that it may behave as an antioxidant. A remarkable amount of experimental work in vivo and in vitro has indeed shown that melatonin can protect cell and tissues from damage initiated by free radicals. These findings opened new perspectives on the biological aspects of this hormone, for which the physiological role in humans has remained elusive, as well as on its therapeutical potential in human pathophysiology.

Some thermodynamic and kinetic requirements must be fulfilled for a compound to act as an effective antioxidant in radical-triggered oxidative processes. First, it must be kept in mind that a reaction, although thermodynamically possible, may not be kinetically feasible (i.e., the rate constant may be so small that the reaction is not biologically significant). In addition, the oxidized, radical form of the scavenger molecule should be relatively harmless (being neither strongly oxidizing nor strongly reducing), react poorly with oxygen, and its kinetic properties should be such that only relatively small amounts are required for it to work as an antioxidant. Finally, it should be recycled, directly or indirectly, by enzyme systems.

This chapter encompasses all the known reactions of melatonin with either strong oxidant or radical species in pure chemical systems, and reports reaction mechanisms and rate constants whenever measured. This information may be of help when considering biological roles of melatonin or may suggest pharmacological applications.

II. REACTION OF MELATONIN WITH REACTIVE OXYGEN SPECIES

A. Hydroxyl Radical

Reactivity of melatonin versus the hydroxyl radical ˙OH was first studied by Tan and colleagues (7), and later by other groups. Two experimental approaches have been used: measurement of the direct reaction with ˙OH generated by radiolysis of H_2O, and competition studies, which analyzed the effect of melatonin in ˙OH-generating systems in the presence of spin traps or chemical probes. By using the UV photolysis of H_2O_2 to generate ˙OH, Tan et al. (7) demonstrated that melatonin competed very efficiently with the spin trap 5,5-dimethylpyrroline N-oxide (DMPO). Increasing concentrations of melatonin (1–100 μM) reduced the formation of DMPO–˙OH adducts, which were identified by high-performance liquid chromatography (HPLC) with electrochemical detection, and confirmed by electron spin resonance (ESR) spectroscopy. Dose–response studies revealed that the concentration required to neutralize 50% of the radicals generated (IC_{50}) was 21 μM. This indicated an effectiveness more than five times higher than that measured for glutathione, and ten times higher than that of mannitol (7).

Matuszak et al. (8) have recently confirmed that melatonin can efficiently reduce DMPO–˙OH adduct formation. They used ESR in conjunction with the spin-trapping technique to evaluate the rate constant for the reaction of melatonin with hydroxyl radicals generated by a Fenton reaction from $FeSO_4$ and H_2O_2. Melatonin reacted with ˙OH with a rate constant of 2.7×10^{10} M^{-1} s^{-1}.

Kinetic competition studies were carried out using the specific radical-trapping reagent 2,2'-azinobis(3-ethylbenzthiazoline-6-sulfonic acid) (ABTS), as a probe for the generation of ˙OH from H_2O_2 and $FeSO_4$ (9). During the coincubation in such a system, melatonin reacted rapidly with ˙OH, which prevented the oxidation of ABTS to its stable thiazoline cation radical, with a calculated rate constant of 0.6×10^{11} M^{-1} s^{-1}.

Hydroxyl radical-scavenging ability of melatonin was investigated by Pahkla et al. (10) using terephthalic acid (THA) as a chemical dosimeter of ˙OH generated by the Fenton reaction from $CuSO_4$ and H_2O_2. Melatonin scavenged ˙OH in a concentration-dependent manner, thereby reducing the fluorescence caused by the formation of the THA–˙OH adduct. The calculated IC_{50} was 11.4 ± 1 μM.

Recently, Chyan et al. (11) performed competition experiments using either 5,5-dimethyl-1-pyrroline N-oxide or ABTS as free radical-trapping agents, to assay the capacity of melatonin at scavenging ˙OH, generated by H_2O_2 exposed to light. The measured reaction constant was 4×10^{10} M^{-1} s^{-1}.

Transient absorption spectra of melatonin radicals, formed during pulse radiolysis of aqueous melatonin N_2O-saturated solutions, were analyzed to study the reaction of melatonin with ˙OH radicals (12). The overall rate constant determined for the pseudo–first-order buildup kinetics was 1.25×10^{10} M^{-1} s^{-1}.

Stasica et al. (13) studied the reaction of melatonin with radiolytically generated radicals. They found that the reaction of melatonin with ˙OH is diffusion-controlled, with a rate constant of 1.2×10^{10} M^{-1} s^{-1}.

Table 1 reports the rate constants calculated for the reaction of melatonin with ˙OH.

B. Peroxyl Radicals

Pieri et al. (14) used a fluorescent assay in which β-phycoerythrin was a fluorescent indicator protein, and the thermal decomposition of the water-soluble 2-2'-azobis(2-amidinopropane) dihydrochloride (AAPH) was the source of peroxyl radicals. Melatonin did not cause clear lag periods at any of the assayed concentrations. However, at 0.5–4.0 μM it delayed the fluo-

Table 1 Reactivity Constants of Melatonin Toward Hydroxyl Radical

Source of ˙OH	Rate constant (M^{-1} s^{-1})	Assay	Ref.
Fe^{2+}/H_2O_2	2.7×10^{10}	EPR-spin trapping	8
Fe^{2+}/H_2O_2	0.6×10^{11}	Kinetic competition with ABTS	44
H_2O_2/UV light	4×10^{10}	Kinetic competition with ABTS or 5,5-dimethyl-1-pirroline-N-oxide	11
Pulse radiolysis of water	1.25×10^{10}	Absorption spectra of melatoninyl radical	12
Pulse radiolysis of water	1.2×10^{10}	Absorption spectra of melatoninyl spectra	13

rescence decay of β-phycoerythrin, showing that it may scavenge the AAPH-derived peroxyl radicals. Trolox, a water-soluble analogue of vitamin E used as a positive control, was less effective (14). However, the issue that melatonin was "twice as effective as vitamin E," as pointed out by the authors, appears as a misinterpretation of the results.

A limited lipoperoxyl radical-scavenging activity of melatonin was observed by other researchers. Marshall and co-workers (15) used ox brain phospholipid liposomes incubated with $FeCl_3$ and ascorbate. Melatonin produced a concentration-dependent inhibition of peroxidation, measured by the thiobarbituric acid (TBA) test, with an IC_{50} value of 210 μM.

Studies on the interaction of melatonin with lipoperoxyl radicals from soybean phosphatidylcholine (PC) liposomes have been carried out (16). With unilamellar liposomes from the nonperoxidable lipid dimirystoyl phosphatidylcholine (DMC) in comparison with soybean PC liposomes, and AAPH as a radical initiator, the authors (16) were capable of distinguishing the reactivity of melatonin with the AAPH-derived peroxyl radicals from that with lipoperoxyl radicals. Fluorescence measurements showed that melatonin was consumed at a rate of 0.13×10^{-8} M^{-1} s^{-1} in the reaction with lipoperoxyl radicals. As a comparison, the rate of disappearance of α-tocopherol in the same assay system, was evaluated as 0.17×10^{-8} M^{-1} s^{-1}. Interaction of melatonin with lipoperoxyl radicals was also observed in multilamellar liposomes induced to undergo peroxidation by a lipophilic azo initiator (16). Although capable of scavenging initiator-derived radicals, and lipoperoxyl radicals as well, the efficacy of melatonin in this liposomal system was very moderate on a concentration–effect basis when compared with that of α-tocopherol.

The lipoperoxyl radical-scavenging activity of melatonin was also checked (17). The assays included peroxidation of linoleic acid micelles by either AAPH (system 1), or Fe^{2+}–EDTA (system 2), and of dilinoleoyl phosphatidylcholine (DLPC) multilamellar liposomes for which peroxidation was induced by Fe^{2-}–EDTA (system 3). The continuous production of conjugated dienes as monitored spectrophotometrically (systems 1 and 2), and a colorimetric assay for reactive aldehydes (system 3), were used to reveal melatonin activity. Although concentrations of melatonin as low as 20 nM were effective in inhibiting the formation of lipid peroxides in systems 2 and 3, no effect was observed in system 1. These results led the authors to conclude that melatonin was poorly effective at scavenging peroxyl radicals, although it was capable of scavenging the ˙OH possibly formed in a Fenton-like reaction. In the micellar system iron-stimulated IC_{50} values of 1.26 μM and 53.4 nM were found for melatonin and vitamin E, respectively. On the other hand, melatonin was more efficient in the inhibition of iron-stimulated peroxidation of multilamellar liposomes ($IC_{50} < 100$ nM), which was suggested by the authors to be the result of a better positioning and orientation of the indolamine in the bilayer. This, however, could also imply that, in addition to acting as a ˙OH scavenger, melatonin can scavenge lipoperoxyl radicals in such a liposomal system (16).

Pahkla and co-workers (10) have recently observed that 42 μM of melatonin inhibited the formation of TBA-reactive substances after incubation of linolenic acid and $FeSO_4$, for 60 min at 37°C, by only 21%.

Several experiments were designed (18) to evaluate the kinetics of lipoperoxyl radical trapping by melatonin. This was checked by monitoring the oxygen uptake in a homogeneous system, using styrene as the autoxidable substrate, and in a heterogeneous micellar system formed with methyl linoleate and di-*tert*-butyl hyponitrite (DBHN) as the azo initiator, dispersed in water with sodium dodecyl sulfate. Finally, experiments were designed to monitor the inhibition by melatonin of the oxidation of phospholipid bilayers induced by either DBHN or AAPH. Vitamin E was assayed as a positive control in all experiments. In accordance with the studies of others (15–17), only a limited activity was observed, and it was concluded that melatonin is "a rather weak and ineffective retarder" of the lipid autoxidation, and not a trap for peroxyl radicals. This would explain, and at the same time would be supported by, the absence of distinct inhibition periods during the lipid oxidation in the presence of melatonin (16,17). Other observations that melatonin acts synergistically with the lipoperoxyl radical-trapping vitamin E in a liposomal system (16) may suggest that melatonin cannot act as a chain-breaking antioxidant in lipid systems. Indeed, antioxidants that act through the same mechanism would show only additive effects when used together.

Melatonin does not possess phenolic hydrogens; its indole hydrogen can more easily undergo electron transfer than hydrogen atom transfer (5). Peroxyl radicals may add to melatonin rather than abstracting hydrogen atoms. Identification of products from the reaction may help establish a mechanism for scavenging lipoperoxyl radicals.

Haloperoxyl radicals possess high reactivity, owing to the highly electron-deficient nature of the halide ions, which makes them capable of oxidizing substrates by electron transfer (19). Marshall et al. (15) established that melatonin is an excellent scavenger of trichloromethylperoxyl radicals. By using radiolysis of an aqueous mixture of propanol-2-ol and CCl_4, they measured the direct reaction of melatonin with $CCl_3OO·$, and calculated a second-order rate constant to be $k = 2.7 \times 10^8$ M^{-1} s^{-1}. In a similar pulse radiolysis system (12) a rate constant of $k = 6 \times 10^8$ M^{-1} s^{-1} was found.

C. Alkoxyl Radicals

Laser flash photolysis was used (20) to cause cleavage of di-*tert*-butoxyl, and di-*tert*-cumyloxyl peroxide into two *tert*-butoxyl radicals (*t*-butO˙) in acetonitrile. Spectrophotometric analysis of the transient spectra was used to provide evidence that melatonin interacted with the photoinduced alkoxyl radical with a rate constant of 3.4×10^7 M^{-1} s^{-1}, generating an indolyl-like radical. Melatonin reacted similarly with di-*tert*-cumyloxyl radicals, with a calculated rate constant of 6.7×10^7 M^{-1} s^{-1}.

tert-Butoxyl radicals were generated on pulse radiolysis of a N_2-bubbled aqueous solution containing *tert*-butanol and *tert*-butyl hydroperoxide, in the presence of melatonin, at pH 7.0 (12). The rate of formation of radical intermediates from melatonin, as evaluated spectrophotometrically, allowed the measurement of a reaction rate with butoxyl radicals of 2.8×10^9 M^{-1} s^{-1}. On the other hand, in recently performed studies (21) melatonin was not capable of quenching the ESR signals in a system in which galvinoxyl radicals in CH_2Cl_2 were used as the hydrogen abstractor.

Table 2 reports on the reactivity constants of melatonin with peroxyl and alkoxyl radicals.

Table 2 Reactivity Constants of Melatonin Toward Peroxyl and Alkoxyl Radicals

Radical	Generation system	Rate constant ($M^{-1}\ s^{-1}$)	Assay	Ref.
$CCl_3OO^{\cdot}$	Radiolysis of aqueous mixture of CCl_4 and propanol-2-ol	2.7×10^8	Measurement of $CCl_3OO^{\cdot}$	15
$CCl_3OO^{\cdot}$	Electron pulse of aqueous mixture of isopropanol, acetone, and CCl_4	6×10^8	Absorption spectra of melatoninyl radical	12
tert-Butoxyl	Laser photolysis of di-tert-butoxyl peroxide in acetonitrile	3.4×10^7	Absorption spectra of melatoninyl radical	20
tert-Butoxyl	Pulse radiolysis of aqueous mixture of tert-butanol and tert-butyl hydroperoxide	2.8×10^9	Absorption spectra of melatoninyl radical	12
tert-Cumyloxyl	Laser photolysis of di-tert-cumyloxyl peroxide in acetonitrile	6.7×10^7	Absorption spectra of melatoninyl radical	20

D. Hydrogen Peroxide

Reaction of melatonin with hydrogen peroxide is controversial. Experiments have been carried out in the laboratory of Livrea and co-workers, by treating ethanol solutions of melatonin in water (0.25% ethanol) with equimolar concentrations of H_2O_2, at 37°C, followed by spectral analysis. No spectral changes of melatonin were observed for 1–10 min. In addition, extraction of the incubation mixture with ethyl acetate, followed by HPLC analysis, did not show any consumption of the indoleamine. This finding confirmed previous observations (22).

Assays in which the reaction of melatonin with H_2O_2 was evaluated after the oxidation of red phenol (23) or guaiacol (24) by horseradish peroxidase in the presence of H_2O_2, must be considered with caution in the light that melatonin could react with the oxoferryl intermediate (see Sec. IV), involved in the catalytic mechanism of this heme enzyme (25).

E. Superoxide Anion Radical

Marshall et al. (15) reported that melatonin did not scavenge superoxide anions. Assays were carried out wherein O_2^- was generated by the hypoxanthine–xanthine oxidase system, in the presence of either cytochrome c or nitroblue tetrazolium, and in the absence or in the presence of melatonin, added in a five times higher concentration than the competitor. Similar findings were described by Chan and Tang (24), who checked the reactivity of melatonin with O_2^- in a competition study in which DL-epinephrine auto-oxidation to adenochrome was stimulated by the xanthine–xanthine oxidase system (26). However, an assay based on the quenching of ESR signals from the species $DMPO-O_2^-$, revealed that melatonin may react with superoxide anions, although with a modest effectiveness (23).

F. Singlet Oxygen

Singlet oxygen is often generated by the photosensitization reaction of substrates such as dyes or biological pigments. Riboflavin catalyzed the oxidation of melatonin on autoxidation induced by irradiation with bright white light (22). In other studies (23), melatonin inhibited singlet oxygen-dependent 2,2,6,6-tetramethyl piperidine oxide (TEMPO) radical formation during rose bengal photodynamic excitation.

G. Hypochlorous Acid

Reaction of melatonin with hypochlorous acid was studied (15) in competition experiments in which the oxidation of 5-thio-2-nitrobenzoic acid (TNB) by HOCl was monitored at a wavelength of 412 nm. Melatonin, at 0.05–0.5 mM, incubated with HOCl before addition of TNB, decreased the loss of absorbance, indicating that it was capable of scavenging HOCl. Further evidence was obtained by monitoring the spectral changes of melatonin after reaction with HOCl.

The absorbance quenching of β-carotene was also used to check the scavenging ability of melatonin with HOCl (24). The results showed that 0.1 μM of melatonin preserved 68% of the β-carotene absorbance.

Recent studies (27) report on the reactivity constant for the reaction of melatonin with HOCl, in phosphate-buffered ethanol–water solution. Melatonin deactivated both HOCl and OCl$^-$, and the relevant constant, at 37°C, and a 23 M water concentration, were of $k_{HOCl} = 7 \pm 1 \times 10^3$ M^{-1} s^{-1}, and $k_{OCl^-} = 6.1 \times 10^2$ M^{-1} s^{-1}.

III. REACTIVE NITROGEN SPECIES

Peroxynitrite (ONOO$^-$) is considered to form from the reaction of superoxide and nitric oxide ($^{\cdot}$NO) (26). At physiological pH, it is rapidly protonated to form peroxynitrous acid (ONOOH), which may oxidize nitrate or hydroxylate biomolecules through a controversial mechanism, involving either homolytic decomposition, with a release of an intermediate with hydroxyl radical-like character (29,30), or isomerization to nitric acid by an activated form of peroxynitrous acid (ONOOH*) (28).

Gilad and co-workers (31) showed the concentration-dependent inhibitory effect of melatonin on the oxidation of dihydrorhodamine 123 by peroxynitrite. The IC$_{50}$ value for the inhibition was 10 μM, similar to that obtained with scavengers of ONOO$^-$, such as glutathione and cysteine. More recently, a paper from Pryor's group reported the spectrum of a melatoninyl radical during the ONOO$^-$–melatonin reaction, providing direct evidence of an initial one-electron transfer from melatonin to ONOO$^-$ (32). Further kinetic studies and product analysis from the same group (33) led to outline a possible mechanism of the reaction (see later discussion). The authors conclude that both peroxynitrous acid (ONOOH) and its anion (ONOO$^-$) are reactive toward melatonin, but at physiological pH most of the reaction of melatonin involves ONOOH and the high-energy intermediate ONOOH*. The second-order rate constant for the reaction with ONOOH was determined as 159 M^{-1} s^{-1}; with the peroxynitrite anion as 5 M^{-1} s^{-1} (33).

The reaction of melatonin with $^{\cdot}$N$_3$ generated by pulse radiolysis was studied spectrophotometrically (12). The transient absorption spectra of the species formed by the azide radical reaction with melatonin allowed the authors to measure a rate constant of 7.5×10^9 M^{-1} s^{-1}.

The $^{\cdot}$NO$_2$ radicals obtained by pulse irradiation of nitrite anions reacted with melatonin to yield a transient spectrum, the absorption of which indicated a rate constant of 3.7×10^6 M^{-1} s^{-1} (12). In addition, a constant of 3×10^7 M^{-1} s^{-1} was measured for the reaction between melatonin and $^{\cdot}$NO radicals generated by pulse radiolysis of a N$_2$-bubbled aqueous solution containing *tert*-butanol and sodium nitrite (12).

Table 3 Reactivity Constants of Melatonin Toward Reactive Nitrogen Species (RNS)

RNS	Generation system	Rate constant (M^{-1} s^{-1})	Assay	Ref.
ONOOH	Ozonation of NaN_3	159	Absorption spectra of melatoninyl radical	33
$ONOO^-$	Ozonation of NaN_3	5	Absorption spectra of melatoninyl radical	33
$·N_3$	Water radiolysis plus N_3^-	7.5×10^9	Absorption spectra of melatoninyl radical	12
$·NO_2$	Pulse irradiation of NO_2^-	3.7×10^6	Absorption spectra of melatoninyl radical	12
$·NO$	Pulse radiolysis of N_2-bubbled aqueous solution of tert-butanol plus $NaNO_2$	3×10^7	Absorption spectra of melatoninyl radical	12

Noda and colleagues (34) have recently shown that melatonin can scavenge ·NO generated by decomposition of 1-hydroxy-2-oxo-3-(N-methyl-3-aminopropyl)-3-methyl-1-triazene (NOC-7).

Table 3 reports on the constants measured for the reaction of melatonin with reactive nitrogen species.

IV. PERFERRYL HEMOGLOBIN

The so-called perferryl-hemoglobin, ·Hb[Fe(IV)=O], as generated from methemoglobin (met-Hb) and H_2O_2 (35), comprises a short-lived radical localized on the globin, possibly an aromatic amino acid radical (36,37), and a Fe(IV)=O oxoferryl heme group (36,38,39), which may be detected by optical spectroscopy. In the laboratory of Livrea and co-workers (40), bovine met-Hb was oxidized by equivalent amounts of H_2O_2 in the absence or in the presence of melatonin. The incubation of methemoglobin (Fig. 1, line 1) with H_2O_2 leads to a rapid loss of the peak at 630 nm within 1 min, with the concomitant evolution of two new peaks at 545 and 580 nm characteristic of the oxoferryl moiety (see Fig. 1, line 2). When the same reaction was carried out in the presence of melatonin, the spectral analysis revealed a markedly reduced amount of Fe(IV)=O after 1 min (see Fig. 1, line 3), and the spectrum recorded after 5 min coincided with the spectrum of met-Hb (see Fig. 1, line 4). An initial reduction rate of 0.4 μM s^{-1} may be calculated from the spectrophotometric data. Consumption of melatonin in the process was evaluated by HPLC (see Fig. 1, inset). Quantification of met-Hb formed per melatonin molecule consumed yielded a 1:1 stoichiometry for the reaction melatonin/perferryl-Hb. As a comparison, Trolox, a water-soluble analogue of vitamin E, which is a powerful reductant of perferryl-Hb (41,42), was capable of regenerating completely met-Hb within 5 min, with a reduction rate of 0.3 μM s^{-1}.

Whether reduction by melatonin was at the oxoferryl moiety or the unpaired electron electrophile center at the globin moiety, or both, is indistinguishable by the spectrophotometric evidence. However, the spectrum of met-Hb induced by melatonin was coincident with the initial met-Hb spectrum before addition of H_2O_2. Although indicating reaction with the oxoferryl moiety, this also suggests that a reduction of the globin radical occurs, otherwise modification of globin residues by the oxidant activity of perferryl-Hb would make the met-

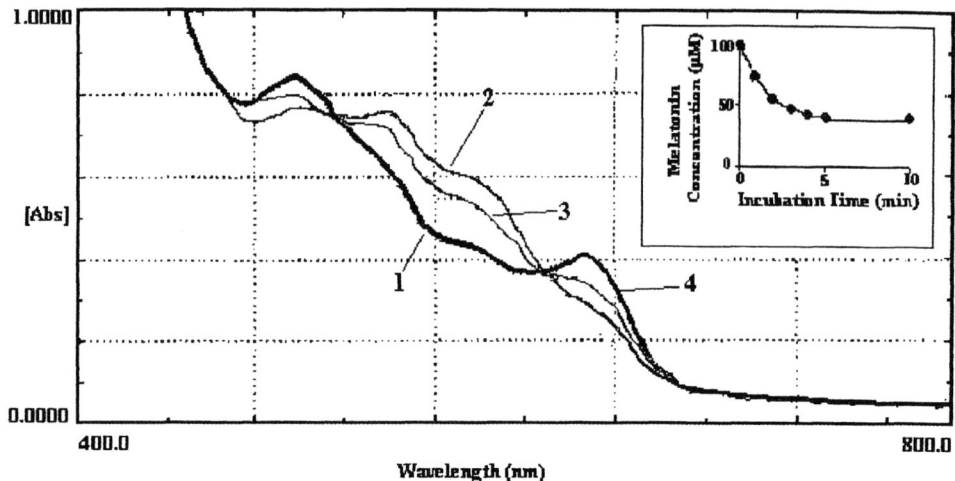

Figure 1 Reduction of perferryl-hemoglobin by melatonin Met-Hb (100 μM, line 1) was converted to perferryl-Hb by a 1-min incubation with H_2O_2 (100 μM) in the absence (line 2) or in the presence (line 3) of melatonin (100 μM). Then, repetitive scans were taken every minute for the following 4 min, the time at which line 4 was recorded.

to ferryl-Hb transformation irreversible (43). This evidence, the observed 1:1 stoichiometry [met-Hb]formed/[melatonin]oxidized, and the identification of the products from melatonin (see later), are consistent with a two-electron oxidation reaction.

V. MISCELLANEOUS REDOX ACTIVITIES OF MELATONIN

Melatonin was capable of scavenging the stable nitrogen-centered cation radical of 2,2′-azino-bis(3-ethylbenzthiazoline-6-sulfonic acid) (ABTS) after it was generated by reaction with the ˙OH radical (44). Under the conditions used, melatonin at 500 μM reduced 91 ± 3% of the ABTS cation radical, as revealed by the decrease of $ABTS^{+\cdot}$ absorbance at 420 nm.

Melatonin scavenged the radicals formed during metal-induced autoxidation of catecholamines (45). The oxidation of the fluorescent protein β-phycoerythrin (β-PE) was used as a probe for the pro-oxidant activity of the free radicals produced from dopamine and L-dopa, during the $CuSO_4$-catalyzed autoxidation. Melatonin at 10 μM markedly reduced the β-PE decay of fluorescence, indicating a reaction with catecholamine radicals. On the other hand, melatonin did not show any effect on the rate of $CuSO_4$-induced oxidation of β-PE, for concentrations ranging from 3 to 100 μM.

An accurate analysis aimed at explaining the protective effects of melatonin in radical-mediated oxidations, has been recently performed (18). Experimental evidence is provided that melatonin can chelate iron, thereby inhibiting metal–ion-catalyzed oxidation processes. This property may account for some activity of melatonin as a preventive antioxidant. In addition, it has been shown (46) that melatonin may form complexes with iron(III).

VI. MELATONIN OXIDATION PRODUCTS

Analysis of products from the reaction of melatonin with strong oxidants or free radicals may be a good strategy to clarify pathways of melatonin oxidation and eventually to distinguish between reactions of various radicals with the indoleamine.

The finding that N-acetyl-N'-formyl 5-methoxykynuramine (AFMK) is formed from melatonin in the rat brain by indole 2,3-dioxygenase, a heme-containing enzyme requiring O_2^- as a substrate (47), and that the same oxidation product was found in a system generating O_2^- by means of xanthine oxidase in the presence of iron–EDTA (48) or hemin (49) as catalysts, led Hardeland et al. (50) to hypothesize that melatonin may trap O_2^-. When AFMK was found among the products from the reaction of melatonin with ·OH generated by UV-irradiation of H_2O_2 (50), a mechanism was suggested in which a one-electron reaction of melatonin with a strong oxidant would produce an indolyl cation radical which, in turn, scavenges O_2^- leading to formation of AFMK (50). This intuition was later confirmed by studies in which the transient formation of the radical from melatonin was shown spectrophotometrically (12,13,20,32), and the formation of AFMK was demonstrated in a biological system generating oxidant species such as heme-derived oxoferryl radicals and O_2^- (40).

Of the two possible reactions—electron or hydrogen atom transfer—that may take place when indole derivatives react with one-electron oxidants in neutral aqueous solution, the electron transfer has appeared as the favored one (5). However, secondary acid–base reactions have an important effect on the overall redox equilibria. The pK_a of indole and substituted indolyl radicals are frequently between 4.5 and 6.5, suggesting that under physiological conditions the neutral form will normally predominate (6,51).

A number of one-electron oxidants, such as $Br_2^{·-}$ and $N_3^·$ were scavenged by melatonin in aqueous solution at pH 7.0 to produce characteristic absorptions at 335 and 500 nm (12), resembling the transient spectra of substituted indolyl neutral radical species (6). At pH 3.0 the protonated form of the transient is formed (12), exhibiting a strong absorption at 450 nm, owing to the interaction of the unpaired electron with the methoxy substituent in C-5 (6), in addition to the typical bands at 330 and 520 nm (3,6). Similar spectra were observed after reaction of melatonin with alkoxyl radicals (20), or with $ONOO^-$ (32).

Stasica et al. (13), and Mahal et al. (12) observed that the spectra after the reaction of melatonin with ·OH match those of the indolyl-type radicals. However, careful analysis of the evolution of the initial absorption spectra indicates that at least one more intermediate, other than the indolyl structure, is involved in the reaction. The authors suggest that this can be formed by ·OH attack at positions on the indole ring other than the indole nitrogen, and formation of adducts (13). This appears in accordance with recent studies of Tan et al. (52), who used HPLC, mass spectral analysis, and proton nuclear magnetic resonance (^{1}H NMR) to isolate and identify the cyclic 3-hydroxy melatonin (1,2,3,3a,8,8a-hexahydro-1-acetyl-5-methoxy-3a-hydroxypyrrolo[2,3-b]indole, according to the IUPAC nomenclature), as a product from the reaction of melatonin with ·OH. According to the authors, the reaction involves the initial addition of one ·OH at the C-3 position of the indole ring.

Products from melatonin oxidation by $ONOO^-$ have been identified using gas chromatography–mass spectrometry and ^{1}H NMR (32,33). Experiments were carried out in aqueous solution, at a physiological pH, either in the absence or in the presence of CO_2. Hydroxylated products such as 6-hydroxymelatonin, the cyclic-1,2,3,3a,8,8a-hexahydro-1-acetyl-5-methoxy-8a-hydroxypyrrolo[2,3-b]indole (cyclic 2-hydroxy melatonin), and 1,2,3,3a,8,8a-hexahydro-1-acetyl-5-methoxy-3a-hydroxypyrrolo[2,3-b]indole (cyclic 3-hydroxy melatonin) were recovered. Spectrophotometric evidence of a melatoninyl radical was found under both conditions, but 6-hydroxymelatonin was not formed in the presence of added bicarbonate. Although ruling out that this compound derives from the melatoninyl radical, this finding suggests that another oxidant species is involved, possibly an activated form of peroxynitrite, formed only in the absence of bicarbonate (53,54). On the other hand, the hydroxypyrrolo[2,3-b]indole products result from the secondary reactions of melatoninyl radicals generated from the reaction of melatonin either with ONOOH and $ONOO^-$, or with reactive species, such as $CO_3^{·-}$ and $·NO_2$

produced from the ONOO$^-$/CO$_2$ reaction. Nitrated products from melatonin were not isolated, either in the absence or in the presence of CO$_2$, although CO$_2$ is known to catalyze nitrations by ONOO$^-$ (55–59). Nitrated species, however, are suggested by the authors as intermediates in the oxidation process (33).

The oxidation products from melatonin after reaction with hemoglobin-derived oxoferryl radicals have been analyzed and identified by gas chromatography–mass spectrometry (40). The cyclic 3-hydroxymelatonin was identified as the major metabolite, whereas minor amounts of AFMK and of a melatonin 2-indolinone derivative [3-(2-acetamidoethyl)-5-

Figure 2 Melatoninyl radical and melatonin metabolites.

methoxy-2-indolinone] were also found. A similar oxindole compound has been proposed (33) as an intermediate to the formation of the cyclic 2-hydroxymelatonin.

Figure 2 reports on structures of the melatonin metabolites identified so far in reactions with radical species or strong oxidants in solution.

VII. PRO-OXIDANT ACTIVITY

There has been only one study that reports the pro-oxidant activity of melatonin. Ianas and colleagues (60) tested the scavenging activity of 0.08–0.5 mM melatonin, in a system consisting of luminol and H_2O_2. They observed that melatonin, at 0.1 mM, develops antioxidant properties only with the increase in peroxide concentrations, whereas at concentrations lower than 0.1 mM it has antioxidative effect. Although puzzling, these results may be related to the assay used, as chemiluminescence of luminol may be enhanced by the presence of ˙OH scavengers in the medium (61).

Marshall et al. (15) reported that melatonin is devoid of pro-oxidative actions, at least in the series of tests they performed. Chyan and co-workers (11) have recently investigated the pro-oxidant activity of melatonin in an ˙OH-generating system consisting of hydrogen peroxide, $FeCl_3$, and EDTA, in the presence of salicylate, and measured the formation of the ˙OH adducts of salicylate. Although ascorbate, Trolox, and glutathione were highly pro-oxidant, leading to the production of the salicylate adduct as high as 200% of control, melatonin led to an increment of the adduct of only 25%.

VIII. REGENERATION OF MELATONIN

Mahal et al. (12) reported regeneration of the one-electron oxidized melatonin radical by ascorbate and urate. By monitoring the first-order decay of the 510-nm transient, they evaluated the rate constant for the regeneration of melatonin as 7×10^7 M^{-1} s^{-1} and 4×10^7 M^{-1} s^{-1} for ascorbate and urate, respectively. Regeneration of melatoninyl radical by such compounds may account for the synergism observed with ascorbate, Trolox, or GSH in assays in which melatonin scavenged ˙OH (9).

IX. MELATONIN ANALOGUES

Several structure–activity studies were carried out with melatonin analogues. In general, it appears that the structural requirements change according to the radicals with which the indole derivatives are interacting.

Tan and co-workers (7) compared the hydroxyl radical-scavenging activity of melatonin with that of the chemically related molecules 5-hydroxytryptamine (serotonin), N-acetylserotonin, and 5-methoxytryptamine. The results suggested that the methyl group at the 5-OH position of the indole nucleus is important for the scavenging function, and the N-acetyl group on the side chain produces a synergistic action. The influence of the methoxy group in the radical-scavenging activity of substituted indoleamines was later investigated by Scaiano (20), in a system generating alkoxyl radicals. 5-Methoxytryptamine and 5-methoxyindole showed reactivity toward tert-butoxyl radicals similar to that of melatonin (20), whereas indole was less effective, confirming the importance of the methoxy group at the C-5 position of the indole ring in the radical-scavenging activity of these substances.

Matuszak et al. (8) determined the rate constants for the reaction of indole derivatives other than melatonin with hydroxyl radicals generated by a Fenton reaction from $FeSO_4$ and

H_2O_2. Interestingly, they observed that serotonin reacts with ·OH with a rate constant that is almost equally as high as melatonin's, a result not in accordance with the findings of Tan et al. (7), who reported that serotonin stimulated ·OH formation. According to the authors, this discrepancy may be explained by considering that Tan et al. (7) generated ·OH by UV irradiation of H_2O_2, which may induce the indoleamine photolysis and produce O_2^- (62,63), which is the precursor of ·OH radicals. On the other hand, Matuszak et al. (8) observed that serotonin may stimulate the generation of ·OH in the presence of Fe^{3+} ions or Fe^{3+}–EDTA. This has been accounted for by the formation of an indoxyl radical during the reduction of Fe^{3+} by the hydroxyl group of serotonin, which may start a sequence leading to the production of ·OH (8). Similar reactivity of serotonin with Fe^{3+} ions was observed by Marshall et al. (15), using the Fe^{3+}–EDTA/H_2O_2–deoxyribose system, and by Chan and Tang (24) and Marshall et al. (15) in the bleomycin assay.

Serotonin was more effective than melatonin in scavenging lipoperoxyl radicals generated in ox brain liposomes (15). Presumably, the phenolic -OH group may positively affect the reactivity of serotonin versus LOO·. However, serotonin was slightly less efficient in scavenging other peroxyl radicals, such as CCl_3OO· (15).

Chan and Tang (24) showed that serotonin scavenged O_2^-, although N-acetylserotonin was ineffective, in a competition study in which DL-epinephrine auto-oxidation to adenochrome was stimulated by the xanthine–xanthine oxidase system (26). As reported in the foregoing, melatonin was ineffective in such a system.

Serotonin and N-acetylserotonin were more effective than melatonin in scavenging HOCl in assays in which the absorbance quenching of β-carotene by HOCl was measured (24).

In contrast to melatonin, N-acetylserotonin showed a hydrogen-donating capacity, as documented by the decrease of the ESR signal of the galvinoxyl radical (21).

Other indole derivatives such as β-carboline (pinoline) or AFMK, and 5-methoxytryptophan, as well as tryptophan, were totally ineffective at scavenging the nitrogen-centered ABTS cation radical (44). Indole-3-propionic acid (IPA), an endogenous melatonin-related compound found in plasma and cerebrospinal fluid of humans, has ·OH-scavenging capacities (11). In competition experiments, a rate constant of 8×10^{10} M^{-1} s^{-1} was calculated.

X. THEORETICAL STUDIES

Various theoretical studies investigated the radical-scavenging activity of melatonin either in the light of structural features of the molecule (64), or from a thermodynamic standpoint (65). As revealed by semiempirical and ab initio quantum mechanical calculations, stabilization of the radical cation of some conformers of melatonin could account for its radical-scavenging properties (64). The same study investigated the possibility for melatonin to form a radical by H-atom abstraction from the indole nitrogen. The most stable radical has a positive heat of formation, suggesting that the direct H-atom abstraction mechanism from the N-atom of the indole moiety is improbable.

Melatonin analogues, including N-acetylserotonin, serotonin, and 5-methoxytryptamine, have a reduced stabilization of the cation radical relative to melatonin (64), which suggests that they should have a lower free radical-scavenging activity. The possibility of an antioxidant mechanism resulting from direct H-atom abstraction was also investigated for N-acetylserotonin and serotonin, as these compounds contain a free -OH group. The value of the relative O–H bond dissociation enthalpy (66) (DH_{abs}) suggests that these compounds should be able to scavenge free radicals by a H-atom-transfer mechanism, but not very efficiently.

The ·OH is not a pure one-electron oxidant. It is also known to abstract hydrogen atoms as well as to add to aromatic nuclei and C=C bond. Computational thermodynamic studies in a vacuum and in a model of aqueous solvation questioned the formation of a indolyl cation radical in the reaction between melatonin and ˙OH, because it was shown that the free-energy change $DG°$ to generate a cation radical in aqueous solution is 8 kcal/mol (65). On the other hand, the abstraction of an indolic hydrogen, with formation of an indolyl neutral radical, proceeds with a $DG°$ of -30 kcal/mol. The possibility that during the process of hydrogen abstraction by the ˙OH to yield a neutral stable indolyl radical, the transition state has a cationic character cannot be ruled out. The same study also shows that an additional mechanism of ˙OH to form 2-hydroxymelatonin turns out to be thermodynamically feasible, with a $DG°$ of -31 kcal/mol (65).

For the structure–antioxidant activity relation, Turjanski et al. (65) calculated that the 5-methoxy and the N-acetyl group of melatonin do not seem to significantly affect its thermodynamic capacity of ˙OH trapping. The global $DG°$ for the reaction of ˙OH with related indoles was very similar to that obtained for melatonin.

XI. SUMMARY AND CONCLUSIONS

The reduction potential (E) is a key thermodynamic property to consider to secure information about the ease with which a redox compound can undergo an electron transfer with an oxidizing radical, and to predict a "pecking order," or hierarchy, for free radical reactions (67). On this basis each oxidized species is capable of stealing an electron, or hydrogen atom, from any reduced species with lower reduction potential or, inversely, each reduced species can donate an electron, or hydrogen atom, to any oxidized species with a higher E. The reduction potential of the couple melatonin˙–melatoninH was determined as 0.95 ± 0.02 V (12). Such a value would predict that melatonin undergoes one-electron oxidation by radicals with a very high oxidation power, such as hydroxyl, alkoxyl, or nitrogen radicals, which indeed has been demonstrated. On the other hand, alkylperoxyl radicals are less reactive, as predicted by their reduction potential ($0.77 < E < 1.4$ V) (68). Although capable of reaction with highly reactive species, melatonin cannot easily reduce peroxyl radicals such as those derived from oxidizing lipids. The regeneration of one-electron oxidized melatonin by urate or ascorbate (12), is also in accordance with the pecking order of the reduction potentials of the radicals involved. Interestingly, in spite of the sufficiently high-reduction potential of the couple melatonin˙–melatoninH, oxidized melatonin does not appear very prone to abstract electrons from the bis-allylic-H of polyunsaturated fatty acid [$E_{(PUFA˙/PUFA-H)} = 0.6$ V] (68), as proved by a number of experiments reporting that melatonin is not pro-oxidant in lipid systems. Final products from the reaction of melatonin with strong oxidants or radicals provide evidence that melatonin easily undergoes a two-electron oxidation, which would suggest that its one-electron oxidation product still has reducing power. In addition, it does not appear to easily react with oxygen to form toxic radicals.

In addition to the thermodynamic properties of the radicals involved, the reaction equilibria will be affected by the actual concentrations of reagents. The pathways involved in melatonin oxidation may easily change according to the reactive species, and their relative abundance, occurring in the system under study. The isolation and identification of products from melatonin may help, in each case, to clarify preferential oxidation pathways in various biological microenvironments.

All information summarized in this chapter unequivocally show that, similar to other indole derivatives, melatonin reacts with a range of strong oxidants and free radicals, including those that can develop in cell and tissues, with high reactivity. Through in vitro as well as in vivo studies, melatonin has been protective in models of Parkinson's and Alzheimer's disease, acute local inflammation, cardiomyopathy, oxidant stress, lipid peroxidation, traumatic brain injury, ischemia–reperfusion, as well as in a number of conditions in which radical species are known to produce cell damage, including ionizing radiation and treatment with carcinogens (for an extensive review see Chap. 28). Being both lipid- and water-soluble (69,70), melatonin can react with radicals formed in all cellular compartments, thus it can virtually protect all biological material. Many questions, however, remain to be solved before deciding about a real role of melatonin in vivo. That melatonin can be a radical scavenger under physiological conditions has not often been shown. With the exception of a few reports (71,72), most of the observed antioxidant effects required what appear supraphysiological concentrations of melatonin, suggesting that these are unlikely mechanisms of action of circulating levels of melatonin in vivo. Certain cells [bone marrow (73)] and fluids (bile) (74) and cerebrospinal fluid (75,76), however, have physiological levels of melatonin several orders of magnitude higher than blood.

Emerging evidence in the latest years showed that reactive oxygen and nitrogen species may act as signal transduction mediators at subtoxic levels (77,78). An intriguing hypothesis may be that the reaction of melatonin with radicals such as $\cdot OH$, $\cdot NO_2$, O_2^-, is not involved in the physiological oxidant defense of cells, but may play a role in redox regulation of cell signaling. Such an activity might require only small amounts of a modulatory factor. Oxidized products from melatonin, found in the urine of rats and humans, are 6-hydroxymelatonin, formed in the liver and excreted as either sulfate or glucuronate conjugate (79); N-acetyl-5-methoxy kynurenamine, a compound formed in the brain through the intermediate AFMK (47); and the cyclic compounds 2-hydroxy- (80) and 3-hydroxymelatonin (52). At any instance, the radical-scavenging properties of the molecule can be pharmacologically exploited. In view of the lack of toxicity of melatonin, the administration of pharmacological doses may significantly improve its efficiency as an antioxidant agent.

REFERENCES

1. Jovanovic SV, Simic MG. (1985) Tryptophan metabolites as antioxidants. Life Chem Rep 3:124–130.
2. Simic M, Jovanovic SV. (1990) Mechanism of inactivation of oxygen radicals by dietary antioxidants and their models. Basic Life Sci 52:127–137.
3. Al-Kazwini AT, O'Neill P, Adams GE, Cundall RB, Jacquet B, Lang G, Junino A. (1990) One-electron oxidation of methoxylated and hydroxylated indoles by azide. 1 Characterization of primary indolic radicals. J Phys Chem 94:6666–6670.
4. Tabor MW, Coats E, Sainsbury M, Shertzer HG. (1991) Antioxidation potential of indoles compounds—structure activity studies. In: Witmer CM, Jollow DD, Kalf GF, Kocsis JJ, Sipes IG, eds. Biological Reactive Intermediates. vol. IV. New York: Plenum Press, pp. 833–836.
5. Solar S, Getoff N, Surdhar PS, Armstrong D, Singh A. (1991) Oxidation of tryptophan and N-methylindole by $N_3 \cdot$, $Br_2 \cdot ^-$, $(SNC)_2 \cdot ^-$ radicals in light and heavy water solutions. A pulse radiolysis study. J Phys Chem 95:3639–3643.
6. Jovanovich S, Steenken S. (1992) Substituent effects on the spectral, acid–base, and redox properties of indolyl radicals: a pulse radiolysis study. J Phys Chem 96:6674–6679.
7. Tan D-X, Chen LD, Poeggeler B, Manchester LC, Reiter RJ. (1993) Melatonin: a potent, endogenous hydroxyl radical scavenger. Endocr J 1:57–60.
8. Matuszak Z, Reszka KJ, Chignell CF. (1997) Reaction of melatonin and related indoles with hydroxyl radicals: EPR and spin trapping investigation. Free Radic Biol Med 23:367–372.
9. Poeggeler B, Reiter RJ, Hardeland R, Sewerynek E, Melchiorri D, Barlow–Walden LR. (1995) Melatonin, a mediator of electron transfer and repair reactions, acts synergistically with the chain-breaking antioxidants ascorbate, Trolox and glutathione. Neuroendocrinol Lett 17:87–91.
10. Pähkla R, Zilmer M, Kullisaar T, Rägo L. (1998) Comparison of the antioxidant activity of melatonin and pinoline in vitro. J Pineal Res 24:96–101.

11. Chyan Y-J, Poeggeler B, Omar RA, Chain DG, Frangione B, Ghiso J, Pappolla MA. (1999) Potent neuroprotective properties against the Alzheimer β-amyloid by an endogenous melatonin-related indole structure, indole-3-propionic acid. J Biol Chem 274:21937–21942.
12. Mahal HS, Sharma HS, Mukherjee T. (1999) Antioxidant properties of melatonin: a pulse radiolysis study. Free Radic Biol Med 26:557–565.
13. Stasica P, Ukanski J, Rosiak JM. (1998) Reactions of melatonin with radicals in deoxygenated aqueous solution. J Radioanal Nucl Chem 232:107–113.
14. Pieri C, Marra M, Moroni F, Recchioni R, Marcheselli F. (1994) Melatonin: a peroxyl radical scavenger more effective than vitamin E. Life Sci 55:271–276.
15. Marshall K-A, Reiter RJ, Poeggeler B, Aruoma OI, Halliwell B. (1996) Evaluation of the antioxidant activity of melatonin in vitro. Free Radic Biol Med 21:307–315.
16. Livrea MA, Tesoriere L, D'Arpa D, Morreale M. (1997) Reaction of melatonin with lipoperoxyl radicals in phospholipid bilayers. Free Radic Biol Med 23:706–711.
17. Longoni B, Salgo MG, Pryor WA, Marchiafava PL. (1998) Effects of melatonin on lipid peroxidation induced by oxygen radicals. Life Sci 62:853–859.
18. Antunes F, Barclay LRC, Ingold KU, King M, Norris JQ, Scaiano JC, Xi F. (1999) On the antioxidant activity of melatonin. Free Radic Biol Med 26:117–128.
19. Valgimigli L, Ingold KU, Lusztyk J. (1996) Antioxidant activities of vitamin E analogues in water and a Kamlet–Taft β-value for water. J Am Chem Soc 118:3545–3549.
20. Scaiano JC. (1995) Exploratory laser flash photolysis study of free radical reactions and magnetic field effects in melatonin chemistry. J Pineal Res 19:189–195.
21. Barsacchi R, Kusmic C, Damiani E, Carloni P, Greci P, Donato L. (1998) Vitamin E consumption induced by oxidative stress in red blood cells is enhanced by melatonin and reduced by N-acetylserotonin. Free Radic Biol Med 24:1187–1192.
22. Poeggeler B, Saarela S, Reiter RJ, Tan D–X, Chen L–D, Manchester LC, Barlow–Walden LR. (1994) Melatonin—a highly potent endogenous scavenger and electron donor: new aspects of the oxidation chemistry of this indole accessed in vitro. Ann NY Acad Sci 738:419–420.
23. Zang L–Y, Cosma G, Gardner H, Vallyathan V. (1998) Scavenging of reactive oxygen species by melatonin. Biochim Biophys Acta 1425:469–477.
24. Chan T–Y, Tang P–L. (1996) Characterization of the antioxidant effects of melatonin and related indoleamines in vitro. J Pineal Res 20:187–191.
25. Halliwell B, Gutteridge JMC. (1999) Free Radicals in Biology and Medicine, 3rd ed. New York: Oxford University Press.
26. Misra HP, Fridovich I. (1972) The role of superoxide anion in the autooxidation of epinephrine and a simple assay for superoxide dismutase. J Biol Chem 247:3170–3175.
27. Dellegar SM, Murphy SA, Bourne AE, DiCesare JC, Purser GH. (1999) Identification of the factors affecting the rate of deactivation of hypoclorous acid by melatonin. Biochem Biophys Res Commun 257:431–439.
28. Squadrito GL, Pryor WA. (1998) Oxidative chemistry of nitric oxide: the roles of superoxide, peroxynitrite, and carbon dioxide. Free Radic Biol Med 25:392–403.
29. Kaur H, Whiteman M, Halliwell B. (1997) Peroxynitrite-dependent aromatic hydroxylation and nitration of salicylate and phenylalanine. Is hydroxyl radical involved? Free Radic Res 26:71–82.
30. Van Der Vliet A, O'Neill CA, Halliwell B, Cross CE, Kaur H. (1994) Aromatic hydroxylation and nitration of phenylalanine and tyrosine by peroxynitrite. Evidence for hydroxyl radical production from peroxynitrite. FEBS Lett 339:89–92.
31. Gilad E, Cuzzocrea S, Zingarelli B, Salzman AL, Szabo C. (1997) Melatonin is a scavenger of peroxynitrite. Life Sci 60:169–174.
32. Zhang H, Squadrito GL, Pryor WA. (1998) The reaction of melatonin with peroxynitrite: formation of melatonin radical cation and absence of stable nitrated products. Biochem Biophys Res Commun 251:83–87.
33. Zhang H, Squadrito GL, Uppu R, Pryor WA. (1999) Reaction of peroxynitrite with melatonin: a mechanistic study. Chem Res Toxicol 12:526–534.
34. Noda Y, Mori A, Liburdy R, Packer L. (1999) Melatonin and its precursors scavenge nitric oxide. J Pineal Res 27:159–163.
35. Patel RP, Svistunenko DA, Darley–Usmar VM, Symons MCR, Wilson MT. (1996) Redox cycling of human methaemoglobin by H_2O_2 yields persistent ferryl iron and protein based radicals. Free Radic Res Commun 25:117–123.

36. McArthur KM, Davies MJ. (1993) Detection and reactions of the globin radical in haemoglobin. Biochim Biophys Acta 1202:173–181.
37. Giulivi C, Cadenas E. (1998) Heme protein radicals: formation fate, and biological consequences. Free Radic Biol Med 24:269–279.
38. Davies MJ. (1988) Detection of peroxyl and alkoxyl radicals produced by reaction of hydroperoxides with heme-proteins by electron spin resonance spectroscopy. Biochim Biophys Acta 964:28–35.
39. Davies MJ. (1991) Identification of a globin free radical in equine myoglobin treated with peroxides. Biochim Biophys Acta 1077:86–90.
40. Tesoriere L, Livrea MA, Avellone G, Ceraulo L, D'Arpa D, Segreto S. (2000) Hemoglobin-dependent oxidation of melatonin in human erythrocytes and in homogeneous solution. Identification of products by gas chromatography–mass spectrometry. (in press).
41. Giulivi C, Romero FJ, Cadenas E. (1992) The interactions of Trolox C, a water-soluble vitamin E analog, with ferrylmyoglobin: reduction of the oxoferryl moiety. Arch Biochem Biophys 299:302–312.
42. Giulivi C, Cadenas E. (1993) Inhibition of protein radical reactions of ferrylmyoglobin by the water-soluble analog of vitamin E, Trolox C. Arch Biochem Biophys 303:152–158.
43. Giulivi C, Cadenas E. (1994) Ferrylmyoglobin: formation and chemical reactivity toward electron-donating compounds. Methods Enzymol 233:189–202.
44. Poeggeler B, Reiter RJ, Hardeland R, Tan D–X, Barlow–Walden LR. (1996) Melatonin and structurally-related, endogenous indoles act as potent electron donors and radical scavengers in vitro. Redox Rep 2:179–184.
45. Miller JW, Selhub J, Joseph JA. (1996) Oxidative damage caused by free radicals produced during catecholamine autoxidation: protective effects of o-methylation and melatonin. Free Radic Biol Med 21:241–249.
46. Limson J, Nyokong T, Daya S. (1998) The interaction of melatonin and its precursors with aluminium, cadmium, copper, iron, lead, and zinc: an adsorptive voltammetric study. J Pineal Res 24:15–21.
47. Hirata F, Hayaishi O, Tokuyama T, Senoh S. (1974) In vitro and in vivo formation of two new metabolites of melatonin. J Biol Chem 249:1311–1313.
48. Uemura T, Kadota K. (1984) Serotonin- and melatonin-dependent light emission induced by xantine oxidase. In: Schlossberger HG, Kochen W, Linzen B, Steinhart H, eds. Progress in Tryptophan and Serotonin Research. Berlin: Walter de Gruyter, pp. 673–676.
49. Hardeland R, Fuhrberg B, Behrmann G, Balzer I. (1993) Sleep-latency reducing pineal hormone melatonin as a scavenger of free radical: hemin-catalysed formation of N^1-acetyl-N^2-formyl-5-methoxykynuramine. Sleep Res 22:621.
50. Hardeland R, Reiter RJ, Poeggeler B, Tan D–X. (1993) The significance of the metabolism of the neurohormone melatonin: antioxidative protection and formation of bioactive substances. Neurosci Biobehav Rev 17:347–357.
51. Merenyi G, Lind J, Shen X. (1988) Electron transfer from indoles, phenol, and sulfite (SO_3^{2-}) to chlorine dioxide (ClO_2). J Phys Chem 92:134–137.
52. Tan D–X, Manchester LC, Reiter RJ, Plummer BF, Hardies LJ, Weintraub ST, Vijayalaxmi, Shepherd AMM. (1998) A novel melatonin metabolite, cyclic 3-hydroxymelatonin: a biomarker of in vivo hydroxyl radical generation. Biochem Biophys Res Commun 253:614–620.
53. Pryor WA, Squadrito GL. (1995) The chemistry of peroxynitrite: a product from the reaction of nitric oxide with superoxide. Am J Physiol 268:L699–L722.
54. Goldstein S, Squadrito GL, Pryor WA, Czapski G. (1996) Direct and indirect oxidations by peroxynitrite, neither involving the hydroxyl radical. Free Radic Biol Med 21:965–974.
55. Lymar SV, Hurst JK. (1995) Rapid reaction between peroxynitrite ion and carbon dioxide: implications for biological activity. J Am Chem Soc 117:8867–8868.
56. Uppu RM, Squadrito GL, Pryor WA. (1996) Acceleration of peroxynitrite oxidations by carbon dioxide. Arch Biochem Biophys 327:335–343.
57. Denicola A, Freeman BA, Trujillo M, Radi R. (1996) Peroxynitrite reaction with carbon dioxide/bicarbonate: kinetics and influence on peroxynitrite mediated oxidations. Arch Biochem Biophys 333:49–58.
58. Gow A, Duran D, Thom SR, Ischiropulos H. (1996) Carbon dioxide enhancement of peroxynitrite mediated protein tyrosine nitration. Arch Biochem Biophys 333:42–48.

59. Lemercier J-N, Padmaja S, Cueto R, Squadrito GL, Uppu RM, Pryor WA. (1997) Carbon dioxide modulation of hydroxylation and nitration of phenol by peroxynitrite. Arch Biochem Biophys 345:160–170.
60. Ianas O, Olinescu R, Badescu I. (1991) Melatonin involvement in oxidative processes. Endocrinologie 29:147–153.
61. Schiller J, Arnhold J, Schwinn J, Sprinz H, Brede O, Arnold K. (1999) Differences in the reactivity of phthalic hydrazide and luminol with hydroxyl radicals. Free Radic Res 30:45–57.
62. Reszka KJ, Jimbow K, Chignell CF. (1992) Free-radical products from UV photolysis of melanogenic compound: hydroxyindoles. Photochem Photobiol 55S:36S.
63. Jimbow K, Reszka KJ, Schmitz S, Salopek T, Thomas P. (1995) Distribution of eu- and pheomelanins in human skin and melanocytic tumors, and their photoprotective vs. phototoxic properties. In: Zeise L, Chedekel MR, Fitzpatrick TB, eds. Melanin: Its Role in Human Photoprotection. Overland Park, KS: Valdenmar, pp. 155–173.
64. Migliavacca E, Ancerewicz J, Carrupt P-A, Testa B. (1998) Theoretical parameters to characterize antioxidants. Part 2. The cases of melatonin and carvedilol. Helv Chim Acta 81:1337–1348.
65. Turjanski AG, Rosenstein RE, Estrin DA. (1998) Reactions of melatonin and related indoles with free radicals: a computational study. J Med Chem 41:3684–3689.
66. Migliavacca E, Carrupt PA, Testa B. (1997) Theoretical parameters to characterize antioxidants. 1. The case of vitamin E and analogs. Helv Chim Acta 80:1613.
67. Buettner GR. (1993) The pecking order of free radicals and antioxidants: lipid peroxidation, α-tocopherol, and ascorbate. Arch Biochem Biophys 300:535–543.
68. Koppenol WH. (1990) Oxyradical reactions: from bond-dissociation energies to reduction potentials. FEBS Lett 264:165–167.
69. Reiter RJ. (1991) Pineal melatonin: cell biology of its synthesis and of its physiological interactions. Endocr Rev 1:109–131.
70. Shida CS, Castrucci AML, Lamy-Freund MT. (1994) High solubility of melatonin in aqueous medium. J Pineal Res 16:198–201.
71. Tan D-X, Reiter RJ, Chen LD, Poeggeler B, Manchester LC, Barlow-Walden LR. (1994) Both physiological and pharmacological levels of melatonin reduce DNA adduct formation induced by carcinogen safrole. Carcinogenesis 15:215–218.
72. Pozo D, Reiter RJ, Calvo JR, Guerrero JM. (1994) Physiological concentrations of melatonin inhibit nitric oxide synthase activity in rat cerebellum. Life Sci 55:PL455–PL460.
73. Tan D-X, Manchester LC, Reiter RJ, Qi W-B, Zhang M, Weintraub ST, Cabrera J, Sainz RM, Mayo JC. (1999) Identification of highly elevated levels of melatonin in bone marrow: its origin and significance. Biochim Biophys Acta 1472:206–214.
74. Tan D-X, Manchester LC, Reiter RJ, Qi W, Hanes MA, Farley NJ. (1999) High physiological levels of melatonin in the bile of mammals. Life Sci 65:2523–2529.
75. Rousseau A, Petren S, Plannthin J, Eklund T, Nordin C. (1999) Serum and cerebrospinal fluid concentrations of melatonin: a pilot study in healthy male volunteers. J Neural Transm 106:883–888.
76. Skinner DC, Malpaux B. (1999) High melatonin concentrations in third ventricular cerebrospinal fluid are not due to Galen vein blood recirculating through the choroid plexus. Endocrinology 140:4399–4405.
77. Suzuki YJ, Forman HJ, Sevanian A. (1997) Oxidants as stimulators of signal transduction. Free Radic Biol Med 22:269–285.
78. Dalton TP, Shertzer HG, Puga A. (1999) Regulation of gene expression by reactive oxygen. Annu Rev Pharmacol Toxicol 39:67–101.
79. Webb SM, Puig-Domingo M. (1995) Role of melatonin in health and disease. Clin Endocrinol 42:221–234.
80. Vakkuri O, Tervo J, Luttinen R, Ruotsalainen H, Rahkamaa E, Leppäluoto J. (1987) A cyclic isomer of 2-hydroxymelatonin: a novel metabolite of melatonin. Endocrinology 120:2453–2459.

30
Selenium: An Antioxidant?

Regina Brigelius-Flohé
German Institute of Human Nutrition, Potsdam–Rehbrücke, Germany

Matilde Maiorino and Fulvio Ursini
University of Padua, Padua, Italy

Leopold Flohé
Technical University of Braunschweig, Braunschweig, Germany

I. INTRODUCTION

Selenium, discovered in 1817 by Berzelius and named after the Greek goddess of the moon *Selene*, is a rare element belonging to main group VI in the periodic table of elements. As a typical chalcogen it shares many properties with its closest relative sulfur. Similar to sulfur it occurs in the oxidation states -2, 0, $+2$, $+4$, and $+6$ (Table 1), which implies that it is prone to release or accept pairs of electrons. Selenium compounds with an uneven number of electrons (i.e., stable selenium radicals) are unknown. Short-lived selenium radicals may, however, be formed. As has also been demonstrated for sulfur amino acids (1,2), complexation of selenols with transition metals may facilitate single-electron transitions resulting in the generation of superoxide in the presence of oxygen. Formation of superoxide, H_2O_2, and OH radicals in aerobic solution of H_2Se or mixtures of selenite and thiols, which lead to the formation of selenide, have indeed been detected (3,4). Inversely, synthetic benzselenazol derivatives, such as ebselen (PZ51), may react with free radicals and, therefore, were discussed as "antioxidants" (5), but the selenium radical thereby produced proved to be reactive enough to propagate a chain reaction instead of terminating it (6). So far, no selenium compound has fulfilled the requirement of a real *antioxidant*, which in its proper definition, is an element or compound that scavenges radicals, is itself transformed into a rather inert radical, and thereby terminates a radical-driven chain reaction (7); nor can selenium be generally rated as an antioxidant in the broader sense of creating a reductive environment in a biological system. Selenate is a stronger oxidant than sulfate; elemental selenium is quite inert. Naturally occurring compounds with selenium, present in low-oxidation states, are reductants, but may generate strong oxidants by reacting with the most abundant oxidant, molecular oxygen (3,4). Similarly, some synthetic

Table 1 Oxidation States of Selenium

Chemical structure	Oxidation state	Name of acid	Name of salts
H_2Se	$-II$	Hydrogen selenide	Selenide
R-SeH	$-II$	Selenol	
Se	0	Selenium	
R-Se-OH	0	Selenenic acid	Selenenate
R-Se(=O)-OH	$+II$	Seleninic acid	Seleninate
HO-Se(=O)-OH	$+IV$	Selenious acid	Selenite (SeO_3^{2-})
HO-Se(=O)(=O)-OH	$+VI$	Selenic acid	Selenate (SeO_4^{2-})

compounds related to ebselen even proved to be pro-oxidants, whereas others, including ebselen itself, reduced peroxides and thus mimicked glutathione peroxidase (8).

Since its discovery as an essential trace element by Schwarz and Foltz in 1957 (9), selenium has been discussed as a constituent of the biological antioxidant defense. Considering the extremely low requirements of the trace element in animals, Schwarz continued stressing the idea that selenium cannot exert its biological role as a simple antioxidant, but rather should, act catalytically as "a cofactor" of an enzymatic process (10). This view was finally supported by the discovery that the H_2O_2-sensitivity of red blood cells from selenium-deficient rats was associated with a decline in glutathione (GSH) peroxidase activity (11,12); by establishing a stoichiometric selenium content of purified glutathione peroxidase (GPx) (13–15); by loss of activity owing to elimination of selenium (16); and by demonstrating the catalytic role of selenium in the enzyme by site-directed mutagenesis (17).

In the meantime selenium has been identified in a wide range of proteins in many taxa of the living kingdom (18–20). Most of these proteins are oxidoreductases, four are peroxidases, and the relevance of the trace element to biological antioxidant defense in mammals has been generally accepted. It might, therefore, appear tempting to redefine selenium as a *biological antioxidant*. The emerging diversity of biological functions of selenium, however, preclude such generalizations. Moreover, selenium overexposure or administration of pharmacological dosages of some selenium compounds is associated with biological phenomena rather reminding one more of the pro-oxidant potential of the element than of a fortified biological antioxidant defense (4).

The aim of this chapter, therefore, is to compile which biological effects of physiological or pharmacological dosages of diverse selenium compounds can be explained by the emerging knowledge on selenium-catalyzed redox biochemistry. To this end, we shall briefly review the bioutilization of nutritionally or pharmacologically relevant selenium compounds, and elaborate in more detail on the mammalian selenoproteins relative to their potential role in biological phenomena, such as antioxidant defense, redox regulation of cytokine function, differentiation, apoptosis, and tumorigenesis.

II. BIOAVAILABILITY AND UTILIZATION OF SELENIUM

The popular talking about the properties of "selenium" is as revealing as talking about "carbon" or "nitrogen" when explaining the toxicity of cyanide or the function of enzymes. The biological effects of selenium compounds depend on their chemical nature and metabolic fate. The literature on absorption, metabolization, and bioutilization of diverse selenium compounds has been amply reviewed elsewhere (21–25); here, it will be presented only as a condensed summary.

Whereas elemental selenium is not bioavailable at all (i.e., it is not taken up), most of the other selenocompounds can be absorbed. Data on the absorption of different selenium species are limited. Naturally occurring organic selenium compounds such as selenomethionine and selenocysteine, are absorbed by transport mechanisms shared with corresponding sulfur amino acids. Selenite absorption occurs by passive diffusion, and selenate is taken up by a sodium-mediated carrier transport (26–28). The different selenium compounds, however, are not equally used for selenoprotein biosynthesis.

The compounds most commonly administered to humans and animals for selenium supplementation are selenomethionine, which is also the major selenium-containing molecule in selenium-yeast (29); selenocysteine, usually as selenocysteyl residue of proteins; and the inorganic salt sodium selenite. Selenite is reduced to hydrogen selenide by glutathione reductase at the expense of GSH (3,4,30,31) or even more efficiently by thioredoxin reductase at the expense of NADPH (32,33). Selenium thereby is reduced from the oxidation state $+4$ to -2 consuming six reduction equivalents per mole of selenite. The rapid oxidation of H_2Se by oxygen leads to further consumption of NADPH by thioredoxin reductase or glutathione reductase if H_2Se concentrations are to be maintained (33). Assimilation of selenate appears to depend on bacterial reduction to selenite before it can be utilized by the mammalian organism. Selenomethionine is either nonspecifically incorporated into proteins instead of methionine (23,34) or transformed into selenocysteine by the transsulfuration pathway (35). Hydrogen selenide is then released from selenocysteine by the selenocysteine-β-lyase (36). Methylation of H_2Se leads to forms of selenium that can be excreted in the urine (trimethyl selenonium cation) or by expiration (mono- and dimethyl selenide) (24,37).

Hydrogen selenide is the key metabolite of selenium metabolism. It is also this form that is used for selenoprotein biosynthesis. The first step is the formation of selenophosphate from H_2Se and ATP by selenophosphate synthetase (38), SelD, being a selenoprotein itself (39). Selenophosphate is required for the synthesis of selenocysteine from serine bound to a specific $tRNA^{(ser)sec}$, SelC, by means of selenocysteine synthase (40) also called SelA. The resulting selenocysteine-loaded $tRNA^{(ser)sec}$ provides selenocysteine for the incorporation into growing peptide chains at the ribosome (41). Selenocysteine is encoded by TGA (42,43), usually meaning stop. Organisms have developed complex mechanisms to differentiate between TGA meaning *stop* and TGA meaning *selenocysteine*. This pathway has been elucidated for prokaryotes (41,43), but is far from being clear for eukaryotes (44). One prerequisite is a characteristic secondary structure in the mRNA called SECIS, for selenocysteine-inserting sequence, which in prokaryotes immediately follows the UGA codon (41,45) and in eukaryotes lies in the 3'-untranslated region (46). In prokaryotes, the mRNA-SECIS, the selenocysteine-loaded $tRNA^{(ser)sec}$, a specific elongation factor SelB, and GTP form a stoichiometric quarternary complex (47). In this complex UGA is recognized as selenocysteine codon and selenocysteine is incorporated into the growing peptide chain. In eukaryotes, the process seems to be similar. It is, however, different enough not to allow expression of eukaryotic selenoproteins in bacteria. Despite major efforts, a mammalian SelB has not yet been unequivocally identified, the role of GTP is unclear, and the formation and stoichiometry of the productive complex has not yet been investigated. Structural analysis of SECIS elements of different mammalian selenoproteins revealed a conserved triple A in the loop plus conserved nucleotides in the stem, first presumed to form bulges at a defined distance from the loop (46,48), but now shown to be paired in a non-Watson–Crick manner (49).

The complex mechanism of selenoprotein biosynthesis offers ample opportunities for regulatory modulation, which contribute to a phenomenon addressed as the *hierarchy of selenoproteins*. At limiting concentrations, selenium is preferentially channeled into some of the selenoproteins, whereas others are less well supplied. In consequence, some selenoproteins respond fast to selenium deficiency with loss of activity, others remain stable in moderate selenium deficiency and decrease only after prolonged and substantial selenium depletion. On the other hand, proteins that slowly respond to selenium deprivation are restored faster after resupplementation than are the fast responders. The factors determining the hierarchy are not fully understood. Loss of activity of selenoproteins from selenium restriction usually is accompanied by a retarded loss of mRNA. This could be explained by a selenium dependency on the stability of the respective selenoprotein mRNA (50–52). The selenium-responsive stabilities of the individual selenoprotein mRNAs differ markedly, as do the efficiencies of the SECIS elements in the translation process (53–56). Therefore, it may be speculated that the SECIS structures play an important role not only as elements required for correct translation of the UGA codon, but also in controlling mRNA stabilities in selenium deficiency (57). Selenium responsiveness of selenoprotein biosynthesis is thus basically regulated by three factors: the availability of selenocysteyl-loaded tRNA$^{(ser)sec}$, the SECIS efficiencies, and the possibly related mRNA stabilities. But this basic concept is open to modulation by transcriptional regulation by external stimuli, hormones, tissue-specific transcription factors or preferential selenium utilization by particular tissues (52,57).

The complexity of selenoprotein biosynthesis and its regulation makes it difficult to choose a particular selenoprotein as a general marker of the selenium status of an organism. Available studies describe mainly the different effects of ingested selenium compounds on cGPx and pGPx activities, or selenoprotein P levels in humans and animals, or on the distinct GPx types or thioredoxin reductase in cultured cells. In vivo, selenite was the most effective precursor for cGPx activity (58), whereas, depending on the experimental design, selenomethionine was either less effective than selenite (59–61) or effective with delay (62,63). Its utilization for selenoprotein biosynthesis depends on the methionine content in the diet (64,65). One study documented an effect of selenomethionine only after cessation of supplementation (6). This shows that degradation of proteins loaded with selenomethionine provides free selenomethionine that can subsequently be used for selenoprotein biosynthesis.

Also, for cultured cells, selenite was the most effective precursor for the expression of glutathione peroxidases. In several cell lines, selenomethionine, although taken up by the cells and increasing the cellular selenium content (67,68), did not enhance GPx activities. Fetal calf serum, supposed to be the main selenium source for cells in culture, was efficiently used for GPx expression only by cells capable of phagocytosis, but was a poor source, for example, endothelial cells, lymphocytes, and hepatocytes (69). The different utilization observed in different cell lines might also be important in vivo.

In contrast to glutathione peroxidases, thioredoxin reductase (TR) activity usually did not respond dramatically to variations in selenium supply. TR activity decreased in some tissues (lung, liver, and kidney) of rats fed a selenium-deficient diet, but remained unaltered in others (70,71). Feeding a highly selenium-enriched diet left GPx activities unchanged, but increased TR activity 2-fold in liver, 3-fold in lung, and 1.3-fold in kidney, before it returned to normal values after prolonged feeding (71). In vitro, TR activity was enhanced 60-fold after 5 days exposure to 10 µM of selenite only in a human colon cancer cell line (72). Interestingly, Se-methylselenocysteine and selenomethionine were much less effective, indicating that they are poor precursors of H_2Se. Whereas in breast, colon, and lung cancer cell lines, TR activity was increased by 1 µM of selenite, cells from lymphoid origin did not respond to the high selenite concentration (73). Jurkat cells responded to selenite with only an increase in TR activity when precultivated in selenium-deficient medium (74).

The differences in the utilization of selenium from different compounds are more pronounced in cell culture studies than in feeding experiments, where the intestinal flora, complementing metabolic capacities of tissues, and interorgan trafficking contribute to selenium assimilation. Despite the obvious differences in potency and speed of bioutilization, bioavailable selenium compounds, such as sodium selenite, selenomethionine, and selenocysteine, are rated as equivalent in common dietary recommendations. For humans, a daily dose of 1 µg of bioavailable selenium per kilogram body weight is suggested to be sufficient to keep GPx activities at optimum (75). The required dosage for optimum activity of other selenoproteins has not been investigated in detail, but selenoprotein P and 5'DI also appear to be at optimum at nutritional selenium levels (76,77). This crude approach may be justified to define dietary allowances, but must not be generalized as a basis for therapeutic measures that aim at a fast normalization of the selenium status or depend on the pharmacological profile of individual selenium compounds.

III. SELENOPROTEINS

Not all species require selenoproteins. Yeast, for instance, has no gene encoding selenocysteyl-tRNA enabling specific selenium incorporation, nor does the entire genome suggest the presence of any selenoprotein. Neither have selenoproteins been convincingly demonstrated in plants. Whenever genes encoding homologues of mammalian selenoproteins (e.g., glutathione peroxidases) were detected in plants, they contained a cysteine codon instead of the selenocysteine-encoding TGA (78,79). Selenoproteins, however, were, amply demonstrated in archaea and eubacteria and in metazoan animals (18–20,80,81). In mammals and insects, one or the other selenoprotein must be of vital importance, because disruption of the selenocysteyl-tRNA gene in mice was lethal (82) as was deletion of the selenophosphate synthetase gene in *Drosophila melanogaster* (83). Likely, these proteins are not those putatively or actually involved in antioxidant defense. Rather, the thioredoxin reductases may be rated as indispensible for survival owing to their pivotal role in DNA biosynthesis (84).

The ten mammalian selenoproteins characterized by sequence and function plus the nine more defined by sequence only are listed in Table 2. Out of those, the four glutathione peroxidases may be particularly relevant to antioxidant defense. But also the thioredoxin reductases need to be discussed in this context, because their product, reduced thioredoxin, feeds some of the peroxiredoxin-type peroxidases (102). Finally, selenoprotein W and selenoprotein P have often been implicated in antioxidant defense, although their precise enzymatic function remains unknown.

A. The Classic Glutathione Peroxidase

Glutathione peroxidase (cGPx, GPx-1) reduces hydroperoxides by the tripeptide GSH. Its enzymology has been studied and reviewed extensively (78,103,104). For the present context it may suffice to recall some basic characteristics. Similar to the other glutathione peroxidases, cGPx contains a catalytic triad consisting of selenocysteine, glutamine, and tryptophan (105–107).

Table 2 Mammalian Selenoproteins Defined by Sequence or Function

Mammalian selenoproteins	Common abbreviations	Refs.
Glutathione peroxidase	GPx	
Cytosolic or classic GPx	cGPx, GPx-1	85
Phospholipid hydroperoxide GPx	PHGPx, GPx-4	86
Plasma GPx	pGPx, GPx-3	87
Gastrointestinal GPx	GI-GPx, GPx-GI, GPx-2	88
Iodothyronine deiodinases		
5'-Deiodinase, type I	5'DI	89,90
5'-Deiodinase, type II	5'DII	91
5-Deiodinase, type III	5-DIII	92
Selenoprotein P	SelP	93
Selenoprotein W	SelW	94
Thioredoxin reductases		
Thioredoxin reductase	TR	95
Mitochondrial thioredoxin reductase	TR-2	96–98
Thioredoxin reductase homologues	SelZf1	99
	SelZf2	99
Selenophosphate synthetase-2		39
15-kDa Selenoprotein (T cells)		100
Selenoprotein R	SelR	101
Selenoprotein T	SelT	101
Selenoprotein X	SelX	99
Selenoprotein N	SelN	99

The selenol group of the selenocysteine therein is activated by hydrogen bonding to react with H_2O_2 or other soluble hydroperoxides at rate constants close to 10^7 M^{-1} s^{-1} (78,103,108,109). Thereby, a selenenic acid derivative is formed that is reduced stepwise by two GSH molecules (103,104). The selenium moiety of the enzyme shuttles between the oxidation state -2 and 0 (Fig. 1). Free radical intermediates are not involved in the catalysis (110) and, correspond-

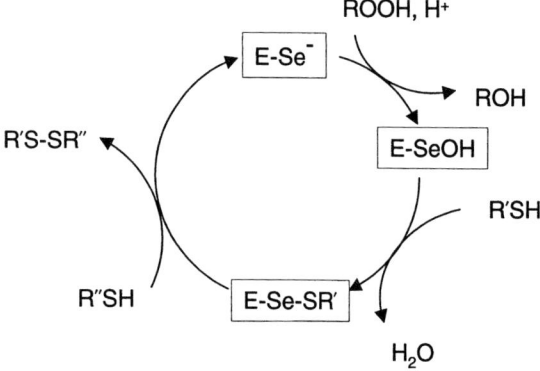

Figure 1 Catalytic cycle common to glutathione peroxidases: R may be H or alkyl. R'SH and R"SH is glutathione in cGPx, it may be glutathione or glutaredoxin for pGPx, and glutathione or protein SH for PHGPx. Specificity of GI-GPx is unclear.

ingly, the stoichiometry of the reaction is surprisingly clean, as opposed to that of many heme peroxidases for which the catalysis involves monovalent redox steps. The peculiarity of GPx is that it reduces hydroperoxides without generating free radicals. Its relevance to free radical metabolism is thus restricted to the prevention of the initiation of propagation of free radical chains by hydroperoxides.

For more than a decade the classic glutathione peroxidase (cGPx), the gene product of *Gpx1*, remained the only known selenoprotein in mammals. Being a highly efficient peroxidase, it seemed to adequately explain the antioxidant effect of alimentary selenium supplementation, and its deficiency was implicated in many pathophysiological phenomena possibly triggered by peroxides (for review see Ref. 103). Needless to state that most of these hypotheses now have to be revised. First of all, it could be ruled out by reverse genetics that cGPx is a vital enzyme. cGPx (−/−) mice developed and grew normally; in fact, they grew faster than control mice (111). Fatal liver necrosis, as seen with combined vitamin E and selenium deficiency by Schwarz and Foltz (9) can, therefore, no longer be discussed as a result of impaired cGPx function.

Unfortunately, the cGPx (−/−) mouse model has not yet been explored extensively enough to scrutinize the realm of ideas related to potential cGPx functions. But the hypothesis claiming cGPx to represent a major antioxidant device was corroborated. cGPx (−/−) mice were more sensitive to poisoning with the redox-cycling herbicides paraquat (112,113) and diquat (114). In fact, the cGPx (−/−) mice died within hours irrespective of selenium supplementation, as did selenium-deficient wild-type mice, whereas selenium-adequate wild-type mice survived. This indicates that none of the other selenoproteins can protect mice against oxidative stress as efficiently as cGPx. Also, bacterial lipopolysaccharides, known to induce oxidative stress by phagocyte activation, were less well tolerated by cGPx −/− mice (115). These findings may be taken to support the original thinking of the discoverer of cGPx, Gordan C. Mills, who considered the enzyme as a protector of red blood cells against oxidative damage by H_2O_2 (85). As amply reviewed elsewhere (78,103,116,117), hydroperoxide removal by cGPx in red blood cells is coupled to glucose metabolism by the pentose phosphate pathway by NADPH-dependent glutathione reductase (Fig. 2). Any defect in this cascade of reactions, be it due to genetic defects or alimentary deficiencies, results in hemolysis of the affected cells when exposed to pro-oxidant drugs or H_2O_2. It was, incidentally, precisely this knowledge that led to the identification of cGPx as a selenoprotein (11,12,118,119). The circumstance that genetic deficiencies in G-6-PDH, which leads to impaired GSH regeneration, became a surprising problem among American soldiers during the Korean war appears particular revealing. These

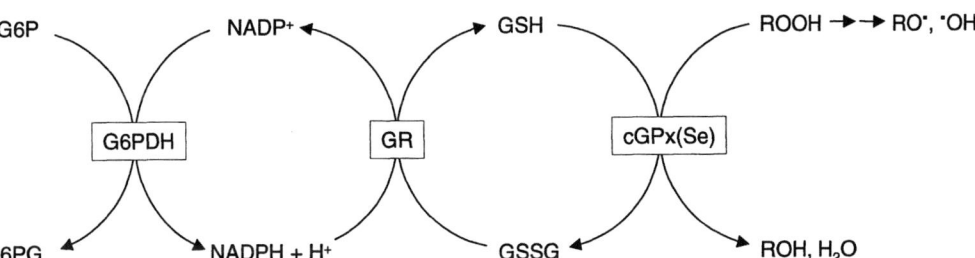

Figure 2 Metabolic context of cGPx in preventing oxidative stress: G6P, glucose-6-phosphate; 6PG, 6-phosphogluconate; G6PDH, glucose-6-phosphate dehydrogenase; GR, glutathione reductase; RO˙, alkoxy radical; ˙OH, hydroxyl radical.

soldiers were perfectly normal youngsters, "they did not show any phenotype" (120), unless they became exposed to pro-oxidant antimalarials. The homology with the cGPx (−/−) mice, of displaying their genetic deficiency only when oxidatively stressed, is striking.

What about the remaining pathophysiological phenomena that were putatively attributed to cGPx deficiency in the past? To say the least, they are less certainly directly related. Admittedly, it is tempting to interpret any pathology seen in small to moderate selenium deficiency to cGPx deficiency, for this enzyme responds fast and substantially to selenium withdrawal (52,57). In the hierarchy of known selenoproteins, biosynthesis of cGPx appears to occupy the lowest position, and the most abundant selenoprotein, cGPx, has even been speculated to represent little else than a selenium store to guarantee the biosynthesis of more important selenoproteins (121). But the selenium-responsiveness of pGPx is similar to that of cGPx, selenoprotein P ranks only slightly higher in the hierarchy, the preferential selenium utilization by any of the remaining 20–30 selenoproteins, known only as ^{75}Se-containing bands from pulse-label experiments, has not been investigated, and the established hierarchy is complicated by organ-specific modulation. In other words, it is not justified to uncritically attribute pathogenic events in low-to-moderate selenium deficiency to cGPx deficiency.

With these precautions in mind, we may first address the potential role of cGPx deficiency and well-documented Se-deficiency diseases such as Keshan disease (122–123) and Kashin–Beck disease (124). In both diseases complicating factors have been envoked, mycotoxin exposure in Kashin–Beck disease (125–127) and coxsackievirus B infection in Keshan disease (128).

Kashin–Beck disease is defined as a chondronecrosis of articular or epiphyseal cartilage leading to secondary osteoarthritis, joint malformations and, if children are affected, to dwarfism. The disease is endemic in selenium-deficient hilly areas of China and southeastern parts of the Soviet Union and reportedly can be ameliorated by selenium supplementation (122,129). The endemic areas overlap, but do not fully coincide with those where the second selenium deficiency disease, Keshan disease, prevails. Kashin–Beck disease appears to predominate in more humid climates, whereas Keshan disease is more frequently observed in semiarid regions. This observation suggested a contribution of additional environmental factors to the manifestation of the diseases. For Kashin–Beck disease exposure to foodborne mycotoxins have been discussed. They are believed to induce inflammatory responses that are not easily managed by the selenium-deficient organism. If we consider the hydroperoxide nature of primary lipoxygenase and cyclooxygenase products and of the secondary oxidative burst products, aggravation of joint inflammation caused by GPx deficiency appears plausible (103), but must still be rated as speculative.

Keshan disease, a cardiomyopathy (129–131), clearly responds to selenium supplementation. It has practically been eradicated by selenium supplementation in the previously endemic regions of China (131). Related symptoms observed with unsupplemented parenteral nutrition (132,133) proved equally selenium-responsive. In the acute form of Keshan disease, the conductive system of the heart is primarily affected (134). This leads to symptoms reminding one of the cardiac side effects of redox-cycling anthraquinone cytostatics (reviewed in Ref. 103). The pathohistology of Keshan disease is equally suggestive of oxidative damage (134). Taken together, Keshan disease may directly result from an impaired hydroperoxide metabolism, be it due to deficiency of cGPx or of another selenium-dependent antioxidant system. More recently, however, the etiology of Keshan disease is being discussed in another context. Based on early histopathological findings (134) and the similarity of the clinical picture to coxsackievirus B-induced cardiomyopathy, a switch in virulence of such viruses is assumed to be facilitated by selenium deficiency. Passage of an avirulent coxsackievirus in selenium-deficient mice indeed resulted in virulent strains causing cardiomyopathy (135,136). Similarly, an avirulent coxsackievirus strain mutated rapidly into virulent ones in cGPx (−/−) mice and caused a cardiomyopathy reminding one of Keshan disease (137). Again, these exciting findings do not rule out that a disturbed hydroperoxide metabolism is ultimately responsible for the disease manifestation. First of all, the mutagenic potential of hydroperoxides might accelerate the generation of virulent strains and, second, the oxidative stress arising from the exposure to the virulent virus might be less well tolerated.

Although a potential link between cGPx deficiency and Keshan disease still appears likely, the hypothetical role of cGPx in the prevention of cancer is loosing attractiveness. Shamberger and Frost (138) were the first to observe a relation between low selenium intake and enhanced risk of cancer. Since then, cancer has long been implicated as partially dependent on selenium deficiency by retrospective epidemiological studies (reviewed in Refs. 21,139). In the meantime, it has become clear from numerous experimental carcinogenesis models (21,24,139–141) and a large-scale prospective clinical trial (142) that cancer incidence is not significantly affected by a selenium supplementation that guarantees optimum cGPx expression. Cancer prevention by pharmacological doses of certain selenium compounds, therefore, must be due to other mechanisms. Emerging knowledge also suggests that the chemical nature of the selenium compounds is relevant to cancer prevention. In most of the human studies, selenium has been administered in the form of selenium-enriched yeast that predominantly contains selenomethionine (29), but also essential amounts of Se-adenosyl-selenohomocysteine (143). Beneficial effects of garlic and selenium-enriched garlic have also been reported (144,145). Chemical forms typical of garlic are the selenium homologues of sulfides, disulfides, and trisulfides (146), and again Se-methylated amino acids and peptides, such as γ-glutamyl-Se-methylselenocysteine and possibly γ-glutamyl-selenomethionine (143). In animal experiments, the best chemopreventive activities were obtained with selenobetaine and Se-methylselenocysteine (24,141). A recent study revealed that selenium-enriched garlic is even more effective than selenium-enriched yeast in the depression of DMBA- and MNU-induced preneoplastic lesions in mammary glands of rats (147). Tentatively, therefore, Se-methylated or alkylated selenium compounds may be rated as more efficient in the chemoprevention of cancer. They are effective irrespective of optimized selenoprotein levels and, thus, are not working through an antioxidant enzyme such as cGPx. In fact, the original view that any increase of cGPx activity by lowering the peroxide tone, should reduce the cancer risk, turned out to be untenable. DMBA-induced and TPA-promoted skin cancer in mice was enhanced, and tumor regression at cessation of promotion was retarded in cGPx overexpressing mice (148). Probably, these findings are due to the prevention of oxidant-triggered apoptosis by the overexpressed cGPx (149–151). Yet, nevertheless, a note of precaution appears mandatory: none of the studies can unequivocally rule out an increased risk of cancerogenesis owing to long-term suboptimal selenium supply and, in consequence, impaired hydroperoxide metabolism.

Subacute selenium deficiency has also been implicated in the etiology of cardiovascular diseases other than Keshan disease (139,152–155). However, a role for cGPx in the prevention of atherosclerosis is not evident either, although pro-oxidant events such as low-density lipoprotein (LDL) oxidation followed by LDL uptake and expression of adhesion molecules are currently implicated in the initial phase of atherogenesis (156,157). cGPx, however, is not in a position to prevent LDL oxidation, simply because it is not present in the extracellular compartment. On uptake of oxidized LDL it probably would not likely reduce LDL-bound lipid hydroperoxides because its specificity is limited to soluble hydroperoxides. In vitro cGPx can silence cyclooxygenase (158) and 5-lipoxygenase (159) that produce lipid mediators with pronounced effects on the cardiovascular system. More recent evidence, however, reveals that this regulatory potential may be common to all selenoperoxidases (160), and PHGPx is probably the one fulfilling this role in vivo (161). Similarly, redox-regulated NF-κB-mediated expression (162) is more likely regulated by PHGPx than by cGPx (163,164). Clearly, in the context, of atherogenesis of pGPx and PHGPx deserve more interest.

In short, cGPx appears to be little else than an emergency device to cope with exposure to high levels of hydroperoxides, as is required in intoxications with redox-cyclers and under serious oxidative stress caused by infections or inflammatory responses. Its antioxidant role is further suggested by the oxygen responsiveness of its gene (165). However, phenomena such as sex-specific cGPx tissue levels (166) or enhanced viral spreading in HIV-infected cells by overexpressed cGPx (167) are not obviously explained by the antioxidant role and demand an open mind for the discovery of additional cGPx functions.

B. Plasma Glutathione Peroxidase, an Orphan Enzyme

The glutathione peroxidase activity detectable in extracellular fluids has long been believed to represent the known GPx released from cells during tissue sampling or natural cell aging, until Takahashi et al. (87,168) demonstrated pGPx to be a distinct gene product. It is expressed as a preprotein equipped with a typical leader sequence targeting the enzyme to the extracellular space. Typical sites of expression are kidney, epididymis, placenta, and the ciliary body of the lens, all known to be involved in protein secretion (52). The specificity of pGPx for hydroperoxides appears to be similar to that of cGPx, but it reportedly also reduces hydroperoxy groups of complex lipids (169). A structural comparison of the glutathione peroxidases (78,170) suggested a less stringent binding of glutathione by pGPx (104), and Björnstedt et al. (171) have identified thioredoxin and glutaredoxin as alternative substrates. But this does not make pGPx less of an orphan in the sense of being an enzyme in search of an appropriate donor substrate. Extracellularly, GSH is present in the low micromolar range (i.e., three orders of magnitude lower than in cellular compartments). The oxidation state of the tiny amounts of extracellular thioredoxin is unknown, and more importantly there is no system known to regenerate the implicated thiol donors outside the cell. Accordingly, pGPx also remains an enzyme in search of any plausible biological role. Therefore, in need of consolidated knowledge one may be allowed to speculate on potential functions of this protein.

Because of the scarcity of extracellular-reducing substrates, pGPx cannot be rated as an efficient antioxidant device, but it might represent an extracellular redox sensor relevant to the regulation of inflammatory responses (Fig. 3). The extracellular peroxide tone has been implicated in the regulation of prostaglandin biosynthesis (158,172) and, also, 5-lipoxygenase, the key enzyme of leukotriene biosynthesis, requires a certain peroxide tone to be active (159). The formation of proinflammatory lipid mediators may thus depend on H_2O_2 previously released by activated phagocytes. Without any balancing system any oxidative burst reaction would be amplified by the activation of lipoxygenases. A broad-spectrum peroxidase such as pGPx could prevent such signal amplification, thereby dampening undue responses to irrelevant inflammatory stimuli. This dampening system, however, would be easily overcome if the initial oxidative burst is pronounced enough to exhaust the limited reduction capacity in the extracellular space. In other words, pGPx being a highly reactive peroxidase yet supported by a tiny capacity of reduction equivalents may be considered the ideal redox buffer to discriminate between relevant and irrelevant inflammatory stimuli. Needless to say, such a role for pGPx would provide a rational for the presumed anti-inflammatory effect of selenium supplementation. Unfortunately, the common use of selenium to treat inflammatory disorders in racing horses or livestock is not supported by any controlled trials, and the recently claimed efficacy of selenium supplementation in serious clinical conditions such as sepsis and pancreatitis is at

SELENIUM

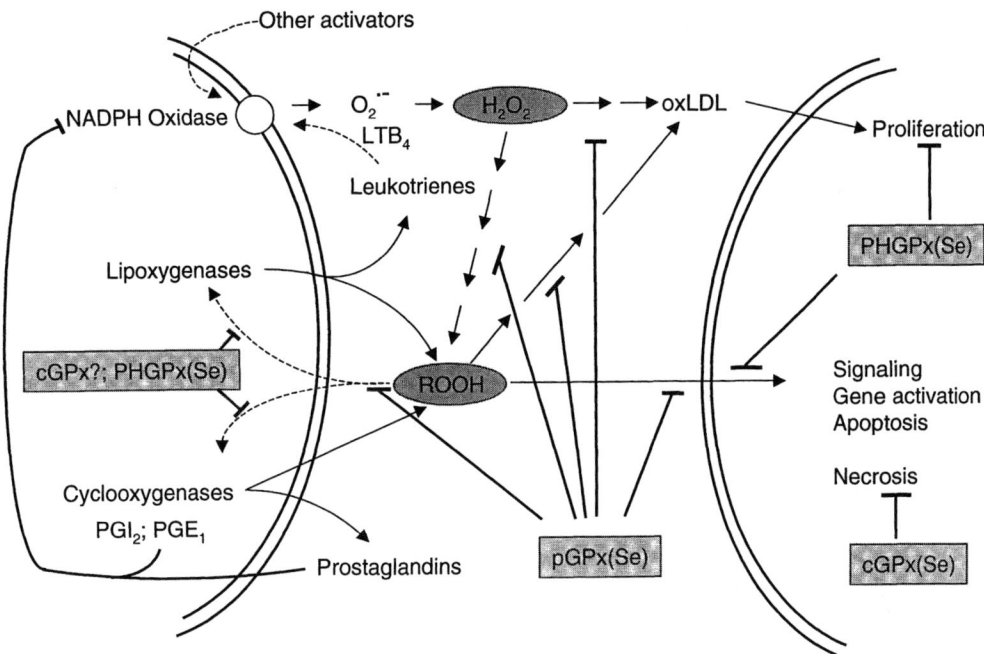

Figure 3 Potential roles of intra- and extracellular glutathione peroxidases in regulating inflammatory responses and cardiovascular disease: Extracellular H_2O_2 is primarily derived from $O_2^{\cdot -}$, which is released from PMNs or macrophages on receptor-mediated activation of NADPH oxidase by inflammatory stimuli such as anaphylatoxin, opsonized microorganisms, bacterial lipopolysaccharides, leukotriene-B_4 (LTB_4), or others. Lipid hydroperoxides are directly formed by activated lipoxygenases and cyclooxygenases and may be released into the circulation or may be generated indirectly by $O_2^{\cdot -}/H_2O_2$-driven unspecific lipid peroxidation. The extracellular hydroperoxide pools can be reduced, although with low reduction capacity, by pGPx. Thereby signal amplification by product activation of lipoxygenases as well as effects of hydroperoxides and oxidized low-density lipoproteins (oxLDL) on target cells (e.g., smooth muscle or endothelial cells) are interrupted. Lipoxygenase activation by lipid hydroperoxides may also be inhibited by intracellular glutathione peroxidases, in particular by PHGPx. Cyclooxygenase activation by hydroperoxides may also lead to inhibition of NADPH oxidase by E- and I-type prostaglandins (PG). Whether PHGPx is relevant to the reduction of oxLDL after scavenger receptor-mediated uptake, remains to be investigated. PHGPx, however, appears to be a key player in redox-modulated signaling cascades. ⟶ and ⟶⟶, direct and indirect pathways; – – →, direct or receptor-mediated activations; ⊣ inhibitory effects of glutathione peroxidases owing to hydroperoxide removal.

best based on controlled pilot trials with limited numbers of patients (173) or on uncontrolled studies (174,175) demanding confirmation.

In the context of atherogenesis, pGPx should not be ignored (see Fig. 3). LDL oxidation can be prevented only by an antioxidant device present in the extracellular space. Of the known selenoproteins, pGPx and selenoprotein P are the only candidates that meet this criterion, and pGPx is the one responding to selenium shortage more rapidly (57). The lipoprotein-bound hydroperoxy lipids are estimated to be in the nanomolar range (176), and the micromolar extracellular thiol level would theoretically be sufficient to support pGPx in keeping them reduced. Presuming a role of pGPx in antagonizing oxLDL-induced atherogenesis, however, does not necessarily depend on the ability of this enzyme to reduce hydroperoxy groups of the oxidized lipoprotein. More importantly, the dampening by pGPx of inflammatory responses, discussed in the foregoing, would inevitably lower the steady-state tone of hydroperoxides that initiate lipid peroxidation in LDL.

C. Another Specialist, GI-GPx?

The gastrointestinal form of GPx, GI-GPx, is the least well-characterized one. In terms of sequence, it most resembles cGPx and presumably displays a similar substrate specificity. For some years it was detected only in the epithelium lining the intestinal tract from the esophagus to the distal colon of the rat (177,178); in humans it was also found in liver (88). In the gut, it prevails in the crypts (179,180). Being the major GPx type of the intestine it has been speculated to protect the organism against hydroperoxides contained in food or formed by intestinal cells or liver after absorption of xenobiotics. More recently, however, GI-GPx was also detected in a retinoic acid-treated cell line derived from human mammary cancer (179). This observation does not speak in favor of a simple barrier function.

Its biological role being unknown, GI-GPx may, nevertheless, be suspected to fulfill some important task, if the ranking within the hierarchy of selenoprotein expression is considered to reflect biological relevance. GI-GPx is not easily depleted by selenium-deprivation, its mRNA does not decline at all in selenium deficiency (55,181), and its biosynthesis resumes much faster than that of cGPx on selenium repletion (55,182).

D. PHGPx, the Moonlighting Selenoprotein

If the term moonlighting proteins is to describe proteins changing their appearance and biological role, it applies to PHGPx in a double sense, historically and physically. It was discovered as a factor preventing lipid peroxidation. As opposed to cGPx, PHGPx proved to reduce hydroperoxy groups of complex lipids integrated in biomembranes (86,183) and has long been considered to build the primary line of defense against oxidative membrane damage (184). Two distinct transcripts of the PHGPx gene were detected (185), the longer one encoding an N-terminal extension which targets the enzyme to mitochondria (186). Atypical tissue distribution (187–190) and hormone-dependence of its activity in testis (187,191) strengthened the idea that PHGPx might be more relevant to cellular regulation or differentiation than to mere antioxidant defense: (1) PHGPx, rather than cGPx, was shown to regulate leukotriene biosynthesis in rat basophilic leukemia cells (161,192); (2) when overexpressed in ECV cells, PHGPx inhibits interleukin (IL)-1-induced NF-κB activation (164); (3) when overexpressed in rabbit aortic smooth-muscle cells, it dampens the proliferative response to oxidized LDL and inhibits apoptosis induced by linoleic acid hydroperoxide (193); (4) mitochondrial PHGPx prevented apoptotic cell death when triggered by deoxyglucose, glucose deprivation, etoposide, staurosporine, UV irradiation, actinomycin D, or cycloheximide, but was ineffective in Fas-mediated or A23187-induced apoptosis (194); (5) PHGPx is present in most cells as a soluble and active peroxidase, and has recently been rediscovered as an enzymatically inactive structural protein in spermatozoa (195).

Beyond any doubt, PHGPx is exceptional among the selenoperoxidases in reducing all kinds of hydroperoxides ranging from H_2O_2 to phosphatidylcholine hydroperoxides and hydroperoxides of cholesterol esters in lipoproteins (196). With this potential and because of the lipophilicity of its surface, PHGPx, in a concerted action with vitamin E, is ideally suited to interrupt a free radical-driven lipid peroxidation chain (197) (Fig. 4). Peroxy radicals, generated by addition of molecular oxygen to alkyl radicals, react fast with tocopherols to generate alkyl hydroperoxides, the substrates of PHGPx. In the absence of PHGPx such hydroperox-

SELENIUM

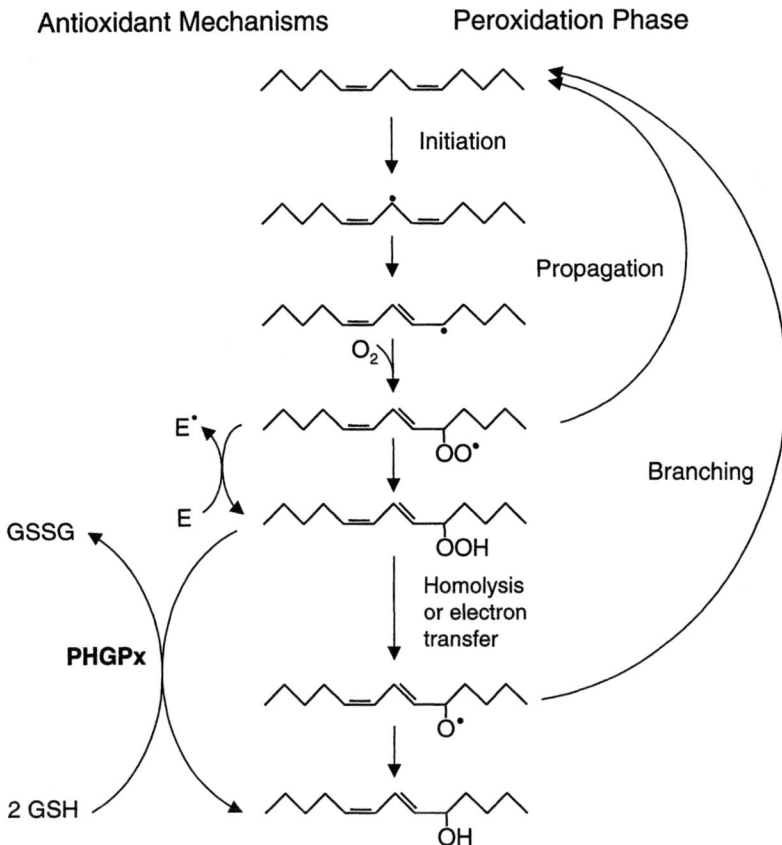

Figure 4 Phases of lipid peroxidation and antioxidant mechanisms: α-Tocopherol (E) suppresses the propagation of radical chain reactions at the stage of the peroxy radical. The hydroperoxides that this give rise to are reduced by PHGPx, whereby the branching of the radical chain is prevented. Efficient suppression of lipid peroxidation is possible only by the concerted action of a chain-breaking antioxidant and a glutathione peroxidase. Depending on the type of lipid and biological compartment, different types of glutathione peroxidases could be involved in the suppression of these radical chain reactions. The scheme refers to membrane lipid peroxidation, thus the enzyme is PHGPx. The reaction principle could also be similarly relevant for the control of inflammation-associated oxidative burst, for the maintenance of integrity of membrane lipids, as well as for the prevention of atherogenesis.

ides, by Fenton-type chemistry, would propagate the free-radical chain via alkoxy or hydroxy radical formation. This scheme attracted considerable interest, because it offered a plausible way to protect biomembranes and also explained the well-documented synergism of selenium and vitamin E (10,198,199). This concept has also been supported by numerous tissue culture studies showing an inverse correlation of PHGPx activity and sensitivity to hydroperoxides (200–202), including phosphatidylcholine hydroperoxide (193). The relevance of these findings for the in vivo situation, however, remains unproved. Monitoring lipid peroxidation markers, such as F_2-isoprostanes and carbonyls (203) in cGPx (−/−) mice with and without selenium supplementation, did not reveal any significant role of PHGPx. Increase of PHGPx activity by selenium supplementation in a cGPx (−/−) background neither improved survival nor markedly blocked the lipid peroxidation markers in mice intoxicated with redox cyclers (112–114,203,204). In these models at least, the initiation of lipid peroxidation by cGPx substrates is obviously more relevant than the propagation of the radical chain by typical PHGPx substrates. Thus, the evidence for an in vivo role of PHGPx in antagonizing unspecific lipid peroxidation is still meager.

In contrast, findings pointing to more specific roles are increasing. The enzymatic nature of PHGPx as a thiol:hydroperoxide oxidoreductase is certainly relevant to all its biological functions. But in some instances at least, PHGPx exerts its biological role by oxidizing thiols at the expense of hydroperoxides, rather than by eliminating peroxides at the expense of thiols. This is not a semantic distinction, as is best exemplified by the "moonlighting" of PHGPx during sperm maturation. PHGPx is abundantly expressed in the seminiferous epithelium of testis (191,205). Its expression and activity in testis depends on the proliferation of the seminiferous epithelium which is regulated by Leydig cell-derived testosterone. In consequence, it is not detectable in testes of prepuberal and hypophysectomized rats (187) and declines on poisoning of Leydig cells (191). At this state of spermatogenesis PHGPx might act as an antioxidant device (e.g., protecting the genome from the mutagenic potential of hydroperoxides). More likely, however, the burst of PHGPx expression in round spermatids serves a different purpose. It has been amply documented that during the transition from spermatids to spermatozoa the redox equilibrium is shifted to a pro-oxidant state that is characterized by an almost complete loss of GSH (206). PHGPx, now deprived of GSH, oxidizes thiols of proteins to create the keratin-like material fixing the mitochondria in the midpiece of sperm. This "mitochondrial capsule" consists of proteins including PHGPx itself, which are cross-linked by disulfide, diselenide, or selenadisulfide bridges (195). Being the most abundant constituent of the capsule, PHGPx accounts for most of the selenium content of sperm. Intriguingly, it is the midpiece of sperm that is affected in selenium deficiency: it displays a fluffy appearance, often looks broken, and in severe cases, the tail becomes disconnected. These disturbances are considered to be responsible for the impaired sperm motility and male infertility observed in selenium deficiency (21,207,208). Definitely this does not result from an impaired antioxidant defense, because, in sperm, PHGPx is enzymatically inactive anyway and can partially be reactivated only from the capsule material by drastic reductive procedures (195). Instead, the role of PHGPx in late sperm maturation is to make use of peroxides to build up a structural element indispensible for appropriate sperm function.

The precise function of PHGPx in signaling processes and other regulatory phenomena is less well understood. But its potential to oxidize protein thiols instead of GSH, as exemplified in the foregoing, offers ample opportunities to modulate the activities of receptors, signaling molecules, and transcription factors. Theoretically, PHGPx, in its oxidized state, could react directly with protein thiols to form a selenadisulfide bridge, in its half-reduced state it could transfer, e.g., glutathionyl residues to protein SH groups, in its reduced state it could even reduce disulfide bonds. In this sense, PHGPx may be considered a "thiol-modifying enzyme." Needless to say that, by such kind of interactions, PHGPx could regulate physiological processes more specifically than by chain breaking of hydroperoxide-driven autoxidation processes.

E. Thioredoxin Reductases

The selenoprotein character of mammalian thioredoxin reductase (TR) had for long been overlooked. It contains a selenocysteyl residue at the penultimate position of the amino acid chain (95–98), and the corresponding TGA codon in the pertinent gene had been considered to represent the stop codon. This interpretation was favored by the seemingly established mechanism of action involving transfer of reduction equivalents from NADPH by the coenzyme FAD to a disulfide bridge near the N-terminus, and from there to the disulfide substrate thioredoxin, a scheme followed almost identically in the homologous enzymes, glutathione reductase and tryparedoxin reductase (209,210). In the meantime it has become clear that the selenocysteine residue is essential in mammalian thioredoxin reductase, although the homologous enzymes of bacteria and plasmodia lack selenocysteine (210–212). As already mentioned, thioredoxin reductase activity in tissue culture cells depends on selenium supplementation (70–74); exchange of the selenocysteyl by a cysteyl residue resulted in loss of activity (213); cleavage of a C-terminal dodecapeptide containing the selenocysteyl residue by trypsin abrogated activity (214), as did treatment with carboxypeptidase (215) and premature chain termination owing to SECIS omission (216). Interestingly, TR isolated from human placenta was resistent to trypsin unless it was reduced by NADPH (214). This observation implies a substantial conformational change during redox transition and suggests an idea for how the selenocysteine contributes to catalysis. Whereas, in homologous enzymes acting on low molecular disulfides, the substrates can be bound to the flavine disulfide reaction center, thioredoxin reductase with its 11-kDa substrate thioredoxin requires a semimobile carrier of reduction equivalents which is the typical Gly-SeCys-Cys-Gly redox center in its C-terminus. In the oxidized state the C-terminus is bound back to the flavin disulfide reaction center (and resistant to tryptic cleavage), after reduction it can reach out to reduce the disulfide active site of thioredoxin (and can be split off by trypsin) (214). A mitochondrial isozyme of TR was also identified as selenoprotein displaying the same C-terminal redox center (96–98). More recently, additional isoforms of TR were detected by screening DNA databases for putative SECIS elements (99). In view of the multiplicity of TR species it is no longer surprising that the response of TR activity to selenium supplementation varies largely between cell lines (see foregoing).

Trying to define the biological role of TR means reviewing thioredoxin, which is definitely beyond the scope of this chapter (Fig. 5). In short, thioredoxins act as reducing substrates for a variety of enzymes such as ribonucleotide reductase, methionine sulfoxide reductase, 3'-phosphoadenosine 5'-phosphosulfate reductase and peroxiredoxin-type peroxidases (102,217,218). They are involved in protein–thiol disulfide exchange reactions, thereby contributing to protein folding and stabilization of the three-dimensional (3-D) structure; they appear to regulate the redox state of redox-sensitive proteins (219) and participate in the activation of transcription factors, in particular of NF-κB (163). Even in well-investigated microorganisms, such as *Escherichia coli*, the individual role of the realm of thioredoxins and thioredoxin-like proteins is far from being clear (218). Therefore, it comes as no surprise that the role of thioredoxin in complex mammalian organisms could not be defined to any satisfactory extend. The typical mammalian thioredoxin has, however, been demonstrated to be of vital importance. Targeted disruption of the thioredoxin gene in mice led to embryonic lethality and resorption before gastrulation (220). If cultured in vitro the inner cell mass of such embryos just did not proliferate. The precise mechanism being unknown, the effect is not easily explained by any antioxidant effect of thioredoxin. More likely it is related to transcriptional control or simply to thioredoxin's role in the biosynthesis of deoxynucleotides.

Certainly, all these biological functions of thioredoxin and, beyond, unknown ones could be disturbed if thioredoxin reductase activity were decreased owing to selenium deficiency. Such decrease is, however, not expected in marginal to moderate selenium deficiency; one or the other thioredoxin reductase isozyme must rank high in the hierarchy of selenoproteins, since total thioredoxin reductase activity usually remains remarkably high even in cell lines grown in unsupplemented media (73,74).

What kind of thioredoxin reductase-dependent pathology can then be envisaged in selenium deficiency? Some effects of prolonged selenium deprivation, such as the complete lack

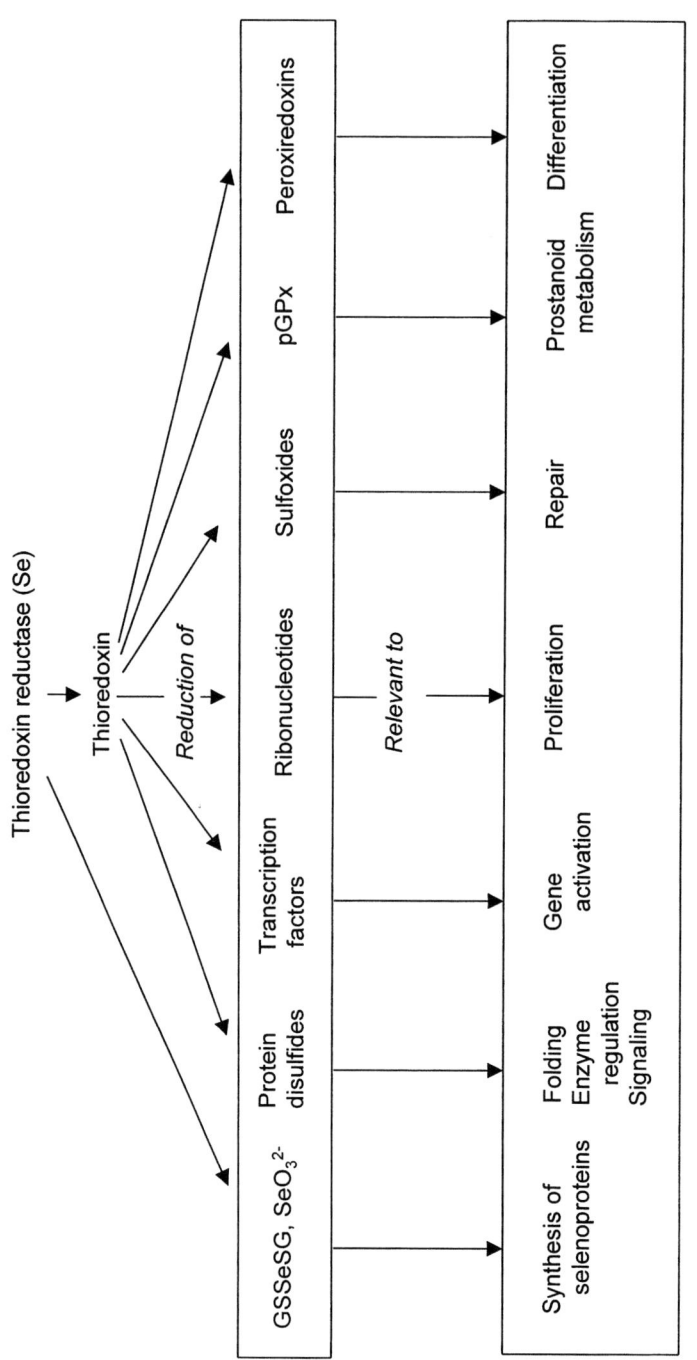

Figure 5 A selection of thioredoxin reductase-dependent events, the majority being unrelated to antioxidant defense.

of spermatogenesis (221,222) in rodents, may be plausibly attributed to the inability to reduce thioredoxin and, in consequence, to build deoxyribonucleotides. Furthermore, disturbances of the delicate redox regulation of signaling cascades could be anticipated. Overexpression of a human thioredoxin peroxidase (AOE 372, Acc. No. U25182), for instance, inhibited activation of *c-jun* N-terminal kinase (JNK) on growth factor stimulation in NIH 3T3 cells and H_2O_2 or TNF-induced NF-κB activation and apoptosis in HeLa cells (223–225), as has been similarly demonstrated with overexpression of cGPx (149,150,226) and PHGPx (see foregoing; 164,194). These observations are in line with the view that some signaling cascades, in particular TNF-induced NF-κB-dependent transcriptional gene activation, are facilitated by a pro-oxidant status of the cytosol (162). As discussed in detail elsewhere (163), a regulation of such processes may be achieved either directly by selenoperoxidases (164,194,226,227) or by selenium-dependent reduction of thioredoxin (223–225,228). Correspondingly, TNF-induced NF-κB activation (229–232) and HIV-1 LTR promoter activity (227,229,230) is reportedly dampened by selenium supplementation. At present, it is, however, not easily decided which of the peroxide-metabolizing selenium-dependent systems is responsible for the selenium-responsiveness of signaling events in a particular cell type. Dampening of NF-κB activation by hydroperoxides in smooth muscle cells and by IL-1 in ECV cells correlated with increased PHGPx (as opposed to cGPx) activity (164), whereas any impact on signaling of the redox status of thioredoxin caused by selenium deprivation remains to be demonstrated. Nevertheless, whenever a signaling cascade responds to supplementation with selenium in the low-nanomolar range, the biosynthesis of each of the selenoproteins relevant to hydroperoxide metabolism may be involved. In contrast, exposure to selenite at the micromolar level may abrogate the transcriptional activation of NF-κB by direct interaction with the vicinal SH groups of thioredoxin (231), which is required for nuclear reduction of the transcription factor (228).

The discovery of selenocysteine as an essential residue in TR has also prompted a reevaluation of the concept of selenium-dependent antioxidant defense (233). This cannot be a surprise after some antioxidant proteins, now renamed peroxiredoxins, had been identified as thioredoxin peroxidases and thus might compete with glutathione peroxidases or catalase for the common hydroperoxide substrates (102). The idea that selenium-dependent antioxidant effects might be mediated by peroxiredoxins is, however, not substantiated by experimental evidence and neither can it be rated as appealing. First of all, the outcome of oxidative challenge in cGPx (−,−) mice, quoted earlier, argues against any significant contribution to antioxidant defense by selenium-dependent enzymes apart from cGPx itself. Second, the peroxiredoxins fall short in efficiency as peroxidases when compared with the selenoperoxidases. Realistic estimates for rate constants of peroxiredoxins with hydroperoxides are available for only two parasitic enzymes: the tryparedoxin peroxidase of *Crithidia fasciculata* (233,234) and *Trypanosoma cruzi* (235). For these enzymes, the rate constants ranged between 3×10^4 M^{-1} s^{-1} and 3×10^5 M^{-1} s^{-1} (i.e., two to three orders of magnitude below those of selenoperoxidases). They were surprisingly similar to those of the sulfur analogues of cGPx (17) and PHGPx (107). A rate constant near 10^5 M^{-1} s^{-1} is obviously the maximum that can be achieved for sulfur-catalyzed hydroperoxide reduction (236). In trypanosomes, for which the peroxiredoxins appear to be the only antioxidant devices (237), this low efficiency is compensated by concentration, reaching for instance in *Crithidia*, 6% of soluble protein (233). Such abundance has never been reported for any of the mammalian peroxiredoxins. This implies that the mammalian peroxiredoxins are probably underestimated when considered as simple antioxidant devices backing up the selenoperoxidases. More likely, they are involved in specific redox regulation of particular pathways, as exemplified earlier for AOE 372. This perspective is also favored by emerging knowledge on the biological contexts in which these proteins are detected: AOP binds to, and is activated by cyclophilin (238); AOP2 is regulated by keratinocyte growth factor (239) and presumed to be involved in wound healing (240), "TRANK" mimics an inflammatory cytokine in activating NF-κB (241) (i.e., it does the opposite of overexpressed AOE 372), and others have been found in distinct differentiation states or stress conditions (242).

The selenoprotein nature of TR has similarly reanimated the discussion of supranutritional selenium dosages in chemoprevention of cancer. Some studies indicated that TR activity can be increased in certain cell lines (72,73) and in vivo (71) by supranutritional selenium supplementation. Yet such increased TR activity is not easily interpreted as a cytostatic effect. Irrespective of the physiological "goals" of TR we consider, an increased TR activity should support tumor growth: by being the cosubstrate of ribonucleotide reductase reduced thioredoxin enables fast proliferation; overexpression of thioredoxin inhibits apoptosis (243), as does any kind of optimization of hydroperoxide metabolism (149,150,193,225,226). Correspondingly, tumor cell lines or malignant tissues are usually characterized by comparatively high TR activity (244,245) and inhibitors of TR or thioredoxin have been discussed and demonstrated to reduce tumor cell proliferation (246,247).

There is, however, one possibility left for how an increased TR activity might generate harmful effects in tumor cells. Being a fairly unspecific enzyme it reduces a variety of selenocompounds such as selenite, selenadiglutathione, and diselenides to the lowest oxidation state (248). The selenols or selenides thus formed are autoxidizable as is evident from an overstoichiometric NADPH consumption when TR tests are performed under aerobic conditions (33). In other words, many selenium compounds commonly used for supplementation become typical redox cyclers by the aid of TR.

Another hypothesis implicating TR in the chemoprevention by selenium, considers TR itself as beneficial to the tumor and the excess of selenium that is not utilized for selenoprotein biosynthesis as kind of subversive TR substrate (24). Organoselenocompounds reduced to alkyl or aryl selenides by TR or the corresponding diselenides or seleninic acid derivatives might interact with the cysteine selenocysteine redox center of TR and, depending on the kind of substitution, cause more or less reversible TR inhibition. The hypothesis appears chemically plausible and is appealing in providing a perspective to understand the superior chemopreventive activities of alkyl and aryl selenides versus selenite. But at present it is supported by little else than the observation that TR activities decline with prolonged supraoptimal selenium supplementation, and TR can be inhibited by diarylselenides or tellurides (246). The specificity of this presumed mechanism may, however, be questioned, since a direct interaction of RSe^-, RSeOH, RSeSeR, or even selenite can be envisaged with a large variety of proteins, depending on redox-active cysteines or selenocysteines. The examples discussed so far, TR (24), thioredoxin (231), and zinc proteins (249), are certainly only the tip of the iceberg.

In brief, then, the identification of selenium in thioredoxin reductases has opened up a fascination chapter of selenium biochemistry, yet there is no compelling evidence for a role of TR in balancing oxidative challenge.

F. Selenoprotein W

The selenoprotein W is the prominent selenoprotein in muscle, but pertinent mRNA was also detected in spleen, testis, and brain (250). The encoding DNA sequences have been determined in five mammalian species including humans. They all contain an in-frame TGA coding for selenocysteine residue in position 13 and a typical SECIS (251). The deduced amino acid sequences comprise 87 or 88 residues complying with the low molecular weight of the isolated proteins.

SELENIUM

The enzymatic function of selenoprotein W is unknown but a participation in glutathione-dependent redox processes may be inferred from a covalently linked glutathionyl residue found in the isolated protein (252). The biological function of selenoprotein W is equally unknown. Because of its predominance in muscle, a link to muscular manifestations of selenium deficiency, such as white muscle disease in lambs and calves (253) or muscle weakness after long-term unsupplemented parenteral nutrition in patients (254), is currently suspected.

G. Selenoprotein P

Selenoprotein P is the most unusual selenoprotein in containing 9 (human) to 12 (bovine) selenocysteines. It is expressed with a leader sequence directing the protein to the extracellular space. The primary source of selenoprotein P appears to be the liver (255,256), but the pertinent mRNA is detected almost ubiquitously. Unexpected high levels of selenoprotein P mRNA were observed in Leydig cells of testis and the Purkinje layer of the cerebellum of mice (256). In the hierarchy of selenoproteins it occupies an intermediate position. The protein is further characterized by one or two histidine-rich clusters and several glycosylation sites. The protein isolated by antibodies still displays a pronounced heterogeneity that may in part result from its glycoprotein nature, in part from premature termination at the in frame UGA codons, most of which are close to the N-terminus (257,258).

The multiple selenocysteine residues of selenoprotein P suggest the ability to catalyze redox functions, yet an enzymatic activity has not yet been identified. Reportedly, selenoprotein P can act as an extracellular glutathione peroxidase (259), but this finding is still being disputed (260). Similar to other selenoproteins (261), selenoprotein P can scavenge peroxynitrite in vitro (262), but the regeneration of reduced protein that is required to close a catalytic cycle remains to be elucidated. Speculations on the biological role of selenoprotein P reach from selenium transport and selenium storage (263), prevention of selenium toxicity (264), up to antioxidant defense (257,264).

An antioxidant role of selenoprotein P was indeed corroborated by in vivo challenge with the redox-cycling herbicide diquat (265). Taking advantage of the differences in speed of recovery of pGPx and selenoprotein P after resupplementation of selenium-deprived rats, lipid peroxidation owing to diquat exposure was monitored within a window characterized by low pGPx and almost normalized selenoprotein P level. Paraquat resistance rather paralleled the reappearance of selenoprotein P than that of pGPx, indicating that the former protein is more relevant to extracellular antioxidant defense than pGPx. These findings seem to conflict with similar experiments performed with cGPx (−/−) mice suggesting irrelevance of any selenoprotein apart from cGPx in this context (see foregoing). There are, however, two differences between the experimental settings, species, and diquat dosage. A cautious interpretation of the findings would attribute the ability to cope with a moderate peroxide generation in the extracellular compartment to selenoprotein P, while balancing a more pronounced and general oxidative stress remains the domain of cGPx. This view is also supported by histochemical investigations showing selenoprotein P bound to the endothelial lining of the vascular system where it can shield the endothelium from bloodborne oxidants (257).

IV. CONCLUDING REMARKS

The fashionable attitude to declare selenium to be an antioxidant irrespective of its being part of an inorganic, organic, or enzymatic entity is misleading and unduly simplifies the multiple role of the essential trace element.

Just because the selenocysteine residue in selenoproteins catalyzes redox reactions, this potential does not justify the label "biological antioxidant." In its proper definition, the *antioxidant defense system* means a set of emergency devices counteracting oxidative stress, as is observed after exposure of the organism to redox-cycling xenobiotics, high oxygen tension, or endogenously produced superoxide radicals and hydroperoxides in infectious or inflammatory diseases (266). Watering down the definition of oxidative stress to comprise all kind of metabolic events involving redox reactions has recently led to the misuse of the term "antioxidant" for any reductant or even redox-inert compound somehow related to metabolic oxidations going on in an absolutely unstressed organism. In a more stringent sense, only few of selenium's known roles in biology can be classified as antioxidant.

1. None of the inorganic or organic selenium supplements currently used exert its physiological effects as a direct antioxidant. Instead, they are utilized as selenium sources for the biosynthesis of selenoproteins.

2. If administered in excess, they are metabolized to neurotoxic dimethylselenide and may induce oxidative tissue damage by autoxidation or redox-cycling as well as other metabolic disturbances.

3. As constituent of selenoperoxidases, selenium reduces H_2O_2 and other hydroperoxides, thereby preventing peroxide-dependent initiation or propagation of free radical chains. There is no experimental evidence whatsoever for any kind of direct radical scavenging by any of the selenoproteins.

4. Experimental evidence for a biologically relevant hydroperoxide detoxification exists only for the classic or cytosolic GPx (GPx1). The biological roles of GI-GPx (GPx2) and pGPx (GPx3) are still undefined. PHGPx (GPx4) appears to be relevant to the regulation of leukotriene biosynthesis and cytokine-induced gene activation. In testis it utilizes oxidants to build up the mitochondrial capsule.

5. The selenoprotein thioredoxin reductase reduces thioredoxin and thus is primarily responsible for DNA biosynthesis. Moreover, it is relevant to the realm of thioredoxin-dependent processes including peroxiredoxin-catalyzed hydroperoxide metabolism. Circumstantial evidence, however, indicates that the peroxiredoxins are involved in specific phenomena of cellular regulation and differentiation, rather than in antioxidant defense.

6. The enzymatic functions of selenoproteins P and W are unknown. A contribution of selenoprotein P to the protection of the vascular endothelium against oxidants, including peroxynitrite, may nevertheless be rated as likely.

7. No theoretical link can be envisaged between antioxidant effects and the deiodinases. They provide or degrade triiodothyronine and thus regulate morphogenesis, sexual maturation, and metabolic rate.

8. Relative to the known selenium-deficiency syndromes, Keshan disease may tentatively be explained by peroxide-induced acquisition of virulence by coxsackieviruses combined with insufficient oxidant defense to cope with virus-induced oxidative stress. Kashin–Beck disease may be partly due to an impaired ability to cope with inflammatory responses to mycotoxins.

9. The relevance of selenium supplementation to the development of cancer is still a matter of debate. Long-lasting subclinical selenium deficiency and resulting low cGPx levels may be anticipated to favor cancer initiation by mutagenic peroxides; this concept, however, cannot yet be experimentally corroborated. Chemoprevention of cancer

by supraoptimum selenium supplementation is mechanistically unclarified but definitely unrelated to antioxidant defense.

10. Epidemiological surveys have suggested an association of atherosclerosis with subacute selenium deficiency and corresponding prooxidant events. Pertinent experimental confirmation is lacking.

This list of summarizing statements is not meant to exhaustively compile the knowns and unknowns in the field of selenium biology. Some medically important aspects such as the possible relevance of the selenium status to neurodegenerative diseases, AIDs manifestation, and the immune system in general, or to critically ill patients were not discussed here in detail, because the links to solid biochemical data were considered too vague. The reader is referred to recent compilations of the pertinent state of knowledge (267–270). It is not very likely that these phenomena can be adequately explained by attaching the label "antioxidant" to selenium. With our steadily growing knowledge, it has become evident that the role of selenium in the antioxidant defense system is just a minor facet of the most diversified and complex selenium biochemistry.

ACKNOWLEDGMENTS

The work was supported by the Deutsche Forschungsgemeinschaft, DFG (INK 26/A/B1-1), the European Community (Biomed II program, PL 963202), and the Volkswagenstiftung (ZN 548).

REFERENCES

1. Bayer E, Giesecke H, Krauss P, Röder A. (1974) Transition metal complexes of thiol compounds. In: Flohé L, Benöhr HC, Sies H, Waller HD, Wendel A, eds. Glutathione. Stuttgart: Georg Thieme, pp. 34–44.
2. Misra HP. (1974) Generation of superoxide free radical during the autoxidation of thiols. J Biol Chem 249:2151–2155.
3. Seko Y, Saito Y, Kitara J, Imura N. (1989) Active oxygen generation by the reaction of selenite with reduced glutathione in vitro. In: Wendel A, ed. Selenium in Biology and Medicine. Berlin: Springer Verlag, pp. 70–73.
4. Seko Y, Imura N. (1997) Active oxygen generation as a possible mechanism of selenium toxicity. Biomed Environ Sci 10:333–339.
5. Schoneich C, Narayanaswami V, Asmus KD, Sies H. (1990) Reactivity of ebselen and related selenoorganic compounds with 1,2-dichloroethane radical cations and halogenated peroxyl radicals. Arch Biochem Biophys 282:18–25.
6. Maiorino M, Roveri A, Ursini F. (1992) Antioxidant effect of ebselen (PZ51): peroxidase mimetic activity on phospholipid and cholesterol hydroperoxides vs. free radical scavenger activity. Arch Biochem Biophys 295:404–409.
7. Cadenas E. (1997) Basic mechanisms of antioxidant activity. Biofactors 6:391–397.
8. Chaudiere J, Yadan J–C, Erdelmeier I, Tailhan–Lomont C, Moutet M. (1994) Design of new selenium-containing mimics of glutathione peroxidase. In: Paoletti R ed. Oxidative Processes and Antioxidants. New York: Raven, pp. 165–184.
9. Schwarz K, Foltz CM. (1957) Selenium as an integral part of factor 3 against dietary necrotic liver degeneration. J Am Chem Soc 79:3292–3293.
10. Schwarz K. (1976) The discovery of the essentiality of selenium, and related topics. (A personnel account). Proceedings of the Symposium on Selenium–Tellurium in the Environment, Notre Dame, Indiana, May 11–13, pp. 349–376.
11. Rotruck JT, Hoekstra WG, Pope AL, Ganther H, Swanson A, Hafeman D. (1972) Relationship of selenium to GSH peroxidase [abstr]. Fed Proc 31:691.
12. Rotruck JT, Pope AL, Ganther HE, Swanson AB, Hafeman DG, Hoekstra WG. (1973) Selenium: biochemical role as a component of glutathione peroxidase. Science 179:588–590.

13. Flohé L, Günzler WA, Schock HH. (1973) Glutathione peroxidase: a selenoenzyme. FEBS Lett 32:132–134.
14. Oh SH, Ganther HE, Hoekstra WG. (1974) Selenium as a component of glutathione peroxidase isolated from ovine erythrocytes. Biochemistry 13:1825–1829.
15. Awasthi YC, Beutler E, Srivastava SK. (1975) Purification and properties of human erythrocyte glutathione peroxidase. J Biol Chem 250:5144–5149.
16. Kraus RJ, Prohaska JR, Ganther HE. (1980) Oxidized forms of ovine erythrocyte glutathione peroxidase. Cyanide inhibition of a 4-glutathione:4-selenoenzyme. Biochim Biophys Acta 615:19–26.
17. Rocher C, Lalanne JL, Chaudière J. (1992) Purification and properties of a recombinant sulfur analog of murine selenium–glutathione peroxidase. Eur J Biochem 205:955–960.
18. Stadtman TC. (1996) Selenocysteine. Annu Rev Biochem 65:83–100.
19. Burk RF, Hill KE. (1999) Orphan selenoproteins. Bioessays 21:231–237.
20. Gladyshev VN, Hatfield DL. (1999) Selenocysteine-containing proteins in mammals. J Biomed Sci 6:151–160.
21. National Research Council (U. S.), Subcommittee on Selenium. (1983) Selenium in Nutrition. Washington DC: National Acadamy Press.
22. Combs GF Jr, Combs SB. (1986) The Role of Selenium in Nutrition. Orlando, FL: Academic Press.
23. Spallholz JE. (1994) On the nature of selenium toxicity and carcinostatic activity. Free Radic Biol Med 17:45–64.
24. Ganther HE. (1999) Selenium metabolism, selenoproteins and mechanisms of cancer prevention: complexities with thioredoxin reductase. Carcinogenesis 20:1657–1666.
25. Barceloux DG. (1999) Selenium. Clin Toxicol 37:145–172.
26. McConnell KP, Cho GJ. (1967) Active transport of L-selenomethionine in the intestine. Am J Physiol 213:150–156.
27. Whanger PD, Pedersen ND, Hatfield J, Weswig PH. (1976) Absorption of selenite and selenomethionine from ligated digestive tract segments in rats. Proc Soc Exp Biol Med 153:295–297.
28. Vendeland SC, Deagen JT, Butler JA, Whanger PD. (1994) Uptake of selenite, selenomethionine and selenate by brush border membrane vesicles isolated from rat small intestine. Biometals 7:305–312.
29. Korhola M, Vainio A, Edelmann K. (1986) Selenium yeast. Ann Clin Res 18:65–68.
30. Ganther HE. (1971) Reduction of the selenotrisulfide derivative of glutathione to a persulfide analog by glutathione reductase. Biochemistry 10:4089–4098.
31. Hsieh HS, Ganther HE. (1977) Biosynthesis of dimethyl selenide from sodium selenite in rat liver and kidney cell-free systems. Biochim Biophys Acta 497:205–217.
32. Björnstedt M, Odlander B, Kuprin S, Claesson H–E, Holmgren A. (1996) Selenite incubated with NADPH and mammalian thioredoxin reductase yields selenide, which inhibits lipoxygenase and changes the electron spin resonance spectrum of the active site iron. Biochemistry 35:8511–8516.
33. Kumar S, Björnstedt M, Holmgren A. (1992) Selenite is a substrate for calf thymus thioredoxin reductase and thioredoxin and elicits a large non-stoichiometric oxidation of NADPH in the presence of oxygen. Eur J Biochem 207:435–439.
34. McConnell KP, Hoffmann JL. (1972) Methionine selenomethionine parallels in liver polypeptide chain synthesis. FEBS Lett 24:60–62.
35. Anwad HK, Adelstein SJ, Potchen EJ, Dealy JB. (1967) The intraconversion and reutilization of injected [75]selenomethionine in the rat. J Biol Chem 242:492–500.
36. Esaki N, Nakamura T, Tanaka H, Soda K. (1982) Selenocysteine lyase: a novel enzyme that specifically acts on selenocysteine. Mammalian distribution and purification and properties of pig liver enzyme. J Biol Chem 257:4386–4391.
37. Ganther HE. (1986) Pathways of selenium metabolism including respiratory excretory products. J Am Coll Toxicol 5:1–5.
38. Veres Z, Kim IY, Scholz TD, Stadtman TC. (1994) Selenophosphate synthetase. Enzyme properties and catalytic reaction. J Biol Chem 269:10597–10603.
39. Guimaraes MJ, Peterson D, Vicari A, Cocks BG, Copeland NG, Gilbert DJ, Jenkins NA, Ferrick DA, Kastalein RA, Bazan JF, Zlotnik A. (1996) Identification of a novel selD homolog from eukaryotes, bacteria, and archea; is there an autoregulatory mechanism in selenocysteine metabolism? Proc Natl Acad Sci USA 93:15086–15091.

40. Mizutani T, Kanaya K, Tanabe K. (1999) Selenophosphate as a substrate for mammalian selenocysteine synthase, its stability and toxicity. Biofactors 9:27–36.
41. Baron C, Böck A. (1995) The selenocysteine-inserting tRNA species: structure and function. In: Söll D, Raj Bhandary U, eds. tRNA: Structure, Biosynthesis, and Function. Washington, DC: American Society for Microbiology, pp. 429–544.
42. Chambers I, Frampton J, Goldfarb P, Affara N, McBain W, Harrison PR. (1986) The structure of the mouse glutathione peroxidase gene: the selenocysteine in the active site is encoded by the "termination" codon, TGA. EMBO J 5:1221–1227.
43. Böck A, Forchhammer K, Heider J, Baron C. (1991) Selenoprotein synthesis: an expansion of the genetic code. Trends Biol Sci 16:463–467.
44. Low SC, Berry MJ. (1996) Knowing when not to stop: selenocysteine incorporation in eukaryotes. Trends Biol Sci. 21:203–208.
45. Heider J, Baron C, Böck A. (1992) Coding from a distance: dissection of the mRNA determinants required for the incorporation of selenocysteine into protein. EMBO J 11:3759–3766.
46. Berry MJ, Banu L, Harney JW, Larsen PR. (1993) Functional characterization of the eukaryotic SECIS elements which direct selenocysteine insertion at UGA codons. EMBO J 12:3315–3322.
47. Tormay P, Sawers A, Böck A. (1996) Role of stoichiometry between mRNA, translation factor SelB and selenocysteyl-tRNA in selenoprotein synthesis. Mol Microbiol 21:1253–1259.
48. Berry MJ, Banu L, Larsen PR. (1991) Type I iodothyronine deiodinase is a selenocysteine-containing enzyme. Nature 349:438–440.
49. Walczak R, Carbon P, Krol A. (1998) An essential non–Watson-Crick base pair motif in 3′UTR to mediate selenoprotein translation. RNA 4:74–84.
50. Saedi MS, Smith C, Frampton J, Chambers I, Harrison PR, Sunde RA. (1988) Effect of selenium status on mRNA levels for glutathione peroxidase in rat liver. Biochem Biophys Res Commun 153:855–861.
51. Bermano G, Arthur JR, Hesketh JE. (1996) Selective control of cytosolic glutathione peroxidase and phospholipid hydroperoxide glutathione peroxidase mRNA stability by selenium supply. FEBS Lett 387:157–160.
52. Brigelius–Flohé R. (1999) Tissue-specific functions of individual glutathione peroxidases. Free Radic Biol Med 27:951–965.
53. Bermano G, Arthur JR, Hesketh JE. (1996) Role of the 3′ untranslated region in the regulation of cytosolic glutathione peroxidase and phospholipid–hydroperoxide glutathione peroxidase gene expression by selenium supply. Biochem J 320:891–895.
54. Weiss SL, Sunde RA. (1997) Selenium regulation of classical glutathione peroxidase expression requires the 3′ untranslated region in Chinese hamster ovary cells. J Nutr 127:1304–1310.
55. Wingler K, Böcher M, Flohé L, Kollmus H, Brigelius–Flohé R. (1999) mRNA stability and selenocysteine insertion sequence efficiency rank gastrointestinal glutathione peroxidase high in the hierarchy of selenoproteins. Eur J Biochem 259:149–157.
56. Kollmus H, Flohé L, McCarthy JE. (1996) Analysis of eukaryotic mRNA structures directing cotranslational incorporation of selenocysteine. Nucl Acids Res 24:1195–1201.
57. Flohé L, Wingender E, Brigelius–Flohé R. (1997) The regulation of glutathione peroxidases. In: Forman H, Cadenas E, eds. Oxidative Stress and Signal Transduction. New York: Chapman & Hall, pp. 415–435.
58. Nève J. (1995) Human selenium supplementation as assessed by changes in blood selenium concentration and glutathione peroxidase activity. J Trace Elem Med Biol 9:65–73.
59. Beilstein MA, Whanger PD. (1988) Glutathione peroxidase activity and chemical forms of selenium in tissues of rats given selenite or selenomethionine. J Inorg Biochem 33:31–46.
60. Butler JA, Whanger PD, Kaneps AJ, Patton NM. (1990) Metabolism of selenite and selenomethionine in the rhesus monkey. J Nutr 120:751–759.
61. Lane HW, Strength R, Johnson J, White M. (1991) Effect of chemical form of selenium on tissue glutathione peroxidase activity in developing rats. J Nutr 121:80–86.
62. Whanger PD, Butler JA. (1988) Effects of various dietary levels of selenium as selenite or selenomethionine on tissue selenium levels and glutathione peroxidase activity in rats. J Nutr 118:846–852.
63. Moksnes K, Norheim G. (1983) Selenium and glutathione peroxidase levels in lambs receiving feed supplemented with sodium selenite or selenomethionine. Acta Vet Scand 24:45–58.
64. Sunde RA, Gutzke GE, Hoekstra WG. (1981) Effect of dietary methionine on the biopotency of selenite and selenomethionine in the rat. J Nutr 111:76–88.

65. Ip C. (1998) Differential effect of dietary methionine on the biopotency of selenomethionine and selenite in cancer chemoprevention. J Natl Cancer Inst 80:258–262.
66. Waschulewski IH, Sunde RA. (1988) Effect of dietary methionine on utilization of tissue selenium from dietary selenomethionine for glutathione peroxidase in the rat. J Nutr 118:367–374.
67. Beilstein MA, Whanger PD. (1987) Metabolism of selenomethionine and effects of interacting compounds by mammalian cells in culture. J Inorg Biochem 29:137–152.
68. Leist M, Maurer S, Schultz M, Elsner A, Gawlik D, Brigelius–Flohé R. (1999) Cytoprotection against lipid hydroperoxides correlates with increased glutathione peroxidase activities, but not selenium uptake from different selenocompounds. Biol Trace Elem Res 68:159–174.
69. Brigelius–Flohé R, Lötzer K, Maurer S, Schultz M, Leist M. (1995/1996) Utilization of selenium from different chemical entities for selenoprotein biosynthesis by mammalian cell lines. Biofactors 5:125–131.
70. Hill KE, McCollum GW, Boeglin ME, Burk RF. (1997) Thioredoxin reductase activity is decreased by selenium deficiency. Biochem Biophys Res Commun 234:293–295.
71. Berggren MM, Mangin JF, Gasdaska JR, Powis G. (1999) Effect of selenium on rat thioredoxin reductase activity. Increase by supranutritional selenium and decrease by selenium deficiency. Biochem Pharmacol 57:187–193.
72. Berggren M, Gallegos A, Gasdaska J, Powis G. (1997) Cellular thioredoxin reductase activity is regulated by selenium. Anticancer Res 17:3377–3380.
73. Gallegos A, Berggren M, Gasdaska JR, Powis G. (1997) Mechanisms of the regulation of thioredoxin reductase activity in cancer cells by the chemopreventive agent selenium. Cancer Res 57:4965–4970.
74. Marcocci L, Flohé L, Packer L. (1997) Evidence for a functional relevance of the selenocysteine residue in mammalian thioredoxin reductase. Biofactors 6:351–358.
75. Levander OA. (1991) Scientific rationale for the 1989 recommended dietary allowance for selenium. J Am Diet Assoc 91:1572–1576.
76. Yang JG, Hill KE, Burk RF. (1989) Dietary selenium intake controls rat plasma selenoprotein P concentration. J Nutr 119:1010–1012.
77. Behne D, and Kyriakopoulos A. (1993) Effects of dietary selenium on the tissue concentrations of type I iodothyronine 5'-deiodinase and other selenoproteins. Am J Clin Nutr 57:310S–312S
78. Ursini F, Maiorino M, Brigelius–Flohé R, Aumann KD, Roveri A, Schomburg D, Flohé L. (1995) Diversity of glutathione peroxidases. Methods Enzymol 252:38–53.
79. Sugimoto M, Sakamoto W. (1997) Putative phospholipid hydroperoxide glutathione peroxidase gene from *Arabidopsis thaliana* induced by oxidative stress. Genes Genet Syst 72:311–316.
80. Maiorino M, Roche C, Kiess M, Koenig K, Gawlik D, Matthes M, Naldini E, Pierce R, Flohé L. (1996) A selenium-containing phospholipid-hydroperoxide glutathione peroxidase in *Schistosoma mansoni*. Eur J Biochem 238:828–844.
81. Buettner C, Harney JW, Berry MJ. (1999) The *Caenorhabditis elegans* homologue of thioredoxin reductase contains a selenocysteine insertion sequence (SECIS) element that differs from mammalian SECIS elements but directs selenocysteine incorporation. J Biol Chem 274:21598–21602.
82. Bösl MR, Takaku K, Oshima M, Nishimura S, Taketo MM. (1997) Early embryonic lethality caused by targeted disruption of the mouse selenocysteine tRNA gene (*Trsp*). Proc Natl Acad Sci USA 94:5531–5534.
83. Alsina B, Corominas M, Berry M, Baguna J, Serras F. (1999) Disruption of selenoprotein biosynthesis affects cells proliferation in the imaginal discs and brain of *Drosophila melanogaster*. J Cell Sci 112:2875–2884.
84. Holmgren A. (1989) Thioredoxin and glutaredoxin systems. J Biol Chem 264:13963–13966.
85. Mills GC. (1957) Hemoglobin catabolism I. Glutathione peroxidase, an erythrocyte enzyme which protects hemoglobin from oxidative breakdown. J Biol Chem 229:189–197.
86. Ursini F, Maiorino M, Valente M, Ferri L, Gregolin C. (1982) Purification from pig liver of a protein which protects liposomes and biomembranes from peroxidative degradation and exhibits glutathione peroxidase activity on phosphatidylcholine hydroperoxides. Biochim Biophys Acta 710:197–211.
87. Takahashi K, Avissar N, Whitin J, Cohen H. (1987) Purification and characterization of human plasma glutathione peroxidase: a selenoglycoprotein distinct from the known cellular enzyme. Arch Biochem Biophys 256:677–686.

88. Chu F-F, Doroshow JH, Esworthy RS. (1993) Expression, characterization, and tissue distribution of a new cellular selenium-dependent glutathione peroxidase, GSH-Px-GI. J Biol Chem 268:2571–2576.
89. Behne D, Kyriakopoulos A, Meinhold H, Köhrle J. (1990) Identification of type I iodothyronine 5'-deiodinase as a selenoenzyme. Biochem Biophys Res Commun 173:1143–1149.
90. Arthur JR, Nicol F, Beckett GJ. (1990) Hepatic iodothyronine deiodinase: the role of selenium. Biochem J 272:537–540.
91. Davey JC, Becker KB, Schneider MJ, Germain GL, Galton VA. (1995) Cloning of a cDNA for the type II iodothyronine deiodinase. J Biol Chem 270:26786–26789.
92. Croteau W, Whittemore SK, Schneider MJ, Germain DL. (1995) Cloning and expression of a cDNA for a mammalian type III iodothyronine deiodinase. J Biol Chem 270:16569–165575.
93. Motsenbocker MA, Tappel AL. (1984) Effect of dietary selenium on plasma selenoprotein P, selenoprotein P1 and glutathione peroxidase in the rat. J Nutr 114:279–285.
94. Vendeland SC, Beilstein MA, Yeh JY, Ream W, Whanger PD. (1995) Rat skeletal muscle selenoprotein W: cDNA clone and mRNA modulation by dietary selenium. Proc Natl Acad Sci USA 92:8749–8753.
95. Tamura T, Stadtman TC. (1996) A new selenoprotein from human lung adenocarcinoma cells: purification, properties, and thioredoxin reductase activity. Proc Natl Acad Sci USA 93:1006–1011.
96. Lee SR, Kim JR, Kwon KS, Yoon HW, Levine RL, Ginsburg A, Rhee SG. (1999) Molecular cloning and characterization of a mitochondrial selenocysteine-containing thioredoxin reductase from rat liver. J Biol Chem 274:4722–4734.
97. Watabe S, Makino Y, Ogawa K, Hiroi T, Yamamoto Y, Takahashi SY. (1999) Mitochondrial thioredoxin reductase in bovine adrenal cortex its purification, properties, nucleotide/amino acid sequences, and identification of selenocysteine. Eur J Biochem 264:74–84.
98. Miranda–Vizuete A, Damdimopoulos AE, Pedrajas JR, Gustafsson J-Å, Spyrou G. (1999) Human mitochondrial thioredoxin reductase. Eur J Biochem 261:405–412.
99. Lescure A, Gautheret D, Carbon P, Krol A. (1999) Novel selenoproteins identified in silico and in vivo by using a conserved RNA structural motif. J Biol Chem 274:38142–38154.
100. Gladyshev VN, Jeang K-T, Wootton JC, Hatfield DL. (1998) A new human selenium-containing protein. J Biol Chem 273:8910–8915.
101. Kryukov GV, Kryukov VM, Gladyshev VN. (1999) New mammalian selenocysteine-containing proteins identified with an algorithm that searches for selenocysteine insertion sequence elements. J Biol Chem 274:33888–33897.
102. Rhee SG, Kang SW, Netto LE, Seo MS, Stadtman ER. (1999) A family of novel peroxidases, peroxiredoxins. Biofactors 10:207–209.
103. Flohé L. (1989) The selenoprotein glutathione peroxidase. In: Dolphin D, Poulson R, Avramovic O, eds. Glutathione: Chemical, Biochemical and Medical Aspects—Part A. New York: John Wiley & Sons, pp. 643–731.
104. Aumann K-D, Bedorf N, Brigelius-Flohé R, Schomburg D, Flohé L. (1997) Glutathione peroxidase revisited. Simulation of the catalytic cycle by computer-assisted molecular modelling. Biomed Environ Sci 10:136–155.
105. Ren B, Huang W, Akesson B, Ladenstein R. (1997) The crystal structure of seleno-glutathione peroxidase from human plasma at 2.9 A resolution. J Mol Biol 268:869–885.
106. Epp O, Ladenstein R, Wendel A. (1983) The refined structure of the selenoenzyme glutathione peroxidase at 0.2-nm resolution. Eur J Biochem 133:51–69.
107. Maiorino M, Aumann KD, Brigelius-Flohé R, Doria D, van den Heuvel J, McCarthy J, Roveri A, Ursini F, Flohé L. (1995) Probing the presumed catalytic triad of selenium-containing peroxidases by mutational analysis of phospholipid hydroperoxide glutathione peroxidase (PHGPx). Biol Chem Hoppe Seyler 376:651–660.
108. Flohé L, Loschen G, Günzler WA, Eichele E. (1972) Glutathione peroxidase, V. The kinetic mechanism. Hoppe Seyler's Z Physiol Chem 353:987–999.
109. Günzler WA, Vergin H, Müller I, Flohé L. (1972) Glutathione peroxidase VI: The reaction of glutathione peroxidase with various hydroperoxides. Hoppe Seyler's Z Physiol Chem 353:1001–1004.
110. Harman LS, Carver DK, Schreiber J, Mason RP. (1986) One- and two-electron oxidation of reduced glutathione by peroxidases. J Biol Chem 261:1642–1648.

111. Ho Y-S, Magneanat JL, Bronson RT, Cao J, Gargano M, Sugawara M, Funk CD. (1997) Mice deficient in cellular glutathione peroxidase develop normally and show no increased sensitivity to hyperoxia. J Biol Chem 272:16644–16651.
112. de Haan JB, Bladier C, Griffiths P, Kelner M, O'Shea RD, Cheung NS, Bronson RT, Silvestro MJ, Wild S, Zheng SS, Beart PM, Hertzog PJ, Kola I. (1998) Mice with a homozygous null mutation for the most abundant glutathione peroxidase, Gpx1, show increased susceptibility to the oxidative stress-inducing agents paraquat and hydrogen peroxide. J Biol Chem 273:22528–22536.
113. Cheng WH, Ho Y-S, Valentine BA, Ross DA, Combs GF, Lei XG. (1998) Cellular glutathione peroxidase is the mediator of body selenium to protect against paraquat lethality in transgenic mice. J Nutr 128:1070–1076.
114. Fu Y, Cheng W-H, Porres JM, Ross DA, Lei XG. (1999) Knockout of cellular glutathione peroxidase gene renders mice susceptible to diquat-induced oxidative stress. Free Radic Biol Med 27:605–611.
115. Jaeschke H, Ho Y-S, Fisher MA, Lawson JA, Farhood A. (1999) Glutathione peroxidase-deficient mice are more susceptible to neutrophil-mediated hepatic parenchymal cell injury during endotoxemia: importance of an intracellular oxidant stress. Hepatology 29:443–450.
116. Flohé L. (1971) Die Glutathionperoxidase: Enzymologie und biologische Aspekte. Klin Wochenschr 49:669–683.
117. Flohé L, Günzler WA, Loschen G. (1979) The glutathione peroxidase reaction: a key to understand the selenium requirement of mammals. In: Kharash N, ed. Trace Metals in Health and Disease. New York: Raven, pp. 263–286.
118. Cohen G, Hochstein P. (1963) Glutathione peroxidase: the primary agent for the elimination of hydrogen peroxide in erythrocytes. Biochemistry 2:1420–1428.
119. Rotruck JT, Pope AL, Ganther HE, Hoekstra WG. (1972) Prevention of oxidative damage to rat erythrocytes by dietary selenium. J Nutr 102:689–696.
120. Beutler E. (1983) Red cell enzyme deficiencies as non-disease. Biomed Biochim Acta 42:S234–S241.
121. Burk RF. (1989) Recent developments in trace element metabolism and function: newer roles of selenium in nutrition. J Nutr 119:1051–1054.
122. Yang GQ, Chen JS, Wen ZM, Ge KY, Zhu LZ, Chen XC, Chen XS. (1984) The role of selenium in Keshan disease. Adv Nutr Res 6:203–231.
123. Gu BQ. (1983) Pathology of Keshan disease. A comprehensive review. Chin Med J (Engl) 96:251–261.
124. Sokoloff L. (1988) Kashin–Beck disease: current status. Nutr Rev 46:113–119.
125. Peng A, Yang C, Rui H, Li H. (1992) Study on the pathogenic factors of Kashin–Beck disease. J Toxicol Environ Health 35:79–90.
126. Peng A, Wang WH, Wang CX, Wang ZJ, Rui HF, Wang WZ, Yang ZW. (1999) The role of humic substances in drinking water in Kashin–Beck disease in China. Environ Health Perspect 107:293–296.
127. Ioannidis N, Kurz B, Hansen U, Schunke M. (1999) Influence of fulvic acid on the collagen secretion of bovine chondrocytes in vitro. Cell Tissue Res 297:141–147.
128. Guanqing H. (1979) On the etiology of Keshan disease: two hypotheses. Chin Med J 92:416–422.
129. Yang GQ, Xia YM. (1995) Studies on human dietary requirements and safe range of dietary intakes of selenium in China and their application in the prevention of related endemic diseases. Biomed Environ Sci 8:187–201.
130. Editorial. (1979) Selenium in the heart of China. Lancet 2:889–890.
131. Cheng YY, Qian PC. (1990) The effect of selenium-fortified table salt in the prevention of Keshan disease on a population of 1.05 million. Biomed Environ Sci 3:422–428.
132. Johnson RA, Baker SS, Fallon JT, Maynard EP 3d, Ruskin JN, Wen Z, Ge K, Cohen HJ. (1981) An accidental case of cardiomyopathy and selenium deficiency. N Engl J Med 304:1210–1212.
133. Reeves WC, Marcuard SP, Willis SE, Movahed A. (1989) Reversible cardiomyopathy due to selenium deficiency. J Parent Enteral Nutr 13:663–665.
134. Ge K, Xue A, Bai J, Wang S. (1983) Keshan disease—an endemic cardiomyopathy in China. Virchows Arch A Pathol Anat Histopathol 401:1–15.
135. Beck MA, Kolbeck PC, Rohr LH, Shi Q, Morris VC, Levander OA. (1994) Benign human enterovirus becomes virulent in selenium-deficient mice. J Med Virol 43:166–170.

136. Beck MA, Shi Q, Morris VC, Levander OA. (1995) Rapid genomic evolution of a non-virulent coxsackievirus B3 in selenium-deficient mice results in selection of identical virulent isolates. Nat Med 1:433–436.
137. Beck MA, Esworthy RS, Ho YS, Chu FF. (1998) Glutathione peroxidase protects mice from viral-induced myocarditis. FASEB J 12:1143–1149.
138. Shamberger RJ, Frost DV. (1969) Possible effect of selenium against human cancer. Can Med Assoc J 100:682.
139. Schrauzer GN. (1998) Selen: neue Entwicklungen aus Biologie, Biochemie und Medizin, 3rd ed. Heidelberg: Johann Ambrosius Barth Verlag.
140. Combs GJ, Gray WP. (1998) Chemopreventive agents: selenium. Pharmacol Ther 79:179–192.
141. Ip C. (1998) Lessons from basic research in selenium and cancer prevention. J Nutr 128:1845–1854.
142. Clark LC, Combs GF, Tumbuli BW, Slate EH, Chalker DK, Chow J, Davis LS, Glover RA, Graham GF, Gross EG, Krongrad A, Lesher JL, Park HK, Sanders BB, Smith CL, Taylor JR. (1996) Effects of selenium supplementation for cancer prevention in patients with carcinoma of the skin. JAMA 25:1957–1985.
143. Kotrebai M, Birringer M, Tyson JF, Block E, Uden PC. (1999) Identification of the principal selenium compounds in selenium-enriched natural sample extracts by ion-pair liquid chromatography with inductively coupled plasma- and electrospray ionization–mass spectrometric detection. Anal Commun 36:249–252.
144. Ip C, Lisk DJ. (1995) Efficacy of cancer prevention by high selenium-garlic is primarily dependent on the action of selenium. Carcinogenesis 16:2649–2652.
145. Ip C, Lisk DJ. (1996) The attributes of selenium-enriched garlic in cancer prevention. In: American Institute Cancer Research, ed. Dietary Phytochemicals in Cancer Prevention and Treatment. New York: Plenum, pp. 179–187.
146. Cai X-J, Uden PC, Block E, Zhang X, Quimby BD, Sullivan JJ. (1994) *Allium* chemistry: identification of natural abundance organoselenium volatiles from garlic, elephant garlic, onion, and Chinese chive using headspace gas chromatography with atomic emission detection. J Agric Food Chem 42:2081–2084.
147. Birringer, personal communication
148. Lu YP, Lou YR, Yen P, Newmark HL, Mirochnitchenko OI, Inouye M, Huang MT. (1997) Enhanced skin carcinogenesis in transgenic mice with high expression of glutathione peroxidase or both glutathione peroxidase and superoxide dismutase. Cancer Res 57:1468–1474.
149. Packham G, Ashmun RA, Cleveland JL. (1996) Cytokines suppress apoptosis independent of increases in reactive oxygen levels. J Immunol 156:2792–2800.
150. Hockenberry DM, Oltavai ZN, Yin X-M, Milliman CL, Korsmeyer SJ. (1993) Bcl-2 functions in an antioxidant pathway to prevent apoptosis. Cell 75:241–251.
151. Hampton MB, Orrhenius S. (1998) Redox regulation of apoptotic cell death. Biofactors 8:1–5.
152. Shamberger RJ, Tytko SA, Willis CE. (1975) Selenium and heart disease. In: Hemphill DD, ed. Trace Substances in Environmental Health—IX. Columbia, MO: University of Missouri Press, pp. 15-22.
153. Shamberger RJ, Gunsch MS, Willis CE, McCormack LJ. (1978) Selenium and heart disease II. Selenium and other trace metal intakes and heart disease in 25 countries. In: Hemphill DD, ed. Trace Substances in Environmental Health—XII. Columbia, MO: University of Missouri Press, pp. 48–52.
154. Shamberger RJ, Willis CE, McCormack LJ. (1979) Selenium and heart disease III. Blood selenium and heart mortality in 19 states. In: Hemphill DD, ed. Trace Substances in Environmental Health—XIII. Columbia, MO: University of Missouri Press, pp. 59–63.
155. Shamberger RJ. (1981) Animal and epidemiological studies relating selenium to heart disease. In: Spallholz JE, Martin JL, Ganther HW, eds. Selenium in Biology and Medicine. Westport, CT: AVI Publishing, pp. 391–394.
156. Steinberg D. (1997) Low density lipoprotein oxidation and its pathobiological significance. J Biol Chem 272:20963–20966.
157. Sevanian A, Hodis H. (1997) Antioxidants and atherosclerosis: an overview. Biofactors 6:385–390.
158. Smith WL, Lands WE. (1972) Oxygenation of polyunsaturated fatty acids during prostaglandin biosynthesis by sheep vesicular gland. Biochemistry 11:3276–3285.
159. Haurand M, Flohé L. (1988) Kinetic studies on arachidonate 5-lipoxygenase from rat basophilic leukemia cells. Biol Chem Hoppe Seyler 369:133–142.

160. Schnurr K, Belkner J, Ursini F, Schewe T, Kühn H. (1996) The selenoenzyme phospholipid hydroperoxide glutathione peroxidase controls the activity of the 15-lipoxygenase with complex substrates and preserves the specificity of the oxygenation products. J Biol Chem 271:4653–4658.
161. Weitzel F, Wendel A. (1993) Selenoenzymes regulate the activity of leukocyte 5-lipoxygenase via the peroxide tone. J Biol Chem 268:6288–6292.
162. Baeuerle PA, Henkel T. (1994) Function and activation of NF-κB in the immune system. Annu Rev Immunol 12:141–179.
163. Flohé L, Brigelius–Flohé R, Saliou C, Traber MG, Packer L. (1997) Redox regulation of NF-κB activation. Free Radic Biol Med 22:1115–1126.
164. Brigelius-Flohé R, Friedrichs B, Maurer S, Schultz M, Streicher R. (1997) Interleukin-1-induced nuclear factor kappa B activation is inhibited by overexpression of phospholipid hydroperoxide glutathione peroxidase in a human endothelial cell line. Biochem J 328:199–203.
165. Cowan DB, Weisel RD, Williams WG, Mickle DAG. (1993) Identification of oxygen responsive elements in the 5′-flanking region of the human glutathione peroxidase gene. J Biol Chem 268:26904–26910.
166. Pinto RE, Bartley W. (1969) The nature of the sex-linked differences in glutathione peroxidase activity and aerobic oxidation of glutathione in male and female rat liver. Biochem J 115:449–456.
167. Sandstrom PA, Murray J, Folks TM, Diamond AM. (1998) Antioxidant defenses influence HIV-1 replication and associated cytopathic effects. Free Radic Biol Med 24:1485–1491.
168. Takahashi K, Akasaka M, Yamamoto Y, Kobayashi C, Mizoguchi J, Koyama J. (1990) Primary structure of human plasma glutathione peroxidase deduced from cDNA sequences. J Biochem 108:145–148.
169. Yamamoto Y, Takahashi K. (1993) Glutathione peroxidase isolated from plasma reduces phospholipid hydroperoxides. Arch Biochem Biophys 305:541–545.
170. Flohé L, Aumann K–D, Brigelius–Flohé R, Schomburg D, Strassburger W, Ursini F. (1993) A structural comparison of the glutathione peroxidases. In: Yagi K, ed. Active Oxygen, Lipid Peroxides, and Antioxidants. Boca Raton, FL: CRC Press, pp. 299–311.
171. Björnstedt M, Xue J, Huang W, Akesson B, Holmgren A. (1994) The thioredoxin and glutaredoxin systems are efficient electron donors to human plasma glutathione peroxidase. J Biol Chem 269:29382–29384.
172. Kulmacz RJ, Lands WEM. (1983) Characteristics of prostaglandin H synthase. In: Samuelsson B, Paoletti R, Ramwell P, eds. Advances in Prostaglandin, Thromboxane, and Leukotriene Research. Vol. 11. New York: Raven Press, pp. 93–95.
173. Gärtner R, Angstwurm M. (1999) Die Bedeutung von Selen in der Intensivmedizin. Klinische Studien bei Patienten mit der SIRS/Sepsis. Med Klin 94:54–57.
174. Wollschläger S, Pätzold K, Bulang T, Meissner D, Porst H. (1999) Einfluss einer prophylaktischen Selensubstitution auf die Entwicklung der ERCP-bedingten akuten Pankreatitis. Med Klin 94:81–83.
175. von Gagern G, Zimmermann T, Albrecht S, Bachmann L, Zwipp H, Saeger HD. (1999) Bedeutung von Selen in der Regulierung der inflammatorischen Antwort durch Transkriptionsfaktoren bei Polytraumapatienten. Eine klinische Studie. Med Klin 94:62–65.
176. Ursini F, Zamburlini A, Cazzolato G, Maiorino M, Bittolo–Bon G, Sevanian A. (1998) Postprandial lipid hydroperoxides: a possible link between diet and atherosclerosis. Free Radic Biol Med 25:250–252.
177. Chu F–F, Esworthy RS. (1995) The expression of an intestinal form of glutathione peroxidase (GSHPx-GI) in rat intestinal epithelium. Arch Biochem Biophys 323:288–294.
178. Esworthy RS, Swiderek KM, Ho YS, Chu FF. (1998) Selenium-dependent glutathione peroxidase-GI is a major glutathione peroxidase activity in the mucosal epithelium of rodent intestine. Biochim Biophys Acta 1381:213–226.
179. Chu F, Esworthy RS, Lee L, Wilczynski S. (1999) Retinoic acid induces *Gpx2* gene expression in MCF-7 human breast cancer cells. J Nutr 129:1846–1854.
180. Brigelius-Flohé R, Wingler K. unpublished data.
181. Wingler K, Brigelius-Flohé R. (1999) Expression of GI-GPx in selenium deficiency [abstr]. Free Radic Biol Med 27:S23.
182. Wingler K, Brigelius-Flohé R. (1999) Gastrointestinal glutathione peroxidase. Biofactors 10:245–249.

183. Ursini F, Maiorino M, Gregolin C. (1985) The selenoenzyme phospholipid hydroperoxide glutathione peroxidase. Biochim Biophys Acta 839:62–70.
184. Ursini F, Bindoli A. (1987) The role of selenium peroxidase in the protection against oxidative damage of membranes. Chem Phys Lipids 44:255–276.
185. Pushpa Rekha TR, Burdsall AI, Oleksa LM, Chisolm GM, Driscoll DM. (1995) Rat phospholipid hydroperoxide glutathione peroxidase. cDNA cloning and identification of multiple transcription and translation start sites. J Biol Chem 270:26993–26999.
186. Arai M, Imai H, Sumi D, Imanaka T, Takano T, Chiba N, Nakagawa Y. (1996) Import into mitochondria of phospholipid hydroperoxide glutathione peroxidase requires a leader sequence. Biochem Biophys Res Commun 227:433–439.
187. Roveri A, Casasco A, Maiorino M, Dalan P, Calligaro A, Ursini F. (1992) Phospholipid hydroperoxide glutathione peroxidase of rat testis. Gonadotropin dependence and immunochemical identification. J Biol Chem 267:6142–6146.
188. Roveri A, Maiorino M, Ursini F. (1994) Enzymatic and immunological measurements of soluble and membrane-bound phospholipid-hydroperoxide glutathione peroxidase. Methods Enzymol 223:202–212.
189. Lei XG, Evenson JK, Thompson KM, Sunde RA. (1995) Glutathione peroxidase and phospholipid hydroperoxide glutathione peroxidase are differentially regulated in rats by dietary selenium. J Nutr 125:1438–1446.
190. Cockell KA, Brash AR, Burk RF. (1996) Influence of selenium status on activity of phospholipid hydroperoxide glutathione peroxidase in rat liver and testis in comparison with other selenoproteins. J Nutr Biochem 7:333–338.
191. Maiorino M, Wissing JB, Brigelius–Flohé R, Calabrese F, Roveri A, Steinert P, Ursini F, Flohé L. (1998) Testosterone mediates expression of the selenoprotein PHGPx by induction of spermatogenesis and not by direct transcriptional gene activation. FASEB J 12:1359–1370.
192. Imai H, Narashima K, Arai M, Sakamoto H, Chiba N, Nakagawa Y. (1998) Suppression of leukotriene formation in RBL-2H3 cells that overexpressed phospholipid hydroperoxide glutathione peroxidase. J Biol Chem 273:1990–1997.
193. Brigelius–Flohé R, Maurer S, Lötzer K, Böl G–F, Kallionpää H, Lehtolainen P, Viita H, Ylä–Herttuala S. (2000) Overexpression of PHGPx inhibits hydroperoxide-induced oxidation, NFκB activation and apoptosis and affects oxLDL-mediated proliferation of rabbit aortic smooth muscle cells. Atherosclerosis 152:307–316.
194. Nomura K, Imai H, Koumura T, Arai M, Nakagawa Y. (1999) Mitochondrial phospholipid hydroperoxide glutathione peroxidase suppresses apoptosis mediated by a mitochondrial death pathway. J Biol Chem 274:29294–29302.
195. Ursini F, Heim S, Kiess M, Maiorino M, Roveri A, Wissing J, Flohé L. (1999) Dual function of the selenoprotein PHGPx during sperm maturation. Science 285:1393–1396.
196. Thomas JP, Maiorino M, Ursini F, Girotti AW. (1990) Protective action of phospholipid hydroperoxide glutathione peroxidase against membrane-damaging lipid peroxidation: in situ reduction of phospholipid and cholesterol hydroperoxides. J Biol Chem 265:454–461.
197. Maiorino M, Coassin M, Roveri A, Ursini F. (1989) Microsomal lipid peroxidation: effect of vitamin E and its functional interaction with phospholipid hydroperoxide glutathione peroxidase. Lipids 24:721–726.
198. Hoekstra WG. (1975) Biochemical function of selenium and its relation to vitamin E. Fed Proc 34:2083–2089.
199. Diplock AT. (1978) The biological function of vitamin E and the nature of the interaction of the vitamin with selenium. World Rev Nutr Diet 31:178–183.
200. Imai H, Sumi D, Sakamoto H, Hanamoto A, Arai M, Chiba N, Nakagawa Y. (1996) Overexpression of phospholipid hydroperoxide glutathione peroxidase suppressed cell death due to oxidative damage in rat basophile leukemia cells (RBL-2H3). Biochem Biophys Res Commun 222:432–438.
201. Yagi K, Komura S, Kojima H, Sun Q, Nagata N, Ohishi N, Nishikimi M. (1996) Expression of human phospholipid hydroperoxide glutathione peroxidase gene for protection of host cells from lipid hydroperoxide-mediated injury. Biochem Biophys Res Commun 219:486–491.
202. Brigelius–Flohé R, Friedrichs B, Maurer S, Streicher R. (1997) Determinants of PHGPx expression in a cultured endothelial cell line. Biomed Environ Sci 10:163–186.

203. Cheng W-H, Fu YX, Porres JM, Ross DA, Lei XG. (1999) Selenium-dependent cellular glutathione peroxidase protects mice against a pro-oxidant-induced oxidation of NADPH, NADH, lipids, and protein. FASEB J 13:1467–1475.
204. Cheng W-H, Combs GF, Lei XG. (1998) Knockout of cellular glutathione peroxidase affects selenium-dependent parameters similarly in mice fed adequate and excessive dietary selenium. Biofactors 7:311–321.
205. Maiorino M, Flohé L, Roveri A, Steinert P, Wissing JB, Ursini F. (1999) Selenium and reproduction. Biofactors 10:251–256.
206. Shalgi R, Seligman J, Kosower NS. (1989) Dynamics of the thiol status of rat spermatozoa during maturation: analysis with the fluorescent labeling agent monobromobimane. Biol Reprod 40:1037–1045.
207. Brown DG, Burk RF. (1973) Selenium retention in tissues and sperm of rats fed a *Torula* yeast diet. J Nutr 103:102–108.
208. Wu AS, Oldfield JE, Shull LR, Cheeke PR. (1979) Specific effect of selenium deficiency on rat sperm. Biol Reprod 20:793–798.
209. Flohé L, Hecht HJ, Steinert P. (1999) Glutathione and trypanothione in parasitic hydroperoxide metabolism. Free Radic Biol Med 27:966–984.
210. Arscott LD, Gromer S, Schirmer RH, Becker K, Williams CH, Jr. (1997) The mechanism of thioredoxin reductase from human placenta is similar to the mechanisms of lipoamide dehydrogenase and glutathione reductase and is distinct from the mechanism of thioredoxin reductase from *Escherichia coli*. Proc Natl Acad Sci USA 94:3621–3626.
211. Muller S, Gilberger TW, Farber PM, Becker K, Schirmer RH, Walter RD. (1996) Recombinant putative glutathione reductase of *Plasmodium falciparum* exhibits thioredoxin reductase activity. Mol Biochem Parasitol 80:215–219.
212. Gilberger TW, Walter RD, Muller S. (1997) Identification and characterization of the functional amino acids at the active site of the large thioredoxin reductase from *Plasmodium falciparum*. J Biol Chem 272:29584–29589.
213. Holmgren A, personal communication.
214. Gromer S, Wissing J, Behne D, Ashman K, Schirmer H, Flohé L, Becker K. (1998) A hypothesis on the catalytic mechanism of the selenoenzyme thioredoxin reductase. Biochem J 332:591–592.
215. Zhong L, Arner ES, Ljung J, Aslund F, Holmgren A. (1998) Rat and calf thioredoxin reductase are homologous to glutathione reductase with a carboxyl-terminal elongation containing a conserved catalytically active penultimate selenocysteine residue. J Biol Chem 273:8581–8591.
216. Fujiwara N, Fujii T, Fujii J, Taniguchi N. (1999) Functional expression of rat thioredoxin reductase: selenocysteine insertion sequence element is essential for the active enzyme. Biochem J 340:439–444.
217. Follmann H, Häberlein I. (1995–1996) Thioredoxins: universal, yet specific thiol–disulfide redox cofactors. Biofactors 5:147–156.
218. Aslund F, Beckwith J. (1999) The thioredoxin superfamily: redundancy, specificity, and gray-area genomics. J Bacteriol 181:1375–1379.
219. Gitler C, Mogyoros M, Kalef E. (1994) Labeling of protein vicinal dithiols: role of protein-S_2 to protein-$(SH)_2$ conversion in metabolic regulation and oxidative stress. Methods Enzymol 233:403–415.
220. Matsui M, Oshima M, Oshima H, Takaku K, Maruyama T, Yodoi J, Taketo MM. (1996) Early embryonic lethality caused by targeted disruption of the mouse thioredoxin gene. Dev Biol 178:179–185.
221. Watanabe T, Endo A. (1991) Effects of selenium deficiency on sperm morphology and spermatocyte chromosomes in mice. Mutat Res 262:93–99.
222. Behne D, Weiler H, Kyriakopoulos A. (1996) Effects of selenium deficiency on testicular morphology and function in rats. J Reprod Fertil 106:291–297.
223. Kang SW, Chae HZ, Seo MS, Kim K, Baines IC, Rhee SG. (1998) Mammalian peroxiredoxin isoforms can reduce hydrogen peroxide generated in response to growth factors and tumor necrosis factor-alpha. J Biol Chem 273:6297–6302.
224. Jin D-Y, Chae HZ, Rhee SG, Jeang KT. (1997) Regulatory role for a novel human thioredoxin peroxidase in NF-kappa B activation. J Biol Chem 272:30952–30961.
225. Zhang P, Liu B, Kang SW, Seo MS, Rhee SG, Obeid LM. (1997) Thioredoxin peroxidase is a novel inhibitor of apoptosis with a mechanism distinct from that of Bcl-2. J Biol Chem 272:30615–30618.

226. Kretz-Remy C, Mehlen P, Mirault ME, Arrigo AP. (1996) Inhibition of I kappa B-alpha phosphorylation and degradation and subsequent NF-kappa B activation by glutathione peroxidase overexpression. J Cell Biol 133:1083–1093.
227. Sappey C, Legrand-Poels S, Best–Belpomme M, Favier A, Rentier B, Piette J. (1994) Stimulation of glutathione peroxidase activity decreases HIV type activation after oxidative stress. AIDS Res Hum Retroviruses 10:1451–1461.
228. Hayashi T, Ueno Y, Okamoto T. (1993) Oxidoreductive regulation of nuclear factor kappa B. Involvement of a cellular reducing catalyst thioredoxin. J Biol Chem 268:11380–11388.
229. Hori K, Hatfield D, Maldarelli F, Lee BJ, Clouse KA. (1997) Selenium supplementation suppresses tumor necrosis factor alpha-induced human immunodeficiency virus type 1 replication in vitro. AIDS Res Hum Retroviruses 13:1325–1332.
230. Makropoulos V, Bruening T, Schulze–Osthoff K. (1996) Selenium-mediated inhibition of transcription factor NF-kappa-B and HIV-1LTR promoter activity. Arch Toxicol 70:277–283.
231. Kim IY, Stadtman TC. (1997) Inhibition of NF-kappaB DNA binding and nitric oxide induction in human T cells and lung adenocarcinoma cells by selenite treatment. Proc Natl Acad Sci USA 94:12904–12907.
232. Tolando R, Jovanovic A, Brigelius–Flohé R, Ursini F, Maiorino M. (2000) Reactive oxygen species and pro-inflammatory cytokine signalling in endothelial cells: effect of selenium supplementation. Free Radic Biol Med 28:979–986.
233. Nogoceke E, Gommel DU, Kiess M, Kalisz HM, Flohé L. (1997) A unique cascade of oxidoreductases catalyzes trypanothione-mediated peroxide metabolism in *Crithidia fasciculata*. Biol Chem 378:827–836.
234. Montemartini M, Kalisz HM, Hecht HJ, Steinert P, Flohé L. (1999). Activation of active site cysteine residues in the peroxiredoxin-type tryparedoxin peroxidase of *Crithidia fasciculata*. Eur J Biochem 264:516–524.
235. Guerrero SA, Lopez JA, Steinert P, Montemartini M, Kalisz HM, Colli W, Singh M, Alves MJM, Flohé L. (2000) His-tagged tryparedoxin peroxidase of *Trypansosma cruzi* as tool for drug screening. Appl Microbiol Biotechnol 53:410–414.
236. Flohé L, Aumann K–D, Steinert P. (1998) Role of selenium in the enzymatic reduction of hydroperoxides. Phosphorous Sulfur Silicon 136–138:25–42.
237. Flohé L. (1998) The Achilles' heel of trypanosomatids: trypanothione-mediated hydroperoxide metabolism. Biofactors 8:87–91.
238. Jäschke A, Mik H, Tropschug M. (1998) Human T cell cyclophilin 18 binds to thiol-specific antioxidant protein AOP-1 and stimulates its activity. J Mol Biol 277:763–769.
239. Frank S, Munz B, Werner S. (1997) The human homologue of a bovine nonselenium glutathione peroxidase is a novel keratinocyte growth factor-regulated gene. Oncogene 14:915–921.
240. Munz B, Frank S, Hübner G, Olsen E, Werner S. (1997) A novel type of glutathione peroxidase: expression and regulation during wound repair. Biochem J 326:579–585.
241. Haridas V, Ni J, Meager A, Su J, Yu G, Zhai Y, Kyaw H, Akama KT, Hu J, van Eldik LJ, Aggarwal BB. (1998) TRANK, a novel cytokine that activates NF-kappa B and c-Jun terminal kinase. J Immunol 161:1–6.
242. Chae HZ, Kang SW, Rhee SG. (1999) Isoforms of mammalian peroxiredoxin that reduce peroxides in presence of thioredoxin. Methods Enzymol 300:219–226.
243. Baker A, Payne CM, Briehl MM, Powis G. (1997) Thioredoxin, a gene found overexpressed in human cancer, inhibits apoptosis in vitro and in vivo. Cancer Res 57:5162–5167.
244. Berggren M, Gallegos A, Gasdaska JR, Gasdaska PY, Warneke J, Powis G. (1996) Thioredoxin and thioredoxin reductase gene expression in human tumors and cell lines, and the effects of serum stimulation and hypoxia. Anticancer Res 16:3459–3466.
245. Gladyshev VN, Factor VM, Housseau F, Hatfield DL. (1998) Contrasting patterns of regulation of the antioxidant selenoproteins, thioredoxin reductase, and glutathione peroxidase, in cancer cells. Biochem Biophys Res Commun 251:488–493.
246. Engman L, Cotgreave I, Angulo M, Taylor CW, Paine–Murrieta GD, Powis G. (1997) Diaryl chalcogenides as selective inhibitors of thioredoxin reductase and potential antitumor agents. Anticancer Res 17:4599–4605.
247. Powis G, Kirkpatrick DL, Angulo M, Baker A. (1998) Thioredoxin redox control of cell growth and death and the effects of inhibitors. Chem Biol Interact 111–112:23–34.

248. Björnstedt M, Kumar S, Bjorkhem L, Spyrou G, Holmgren A. (1997) Selenium and the thioredoxin and glutaredoxin systems. Biomed Environ Sci 10:271–279.
249. Jacob C, Maret W, Vallee BL. (1999) Selenium redox biochemistry of zinc–sulfur coordination sites in proteins and enzymes. Proc Natl Acad Sci USA 96:1910–1914.
250. Yeh JY, Vendeland SC, Gu Q, Butler JA, Ou BR, Whanger PD. (1997) Dietary selenium increases selenoprotein W levels in rat tissues. J Nutr 127:2165–2172.
251. Whanger PD, Vendeland SC, Gu QP, Beilstein MA, Ream LW. (1997) Selenoprotein W cDNAs from five species of animals. Biomed Environ Sci 10:190–197.
252. Beilstein MA, Vendeland SC, Barofsky E, Jensen ON, Whanger PD. (1996) Selenoprotein W of rat muscle binds glutathione and an unknown small molecular weight moiety. J Inorg Biochem 61:117–124.
253. Schubert JR, Muth OH, Oldfield JE, Remmert LF. (1961) Experimental results with selenium in white muscle disease of lambs and calves. Fed Proc 20:689–694.
254. Brown MR, Cohen HJ, Lyons JM, Curtis TW, Thunberg B, Cochran WJ, Klish WJ. (1986) Proximal muscle weakness and selenium deficiency associated with long term parenteral nutrition. Am J Clin Nutr 43:549–554.
255. Hill KE, Lloyd RS, Burk RF. (1993) Conserved nucleotide sequences in the open reading frame and 3′-untranslated region of selenoprotein P mRNA. Proc Natl Acad Sci USA 90:537–541.
256. Steinert P, Bachner D, Flohé L. (1998) Analysis of the mouse selenoprotein P gene. Biol Chem 379:683–691.
257. Hill KE, Burk RF. (1997) Selenoprotein P: recent studies in rats and humans. Biomed Environ Sci 10:198–208.
258. Steinert P, Ahrens M, Gross G, Flohé L. (1997) cDNA and deduced polypeptide sequence of a mouse selenoprotein P. Biofactors 6:311–319.
259. Saito Y, Hayashi T, Tanaka A, Watanabe Y, Suzuki M, Saito E, Takahashi K. (1999) Selenoprotein P in human plasma as an extracellular phospholipid hydroperoxide glutathione peroxidase. Isolation and enzymatic characterization of human selenoprotein P. J Biol Chem 274:2866–2871.
260. Burk RF. personal communication.
261. Sies H, Klotz LO, Sharov VS, Assmann A, Briviba K. (1998) Protection against peroxynitrite by selenoproteins. Z Naturforsch 53:228–232.
262. Arteel GE, Mostert V, Oubrahim H, Briviba K, Abel J, Sies H. (1998) Protection by selenoprotein P in human plasma against peroxynitrite-mediated oxidation and nitration. Biol Chem 379:1201–1205.
263. Burk RF. (1989) Recent developments in trace element metabolism and function: newer roles of selenium in nutrition. J Nutr 119:1051–1054.
264. Wilson DS, Tappel AL. (1993) Binding of plasma selenoprotein P to cell membranes. J Inorg Biochem 51:707–714.
265. Burk RF, Hill KE, Awad JA, Morrow JD, Kato T, Cockell KA, Lyons PR. (1995) Pathogenesis of diquat-induced liver necrosis in selenium-deficient rats: assessment of the roles of lipid peroxidation and selenoprotein P. Hepatology 21:561–569.
266. Sies H. (1985) Oxidative Stress. New York: Academic Press.
267. Baum MK, Shor-Posner G. (1998) Micronutrient status in relationship to mortality in HIV-1 disease. Nutr Rev 56:S135–S139.
268. Dworkin BM. (1994) Selenium deficiency in HIV infection and the acquired immunodeficiency syndrome (AIDS). Chem Biol Interact 91:181–186.
269. McKenzie RC, Rafferty TS, Beckett GJ. (1998) Selenium: an essential element for immune function. Immunol Today 19:342–345.
270. Emard JF, Thouez JP, Gauvreau D. (1995) Neurodegenerative diseases and risk factors: a literature review. Soc Sci Med 40:847–858.

31

Selenium Status and Prevention of Chronic Diseases

Paul Knekt
National Public Health Institute, Helsinki, Finland

I. INTRODUCTION

Selenium (Se) is an essential trace element found in grains, meat, seafood, and certain vegetables. It is a cofactor of the antioxidant enzyme glutathione peroxidase, which plays a key role in cellular defense against oxidative damage (1). Because oxygen free radicals and lipid peroxidation might be involved in several pathological conditions, such as atherosclerosis, cancer, and chronic inflammation, selenium may provide protection against several chronic diseases.

The effect of selenium status on risk of chronic diseases in humans has been studied in prospective, observational, epidemiological studies (cohort studies and nested case–control studies); retrospective observational studies (case–control studies); ecological studies; and in randomized trials. In the prospective studies, selenium status has been determined mainly from serum or plasma. Less frequently used is the selenium concentration in toenails or dietary intake of selenium. Dietary intake of selenium cannot be considered a feasible indicator of selenium status owing to wide variation in the selenium content of food from different geographical areas (2). In case–control studies selenium has also been determined from hair and urine.

Blood selenium levels decrease with progression of disease (3), and cancer treatment may also lower plasma selenium levels (4). Retrospective studies, therefore, cannot determine whether a reduction in tissue selenium status is a cause of chronic disease, or whether the selenium levels measured were caused by disease. In ecological studies, which are not based on measurements on an individual basis, it is difficult to adequately adjust for confounding factors. For these reasons this presentation, which describes the predictive value of selenium status on subsequent occurrence of selected chronic diseases, is mainly based on evidence derived from prospective observational studies and randomized trials. The chronic diseases considered are cancer, cardiovascular disease, diabetes, rheumatoid arthritis, cataract, and asthma.

II. CANCER

Antioxidants provide protection against reactive oxygen species (ROS), which have been implicated in the initiation, promotion, and progression stages of carcinogenesis (5). Selenium may thus be an anticarcinogenic agent, owing to its role as an essential component of selenium-dependent glutathione peroxidase. Selenium supplementation has been demonstrated to provide protection against cancer in several anatomical sites in a wide variety of animal models (6,7). Most of the animal studies have provided evidence for an anticancer role at very high selenium levels. However, at high levels any protective effect of selenium is apparently unrelated to its antioxidant role. Selenium is thus apparently also anticarcinogenic, owing to mechanisms that include alleviation of carcinogen-induced oxidative damage, alteration of carcinogen metabolism, inhibition of cellular proliferation, and stimulation of the immune system (8). The results from studies focusing on the effect of selenium deficiency on cancer in animals have suggested effects for some cancers (8). The findings in human studies have been inconsistent (2,9). In the following we update previous findings.

A. All Sites Combined

Prospective studies on the association between baseline selenium status (determined from serum, plasma, or toenails) and subsequent cancer risk have reported both an inverse association and no association (Table 1). The Hypertension Detection and Follow-up Program, carried out in the United States, was based on 10,940 men and women 30–69 years of age (10). During a 5-year follow-up, 111 cancer cases occurred. Based on these cases and 210 cancer-free controls matched for age, race, sex, and smoking history, the relative risk of cancer between the highest and lowest quintiles of serum selenium was 0.5 (95% confidence interval [CI] = 0.3–0.9). Adjustment for geographical area and serum levels of lipids, vitamins A and E, and carotene did not alter the relation. Other studies from the United States did not confirm this finding, however. The Evans County study (11), one study among Japanese men in Hawaii (12), one study from Washington State (13), and the Nurses' Health Study (14) gave relative risks between higher and lower selenium status of 0.8–1.2 (see Table 1). In accordance a significant case–control difference was absent in the Lipid Research Clinics Prevalence and Follow-up Studies, carried out in ten North American populations (15).

Studies from Europe have, in general, presented a significant inverse association between selenium status and subsequent cancer occurrence, with relative risks of 0.2–0.4 among persons with higher versus lower selenium status. In one study from eastern Finland, 8113 men and women, 31–59 years of age, were followed for 6 years (16). During that time 128 new cancer cases were identified. One control per case was selected by matching for age, sex, smoking status, and serum cholesterol concentration. In this study population the relative risk of cancer between serum selenium ≥ 45 μg/L and < 45 μg/L was 0.3 (CI = 0.1–0.7; see Table 1). The Eastern Finland Heart Survey comprised 12,155 men and women, 30–64 years of age (17). During a 4-year follow-up 51 persons died of cancer. The relative risk of cancer between subjects in the higher tertiles in comparison with the lowest tertile among these cases and controls, matched for sex, age, and smoking status, was 0.2 (CI = 0.0–0.8). One Swedish study based on 10,000 men, 46–48 years of age, reported that 35 men with plasma samples available died of cancer during a 3.5- to 8-year follow-up (18). Two age-matched living controls per case were selected. The relative risk of cancer between the highest and lowest quintiles of plasma selenium was 0.3 (p-value for trend < 0.05). One Dutch study based on 10,532 persons 5 years of age or older from Zoetermeer noted 69 deaths from cancer during a maximum follow-up time of 9 years (19). A total of 138 cancer-free controls were selected by matching for sex,

Table 1 Prospective Studies[a] on the Association Between Selenium Status and Cancer Occurrence

Reference, country	Site of cancer	No of cases[b]	Exposure type	Category	RR	(95% CI)[c]	p Value for trend	Control mean (μg/L)	Difference[d] (%)
Willett et al. (1983) USA (10)	All	111 M/F	Serum	Quintile[e]	0.5	(0.3–0.9)	—	136	−5*
Salonen et al. (1984) Finland (16)	All	128 M/F	Serum	Decile[f]	0.3	(0.1–0.7)	< 0.01	54	−7*
Peleg et al. (1985) USA (11)	All	130 M/F	Serum	Quartile	1.0	—	—	115	+1
Salonen et al. (1985) Finland (17)	All	51 M/F	Serum	Tertile[g]	0.2	(0.0–0.8)	—	61	−12*
Fex et al. (1987) Sweden (18)	All	35 M	Plasma	Quintile	0.3	—	< 0.05	88	−5*
Kok et al. (1987) Holland (19)	All	40 M 29 F	Serum	Quintile[g]	0.4 0.7	(0.2–0.8) (0.2–2.0)	— —	126 129	−8* +1
Nomura et al. (1987) USA (12)	All[h]	280 M	Serum	Quintile	0.8	—	0.61	125	−1
Virtamo et al. (1987) Finland (21)	All	109 M	Serum	Tertile	0.9	(0.5–1.5)	—	56	−5
Coates et al. (1988) USA (13)	All	154 M/F	Serum/ plasma	Quintile	1.0	(0.5–1.8)	—	160	0
Ringstad et al. (1988) Norway (22)	All	60 M/F	Serum	Quartile[e]	0.7	(0.3–1.7)	—	129	−4
Knekt et al. (1990) Finland (20)	All	597 M 499 F	Serum	Quintile	0.41 0.86	— —	< 0.001 0.60	63 64	−6*** −1
Garland et al. (1995) USA (14)	All[i]	934 F	Toenails	Quintile	1.24	(0.93–1.65)	0.10	—	0[j]
Menkes et al. (1986) USA (36)	Lung	99 M/F	Serum	Quintile	1.47	—	0.07	110	+3

(continued)

Table 1 (Continued)

Reference, country	Site of cancer	No of cases[b]	Exposure type	Category	RR	(95% CI)[c]	p Value for trend	Control mean (μg/L)	Difference[d] (%)
Nomura et al. (1987) USA (12)	Lung	71 M	Serum	Quintile	0.91	—	0.46	125	0
Coates et al. (1988) USA (13)	Lung	11 M/F	Serum/plasma	Tertile	0.8	—	0.73	—	—
Knekt et al. (1990) Finland (20)	Lung	189 M	Serum	Quintile	0.30	—	0.001	61	−7**
Knekt et al. (1991) Finland (31)	Lung	117 M	Diet	Tertile	1.03[k] 0.83[l]	— —	0.63 0.63	— —	−4 —
van den Brandt et al. (1993) Holland (33)	Lung	317 M/F	Toenails	Quintile	0.50	(0.30–0.81)	0.006	—	—
Kabuto et al. (1994) Japan (34)	Lung	77 M/F	Serum	Quartile	0.6	(0.2–1.4)	—	108[m]	−4
Garland et al. (1995) USA (14)	Lung	47 F	Toenails	Tertile	4.33	(0.54–34.6)	0.17	—	−10*
Comstock et al. (1997) USA (35)	Lung	258 M/F	Serum	Quintile	0.65	—	0.08	—	−2
Knekt et al. (1998) Finland (32)	Lung	95 M/F	Serum	Tertile	0.41	(0.17–0.94)	0.05	58	−8
Coates et al. (1988) USA (13)	Gastrointestinal	28 M/F	Serum/plasma	Tertile	1.0	—	0.89	—	—
Knekt et al. (1990) Finland (20)	Colorectal	32 M 59 F	Serum	Quintile	0.53 0.80	— —	0.64 0.72	64 65	−1 −2
Garland et al. (1995) USA (14)	Colorectal	89 F	Toenails	Tertile	2.04	(0.88–4.75)	0.12	—	+2
Nomura et al. (1987) USA (12)	Colon	82 M	Serum	Quintile	0.56	—	0.33	125	−2

Reference	Site	N/sex	Sample	Grouping	Ratio	(CI)	p	Se level	Diff
Schober et al. (1987) USA (38)	Colon	72 M/F	Serum	Quintile	0.71	(0.29–1.67)	—	115	−4
van den Brandt et al. (1993) Holland (40)	Colon	116 M 100 F	Toenails	Quintile	0.82 0.77	(0.43–1.58) (0.41–1.45)	0.33 0.13	— —	— —
Bostick et al. (1993) USA (39)	Colon	212 F	Supplement	Use	0.60	(0.27–1.32)	—	—	—
Nelson et al. (1995) USA (41)	Colon	25 M/F	Serum	Quartile	1.7	(0.5–5.9)	—	—	—
Nomura et al. (1987) USA (12)	Rectum	32 M	Serum	Quintile	0.63	—	0.66	125	0
van den Brandt et al. (1993) Holland (40)	Rectum	70 M 32 F	Toenails	Quintile	0.91 1.58	(0.41–2.00) (0.59–4.22)	0.73 0.27	— —	— —
Nomura et al. (1987) USA (12)	Stomach	66 M	Serum	Quintile	1.1	—	0.88	125	−2
Knekt et al. (1990) Finland (20)	Stomach	58 M 37 F	Serum	Quintile	0.90 0.27	— —	0.002 0.15	65 65	−11** −6
van den Brandt et al. (1993) Holland (40)	Stomach	32 M 20 F	Toenails	Quintile	0.40 1.68	(0.17–0.96) (0.43–6.54)	0.14 0.25	— —	— —
Kabuto et al. (1994) Japan (34)	Stomach	202 M/F	Serum	Quartile	1.0	(0.5–2.0)	—	116	−1
Burney et al. (1989) USA (42)	Pancreas	22 M/F	Serum	Tertile	0.22	—	< 0.02	112	−9*
Knekt et al. (1990) Finland (20)	Pancreas	22 M 23 F	Serum	Quintile	0.0 3.49	— —	0.01 0.49	63 63	−20** +4
Knekt et al. (1991) Finland (43)	Esophagus	9 M/F	Serum	Standard unit[a]	0.41	—	0.08	72	−16
Knekt et al. (1991) Finland (43)	Liver and gall-bladder	12 M/F	Serum	Standard unit[a]	0.76	—	0.66	62	−3
van Noord et al. (1987) Holland (47)	Breast	27 F	Toenails	Quartile	1.1	(0.5–2.9)	—	—	—

(continued)

Table 1 (Continued)

Reference, country	Site of cancer	No of cases[b]	Exposure type	Category	RR	(95% CI)[c]	p Value for trend	Control mean (μg/L)	Difference[d] (%)
Coates et al. (1988) USA (13)	Breast	20 F	Serum/plasma	Tertile	3.4	—	0.09	—	—
Hunter et al. (1990) USA (48)	Breast	434 F	Toenails	Quintile	1.10	(0.70–1.72)	—	—	0
Knekt et al. (1990) Finland (20)	Breast	90 F	Serum	Quintile	0.64	—	0.45	66	−2
Overvad et al. (1991) England (49)	Breast	46 F	Plasma	Quartile	1.3	(0.5–3.4)	—	103	+6
van den Brandt et al. (1994) Holland (50)	Breast	355 F	Toenails	Quintile	0.84	(0.55–1.27)	0.31	—	−1
Dorgan et al. (1998) USA (51)	Breast	105 F	Serum	Quartile	0.9	(0.4–1.8)	0.99	—	—
Garland et al. (1995) USA (14)	Ovary	58 F	Toenails	Tertile	1.22	(0.44–3.38)	0.52	—	+3
Helzlsouer et al. (1996) USA (52)	Ovary	35 F	Serum	Tertile	0.23	(0.1–0.9)	0.02	111	−5
Knekt et al. (1996) Finland (53)	Ovary	24 F	Serum	Tertile	0.87	(0.25–5.26)	—	61	−2
Coates et al. (1988) USA (13)	Cervix	12 F	Serum/plasma	Tertile	1.1	—	0.79	—	—
Baticha et al. (1993) USA (54)	Cervix	50 F	Serum	Tertile	0.89	(0.40–2.00)	0.78	—	−2
Garland et al. (1995) USA (14)	Uterine	91 F	Toenails	Tertile	1.38	(0.62–3.08)	0.46	—	−1
Coates et al. (1988) USA (13)	Prostate	13 M	Serum/plasma	Tertile	0.3	—	0.18	—	—

Study	Cancer	N	Sample	Quantile	RR	CI	p	Se	Δ
Knekt et al. (1990) Finland (20)	Prostate	51 M	Serum	Quintile	1.15	—	0.71	58	+2
Hartman et al. (1998) Finland (55)	Prostate	190 M[o] 127 M[p]	Intake	Quartile	1.27 0.84	(0.70–2.20) (0.43–1.67)	0.49 0.64	— —	— —
Yoshizawa et al. (1998) USA (56)	Prostate	181 M	Toenails	Quintile	0.35	(0.16–0.78)	0.03	—	−15
Knekt et al. (1990) Finland (20)	Skin, basal cell	64 M 62 F	Serum	Quintile	0.54 1.55	— —	0.43 0.74	62 63	−2 0
Knekt et al. (1991) Finland (43)	Melanoma	10 M/F	Serum	Standard units[n]	0.79	—	0.68	61	−2
Breslow et al. (1995) USA (58)	Melanoma skin Basal cell skin Squamous cell	23 M/F 32 M/F 37 M/F	Serum	Tertile	0.9 0.8 0.6	(0.3–2.5) (0.1–4.5) (0.2–1.5)	— — 0.23	115 117 114	+1 −2 −1
Garland et al. (1995) USA (14)	Melanoma	63 F	Toenails	Tertile	1.66	(0.71–3.85)	0.21	—	+6
Karagas et al. (1997) USA (59)	Skin, squamous cell	131 M/F	Plasma	Quartile	0.86	(0.47–1.58)	0.89	—	−1
Nomura et al. (1987) USA (12)	Bladder	29 M	Serum	Quintile	0.32	—	0.12	125	−3
Helzlsouer et al. (1989) USA (60)	Bladder	35 M/F	Serum	Tertile	0.49	(0.16–1.49)	0.03	117	−5*
Knekt et al. (1991) Finland (43)	Bladder	15 M/F	Serum	Standard units[n]	1.24	—	0.52	70	+6
Glattre et al. (1989) Norway (61)	Thyroid	43 M/F	Serum	Three groups	0.13	(0.02–0.77)	—	116	−5*
Coates et al. (1988) USA (13)	Leukemia/lymphoma	12 M/F	Serum/plasma	Tertile	0.6	—	0.55	—	—
Knekt et al. (1991) Finland (43)	Kidney	20 M/F	Serum	Standard units[n]	0.51	—	0.07	64	−9

(continued)

Table 1 (*Continued*)

Reference, country	Site of cancer	No of cases[b]	Exposure type	Category	RR	(95% CI)[c]	p Value for trend	Control mean (μg/L)	Difference[d] (%)
Knekt et al. (1991) Finland (43)	Oral and pharynx	20 M/F	Serum	Standard units[n]	1.60	—	0.19	61	+7
Zheng et al. (1993) USA (62)	Oral and pharynx	28 M/F	Serum	Tertile	4.30	—	0.04	100	+4
Knekt et al. (1991) Finland (43)	Larynx	11 M/F	Serum	Standard units[n]	0.68	—	0.39	68	−9
Knekt et al. (1991) Finland (43)	Brain	18 M/F	Serum	Standard units[n]	0.38	—	0.05	72	−10

[a] Including studies reporting relative risks.
[b] M, male; F, female.
[c] RR (95% CI), relative risk for highest versus lowest category (95% confidence interval).
[d] Difference between cases and controls: estimated as [(case mean − control mean)/control mean] *100; test for difference from zero: * $p < 0.05$; ** $p < 0.01$; *** $p < 0.001$.
[e] Highest three vs. lowest.
[f] Higher deciles vs. three lowest deciles.
[g] Higher vs. lowest.
[h] Bladder, colon, rectum, lung, and stomach cancers combined.
[i] Excluding nonmelanoma skin cancer.
[j] Excluding breast cancer and nonmelanoma skin cancer.
[k] Nonsmoker.
[l] Smoker.
[m] ng/mL.
[n] Difference for mean divided by standard deviation.
[o] Not supplemented with α-tocopherol.
[p] α-Tocopherol supplementation group.

age, and smoking status. The relative risk of cancer in higher quintiles of serum selenium in comparison with the lowest after adjustment for age, smoking status, serum cholesterol, serum vitamins A and E, blood pressure, body mass index, and education, was 0.4 (CI = 0.2–0.8) for men, but 0.7 (CI = 0.2–2.0) for women. The Finnish Mobile Clinic Health Examination Survey, which was based on 39,268 men and women 15 years of age and older reported a similar result (20). During a median 10-year follow-up time, 1096 new cancer cases occurred and 2 sex-, age-, and municipality-matched controls were selected per case. The relative risk of cancer between the highest and lowest quintiles of serum selenium was 0.41 (p-value for trend < 0.001) for men and 0.86 for women (p-value for trend = 0.60). Of the studies carried out in Europe, one from eastern and southwestern Finland (21) and one from Norway (22) failed to find any significant association (see Table 1).

The Nutritional Prevention of Cancer Trial, based on a total of 1312 patients with a history of basal cell or squamous cell carcinoma of the skin, was a double-blind, randomized, placebo-controlled cancer prevention trial (23). In this study, 200 μg of selenium or placebo was administered daily. Individuals receiving selenium supplements for an average period of 4.5 years had a reduced risk of all cancers combined, the relative risk being 0.63 (CI = 0.47–0.85). In the Nutrition Intervention Trial in Linxian, China, which was also a double-blind, randomized, placebo-controlled trial, one treatment group received a supplement including 15 mg β-carotene, 50 μg selenium, and 30 mg α-tocopherol (24). The relative risk for mortality from all sites of cancer combined related to this supplement in comparison with the placebo group was 0.87 (CI = 0.75–1.00).

In summary, although the protective effect observed in the Linxian trial is not necessarily attributable to the selenium content of the supplement and although some of the prospective studies failed to reveal reduced risk at higher selenium levels, there are strong suggestions that selenium may provide protection against cancer. This possible protection may be concentrated in subgroups of populations (e.g., in males) (19,20) and at specific cancer sites.

B. Lung Cancer

Case–control studies on selenium status and lung cancer risk have given contradictory results that suggest both a significant inverse association (25–27) and no association (28,29). Several follow-up studies, based on a small number of lung cancer cases (varying from 7 to 38), generally found no significant differences in serum selenium levels between lung cancer cases and controls (10,11,15,16,21,22,30). The only exception was the Eastern Finland Heart Survey, which reported 15% lower mean serum selenium values in subsequent respiratory cancer cases than in controls (17). The results from follow-up studies based on larger numbers of lung cancer cases are contradictory (see Table 1). Of three studies based on subpopulations of the Finnish Mobile Clinic Health Examination Survey, one using dietary intake of selenium as exposure found no association (31), and two studies based on serum selenium found a strong inverse association (20,32). The large Netherlands Cohort Study (33) also found a strong association, in which the population comprised 120,852 men and women, 55–69 years of age. After 3.3 years of follow-up, 370 incident cases of lung cancer carcinoma with toenail selenium data available were detected. A subcohort of 2,459 individuals was randomly selected as a control population. The relative risk of lung cancer between the highest and lowest quintiles of toenail selenium after adjustment for age, sex, smoking status, and education was 0.50 (CI = 0.30–0.81). A study based on a cohort of approximately 20,000 atomic bomb survivors from Hiroshima and Nagasaki (34) and a study from Washington County (35) reported a nonsignificant inverse association. Two contradictory studies reported a nonsignificantly elevated risk of lung cancer at higher serum or toenail selenium levels (14,36) and two studies found no association (12,13).

The Nutritional Prevention of Cancer Trial reported a reduced risk of lung cancer among individuals receiving selenium supplements in comparison with individuals receiving placebo; the relative risk was 0.54 (CI = 0.30–0.98) (23).

The discrepant results observed may partly be due to methodological issues. Repeatability of both toenail selenium and serum selenium is apparently poor, leading to conservative estimates of the relative risks (32,37). Furthermore, a reduced risk of lung cancer at higher selenium levels may be present only in subpopulations of smokers, persons with higher levels of serum orosomucoid or serum copper, or among individuals with lower levels of serum α-tocopherol (32). The power to reveal associations has apparently not been strong enough in some studies, because of the small number of lung cancer cases. The finding that 12 of the 15 studies reporting case–control differences found lower levels in subsequent lung cancer cases, but that only three of the differences were significant, is in agreement with the hypothesis. To summarize, it cannot be excluded that selenium provides protection against lung cancer both at very high levels and at dietary levels.

C. Gastrointestinal Cancer

Several case–control studies have reported significantly lower selenium levels among combined cases of gastrointestinal cancer, compared with controls (2). In such studies, however, prediagnostic symptoms may have influenced dietary habits, thus biasing the results. Therefore, conclusions about possible associations between selenium status and risk of gastrointestinal cancer should be based on prospective studies. Small prospective nested case–control studies (number of cancer cases less than 30) reporting the mean selenium difference between gastrointestinal cases and corresponding controls generally found nonsignificantly smaller selenium values in cases than in controls (10,11,14–17,21,22). One nested case–control study, based on a small number of combined gastrointestinal cancers, found no association with serum selenium concentration at baseline (13) (see Table 1).

Prospective studies on selenium status and subsequent occurrence of colorectal cancer have failed to find any significantly reduced risk at higher selenium levels (see Table 1). One study from Finland reported a nonsignificantly reduced risk at higher serum selenium levels among men (20), whereas, in contrast, one study from the United States reported strong but nonsignificantly elevated risks at higher toenail selenium levels (14). The Nutritional Prevention of Cancer Trial reported a significantly reduced risk of colorectal cancer among patients receiving selenium supplements (23); the relative risk was 0.42 (CI = 0.18–0.95). Two studies based on serum selenium (12,38)—one based on selenium supplement use (39) and one based on toenail selenium (40)—found a nonsignificantly reduced risk of colon cancer, whereas one serological study reported a nonsignificantly elevated risk (41). The results on rectal cancer were also contradictory, giving nonsignificant effects in both directions (12,40).

Two studies on selenium status and stomach cancer reported significantly reduced risk in males, but not in females (20,40) (see Table 1). The relative risks between higher and lower selenium status in men were 0.09 (p value for trend = 0.002) and 0.40 (CI = 0.17–0.96), respectively. These findings were in agreement with those from the Linxian trial, which reported a relative risk of 0.79 (CI = 0.64–0.99) between the selenium-supplemented and the placebo group (24). One study based on Japanese men in Hawaii (12), and one based on atomic bomb survivors in Hiroshima and Nagasaki (34) failed to find any association. One study from Washington County and one from the Finnish Mobile Clinic Health Examination Survey on pancreatic cancer found a reduced risk at higher levels in men, but not in women (20,42). A small study on liver and gallbladder cancer revealed no association (43).

An inverse association between serum selenium level and esophageal cancer incidence was reported in one prospective study based on a small number of cancer cases (43) (see Table 1). The Nutritional Prevention of Cancer Trial reported a similar result (23). The relative risks were 0.41 (p-value for trend = 0.08) and 0.33 (CI = 0.03–1.84), respectively. The Nutrition Intervention Trial in Linxian, however, found no association between intake of the selenium supplement and occurrence of esophageal cancer (24), the relative risk being 0.96 (CI = 0.78–1.18).

To summarize, high selenium intake appears to provide protection against colorectal cancer. No notable beneficial effects, however, have been observed at common dietary levels. The few studies on other gastrointestinal cancers suggest a reduced risk of stomach and pancreatic cancer at higher dietary selenium levels.

D. Female Cancers

The association between selenium status and breast cancer has been widely studied in case–control studies of which some have recorded significantly lower blood selenium levels in cases than in controls (2). However, recent studies have failed to reveal any association (29,44–46).

Prospective studies on selenium status and occurrence of breast cancer have revealed no significant associations. Studies that reported only case–control differences in selenium status found only negligible values (10,11,22), and studies that estimated the relative risk between higher and lower intakes gave, with one exception, values of 0.64–1.3 (20,47–51) (see Table 1). A small study from the United States found a nonsignificantly elevated risk related at higher serum and plasma levels, with a relative risk of 3.4 (p value for trend = 0.09) (13). In accordance with this study, the Nutritional Prevention of Cancer Trial reported a nonsignificantly elevated risk of breast cancer related to selenium supplementation, with a relative risk of 2.88 (CI = 0.72–16.5) (23).

The study from Washington County reported a significantly reduced risk of ovarian cancer among women in the highest tertile of serum selenium; the relative risk was 0.23 (CI = 0.1–0.9) (52) (see Table 1). Two other studies failed to confirm these results (14,53). None of the few existing studies on cervical or uterine cancer found any significant association (13,14,54) (see Table 1).

To summarize, no notable evidence for a reduced risk of female cancers at higher selenium levels has been reported thus far.

E. Prostate Cancer

Selenium is involved in the biosynthesis of testosterone and can stimulate the production of pituitary and adrenal hormones. Thus, selenium can also be linked to prostate carcinogenesis (23). However, the results on the association between selenium status and prostate cancer from case–control studies are contradictory (2).

Four prospective studies from the United States based on small numbers (from 6 to 14) of prostate cancer cases (10,11,13,15) did not report a reduced risk of prostate cancer associated with higher plasma or serum selenium status. The larger Mobile Clinic Health Examination Survey and the large Alpha-Tocopherol, Beta-Carotene Cancer Prevention Study, both carried out in Finland, also failed to find any association (20,55) (see Table 1). The relative risk of prostate cancer between the highest and lowest quintiles of serum selenium in the Mobile Clinic Health Examination Cohort was 1.15 (p for trend = 0.71) (20). In the Alpha-Tocopherol, Beta-Carotene Cancer Prevention Study based on 29,133 smoking men the relative risk of prostate cancer for prestudy selenium supplement use was 1.36 (CI = 0.98–1.90). No significant synergistic effect of vitamin E and selenium intake was found in this study. The relative risk between the highest (> 111 μg/day) and lowest (< 72 μg/day) quartiles of intake of selenium (including supplements) was 1.27 (CI = 0.70–2.20) among those not receiving α-tocopherol supplementation during the follow-up, compared with 0.84 (CI = 0.43–1.67) in the group receiving the supplement (55). In contrast, the Health Professionals Follow-Up Study reported an association between higher selenium levels in toenails and a reduced risk of prostate cancer (56). The population of this study consisted of 33,737 male health professionals who provided toenail clippings. During a 5-year follow-up period, 181 new cases of advanced prostate cancer cases were reported. One control subject was selected for every case by matching for age and smoking status. The mean levels of selenium in toenails were 0.82 μg/g in cases and 0.96 μg/g in controls. The relative risk of prostate cancer between the highest and lowest quintiles of selenium was 0.35 (CI = 0.16–0.78; p value for trend = 0.03). Even more provocative evidence for a protective effect of selenium in prostate cancer comes from the Nutritional Prevention of Cancer Trial (57). In this study the relative risk of prostate cancer was 0.37 between those groups receiving selenium supplementation and placebo (p value for difference from unity = 0.002). The strongest benefit was observed in the subpopulation with low plasma selenium at baseline. The relative risk was 0.08 (p value for difference from unity = 0.002) in the lowest plasma selenium tertile (< 106 ng/mL) compared with 0.85 (p value for difference from unity = 0.75) in the highest (> 121 ng/mL).

To summarize, the results suggest a protective effect of selenium at very high levels, whereas at dietary levels, the results are controversial.

F. Skin Cancer

Case–control studies have reported an inverse association between selenium status and skin cancer occurrence (2). However, two prospective studies based on a small number of combined skin and skeletal cancers (16,21) and one study on skin cancer (11) found no significant difference in serum selenium levels between cases and corresponding controls.

None of the three studies on selenium status and melanoma occurrence revealed any significant associations. In one study by Knekt et al. (43) the relative risk was 0.79 (p value for trend = 0.68), whereas in another by Breslow et al. (58) it was 0.9 (CI = 0.3–2.5), and in a third study it was 1.66 (CI = 0.71–3.85) (14) (see Table 1). The Nutritional Prevention of Cancer Trial gave a similar result, with a relative risk of 0.97 (CI = 0.32–2.96) (23). One study reported an inverse associated between serum selenium and basal cell carcinoma risk in men, but not in women (20). The relative risk between the four higher and the lowest quintile of serum selenium was 0.32 (p value for difference from unity < 0.05) and 1.73, respectively. Another study also failed to find any association with a relative risk of 0.8 (CI = 0.1–4.5) (58). Two studies on squamous cell carcinoma of the skin gave no significant associations with relative risks of 0.6 (CI = 0.2–1.5) (58) and 0.86 (CI = 0.47–1.58) (59).

In summary, selenium status is apparently not predictive of occurrence of skin cancer.

G. Other Cancers

A study from the Washington County population based on a small number of bladder cancer cases and corresponding controls reported an inverse association with serum selenium (60) (see Table 1). The relative risk between the highest and lowest tertiles was 0.49 (CI = 0.16–1.49; p value for trend = 0.03). Another small-scale study from the United States reported a nearly significant association with a relative risk of 0.32 (p value for trend = 0.12) (12). A third study based on the Finnish Mobile Clinic study population found no association for bladder cancer, the relative risk being 1.24 (p value for trend = 0.52) (43), or for all cancers of the urinary tract combined (20). Although the majority of the small-scale studies reporting mean levels of selenium in cases of urogenital cancer or cancer of the urinary tract and controls have reported lower levels in cases than in controls, none of the associations were significant (11,14–16,21,22).

The Norwegian JANUS study reported an inverse association between serum selenium and subsequent development of thyroid cancer (61). The relative risk between higher (≥ 130 μg/L) and lower (< 99 μg/L) levels was 0.15 (CI = 0.02–0.77). A study by Garland et al. (14) found no similar associations. One small study reported significantly lower (13% mean levels of serum selenium in cases of hematological cancer (22), and one study reported a nonsignificant relative risk of 0.6 (13). None of the other small studies published found any associations (10,14–16,21,22). One study, based on a small amount of data, found an inverse association between serum selenium level and kidney cancer occurrence, with a relative risk of 0.51 (p value for trend = 0.07) (43). A study from Washington County based on a small number of oral and pharyngeal cancer cases reported an elevated risk at higher serum selenium levels (62). The relative risk between higher and lower serum selenium levels was 4.30 (p value for trend = 0.04). No associations were found in other studies for oral and pharyngeal (14,43) or laryngeal cancer (43). Knekt et al. (43) reported a significant inverse association between serum selenium level and brain cancer occurrence. The relative risk was 0.38 (p value for trend = 0.05). In contrast, Garland et al. (14) found no significant association.

To summarize, no consistent evidence exists for a reduced risk of bladder, liver, thyroid, hematological, pharyngeal, or brain cancer associated with high selenium status.

III. CARDIOVASCULAR DISEASE

Low selenium status is linked to cardiovascular diseases based on roles played by free radicals, increased lipid peroxidation, and oxidative low-density lipoprotein (LDL) modification, changes in prostaglandin metabolism, and reduced protection against cardiotoxic heavy metals (1,63). Low selenium status has also been reported to be associated with increased platelet aggregation, low high-density lipoprotein (HDL) cholesterol levels, and elevated blood pressure (1).

A. Coronary Heart Disease

Several case-control studies have reported lower selenium status in coronary heart disease patients than in matched controls. One study conducted in New Zealand comprised 252 men and women with acute myocardial infarction and 838 controls matched for sex and age (64). The cases had significantly lower serum selenium levels than the controls. The relative risk of myocardial infarction in participants with selenium levels above the median (≥ 85 μg/L) in comparison with persons below the median were 0.6 (CI = 0.5–0.9) and 0.6 (CI = 0.3–1.1) in men and women, respectively. The association between selenium and myocardial infarction was confined to cigarette smokers. Another case-control study, carried out in Rotterdam, Holland, was based on 91 patients having more than 85% stenosis in at least one coronary artery and 72 control patients having less than 50% stenosis in all three vessels (65). Plasma selenium was significantly lower in cases (95.1 μg/L) than in controls (108.8 μg/L) (p-value for difference < 0.01). The ratio between serum selenium and total polyunsaturated fatty acids was significantly lower in cases than controls in the subpopulation with low plasma α-tocopherol, but not in the subpopulation with higher α-tocopherol, suggesting that high levels of polyunsaturated fatty acids, when insufficiently protected by antioxidants against peroxidation, may be indicative of a higher risk of atherosclerosis. The relation between selenium in toenails and first acute myocardial infarction was studied in the EURAMIC case-control study in ten centers from Europe and Israel, in 683 male cases and 729 controls matched for age (66). Median toenail selenium content was 0.553 µg/g for cases and 0.590 µg/g for controls. The odds ratio for myocardial infarction between the highest and lowest quintiles of toenail selenium was 0.59 (CI = 0.34–1.02; p value for trend = 0.05) after adjustment for age, center, smoking, and vitamin E status. Analyses of subgroups in the study population showed a significant association in former smokers, but not in current smokers or never smokers.

Prospective studies (cohort studies and nested case-control studies) have reported inconsistent results. A nested case–control study carried out in two counties in eastern Finland in 1972 and based on a random sample of 8113 men and women, 35–59 years of age, found an inverse association between serum selenium concentration and both cardiovascular death and incidence of myocardial infarction (67) (Table 2). In this study 131 persons died of cardiovascular disease and 95 of coronary heart disease (CHD) during a 7-year follow-up. A total of 252 persons were admitted to the hospital for acute myocardial infarction. The mean concentration of serum selenium was 51.8 µg/L for all disease cases and 55.3 µg/L for controls matched for sex, age, smoking status, serum cholesterol, blood pressure, and history of angina pectoris (p value for difference < 0.01). The relative risk of CHD deaths between persons with serum selenium ≥ 45 µg/L in comparison with lower levels was 0.3 (CI = 0.2–0.7; p value for trend < 0.001). The corresponding value for cardiovascular disease deaths was 0.5 (CI = 0.3–0.8, p value for trend < 0.01) and for myocardial infarction 0.5 (CI = 0.3–0.7; p value for trend < 0.01). A Danish cohort study comprising 3387 employed men 53–74 years of age from Copenhagen, carried out in 1985–1986, also found a similar relation for ischemic heart disease (68). Among the participants free of cardiovascular disease at baseline, 107 new ischemic heart disease events occurred. The relative risk of ischemic heart disease adjusted for known cardiovascular risk factors at levels more than 80 µg/L in comparison with lower levels (approximately the lowest tertile) was 0.6 (CI = 0.4–1.0).

Later studies from Finland failed to confirm the findings by Salonen et al. (67) (see Table 2). During a 5- to 7-year follow-up starting from 1974–1975, 33 men experienced fatal or nonfatal myocardial infarction in a population of 1222 middle-aged men mainly from southwestern Finland (69). For these cases and 64 controls, matched for age and several risk factors of cardiovascular disease, the mean serum selenium concentration did not differ significantly (71.6 µg/L and 72.9 µg/L, respectively). The Eastern Finland Heart Survey carried out in 1977 among 12,155 men and women, 30–64 years of age, also failed to find any association (70). In this study the association between serum selenium and death from coronary artery disease (CAD) was investigated in 92 persons with no previous myocardial infarction, who died of CAD during a 5-year follow-up, and 92 controls individually matched for sex, age, smoking status, serum cholesterol, blood pressure, and history of cardiovascular diseases. The mean selenium levels were 62 µg/L in cases and 68 µg/L in controls. The relative risk of CAD between persons with serum selenium ≥ 45 µg/L in comparison with persons with lower values was 0.8 (CI = 0.1–3.3). The corresponding value in the subpopulation with no chest pain on effort was 0.3 (CI = 0.1–1.7). One study based on 1110 men, 55–74 years of age, in one cohort from eastern and one from southwestern Finland also failed to find any significant associations for coronary heart disease or myocardial infarction (71). During a 5-year follow-up from 1974 a total of 141 cardiovascular deaths occurred, of which 105 were coronary deaths, and 135 incident myocardial cases. The risk of cardiovascular disease was significantly lower among individuals with higher (≥ 45 µg/L) serum selenium levels. The relative risk, adjusted for cardiovascular risk factors, between higher and lower levels was 0.6 (CI = 0.4–0.9; p value < 0.05). The corresponding values for coronary heart disease mortality and myocardial infarction incidence were, however, a nonsignificant 0.8 (CI = 0.5–1.3) and 0.9 (0.6–1.4), respectively.

Table 2 Prospective Studies on the Association Between Selenium Status and Cardiovascular Disease Occurrence

Reference, country		No of[a] cases	Exposure type	Category[b]	RR (95% CI)[c]	p Value for trend	Control mean (μg/L)	Difference (%)[d]
Salonen et al. (1982) Finland (67)	CHD death	95 M/F	Serum	≥ 45 μg/L	0.3 (0.2–0.7)	< 0.01	—	—
	CVD death	131 M/F			0.5 (0.3–0.8)	< 0.01		
	MI	252 M/F			0.5 (0.3–0.7)	< 0.001	55	-6^*
	All	283 M/F					73	-2
Miettinen et al. (1983) Finland (69)	MI incidence	33 M	Serum	—	—	—	—	—
Salonen et al. (1985) Finland (70)	CAD death	92 M/F	Serum	≥ 45 μg/L	0.8 (0.1–3.3)	—	68	-9
Virtamo et al. (1985) Finland (71)	CVD death	141 M	Serum	≥ 45 μg/L	0.6 (0.4–0.9)	—	55.0	—
	CHD death	105			0.8 (0.5–1.3)			
	MI incidence	135			0.9 (0.6–1.4)			
	Stroke death	19			0.3 (0.1–1.0)			
Kok et al. (1987) Holland (72)	CVD death	84 M/F	Serum	≥ 105 μg/L	0.6 (0.3–1.3)	—	126.5	-1
	CHD death	56 M/F			0.9 (0.4–2.0)			
	Stroke death	15 M/F			0.3 (0.1–1.3)			
Ringstad et al. (1987) Norway (73)	MI incidence	59 M	Serum	≥ 114 μg/L	1.0 (0.4–2.5)	—	127	-2
Suadicani et al. (1992) Denmark (68)	IHD incidence	107 M	Serum	≥ 80 μg/L	0.6 (0.4–1.0)	—	94	-2
Salvini et al. (1995) USA (74)	MI incidence	251 M	Plasma	Quintile[e]	1.5 (0.6–3.8)	—	113[f]	$+1$

[a]M, male; F, female.
[b]The category vs. the lower category.
[c]RR (95% CI), relative risk between categories (95% confidence interval).
[d]Difference between cases and controls: estimated as [(case mean − control mean)/control mean] *100; test for difference from zero: * $p < 0.05$; ** $p < 0.01$; *** $p < 0.001$.
[e]Highest vs. lowest quintile.
[f]ng/g

IHD, ischemic heart disease; CHD, coronary heart disease; CVD, cardiovascular disease; MI, myocardial infarction; CAD, coronary artery disease.

One nested case-control study each from the Netherlands, Norway, and the United States failed to find any significant association between serum selenium status and heart disease (see Table 2). In the Dutch study, which was carried out in 1975–1978 in the town of Zoetermeer, a total of 10,532 men and women participated (72). During a 6- to 9-year follow-up, 84 cardiovascular deaths occurred (56 from CHD and 15 from stroke). The mean level of serum selenium was 125.1 μg/L in the cardiovascular disease cases, 129.2 μg/L in the CHD cases, and 126.5 μg/L in the controls matched for sex and age. The relative risk of CHD between higher quintiles and the lowest quintile (< 105.0 μg/L) of serum selenium was 0.9 (CI = 0.4–2.0) after adjustment for cardiovascular risk factors. The Tromso Heart Study, carried out in 1979–1980, comprised 9364 men and women, 20–54 years of age (73). A total of 59 men, initially free of disease at the baseline examination, experienced a fatal or nonfatal myocardial infarction during a 6-year follow-up. One healthy control was selected per case, using individual matching for sex, age, smoking status, and place of residence. No significant differences were observed between serum selenium in myocardial infarction cases or controls. The mean levels were 124 μg/L and 127 μg/L, respectively (p value for difference = 0.34). The relative risk for myocardial infarction among persons above or equal to 114 μg/L compared with other persons was 1.00 (CI = 0.4–2.5). The Physicians' Health Study, a randomized trial of aspirin and β-carotene, included 22,071 male physicians from the United States, 40–84 years of age at baseline (74). During a 5-year follow-up, 251 cases of first myocardial infarction occurred. The mean plasma serum level at baseline examination was 114.4 ng/g in future cases and 113.2 ng/g in controls selected by matching for age, smoking status, and time for randomization (p value for difference = 0.35). The relative risk of myocardial infarction between the highest and lowest quintiles of serum selenium was 1.53 (CI = 0.61–3.84) after adjustment for other cardiovascular risk factors. In the Nutritional Prevention of Cancer Trial, 93 deaths attributable to cardiovascular and cerebrovascular disease occurred during a 6-year follow-up (23). No reduced risk was observed in the group receiving selenium supplementation. The relative risk between this group and that of those receiving placebo was 1.00 (CI = 0.66–1.55).

B. Stroke

Two nested case-control studies, based on a small number of stroke cases, suggested a possible prediction of serum selenium level on subsequent stroke occurrence (see Table 2). In the Zoetermeer study 15 stroke deaths occurred during the follow-up (72). The mean serum selenium level in the stroke cases was 115.0 μg/L and in the controls 126.5 μg/L. The relative risk of stroke between higher quintiles of serum selenium and the lowest quintile (< 105 μg/L) was 0.3 (CI = 0.1–1.3) after adjustment for several cardiovascular risk factors. In the study from southwestern and eastern Finland, 19 stroke death cases occurred in the subpopulation free of stroke at baseline (71). In this population, low serum selenium was significantly associated with stroke mortality. The relative risk adjusted for cardiovascular risk factors was 0.3 (CI = 0.1–1.0) among men with serum selenium level ≥ 45 μg/L in comparison with men with lower levels. A small case-control study based on 36 ischemic stroke patients and 21 controls in Taiwan did not confirm these findings, however (75). The intervention trial in Linxian reported a nonsignificantly reduced risk of stroke among individuals receiving the supplement including selenium, α-tocopherol, and β-carotene. The relative risk of death from cerebrovascular disease to these persons in comparison with those receiving placebo was 0.90 (CI = 0.76–1.07) (24).

To summarize, although few studies on stroke do not disagree with the hypothesis of a protective effect of selenium, no notable overall evidence exists from prospective studies that selenium provides protection against cardiovascular diseases.

IV. OTHER DISEASES

A. Diabetes

Oxygen-derived free radicals have been implicated in the pathogenesis of diabetes as well as in development of complications of the disease (76). Free radicals contribute to autoimmune destruction of beta cells, leading to insulin-dependent diabetes mellitus (IDDM). Accordingly, antioxidants may provide protection against IDDM. The hypothesis that selenium status predicts the occurrence of IDDM was investigated in a nested case-control study carried out by the Finnish Mobile Clinic (77). The cohort comprised 7526 men 20–99 years of age and free of IDDM. During a follow-up from baseline examination in 1973–1976 to the late 1994, 19 IDDM cases occurred. Three controls per case were selected by individual matching for age. No significant differences between mean serum selenium levels in cases (55.4 $\mu g/L$) and controls (55.8 $\mu g/L$) were observed (p value for difference = 0.90). Another nested case-control study on non–insulin-dependent diabetes mellitus (NIDDM) was carried out based on the same study population (78). A total of 106 male and female NIDDM cases occurred during an 18-year follow-up, and two controls per diabetes case were selected. Serum selenium was not associated with NIDDM; the mean level for cases was 64.8 $\mu g/L$ and for controls 64.0 $\mu g/L$ (p value for difference = 0.47). A case-control study on cardiovascular risk factors in NIDDM, carried out among 30- to 69-year-old persons from the general population of Singapore, also found no differences in serum selenium levels between 126 cases and 530 controls (79). The mean difference was 1%.

To summarize, the few studies addressing selenium status and subsequent occurrence of diabetes do not support the hypothesis that selenium provides protection against the disease.

B. Rheumatoid Arthritis

Rheumatoid arthritis (RA) is a chronic inflammatory disease, or unknown cause, resulting in joint deformities through the destruction of articular tissues. Free oxygen radicals have been implicated as mediators of tissue damage in inflammatory disease of the joints (80). Thus it is possible that selenium acting as an antioxidant and free radical scavenger provides protection against RA. In a small nested case-control study in Finland, based on the Mobile Clinic cohort and comprising 27 incident RA patients and 51 matched controls, a nonsignificant inverse association between serum selenium level and incidence of the RA was observed (81). The relative risk of RA between individuals in the highest serum selenium tertile in comparison with those in the lowest was 0.61 (CI = 0.21–1.75; p value for trend = 0.11). A similar but larger study based on another subpopulation from the same Finnish cohort, comprising 122 cases and 357 matched controls, also gave a nonsignificantly reduced risk of RA among persons with higher serum selenium levels. The relative risk of RA between the highest and lowest tertiles of serum selenium was 0.65 (CI = 0.36–1.16; p value for trend = 0.41) (82). The association was significant for rheumatoid factor (RF)-negative, but not for RF-positive RA. The relative risks adjusted for smoking status and serum cholesterol were 0.16 (CI = 0.04–0.69; p value for trend = 0.02) and 0.96 (CI = 0.49–1.90; p value for trend = 0.70), respectively.

To summarize, it cannot be excluded that selenium status predicts occurrence of RF-negative RA; therefore, this question needs further study.

C. Cataract

Age-related cataract is the common cumulative response to various damaging influences attacking the capsule, epithelium, and constituent fibers of the lens of the eye. The oxidation of lens proteins by free radicals is believed to play an important role in the multifactorial process leading to cataract (83). This process may be modified by micronutrients with antioxidant capacity, such as selenium. The hypothesis that selenium deficiency may be a risk factor for cataract is supported by animal experiments (83). On the other hand, excess selenium has been demonstrated to result in elevated risk in other animal studies (83). Case-control studies in humans have also given contradictory results, indicating no association (84), a reduced risk at higher selenium levels (85), and an elevated risk at higher selenium levels (86).

A longitudinal, nested case-control study on the predication of serum selenium in cataract occurrence was conducted in Finland based on 40- to 83-year-old men and women from the Mobile Clinic study population (87). During a 15-year follow-up, 47 patients admitted to ophthalmological wards for senile cataract and two healthy controls per case were selected. No association between serum selenium level and subsequent incidence of senile cataract was revealed. The serum selenium levels in cases and controls were 62.5 μg/L and 63.5 μg/L, respectively (p value for difference = 0.77). The relative risk between higher tertiles and the lowest tertile of serum selenium was 0.77 (CI = 0.3–2.0). The Nutrition Intervention Trial in the general population of Linxian compared cataract occurrence between individuals receiving the supplement including selenium, α-tocopherol, and β-carotene, and persons receiving placebo (88); no beneficial effect of the supplement was noted in this study. The relative risk for nuclear cataract was 1.19 (CI = 0.90–1.59). Analyses of cortical cataract showed no significant treatment effect on cataract prevalence with a relative risk of 0.96 (CI = 0.82–1.13). For posterior subscapsular cataract, the relative risk was 1.56 (CI = 0.81–3.00).

To summarize, the effect of selenium on cataract development in humans has been rarely studied and there is no evidence thus far suggesting any protective effect of the micronutrient.

D. Asthma

Asthma is characterized by inflammation of the airways. Oxidative stress has been suggested to result in inflammation and tissue damage in the respiratory system, and accordingly selenium, as a component of glutathione peroxidase, can protect membranes in airways from damage, thus providing protection against the disease (89).

The concentration of selenium in plasma or serum of asthma patients and corresponding controls has been measured in several case–control studies. In one study, significantly reduced plasma selenium levels were observed in 22 intrinsic asthma patients (50.5 μg/L) in comparison with 33 controls (58.4 μg/L) (90). Another case–control study, based on 56 asthma patients and 59 healthy controls, reported a relative risk of asthma of 0.6 (CI = 0.2–2.0) in subjects with higher serum selenium levels ($\geq$70 ng/mL) in comparison with those with lower levels (< 50 ng/mL) (91). One case-control study based on 40 asthma patients and 20 controls reported no differences between case and control intake of selenium (92).

A nested case-control study based on 26 children 8–13 years of age who were suffering from asthma symptoms and 61 controls of children who had not experienced asthma symptoms at any time in their lives reported a relative risk of 0.3 (CI = 0.1–1.1; p value for trend = 0.05) between individuals with higher serum selenium levels ($\geq$ 70 μg/L) in comparison with those with lower levels (< 50 μg/L) (93). The Mini-Finland Health Survey followed occurrence of asthma in 7217 men and women, 30–65 years of age, for 17 years (94). During this follow-up period, 219 new asthma cases occurred. The relative risk of asthma between the highest and lowest quartiles of serum selenium in these cases and corresponding controls matched for sex and age was 0.64 (CI = 0.31–1.31; p value for trend = 0.02).

To summarize, more studies are needed to conclude whether higher intake of selenium predicts a reduced risk of asthma.

V. CONCLUSIONS

Although the results from prospective human studies on selenium status and cancer occurrence are inconsistent, there are strong suggestions that selenium may provide protection against cancer. Some of the discrepancies in the reported results may be due to methodological issues. The reproducibility of selenium status measured at baseline of prospective studies is apparently low, leading to conservative estimates of the strength of association between selenium status and cancer occurrence. The preventive effect may also be present only under specific conditions and thus be revealed only in subgroups of the populations considered. It is also apparent that selenium may provide protection against only some cancer sites. The results for lung cancer are contradictory. Despite this controversy, it cannot be excluded that selenium provides protection against the disease both at the dietary and pharmacological levels. Selenium intake at pharmacological levels may provide protection against colorectal cancer. However, no notable beneficial effects were observed at dietary levels. The few studies on other gastrointestinal cancers suggest a reduced risk of stomach and pancreatic cancer at higher dietary selenium levels. Selenium does not appear to provide protection against female cancers. Although case–control studies have suggested an inverse association between selenium status and skin cancer occurrence, the prospective studies and an intervention trial did not confirm these findings. The data from prospective studies for other cancer sites are too limited for any conclusions to be made.

No notable evidence exists from prospective studies on that selenium provides protection against cardiovascular diseases. The few prospective studies addressing selenium status and subsequent occurrence of diabetes or cataract also do not support the hypothesis of a protective effect. Although selenium status predicted the occurrence of RF-negative RA in one study and an inverse association between selenium status and asthma risk was reported in some studies, more results are needed before any conclusions can be made.

Chemoprevention trials are necessary for providing valuable information on the hypothesis of a protective effect of selenium intake on occurrence of cancer and other chronic diseases. Because selenium has toxic effects at higher levels, very careful attention must be paid to dosage. Large prospective studies are also warranted to give more information on selenium status at dietary levels and risk of chronic diseases.

REFERENCES

1. Foster LH, Sumar S. (1997) Selenium in health and disease: a review. Crit Rev Food Sci Nutr 37:211–228.
2. Garland M, Stampfer MJ, Willett WC, Hunter DJ. (1994) The epidemiology of selenium and human cancer. In: Frei B, ed. Natural Antioxidants in Human Health and Disease. San Diego: Academic Press, pp. 263–286.
3. Robinson MF, Godfrey PJ, Thomson CD, Rea HM, van Rij AM. (1979) Blood selenium and glutathione peroxidase activity in normal subjects and in surgical patients with and without cancer in New Zealand. Am J Clin Nutr 32:1477–1485.
4. Pothier L, Lane WW, Bhargava A, Michielson C, Douglas HO, Jr. (1987) Plasma selenium levels in patients with advanced upper gastrointestinal cancer. Cancer 60:2251–2260.
5. Trush MA, Kensler TW. (1991) An overview of the relationship between oxidative stress and chemical carcinogenesis. Free Radic Biol Med 10:201–209.
6. Strain JJ. (1994) Putative role of dietary trace elements in coronary heart disease and cancer. Br J Biomed Sci 51:241–251.
7. Ip C. (1998) Lessons from basic research in selenium and cancer prevention. J Nutr 128:1845–1854.
8. Combs GF, Jr, Clark LC. (1985) Can dietary selenium modify cancer risk? Nutr Rev 43:325–331.

9. Comstock GW, Bush TL, Helzlsouer K. (1992) Serum retinol, beta-carotene, vitamin E, and selenium as related to subsequent cancer of specific sites. Am J Epidemiol 135:115–121.
10. Willett WC, Polk BF, Morris JS, Stampfer MJ, Pressel S, Rosner B, Taylor JO, Schneider K, Hames CG. (1983) Prediagnostic serum selenium and risk of cancer. Lancet 2:130–134.
11. Peleg I, Morris S, Hames CG. (1985) Is serum selenium a risk factor for cancer? Med Oncol Tumor Pharmacother 2:157–163.
12. Nomura A, Heilbrun LK, Morris JS, Stemmermann GN. (1987) Serum selenium and the risk of cancer, by specific sites: case–control analysis of prospective data. J Natl Cancer Inst 79:103–108.
13. Coates RJ, Weiss NS, Daling JR, Morris JS, Labbe RF. (1988) Serum levels of selenium and retinol and the subsequent risk of cancer. Am J Epidemiol 128:515–523.
14. Garland M, Morris JS, Stampfer MJ, Colditz GA, Spate VL, Baskett CK, Rosner B, Speizer FE, Willett WC, Hunter DJ. (1995) Prospective study of toenail selenium levels and cancer among women. J Natl Cancer Inst 87:497–505.
15. Criqui MH, Bangdiwala S, Goodman DS, Blaner WS, Morris JS, Kritchevsky S, Lippel K, Mebane I, Tyroler HA. (1991) Selenium, retinol, retinol-binding protein, and uric acid. Associations with cancer mortality in a population-based prospective case–control study. Ann Epidemiol 1:385–393.
16. Salonen JT, Alfthan G, Huttunen JK, Puska P. (1984) Association between serum selenium and the risk of cancer. Am J Epidemiol 120:342–349.
17. Salonen JT, Salonen R, Lappeteläinen R, Mäenpää PH, Alfthan G, Puska P. (1985) Risk of cancer in relation to serum concentrations of selenium and vitamins A and E: matched case–control analysis of prospective data. Br Med J (Clin Res Ed) 290:417–420.
18. Fex G, Pettersson B, Akesson B. (1987) Low plasma selenium as a risk factor for cancer death in middle-aged men. Nutr Cancer 10:221–229.
19. Kok FJ, de Bruijn AM, Hofman A, Vermeeren R, Valkenburg HA. (1987) Is serum selenium a risk factor for cancer in men only? Am J Epidemiol 125:12–16.
20. Knekt P, Aromaa A, Maatela J, Alfthan G, Aaran RK, Hakama M, Hakulinen T, Peto R, Teppo L. (1990) Serum selenium and subsequent risk of cancer among Finnish men and women. J Natl Cancer Inst 82:864–868.
21. Virtamo J, Valkeila E, Alfthan G, Punsar S, Huttunen JK, Karvonen MJ. (1987) Serum selenium and risk of cancer. A prospective follow-up of nine years. Cancer 60:145–148.
22. Ringstad J, Jacobsen BK, Tretli S, Thomassen Y. (1988) Serum selenium concentration associated with risk of cancer. J Clin Pathol 41:454–457.
23. Clark LC, Combs GF, Jr, Turnbull BW, Slate EH, Chalker DK, Chow J, Davis LS, Glover RA, Graham GF, Gross EG, Krongrad A, Lesher JL, Jr, Park HK, Sanders BB, Jr, Smith CL, Taylor JR. (1996) Effects of selenium supplementation for cancer prevention in patients with carcinoma of the skin. A randomized controlled trial. Nutritional Prevention of Cancer Study Group. JAMA 276:1957–1963.
24. Blot WJ, Li JY, Taylor PR, Guo W, Dawsey S, Wang GQ, Yang CS, Zheng SF, Gail M, Li GY. (1993) Nutrition intervention trials in Linxian, China: supplementation with specific vitamin/mineral combinations, cancer incidence, and disease-specific mortality in the general population. J Natl Cancer Inst 85:1483–1492.
25. Miyamoto H, Araya Y, Ito M, Isobe H, Dosaka H, Shimizu T, Kishi F, Yamamoto I, Honma H, Kawakami Y. (1987) Serum selenium and vitamin E concentrations in families of lung cancer patients. Cancer 60:1159–1162.
26. Zachara BA, Marchaluk–Wisniewska E, Maciag A, Peplinski J, Skokowski J, Lambrecht W. (1997) Decreased selenium concentration and glutathione peroxidase activity in blood and increase of these parameters in malignant tissue of lung cancer patients. Lung 175:321–332.
27. Zhou B, Wang T, Sun G, Guan P, Wu JM. (1999) A case–control study of the relationship between dietary factors and risk of lung cancer in women of Shenyang, China. Oncol Rep 6:139–143.
28. Tominaga K, Saito Y, Mori K, Miyazawa N, Yokoi K, Koyama Y, Shimamura K, Imura J, Nagai M. (1992) An evaluation of serum microelement concentrations in lung cancer and matched non-cancer patients to determine the risk of developing lung cancer: a preliminary study. Jpn J Clin Oncol 22:96–101.
29. Piccinini L, Borella P, Bargellini A, Medici CI, Zoboli A. (1996) A case–control study on selenium, zinc, and copper in plasma and hair of subjects affected by breast and lung cancer. Biol Trace Elem Res 51:23–30.

30. Kok FJ, van Duijn CM, Hofman A, Vermeeren R, de Bruijn AM, Valkenburg HA. (1987) Micronutrients and the risk of lung cancer [letter]. N Engl J Med 316:1416.
31. Knekt P, Järvinen R, Seppänen R, Rissanen A, Aromaa A, Heinonen OP, Albanes D, Heinonen M, Pukkala E, Teppo L. (1991) Dietary antioxidants and the risk of lung cancer. Am J Epidemiol 134:471–479.
32. Knekt P, Marniemi J, Teppo L, Heliövaara M, Aromaa A. (1998) Is low selenium status a risk factor for lung cancer? Am J Epidemiol 148:975–982.
33. van den Brandt PA, Goldbohm RA, van't Veer P, Bode P, Dorant E, Hermus RJ, Sturmans F. (1993) A prospective cohort study on selenium status and the risk of lung cancer. Cancer Res 53:4860–4865.
34. Kabuto M, Imai H, Yonezawa C, Neriishi K, Akiba S, Kato H, Suzuki T, Land CE, Blot WJ. (1994) Prediagnostic serum selenium and zinc levels and subsequent risk of lung and stomach cancer in Japan. Cancer Epidemiol Biomarkers Prev 3:465–469.
35. Comstock GW, Alberg AJ, Huang HY, Wu K, Burke AE, Hoffman SC, Norkus EP, Gross M, Cutler RG, Morris JS, Spate VL, Helzlsouer KJ. (1997) The risk of developing lung cancer associated with antioxidant in the blood: ascorbic acid, carotenoids, alpha-tocopherol, selenium, and total peroxyl radical absorbing capacity. Cancer Epidemiol Biomarkers Prev 6:907–916.
36. Menkes MS, Comstock GW, Vuilleumier JP, Helsing KJ, Rider AA, Brookmeyer R. (1986) Serum beta-carotene, vitamins A and E, selenium, and the risk of lung cancer. N Engl J Med 315:1250–1254.
37. Garland M, Morris JS, Rosner BA, Stampfer MJ, Spate VL, Baskett CJ, Willett WC, Hunter DJ. (1993) Toenail trace element levels as biomarkers: reproducibility over a 6-year period. Cancer Epidemiol Biomarkers Prev 2:493–497.
38. Schober SE, Comstock GW, Helsing KJ, Salkeld RM, Morris JS, Rider AA, Brookmeyer R. (1987) Serologic precursors of cancer. I. Prediagnostic serum nutrients and colon cancer risk. Am J Epidemiol 126:1033–1041.
39. Bostick RM, Potter JD, McKenzie DR, Sellers TA, Kushi LH, Steinmetz KA, Folsom AR. (1993) Reduced risk of colon cancer with high intake of vitamin E: the Iowa Women's Health Study. Cancer Res 53:4230–4237.
40. van den Brandt PA, Goldbohm RA, van't Veer P, Bode P, Dorant E, Hermus RJ, Sturmans F. (1993) A prospective cohort study on toenail selenium levels and risk of gastrointestinal cancer. J Natl Cancer Inst 85:224–229.
41. Nelson RL, Davis FG, Sutter E, Kikendall JW, Sobin LH, Milner JA, Bowen PE. (1995) Serum selenium and colonic neoplastic risk. Dis Colon Rectum 38:1306–1310.
42. Burney PG, Comstock GW, Morris JS. (1989) Serologic precursors of cancer: serum micronutrients and the subsequent risk of pancreatic cancer. Am J Clin Nutr 49:895–900.
43. Knekt P, Aromaa A, Maatela J, Alfthan G, Aaran RK, Nikkari T, Hakama M, Hakulinen T, Teppo L. (1991) Serum micronutrients and risk of cancers of low incidence in Finland. Am J Epidemiol 134:356–361.
44. Antila E, Mussalo-Rauhamaa H, Kantola M, Atroshi F, Westermarck T. (1996) Association of cadmium with human breast cancer. Sci Total Environ 186:251–256.
45. van't Veer P, Strain JJ, Fernandez-Crehuet J, Martin BC, Thamm M, Kardinaal AF, Kohlmeier L, Huttunen JK, Martin-Moreno JM, Kok FJ. (1996) Tissue antioxidants and postmenopausal breast cancer: the European Community Multicentre Study on Antioxidants, Myocardial Infarction, and Cancer of the Breast (EURAMIC). Cancer Epidemiol Biomarkers Prev 5:441–447.
46. Strain JJ, Bokje E, van't Veer P, Coulter J, Stewart C, Logan H, Odling-Smee W, Spence RA, Steele K. (1997) Thyroid hormones and selenium status in breast cancer. Nutr Cancer 27:48–52.
47. van Noord PA, Collette HJ, Maas MJ, de Waard F. (1987) Selenium levels in nails of premenopausal breast cancer patients assessed prediagnostically in a cohort-nested case–referent study among women screened in the DOM project. Int J Epidemiol 16:318–322.
48. Hunter DJ, Morris JS, Stampfer MJ, Colditz GA, Speizer FE, Willett WC. (1990) A prospective study of selenium status and breast cancer risk. JAMA 264:1128–1131.
49. Overvad K, Gron P, Langhoff O, Tarp U, Foldspang A, Thorling EB. (1991) Selenium in human mammary carcinogenesis: a case–referent study. Eur J Cancer Prev 1:27–30.
50. van den Brandt PA, Goldbohm RA, van't Veer P, Bode P, Dorant E, Hermus RJ, Sturmans F. (1994) Toenail selenium levels and the risk of breast cancer. Am J Epidemiol 140:20–26.
51. Dorgan JF, Sowell A, Swanson CA, Potischman N, Miller R, Schussler N, Stephenson HE, Jr. (1998) Relationships of serum carotenoids, retinol, alpha-tocopherol, and selenium with breast cancer risk:

results from a prospective study in Columbia, Missouri (United States). Cancer Causes Control 9:89–97.
52. Helzlsouer KJ, Alberg AJ, Norkus EP, Morris JS, Hoffman SC, Comstock GW. (1996) Prospective study of serum micronutrients and ovarian cancer. J Natl Cancer Inst 88:32–37.
53. Knekt P, Aromaa A, Alfthan G, Maatela J, Hakama M, Hakulinen T, Teppo L. (1996) Prospective study of serum micronutrients and ovarian cancer [letter]. J Natl Cancer Inst 88:1408.
54. Batieha AM, Armenian HK, Norkus EP, Morris JS, Spate VE, Comstock GW. (1993) Serum micronutrients and the subsequent risk of cervical cancer in a population-based nested case–control study. Cancer Epidemiol Biomarkers Prev 2:335–339.
55. Hartman TJ, Albanes D, Pietinen P, Hartman AM, Rautalahti M, Tangrea JA, Taylor PR. (1998) The association between baseline vitamin E, selenium, and prostate cancer in the alpha-Tocopherol, beta-Carotene Cancer Prevention Study. Cancer Epidemiol Biomarkers Prev 7:335–340.
56. Yoshizawa K, Willett WC, Morris SJ, Stampfer MJ, Spiegelman D, Rimm EB, Giovannucci E. (1998) Study of prediagnostic selenium level in toenails and the risk of advanced prostate cancer. J Natl Cancer Inst 90:1219–1224.
57. Clark LC, Dalkin B, Krongrad A, Combs GF, Jr, Turnbull BW, Slate EH, Witherington R, Herlong JH, Janosko E, Carpenter D, Borosso C, Falk S, Rounder J. (1998) Decreased incidence of prostate cancer with selenium supplementation: results of a double-blind cancer prevention trial. Br J Urol 81:730–734.
58. Breslow RA, Alberg AJ, Helzlsouer KJ, Bush TL, Norkus EP, Morris JS, Spate VE, Comstock GW. (1995) Serological precursors of cancer: malignant melanoma, basal and squamous cell skin cancer, and prediagnostic levels of retinol, beta-carotene, lycopene, alpha-tocopherol, and selenium. Cancer Epidemiol Biomarkers Prev 4:837–842.
59. Karagas MR, Greenberg ER, Nierenberg D, Stukel TA, Morris JS, Stevens MM, Baron JA. (1997) Risk of squamous cell carcinoma of the skin in relation to plasma selenium, alpha-tocopherol, beta-carotene, and retinol: a nested case–control study. Cancer Epidemiol Biomarkers Prev 6:25–29.
60. Helzlsouer KJ, Comstock GW, Morris JS. (1989) Selenium, lycopene, alpha-tocopherol, beta-carotene, retinol, and subsequent bladder cancer. Cancer Res 49:6144–6148.
61. Glattre E, Thomassen Y, Thoresen SO, Haldorsen T, Lund–Larsen PG, Theodorsen L, Aaseth J. (1989) Prediagnostic serum selenium in a case–control study of thyroid cancer. Int J Epidemiol 18:45–49.
62. Zheng W, Blot WJ, Diamond EL, Norkus EP, Spate V, Morris JS, Comstock GW. (1993) Serum micronutrients and the subsequent risk of oral and pharyngeal cancer. Cancer Res 53:795–798.
63. Korpela H. (1993) Selenium in cardiovascular disease. J Trace Elem Electrolytes Health Dis 7:115.
64. Beaglehole R, Jackson R, Watkinson J, Scragg R, Yee RL. (1990) Decreased blood selenium and risk of myocardial infarction. Int J Epidemiol 19:918–922.
65. Kok FJ, van Poppel G, Melse J, Verheul E, Schouten EG, Kruyssen DH, Hofman A. (1991) Do antioxidants and polyunsaturated fatty acids have a combined association with coronary atherosclerosis? Atherosclerosis 31:85–90.
66. Kardinaal AF, Kok FJ, Kohlmeier L, Martin–Moreno JM, Ringstad J, Gomez–Aracena J, Mazaev VP, Thamm M, Martin BC, Aro A, Kark JD, Delgado–Rodriguez M, Riemersma RA, van't Veer P, Huttunen JK. (1997) Association between toenail selenium and risk of acute myocardial infarction in European men. The EURAMIC Study. European Antioxidant Myocardial Infarction and Breast Cancer. Am J Epidemiol 145:373–379.
67. Salonen JT, Alfthan G, Huttunen JK, Pikkarainen J, Puska P. (1982) Association between cardiovascular death and myocardial infarction and serum selenium in a matched-pair longitudinal study. Lancet 2:175–179.
68. Suadicani P, Hein HO, Gyntelberg F. (1992) Serum selenium concentration and risk of ischaemic heart disease in a prospective cohort study of 3000 males. Atherosclerosis 96:33–42.
69. Miettinen TA, Alfthan G, Huttunen JK, Pikkarainen J, Naukkarinen V, Mattila S, Kumlin T. (1983) Serum selenium concentration related to myocardial infarction and fatty acid content of serum lipids. Br Med J (Clin Res Ed) 287:517–519.
70. Salonen JT, Salonen R, Penttila I, Herranen J, Jauhiainen M, Kantola M, Lappeteläinen R, Mäenpää PH, Alfthan G, Puska P. (1985) Serum fatty acids, apolipoproteins, selenium and vitamin antioxidants and the risk of death from coronary artery disease. Am J Cardiol 56:226–231.
71. Virtamo J, Valkeila E, Alfthan G, Punsar S, Huttunen JK, Karvonen MJ. (1985) Serum selenium and the risk of coronary heart disease and stroke. Am J Epidemiol 122:276–282.

72. Kok FJ, de Bruijn AM, Vermeeren R, Hofman A, van Laar A, de Bruin M, Hermus RJ, Valkenburg HA. (1987) Serum selenium, vitamin antioxidants, and cardiovascular mortality: a 9-year follow-up study in the Netherlands. Am J Clin Nutr 45:462–468.
73. Ringstad J, Jacobsen BK, Thomassen Y, Thelle DS. (1987) The Tromso Heart Study: serum selenium and risk of myocardial infarction a nested case–control study. J Epidemiol Community Health 41:329–332.
74. Salvini S, Hennekens CH, Morris JS, Willett WC, Stampfer MJ. (1995) Plasma levels of the antioxidant selenium and risk of myocardial infarction among U. S. physicians. Am J Cardiol 76:1218–1221.
75. Chang CY, Lai YC, Cheng TJ, Lau MT, Hu ML. (1998) Plasma levels of antioxidant vitamins, selenium, total sulfhydryl groups and oxidative products in ischemic-stroke patients as compared to matched controls in Taiwan. Free Radic Res 28:15–24.
76. Oberley LW. (1988) Free radicals and diabetes. Free Radic Biol Med 5:113–124.
77. Knekt P, Reunanen A, Marniemi J, Leino A, Aromaa A. (1999) Low vitamin E status is a potential risk factor for insulin-dependent diabetes mellitus. J Intern Med 245:99–102.
78. Reunanen A, Knekt P, Aaran RK, Aromaa A. (1998) Serum antioxidants and risk of noninsulin dependent diabetes mellitus. Eur J Clin Nutr 52:89–93.
79. Hughes K, Choo M, Kuperan P, Ong CN, Aw TC. (1998) Cardiovascular risk factors in non–insulin-dependent diabetics compared to non-diabetic controls: a population-based survey among Asians in Singapore. Atherosclerosis 136:25–31.
80. Halliwell B, Hoult JR, Blake DR. (1988) Oxidants, inflammation, and anti-inflammatory drugs. FASEB J 2:2867–2873.
81. Heliövaara M, Knekt P, Aho K, Aaran RK, Alfthan G, Aromaa A. (1994) Serum antioxidants and risk of rheumatoid arthritis. Ann Rheum Dis 53:51–53.
82. Knekt P, Heliövaara M, Aho K, Alfthan G, Marniemi J, Aromaa A. (2000) Serum selenium, serum alpha-tocopherol, and the risk of rheumatoid arthritis. Epidemiology 11:402–405.
83. Bunce GE, Kinoshita J, Horwitz J. (1990) Nutritional factors in cataract. Annu Rev Nutr 10:233–254.
84. Leske MC, Wu SY, Hyman L, Sperduto R, Underwood B, Chylack LT, Milton RC, Srivastava S, Ansari N. (1995) Biochemical factors in the lens opacities. Case–control study. The Lens Opacities Case–Control Study Group. Arch Ophthalmol 113:1113–1119.
85. Karaküçük S, Ertugrul Mirza G, Faruk Ekinciler Ö, Saraymen R, Karaküçük I, Üstdal M. (1995) Selenium concentrations in serum, lens and aqueous humour of patients with senile cataract. Acta Ophthalmol Scand 73:329–332.
86. Jacques PF, Hartz SC, Chylack LT, Jr, McGandy RB, Sadowski JA. (1988) Nutritional status in persons with and without senile cataract: blood vitamin and mineral levels. Am J Clin Nutr 48:152–158.
87. Knekt P, Heliövaara M, Rissanen A, Aromaa A, Aaran RK. (1992) Serum antioxidant vitamins and risk of cataract. Br Med J 305:1392–1394.
88. Sperduto RD, Hu TS, Milton RC, Zhao JL, Everett DF, Cheng QF, Blot WJ, Bing L, Taylor PR, Li JY. (1993) The Linxian cataract studies. Two nutrition intervention trials. Arch Ophthalmol 111:1246–1253.
89. Monteleone CA, Sherman AR. (1997) Nutrition and asthma. Arch Intern Med 157:23–34.
90. Kadrabova J, Mad'aric A, Kovacikova Z, Podivinsky F, Ginter E, Gazdik F. (1996) Selenium status is decreased in patients with intrinsic asthma. Biol Trace Elem Res 52:241–248.
91. Flatt A, Pearce N, Thomson CD, Sears MR, Robinson MF, Beasley R. (1990) Reduced selenium in asthmatic subjects in New Zealand. Thorax 45:95–99.
92. Baker JC, Tunnicliffe WS, Duncanson RC, Ayres JG. (1999) Dietary antioxidants and magnesium in type 1 brittle asthma: a case control study. Thorax 54:115–118.
93. Shaw R, Woodman K, Crane J, Moyes C, Kennedy J, Pearce N. (1994) Risk factors for asthma symptoms in Kawerau children. NZ Med J 107:387–391.
94. Knekt P, Heliövaara M, Reunanen A, Aromaa A, Health and Disability Dept. (1999) The epidemiology of selenium; Finnish experience. In: First STDA symposium on human health related aspects of selenium research in Europe, Brussels, Belgium, pp. 15, STDA, 27.11.1999.

32
Antioxidant Properties of Nitric Oxide

Homero Rubbo and Rafael Radi
Universidad de la República, Montevideo, Uruguay

I. INTRODUCTION

Nitric oxide (·NO) is an endogenously synthesized free radical first characterized as a component of the endothelial-derived relaxation factor (EDRF) (1,2). The physiological actions of ·NO range from mediating vasodilation and neurotransmission, inhibiting platelet adherence and aggregation, and the macrophage and neutrophil killing of pathogens (3,4). The broad distribution of sites of production of ·NO, combined with its facile reactions with metalloproteins and radical species, determines that ·NO plays an important role in regulating critical oxidant reactions. The influence of ·NO in redox and free radical processes extends beyond its recognized ability to mediate signal transduction by stimulation of guanylate cyclase-mediated cGMP synthesis (5,6). Chemical reaction systems, cell and animal models, and clinical studies have recently revealed an ability of ·NO to modulate reactions and pathological processes associated with the excess production and biological effects of reactive oxygen species (ROS). The focus of this chapter will be to analyze the antioxidant properties of ·NO in the context of the current knowledge on the target molecule reactivities of this free radical species. This biochemical foundation provides the rationale to understand many cytoprotective actions of ·NO, which are due to its ability to redirect the reactivity of partially reduced oxygen and nitrogen species and opens the possibility of pharmacological developments directed at inhibiting oxidative processes involving the delivery of ·NO.

II. CHEMICAL PROPERTIES OF NITRIC OXIDE

Nitric oxide is a free radical species as it contains an odd number of electrons—15—of which 7 are located in the outer shell. The molecular orbital electronic configuration of ·NO is $(Be)_2(2p\sigma)^2(2p\pi)^4(2p\pi^*)^1$. This results in the presence of the last electron in a π^*-antibonding molecular orbital and an overall bond order between the nitrogen and oxygen atoms of 2.5 (7).

Nitric oxide has proved to be a ubiquitous signal transduction molecule and mediator of tissue physiology and pathology because of its chemical properties, which include (1) relatively

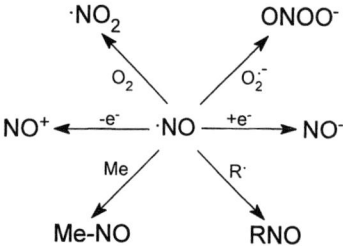

Figure 1 Nitric oxide chemistry: One-electron redox (to NO^+ or NO^-), pro-oxidant (to NO_2 or $ONOO^-$) and antioxidant reactions (to Me-NO or RNO) are shown. Me, transition metal center (e.g., iron or copper); R·, organic radical.

low reactivity for a free radical species, resulting in a biological half-life in the range of seconds; (2) charge neutrality; (3) a small molecular radius; (4) hydrophobicity; (5) selective reactivity with heme and iron–sulfur proteins; and (6) facile reaction with free radicals (e.g., superoxide anion, $O_2^{·-}$ and organic-derived free radicals) (8).

Nitric oxide readily crosses biological membranes and can concentrate in hydrophobic compartments, being able to participate in chemical reactions both in aqueous and lipid phases. However, although being a free radical, ·NO does not readily react with most organic molecules. In fact, ·NO is neither a strong oxidant nor a strong reductant. The one-electron reduction of ·NO to nitroxyl anion (NO^-) occurs with a standard one-electron redox potential of $+0.38$ V, whereas one-electron oxidation to nitrosonium (NO^+) is $+1.21$ V (7,8). However, ·NO rapidly reacts with both organic and oxygen-centered radicals to yield a variety of reactive intermediates and with transition metal centers (e.g., iron and copper) (Fig. 1). Nitric oxide can also be oxidized under aerobic conditions to form nitrogen dioxide (·NO_2), an oxidant and nitrating agent (8,9).

III. PRO-OXIDANT PROPERTIES OF NITRIC OXIDE

A. Nitric Oxide-Derived Oxidants

Although under physiological concentrations (~ 1–100 nM) ·NO predominantly elicits antioxidant actions, excess ·NO formation (~ 1–10 μM) observed under different pathological states, owing to either excessive activation of constitutive nitric oxide synthase (cNOS) or expression of inducible nitric oxide synthase (iNOS) can result in the formation of ·NO-derived oxidants that cause biological damage. It is important to emphasize that ·NO itself is not an efficient oxidant, and its pro-oxidant activity depends on the formation of more reactive intermediates such as ·NO_2 or peroxynitrite, by its reactions with molecular oxygen or $O_2^{·-}$, respectively (8,9).

The formation of ·NO_2 from ·NO is a relatively slow process in biology because the concentration of ·NO is typically in the nanomolar or submicromolar range and the peculiar mechanism of reaction with molecular oxygen, which involves a termolecular reaction being second-order in ·NO ($k = 2 \times 10^6$ M^{-2} s^{-1}) (10). This reaction may be relevant in the interior of biological membranes where ·NO and oxygen can concentrate severalfold. Nitrogen dioxide can be also formed secondary to the decomposition and target molecule reactions of peroxynitrite and heme–peroxidase-dependent oxidation of nitrite (9,11). Nitrogen dioxide is a strong one-electron oxidant ($E^\circ = +0.99$ V), it crosses membranes readily, and at low concentrations, efficiently initiates free radical oxidation reactions, whereas at higher concentrations it will further react with most organic radicals at near diffusion-limited rates to form nitroderivatives (R-NO$_2$) (9,12).

Nitric oxide reacts at diffusion-limited rates with O$_2^{\cdot-}$ to form peroxynitrite ($k \sim 10^{10}$ M^{-1} s^{-1}) (13–15), a reactive nitrogen species with strong oxidizing properties. In contrast to extremely reactive biological oxidants, such as the hydroxyl radical ($^\cdot$OH), for which the high rate of reaction with most molecules ($> 10^9$ M^{-1} s^{-1}) determines that it will react nonspecifically and close to its site of formation, peroxynitrite reactions are typically much slower and more selective. Peroxynitrite's biological half-life can be estimated in the range of 10–100 ms (16); therefore, at a cellular–tissue level, it could potentially diffuse some distance before enacting target molecule reactions. Mechanisms for transmembrane diffusion of both the anionic and protonated forms of peroxynitrite have been recently revealed (16,17).

Peroxynitrite anion (ONOO$^-$) is in rapid protonation equilibrium with peroxynitrous acid (ONOOH) (p$K_a = 6.8$) and both species have unique reactivities toward biomolecules (18–24). Relevant biological reactions include oxidations and nitrations [Eqs. (1–3)], with many biological reactions of peroxynitrite being catalyzed or mediated through transition metal centers or carbon dioxide (9).

$$\text{ONOO}^- + \text{H}^+ \rightleftarrows \text{ONOOH} \tag{1}$$

$$\text{ONOOH} + \text{RH} \rightarrow \text{R}^\cdot + \text{H}_2\text{O} + {}^\cdot\text{NO}_2 \tag{2}$$

$$\text{R}^\cdot + {}^\cdot\text{NO}_2 \rightarrow \text{RNO}_2 \tag{3}$$

Recently, it has been shown that different peroxidases including myeloperoxidase and eosinophil peroxidase promote nitration reactions by peroxidase–hydrogen peroxide-dependent oxidation of nitrite, presumably through $^\cdot$NO$_2$ formation (25).

B. Biological Nitration as a Marker of $^\cdot$NO-Derived Oxidants

Nitration of tyrosine residues in proteins has been detected following $^\cdot$NO-derived oxidant formation by cells and tissues (11,26–28). In addition to tyrosine, other residues can be nitrated including other aromatics, such as tryptophan and guanine, and aliphatic residues, including sugars and fatty acids (9,29). For instance, the reaction of peroxynitrite with unsaturated fatty acids yields significant amounts of nitrogen-containing lipid species as well as oxidation products (30,31).

C. Nitric Oxide-Derived Oxidants and Atherosclerosis

Oxidation of low-density lipoprotein (LDL) is a critical event in the pathogenesis of atherosclerosis. Peroxynitrite oxidizes and nitrates LDL, converting it to a form readily recognized by macrophage scavenger receptors and potentially atherogenic, which causes rapid depletion of LDL antioxidants such as α-tocopherol (32–36). Detection of nitrotyrosine in both the protein moiety of LDL and atherosclerotic plaques indicates $^\cdot$NO-derived oxidant-dependent reactions during both early and chronic stages of atherosclerotic disease, which result in the formation of highly immunogenic and potentially proinflammatory protein oxidation products. Antibodies to nitrotyrosine show immunoreactivity in fatty streaks of coronary arteries in close association with foam cells, vascular endothelium, and in the neointima of atherosclerotic lesions (26). In addition, measurements of 3-nitrotyrosine in LDL isolated from human atherosclerotic lesions show that there is a striking 90-fold increase compared with circulating LDL (37). As an additional mechanism for LDL nitration, myeloperoxidase-generated reactive nitrogen species has been recently proposed as a physiologically plausible pathway for converting LDL into an atherogenic form (38).

IV. ANTIOXIDANT PROPERTIES OF NITRIC OXIDE

A. Nitric Oxide Reaction with Metals

The interactions of ˙NO with metalloproteins constitute relevant molecular mechanisms accounting for signal transduction and modulation of free radical chemistry. Nitric oxide can exert a protective role toward metal complex and metalloprotein-catalyzed oxidations (e.g., lipid oxidation), by formation of catalytically inactive metal–nitrosyl complexes (e.g., iron–nitrosyl), thereby modulating the pro-oxidant effects of iron and other transition metals (7,39–41). Transition metals, in particular iron and copper, play critical roles in promoting or catalyzing oxidative reactions through a combination of molecular mechanisms, including the (1) Fenton reaction, (2) Haber–Weiss cycle, (3) reduction of hydroperoxides, and (4) reactivity of ferryl intermediates (42).

Nitric oxide can reversibly interact with ferrous (Fe^{2+}) or ferric (Fe^{3+}) iron of various hemeproteins that have an accessible 6th coordination position (7,40), resulting in antioxidant activity. Moreover, ˙NO can even react and reduce higher-oxidation states of the heme iron, such as the ferryl form (Fe^{4+}=O) (Fig. 2).

Nitric oxide reacts with the ferrous state of heme proteins typically faster ($\sim 10^7$ M^{-1} s^{-1}) than with the ferric state (10^2–10^7 M^{-1} s^{-1}) (7). Once formed, the ferrous or ferric, heme–nitrosyl complex is typically fairly stable and dissociates slowly: the dissociation is usually faster for the ferric- ($\sim 10^1$–10^2 s^{-1}) than for the ferrous–heme nitrosyl complex ($\sim 10^4$–10^5 s^{-1}) (7). For some hemoproteins, such as myoglobin and hemoglobin, the $heme^{3+}$-nitrosyl complex can also undergo internal electron transfer to yield a ˙NO–$heme^{2+}$ complex, which can either hydrolyze to nitrite and $heme^{2+}$, or transfer the NO^+ moiety to acceptor nucleophiles, such as thiols (41). Electron transfer from ˙NO to the $heme^{3+}$ more readily occurs in those proteins having a more positive redox potential of the iron (7). The formation of complexes between ˙NO and heme can be evidenced both by optical and electron paramagnetic resonance (EPR) studies (7,40). The formation of a ˙NO–$heme^{2+}$ complex results in an EPR signal of $g = 2.0$, indicating an iron complex with rhombic symmetry. On the other hand, the ˙NO–$heme^{3+}$ complex is diamagnetic and, therefore, the EPR spectrum is flat (40).

While guanylate cyclase is activated by low ˙NO concentrations through the formation of an iron–nitrosyl complex (43,44), heme proteins participating in metabolic redox processes, such as cytochrome P450 (45,46) and cytochrome oxidase (47), are inhibited by ˙NO. Similarly, the mammalian NOS, which utilizes heme as a cofactor, may also be inhibited by ˙NO (40).

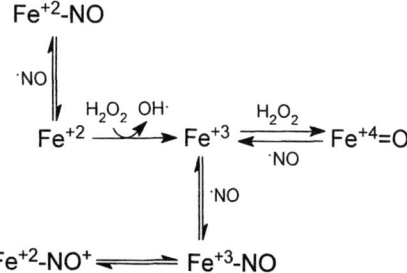

Figure 2 Nitric oxide reactions with iron: Nitric oxide inhibits pro-oxidant actions of iron by formation of stable iron–nitrosyl complexes (Fe–NO), which precludes further redox chemistry, or by reduction of highly oxidizing oxo-ferryl iron intermediates.

Cyclooxygenase is a heme protein that is activated by ˙NO (48). However, the mechanism for activation does not appear to be mediated through interactions of ˙NO with the ferric heme of this enzyme (48). It is hypothesized that ˙NO augments its activity by acting as an antioxidant through removing of $O_2^{˙-}$ generated during cyclooxygenase activation, thus preventing its autoinactivation and promoting peroxynitrite formation that directly activates cyclooxygenase (49). In spite of the general antioxidant action of ˙NO by formation of heme–nitrosyl complexes in redox enzymes, there is one case in which ˙NO–heme interactions can result in pro-oxidant effects: the binding and inhibitory action of ˙NO on catalase, a critical hydrogen peroxide-detoxifying enzyme (50), the relevance of which in vivo remains to be shown.

Nonheme pro-oxidant iron proteins, such as lipoxygenase (51–53) and xanthine oxidase (54), are inhibited by ˙NO, albeit minimally or at much greater concentrations of ˙NO than are biologically achievable. This is in line with the fact that nonheme iron enzymes bind ligands at the iron site less tightly than hemoproteins (40). At biologically relevant ˙NO concentrations, reaction of ˙NO with the reduced form of lipoxygenase leads to reversible enzyme inhibition, resulting in further inhibition of its redox–free radical chemistry (53). For xanthine oxidase, ˙NO reacts with an essential sulfur of the reduced molybdenum center to produce a desulfo-type inactive enzyme (55).

Heme and nonheme iron–nitrosyl complexes have been evidenced in cells, tissues, and blood secondary to endogenous ˙NO production or exogenous exposure, confirming the relevance of these reactions in living systems (7).

In addition to interacting with iron, ˙NO also act as a ligand of copper. Thus, ˙NO has been used to study the binuclear copper centers in hemocyanin and tyrosinase; the iron/copper center in cytochrome oxidase; the multicopper oxidases ceruloplasmin, ascorbate oxidase, and laccase; the blue copper type-1 enzymes halocyanin and azurin; and the type-2 copper enzymes galactose oxidase and diamine oxidase (56). Even when copper often forms an essential part of the catalytic sites of all these enzymes, a potential antioxidant role of ˙NO on those catalyzing redox reactions has not yet been described. Of note, is that ˙NO neither reacts nor inhibits the type-2 copper antioxidant enzyme Cu–Zn superoxide dismutase (9).

B. Nitric Oxide Reaction with Lipid Radicals

Nitric oxide plays a critical role in regulating lipid oxidation induced by reactive oxygen and nitrogen species. Nitric oxide crosses cell membranes and concentrates in lipophilic milieu by virtue of its low molecular mass and relatively high lipid/water partition coefficient (n-octanol:water partition coefficient of 6–8:1) (57,58), implying that both lipid peroxidation processes and reactions of lipophilic antioxidants will be influenced by local ˙NO concentrations. Nitric oxide inhibits lipid peroxidation by scavenging alkoxyl (LO˙) and peroxyl (LOO˙) radicals involved in the chain-propagation steps to yield nitrated and nitrosylated lipid derivatives as shown by the following equations:

$$LOO˙ + ˙NO \rightarrow LOONO \tag{4}$$

$$LOONO \rightarrow\rightarrow LONO_2, L[O]NO_2, LNO_2, LOOH \tag{5}$$

$$LO˙ + ˙NO \rightarrow LONO \tag{6}$$

The almost diffusion-limited reaction of ˙NO with LOO˙ (3×10^9 M^{-1} s^{-1}) (59) will be significantly more facile than the initiation of secondary peroxidation propagation reactions by LOO˙ with vicinal unsaturated lipids ($k = 30–200$ M^{-1} s^{-1}). The importance of Eqs. (4–6) are underscored by the fact that these reactions are significantly faster than the reaction of ˙NO with most metal centers; therefore it plays a critical role in limiting the propagation of radical chain oxidant processes.

Both ˙NO$_2$ and ˙NO can react with peroxyl radicals giving rise to nonradical end products of lipid peroxidation. With linolenic acid, these products have been tentatively identified from their molecular weight as a nitrosoperoxolinolenate, hydroxylnitrosoperoxolinolenate, and hydroperoxonitrosoperoxolinolenate (30). Some nitrogen-containing lipid intermediates appear to be highly unstable and may decompose to reinitiate radical processes. In fact, the product of the LOO˙/˙NO combination reaction (LOONO) has several fates: 1) internal rearrangement to give the more stable LONO$_2$ and LNO$_2$, 2) homolytic cleavage to LO˙ and ˙NO$_2$, with rearrangement of LO˙ to an epoxyallylic acid radical L(O)˙, followed by recombination of L(O)˙ with ˙NO$_2$ to L[O]NO$_2$, and 3) hydrolysis to yield the hydroperoxide (LOOH) (31).

Nitric oxide has been reported to have protective effects on LDL oxidation. For both macrophage and endothelial cell model systems, increased rates of cell ˙NO production by cytokine-mediated stimulation of inducible macrophage nitric oxide synthase gene expression and activity of exogenous addition of ˙NO inhibits cell and $O_2^{˙-}$-mediated lipoprotein oxidation (52,60–63). Nitric oxide causes a prolongation of the lag time and inhibition of the propagation phase of LDL oxidation (52,61). Fragmentation of apolipoprotein B by oxidants, loss of tryptophan, and protein–lipid fluorescent adducts formation is prevented by ˙NO (52,64,65). The formation of lipid peroxidation-dependent antigenic epitopes in oxidized LDL is also inhibited by ˙NO (66).

Because 15-lipoxygenase is present in the subendothelial layer of atherosclerotic lesions, it is relevant to investigate whether lipid peroxidation reactions generated by this enzyme can be influenced by ˙NO. In fact, ˙NO can diffuse into the active site of lipoxygenase, and the reaction of ˙NO with enzyme-derived LOO˙ is highly plausible, followed by hydrolysis of the LOONO generated at the active site. We have demonstrated the formation of LONO$_2$, LNO$_2$, LOOH(NO$_2$), and LOH(NO$_2$) during the oxidation of phosphocholine liposomes by lipoxygenase in the presence of ˙NO (52). Inhibition of lipoxygenase by ˙NO may contribute to the antiatherogenic properties of ˙NO that have been observed in both animal and human models.

The ˙NO radical–radical termination reaction with lipid radicals occurs both in vitro and in vivo. Indeed, in lipid extracts of atherosclerotic vascular lesions, the major oxidizable lipid in LDL, cholesteryl linoleate, yields nitrogen-containing oxidized lipid derivatives (unpublished data). These observations, when taken together with the fact that ˙NO can readily diffuse into the hydrophobic core of the LDL particle (67), are in agreement with our hypothesis that ˙NO can represent a major lipophilic antioxidant in LDL.

C. Nitric Oxide Fluxes and Antioxidant Action

Many biological effects of ˙NO are critically related to the rate of ˙NO formation, and, therefore, timing of flux or delivery of ˙NO becomes a key variable that determines the extent of antioxidant action and even the pro-oxidant actions of ˙NO (30,68,69). An optimal rate of ˙NO release is required for maximal suppression of fatty acid and LDL oxidation that depends on the rate and the mechanism of lipid oxidation. As lipid oxidation involves a propagation phase by which initial radical reactions are amplified severalfold, effective ˙NO-mediated inhibition requires a threshold ˙NO flux (and steady-state concentration) under which propagation reactions predominate over inhibition. In fact, during azo–compound-initiated lipid oxidation (68), lag times correlated well with the presence of ˙NO levels (Fig. 3a) above a critical threshold.

ANTIOXIDANT PROPERTIES OF NO

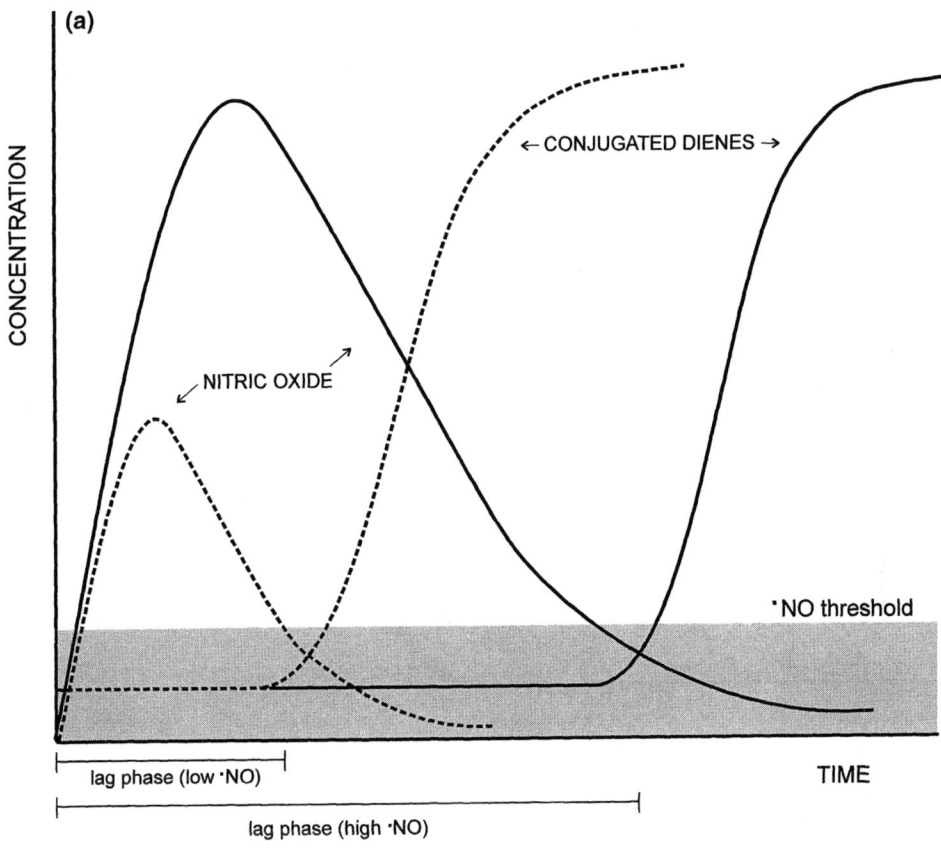

Figure 3 Nitric oxide and lipid oxidation: (a) The presence of ˙NO inhibits conjugated diene formation. Lipid oxidation propagation starts after ˙NO is consumed below threshold levels.

Current evidence with model systems support the concept that permanent generation of low levels of ˙NO by vascular endothelium represent a continuous source of antioxidant, playing an integral role in suppressing oxidative reactions within the vasculature.

1. Nitric Oxide Donors

Experimentally, to achieve various fluxes and timing of ˙NO delivery, a series of compounds generally named ˙NO donors can be used. These include (1) solutions of ˙NO gas, which exhibit antioxidant activity, added either as a bolus at submicromolar concentrations or by slow continuous infusion, to avoid the production of higher oxides of nitrogen from the reaction between ˙NO and oxygen; (2) S-nitrosothiols, for which the rate of ˙NO release depends on the structure of the S-nitrosothiol (e.g., S-nitrosoacetylpenicillamine and S-nitrosoglutathione), and other factors such as the concentration of metals (iron or copper) and other reductants (e.g., thiols or ascorbate) in the solution, and light exposure; and (3) NONOates (diazeniumdiolates), that release ˙NO thermolytically and do not require light or catalysis by enzymes or metal ions (70). NONOates are currently first choice for performing experiments at controlled ˙NO fluxes and a variety of them, with a wide range of decomposition half-lives, exist. As an example, at pH 7.4 and 37°C the NONOates DEA NONOate, PAPA NONOate, spermine NONOate, and

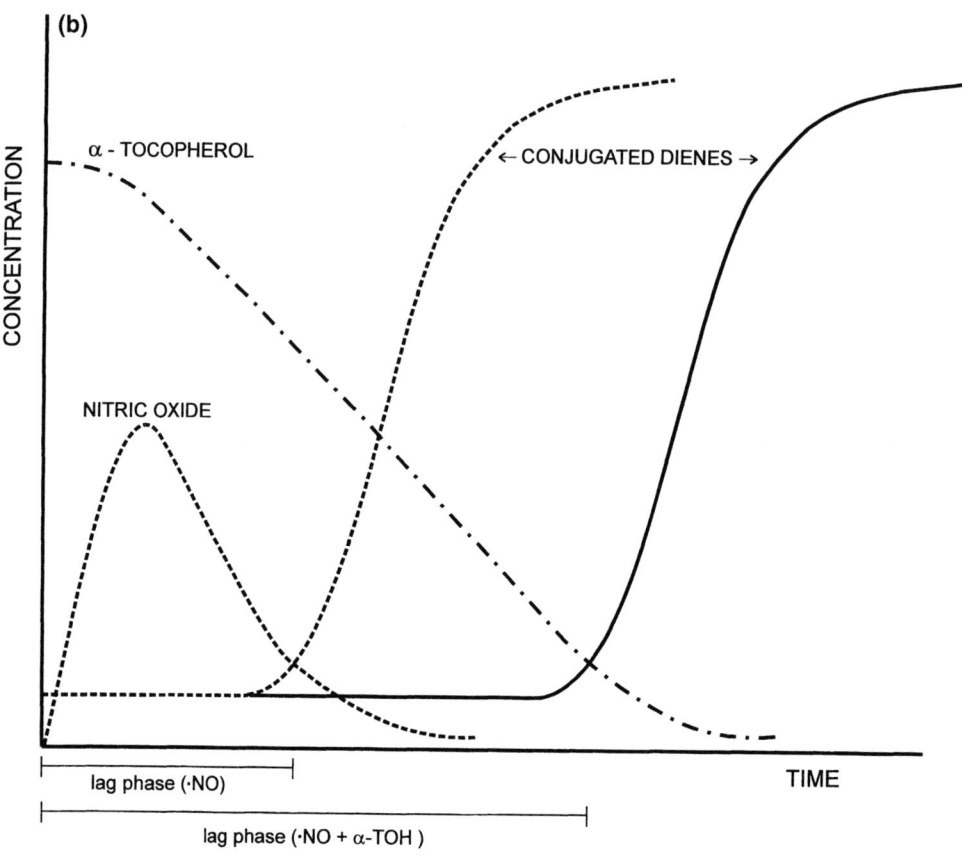

Figure 3 (b) Nitric oxide spares α-tocopherol during lipid oxidation. Both antioxidants cooperatively increase the lag phase of initiation of conjugated diene formation.

DETA NONOate have $t_{1/2}$ of about 2 min, 15 min, 39 min, and 20 h, respectively. Importantly, after choosing the appropriate NONOate to fit the time course of a given experiment, the values of $t_{1/2}$ provided in the literature are always approximate and the rate of ˙NO release must be precisely quantitated in each particular system by the use of ˙NO detection methods. As release rates and half-times are affected by reaction conditions, it is important to establish the rate of ˙NO release in the particular experimental system. In addition, control studies must be performed in the presence of both the decayed compound and the secondary amine backbone. Finally, we do not recommend the use of the ˙NO donor sodium nitroprusside because of its poorly controlled decomposition, formation of redox active products, such as ferricyanide, and toxic effects of both reactants and products.

2. Nitric Oxide–Superoxide Fluxes: Pro- Versus Antioxidant Effects

Although the biological reaction of ˙NO with $O_2^{˙-}$ to form peroxynitrite in vivo is well established (8,9,71), under some circumstances this interaction has been proposed to exert protective actions (72,73). This places a paradox because peroxynitrite is a much stronger oxidant than its precursors. However, (1) the more limited diffusibility and shorter half-life of peroxynitrite relative to ˙NO, which may limit the reactions of peroxynitrite in critical biological compartments; (2) the efficient scavenging of low levels of peroxynitrite by intracellular glutathione; (3) the relative fluxes of ˙NO and $O_2^{˙-}$; and (4) direct toxic actions of ˙NO by oxidant-independent mechanisms, are variables that may account for a limited number of observations that found the ˙NO plus $O_2^{˙-}$ interaction as cytoprotective in some experimental models. In spite of this, there is a large body of evidence affirming that peroxynitrite is a more reactive and damaging species than ˙NO and $O_2^{˙-}$ in biology, and that many of the toxic effects previously ascribed to ˙NO are, in fact, due to peroxynitrite formation (8,9,74,75).

D. Nitric Oxide–α-Tocopherol–Ascorbate Interactions During Lipid Oxidation

α-Tocopherol, a key lipophilic, chain-breaking antioxidant in biological membranes and lipoproteins acts by donating hydrogen atoms to chain-propagating LOO˙ to form the corresponding hydroperoxide (LOOH). Because the reaction of LOO˙ with α-tocopherol ($k = 2.5 \times 10^6$ M^{-1} s^{-1}) occurs with a rate constant three orders of magnitude less than that for the reaction of LOO˙ with ˙NO, and may have access to hydrophobic sites where α-tocopherol is not present (76), ˙NO could act more readily than or in concert with α-tocopherol as an antioxidant defense against oxygen radical-derived oxidized lipid species.

We have just demonstrated that ˙NO represents a key lipid-soluble chain-breaking antioxidant protecting α-tocopherol from oxidation (68). Indeed, ˙NO serves to spare α-tocopherol, which is not consumed during lipid oxidation reactions until ˙NO concentrations fall under a critical level (see Fig. 3b). Thermodynamic predictions suggest ˙NO to be capable of limiting α-tocopherol oxidation, by the one-electron reduction of α-tocopheroxyl radical to α-tocopherol. However, pulse radiolysis analysis revealed that ˙NO does not undergo direct reaction with the phenoxyl radical of α-tocopherol (68), implying that LOO˙ termination reactions are the principal lipid-protective mechanism mediated by physiologically relevant (nM) concentrations of ˙NO, thus preventing α-tocopherol loss.

In addition, α-tocopherol and ˙NO can act cooperatively to inhibit lipid peroxidation processes, exhibiting greater antioxidant capacity than the pair α-tocopherol–ascorbate (68). This cooperative action of α-tocopherol and ˙NO results in increased lag times before the onset of autocatalytic peroxidative propagation reactions (see Fig. 3). Ascorbate can both directly reduce α-tocopheroxyl radical to α-tocopherol with a rate constant of 1.5×10^6 M^{-1} s^{-1} and LOO˙ to LOOH at the slower rate constant of $k = 7.5 \times 10^4$ M^{-1} s^{-1} (68). When both antioxidants are present, ascorbate is consumed first, and after ascorbate depletion, α-tocopherol becomes oxidized, because LOO˙ preferentially reacts with α-tocopherol and ascorbate preferentially reduces α-tocopheroxyl radical, rather than LOO˙. Because lipid radicals formed in lipophilic milieu do not readily partition into the bulk aqueous medium (where ascorbate is present) and ˙NO has access to hydrophobic sites, it is conceivable that the pair ˙NO–α-tocopherol would be more efficient than ascorbate–α-tocopherol in the inhibition of lipid peroxidation (Fig. 4). The reduction of α-tocopheroxyl radical by ascorbate represents a comparatively less efficient mechanism for preserving α-tocopherol than the ˙NO-mediated termination reaction with LOO˙, owing to slower reaction kinetics and limited transfer of reducing equivalents from the aqueous phase (68).

E. Nitric Oxide Reaction with Protein Radicals

In addition to its fast reaction with lipid radicals, ˙NO rapidly reacts with aminoacyl radicals, including cysteinyl (and glutathionyl), tyrosyl, and tryptophanyl-derived radicals of free amino acids, peptides, and proteins, with rate constants of $\sim 10^9$ M^{-1} s^{-1} (77,78) to yield the

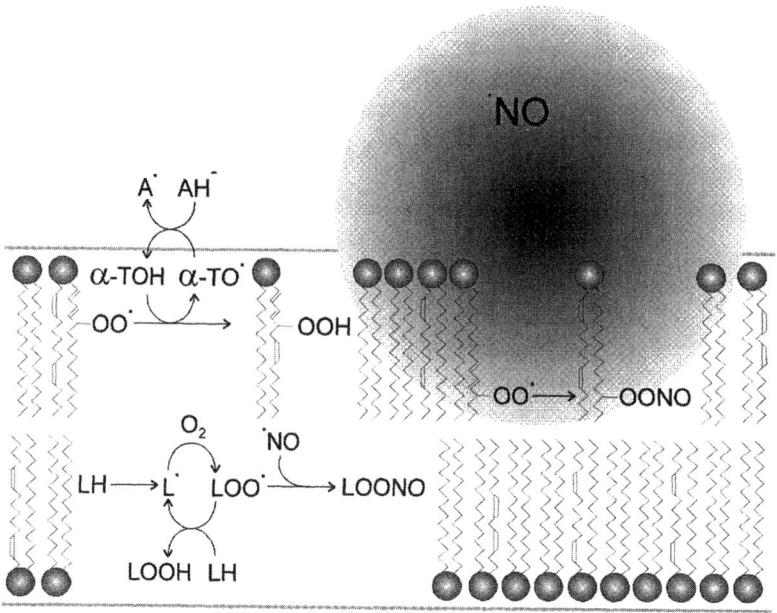

Figure 4 Antioxidant reactions of nitric oxide in membranes: Nitric oxide can readily diffuse and concentrate to the interior of the biomembranes and lipoproteins to terminate lipid peroxidation processes. The antioxidant action of α-tocopherol and the recycling by ascorbate may be relatively limited to the more superficial oxidizable lipid moieties. α-TOH, α-tocopherol; α-TO˙, α-tocopheroxyl radical; AH⁻, ascorbate; A˙, ascorbyl radical; LH, unsaturated fatty acid; LOOH, lipid hydroperoxide; L˙, lipid radical; LOO˙, peroxyl radical.

corresponding nitrosocompounds [Eqs. (7 and 10)] and stop propagation reactions [Eqs. (8,9, and 11)]:

1. *Thiyl Radical Reactions*

$$˙NO + RS˙ \rightarrow RSNO \tag{7}$$

$$RS˙ + RS^- \rightarrow RSSR˙^- \tag{8}$$

$$RSSR˙^- + O_2 \rightarrow RSSR + O_2˙^- \Rightarrow \text{Propagation} \tag{9}$$

2. *Tryptophanyl Radical Reactions*

$$˙NO + Trp˙ \rightarrow Trp\text{-}NO \tag{10}$$

$$Trp˙ + O_2 \rightarrow TrpOO˙ \Rightarrow \text{Propagation} \tag{11}$$

Although the reactions of ˙NO with thiyl and tryptophanyl radicals lead to the formation of stable *S*-nitrosothiol (RSNO) and nitrosotryptophan (Trp-NO), respectively, the reaction with tyrosyl radical transiently yields nitrosotyrosine, which then decomposes into secondary products (78).

The oxidative changes occurring during LDL oxidation in its protein moiety, apoprotein B-100, are considered to result from the interaction of lipid oxidation products with amino acids residues. The formation of tryptophan-centered radicals during the oxidation of both LDL and apoB-100 have recently been demonstrated (79), raising the possibility that tryptophan-centered and tryptophan-peroxyl radicals may initiate lipid oxidation. In this context, ˙NO reaction with tryptophan-centered radicals in LDL may represent a novel antioxidant role of ˙NO during copper-mediated LDL oxidation. In addition, nitrosation of tryptophan may preserve the salutary actions of ˙NO, as nitrosotryptophan in serum albumin and peptides exhibits ˙NO-like vasorelaxation and antiplatelet activity (80).

V. ANTIOXIDANT ROLES OF NITRIC OXIDE AND CYTOPROTECTION

The concept of ˙NO-mediated cytoprotection from oxidative stress was affirmed by the seminal observation that rodent lung fibroblasts (V79 cells) and dopaminergic mesencephalic neuronal cells were protected from toxicity induced by either purine plus xanthine oxidase or addition of hydrogen peroxide to culture medium, when ˙NO was introduced by the release of NONOates (81). Subsequently, it was observed that V79 cells (82) and cardiomyocytes (83) also became more resistant to the toxicity of LOOH added to culture medium if chemical sources of ˙NO were present. Importantly, when peroxides enter a cell, they react with metalloproteins, forming complexes, which can lead to lipid peroxidation. Nitric oxide can rapidly react with these metalloproteins, preventing their oxidative reactions and limiting intracellular damage mediated by oxidative stress (82).

Exogenous ˙NO is cytoprotective to both the endothelium (84) and the intestinal epithelium (85) in the presence of oxidants through a reduction of lipid peroxidation processes. In addition, ˙NO protected human leukemia cells from iron-induced lipid peroxidation (86). Endogenous cell ˙NO production can also be cytoprotective toward exogenously and endogenously generated reactive oxygen species added to cultures of pulmonary epithelial cells (87). Furthermore, either hepatocytes (88) or leukocytes (89) treated with ˙NO became resistant to oxidative injury. In addition to protecting against oxidative stress at the cellular level, ˙NO can participate at the organ level, which can result in protection against tissue injury (i.e., ischemia–reperfusion and septic shock) by a combination of physiological mechanisms, one of which is its antioxidant actions (70).

VI. ANTIATHEROGENIC EFFECTS OF NITRIC OXIDE

Nitric oxide has many physiological actions that can be interpreted to be potentially antiatherosclerotic (90–92): it inhibits (1) platelet aggregation and adherence to endothelial cells, (2) monocyte adherence to endothelial cells, (3) the expression of the monocyte chemoattractant protein, (4) vascular smooth-muscle cell migration and proliferation, and (5) the in vivo intimal proliferative response to balloon injury. The atherogenic process involves a pathogenic role for oxidant injury and a number of model systems indicate that either endogenous ˙NO biosynthesis or exogenous supplementation with sources of ˙NO inhibit oxidant-dependent damage at both molecular and tissue functional levels. Nitric oxide reduces oxidant stress in the vascular wall which, in turn, may lower the rate of LDL oxidation and the expression of redox-sensitive genes that contribute to atherogenesis.

A. Macrophage and Endothelial Cell Inhibition of LDL Oxidation

Nitric oxide represents an important radical intermediate participating in macrophage-dependent LDL oxidation processes. Macrophages express the iNOS on immunological stimuli with inflammatory mediators such as interferon (IFN)-γ and tumor necrosis factor (TNF)-α (93).

Although endothelial nitric oxide synthase (eNOS) has been reported to be expressed in the endothelial cells of normal and atherosclerotic vessels, iNOS is also expressed in macrophages in the core of atheromatous plaques (94). In addition, macrophage-rich areas are positive for epitopes characteristic of oxidized LDL and ˙NO-derived oxidant-modified proteins (95).

However, in cell culture systems, ˙NO mainly limits macrophage-dependent LDL oxidation owing to its termination reactions with LOO˙ (96,97). Oxidized LDL inhibits ˙NO production in both macrophages and endothelial cells, but the components in oxidized LDL responsible for the inhibition of ˙NO production are unclear. Recent data showed that either oxysterols or LOOH in oxidized LDL may be responsible for the inhibition of iNOS-induced ˙NO production in stimulated macrophages (98,99). Importantly, inhibition of ˙NO production by oxidized LDL blocks the potential antioxidant role of cell-derived ˙NO, facilitating further oxidation by oxygen radicals (100).

B. Nitric Oxide and Gene Regulation

The redox-sensitive modulation of the expression and function of vascular genes appears to play a central role in the initiation and propagation of atherosclerosis (101). The oxidative modification of LDL by reactive oxygen species and enzymes, such as lipoxygenase, will generate novel epitopes on LDL, yielding minimally modified and further-oxidized species of LDL. Another critical oxidative event in atherogenesis is the activation of proinflammatory gene transcription by oxidized lipids (102). Specifically, fatty acid hydroperoxides found in oxidized LDL (e.g., 13-hydroperoxy-octadecadienoic acid) activate (at least) NF-κB, with this transcription factor then mediating gene expression of an integrin termed vascular cell adhesion molecule-1 (VCAM-1). In both oxidized lipid and cytokine-mediated activation of VCAM-1 gene expression, ˙NO serves an inhibitory role to both oxidative activation of NF-κB and the ultimate gene expression of VCAM-1 (103). Additionally, ˙NO indirectly inhibits NF-κB-mediated gene expression by inducing the expression of and stabilizing the inhibitory protein for NF-κB, I-κBα (104). A final oxidant-protective event that ˙NO mediates in vascular injury mechanisms is a consequence of ˙NO-mediated inhibition of integrin gene expression (105).

C. Nitric Oxide, Antioxidants, and Endothelial-Dependent Vasodilation

The changes that occur during atherosclerosis include loss of the control of vascular tone, an ˙NO-dependent event (106). The mechanisms accounting for endothelial dysfunction in hypercholesterolemia have not been completely elucidated, but may be explained by decreased bioavailability of ˙NO owing to decreased expression of the eNOS, decreased substrate availability, presence of an endogenous eNOS inhibitor, or increased ˙NO degradation by reactive oxygen species (107). In addition, consumption of ˙NO by the 15-lipoxygenase present in atherosclerotic lesions, could then contribute to the reduced vascular responses to ˙NO and increased degradation of EDRF activity seen during hypercholesterolemia.

Increasing the availability of the substrate L-arginine for ˙NO synthesis will restore vascular function, whereas inhibiting ˙NO synthesis is proatherogenic (108–112). In fact, both animal models and clinical studies are showing that chronic administration of L-arginine improves endothelial-dependent relaxation, decreases inflammatory cell accumulation at the vessel wall, and reduces intimal hyperplasia, all hallmarks of atherosclerotic disease (108–117). Furthermore, balloon angioplasty is often used to treat atherosclerotic vaso-occlusive problems. Both administration of ˙NO donors as well as transfection of cNOS to balloon-injured vessels reduces the intimal cell hyperplasia, often the cause for repeat angioplasty, aortocoronary bypass graft surgery, or myocardial infarction. In vivo transfection of the gene for eNOS to the vessel wall after balloon-induced denudation of the rat carotid artery not only restored ˙NO production and vasorelaxation, but also inhibited neointima formation, providing direct evidence that ˙NO is an endogenous inhibitor of intimal hyperplasia and suggesting that transfection of the eNOS gene is a potential therapeutic approach to test restenosis after balloon angioplasty (118).

Antioxidants can improve endothelium-dependent vasodilation in humans with atherosclerosis, as documented by coronary angiography. In fact, acute administration of superoxide dismutase (SOD) (119) or a combination of lovastatin with probucol during 1 year (120) reverses the abnormal vasoconstrictor response of the coronary arteries to acetylcholine in atherosclerotic patients. In essential hypertensive patients, impaired endothelial vasodilation can also be improved by intrabrachial administration of ascorbic acid (vitamin C), an effect that can be reversed by NOS inhibitors, supporting the hypothesis that ˙NO inactivation by oxidant species contributes to endothelial dysfunction (121). In addition, administration of ascorbic acid improves endothelium-dependent vasodilation in patients with hypercholesterolemia in the absence of clinical evidence of atherosclerosis (122). Because intracellular ascorbic acid is able to enhance ˙NO synthesis in endothelial cells, this may also explain part of its beneficial vascular effects (123–125). Similarly, administration of vitamin E (500 UI/day) has also shown the same beneficial vascular effects (126,127). These clinical data (120–127) support the general idea that ˙NO–oxidant interactions play central roles in the physiology and pathology of the cardiovascular and other organ systems and that future therapies will take advantage of both the direct signal transduction and antioxidant properties of ˙NO for the prevention and treatment of human diseases.

ACKNOWLEDGMENTS

This work has been supported by CONICYT (Uruguay) and FOGARTY-NIH (USA) to HR and ICGEB (Italy), SAREC (Sweden), FOGARTY-NIH (USA) and the Howard Hughes Medical Institute (USA) to RR.

REFERENCES

1. Palmer RMJ, Ferrige AG, Moncada S. (1987) Nitric oxide release accounts for the biological activity of endothelium-derived relaxing factor. Nature 327:524–526.
2. Ignarro LJ, Buga GM, Wood KS, Byrns RE, Chaudhuri G. (1987) Endothelium-derived relaxing factor produced and released from artery and vein is nitric oxide. Proc Natl Acad Sci USA 84:9265–9269.
3. Moncada S, Higgs EA. (1991) Endogenous nitric oxide: physiology, pathology and clinical relevance. Eur J Clin Invest 21:361–374.
4. Wink DA, Mitchell JB. (1998) Chemical biology of nitric oxide: insights into regulatory, cytotoxic, and cytoprotective mechanisms of nitric oxide. Free Radic Biol Med 25:434–456.
5. Lincoln TM, Cornwell TL. (1993) Intracellular cyclic GMP receptor proteins. FASEB J 7:328–338.
6. McDonald LJ, Murad F. (1995) Nitric oxide and cGMP signaling. Adv Pharmacol 34:263–275.
7. Radi R. (1996) Reactions of nitric oxide with metalloproteins. Chem Res Toxicol 9:828–835.
8. Beckman JS, Koppenol WH. (1996) Nitric oxide, superoxide, and peroxynitrite: the good, the bad and the ugly. Am J Physiol 271:C1424–C1437.
9. Radi R, Denicola A, Ferrer G, Alvarez B, Rubbo H. (2000) The biological chemistry of peroxynitrite. In: Ignarro L, ed. Nitric Oxide Biology and Pathobiology, Advances in Pharmacology. San Diego, CA: Academic Press: 57–82.
10. Ford PC, Wink DA, Stanbury DM. (1993) Autoxidation kinetics of aqueous nitric oxide. FEBS Lett 326:1–3.
11. Ischiropoulos H. (1998) Biological tyrosine nitration: a pathophysiological function of nitric oxide and reactive oxygen species. Arch Biochem Biophys 356:1–11.

12. Prutz WA, Monig H, Butler J, Land EJ. (1985) Reactions of nitrogen dioxide in aqueous model systems: oxidation of tyrosine units in peptides and proteins. Arch Biochem Biophys 243:125–134.
13. Kissner R, Nauser T, Bugnon P, Lye PG, Koppenol WH. (1997). Formation and properties of peroxynitrite as studied by laser flash photolysis, high-pressure stopped-flow technique, and pulse radiolysis. Chem Res Toxicol 10:1285–1292.
14. Goldstein S, Czapski G. (1995) The reaction of NO$^{\bullet}$ with $O_2^{\bullet-}$ and $HO_2^{\bullet}$: a pulse radiolysis study. Free Radic Biol Med 19:505–510.
15. Huie RE, Padmaja S. (1993) The reaction of NO with superoxide. Free Radic Res Commun 18:195–199.
16. Denicola A, Souza J, Radi R. (1998) Peroxynitrite diffusion across erythrocyte membranes. Proc Natl Acad Sci USA 95:3566–3571.
17. Marla SS, Lee J, Groves JT. (1997) Peroxynitrite rapidly permeates phospholipid membranes. Proc Natl Acad Sci USA 94:14243–14248.
18. Radi R, Beckman JS, Bush K, Freeman BA. (1991) Peroxynitrite oxidation of sulfhydryls: the cytotoxic potential of endothelial-derived superoxide and nitric oxide. J Biol Chem 266:4244–4250.
19. Quijano C, Alvarez B, Gatti RM, Augusto O, Radi R. (1997) Pathways of peroxynitrite oxidation of thiol groups. Biochem J 322:167–173.
20. Castro L, Rodriguez M, Radi R. (1994) Aconitase is readily inactivated by peroxynitrite, but not by its precursor, nitric oxide. J Biol Chem 269:29409–29415.
21. MacMillan–Crow LA, Crow JP, Kerby JD, Beckman JS, Thompson JA. (1996) Nitration and inactivation of manganese superoxide dismutase in chronic rejection of human renal allografts. Proc Natl Acad Sci USA 93:11853–11858.
22. Briviba K, Kissner R, Koppenol WH, Sies H. (1998) Kinetic study of the reaction of glutathione peroxidase with peroxynitrite. Chem Res Toxicol 11:1398–1401.
23. Radi R, Beckman JS, Bush K, Freeman BA. (1991) Peroxynitrite-induced membrane lipid peroxidation: the cytotoxic potential of superoxide and nitric oxide. Arch Biochem Biophys 288:481–487.
24. Burney S, Caulfield JL, Niles JC, Wishnok JS, Tannenbaum SR. (1999) The chemistry of DNA damage from nitric oxide and peroxynitrite. Mutat Res 424:37–49.
25. Eiserich JP, Hristova M, Cross CE, Jones AD, Freeman BA, Halliwell B, van der Vliet A. (1998) Formation of nitric oxide-derived inflammatory oxidants by myeloperoxidase in neutrophils. Nature 391:393–397.
26. Beckmann JS, Ye YZ, Anderson PG, Chen J, Accavitti MA, Tarpey MM, White CR. (1994) Extensive nitration of protein tyrosines in human atherosclerosis detected by immunohistochemistry. Biol Chem Hoppe Seyler, 375:81–88.
27. Brito C, Naviliat M, Tiscornia AC, Vuillier F, Gualco G, Dighiero G, Radi R, Cayota AM. (1999) Peroxynitrite inhibits T lymphocyte activation and proliferation by promoting impairment of tyrosine phosphorylation and peroxynitrite-driven apoptotic death. J Immunol 162:3356–3366.
28. Estevez AG, Spear N, Manuel SM, Radi R, Henderson CE, Barbeito L, Beckman JS. (1998) Nitric oxide and superoxide contribute to motor neuron apoptosis induced by trophic factor deprivation. J Neurosci 18:923–931.
29. Alvarez B, Rubbo H, Kirk M, Barnes S, Freeman BA, Radi R. (1996) Peroxynitrite-dependent tryptophan nitration. Chem Res Toxicol 9:390–396.
30. Rubbo H, Radi R, Trujillo M, Telleri R, Kalyanaraman B, Barnes S, Kirk M, Freeman BA. (1994) Nitric oxide regulation of superoxide and peroxynitrite-dependent lipid peroxidation: formation of novel nitrogen-containing oxidized lipid derivatives. J Biol Chem 269:26066–26075.
31. O'Donnell VB, Eiserich JP, Chumley P, Jablonsky MJ, Rama Krishna N, Kirk M, Barnes S, Darley–Usmar V, Freeman BA. (1999) Nitration of unsaturated fatty acids by nitric oxide-derived reactive nitrogen species peroxynitrite, nitrous acid, nitrogen dioxide and nitronium ion. Chem Res Toxicol 12:83–92.
32. Graham A, Hogg N, Kalyanaraman B, O'Leary VJ, Darley–Usmar V, Moncada S. (1993) Peroxynitrite modification of low density lipoprotein leads to recognition by the macrophage scavenger receptor. FEBS Lett 330:181–185.
33. Hogg N, Darley–Usmar VM, Wilson MT, Moncada S. (1993) The oxidation of α-tocopherol in human low density lipoprotein by the simultaneous generation of superoxide and nitric oxide. FEBS Lett 326:199–203.

34. White R, Brock T, Chang L, Crapo J, Briscoe P, Ku D, Bradley W, Gianturco S, Gore J, Freeman BA, Tarpey MM. (1994) Superoxide and peroxynitrite in atherosclerosis. Proc Natl Acad Sci USA 91:1044–1048.
35. Hogg N, Darley–Usmar V, Graham A, Moncada S. (1993) Peroxynitrite and atherosclerosis. Biochem Soc Trans 21:358–361.
36. Thomas SR, Davies MJ, Stocker R. (1998) Oxidation and antioxidation of human low-density lipoprotein and plasma exposed to 3-morpholinosydnonimine and reagent peroxynitrite. Chem Res Toxicol 11:484–494.
37. Leeuwenburgh C, Hardy MM, Hazen SL, Wagner P, Oh-ishi S, Steinbrecher UP, Heinecke JW. (1997) Reactive nitrogen intermediates promote low-density lipoprotein oxidation in human atherosclerotic intima. J Biol Chem 272:1433–1436.
38. Podrez EA, Schmitt D, Of HF, Hazen SL. (1999) Myeloperoxidase-generated reactive nitrogen species convert LDL into an atherogenic form in vitro. J Clin Invest 103:1547–1560.
39. Kanner J, Harel S, Granit R. (1991) Nitric oxide as an antioxidant. Arch Biochem Biophys 289:130–136.
40. Cooper CE. (1999) Nitric oxide and iron proteins. Biochim Biophys Acta 1411:290–309.
41. Sharma VS, Taylor TG, Gardiner R. (1987) Reaction of nitric oxide with heme proteins and model compounds of hemoglobin. Biochemistry 26:3837–3843.
42. Goldstein S, Meyerstein D, Czapski G. (1993) The Fenton reagents. Free Radic Biol Med 15:435–445.
43. Drewett JG, Garners DL. (1994) The family of guanyl cyclase receptors and their ligands. Endocr Rev 15:135–162.
44. Ignarro LJ, Degnan J, Baricos W, Kadowitz P, Wolin MS. (1982) Activation of purified guanylate cyclase by nitric oxide requires heme: comparison of the heme-deficient, heme-reconstituted and heme-containing forms of soluble enzyme from bovine lung. Biochim Biophys Acta 718:49–59.
45. Wink DA, Osawa Y, Darbyshire J, Jones CR, Eshenaur S, Nims RW. (1993) Inhibition of cytochromes P450 by nitric oxide and a nitric oxide-releasing agent. Arch Biochem Biophys 300:115–123.
46. Hori H, Masuya F, Tsubaki M, Yoshikawa S, Ichikawa Y. (1992) Electronic and stereochemical characterizations of intermediates in the photolysis of ferric cytochrome P450 nitrosyl complexes. J Biol Chem 267:18377–18381.
47. Cassina A, Radi R. (1996) Differential inhibitory action of nitric oxide and peroxynitrite on mitochondrial electron transport. Arch Biochem Biophys 328:309–316.
48. Salvemini D. (1997) Regulation of cyclooxygenase enzymes by nitric oxide. CMLS Cell Mol Life Sci 53:576–582.10.
49. Landino LM, Crews BC, Timmons MD, Morrow JD, Marnett LJ. (1996) Peroxynitrite, the coupling product of nitric oxide and superoxide, activates prostaglandin biosynthesis. Proc Natl Acad Sci USA 93:15069–15074.
50. Brown GC. (1995) Reversible binding and inhibition of catalase by nitric oxide. Eur J Biochem 232:188–191.
51. Kanner J, Harel S, Granit R. (1992) Nitric oxide, an inhibitor of lipid oxidation by lipoxygenase, cyclooxygenase and hemoglobin. Lipids 27:46–49.
52. Rubbo H, Parthasarathy S, Kalyanaraman B, Barnes S, Kirk M, Freeman BA. (1995) Nitric oxide inhibition of lipoxygenase-dependent liposome and low density lipoprotein oxidation: termination of radical chain propagation reactions and formation of nitrogen-containing oxidized lipid derivatives. Arch Biochem Biophys 324:15–25.
53. O'Donnell VB, Taylor KB, Parthasarathy S, Kuhn H, Koesling D, Friebe A, Bloodsworth A, Darley–Usmar V, Freeman BA. (1999) 15-Lipoxygenase catalytically consumes nitric oxide and impairs activation of guanylate cyclase. J Biol Chem 274:20083–20091.
54. Houston M, Chumley P, Radi R, Rubbo H, Freeman BA. (1998) Xanthine oxidase reaction with nitric oxide and peroxynitrite. Arch Biochem Biophys 355:1–8.
55. Ichimori K, Fukahori M, Nakazawa H, Okamoto K, Nishino T. (1999) Inhibition of xanthine oxidase and xanthine dehydrogenase by nitric oxide. J Biol Chem 274:7763–7768.
56. Torres J, Wilson MT. (1999) The reactions of copper proteins with nitric oxide. Biochim Biophys Acta 1411:310–322.
57. Denicola A, Souza JM, Radi R, Lissi E. (1996) Nitric oxide diffusion in membranes determined by fluorescence quenching. Arch Biochem Biophys 328:208–212.

58. Liu X, Miller MJ, Joshi MS, Thomas DD, Lancaster JR, Jr. (1998) Accelerated reaction of nitric oxide with oxygen within the hydrophobic interior of biological membranes. Proc Natl Acad Sci USA 95:2175–2179.
59. Padmaja S, Huie RE. (1993) The reaction of nitric oxide with organic peroxyl radicals. Biochem Biophys Res Commun 195:539–544.
60. Hogg N, Kalyanaraman B, Joseph J, Struck A, Parthasarathy S. (1993) Inhibition of low-density lipoprotein oxidation by nitric oxide. Potential role in atherogenesis. FEBS Lett 334:170–174.
61. Goss SP, Hogg N, Kalyanaraman B. (1995) The antioxidant effect of spermine NONOate in human low density lipoprotein. Chem Res Toxicol 8:800–806.
62. Malo–Ranta U, Yla–Herttuala S, Metsa–Ketela T, Jaakkola O, Moilanen E, Vuorinen P, Nikkari T. (1994) Nitric oxide donor GEA 3162 inhibits endothelial cell-mediated oxidation of low density lipoprotein. FEBS Lett 337:179–183.
63. Bolton EJ, Jessup W, Stanley K, Dean RT. (1994) Enhanced LDL oxidation by murine macrophage foam cells and their failure to secrete nitric oxide. Atherosclerosis 106:213–223.
64. Seccia M, Perugini C, Albano E, Bellomo G. (1996) Inhibition of copper-induced LDL oxidation by nitric oxide: a study using donors with different half-time of nitric oxide release. Biochem Biophys Res Commun 220:306–309.
65. Yamanaka N, Oda O, Nagao S. (1996) Nitric oxide released from zwitterionic polyamine/nitric oxide adducts inhibits copper-induced LDL oxidation. FEBS Lett 398:53–56.
66. Seccia M, Perugini C, Bellomo G. (1997) The formation of some antigenic epitopes in oxidized human LDL is inhibited by nitric oxide. Biochem Biophys Res Commun 232:613–617.
67. Denicola A, Rubbo H, Batthyány C, Freeman BA, Radi R. (1999) Diffusion of nitric oxide in native and oxidized low density lipoprotein. Free Radic Biol Med 27(supp 1):S74.
68. Rubbo H, Radi R, Anselmi D, Kirk M, Barnes S, Eiserich J, Freeman BA. (2000) Nitric oxide reaction with lipid peroxyl radicals spares α-tocopherol during lipid peroxidation: greater oxidant protection from the pair nitric oxide/α-tocopherol than α-tocopherol/ascorbate. J Biol Chem 275:10812–10818.
69. Goss S, Hogg N, Kalyanaraman B. (1997) The effect of nitric oxide release rates on the oxidation of human LDL. J Biol Chem 272:21647–21653.
70. Maragos CM. (1991) Complexes of nitric oxide with nucleophiles as agents for the controlled biological release of nitric oxide. J Med Chem 34:3242–3247.
71. Estévez AG, Crow JP, Sampson J, Reiter C, Zhuang Y, Richardson G, Tarpey MM, Barbeito B, Beckman JS. (1999) Induction of nitric oxide-dependent apoptosis in motor neurons by zinc-deficient superoxide dismutase. Science 286:2498–2500.
72. Wink DA, Vodovotz Y, Grisham MB, Degraff W, Cook JC, Pacelli R, Krishna M, Mitchell JB. (1999) Antioxidant effects of nitric oxide. Methods Enzymol 301:413–424.
73. Brune B, Messmer UK, Sandau K, Hirvonen MR, Lapetina EG. (1997) Superoxide formation and macrophage resistance to nitric oxide-mediated apoptosis. J Biol Chem 272:7253–7258.
74. Goldstein S, Czapski G, Lind J, Merényi G. (2000) Tyrosine nitration by simultaneous generation of nitric oxide and superoxide. J Biol Chem 275:3031–3036.
75. Reiter C, Teng R, Beckman JS. (2000) Superoxide reacts with nitric oxide to nitrate tyrosine at physiological pH via peroxynitrite. J Biol Chem 275:32460–32466.
76. O'Donnell VB, Chumley P, Hogg N, Bloodsworth A, Darley–Usmar V, and Freeman BA. (1997) Nitric oxide inhibition of lipid peroxidation: kinetics of reaction with lipid peroxyl radicals and comparison with α-tocopherol. Biochemistry 36:15216–15223.
77. Eiserich JP, Butler J, van der Vliet A, Cross CE, Halliwell B. (1995) Nitric oxide rapidly scavenges tyrosine and tryptophan radicals. Biochem J 310:745–749.
78. Goodwin DC, Gunther MR, His LC, Crews B, Eling T, Mason RP, Marnett LJ. (1988) Nitric oxide trapping of tyrosyl radicals generated during prostaglandin endoperoxide synthase turnover. J Biol Chem 273:8903–8909.
79. Batthyány C, Santos C, Botti H, Cerveñansky C, Radi R, Augusto O, Rubbo H. (2000) Direct evidence for apo B-100-mediated copper reduction during LDL oxidation: studies with purified apo B-100 and detection of tryptophanyl radicals in LDL. Arch Biochem Biophys 384:335–340.
80. Yi Zhang Y, Ming A, Nomen M, Walsh M, Keaney JF, Loscalzo J. (1996) Nitrosation of tryptophan residues in serum albumin and model dipeptides. J Biol Chem 271:14271–14279.
81. Wink DA, Hanbauer I, Krishna MC, DeGraff W, Gamson J, Mitchell JB. (1993) Nitric oxide protects against cellular damage and cytotoxicity from reactive species. Proc Natl Acad Sci USA 90:8913–9817.

82. Wink DA, Cook J, Krishna MC, Hanbauer I, DeGraff W, Gamson J, Mitchell JB. (1995) Nitric oxide protects against alkyl peroxide-mediated cytotoxicity: further insight into the role nitric oxide plays in oxidative stress. Arch Biochem Biophys 319:402–407.
83. Gorbunov NV, Tyurina YY, Salama G, Day B, Claycamp HG, Argyros G, Elsayed NM, Kagan VE. (1998) Nitric oxide protects cardiomyocytes against tert-butyl hydroperoxide-induced formation of alkoxyl and peroxyl radicals and peroxidation of phosphatidylserine. Biochem Biophys Res Commun 244:647–651.
84. Degnim AC, Morrow SE, Ku J, Zar HA, Nakayama DK. (1998) Nitric oxide inhibits peroxide-mediated endothelial toxicity. J Surg Res 75:127–134.
85. Chamulitrat W. (1998) Nitric oxide inhibited peroxyl and alkoxyl radical formation with concomitant protection against oxidant injury in intestinal epithelial cells. Arch Biochem Biophys 355:206–214.
86. Kelley EE, Wagner BA, Buettner GR, Burns CP. (1999) Nitric oxide inhibits iron-induced lipid peroxidation in HL-60 cells. Arch Biochem Biophys 370:97–104.
87. Gutierrez H, Nieves B, Chumley P, Rivera A, Freeman BA. (1996) Nitric oxide regulation of superoxide-dependent lung cell injury: oxidant-protective actions of endogenously produced and exogenously administered nitric oxide. Free Radic Biol Med 21:43–52.
88. Muriel P. (1998) Nitric oxide protection of rat liver from lipid peroxidation, collagen accumulation and liver damage induced by carbon tetrachloride. Biochem Pharmacol 56:773–779.
89. Rubanyi GM, Ho E, Cantor E, Lumma W, Parker LH. (1991) Cytoprotective function of nitric oxide: inactivation of superoxide radicals produced by human leukocytes. Biochem Biophys Res Commun 181:1392–1397.
90. Bult H. (1996) Nitric oxide and atherosclerosis: possible implications for therapy. Mol Med Today 2:510–518.
91. Boger RH, Bode–Boger S, Kienke S. (1998) Dietary L-arginine decreases myointimal cell proliferation and vascular monocyte accumulation in cholesterol-fed rabbits. Atherosclerosis 136:67–77.
92. Maxwell AJ, Tsao PS, Cooke JP. (1998) Modulation of the nitric oxide synthase pathway in atherosclerosis. Exp Physiol 83:573–584.
93. Maxwell AJ, Tsao PS, Cooke JP. (1998) Modulation of the nitric oxide synthase pathway in atherosclerosis. Exp Physiol 83:573–584.
94. Esaki T, Hayashi T, Muto E, Yamada K, Kuzuya M, Iguchi A. (1997) Expression of inducible nitric oxide synthase in T lymphocytes and macrophages of cholesterol-fed rabbits. Atherosclerosis 128:39–46.
95. Luoma JS, Stralin P, Marklund SL, Hiltunen TP, Sarkioja T, Yla–Herttuala S. (1998) Expression of extracellular SOD and iNOS in macrophages and smooth muscle cells in human and rabbit atherosclerotic lesions. Arterioscler Thromb Vasc Biol 18:157–167.
96. Hogg N, Struck A, Goss SP, Santaman N, Joseph J, Parthasarathy S, Kalyanaraman B. (1995) Inhibition of macrophage-dependent LDL oxidation by nitric oxide donors. J Lipid Res 36:1756–1762.
97. Rikitake Y, Hirata K, Kawashima S, Akita H, Yokoyama M. (1998) Inhibitory effect of inducible type nitric oxide synthase on oxidative modification of LDL by vascular smooth muscle cells. Atherosclerosis 136:51–57.
98. Liu S, Chen Y, Zhou M, Wan J. (1998) Oxidized cholesterol in oxidized LDL may be responsible for the inhibition of LPS-induced nitric oxide production in macrophages. Atherosclerosis 136:43–49.
99. Huang A, Li C, Kao R, Stone WL. (1999) Lipid hydroperoxides inhibit nitric oxide production in Raw264.7 macrophages. Free Radic Biol Med 26:526–537.
100. Yang X, Cai B, Sciacca A, Cannon PJ. (1994) Inhibition of inducible nitric oxide synthase in macrophages by oxidized LDL. Circ Res 74:318–328.
101. Khan BV, Parthasarathy S, Alexander RW, Medford RM. (1995) Modified low density lipoprotein and its constituents augment cytokine-activated vascular cell adhesion molecule-1 gene expression in human vascular endothelial cells. J Clin Invest 95:1262–1270.
102. Marui N, Offermann M, Swerlick R, Kunsch C, Ahmad M, Alexander RW, Medford RM. (1993) VCAM-1 gene transcription and expression are regulated through an antioxidant-sensitive mechanism in human vascular endothelial cells. J Clin Invest 92:1866–1874.
103. De Caterina R, Libby P, Peng H, Thannickal V, Rajavashisth T, Gimbrone MA Shin W, Liao JK. (1995) Nitric oxide decreases cytokine-induced endothelial activation: nitric oxide selectively

reduces endothelial expression of adhesion molecules and proinflammatory cytokines. J Clin Invest 96:60–68.
104. Peng H-B, Libby P, Liao JK. (1995) Induction and stabilization of IκBα by nitric oxide mediates inhibition of NF-κB. J Biol Chem 270:14214–14219.
105. Fujita H, Morita I, Murota S. (1994) A possible mechanism for vascular endothelial cell injury elicited by activated leukocytes: a significant involvement of adhesion molecules, CD11/CD18, and ICAM-1. Arch Biochem Biophys 309:62–69.
106. Flavahan NA. (1992) Atherosclerosis or lipoprotein-induced endothelial dysfunction. Potential mechanisms underlying reduction in EDRF/nitric oxide activity. Circulation 85:1927–1938.
107. Busse R, Fleming I. (1996) Endothelial dysfunction in atherosclerosis. J Vasc Res 33:181–194.
108. Cooke JP, Singer AH, Tsao P, Zera P, Rowan R, Billingham ME. (1992) Antiatherogenic effects of L-arginine in the hypercholesterolemic rabbit. J Clin Invest 90:1168–1172.
109. Wang B, Singer AH, Tsao P, Drexler H, Kosek J, Cooke JP. (1994) Dietary arginine prevents atherogenesis in the coronary artery of the hypercholesterolemic rabbit. J Am Coll Cardiol 23:452–458.
110. Davies MG, Dalen H, Kim J, Barber L, Svendsen E, Hagen P. (1995) Control of accelerated vein graft atheroma with the nitric oxide precursor L-arginine. J Surg Res 59:35–42.
111. Drexler H, Zeiher A, Meinzer K, Just H. (1991) Correction of endothelial dysfunction in coronary microcirculation of hypercholesterolaemic patients by L-arginine. Lancet 338:1546–1550.
112. Drexler H, Fischell T, Pinto F, Chenzbraun A, Botas J, Cooke JP, Alderman EL. (1994) Effect of L-arginine on coronary endothelial function in cardiac transplant recipients. Circulation 89:1615–1623.
113. Cooke JP, Tsao PS. (1993) Cytoprotective effects of nitric oxide. Circulation 88:2451–2454.
114. Boger RH, Bode–Boger S, Kienke S. (1998) Dietary L-arginine decreases myointimal cell proliferation and vascular monocyte accumulation in cholesterol-fed rabbits. Atherosclerosis 136:67–77.
115. Cooke JP. (1998) Is atherosclerosis an arginine deficiency disease? J Invest Med 46:377–380.
116. Clarkson P, Adams M, Powe A. (1996) Oral L-arginine improves endothelium-dependent dilation in hypercholesterolemic young adults. J Clin Invest 97:1989–1994.
117. Hayward R, Lefer AM. (1998) L-Arginine attenuates endothelial dysfunction and prolongs survival in rats subjected to traumatic shock. Endothelium 6:71–79.
118. von der Leyen HE. (1995) Gene therapy inhibiting neointimal vascular lesion: in vivo transfer of endothelial cell nitric oxide synthase gene. Proc Natl Acad Sci USA 92:1137–1141.
119. Meredith UT, Anderson IJ. (1993) Superoxide dismutase restores endothelial vasodilator function in human coronary arteries in vivo. Circulation 88:1–467.
120. Anderson TJ, Meredith IT. (1995) The effect of cholesterol lowering and antioxidant therapy on endothelium-dependent coronary vasomotion. N Engl J Med 332:488–493.
121. Taddei S, Virdis A, Ghiadoni L, Magagna A, Salvetti A. (1998) Vitamin C improves endothelium-dependent vasodilation by restoring nitric oxide activity in essential hypertension. Circulation 97:2222–2229.
122. Ting H, Timini F. (1997) Vitamin C improves endothelium-dependent vasodilation in forearm resistance vessels of humans with hypercholesterolemia. Circulation 95:2617–2622.
123. Heller R, Munscher F, Grabner R, Till U. (1999) L-Ascorbic acid potentiates nitric oxide synthesis in endothelial cells. J Biol Chem 274:8254–8260.
124. Huang A, Vita J, Venema R, Keaney JF. (2000) Ascorbic acid enhances endothelial nitric oxide synthase activity by increasing intracellular tetrahydrobiopterin. J Biol Chem 275:17399–17406.
125. May JM. (2000) How does ascorbic acid prevent endothelial dysfunction? Free Rad Biol Med 28:1421–1429.
126. Green D, O'Driscoll G, Rankin JM, Maiorana A, Taylor RR. (1998) Beneficial effect of vitamin E administration on nitric oxide function in subjects with hypercholesterolaemia. Clin Sci 95:361–367.
127. Pryor WA. (2000) Vitamin E and heart disease: basic science to clinical intervention trials. Free Rad Biol Med 28:141–164.

Index

Aging,
   free radical theory, 489
     and lipoic acid, 491
Aloe, 452
Anise, 453
Anthocyanins, 412
Antioxidants,
   assays, 5
   in Asian cooking, 6
   chain-breaking, 1
   characterization in vitro, 5
   definition, 3
   effects on,
     glucose metabolism, 538
     lipid peroxidation, 19
     lipoxygenase, 18
     phagocytes, 27
   food-derived, 1
Ascorbic acid (see Vitamin C)
Atherosclerosis, 303

Benzoic acids, 406
Black tea polyphenols, 376
   cognitive effects, 386, 387
   role of caffeine, 385

Caffeic acid, 279
   bioavailability, 291
   cellular effects,
     cell signaling, 292
     mutagenicity, 293
   chemical structures, 280
   in atherosclerosis, 286
   in LDL oxidation, 286

[Caffeic acid]
   mechanisms of antioxidant activity,
     metal interaction, 285
     radical scavenging, 284
     redox cycling, 286
   radical decay pathways, 282
   reactions with,
     tocopherol, 287
     ascorbate, 287
   redox potentials, 283
   scavenging rate constants, 281
Cardiovascular diseases,
   oxidative processes, 148
Carotenoids, 189
   absorption and metabolism, 198
     tissue accumulation, 203
     transport, 200
   antioxidant effects, 223
   bioavailability, 265
     absorption and metabolism, 266
     factors relative to, 269
     measurement of, 266
   chemical structures, 190, 191
     basic molecular features, 191
     geometric isomers, 192
   chemistry and biological effects, 191
   interactions with food components,
     dietary fat, 273
     dietary fiber, 273
   oxidative breakdown, 235
     consequences, 239
     inhibition of Na,K,ATPase, 242
     methodology, 237
     toxicity, 245

[Carotenoids]
   properties,
      antioxidant activity, 195, 236, 252
      effects in biological systems, 197
      effects in membranes, 197
      light absorption, 194
      prooxidative effects, 241
   roles in,
      age-related macular degeneration, 225
      cardiovascular disease, 208
      cataract, 227
      development of visual function, 253
      the eye, 206
      immune response, 210, 252
      infant nutrition, 251
      lung cancer, 204
      nutrition of neonates, 254
      nutrition of older infants, 257
      prostate cancer, 205
      skin, 207, 228
   supplementation in infancy, 258
Cataracts, 482, 501
Chain-breaking antioxidants, 1, 18
   prooxidant effects, 18
Crocetin, 454

Diabetes,
   oxidative stress, 511
   role of antioxidants, 511
   vascular complications, 511, 515
      activation of PKC, 515
      extracellular matrix, 521
      vascular blood flow, 519
      vascular permeability, 521
Dihydroascorbate,
   transporters, 127
DNA,
   oxidative damage, 30

Ellatic acid, 455
Endothelium-dependent vasodilation, 154
   effects of vitamin C, 154

Ferulic acid, 419
Flavanols, 408
Flavonoids,
   antioxidant activity, 309
   classification, 306
   content in foods, 307
   structure, 306
Flavonols, 411

F_2-isoprostane,
   quantification, 66
      in models of oxidative stress, 66
      in oxidant injury in human diseases, 68

Garlic, 326, 450
Ginger, 324, 452
Gingko biloba,
   and peroxynitrite scavenging, 362
Glabridin,
   antioxidative effects, 316
   chemical structure, 315
Glucose metabolism,
   effect of lipoic acid, 539
Glutathione,
   bioavailability, 549
   effect on,
      glutathione S transferase, 555
      influenza, 556
      pharyngeal cancer, 555
   in foods, 551
      content, 552
      utilization, 551
   metabolism, 549
   oral supply, 551
   redox state, 558
   utilization in GI tract, 553
Grape seed extracts,
   and peroxynitrite scavenging, 362
Green tea polyphenols, 376

Heme proteins, 28
Hydrogen peroxide,
   assay, 10
   scavenging, 10
Hydrolyzable tannins, 406
Hydroxycinnamates, 405
Hydroxyl radical, 11
   assessment, 12
   detection, 13, 15, 16
   effects of antioxidants, 12
   reactions of, 11

Isoprostanes, 57
   as index of endogenous lipid peroxidation, 63
   basic levels in body fluids, 62
   in vitro studies, 65
   measurement, 64
   mechanisms of formation, 59
   quantification, 57
   relevance, 62

Index

Kashin-Beck disease, 640
Keshan disease, 640, 641

LDL, 30
  atherogenic modifications, 305
  oxidatively modified, 149
Licorice, 313
Lignan,
  and cancer, 340
  content of foods, 339
Lipid peroxidation, 2
  assays, 19, 20, 21, 22, 23
    diene conjugation, 24
    ethane/pentane, 24
    in vivo, 31
    isoprostanes, 26
    loss of substrates, 19
    measurement of peroxides, 24
    thiobarbituric acid, 25
    total, 31
  phases, 645
Lipoic acid,
  and aging, 489, 491
    apoptosis, 494
    atherosclerosis, 498
    cataracts, 482, 501
    heart dysfunction, 495
  antioxidant activity, 146
  as antidiabetic neuropathy agent, 479
  as hypoglycemic agent, 478
  biochemistry, 491
  in bioenergetics, 473
  in cataract, 482, 501
  cofactor of pyruvate dehydrogenase, 475
  effects on,
    apoptosis, 481
    cell adhesion, 481
    gene expression, 480
    NF-κB, 480
  functions,
    free radical scavengers, 493
    metal chelator, 493
    reducing agent, 492
    in glucose metabolism, 478
    in regulation of aging, 480
  molecular structures, 474
  therapeutic effects, 535

Melatonin,
  analogs, 625
  antioxidative capacity, 565

[Melatonin]
  effects on,
    chemical toxins, 593
    drugs, 591
    exercise, 589
    excitotoxicity, 579
    heavy metal toxicity, 585
    ionizing radiation, 582
    ischemia reperfusion injury, 567
    mitochondrial dysfunction, 596
    neurodegenerative diseases, 575
    traumatic brain injury, 583
  oxidation products, 622
  prooxidant activity, 625
  reaction with,
    alkoxyl radical, 618
    hydrogen peroxide, 619
    hydroxyl radical, 616
    hypochlorous acid, 620
    perferryl hemoglobin, 621
    peroxyl radical, 616
    reactive nitrogen species, 620
    singlet oxygen, 619
    superoxide anion, 619
  regeneration, 625

Nitric oxide, 2
  antiatherogenic effects,
    gene regulation, 700
    inhibition of LDL oxidation, 699
    vasodilation, 700
  antioxidant properties, 689
  chemical properties, 689
  cytoprotection, 699
  interaction with antioxidants, 697
  prooxidant effects, 690
    derived prooxidants, 690
    in atherosclerosis, 691
  reaction with,
    lipid radicals, 693
    metals, 692
    protein radicals, 697

Olive oil, 321

Peroxyl radicals, 14
  assessment of scavenging, 17
  scavenging, 14
Peroxynitrite,
  and NADH oxidation, 352
  chemistry, 8

[Peroxynitrite]
  inactivation of antiprotease, 8
  interaction with,
    flavonoids, 349
    hydroxycinnamates, 361
    plant extracts, 361
    mitochondrial reductants, 354
      rate constants, 354
    scavenging kinetics, 352
    tyrosine nitration, 8, 357
      effect of plant polyphenols, 363
Phenoxyl radicals, 1
Phytoestrogens, 337
  and risk of cancer, 339
    breast cancer, 341
    colorectal cancer, 344
    endometrial cancer, 342
    lung cancer, 345
    prostate cancer, 343
    stomach cancer, 344
  content in foods, 338
  definition, 337
Plant extracts, 2
Plant polyphenols, 351
  peroxynitrite scavenging, 351
Polyphenols,
  antioxidant activity, 309
  classification, 306
  content in foods, 307
  effects on,
    LDL oxidation, 309
    LDL protection, 311
  rich nutrients,
    garlic, 326
    ginger, 324
    licorice, 313
    olive oil, 321
    pomegranate, 319
    red wine, 311
    rosemary, 326
    soy bean, 317
    tea, 318
  structure, 306
Proteins,
  oxidative damage, 32
    carbonyl assay, 32
    rate of total protein damage, 33
Pycnogenol, 417
  binding to proteins, 424
  bioavailability, 418
  cardiovascular effects, 425
  free radical scavenging activity, 420

[Pycnogenol]
  inflammatory response, 428
  in the antioxidant network, 422

Raisins, 456
Reactive chlorine species, 3
  hypochlorous acid, 27
    assays for scavengers of, 27
Reactive nitrogen species, 3
  scavenging, 7
Reactive oxygen species, 3
  scavenging, 9
Red pepper, 447
Red wine, 311
Rosemary, 326

Saffron, 454
Selenium,
  asthma, 682
  bioavailability, 635
  cancer, 666–673
    gastrointestinal cancer, 674
    lung cancer, 673
    prostate cancer, 675
    skin cancer, 676
  cardiovascular disease,
    coronary heart disease, 677
    stroke, 680
  cataract, 681
  diabetes, 681
  oxidation states, 634
  rheumatoid arthritis, 681
Seneloproteins,
  gastrointestinal peroxidase, 644
  glutathione peroxidase, 637
  mammalian, 638
  phospholipid glutathione peroxidase, 644
  plasma glutathione peroxidase, 642
  selenoprotein P, 651
  selenoprotein W, 650
  thioredoxin reductases, 646
Singlet oxygen, 28
Soy bean, 317
Spices, 437
  aloe, 452
  anise, 453
  biological effects, 442
  chemical composition, 438
  crocetin, 454
  ellatic acid, 455

Index

[Spices]
  garlic, 450
  ginger, 452
  propolis, 451
  raisins, 456
  red pepper, 447
  saffron, 454
  turmeric, 441
Stilbenes, 406
Superoxide anion,
  scavenging, 9

Tea, 371
  flavonoid composition, 371
  production and consumption, 376
Tea flavonoids,
  bioavailability, 379
  epidemiology, 388
    cancer, 391
    cardiovascular diseases, 388
    chronic diseases, 391
  functions in,
    animal models, 380
    cardiovascular disease, 38
    cell culture, 380
    humans, 383
  physicochemical properties, 377
Tocotrienols,
  absorption and distribution, 111
  antioxidant activity, 111
  biological activity, 109
  effects on,
    cancer, 113
    cholesterol synthesis, 112
    LDL oxidation, 112
    nervous system, 113
    skin, 113
Total antioxidant capacity, 5, 47
  application in,
    nutritional studies, 50
    clinical studies, 50
  automated procedure, 51
  factors, 53
  interpretation, 53
  manual procedure, 52
  overview of methodology, 48, 49
Trolox equivalents antioxidant capacities, 6
Turmeric, 441

Vitamin C,
  and nitric oxide, 150

[Vitamin C]
  bioavailability, 134
  biochemical function, 128
  cellular mechanisms,
    decrease of oxidant production, 153
    reduction of cellular adhesion, 154
  deficiency, 117
  depletion-repletion studies, 130
  diet, 133
  effect on coronary heart mortality, 523
  epidemiological studies, 156, 167
  food sources, 138
  intake, 129
    in the United States, 139
  nonenzymic functions, 120
  physiology, 122
    tissue distribution, 122
    transport and accumulation, 122, 125
  plasma concentration, 129
  properties as, 118
    cofactor, 120
    electron donor, 119
    vitamin, 118
    water-soluble antioxidant, 147
  recommended dietary allowance, 139
  recycling, 128
  scurvy, 118
  studies in humans, 169
  urinary excretion, 136
    in cancer, 167, 171–176
    in cardiovascular disease, 148
    in endothelium-dependent vasodilation, 154
    in lipid peroxidation, 151
      in vitro, 151
      in vivo, 152
Vitamin E,
  bioavailability, 99
    intestinal absorption, 100
    hepatic tocopherol transfer protein, 101
    plasma transport, 101
  biokinetics, 102
  clinical deficiency states, 76
  content in oils, 110
  distribution to tissues, 102
    delivery, 102
    tissue, 103
  effect on coronary heart mortality, 523
  efficacy in humans, 75
  functions, 75
  in aging, 85
  in air pollution, 88

[Vitamin E]
- in cancer, 77–80
- in cardiovascular disease, 83
- in cataracts, 86, 87
- in strenuous exercise, 89
- isoforms, 109
- metabolism,
  - chroman ring oxidation, 103
  - unoxidized metabolites, 103
- requirements, 76

Wine flavonoids,
- anthocyanins, 412
- flavanols, 408
- flavonols, 411

Wine phenols,
- basic antioxidant activity, 403
- definitions, 401
- levels in,
  - grapes, 103
  - wines, 404

RB
120
.H36

Ref
RB
170
.H36

2988